Praise for the

Harvard Medical School Family Health Guide

"Photos, helpful illustrations, and easy-to-read type with
information on hundreds of health problems make [this]
a welcome addition to any home library."
—*The Cincinnati Enquirer*

"A massive, basic, and complete guide to family
health matters—staying well, diagnostic problems, finding
help, dealing with the health care and insurance systems—
it's all here."
—*Kirkus Reviews*

"This comprehensive resource offers tips on prevention,
diagnosis, and treatment for a range of diseases and disorders."
—*Country Living*

"You need this book."
—*Jane*

"Is there a doctor in your house? If not, the next best
thing is the *Harvard Medical School Family Health Guide*."
—*The Times-Picayune* (New Orleans)

Harvard Medical School Family Health Guide

Anthony L. Komaroff, MD, *Editor in Chief*

Free Press

NEW YORK · LONDON · TORONTO · SYDNEY

FREE PRESS
A Division of Simon & Schuster, Inc.
1230 Avenue of the Americas
New York, NY 10020

First Free Press trade paperback edition 2005

FREE PRESS and colophon are trademarks of Simon & Schuster, Inc.

For information regarding special discounts for bulk purchases, please contact Simon & Schuster Special Sales: 1-800-456-6798 or business@simonandschuster.com

Designed by Martin Lubin Graphic Design

Additional typesetting by Dana Hayward, Angela Taormina, Brad Walrod, High Text Graphics

Art on the following pages is copyright © Harriet R. Greenfield, Newton, Mass: 38, 45 (a), 45 (b), 52, 72, 73 (a), 73 (b), 75 (a), 75 (b), 78, 127, 133, 169, 338, 340, 341, 343 (a), 343 (b), 345 (a), 345 (b), 347, 350, 365, 369, 371, 372, 386, 388, 389, 398, 415, 416, 421, 425 (a), 425 (b), 428, 433, 436, 438 (a), 438 (b), 441, 442, 443, 446, 454, 460, 465, 475, 476, 484, 490, 528, 534, 540, 541, 553, 554 (a), 554 (b), 555, 557, 582, 594, 598, 599, 601, 603, 605, 607, 612, 614, 617, 620 (a), 620 (b), 621, 623 (a), 623 (b), 625, 627, 629, 630, 632, 637, 640, 644, 661, 662, 664, 685, 696, 700, 702, 734, 743, 747, 748 (a), 748 (b), 753, 755, 772, 774, 781, 785 (a), 785 (b), 787, 795, 796, 798, 801, 822, 827, 845, 869, 881, 883, 897, 905, 913, 917, 1040 (a), 1040 (b), 1043, 1048, 1050, 1055 (a), 1055 (b), 1061 (a), 1061 (b), 1061 (c), 1061 (d), 1068, 1071, 1074 (a), 1074 (b), 1075, 1076, 1086, 1098, 1101 (a), 1101 (b), 1104, 1107, 1108, 1115, 1129.

Art on the following pages prepared by Jacqueline Heda, Charlotte, NC: 97–120, 1219–20.

Additional illustrations prepared by Hilda Muinos, Weehawken, NJ.

Photo credits appear on p. 1312.

Manufactured in the United States of America

10 9 8 7 6 5 4 3 2

Library of Congress Cataloging-in-Publication Data

Harvard Medical School family health guide / Anthony L. Komaroff
    p.   cm.
1. Medicine, Popular, 2. Health. I. Komaroff, Anthony L. II. Harvard Medical School. III. Title: Family health guide.
RC81.H38   1999   99-27223
610—ac21   CIP

ISBN 0-684-86373-1

CONTENTS

WELCOME TO THE HARVARD MEDICAL SCHOOL FAMILY HEALTH GUIDE

I am proud to introduce you to the *Harvard Medical School Family Health Guide*. For more than 200 years, the Harvard Medical School has provided state-of-the-art health care to millions of people from New England and all over the world.

First and foremost, the 7,000 doctors on the faculty take care of patients. Harvard Medical School faculty staff some of the world's most distinguished hospitals and health care systems (see p.14). We teach our patients how to stay healthy. And every day we are there to care for them when medical problems develop, whether they have a bad cold or need emergency surgery.

We also teach the next generation of doctors and conduct the largest medical research program in the world. At Harvard Medical School:

■ Anesthesia was discovered. Can you imagine having to undergo major surgery without anesthesia?

■ The virus that causes polio was discovered, leading to the development of the polio vaccine. If you are over 60, you will remember what it was like to live with the fear that you might be the next victim of polio and paralyzed for the rest of your life.

■ The cure for pernicious anemia was discovered.

■ The transplantation of organs was first performed.

■ The use of the artificial kidney was pioneered.

■ The field of brain surgery was started.

Harvard Medical School today is home to the largest and longest ongoing study of women's health—the famous Nurses' Health Study—and three of the largest and longest studies of men's health. We are very proud of what we have done to help people lead longer and healthier lives.

We also make house calls, all over the world. For more than 20 years, Harvard Medical School has been publishing health information for the public in our newsletters. Now we are publishing books.

The members of the faculty who edited this book care for patients every day. We know that people are faced with many confusing choices and with more health information than ever before. We also know that the face-to-face time you have with your doctor can be limited.

This book gives you the latest information—what you need to know to keep yourself healthy and to cope with illness. It also provides you with the information you need to navigate the sometimes confusing and frustrating world of managed care.

To deal with the world of medicine, you need information that is clear, accurate, easily understandable, and accessible.

This book provides that information, sometimes presented in special features, many of which cannot be found in other books. These features include:

Symptom charts What do you do when you develop a particular symptom, such as sudden pain in your abdomen? Is there a home remedy, valid alternative medicine treatment, or over-the-counter medicine you can get at the drugstore? When do you need to contact the doctor? Along with several other colleagues, about 30 years ago I first developed the idea of outlining medical logic in the form of symptom charts (see p.171). When you or a member of your family has a new symptom, the logically organized charts in this book will help you determine how you may be able to care for yourself, and when you need to contact the doctor.

Advice for when you visit your doctor Today, more than ever, you need to know what questions to ask your doctor. And you need to know what your doctor should be doing for you. You should be getting the best medical care. For many common illnesses, we provide information about what should happen when you visit your doctor—what issues you should discuss and what kind of a physical examination and laboratory tests your doctor should perform regularly. Think about and write down questions to discuss with your doctor before your visit. Knowing what to expect when you see your doctor can also help you judge how thorough your care has been. For an example of the kinds of questions to ask, see p.899.

Advice on understanding medicines Your doctor may be too busy to fully explain all about your medicine, its benefits, and its possible side effects. In the chapter Medicines (see p.1148), we describe the major types of medicines that doctors prescribe today, and what they are used for.

Advice on drug-drug interactions The Medicines chapter also has an extensive chart of possible adverse reactions between different drugs. If you are taking more than one medication, you need to know if there might be a dangerous interaction between them (see p.1167).

Home remedies You don't always need a doctor. In this book, we offer home remedies that can give you relief from common symptoms. For an example of home remedies for the common cold, see p.461.

Alternative medicine treatments A variety of alternative medicine treatments are being seriously studied at Harvard Medical School and elsewhere, and a number have been found to be beneficial. We present them in this book. Conventional medicine has been too slow to study alternative medicine treatments, some of which have won the confidence of healers and patients for thousands of years; it is wrong to reject them out of hand. Alternative medicine treatments, like new conventional treatments, need to be studied scientifically to determine their benefits and risks. For an example of an alternative treatment for chronic low back pain, see p.621.

Understanding diagnostic tests Modern medicine uses many diagnostic tests. In the section called Diagnostic Tests (see p.153), we describe what these tests are and what they are used for. In the Guide to Imaging, we show you the most sophisticated tests available. Take a look at the remarkable imaging procedures on p.135 that produce pictures of the inside of your body without causing you pain. We also describe many other tests performed in your doctor's office or that can be performed by you at home (see p.79).

Benefit and risk-assessment graphs There is so much health information available and, often, more than one treatment for a problem. How do you choose among them? We provide information about the benefits and risks of various diagnostic tests and treatments, and the benefits of adapting certain lifestyle changes designed to preserve your health. This numerical information is provided in easy-to-grasp graphs. An example, showing the benefits and risks of blood-thinning treatment, can be found on p.348.

Advice from Harvard doctors Some of the best doctors on the Harvard Medical School faculty have provided personal words of advice based on their experience—the advice they give their own patients. For example, take a look at Dr Brazelton's advice on the developmental touchpoints in your young child (see p.954), Dr Lipson's advice on back surgery (see p.623), Dr Samuels' advice on preventing strokes (see p.344), Dr Benson's advice on the relaxation response (see p.90), and Dr Ferber's advice on helping your young child learn healthy sleep habits (see p.960).

First-person stories We present the personal statements of people who have suffered from an illness, and sometimes how they have coped with it. For example, author John Updike describes what it is like to live with psoriasis (see p.551), the actress Patty Duke describes her experience with bipolar disorder (see p.401), and an anonymous person—perhaps someone like you—talks about living with gout (see p.604).

Advice on understanding how your body works Other books describe how your body is *built*. We show you how your body *works*—in colorful art (see p.97) that clearly depicts how you see, hear, move, digest food, circulate blood, and so forth. To better understand what can go wrong with your body, it is important to understand how your body works when it is healthy.

Advice on finding health care resources In the Appendix, we provide the names, addresses, phone numbers, and (when available) Internet addresses of the agencies and organizations that can help you with many different problems, particularly community support services.

Glossary A glossary defining various medical terms is found on p.1221.

Advice on dealing with the health care system Dealing with the health care system can be a pain in the neck. The many different kinds of health insurance policies and managed care programs can be very confusing. Also, doctors are under increased pressure to see more patients— which means they have less time to spend with you.

Throughout this book, we provide information that will enable you to be your own advocate in obtaining the best health care. In Navigating the Health Care System (see p.15), we specifically discuss managed care, health insurance, ways to get information about the quality of care in various health care systems, and the quality of care by doctors.

Having this book on a shelf in your home can help you stay healthy, cope with illness, and deal with the health care system, particularly the world of managed care. My colleagues and I have spent literally thousands of hours putting this book together. I have personally written or edited every word and the captions for every drawing or picture. For some of us, you might even call this book an obsession. Just ask my wife.

We wanted to give you the clearest, most current, and most complete information possible—information you can use today, when you or a loved one is faced with a frightening symptom, a new diagnosis, or a recommendation to have a test or a treatment that may have risks as well as benefits. With this book, the other books that will follow, and our newsletters, we think we have done that; we hope that you agree.

ACKNOWLEDGMENTS

Harvard Medical School More than 165 members of the Harvard Medical School faculty participated in the writing and editing of this book. I am enormously grateful to the associate editors who pulled together many of the book's chapters, as well as to the many contributing editors who gave generously of their time, experience, and wisdom.

My special thanks go to deans Daniel Tosteson, MD, and Joseph Martin, MD, PhD; executive deans David Bray and Paul Levy, and colleagues dean Daniel Moriarty, Elizabeth Allison, PhD, Robert Donin, and Cynthia Glott, without whom the Harvard Health Publications program would not have become a reality.

I must also thank my wife, Lydia Villa-Komaroff, and my colleagues at Harvard Medical School who, through observing my occasional absences from the normal activities of life, came to appreciate how editing a book of this size and complexity can become all-consuming. Thank you for your patience.

Simon & Schuster It was a great pleasure to work directly with Simon & Schuster and the Stonesong Press as the book was taking shape. I am especially grateful to Roslyn Siegel and William Rosen at Simon & Schuster for their ongoing support and superb editorial advice; to Paul Fargis, Ellen Scordato, Martin Lubin, and their colleagues at The Stonesong Press and Martin Lubin Graphic Design for their great skill in producing a beautiful-looking book; and to Robin Husayko for her remarkably careful and thoughtful copy-editing.

Finally, my eternal gratitude to editorial director Heidi Hough of Heidi Hough & Associates Inc, who worked tirelessly and skillfully to organize this enormous project, and to make sure that everything in it was clear and comprehensible. We couldn't have created this book without the help and involvement of everyone, especially Heidi Hough.

Anthony L. Komaroff

ANTHONY L. KOMAROFF, MD
Editor in Chief
Professor of Medicine, Harvard Medical School
Editor in Chief, Harvard Health Publications
Boston, Massachusetts
September 1999

EDITORIAL STAFF

Editor-in-Chief

ANTHONY L. KOMAROFF, MD
Professor of Medicine, Harvard Medical School;
Senior Physician, Brigham and Women's Hospital

Deputy Editors for Paperback Edition

STUART B. MUSHLIN, MD
Assistant Professor of Medicine, Harvard Medical School; Physician, Brigham and Women's Hospital

ISAAC SCHIFF, MD
Joe Vincent Meigs Professor of Gynecology, Harvard Medical School; Chief of Vincent Memorial Obstetrics and Gynecology Service, Massachusetts General Hospital

HENRY H. BERNSTEIN, DO
Associate Professor of Pediatrics, Harvard Medical School; Director, Children's Hospital Primary Care Center

Associate Editors

JERRY AVORN, MD
Associate Professor of Medicine, Harvard Medical School; Chief, Division of Pharmacoepidemiology and Pharmacoeconomics, Brigham and Women's Hospital

HENRY H. BERNSTEIN, DO
Associate Professor of Pediatrics, Harvard Medical School; Associate Chief, Division of General Pediatrics, Director of Primary Care, Children's Hospital

ALICE Y. CHANG, MD
Clinical Instructor in Medicine, Harvard Medical School; Harvard Pilgrim Health Care

SARA FORMAN, MD
Instructor in Pediatrics, Harvard Medical School; Children's Hospital

MURIEL R. GILLICK, MD
Assistant Professor of Medicine, Harvard Medical School; Hebrew Rehabilitation Center for Aged; Beth Israel Deaconess Medical Center

SUSAN HAAS, MD, MSc
Assistant Professor of Obstetrics, Gynecology, and Reproductive Biology, Harvard Medical School; Chief, Harvard Vanguard Medical Associates; Division of Obstetrics/Gynecology, Brigham and Women's Hospital

SERENA P. KOENIG, MD
Instructor in Medicine, Harvard Medical School; Brigham and Women's Hospital

EDWARD MARCANTONIO, MD
Instructor of Medicine, Harvard Medical School; Director of Quality Assurance and Outcomes Research, Hebrew Rehabilitation Center for Aged

MALLIKA JOY MARSHALL, MD
Clinical Fellow in Medicine and Pediatrics, Harvard Medical School; Massachusetts General Hospital; and Brigham and Women's Hospital

VICTORIA MCEVOY, MD
Assistant Professor of Pediatrics, Harvard Medical School; Medical Director, Massachusetts General West; Chief of Pediatrics, General Medical Associates; Massachusetts General Hospital

SYLVIA MCKEAN, MD
Instructor in Medicine, Harvard Medical School; Medical Director of the Hospitalist Services, Brigham and Women's Hospital

BARBARA OGUR, MD
Instructor in Medicine, Harvard Medical School; Cambridge Hospital

SUSAN PAUKER, MD, FACMG
Assistant Clinical Professor of Pediatrics, Harvard Medical School; Chief, Genetics Department, Harvard Vanguard Medical Associates; Director, Genetics Clinic, Massachusetts General Hospital

NANCY A. RIGOTTI, MD
Assistant Professor of Medicine, Harvard Medical School; Massachusetts General Hospital

ROBERT H. SHMERLING, MD
Assistant Professor of Medicine, Harvard Medical School; Firm Chief and Associate Physician, Beth Israel Deaconess Medical Center

HARVEY B. SIMON, MD
Associate Professor of Medicine, Harvard Medical School; Massachusetts General Hospital; Member, Health Sciences Technology Faculty, Massachusetts Institute of Technology

WILLIAM C. TAYLOR, MD
Associate Professor of Medicine and Associate Master, W. B. Castle Society, Harvard Medical School; Division of General Medicine and Primary Care, Beth Israel Deaconess Medical Center

RON M. WALLS, MD
Associate Professor of Medicine, Division of Emergency Medicine, Harvard Medical School; Chairman, Department of Emergency Medicine, Brigham and Women's Hospital

ROY D. WELKER, MD
Instructor in Medicine, Harvard Medical School; Medical Director, Brigham Primary Physicians, Brigham and Women's Hospital

Contributing Editors

ABUL KHAIR ABBAS, MB, BS
Professor of Pathology, Harvard Medical School; Brigham and Women's Hospital

JOHN ANDERSON, MD
Instructor in Medicine, Harvard Medical School; Chief, Division of Geriatric Medicine, Mount Auburn Hospital

RONALD J. ANDERSON, MD
Associate Professor of Medicine, Harvard Medical School; Physician, Brigham and Women's Hospital

JOSEPH H. ANTIN, MD
Associate Professor of Medicine, Harvard Medical School; Brigham and Women's Hospital and Dana Farber Cancer Institute

RONALD ARKY, MD
Charles S. Davidson Professor of Medicine, Harvard Medical School; Beth Israel Deaconess Medical Center

ABDUL CADER ASMAL, MD, PhD
Assistant Clinical Professor of Medicine, Harvard Medical School; Beth Israel Deaconess Medical Center

ANN M. BAJART, MD, FACS
Clinical Instructor in Ophthalmology, Harvard Medical School; Massachusetts Eye and Ear Infirmary; Boston Eye Surgery and Laser Center

MICHAEL BARRY, MD
Associate Professor of Medicine, Harvard Medical School; Chief, General Medicine Unit, Massachusetts General Hospital

VANESSA A. BARSS, MD
Associate Professor of Obstetrics, Gynecology, and Reproductive Biology, Harvard Medical School; Director of Maternal-Fetal Medicine, Harvard Vanguard Medical Associates; Brigham and Women's Hospital

DAVID BATES, MD
Associate Professor of Medicine, Harvard Medical School; Chief, Division of General Medicine, Brigham and Women's Hospital

HERBERT BENSON, MD
President, Mind/Body Medical Institute; Beth Israel Deaconess Medical Center; Associate Professor of Medicine, Harvard Medical School

BONNIE LEE BERMAS, MD
Clinical Instructor in Medicine, Harvard Medical School; Associate Director of Clinical Affairs for Women's Health, Brigham and Women's Hospital

DON C. BIENFANG, MD
Assistant Professor of Ophthalmology, Harvard Medical School; Brigham and Women's Hospital

MICHAEL F. BIERER, MD, MPH
Instructor in Medicine, Harvard Medical School; Director, Boston Health Care for the Homeless Program, Massachusetts General Hospital

DAVID BLUMENTHAL, MD
Associate Professor of Medicine and Associate Professor of Health Policy, Harvard Medical School; Physician and Director, Institute for Health Policy, Massachusetts General Hospital/Partners Healthcare System, Inc.

DAVID H. BOR, MD
Charles S. Davidson Associate Professor of Medicine, Harvard Medical School; Chief of Medicine, Cambridge Health Alliance

JONATHAN F. BORUS, MD
Professor of Psychiatry, Harvard Medical School; Psychiatrist-in-Chief, Brigham and Women's Hospital

MALCOLM P. ROGERS, MD
Associate Professor of Psychiatry, Harvard Medical School; Brigham and Women's Hospital

PABLO R. ROS, MD, MPH
Professor of Radiology, Harvard Medical School; Executive Vice Chair, Department of Radiology, Brigham and Women's Hospital

MARTIN A. SAMUELS, MD
Professor of Neurology, Harvard Medical School; Neurologist-in-Chief and Chair, Department of Neurology, Brigham and Women's Hospital; Co-Chair, Partners Neurology

BRUCE E. SANDS, MD
Instructor in Medicine, Harvard Medical School; Director, Clinical Inflammatory Bowel Disease Research, Massachusetts General Hospital

PAUL E. SAX, MD
Assistant Professor of Medicine, Harvard Medical School; Brigham and Women's Hospital

ASSAAD JEAN SAYAH, MD
Instructor in Medicine, Harvard Medical School; Brigham and Women's Hospital

ISAAC SCHIFF, MD
Joe Vincent Meigs Professor of Gynecology, Harvard Medical School; Chief of the Vincent Memorial Obstetrics and Gynecology Service, Massachusetts General Hospital

JEREMY DAN SCHMAHMANN, MD
Associate Professor of Neurology, Harvard Medical School; Director, Ataxia Unit, Massachusetts General Hospital

ERIC C. SCHNEIDER, MD, MSc
Instructor in Medicine, Harvard Medical School; Brigham and Women's Hospital

RICHARD M. SCHWARTZSTEIN, MD
Assistant Professor of Medicine, Harvard Medical School; Clinical Director, Division of Pulmonary and Critical Care Medicine, Beth Israel Deaconess Medical Center

JULIAN L. SEIFTER, MD
Associate Professor of Medicine, Harvard Medical School; Brigham and Women's Hospital

STEVEN E. SELTZER, MD
Philip H. Cook Professor of Radiology, Harvard Medical School; Chair, Department of Radiology, Brigham and Women's Hospital

MICHAEL W. SHANNON, MD, MPH
Associate Professor of Pediatrics, Harvard Medical School; Director, The Pediatric Environmental Health Center, Children's Hospital

JUDITH S. SHAW, RN, MPH
Director, Injury Prevention Program, Children's Hospital

STEVEN J. SHIELDS, MD
Instructor in Medicine, Harvard Medical School; Brigham and Women's Hospital

JANE S. SILLMAN, MD
Instructor in Medicine, Harvard Medical School; Director, Primary Care Residency, Brigham and Women's Hospital

CAREN SOLOMON, MD
Assistant Professor of Medicine, Harvard Medical School; Brigham and Women's Hospital

ANDREW SONIS, DMD
Associate Clinical Professor of Pediatric Dentistry, Harvard Medical School; Children's Hospital

STEPHEN T. SONIS, DMD, DMSc
Professor of Oral Medicine, Harvard School of Dental Medicine; Chief, Division of Oral Medicine, Oral and Maxillofacial Surgery and Dentistry, Brigham and Women's Hospital

ROBERT S. STERN, MD
Professor of Dermatology, Harvard Medical School; Beth Israel Deaconess Medical Center

DAVID J. SUGARBAKER, MD
Associate Professor of Surgery, Harvard Medical School; Vice Chairman, Department of Surgery and Chief, Division of Thoracic Surgery, Brigham and Women's Hospital

CRAIG A. THOMPSON, MD
Clinical and Research Fellow in Cardiovascular Medicine, Harvard Medical School; Brigham and Women's Hospital

PETER V. TISHLER, MD
Associate Professor of Medicine, Harvard Medical School; Brockton/West Roxbury Veterans Affairs Medical Center

MARY M. TORCHIA, MD
Instructor in Pediatrics, Harvard Medical School; Assistant in Medicine, Children's Hospital

JACQUES VAN DAM, MD, PhD
Assistant Professor of Medicine, Harvard Medical School; Associate Director of Endoscopy, Brigham and Women's Hospital

STEVEN E. WEINBERGER, MD
Professor of Medicine, Harvard Medical School; Chief, Pulmonary and Critical Care Division, Beth Israel Deaconess Medical Center

MICHAEL ELLIOTT WEINBLATT, MD
Professor of Medicine, Harvard Medical School; Director of Clinical Rheumatology, Brigham and Women's Hospital

NEIL J. WEINER, MD
Clinical Instructor in Medicine, Harvard Medical School; Section of Hematology, Lahey Clinic

MARY E. WILSON, MD
Assistant Clinical Professor of Medicine, Harvard Medical School; Chief of Infectious Diseases, Mount Auburn Hospital

JOHN W. WINKELMAN, MD, PhD
Instructor in Medicine, Harvard Medical School; Brigham and Women's Hospital

MARY ELLEN WOHL, MD
Professor of Pediatrics, Harvard Medical School; Chief, Division of Respiratory Diseases, Children's Hospital

JACQUELINE WOLF, MD
Associate Professor of Medicine, Harvard Medical School; Physician, Brigham and Women's Hospital

ALAN D. WOOLF, MD, MPH
Associate Professor of Pediatrics, Harvard Medical School; Children's Hospital

JOHN D. YEE, MD, MPH
Instructor in Pediatrics, Harvard Medical School; Director of Community Medicine, Children's Hospital

MICHAEL ZINNER, MD
Moseley Professor of Surgery, Harvard Medical School; Surgeon-in-Chief, Brigham and Women's Hospital

EDITORIAL DIRECTOR
HEIDI HOUGH
Heidi Hough & Associates Inc

BOOK DEVELOPMENT
PAUL FARGIS
ELLEN SCORDATO
The Stonesong Press, Inc

WRITERS
MARIETTA ABRAMS BRILL
CATHERINE DOLD
HEIDI HOUGH
KATHY KAYE
ANTHONY L. KOMAROFF, MD
DAVID LAHODA
EILEEN C. NORRIS
TED E. PALEN, MD, PhD, MSPH
STEPHANIE SLON

EDITOR
ROBIN FITZPATRICK HUSAYKO

DESIGN
MARTIN LUBIN
Martin Lubin Graphic Design

LINE ART
HARRIET GREENFIELD
HILDA MUINOS

COLOR ART AND REPLACEABLE BODY PARTS
JACQUELINE HEDA

ACKNOWLEDGMENTS

Roberta Miller provided critical support in the handling and indexing of the pieces of the book as they were developed and reviewed. Sally Edwards and Marianna Jakab provided critical images. The American Society of Plastic & Reconstructive Surgeons provided valuable material. Sharon Kidd provided valuable help in jacket design.

HOSPITALS AND HEALTH CARE INSTITUTIONS AFFILIATED WITH HARVARD MEDICAL SCHOOL

Beth Israel Deaconess Medical Center
Brigham and Women's Hospital
Cambridge Hospital
Center for Blood Research
Children's Hospital
Dana Farber Cancer Institute
Harvard Pilgrim Health Care
Joslin Diabetes Center
Judge Baker Children's Center
Massachusetts Eye and Ear Infirmary
Massachusetts General Hospital
Massachusetts Mental Health Center
McLean Hospital
Mount Auburn Hospital
Schepens Eye Research Institute
Spaulding Rehabilitation Hospital
VA Boston Healthcare System

Navigating the Health Care System

THE SYSTEM 100 YEARS AGO

Consider what our health care system was like 100 years ago as we entered the 20th century. Like life itself, health care was much simpler then—simpler, but not necessarily better.

Few doctors could be called specialists. Hospitals were places where you went to die or to live the rest of your life with an incurable disease, separated from society and often separated from your family.

There was no such thing as health insurance. You paid for your care with your own money, or you bartered for your care, trading some food from your garden or a pie you had baked for medical care. If you had no money or things to barter, you were considered a "charity case." And if you were the average person, you died before you were 50.

One explanation for the way things were 100 years ago—for the short life span, the lack of specialists, and the scarcity of hospitals—is that there was very little medical knowledge.

Although doctors were able to give you their undivided attention, a careful examination, and an explanation of what they thought was wrong, they could do virtually nothing to help you get better.

The doctor would come to the home of a dying child, perform a brief exam, and perhaps hold the child's hand. This was all the doctor had to offer. How sad that must have been—for the parents, the child, and the doctor.

THE SYSTEM TODAY

Triumphs of 20th Century Medicine

The 20th century brought breathtaking advances in medical knowledge. We have learned an enormous amount about how the body functions.

We have learned what genes are, how we inherit them from our parents, and how they work. We are learning how to identify defective genes and how to repair them.

We have invented machines that can "see" deep inside the body without causing pain—and without cutting. Science has discovered and created miraculous medicines that lower blood pressure and cholesterol, kill many infections, cure some cancers, and provide the life-preserving hormones our bodies no longer produce.

These and other advances have brought about a 60% increase in the average life span—to about 80 years—in just one century, an event unparalleled in human history.

Moreover, most people today have health insurance to protect them against financial calamity from a serious health problem, whereas virtually no one had such insurance a century ago.

Most people also have their own doctor, and people see doctors much more often than their ancestors did a century ago. Today we know a lot more about how to prevent illness and promote health, not just how to cure disease once it occurs.

Problems of 20th Century Medicine

THE POWER TO DO HARM

The explosion of medical knowledge in the 20th and 21st centuries has also caused problems. Powerful technologies can do harm as well as good. Tests and treatments can cause side effects. Strong, effective drugs can cause problems if they interact poorly.

Sometimes these negative effects are predictable and preventable and sometimes they are not. In addition to the risks posed by modern medicine, many studies have found that not all doctors are making use of the latest and best practices and technologies, possibly because not all doctors keep up with the latest knowledge.

EXPENSE

Another major issue with the medical care system today—particularly in the United States—is its size and expense. There are approximately 6,200 hospitals and 738,000 physicians in the United States, more than half of them specialists.

Our health care system is the world's most expensive, costing more than $1 trillion per year and constituting 15% of our total economy. In other developed nations, total health care expenditures are 25% to 50% less than they are here.

Compared to other countries, we spend a much greater fraction of our wealth on health care, and a dollar spent on health care is one that is no longer available for other important goals, such as building homes, libraries, universities, and places of worship.

High health costs can also be a drain on U.S. companies, leaving them less able to compete in a global marketplace. Companies in Japan or Germany typically spend much less on employee health costs than US employers spend. Such high costs can be a real problem for a company's leadership, stockholders, and employees, and for labor unions.

Since the 1960s, the state and federal government have greatly expanded their support for health insurance, largely through the Medicare and Medicaid programs, which are supported by tax dollars. As the cost of health care has risen, governments and taxpayers alike have become increasingly concerned.

SIZE, COMPLEXITY, AND IMPERSONALITY

Many people, particularly older people who remember what health care was like 30 to 60 years ago, view the current system as complex, confusing, and impersonal.

Although many more people have health insurance today than 50 years ago, insurance has become complicated; determining the amount that is covered by your insurance and the fraction you must pay can be confusing. Also, as the health care system has grown into a trillion-dollar-a-year business, many people believe it has become less personal.

Doctors today must arrange so many tests and treatments that they have less and less time to talk to patients. In addition, they often are part of large organizations that set limits on the amount of time physicians can spend with patients.

In some systems, the participants are no longer called "doctors" and "patients"; they are called "providers" and "clients."

The health care system today is much more adept at diagnosing and treating your health problems, but to many people it does not feel as warm and caring as it once did.

YOUR RIGHTS

When visiting the doctor or being admitted to a hospital, some people want to "put themselves in the doctor's hands" and do not choose to participate in decisions about their care. Many others, however, prefer to take an active role in all important decisions surrounding their care. If you

purchased this book, this is probably true of you. In either case, you need to know your rights.

Informed Consent

Physicians and health care workers are legally required to inform you about the risks and benefits of all proposed treatments, as well as any reasonable alternatives to those treatments. Your consent is required before any treatment or diagnostic test.

Informed consent also requires that no physician treat you without having first obtained your consent. If a person is unable to make such decisions, a family member or friend typically serves as a proxy. If the proposed treatment poses a considerable risk, such as surgery, you are required to give your informed consent in writing.

Your Right to Privacy

It may seem obvious, but you have control of your privacy. That is, you have the right to say whatever you want to your doctor or any health care professional, and you have the right to refrain from saying anything you do not want to say.

However, because it is often essential for your doctor to know certain things in order to give you the best care, it is in your best interest to develop a relationship with your doctor in which you feel free to discuss private matters.

Other doctors who become involved in your care—such as in an emergency situation, when your doctor is away, or when you switch doctors—will also need to know and will have

Working with Your Child's Doctor to Improve the System: Dr Brazelton's Advice

Present health systems are too often crisis-driven, deficit-oriented, and unwelcoming to parents. Instead, the system should focus on the passion of parents and how it can be captured to enhance the development of their children, and on how to preserve good health and promote child development. Our society should be investing in improved education about promoting health instead of having the vast majority of our health care investments going to treat disease after it has occurred. Caring health professionals should join parents as allies in the system of care for their children.

T. BERRY BRAZELTON, MD
CHILDREN'S HOSPITAL MEDICAL CENTER
HARVARD MEDICAL SCHOOL

access to private information in your medical record.

If you are an adult, your doctor is legally required to keep private anything you reveal, but there are some exceptions. Some diseases (typically infections that can be transmitted from one person to another) must, by law, be reported to state health authorities.

Recently passed federal legislation, called the Health Insurance Portability and Accountability Act (HIPAA), has made the protection of your medical information more prominent, and includes protections for your privacy even in such places as your local pharmacy. Most physicians' offices have written documents in compliance with HIPAA legislation to show you your rights to confidentiality.

Also, in a legal proceeding, if a judge determines that medical information is relevant to a case, that information can be subpoenaed and disclosed. The law also allows an insurance company to disclose information about you to another insurance company.

For some kinds of insurance, such as life insurance, the insurance company may require that you authorize your doctor to send the company certain medical information. You can refuse, but the insurance company can then refuse to insure you.

Your Right to Medical Care

If you have a medical emergency and have no health insurance, the law requires that any hospital that has an emergency department (not all do) must care for you, if sending you to another hospital would put you at serious risk.

If your condition is judged to be not a true emergency, the hospital is allowed to transfer you to a public hospital (often a city or county hospital) that is funded, in part, to care for those without insurance.

Your Right to Make Decisions

You are in charge of all decisions about your medical care. When it comes to your health, you are the boss, and no one else. You are not required to follow the advice your doctor gives you. Indeed, if you have any doubts about treatment, a good doctor will encourage you to obtain a second medical opinion before you decide on a course of treatment.

Any person may refuse to take a medicine, have a test, or undergo an operation. You can discharge yourself from a hospital even if your doctor does not agree (although you must sign a statement that you are doing so).

In some situations (although it is hoped this occurs only rarely), you might choose not to follow your doctor's recommendations because you do not trust his or her advice. In other cases, you might find that you and your physician view a procedure from different vantage points.

For example, you may choose not to undertake the short-term risks of surgery, even if you trust the doctor's judgment that the operation will help you function better a year from now.

If You Are Unable to Make Decisions

The only people who are not in direct control of decisions about their health care are minors and adults who have been judged not to be competent enough to make health care decisions—for example, people who are in a coma or have dementia (see p.362) and cannot express themselves or think clearly.

In such cases, your closest relative or a health care proxy (see p.1245) designated by you will be asked to make decisions for you. Be sure to discuss your wishes with your family and the health care proxy while you are able to do so. (See p.1142 for a broader discussion of this issue, including living wills.)

DOCTORS

How to Choose and Evaluate a Doctor

Finding a high-quality doctor for yourself or a member of your family is not an easy task. What makes a good doctor?

A good doctor has excellent knowledge and judgment, as well as excellent personal qualities, such as the ability to listen and explain. If the doctor performs diagnostic or treatment procedures, he or she also needs to be skilled in those areas.

You may place a different importance on the different elements than someone else may. Some people choose doctors who they think are knowledgeable and technically proficient, even if they do not find those doctors to be personally warm. Others put primary emphasis on a doctor's personal qualities. Still others look for a balance of the two.

As recently as 20 years ago, there was very little information available to help people select a doctor. Today, however, you can easily have access to valuable information, such as board certifications, medical school history, and professional affiliations.

If you are enrolling in a managed care health plan (see p.22), your choices may be restricted to

certain doctors. You might want to consider the doctors that are available through a plan before you enroll.

BOARD CERTIFICATION

The American Board of Medical Specialties (ABMS) recognizes 24 areas of medical specialty, such as cardiology and anesthesiology. Each of these specialties is overseen by a board, which is an organization that certifies doctors as specialists in that area.

Once a doctor has completed his or her residency training, the doctor is eligible to take a comprehensive exam sponsored by the board in the chosen specialty. At that point, the doctor is considered "board-eligible." Those who pass the exam are called "board-certified."

Board certification means that a doctor has been judged by a board of experts and found to be knowledgeable and skilled in the specialty of that board of experts. Some outstanding doctors choose not to take board examinations; this does not necessarily mean that they are less knowledgeable than board-certified doctors.

On the other hand, doctors who are many years out of training and are still listed as "board-eligible" may have taken the exam but failed it.

You can determine if a physician is board certified by calling the ABMS at 1-800-776-CERT or by checking the ABMS Public Education Web site (www. certifieddoctor.org/verify).

MEDICAL SCHOOL AND RESIDENCY TRAINING

Where a doctor was trained also provides some information about the quality of his or her knowl-

edge and skills. You can find this information on the AMA's Web site (www.AMA-assn.org/aps).

The AMA's free Physician Select Service (at the Web site given above) allows you to search for any physician by name and specialty and provides data on the physician's location, gender, medical school, year of graduation, residency training, board certification, and specialty.

United States versus foreign medical schools The medical school a physician attended is not an absolute indication of his or her abilities, but those who completed medical school in the United States may have completed a more standardized course of study (set by national medical education boards) than those who attended foreign medical schools. Many overseas medical schools provide an excellent education, but there is great variability in quality. Knowing which medical school a person graduated from does not tell you how well they performed in school.

Residency training programs Programs that are closely affiliated with medical schools, such as residency programs in teaching hospitals, usually are more rigorous and difficult to gain entry to. Thus, while training in such a program is not an absolute indication of quality, it does signal that the individual's performance in medical school was judged to be very good (or he or she would not have been chosen for the residency program) and that the training received was likely to have been rigorous.

PHYSICIAN REPORT CARDS

Various reports about physicians are being developed. They are all somewhat rudimentary, but they are a step in the right direction. And many are now available.

Like the AMA Physician Select Service (see left), the databases often include information about physician demographics, education, training, awards, works published, disciplinary actions (such as whether a physician's hospital privileges have ever been suspended or revoked), and paid malpractice claims.

As of 1999, 16 states (Arizona, California, Colorado, Iowa, Kansas, Maine, Maryland, Massachusetts, Minnesota, North Carolina, Ohio, Oklahoma, Oregon, Rhode Island, Texas, and Vermont) had made data about physicians available to consumers at a Web site (www. docboard.org).

MALPRACTICE CLAIMS HISTORY

In the United States, many doctors get sued for malpractice. Most cases are won by the doctors, and many are simply thrown out of court as frivolous. In addition, different specialties of medicine experience different rates of malpractice suits.

The fact that a doctor has been sued for malpractice does not, in itself, say anything about the quality of the doctor. However, if you find that a physician has a pattern of many large paid claims, you probably have cause for concern.

A Web site (www.docboard. org), as well as state licensing boards and state insurance departments, may be able to provide you with this information.

A DOCTOR'S AFFILIATIONS

No doctor practices alone, and no doctor can be considered a good doctor if he or she acts alone. A good physician needs colleagues to consult with, outstanding facilities and equipment in the office and in the hospital, and capable teams of other health professionals to assist in your care.

The reputation of the hospitals that a doctor is affiliated with often says something about the quality of the doctor. Top-flight hospitals permit on their staffs only those doctors they consider to be the best. Selecting a doctor who is affiliated with the best hospitals also means that you will have access to a respected hospital should you ever need it.

"BEST DOCTOR" LISTS

Several magazines and newspapers annually publish lists of what they consider to be the best doctors and hospitals. These lists are usually based on surveys that ask doctors about other doctors, but they are not always scientifically valid.

Relatively few doctors are polled, and they are not selected at random. The listings also tend to highlight doctors who are more famous for their research than for their skill at caring for people.

EVALUATING A DOCTOR'S PERSONAL QUALITIES

Evaluating a doctor's interpersonal skills is a highly subjective task. It often boils down to whether or not two people feel any "chemistry" between them, and whether or not they are comfortable building a doctor-patient relationship.

There is no authority you can turn to for an assessment of a doctor's interpersonal skills. To find a good doctor, many people rely on the recommendations of family and friends. Ask people whose opinion you respect for a recommendation to a caring, skilled physician.

Primary Care Doctors and Specialists

The tremendous growth of medical knowledge has resulted in the creation of many different medical specialties and specialists. There are even subspecialists within some specialties. For example, some cardiologists (heart doctors) are experts on congestive heart failure, while others are experts on heart rhythm disturbances.

Paradoxically, the explosion of knowledge that created so many specialties also has led to a need for good generalists, also called primary care doctors. Many insurance companies now require that you have one.

Everyone should have a primary care doctor. Here are several reasons why:

■ You need a doctor who knows your complete medical history. A specialist will focus on only one area but you may have several medical problems.

■ You need a doctor who will get to know you. A doctor who knows what type of person you are is better able to understand your concerns, to know how your personal life may affect your illness (and vice versa), and to explain things to you.

■ You need a doctor who is trained to determine whether you need a specialist and, if so, which kind. Even if you are healthy, or have just one medical problem, new symptoms and problems can always emerge. Many symptoms do not obviously fall into one specialty area. For example, a pain in the chest can reflect a problem with your heart, stomach, ribs, nerves, or lungs.

■ You need a doctor who oversees all of your care and, when necessary, works in conjunction with specialists, particularly if you have a number of different medical problems and are taking a variety of medicines.

■ You need a doctor who attends to all the screening tests you need to stay healthy and prevent disease.

Primary care doctors come from many different educational backgrounds:

General internists have at least 3 years of training in internal medicine and typically do not care for children, deliver babies, or perform surgery. They do give basic gynecologic care (such as a Pap smear and pelvic exam), but do not perform gynecologic surgery.

Family physicians have at least 3 years of training in a mix of internal medicine, pediatrics, obstetrics, and surgery. They take care of children and adults, provide basic gynecologic care, and sometimes perform surgical procedures or deliver babies.

General pediatricians have at least 3 years of training in pediatrics and care for only children and adolescents.

Internal medicine/pediatricians have 4 years of training in both internal medicine and pediatrics but not in surgery or obstetrics. The breadth of their training is greater than that of general internists and pediatricians, but less than that of family

physicians. However, they undergo more internal medicine and pediatric training than family physicians do.

Gynecologists may provide primary care for women; however, they are not trained to care for nongynecologic problems.

How Doctors Practice

In the first half of the 20th century, most doctors were in solo practice—they were independent, self-employed professionals. Most physicians now work in larger groups. Most of these group practices are independent entities; the doctors are employees and, usually after several years, co-owners of the practice.

Many group practices are affiliated with hospitals, integrated health care systems, or managed care plans, and some are owned outright by such organizations. Doctors today also increasingly practice side-by-side with other health professionals, such as nurse practitioners and midwives, as the complexity of modern medical care requires the use of many different skills and technologies.

It will come as no surprise to hear that doctors rarely make house calls anymore. That change has come about both because house calls are thought to be an inefficient use of doctor time and because many tests cannot be done at home.

Finally, there is a growing trend for primary care doctors to remain in their offices and to have hospital-based doctors (specialists and a new breed of doctors called "hospitalists") care for you when you are hospitalized, remaining in close touch with your primary care doctor.

HOSPITALS

There are many different types of hospitals (see Going to the Hospital, p.163). Like doctors, hospitals traditionally have been independent entities. Most are privately owned, sometimes by religious organizations, while others are owned and run by the federal government (such as Veterans Administration hospitals) or a local government (such as city or county hospitals).

Also like doctors, hospitals in recent years have begun to band together. Some hospitals choose to affiliate with one another, others merge with each other and become one organization, and still others are purchased by large chains of hospitals.

Traditionally, hospitals have been not-for-profit institutions, but increasingly they are owned by for-profit companies, many of which have stockholders who expect a good profit. In most cases, a hospital employs all the health professionals who work there, with the exception of the doctors, who are "affiliated" with a hospital. (Academic medical centers are an exception, employing many of their doctors.)

Hospitals that do not employ doctors directly nevertheless do determine who will practice within their walls, by granting doctors "hospital privileges." Many physicians have privileges at more than one hospital. The reputations of doctors and hospitals are intertwined. Hospitals seek to provide privileges to the top physicians, and physicians compete to have privileges at the finest hospitals.

Only a doctor can admit you to the hospital. The hospital itself cannot admit you, and you cannot "check yourself into" a hospital.

Hospital Quality

Studies of the quality and cost of care in a variety of hospitals have revealed some striking differences. As a general rule, academic medical centers have been found to give the highest quality of care, but many community hospitals are outstanding as well.

With hospitals as with doctors, experience counts (see Choosing a Hospital, p.164). The more often a hospital and its staff have dealt with a particular medical problem or performed a procedure, the more likely they are to do it well.

The Joint Commission on Accreditation of Healthcare Organizations (JCAHO) inspects hospitals regularly to determine whether they are meeting minimal standards. A hospital that has specific quality problems may be denied accreditation or it may be given a provisional accreditation in which certain deficiencies must be corrected before full accreditation is awarded.

Accreditation status of hospitals is available at the JCAHO Web site (www.jcaho.org).

HEALTH INSURANCE

Many more people today have health insurance than in years past. This has been accomplished through a patchwork of private insurance (from hundreds of different companies) and government-sponsored programs.

Most people younger than age 65 receive their health insurance through their employer (or a par-

ent's, spouse's, or partner's employer), which pays most or all of the cost. People 65 years or older usually receive health insurance through Medicare (see p.27), while some lower-income people are insured through Medicaid (see p.28).

Although insurance is more common today, there are still more than 40 million people in the United States who have no health insurance. Most of these people are employed in small businesses that do not provide insurance to their employees; millions of the uninsured are children.

Among all of the industrialized countries in the world, the United States is one of only two nations (the other is South Africa) that lacks a broad nationally sponsored health insurance program.

Fee-for-Service

The first type of health insurance was called fee-for-service, or indemnity, insurance. Most people had this type of insurance until the late 1980s.

In this system, people were free to seek care from any doctor they chose and to see doctors as often as they wanted. If their insurance covered most or all of their medical expenses, their care cost them little or nothing. Doctors were free to order tests, make referrals, or hospitalize someone without any questions being asked, and were promptly paid by the insurance company for their services.

People expected, and physicians tended to provide, any service that might be of benefit, no matter how small the benefit or what the cost. People enjoyed

Paying for Your Health Care

There are many different elements to paying for your health care, depending on what type of insurance you have:

- **Premium** The monthly amount paid to a health plan to pay for covered services. Employers often cover a portion of this cost.

- **Co-payment** A relatively small, fixed-dollar payment (often $5 to $10) that you make with every doctor visit or prescription.

- **Co-insurance** A fixed percentage of the physician or hospital charges that you must pay, up to a certain limit.

- **Deductible** The amount of covered expenses you must pay before any charges are paid by the health plan. For example, each year you might be responsible for the first $200 of medical expenses; after that, your insurance begins to cover expenses.

- **Annual and lifetime limits** The maximum amount of charges a health plan will cover for a particular person or family in a given year or over a lifetime.

the service, attention, and low cost (to them) of their health care, and physicians saw their incomes increase in a dramatic fashion. Not surprisingly, it was a very popular system with patients, doctors, and hospitals.

However, the fee-for-service system greatly increased the costs of medical care, which doubled nearly every 5 years, growing much faster than the rest of the economy.

Another factor that contributed to this rapid rise in health care costs was the broad array of new scientific advances that were introduced and adopted with ever-increasing speed.

If all of these new expenditures and technologies had led to greatly improved health, society might have been willing to accept the expense. However, studies began to show that many diagnostic tests and treatments were being performed with little or no benefit to the patient. In a few cases, the widespread use of new technologies actually caused more harm than good. More, it turned out, was not always better.

In the early 1980s, the organizations that pay for health insurance—employers, stockholders, employees, governments, and taxpayers (in short, nearly everybody)—began to become concerned. The perception was that the health care system was too lax and that it should be more tightly managed.

The focus shifted to controlling health care costs while improving the quality of health care even more. The stage was set for the introduction of managed care.

Managed Care

"Managed care" is a catchall term that refers to any attempt by a health care insurance company or health care provider (such as doctors or hospitals) to influence the quality or cost of medical services. The goal is to control the use of medical resources, directing them to where they are most clearly needed.

Currently, more than 75% of privately insured individuals are enrolled in one of the many different forms of managed care.

One very good thing that managed care plans have done is to pay for "wellness" care such as preventive medicine services; the old fee-for-service system rarely paid for such services.

Managed care plans have also created systems to ensure that your doctor is providing you with these preventive services and making sure you receive appropriate care for common medical illnesses. The systems that currently do this are rudimentary, but they are a start.

Managed care plans have produced great anger and frustration when they have attempted to limit the doctors you can see and the number of medical services you can request. The fewer restrictions a plan places on you, the more expensive the plan is likely to be.

Managed care plans also place restrictions on doctors and hospitals, monitoring the expense of the care they provide and placing financial pressure on doctors to conserve on cost. These pressures range from mild to severe and affect the doctors' and hospitals' income and sometimes the treatment you are able to receive.

An important part of most managed care plans is the role of the primary care doctor. Many plans require that you have a primary care doctor, and that he or she be the one to organize your medical care, acting as a "gatekeeper."

For example, under such a system you cannot consult with a specialist, or go to an emergency department for nonemergency problems, without the approval of your primary care physician.

The rationale behind this system is that under the old fee-for-service plans, many people sought a lot of unneeded, very expensive medical care.

Many people are not happy with the constraints imposed by the gatekeeper system. Open access plans, which allow patients direct access to specialists, are becoming popular. However, they are more costly.

In addition, some managed care plans now allow people who have chronic diseases to see a specialist on a recurring basis, without the need to gain the approval of a primary care doctor each time.

TWO APPROACHES TO PAYING

Although there are many different forms of managed care, there are two general approaches by which doctors and hospitals are paid. Both place financial pressure on your doctor to use medical resources efficiently.

Managed fee-for-service In this approach, as in the old fee-for-service system, the cost of covered services is paid for by the insurer after services have been received. There are several differences from the old system, however.

First, the insurance company that offers managed fee-for-service often sets limits on the amount a doctor or hospital can charge for your care.

Second, the insurer may have a system to check that you truly do need something that has been ordered for you (such as tests, consultations, or hospitalization). The insurance company might have written guidelines that direct such decisions or it might seek a second opinion from another doctor.

Third, this system often withholds from your doctor some of the amount that is due for each service. Then, at the end of the year, if the insurance company determines that your doctor has used too many medical resources in caring for you and for others, the company keeps some or all of what it has withheld from the doctor.

This places financial pressure on the doctor to use fewer medical resources. Such pressure is not necessarily bad; there is evidence that, traditionally, more tests and treatments have been performed than are needed, and that some of these unnecessary tests and treatments put patients at some risk.

Nevertheless, this system may also encourage some doctors to refrain from ordering services that are truly needed.

Capitation In this system, doctors and hospitals receive a set amount of money to cover all the medical care that you are expected to need over the course of a year. In contrast to the managed fee-for-service system described above, doctors and hospitals are paid a set amount for each patient, each month, regardless of what care they have provided.

This system, too, places financial pressure on doctors and hospitals to use fewer medical resources. If the doctors and hospitals spend less money caring for a patient than they have received, they keep the difference.

Health maintenance organizations (HMOs) have used capitation for 50 years. In the oldest and most established HMOs (which

are usually not-for-profit organizations), there is little evidence that such financial pressures have led to substandard care.

However, there are examples of newer HMOs that have cut too many corners and delivered poor-quality care. Some people are concerned that the many HMOs formed in recent years on a for-profit basis may do the same.

Many HMOs and capitated health plans also provide incentives to ensure that doctors deliver the best possible care. They set standards for high-quality care, assess whether doctors and hospitals are meeting those standards, actively measure patient satisfaction, and monitor patient complaints and grievances.

Different HMOs and capitated plans vary considerably in how much of the financial pressure from capitation is placed directly on the individual physician.

PHYSICIAN AND HOSPITAL ORGANIZATIONS

Managed care organizations come in many different shapes. Some are loosely organized groups of independent doctors and hospitals, others are more tightly linked, and some are literally one organization.

Preferred provider organization (PPO) PPOs are groups of doctors, other health professionals, and hospitals that have been identified by an employer to provide care to its employees. A PPO is typically a loose organization of independent doctor groups and institutions, all of which are paid on a managed fee-for-service basis (see p.22), according to a specific fee schedule. Usually, a health insurance

company takes premium payments from the employer and then pays the doctors and hospitals. Sometimes, employers contract directly with doctors and hospitals.

Physician group organization In this increasingly popular option, large groups of doctors form a group that employs them all, and then contracts with (and sometimes buys) local hospitals. These groups may work with a local health insurance company or they may try to form their own insurance organization. The attraction of this model, for the doctors involved and for many of their patients, is that the organization is more clearly run by doctors than most health plans. However, these physician group organizations are under the same pressure as are all other managed care organizations to cut costs, and it has not been shown that they are any better at maintaining quality of care.

Health maintenance organization (HMO) HMOs are health plans that are both an insurance company and a provider organization (see left). An HMO often owns its own hospitals and other institutions. It often employs its doctors and other health professionals, although sometimes it provides care through a large doctor group that is legally independent from the HMO but closely bound to it. Some HMOs develop looser relationships with independent doctor groups; these are called independent practice associations (IPAs). In most HMOs, patients are required to use participating providers and are enrolled for specified periods of time.

The Care of the Poor: Dr Coles' Observations

For many years, in the rural South, and later, in northern cities such as Boston, I have worked with poor, vulnerable families, with the children of migrant farmers, with boys and girls growing up in troubled, relatively impoverished neighborhoods (as compared to what I myself experience as a resident of a suburban town).

Often I have noted a particular medical problem, a child ailing for one reason or another—and yet no pediatrician has been called or visited. I wonder why, of course, and have done so aloud, under some circumstances with parents or grandparents I've known well.

Soon enough, I discover the medical reality that the young ones and their mothers, fathers, and grandparents know: they don't "have" a pediatrician, don't have the money or even the means (a car) that enables ready access to a physician. Nor do such individuals sometimes know where they might go to secure medical assistance—even as they fear that, were they to go to a clinic or a hospital, they would be unwelcome.

All of the above is meant to convey the obvious—that some people in America are at a substantial remove from doctors and from medical institutions. Here is a public health nurse describing her own difficulties in being of help to migrant farm families in Florida, not to mention the difficulties those people face when illness arrives: "My job is to try to find migrants who are sick, and need to see a doctor, but they live in another world, you could say—they're on the move all the time, and I can't just go and talk with them. The growers don't want us 'poking around,' and the migrants, they're scared when they see us coming. I told the doctors they should go out and try to do their work where the folks are, but that would get the growers down on us!"

She was in her own direct, melancholy way bringing up, by implication, many of those "socioeconomic variables" that are mentioned in academic papers and discussions—the way "marginality" bears down on a family's and a child's life.

When she and a public health physician did their work, made their efforts to connect with migrant families, many obstacles became all too evident, to the point that perplexity and discouragement were quickly felt: "We try to go where they [migrant families] live or work, but we're not allowed [by the grow-ers or crew leaders] to get near, and the migrants are afraid we bring trouble, because they'll be punished for talking with us."

Of course, many Americans are not separated from the health care system in this way. Still, I worked for 7 years in a Boston neighborhood not too far from any of the city's three medical schools and its teaching hospitals, and I noted some children clearly in trouble medically (with anemia, asthma, gastrointestinal difficulties, and other symptoms) who weren't getting the kind of regular medical attention and care they needed.

An "informant," a woman who at 42 was already a grandmother, sums it up: "I know when a child is sick, but where to go and how to go, that's my question! I work all day and I'm beat when I come home, and my daughter, too, she has a job, and it's a haul on the bus, and you get there, to a hospital, and you can get lost, for hours, because they speak one language and you another!"

Once I went with her, her daughter, and two of her grandchildren to a Boston hospital, sat with them as they sat, listened to them and others trying to get past various bureaucratic hurdles—felt irritated by the length of time taken, the delays and more delays, the confusion (and miscommunication) that reigned in corridors, at desks, on crowded benches, and realized how different it had gone for me and my wife and our sons, when our children were sick: the respect we'd received, the dispatch with which we were attended.

I recall thinking, then, that with some other doctors, with medical students and nurses, working in a neighborhood health clinic, things might be different "there," in that stretch of streets where that grandmother and her family lived. "We" might, then, be with "them." Some of the medical, social, cultural, racial, and educational differences would be diminished.

Our own lives as doctors or doctors-to-be would be distinctly enhanced: people in need of us now would be able to call upon us, see us, and be "seen" by us.

ROBERT COLES, MD
HARVARD UNIVERSITY HEALTH SERVICES
HARVARD MEDICAL SCHOOL

Point-of-service plan In this type of plan, patients enroll with an HMO and its providers but have the option to receive services from providers who are not part of the HMO's panel. The price for such freedom is higher costs to you—higher deductibles, higher co-payments, or the need for co-insurance.

How to Choose a Health Plan

A health plan is basically a health insurance program that is connected to certain doctors and hospitals. If you have one or more doctors and hospitals that you know well, and those doctors and hospitals are affiliated with a plan that you can afford, you are lucky. Choosing a plan may be easy for you.

Another approach to choosing a health plan is to ask friends for their recommendations. Or, if you like a particular hospital but do not know any doctors there, you can call the hospital (or check its Web site) to find out which health plans they use and for help in finding and making an appointment with one of their affiliated doctors.

If you must choose from plans that have doctors and hospitals you are not familiar with, then you will need to do some homework. Some of the important issues you should consider and some of the questions you should ask when evaluating health plans are discussed below.

Affiliated doctors and hospitals Every health plan is required to give you lists of its affiliated doctors and hospitals. If a plan has doctors you would like to use, check to see whether they are

taking new patients. The plan's literature should tell you this. Also consider checking on the quality of the doctors (see p.18) and the hospitals (see p.20).

Rating the quality of the plans Several organizations now investigate and evaluate health plans and make the information available to consumers (see Rating the Quality of Health Plans, p.26).

Price versus choice As discussed on p.21, the plans that give you the greatest freedom of choice—of doctors and hospitals and of how often you can seek medical care—are usually the most expensive. Think carefully about what you can afford, and what you want to pay for. Find out what types of payments will be expected of you by reading the literature sent to you by each plan. Call and ask questions if there is anything you do not understand.

Range of benefits The benefits offered by various health insurance plans vary considerably. You will need to determine which benefits are most important to you, given the illnesses or special needs that you or your family have. Some questions to ask:

■ Does the plan pay for drugs? If so, is there a limit on how much?

■ Does the plan place limits on the total amount of services you can have? This is often the case with psychiatric care.

■ Are you covered if you become ill in another state or country and need medical care there? If so, is this only for emergencies? How does the plan define an emergency?

■ Does the plan pay for any dental or eye care?

■ Does the plan allow a specialist to be your primary care doctor? For example, if you have asthma but are otherwise healthy, can a lung specialist be your primary care doctor? This is useful for those who have a single chronic illness that falls into the area of a particular specialty.

Determining financial pressures on doctors and hospitals The literature you get from a plan usually does not give you the answers to the questions below. You will have to call the plan administrators and press for answers.

You should ask two questions:

■ Under the plan, does your doctor have a financial incentive to see you more often or to perform more tests or treatments? If so, it increases the possibility that you might have medically unnecessary tests and treatments, some of which could cause harm.

■ Under the plan, does your doctor have a financial incentive to see you less often, or to perform fewer tests and treatments? If so, it increases the chance that you might not get medically necessary care.

Determining financial pressures on the plan Increasingly, managed care plans are owned by for-profit companies that must share their earnings with stockholders. Some experts believe that such companies spend too little of the money they get on your care, and use too much of it to support administration and to pass on as profits.

Many for-profit managed care plans provide high-quality care, but they have pressures on them that are different than the pressures on not-for-profit plans.

Determining your right to appeal plan decisions Any managed care plan you choose will impose some restraints on your health care. If you have already joined a plan, appealed a decision made about your care, and are not satisfied with the resolution, there are other avenues to pursue. You can contact your employee benefits manager, the state insurance commission, or the state department of health.

You need to determine how you can appeal any decision that you believe compromises your care. Find out if and how you can appeal the following types of decisions and what the process is for making that appeal:

■ If the plan refuses to pay for care you have received because the plan says it is not covered.

■ If your primary care doctor does not want to refer you to a specialist for consultation.

■ If you are not satisfied with the quality of the care you receive.

■ If you are not satisfied with the plan and its appeals process, how easily can you leave the plan altogether? Is there a waiting period and, if so, how long? Does the process for appealing sound fair to you? No plan is going to approve every appeal, but you should at least be given a fair hearing.

Comparing insurance policies When there are two people working (married couples or domestic partners) in a household, often each is entitled to health insurance through an employer. If this is the case in your family, look carefully at the choices for health plans that each of you has and consider what each plan has to offer as cover-

age for individuals versus coverage for families.

Health insurance for a family is always more expensive than it is for an individual. If you have no dependent children, the best option might be for each of you to take an individual policy. In addition, if your policy covers dental treatment but your partner's does not, you will want to consider adding your partner to this portion of your insurance plan, if possible.

Congress has recently passed legislation that facilitates people starting Medical Savings Accounts. These accounts are tax deductible when medical expenses are paid from the account. There is backup insurance available at low cost to kick in once the expenses for the MSA are depleted. Congress enacted this legislation to encourage people to inform themselves about health care expenses and to budget for them. All of the money set aside for an MSA in a given year must be spent or the remainder in the account is forfeited.

RATING THE QUALITY OF HEALTH PLANS

If you must choose from among plans that include doctors and hospitals you are not familiar with, collect information about their quality. See p.18 for a discussion of how to collect information about individual doctors.

Health plans are evaluated by various organizations. The evaluations typically assess issues such as the overall cost of the plan, choice of physicians, and range of benefits.

One organization that rates health plans is the National Committee on Quality Assurance (NCQA), a private, nonprofit

organization that assesses and reports on the quality of managed care plans.

NCQA provides the names of health plans it has examined and accredited. If a plan has not been accredited by NCQA, find out whether NCQA has simply not yet surveyed the plan and intends to do so in the future, or whether the plan has previously sought accreditation and failed to obtain it.

The NCQA collects information about a plan's actual medical practices and a consumer's ability to obtain care, rather than about the reputations of its doctors and hospitals. This information is compiled in the Health Plan Employer Data and Information Set (HEDIS).

Included in HEDIS is such information as the immunization rate of children within the health plan and the percentage of diabetics in the plan who have their eyes examined. The HEDIS scorecard also provides information about how the plan is helping to maintain and improve the health care of its population.

The NCQA also can give you the following information about each plan:

■ Member satisfaction with the care provided

■ Percentage of patients who leave a plan

■ Percentage of physicians who leave a plan

■ Specific health care options, such as language translation services or education of new members

■ Proportion of physicians within a plan who are board certified and the way in which a plan periodically reviews the qualifications of its physicians

Organizations That Rate Health Plans

The following organizations provide information on various health plans:

National Committee on Quality Assurance (NCQA)
Web site: www.NCQA.org/consumer
Toll-free phone: 888–275–7585

California Consumer Health Scope
Web site: www.healthscope.org
Toll-free phone: 888–244–2124

Agency for Health Care Research and Quality (AHRQ)
Web site: www.ahrq.gov/consumer
Toll-free phone: 800-358-9295

■ Financial incentives attached to the salaries of the plan's physicians that may influence their ability to order tests or specialized services

The Agency for Health Care and Quality Research (AHRQ), a part of the US Public Health Service, also provides important consumer information on health plans, as well as links to other useful databases and preventive services information for patients.

While the information provided will not necessarily suggest which plan is best for you, it does review specific factors that will help you identify those that better suit your needs. Such factors include the cost of various plans as well as how difficult it is to gain access to services.

Medicare

Medicare is the federal government's health insurance program for people aged 65 and older and for some younger people who have chronic disabilities such as end-stage kidney disease.

Traditionally, Medicare has been an "old-style" fee-for-service system (see p.21). Inpatient care in hospitals or skilled nursing facilities, home health care, and hospice care are paid for by Medicare under a program called Part A, for which you pay nothing.

Outpatient services, laboratory tests, mental health care, and durable medical equipment such as wheelchairs and hospital beds are paid for by Medicare under Part B. The federal government pays for most but not all of Part B; you must pay a monthly premium (which in 1999 was about $45 a month).

Long-term care (such as nursing home care) and medicine prescribed outside of a hospital are not paid for by traditional Medicare. Medicare also requires patients to pay co-payments and deductibles (see p.21).

Because of these expenses, as well as the expense of the Part B monthly premium and the services that Medicare does not cover, many people purchase supplemental Medicare, or "Medigap" insurance.

There are different kinds of Medigap policies, with different costs and benefits. The more you can pay, the more benefits you will typically receive. However, even if you have this policy, you will still have to pay for some expenses out-of-pocket.

MEDICARE AND MANAGED CARE

Medicare has introduced a managed care option as a voluntary alternative to the traditional program. Under Medicare managed care, you enroll in a private health maintenance organization (HMO) that is paid a fixed monthly fee from Medicare in exchange for providing all covered, medically necessary care. Enrollees must still pay the Part B premium to the government.

The advantages of Medicare managed care plans are:

■ Enrollees usually get additional benefits, such as coverage for cost of medicines and eyeglasses.

■ Because the care is pre-paid, there are no deductibles and usually only small co-payments.

■ There may be fewer administrative details to monitor, such as the multitude of bills from different doctors and hospitals that can occur with traditional Medicare.

■ Enrollees sometimes have access to special services, such as transportation to and from home.

■ Unlike commercial managed care plans, enrollees may not need to wait for open-enrollment periods to change plans.

The disadvantages of Medicare managed care plans are:

■ Like commercial managed care plans, most Medicare HMOs limit your choice of doctors and hospitals and limit the number of visits for certain problems, such as mental health.

■ You may not have the same freedom that you had with traditional Medicare to visit any doctor you choose.

If you are selecting a Medicare managed care health plan, recognize that quality may vary widely among some of the newer Medicare HMOs. Find out whether the plan is accredited by the National Committee on Quality Assurance (see above left); also ask for "report card" information, which may help you determine how members within these plans report on their health care. In addition, read How to Choose a Health Plan (see p.25).

Medicaid

Medicaid is a joint federal and state program that provides care for more than 38 million low-income people who would otherwise be uninsured. While the federal government sets broad overall guidelines for Medicaid, each state runs its own program with its own set of rules and regulations.

Traditionally, people on welfare are eligible for Medicaid. Welfare programs usually cover pregnant women and children eligible for Aid to Families with Dependent Children (AFDC) and the disabled. Low-income people who are also older than 65 may be covered by both Medicaid and Medicare.

Medicaid covers several items that Medicare does not, such as drugs, the deductibles and co-payments of traditional Medicare plans, and long-term care (such as nursing homes).

Senior citizens who are seeking Medicaid coverage in addition to Medicare (for example, to cover nursing home expenses) are required by law to "become poor" in order to qualify for Medicaid.

MEDICAID AND MANAGED CARE

Like private insurance and Medicare, Medicaid is rapidly moving to adopt managed care. As of 1997, approximately 50% of all Medicaid beneficiaries were in some form of managed care.

However, unlike Medicare (in which enrollees can choose to convert to managed care or not), many Medicaid programs require enrollees to take the managed care plan.

Veterans Administration and Military Hospitals

For current or past members of the US armed forces, government hospitals may be available to provide care. Not all veterans are eligible for care in the Veterans Administration (VA) hospital system; however, all members of the armed forces on active duty are eligible for care at military hospitals.

Both veterans hospitals and military hospitals are forming relationships with local private, nonfederal physicians and hospitals to provide some services. If you have served in the armed forces and are not sure if you are eligible for care in the VA system, call the local office and find out; it could save you considerable expense.

MEDICAL MALPRACTICE

The practice and technology of medicine are not perfect; neither is the care given to you by doctors and hospitals. Even when care is rendered in the best possible manner, complications can arise.

Sometimes complications are unavoidable; sometimes they can be predicted and prevented. The medical malpractice system addresses the injuries that are suffered because of a health care worker's negligence or carelessness.

The purpose of the malpractice system is to:

■ Fairly compensate someone for injury that has resulted from malpractice.

■ Serve as a deterrent toward future malpractice, thus improving quality of care.

To prove malpractice, you must be able to show that:

■ The doctor, other health professional, or institution was responsible for your care.

■ The doctor, health professional, or institution was negligent in the care given, either through inaction or action.

■ The negligence caused real damages. If there was no harm done to you, there is no malpractice, even in cases of gross negligence.

The malpractice system does not appear to work very well. A Harvard Medical School study found that the majority of negligent acts never come to the attention of the malpractice system and, conversely, the majority of malpractice awards and settlements are for cases with poor outcomes that were not the result of negligent care.

Also, only about 40% of malpractice awards actually go to the person who was allegedly injured; the rest (60%) pays for attorney fees and other administrative costs.

Various reforms that might correct some of these shortcomings, such as a no-fault system, are currently under consideration. However, there appears to be no perfect solution.

Taking Charge of Your Health

HOW TO STAY HEALTHY

Do you lack advice on how to stay healthy? Probably not. TV, newspapers, magazines, and the Internet offer a steady stream of new theories on how to change your diet or exercise regimen, or how often to get tested for various diseases. Well-meaning friends and family members may urge you to accept their own theories.

Pap smears and mammograms for women, prostate cancer screenings for men, preventive medicines such as aspirin and vitamin and mineral supplements, advice on diet and exercise, new herbal preparations and other forms of alternative therapy—What should you do? Merely deciding which of these to incorporate into your life, let alone actually incorporating them, could be a full-time job.

While a lot of the advice you will hear from friends or the media is unproven, the fact is that in the past 50 years scientists have learned many ways to reduce the chance of suffering or premature death. The knowledge has paid off; in developed nations like the United States, the average life expectancy has gone up 60% in the twentieth century.

This chapter explains how medical studies teach you to stay healthy. It also provides a guide for how to take responsibility for your health, so that you can spend less of your time figuring out how to maintain your health, and more of your time enjoying life in good health.

Life Expectancy

The chart below shows the number of years that black and white men and women have left to live at different ages, on average. (These U.S. Census Bureau statistics are from 1994.) For example, a 30-year-old black woman could expect to live another 46 years—to age 76. A white woman the same age could expect to live another 50 years—to age 80. On average, whites have longer life expectancies than blacks, and women of both races outlive men.

AGE	WHITE MALE	WHITE FEMALE	BLACK MALE	BLACK FEMALE
Birth	73	79	65	74
20	54	60	47	55
30	45	50	38	46
40	36	41	30	37
50	27	32	23	28
60	19	23	16	20
70	12	15	11	14
80	7	9	7	8

Interpreting Medical Studies

To determine what healthy lifestyle practices, tests, or treatments are worthwhile, doctors

Gains in Life Expectancy From Healthy Lifestyle Practices

The following figures present reasonable estimates of how many additional months of life the average person might gain from making healthy lifestyle choices, based on studies of large numbers of people. For example, the average gain in life expectancy for 1,000 35-year-old men who engage in a regular exercise program over 30 years is estimated to be 6.2 months. For some people, the gain will be 1 month; for others, 30 months. These figures can give you a sense of the relative value of adopting various healthy lifestyle practices.

REDUCING YOUR BLOOD PRESSURE TO NORMAL IF YOUR DIASTOLIC BLOOD PRESSURE (SEE P.646) IS GREATER THAN 105 MILLIMETERS OF MERCURY (MM HG)

Men: 64 months

Women: 68 months

REDUCING YOUR BLOOD PRESSURE TO NORMAL IF YOUR DIASTOLIC BLOOD PRESSURE IS 90 TO 94 MM HG

Men: 13 months

Women: 11 months

REDUCING YOUR CHOLESTEROL TO 200 MILLIGRAMS PER DECILITER (MG/DL), IF YOUR LEVEL IS OVER 300 MG/DL

Men: 50 months

Women: 76 months

QUITTING CIGARETTE SMOKING (SEE P.59) IF YOU ARE 35 YEARS OLD

Men: 28 months

Women: 34 months

REDUCING YOUR WEIGHT TO NORMAL IF YOU ARE MORE THAN 30% ABOVE YOUR IDEAL BODY WEIGHT (SEE P.51)

Men: 20 months

Women: 13 months

HAVING A PAP SMEAR (SEE P.1067) EVERY 3 YEARS IF YOU ARE 20 YEARS OLD OR OLDER

Women: 3.1 months

EXERCISING VIGOROUSLY FOR 30 YEARS DURING YOUR LIFETIME

Men: 6.2 months

Women: No information

HAVING A FECAL OCCULT BLOOD TEST (SEE P.791) AND BARIUM ENEMA OR COLONOSCOPY EVERY 5 YEARS IF YOU ARE 50 YEARS OLD

Men: 2.5 months

Women: 2.2 months

HAVING A MAMMOGRAM (SEE P.82) EVERY 2 YEARS FOR 10 YEARS IF YOU ARE 50 YEARS OLD

Women: 0.8 months

perform studies. Not all studies are of equally strong quality. And not all good studies of a single subject reach the same conclusion. When you hear about a new study, learn more about how it was performed so that you can judge how trustworthy the results are likely to be.

There are a great many factors that affect the strength of a study. Here are a few of the most important.

SIZE OF STUDY

The greater the number of subjects (people) in a study, the greater the likelihood that the study will produce results that are applicable to large numbers of people.

There are two reasons for this. First, not all people are alike, and the larger the number of subjects in a study, the greater the likelihood that the results will be applicable to most people. Second, the greater the number of subjects, the greater the likelihood that the results of the study did not occur merely by chance.

Nevertheless, even very large studies that involve thousands of people can contain flaws, and occasionally very small studies are so striking that many scientists believe the results.

CONTROLLING FOR CHANCE

Chance can affect the results of any study. Suppose a study finds that people who take a vitamin pill every day live longer than people who do not. Before doctors conducting the study can conclude that taking a vitamin every day will lengthen your life, they must ask whether the findings of the study could have occurred by chance.

They ask themselves the likelihood that the result (for example, living longer) is due to chance and not to (in this instance) taking a daily vitamin. Statistical tests give the answer. Doctors generally agree that, if the likelihood that the result occurred by chance is less than 5%, it is probably valid (or "statistically significant").

In certain circumstances, the threshold for statistical significance is set lower, such as at 1%. In general, the more subjects there are in a study, the more likely it is that a difference between subjects receiving the treatment and those not receiving the treatment will be found to be statistically significant. That is how the size of a study helps control for chance.

The same logic applies in reverse. Suppose the study finds that people who take a daily vitamin live 2 months longer than those who do not, but the statistical tests find that this result is not statistically significant. Before concluding that taking a daily vitamin does not lengthen life, the doctors must perform another kind of statistical test.

They must consider the likelihood that there really is a benefit in extending life from taking a daily vitamin but that this study might not have been large enough to detect it.

In summary, sometimes studies that seem to show a positive result (that a practice is beneficial) are a fluke; the apparent benefit occurred because of chance. And sometimes studies that seem to show a negative result (because the result was not statistically significant) are also wrong. A high-quality study evaluates the likelihood that a positive or negative result was the result of chance.

DURATION OF STUDY

Some medical treatments give immediate results. For example, antibiotics cure most infections in a matter of days. Other medical treatments, and almost all of the things that are currently recommended to maintain your health, took many years to achieve their benefits.

Therefore, studies must be conducted over many years to determine if a practice (such as a screening test, changing your diet, or taking a daily vitamin) is beneficial.

TYPE OF STUDY

There are various types of studies that can be performed. Not surprisingly, the ones that can be done most easily and inexpensively are the ones that lead to the least valid results. And vice versa.

Randomized, controlled trial (RCT) The very best kind of study, the one that provides the strongest evidence, is an RCT that is "double blind" (see explanation below). This is particularly true if it leads to a statistically significant conclusion.

However, unless an RCT is unusually large, involves a very diverse group of people, had few weaknesses in its design, and produces a result that is highly statistically significant, doctors are unlikely to change their beliefs and practices on the basis of a single study.

The main features of an RCT are:

■ Some participants are assigned to receive a treatment and other

Nine Choices for Good Health

Doctors can help protect you from some illnesses by giving you screening tests and immunizations. But the impact of what your physician can do is small compared to what you can do for yourself by eating a nutritious diet, exercising, not using addicting substances, and engaging only in safe sex.

You may decide to make changes slowly, integrating healthy practices into your life one at a time. One thing we can tell you with confidence. If you are currently healthy and want to stay that way, following the advice in this chapter is the best way to protect your health.

Life is a series of choices. Some turn out to matter, and some do not. Your choices can have a profound impact on your health. If you follow the advice in this chapter, you will truly be taking charge of your health—and on your way toward the best possible chance for a long, healthy life.

EAT A HEALTHY DIET

There are "good" foods and "bad" foods, but they are only good or bad if they are consumed regularly, over a long period of time. It is a matter of balance, but is actually even more complicated than this.

Some foods appear to be good for you when consumed in moderation, but bad if consumed in excess. A prime example is red meat, which contains valuable iron but also often contains a great deal of saturated fat. It should be eaten in moderation.

Just about everyone eats some less-than-healthful foods occasionally, and there is nothing wrong with this. These foods are not like a fast-acting poison: one bite and you become ill. Let the person who has never consumed a big piece of chocolate cake cast the first stone.

The point is that the regular food choices you make over months and years can affect your health. It really is true that a diet rich in wholesome foods such as vegetables, grains, and fruits, which contain fiber and valuable vitamins and minerals, benefits your health.

EXERCISE

Make exercise a part of your life every day. Moderate activity—such as taking the stairs instead of the elevator or walking to the store instead of driving—offers substantial health benefits, even if the activity lasts for only 5 to 15 minutes.

While 30 minutes of exercise every day continues to be optimal, you do not need to join a health club or own a leotard to work out. Begin by stretching for 10 minutes each day (see p.56) and build in a 20-minute brisk walk in the morning, on your lunch hour, or at the end of the day.

The key is to get moving and integrate regular exercise into your daily routine. Vigorous exercise is even more beneficial. In short, exercising can help you live better, as well as longer.

DO NOT USE ADDICTING SUBSTANCES

Smoking is the leading preventable cause of death in the United States, responsible for more than 400,000 deaths per year. And while there is a decline in the overall number of smokers (largely due to adults who quit), there is an alarming increase in the number of teenage smokers, as well as a surge in those who smoke cigars and pipes.

Most smokers start before age 20, which is why it is so important for younger people never to start. Even if you have smoked for a long time, your body begins to heal much of the damage as soon as you stop. It is never too late to quit.

When used in more than moderate doses, alcohol can also be addicting. Addicting illicit substances such as cocaine or morphine have absolutely no benefit when used for "recreational purposes" (as contrasted to their medical use).

Like addiction to alcohol, once you are "hooked," the only pleasure you get is from avoiding the pain of withdrawal symptoms.

ENGAGE ONLY IN SAFE SEX

Unsafe sex can lead to unwanted pregnancy and sexually transmitted diseases (STDs). There are at least 25 STDs, including infection with the virus that causes cancer of the cervix and the human immunodeficiency virus (HIV), which causes AIDS.

p.76

The best way to prevent STDs is by using a male or female condom (see p.71). The fewer sexual partners you have, the less risk you have of contracting an STD. Other than abstaining from sex, the safest behavior is to have a monogamous relationship with one monogamous partner.

Because many teenagers in the United States are sexually active, it is important for parents to talk to their children at a younger age about sex and the risks of sexual activity. If you find this difficult, read the chapter Health of Adolescents (see p.1021) with your child.

HAVE REGULAR MEDICAL CHECKUPS (AND CHECK YOURSELF)

To identify health problems early, you need to have certain parts of your body examined and certain screening tests performed regularly. However, regular exams are not something only your doctor performs; there are some self-examinations, including those of the skin, breasts, and testicles, that you should perform regularly. There are also some screening tests, such as for blood pressure, that you can do yourself.

p.77

If you have a chronic (long-term) condition, such as diabetes, it too needs to be monitored. Your doctor will periodically check your condition, but it is equally important for you to monitor yourself using the home tests recommended by your physician.

PREVENT INJURY

Injuries account for a significant percentage of suffering and premature deaths. Even your home, usually considered a safe haven, can contain numerous threats to health and safety. Medicine has learned a lot about how to prevent injuries. Educate yourself about the steps you can take to keep your family safe.

p.86

MANAGE STRESS

Very few lives are free of stress, and not all stress is bad for you. However, excessive stress can lead to disturbing symptoms that have health implications. Learn the techniques for reducing the adverse effects of stress.

p.89

GET IMMUNIZED

Immunizations to many terrible diseases have had a profound positive impact on health in the past 50 years. It is easy to take that impact for granted, and many people do. You should not. It is essential for children to have the required immunizations (see p.947). Adults also require regular immunizations.

p.94

MAINTAIN IDEAL BODY WEIGHT

If you can maintain an ideal body weight, through whatever combination of diet and exercise (see pp.37–55), you can do more to protect your health than any doctor's pill. Being overweight or obese (see pp.853–855) increases your risk of getting heart disease, diabetes, and several forms of cancer.

p.47

participants are assigned to receive a harmless, fake treatment (a placebo).

■ The study (not the people in the study or their doctors) controls which subjects get the real treatment and which subjects get the placebo, and chooses these people by a random process. This approach describes the term "randomized, controlled trial."

■ Usually the subjects do not know whether they are getting the real treatment or a placebo; they are "blind" to that knowledge. Often the doctors also do not know, since they could unintentionally influence the outcome. When both the people in the study and the doctors involved in the study do not know who is getting the real treatment and who is getting the placebo, the study is called a "double-blind" study.

■ Specific information about the subjects that is relevant to the study—for example, their weight, whether they smoked, or what diseases they develop over time—is carefully collected before, during, and after completion of the study.

While RCTs are generally regarded as the best kind of study, they may contain weaknesses that make them less convincing. For example, they may enroll only a narrow spectrum of subjects (such as only the most severely affected people with a disease, not the average person), may have many subjects drop out of the study before it is completed, or may not use the most accurate diagnostic tests.

Sometimes, such studies are just plain impractical. For example, suppose doctors wanted to do an RCT to study whether eating broccoli could protect people from getting colon cancer. For a perfect RCT, they would have to make sure that subjects assigned to eat broccoli were willing to eat broccoli (no small task).

For the placebo group they would have to create something that looked and tasted like broccoli but which was not broccoli. And they would have to make sure that the subjects assigned to eat the fake broccoli (the placebo) could not distinguish it from real broccoli. You begin to see the problem.

Even when such practical difficulties are not present, most RCTs require large numbers of people, take a long time, and are very expensive.

Therefore, doctors sometimes conduct different kinds of studies that are easier, faster, and less expensive to perform, even though the studies may not provide evidence that is as strong as that obtained from an RCT.

Cohort study This kind of study provides evidence that is not as strong as the evidence from an RCT, but it avoids some of the practical problems of RCTs. The main features of cohort studies are:

■ As in RCTs, specific information about the participants that is relevant to the study is carefully collected before, during, and after completion of the study.

■ Unlike RCTs, there is no control over whether a subject takes a particular medicine or eats a particular food. But (continuing with the fictional broccoli study)

whether or not they eat broccoli or not is carefully measured.

■ When the study is finished, researchers determine if the subjects who ate broccoli were less likely than the subjects who did not eat it to get colon cancer—and if the more broccoli the subjects ate, the lower the risk they had of colon cancer.

■ However, because the study does not control which subjects ate broccoli, it is not known for certain if the lower rates of colon cancer in subjects who ate broccoli were because they ate broccoli, or because of some other factor. For example, perhaps the same subjects who ate broccoli also exercised regularly and ate lots of fruits and other vegetables, and it was these factors that protected them against colon cancer, not the broccoli.

Case-control study This kind of study provides the least amount of strong evidence, but is the easiest and fastest to perform because it is done by retroactively reviewing information that has already been collected in medical records or elsewhere. The main features of case-control studies are:

■ People who have had a particular disease diagnosed (such as colon cancer) are identified from medical records.

■ People who have not had the disease diagnosed (and therefore are not likely to have it) are identified from medical records.

■ Various other aspects of lifestyle (such as eating certain foods or exercising) and medical history are obtained.

■ The study measures if people

who have had the disease were less likely to have followed certain lifestyle habits (such as eating certain foods or exercising).

The problem with case-control studies is that the information in medical records may not be entirely accurate for purposes of a study because it was not originally collected as part of a study. Also, the needed information (such as whether someone eats certain foods, and how much) may not have been routinely recorded in the medical record.

Other kinds of studies There are other kinds of studies and variants of the three types of studies described here. In general, these three types are the ones that doctors pay most attention to.

When you learn about a new study, keep in mind which of these kinds of studies it was. If it was an RCT, there is a higher likelihood that it is accurate. In addition, find out if the subjects included in the study resemble you or the person you are concerned about. Finally, ask your doctor for his or her opinion of the study and its conclusions.

Selective Benefits of Preventive Practices

Not every good thing is equally good for everybody. Consider screening tests that are designed to detect disease at an early stage—before the disease has produced symptoms. The higher the risk of the disease to begin with, the more likely the test will be useful.

The risk of having a disease varies with age, gender, occupation, history of the disease in other family members, and other factors.

For example, no medical authority recommends that women below age 35 routinely have mammograms because it is rare for young women to get breast cancer. No one recommends that men of any age get mammograms because it is extremely rare for men to get breast cancer.

On the other hand, people in health care occupations are more likely to come into contact with people who have tuberculosis, so health care professionals are regularly screened for tuberculosis with a skin test.

For most other people in the United States, however, the chance of having a tuberculosis infection is too low to justify screening tests. These tests are nevertheless sometimes performed by institutions where people live in particularly close quarters, such as school dormitories.

Screening tests are not ordered routinely for people whose risk of the disease is very small to begin with because the tests can generate risks that outweigh the benefits. The tests are also expensive.

Recommendations for a healthy lifestyle can also vary by age, gender, and other factors. Preventive activities such as reducing cholesterol to lower the risk of heart disease are clearly beneficial in many middle-aged men with elevated cholesterol levels.

Yet, testing cholesterol levels is not recommended for people who are very old or sick with diseases such as cancer because the potential benefit is small.

SCREENING TESTS: THE POSITIVES AND NEGATIVES

It is possible through screening tests to diagnose serious diseases early, and to treat them before they cause damage.

Although many scientific studies have proven the value of screening tests, there is still controversy over who should get a particular screening test, and how often. Read What Screening Tests Should I Have? (see p.80) to find out which tests are recommended for you and your family.

For a screening test to be useful:

■ The test must be accurate. When the test result is abnormal (a positive test result), there should be a high likelihood that the person who had the test really has the disease being screened for. When the test result is normal (a negative test result), there should be a high likelihood that the person does not have the disease.

■ The test should be able to detect the disease early enough so that the disease can be cured, or so that suffering from the disease can be reduced.

■ The screening test itself should not have any adverse effects on the person being tested.

No test is perfectly accurate; all have some degree of error. When a test is "falsely positive" (the test result is abnormal, but the person who had the test does not have the disease), unnecessary (and sometimes painful or risky) additional tests may be ordered. In addition, the person with a false-positive test result is unnecessarily worried.

A Harvard study of women

having mammograms estimated that, over a 10-year period, nearly half of the women would have at least one falsely positive mammogram, and that about 20% would undergo a biopsy that, in retrospect, was unnecessary.

When a screening test is "falsely negative" (the test result is normal, but the person who had the test really does have the disease), the person is falsely reassured. The person might dismiss symptoms of the disease and not seek further treatment, because the results of the recent screening test showed that nothing was wrong.

Not every screening test can detect disease early enough to improve your health. An example is using chest x-rays to screen for lung cancer.

In other cases, a screening test may detect a disease that, though sometimes serious, does not always require treatment. An example is some cases of prostate cancer.

In older men, when the cancer in the prostate is very small, is causing no symptoms, and has not spread (and is unlikely to spread in the man's lifetime), diagnosis and treatment can cause anxiety and more problems than if the disease had never been diagnosed in the first place.

Chest x-ray: a screening test failure In the case of chest x-rays to screen for lung cancer, the negatives exceeded the positives. For many years, regular

Benefits of Pap Smears for Detecting Cervical Cancer

The incidence of invasive cancer of the cervix has dropped significantly since the 1940s. This is due primarily to the advent of regular screening with Pap smears. Having a regular Pap smear significantly lowers a woman's chance of developing (and subsequently dying of) invasive cancer of the cervix.

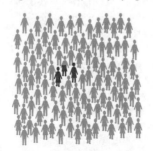 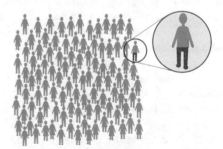

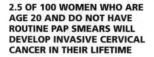

2.5 OF 100 WOMEN WHO ARE AGE 20 AND DO NOT HAVE ROUTINE PAP SMEARS WILL DEVELOP INVASIVE CERVICAL CANCER IN THEIR LIFETIME

0.3 OF 100 WOMEN WHO ARE AGE 20 AND HAVE ROUTINE PAP SMEARS WILL DEVELOP INVASIVE CERVICAL CANCER IN THEIR LIFETIME

chest x-rays were recommended for smokers as a way to detect lung cancer before it had spread (metastasized) to other parts of the body. Millions of people got regular chest x-rays.

Then it was discovered that most lung cancers had spread by the time they could reliably be seen on a chest x-ray. So, by the time the chest x-rays did reveal lung cancer, it was usually too late for treatment.

Furthermore, sometimes the x-rays revealed suspicious abnormalities that caused the person to undergo further tests and even surgery, only to discover nothing serious. On very rare occasions, people died of complications of

the surgery. A test that seemed sensible caused more harm than good.

Pap smear: a screening test success The screening test for cervical cancer—the Pap smear—is an example of the ideal screening test. It can detect abnormal cells in the cervix well before any symptoms appear, and it can detect them early enough so that the vast majority of women with early-stage cervical cancer can be completely cured.

There is virtually no risk in having the test done. It is also relatively inexpensive and simple to perform. The Pap smear has greatly reduced deaths from cervical cancer in the past 40 years.

DIET AND NUTRITION

Your body relies on at least 40 nutrients found in food for life-sustaining functions. As you digest food, it is broken down into nutrients, which are absorbed into your bloodstream and carried to every cell in your body. Nutrients and other essential food components, such as fiber, are classified into six groups:

Water

Water makes up almost 70% of the weight of your body. People tend not to think of it as a nutrient, but it is one, and it is critical to your health. Water is the major component of most cells. It carries nutrients to your cells and takes away waste products. Water also helps regulate your body temperature.

Your body loses water every day, through urine, bowel movements, sweat, and the moisture you expel into the atmosphere when you exhale. To make up for that loss, men require about 15½ cups a day and women about 11½ cups a day. Remember, that includes beverages other than water and the water contained in food. For example, a small tossed salad contains nearly one cup of water.

Caffeine-containing beverages such as coffee, tea, and some colas act as diuretics, drawing water out of your body. Alcohol has the same effect.

If you exercise vigorously, are pregnant or breast-feeding, or are exposed to hot temperatures regularly, you should drink even more water. Drinking water is a good habit; substitute water for soft drinks or coffee. Sparkling water is a good substitute for alcohol if you cannot drink it or want to reduce the amount you drink.

Carbohydrates

Carbohydrates are the starches or sugars found in foods such as bread, pasta, rice, dried beans and peas, potatoes, cereals, and sugars. They should be your main source of energy, or calories.

Carbohydrates come in two forms: simple (found in all sugars, including honey, corn syrup, and fruits) and complex (found in the starchy foods listed above).

Foods rich in complex carbohydrates also contain vitamins, minerals, and fiber.

Fruit contains simple carbohydrates and also provides valuable vitamins, minerals, and fiber.

Fiber

Fiber is not a nutrient (because it is not digested and absorbed into the body) but is helpful because it provides the bulk necessary to help the large intestine move waste out of your system.

Dietary fiber is found only in plant foods; it is the part of the whole grains, fruits, vegetables, beans, nuts, and seeds that humans cannot digest.

A diet high in fiber prevents constipation and may lower the risk of heart disease (see p.652), type 2 diabetes (see p.833), and diverticular disease (see p.783). Most studies have not found that

High-Fiber Foods

The chart shows selected foods and their fiber content. Start by taking in about 8 grams of fiber a day and work up to about 25 grams per day.

FOOD	AMOUNT	TOTAL FIBER (GRAMS)
100% bran cereal	½ cup	10.0
Peas (cooked)	½ cup	5.2
Kidney beans	½ cup	4.5
White beans	½ cup	4.2
Apple with skin	1 medium	3.9
Whole-wheat bread	2 slices	3.9
Potato	1 small	3.8
Popcorn	3 cups popped	2.8
Broccoli (cooked)	½ cup	2.6
Pear	1 medium	2.5
Tangerine	1 medium	1.6

fiber protects against colon cancer, although this remains unclear. Take in at least 25 grams of fiber every day.

There are two types of fiber: **Insoluble fiber** is found in foods such as wheat bran, whole grains, and vegetables. It does not dissolve in water. Water-insoluble fiber helps you digest food and eliminate wastes by encouraging stools to move through and out of the large intestine.

Soluble fiber is found in beans, oats, barley, and some fruits and vegetables. It dissolves in water and lowers blood cholesterol in some people by forming a gel in the intestines that binds to cholesterol and carries it out of the body.

Fats and Oils

Fat (which is solid) and oil (which is liquid) are energy-dense, meaning they contain many calories per serving—more, in fact, than any other food at about 135 calories per tablespoon. (A tablespoon of a carbohydrate or protein contains about 60 calories.)

You should consume only in small amounts foods that are rich in cholesterol and saturated fats. The nutrition-facts label (see p.50) on foods tells you how much cholesterol and saturated fat a serving of food contains. By subtracting the amount of saturated fat from the total fats (also on the label), you can estimate how much polyunsaturated fat and monounsaturated fat the food contains.

Transunsaturated fatty acid, also known as trans fat, was created by food chemists a century ago as a cheap alternative to

Integrating Fiber Into Your Diet

Consider these recommendations to integrate fiber into your daily diet.

■ Choose bran and whole-grain breads, cereals, and pastas over white-flour versions.

■ Eat fresh fruits and vegetables rather than drinking juice, which contains much less fiber.

■ Eat the skin and membranes of fruits and vegetables such as apples, peaches, tomatoes, and carrots (wash them well first). Much of the fiber is in the skin.

■ Integrate fiber gradually into your diet to give your body time to adjust. Suddenly increasing the amount of fiber you eat can cause gas, bloating, or diarrhea. Start with about 8 grams of fiber a day and work up to about 25 grams per day.

■ Drink lots of water. For fiber to be beneficial, you must drink an adequate amount of fluids. Increasing your intake of insoluble fiber without increasing your intake of fluids can cause constipation rather than prevent it.

Fiber Intake and Reduction in Heart Attack Risk

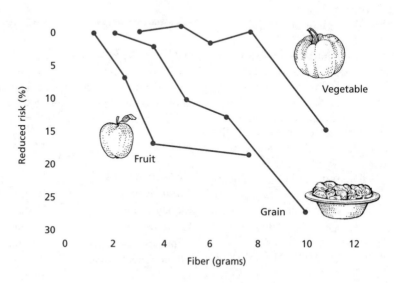

A 6-year Harvard study of 40,000 men strengthens the case for eating a high-fiber diet. As fiber consumption increased, the risk of having a heart attack dropped. This was true whether the fiber came from fruits, grains, or vegetables. The men who ate the most fiber had a risk of heart attack that was about 30% lower than the risk of the men who ate the least amount of fiber.

Types of Fat

There are different kinds of dietary fats. Some are clearly better for your health than others. Most of the fats you eat should be in the healthy forms shown below.

TYPE OF DIETARY FAT	INFORMATION	FOODS	
Polyunsaturated fat	Needed by the body to help form the membranes covering every cell	Natural vegetable oils; soft (tub) margarine	BETTER FOR YOU
Monounsaturated fat	Needed by the body to help form the membranes covering every cell	Natural vegetable oils; soft (tub) margarine	
Cholesterol	Raises blood cholesterol (by adding to cholesterol made by the body); harmful if eaten in large amounts	Animal fats (fatty meats, butter, lard, whole milk, poultry skin)	
Saturated fat	Raises blood cholesterol even more than cholesterol in diet; harmful if eaten in large amounts	Animal fats (fatty meats, butter, whole milk, poultry skin); some vegetable oils	
Transunsaturated fat	A type of unsaturated fat that has recently been found to raise cholesterol and to be harmful	Animal fats; stick (hard) margarine	WORSE FOR YOU

Comparing Fats and Oils

Different oils contain different amounts of the various types of fats, as shown below. Use oils and fats that are high in monounsaturated fat (such as olive and canola oils) or polyunsaturated fat (such as safflower oil). Use saturated fats (such as butter) only in moderation.

OIL OR FAT	% SATURATED FAT	% MONO-UNSATURATED FAT	% POLY-UNSATURATED FAT	
Olive oil	14	70	11	BETTER FOR YOU
Canola oil	6	62	31	
Sunflower oil	13	32	50	
Peanut oil	20	45	35	
Soybean oil	15	43	38	
Safflower oil	10	20	66	
Corn oil	13	24	59	
Soft (tub) margarine	14	32	31	
Chicken fat	30	45	21	
Lard	39	45	21	
Butter	62	29	4	WORSE FOR YOU
Coconut oil	87	6	2	

butter. It is now used in many packaged and convenience foods such as cookies, cakes, and chips to improve taste and preserve freshness. Small amounts of natural trans fats are also found in meat and dairy products. Trans fat is the worst kind of fat—worse even than saturated fat—because it raises LDL ("bad") cholesterol and lowers HDL ("good") cholesterol, increasing the risk of heart disease, heart attacks, strokes, and premature death.

As of January 1, 2006, the FDA will require food manufacturers to include trans fat on the nutrition-facts labels of all products. Until then, you can still look to the label for help figuring out how much trans fat a product contains. If the label lists "shortening," "partially hydrogenated," or "hydrogenated oil" as one of its first ingredients, it has a lot of trans fat. Eat only very small amounts.

Hard (stick) margarine contains high concentrations of this unhealthy kind of fat. However, soft (tub) margarine contains mainly polyunsaturated and monounsaturated fats.

Some fats are rich in a chemical called omega-3 fatty acids. These fatty acids are found mainly in fish and linseed oil. They may have protective effects against atherosclerosis and some inflammatory diseases, such as arthritis.

Proteins

Proteins supply amino acids, which build, repair, and maintain body tissue and are vital to everyday body function. The body needs a constant supply of protein to repair body cells as they wear out and to help regulate body processes.

Protein is found in meat, poultry, fish, eggs, milk, cheese, yogurt, and soy products, as well as beans, seeds, nuts, and, in smaller amounts, grain products and many vegetables. Protein-rich foods that contain high levels of fat, such as meats and cheeses, should be eaten in moderation.

Most people eat more protein than they need; protein should not represent more than 10% to 15% of your total caloric intake every day. For an adult, this is about 50 grams per day, or a chicken breast the size of a deck of cards. Extra protein is not used to build extra muscle unless you exercise; it leaves the body in urine.

Vitamins and Minerals

Vitamins are substances that your body needs but cannot make. They facilitate chemical reactions in body cells and help you process the food you eat. Each vitamin has a specific role (see Vitamins and Minerals in Foods, p.42) and regulates different body processes. There are 13 essential vitamins divided into two categories—fat-soluble and water-soluble.

The best way to get the vitamins you need is by eating a wide variety of whole, natural foods—vegetables, fruits, and whole grains. Although vitamin supplements (see right) are useful for some people, most nutrition experts recommend eating healthy foods as the main source of vitamins and minerals.

There is strong evidence that people who have a high intake of vitamin-rich foods are healthier than those who do not. There is no absolute proof that such a diet is the cause of their better health, but it is very likely. Increase your intake of vitamins by increasing the amount of vitamin-rich foods you eat every day.

Minerals help regulate fluid balance, muscle contractions, and nerve impulses, and are essential to the healthy development of bones and teeth. There are at least 20 minerals in a balanced diet, including calcium, magnesium, sodium, iron, potassium, and phosphorus.

Major minerals, such as calcium, are needed to build bones in childhood and slow the rate of bone loss in adulthood to prevent the bone-thinning condition osteoporosis (see p.596).

Like vitamins, the best way to get the minerals you need for health is by eating a balanced diet rich in fruits, vegetables, and whole grains.

Women, who are especially vulnerable to osteoporosis, should eat enough calcium-rich foods to take in from 1,000 to 1,500 milligrams of calcium (see p.44) every day; calcium supplements are recommended if you cannot get enough from your diet.

SUPPLEMENTS

As summarized above, there is a great deal of evidence that it is beneficial for you to eat vitamin-rich foods. The question is whether it is also good for you to take these same vitamins and minerals in pill or liquid form.

For many years doctors believed that almost everyone in

the world's developed nations received enough vitamins and minerals from the food they ate, and that there was therefore little value in taking supplements.

In recent years, however, it has been discovered that the traditional definition of the minimum daily requirements for some vitamins may have been too low. A prime example is folic acid. It is now known that the daily amounts of this vitamin that were recommended as recently as the 1970s were too low. Especially in women of child-bearing age, much more folic acid is needed to reduce the risk of neural tube defects (see p.985).

There is some evidence that folic acid may also help reduce the risk of colon cancer and breast cancer, atherosclerosis, and osteoporosis—although this has not been proven.

The following general recommendations can be made, although much research is under way and they could change in the future. Since most of these recommendations are controversial, or may not apply in your situation, ask your doctor for his or her advice on taking a supplement.

INFANTS

■ If you are breast-feeding your baby, he or she may benefit from a vitamin D supplement.

■ If your baby is older than 6 months and feeds predominantly on "ready-to-feed" formulas or liquids that are prepared with distilled water or spring water (that are not fluoridated, like the tap water in most communities), your baby may also need a fluoride supplement.

■ If your baby is 6 months to 1 year or is bottle-fed, iron supplements are sometimes recommended.

MENSTRUATING GIRLS AND WOMEN

■ If you are menstruating, you lose a lot of iron in menstrual blood. Eating iron-rich foods is the best way to replace lost iron. If tests show your iron is low despite including more iron in your diet, an iron supplement may be beneficial. Prescription iron pills are stronger than nonprescription iron supplements. Check with your doctor.

■ Adequate calcium intake (1,000 to 1,500 milligrams [mg]/day) throughout adolescence and young adulthood helps ensure strong bones before menopause, when bones slowly begin to thin. Calcium supplements are recommended if you cannot get enough from your diet.

■ Folic acid is recommended for all menstruating girls and women (see below).

WOMEN WHO ARE PREGNANT OR TRYING TO BECOME PREGNANT

■ We strongly recommend that all women of childbearing age get at least 400 micrograms [μg]/day of folic acid. This can greatly reduce the chance of a birth defect called neural tube defect (see p.985). You can get the folic acid you need in fortified cereals or in folic acid supplements.

■ You need extra iron (15 to 30 mg/day) and calcium (1,200 mg/day) if you are now or will soon be pregnant.

BREAST-FEEDING WOMEN

■ You need extra calcium (1,200 mg/day) if you are breast-feeding; many doctors also recommend taking a multivitamin.

MENOPAUSAL WOMEN

■ You need extra calcium (1,500 mg/day if you are not on hormone therapy and 1,000 mg/day if you are) to slow bone loss from osteoporosis (see p.596); many doctors also recommend taking a multivitamin to ensure you have enough vitamin D as well.

PEOPLE OVER AGE 60

■ You may benefit from a daily multivitamin to ensure adequate nutritional intake. Many older people consume a diet poor in nutrients. Furthermore, some nutrition experts believe the body's ability to absorb certain nutrients declines with age.

■ For people over age 50 who are not out in the sun regularly, daily supplements of vitamin D (400 international units [IU] per day) are recommended. Avoid doses in excess of 50,000 units per day; they are toxic.

SOME VEGETARIANS

■ If you do not eat any meat, dairy, or animal products, you may need extra calcium, iron, zinc, and vitamins B_{12} and D.

GENERAL ADULT POPULATION

■ For people who do not eat adequate amounts of vegetables and fruits, which are the best sources of most vitamins, an inexpensive standard multivitamin pill

Vitamins and Minerals in Foods

The best way to get all the nutrients you need is to eat a variety of foods, including whole grains, vegetables, fruits, and modest portions (2 to 3 ounces per meal) of lean meats, skinless poultry, or fish.

VITAMIN OR MINERAL	FOOD SOURCES	ACTION
Fat-soluble vitamins		
Vitamin A	Fortified milk; eggs; cheeses; liver; fish oil	Keeps eyes healthy; essential for growth and health of cells in organs, skin, and hair; works as an antioxidant (protects cells from damage). Excess retinol, the active version of vitamin A, may cause decreased bone strength and a greater risk of fracture. The other form of vitamin A, beta carotene, is not associated with increased fracture risk.
Vitamin D	Fortified milk	Promotes absorption of calcium; helps form bones and teeth; supports function of nervous system and muscles
Vitamin E	Vegetable oils; nuts; seeds; wheat germ; leafy green vegetables	Works as an antioxidant (protects cells from damage); plays a part in formation of blood cells
Vitamin K	Spinach; broccoli; milk; eggs; cereals	Essential for production of proteins that permit blood clotting
Water-soluble vitamins		
Vitamin B$_1$ (thiamin)	Pork; legumes; seeds; nuts; fortified grains; cereals	Converts food into energy; essential for the function of muscles and nervous system
Vitamin B$_2$ (riboflavin)	Milk; yogurt; meats; leafy green vegetables; whole-grain breads and cereals	Helps release energy from food; regulates hormones and helps maintain healthy eyes, skin, and nerve function
Vitamin B$_3$ (niacin)	Meats; fish; legumes; nuts; whole-grain and enriched breads and cereals	Helps convert food into energy; aids in the formation of red blood cells; essential for the body's use of some hormones
Vitamin B$_6$ (pyridoxine)	Chicken; fish; eggs; brown rice; whole-wheat products	Needed for formation of red blood cells; helps the body make proteins; assists in fighting infection; may reduce risk of atherosclerosis
Vitamin B$_{12}$	Meats; fish; poultry; eggs; milk	Helps make red blood cells; maintains nervous system; may reduce risk of atherosclerosis
Vitamin C	Citrus fruits; green vegetables; fortified cereals	Works as an antioxidant (protects cells from damage); necessary for healthy skin; regulates metabolism during stress or illness

VITAMIN OR MINERAL	FOOD SOURCES	ACTION
Water-soluble vitamins		
Folic acid (folate)	Fortified cereals; dark green leafy vegetables; fruits; legumes; yeast breads; wheat germ	Helps make new body cells; before pregnancy and in first 3 months of pregnancy helps prevent birth defects; helps in red blood cell formation; may reduce risk of atherosclerosis and possibly help protect bone strength.
Minerals		
Calcium	Milk and dairy products; green leafy vegetables; tofu; sardines and salmon with bones; calcium-fortified orange juice	Essential for formation and maintenance of bones and teeth; contraction of muscles (including the heart muscle); supports normal nerve function; aids blood clotting; may reduce risk of colon cancer
Chromium	Whole-grain products; bran cereals; brewer's yeast; calf's liver; American cheese; wheat germ	Works with insulin to convert carbohydrates and fat into energy
Copper	Shellfish; nuts; seeds; legumes; liver; whole grains	Essential in formation of skin and connective tissue; needed for many chemical reactions related to energy; essential for heart function
Iron	Meats; poultry; fish; cereals; fruits; green vegetables; whole-grain products	Helps carry oxygen in the bloodstream; essential for formation of red blood cells
Magnesium	Nuts; legumes; whole grains; green vegetables; bananas	Works in hundreds of chemical reactions in the body that metabolize food and transmit messages between cells
Phosphorus	Milk; meats; poultry; fish; cereals; legumes; fruits	Needed for strong bones and teeth; involved in helping the body release energy
Potassium	Fruits; vegetables; legumes; meats	Helps transmit nerve impulses; contraction of muscles (including the heart muscle); may help maintain normal blood pressure
Selenium	Seafood; kidney; liver; cereals; grains	Works as an antioxidant (protects cells from damage); essential for healthy heart muscle
Sodium	Table salt; vegetables; many prepared foods; some bottled water	Maintains fluids in body; helps in nerve transmission and muscle contraction; helps control rhythm of heart muscle
Zinc	Meats; poultry; oysters; eggs; legumes; nuts; milk; yogurt; whole-grain cereals	Used in sperm production; needed for growth and production of energy; helps immune function and blood clotting

Sources of Calcium

The best food sources of calcium are dairy products, which also contain the vitamin D your body needs to absorb calcium. Choose skim milk, low-fat or nonfat yogurt, and low-fat cheeses to maximize your calcium intake without adding fat to your diet.

People who cannot digest the sugars in dairy products (see Lactose Intolerance, p.798) can obtain calcium from lactose-free dairy products, calcium-enriched orange juice, calcium supplements, and the other nondairy sources listed here.

FOOD SOURCE	AMOUNT	CALCIUM (MILLIGRAMS)
Sardines with bones	3 ounces	325
Dry milk	1/3 cup	300
Nonfat or low-fat yogurt (plain)	1 cup	300
Cheddar cheese	1½ ounces	300
Skim or low-fat milk	1 cup	300
Spinach (cooked)	1¼ cups	300
Collard greens (cooked)	2 cups	300
Black beans	1 cup	125

HOW MUCH CALCIUM DO I NEED?

Of all the minerals you need in your diet, you should pay particular attention to iron and calcium. This chart shows how much calcium you should consume every day.

If you find that you cannot eat or drink enough calcium-containing foods to reach the recommended levels, take a calcium supplement. Calcium supplements contain varying amounts of pure (elemental) calcium, depending on the elements with which they are combined. Look for the amount of elemental calcium on the package; this is the number that you should match to your requirements, as listed below.

AGE OR CONDITION	CALCIUM (MILLIGRAMS/DAY)
6 to 10 years	800–1,200
11 to 24 years	1,200–1,500
Men, 25 to 65 years	1,000
Women, 25 to 50 years	1,000
Pregnant or breast-feeding women	1,200
Postmenopausal women taking estrogen	1,000
Postmenopausal women not taking estrogen	1,500
65 years and older	1,500

once daily may be beneficial, and will not cause problems.

■ For people with a family history (parents or siblings) of coronary artery disease at a young age (men under age 50; women under age 60), regular intake of folic acid (400 µg/day) and possibly vitamin B_6 (100 mg) and vitamin B_{12} (100 mg) may protect against heart disease. This is unproven, but indirect evidence leads some doctors to recommend it, and at these doses the vitamins are not harmful.

■ Daily supplements of vitamin C (500 mg) and vitamin E (400 international units [IU]) may have some protective effect against atherosclerosis and some cancers. This is unproven, but indirect evidence leads some doctors to recommend it, and at these doses the vitamins are not harmful.

■ Regularly taking more than 20,000 IU/day of vitamin A or more than 5,000 IU/day of vitamin D can be toxic, and should be avoided.

A healthy diet is not just about balancing your food choices and avoiding deficiencies. It's about eating the foods that improve health and avoiding those that raise the risk for illnesses such as heart disease, cancer, and diabetes. We need a mix of proteins, carbohydrates, and fats—that has not changed—but research has shown that some choices within these categories are better than others. Here are some guidelines to help you make healthy choices in your diet:

Eat fewer "bad" fats and more "good" fats. Not all fats are bad. The two types of unhealthy fat—saturated and trans fats—raise your total cholesterol. These are found in highest amounts in

Understanding the Healthy Eating Pyramid

This healthy eating pyramid was created by Harvard scientists, who concluded—based on years of research—that it represented a more healthy diet than the familiar U.S. Department of Agriculture (USDA) food pyramid, which had been devised in 1992. (The USDA is working on a revision of its food pyramid that will take into consideration more recent research.)

In the healthy eating pyramid, the widest part at the bottom represents the most important category—daily exercise and weight control. The foods in the top section, at the tip of the pyramid, should be eaten as little as possible. Healthy

Use sparingly

Sweets, potatoes, white rice, white bread, and pasta

Alcohol in moderation (unless contraindicated)

Red meat; butter

Dairy or calcium supplement, 1–2 times a day

Fish, poultry, and eggs, 0–2 times a day

Multiple vitamins for most

Nuts and legumes, 1–3 times a day

Vegetables, in abundance

Fruits, 2–3 times a day

Whole grains at most meals

Plant oils, including canola, corn, and olive

Daily exercise and weight control

fats, including polyunsaturated, monounsaturated, and omega-3, are in a wider section of the new pyramid, indicating that they are healthy. Carbohydrates such as white bread and white rice are in the top part because you should eat these in moderation. Eat red meat sparingly, opting instead for healthier choices such as fish, poultry, and eggs.

The healthy eating pyramid has shown results. In 2002, a study was published showing that the healthy eating pyramid nutrition plan was nearly twice as effective as that of the USDA food pyramid in reducing the risk for major diseases. The study examined the diets of more than 100,000 adults. It found that men who followed the healthy eating pyramid lowered their overall risk of certain diseases by 20% versus 11% of men following the USDA pyramid. Women in the study who followed the healthy eating pyramid lowered their overall risk by 11% versus just 3% of women following the USDA food pyramid.

From: *Eat, Drink, and Be Healthy: The Harvard Medical School Guide to Healthy Eating,* by Walter C. Willett, MD, published by Free Press, 2003.

Serving Sizes and Food Choices

FOOD GROUP

ONE SERVING SIZE

Whole grain foods
1 slice bread; 1/2 cup cooked cereal, brown rice, or wheat pasta; 1 ounce ready-to-eat cereal

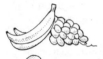

Vegetable
1 cup raw, leafy vegetables; 1/2 cup other vegetables (cooked or raw); 3/4 cup vegetable juice

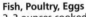

Fruit
1 medium apple, banana, or orange; 1/2 cup chopped, cooked, or canned fruit; 3/4 cup fruit juice

Fish, Poultry, Eggs
2–3 ounces cooked lean meat, poultry, or fish (1 egg or 2 tablespoons peanut butter counts as 1 ounce of meat); 1/2 cup cooked dry beans

Dairy
1 cup milk or yogurt; 1 1/2 ounces cheese; 2 ounces processed cheese

Eating according to the healthy eating pyramid may take some adjustment. Learn to think of grains, fruits, and vegetables as a primary portion of your diet and be aware of hidden fats in meat and dairy products. The servings described are generally smaller than the average American helping.

red meats, butter, whole milk and other dairy products, beef, and prepackaged foods such as cookies and cakes. You've heard for years that saturated fat is bad for you. You may not have heard that trans fat is worse, but it is.

But you should not avoid *all* kinds of fat. Some kinds of fat have powerful positive health effects. Indeed, some dietary fats are essential for your health, since your body needs them and cannot make them. These "good fats"—polyunsaturated and monounsaturated fats—come from vegetable and fish products. So, it's okay if more than 30% of your daily calories come from good fats.

Two particularly important "good fats" are the omega-3 (or n-3) fatty acids, and the omega-6 (or n-6) fatty acids. The n-3 fatty acids are found predominantly in fish, nuts, flaxseed, canola oil, and unhydrogenated soybean oil. There is strong evidence that the omega-3 fatty acids protect against atherosclerosis (and, hence, against heart disease and stroke, two of the biggest killers), against abnormal heart rhythms that can cause sudden death, and possibly against autoimmune diseases such as lupus and rheumatoid arthritis. The omega-6 fatty acids are also healthy for you.

The emphasis on eating a low-fat diet during the 1980s and 1990s led many people to avoid foods that contained good fats—like nuts—and to substitute foods that contained more carbohydrates, like chips. That was a big mistake, because the carbohydrates that most people binged on were refined-grain carbohydrates, often coated with bad fats.

Caffeine and Your Health

Caffeine is an addictive drug, but there is no evidence that clearly links consuming a moderate amount of caffeine (about 3 cups of brewed coffee per day) to disease. Caffeine does not raise cholesterol levels, although boiled or percolated (but not filtered) coffee contains chemicals that may raise cholesterol levels.

In some people, however, caffeine causes heartburn, nervousness, irritability, sleeplessness, and the jitters. If you experience these symptoms, gradually cut down on your caffeine intake.

Pain-relieving drugs often contain caffeine because caffeine can slightly strengthen the effect of the pain relievers. The caffeine in the medication can also alleviate the symptoms of caffeine withdrawal, which, in some instances, may be causing the pain (particularly headache pain).

If you decide to stop consuming your daily amount of caffeine, be prepared for a few days of withdrawal symptoms, including headache, depression, dizziness, or anxiety. The chart shows some examples of the amount of caffeine in various beverages, food, and medicines.

CAFFEINE-CONTAINING SUBSTANCE	SERVING SIZE OR DOSE	CAFFEINE CONTENT (MILLIGRAMS)
Brewed coffee	6 ounces	105 to 150
Instant coffee	6 ounces	65 to 100
Decaffeinated coffee	6 ounces	1 to 5
Tea	6 ounces	28 to 100
Colas	8 ounces	24 to 31
Milk chocolate	1 ounce	1 to 15
Chocolate cake	1 slice	20 to 30
Many pain-relievers and headache preparations	1 dose	33
Drugs to maintain alertness	1 dose	100 to 130

Eat fewer refined-grain ("bad") carbohydrates and more whole-grain ("good") carbohydrates. Like fats, carbohydrates also come in good and bad varieties. The healthy kind, and the kind that most of your daily carbohydrate intake should encompass, come from whole-grain foods, vegetables, and fruits.

White bread, white rice, most pasta, and potatoes are chock-full of bad carbohydrates. They have a high glycemic load, which means they are very rapidly absorbed and cause sudden high levels of sugar in the blood. A diet that regularly contains foods with a high glycemic load can increase your risk of diabetes and heart disease, and increases your tendency to gain weight.

Choose healthier sources of protein. It has been recognized for a long time that eating red meat frequently as a source of protein is a bad idea, since red meat also contains a lot of saturated ("bad") fat. Scientists are currently working to find out if protein from vegetable sources—such as soy, lentils, beans, and nuts—is healthier than protein from meat. While there is not enough evidence to prove that vegetable protein in itself is better for you than meat protein, there are still reasons to choose protein-rich vegetables.

Eat plenty of fruits and vegetables—but not potatoes! A diet rich in fruits and vegetables offers countless health benefits, including lower blood pressure, a decreased risk of heart attacks and stroke, and protection against a variety of cancers. However, potatoes do not offer the same advantages because they have a high glycemic load.

Use alcohol in moderation. Research suggests that a drink a day for women, and one or two for men, cuts the chances of having a heart attack or dying from heart disease by about a third. However, regularly drinking more than this can increase your risk for various cancers, high blood pressure, stroke, and heart disease.

ANTIOXIDANTS

Your tissues make chemicals called oxygen-free radicals that cause the chemical process oxidation, which can injure tissues. Various substances in food (antioxidants) fight the oxidation. Several vitamins are antioxidants, including beta carotene, vitamin C, and vitamin E.

Beta carotene, which is found in dark green and deep yellow fruits and vegetables, is converted into vitamin A in the body (vitamin A is found in animal products such as liver, eggs, and milk).

Vitamin C is contained in citrus fruits such as oranges, grapefruits, and lemons (and their juices). It also can be found in strawberries, kiwi, tomatoes, broccoli, cabbage, potatoes, and some dark green, leafy vegetables like spinach and mustard greens.

Vitamin C is a water-soluble vitamin. Vitamins A and E are fat-soluble and require some fat in the diet in order to be absorbed by the digestive system.

Most cancers start when DNA in a cell is damaged, such as by oxidation. In theory, antioxidants could prevent this damage and reduce the risk of cancer.

The oxidation of low-density lipoprotein (LDL) cholesterol plays an important role in atherosclerosis (see p.653), which can lead to strokes and heart attacks. In theory, antioxidant vitamins could provide this benefit, whether they are consumed in the diet or taken as vitamin pills.

People who eat diets rich in antioxidant vitamins have lower rates of cancer and atherosclerosis. However, it has not been proven that it is the antioxidants in the diet that cause the lower rates.

There is currently no evidence that any of the antioxidant vitamins actually prevent cancer, though only beta carotene and vitamin E have been studied closely.

In fact, one study showed that beta carotene may increase the risk of lung cancer. With regard to preventing atherosclerosis, there has been no benefit shown by taking either beta carotene or vitamin C.

Some studies do suggest that vitamin E pills, in relatively high supplemental doses, may be beneficial in slowing atherosclerosis; other studies, however, have not shown a benefit. Better and larger studies of this important question are underway.

At present, there is not enough evidence to either strongly encourage or discourage the use of vitamin E supplements to prevent heart disease.

HEALTHY AND UNHEALTHY WEIGHT— AND SHAPE

More than 1 of 3 American adults are at an unhealthy weight, and their risk of developing certain diseases is greater because of the excess weight.

There are five classes of weight: underweight, acceptable weight, overweight, obesity, and morbid obesity (the most overweight class).

This classification system has been created because there is strong scientific evidence that people in classes other than "acceptable weight" are more likely to have health problems.

For example, being overweight, obese, or morbidly obese increases the chance you will develop type 2 diabetes (see p.833) and high blood pressure. The more overweight you are, the greater the risk. In addition, developing diabetes or high blood pressure can increase your risk of heart disease and stroke.

AM I OVERWEIGHT?

The best way to check whether you are at a healthy or unhealthy

"Apples" and "Pears"

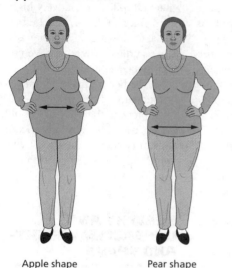

Apple shape   Pear shape

People who are built like apples (also known as "barrel-shaped")—who carry their weight around their midsection—are at greater health risk than people who carry the same amount of weight mainly around their hips, buttocks, and thighs.

weight is to determine your body mass index (see p.51). Using height and weight charts are another method. These guides are generally good, but they are not foolproof. For example, muscle weighs more than fat, so it is possible to be extremely fit and have a weight at the top of the weight charts for your height.

AM I AN "APPLE" OR A "PEAR"?

Not only your weight but also your shape affects your risk. If you have excess fat, it matters where on your body you are carrying it.

If you carry excess fat in the abdominal area around your waist (giving you an applelike shape), you are at higher risk for heart disease, high blood pressure, and diabetes.

In contrast, if you carry excess weight below the waist in the hips, buttocks, and thighs (giving you a pearlike shape), the risk

of disease is lower. There are some theories as to why it is better to be shaped like a pear rather than an apple, but it remains a mystery.

WHY IS THE U.S. POPULATION GETTING HEAVIER?

Over the past 20 years, people have increasingly used sugar-free sweeteners and cut down on the percentage of total calories that come from fat. In addition, various fat substitutes have become available. You would think this would mean that the average weight of the population is going down. In fact, it continues to go up.

Why is this? The simple explanation is that we are eating more. Though more of the food being eaten may be sugar-free or low-fat, the total number of calories being consumed is going up. Though we are using lots of sugar-free foods, we are eating

more sugar; and though we are eating more low-fat foods, we are eating more total fat.

Experts speculate that sugar-free foods have increased our appetite for sweets—real, sugar-rich sweets. We also tend to fool ourselves into thinking that sugar-free or fat-free foods have no calories.

While that is nearly true for some sugar-free soft drinks, it is not true for puddings, crackers, coffee cakes, and other foods that are sugar-free or fat-free.

People are also eating in restaurants more frequently, and restaurant meals typically contain many more total calories (and more fat) than home-cooked meals.

Losing Weight

The best approach to achieving and maintaining a healthy weight is to use common sense. To lose weight, you need to take in fewer calories than you burn. Incorporating exercise into your everyday life (see p.53) and eating a diet of mostly healthy foods—such as fruits, vegetables, and grains chosen for variety, balance, and moderation—will help you maintain a healthy weight.

If you need to lose weight, look for a program that emphasizes slow weight loss (no more than 2 pounds per week). For more information on weight-loss techniques, see p.855.

Cholesterol and Diet

The amount of cholesterol in your blood is determined partly by your genes and partly by how much saturated fat you eat. Cholesterol is a chemical that is not

What Do Scientific Studies Say Are the Best Weight-Loss Diets?

Many people have made millions of dollars writing books touting their theories about weight-loss programs. Rarely have these weight-loss programs been studied scientifically, to see if they really are effective—in the short term and, more important, in the long term.

As this book goes to press, probably the most popular weight-loss programs in the U.S. are low-carbohydrate ("low-carb") diets. Low-carb diets are relatively rich in fat. As originally proposed by Dr Robert Atkins, his low-carb diet allowed not only a diet rich in fat, but a diet rich in bad fats (see p.39).

More recent versions of the Atkins diet still recommend that the diet be low in carbohydrates, but add that it is best for these to be the good carbohydrates (see p.37). They also suggest that most of the fat in the high-fat diet they recommend be the good fats (see p.39). The same is true of another popular low-carb diet, the South Beach Diet.

What evidence is there that low-carb, high-fat diets are more effective for weight loss than low-fat, high-carb diets? Until recently, there was none. However, several studies published in 2003 and 2004 found that the low-carb, high-fat diets probably *are* more effective for weight loss—for 6–12 months. But after a year, the results tend to be the same as for low-fat, high-carb diets, mainly because people on both types of diet tend to gain weight again. One of the surprising findings in these studies was that the low-carb, high-fat diets do not increase blood levels of harmful fats like bad cholesterol, which many had predicted.

What is the reason that low-carb diets may be superior to low-fat diets for short-term weight loss? One widely-held theory is that many people who try to lose weight on low-fat, high-carb diets eat foods rich in bad carbo-hydrates that have a high glycemic load (see p. 000). Rapidly digested foods flood your bloodstream with a lot of sugar all at once. Sudden, high spikes of blood sugar levels set off a surge of insulin to clear out the sugar from your blood. But this quick surge can leave your blood sugar too low after just a few hours. And when blood sugar is too low, you feel hungry. So if it's low soon after a meal, you're likely to overeat. Said another way, the low-carb, high-fat diets may do a better job of curbing your appetite.

Based on current evidence, here are the facts:

■ It still is true that the only way to lose weight is to burn off more calories through exercise than are contained in the food you eat. For a weight-loss program to be successful, even in the short term, you must reduce your caloric intake and increase exercise.

■ It may be true that low-carb, high-fat diets make it easier for you to lose weight than low-fat, high-carb diets—in the short term. However, no diet has been shown to be successful for most people following it after about a year.

■ If you are going to try a low-carb, high-fat diet, be sure that the few carbs you eat are in the form of good carbs and that the fats you eat are good fats.

truly a fat but is related to fats (see p.39). Your body manufactures all the cholesterol it needs for the functioning of cells and hormones.

A high cholesterol level may reflect a diet high in cholesterol and high in saturated fats. It puts you at greater risk for developing atherosclerosis, in which a buildup of deposits on the walls of blood vessels narrows and stiffens them, leading to heart disease, strokes, and other similar conditions.

Simply avoiding saturated fats in foods such as meats, full-fat dairy products, and tropical oils (palm and coconut oil) is not the full answer, however. Eating a diet that is high in any kind of fat can result in higher quantities of low-density lipoprotein cholesterol (LDL—the "bad" cholesterol) in your bloodstream. People who have high levels of LDL in their blood are at greatest risk of heart disease.

Eating a varied diet that includes polyunsaturated fats, such

How to Read a Food Label

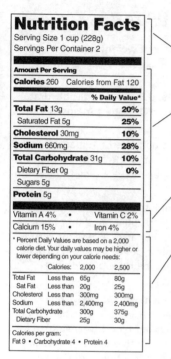

Nutrition Facts

Serving Size 1 cup (228g)
Servings Per Container 2

Amount Per Serving	
Calories 260	Calories from Fat 120

	% Daily Value*
Total Fat 13g	**20%**
Saturated Fat 5g	**25%**
Cholesterol 30mg	**10%**
Sodium 660mg	**28%**
Total Carbohydrate 31g	**10%**
Dietary Fiber 0g	**0%**
Sugars 5g	
Protein 5g	

Vitamin A 4%	•	Vitamin C 2%
Calcium 15%	•	Iron 4%

* Percent Daily Values are based on a 2,000 calorie diet. Your daily values may be higher or lower depending on your calorie needs:

	Calories:	2,000	2,500
Total Fat	Less than	65g	80g
Sat Fat	Less than	20g	25g
Cholesterol	Less than	300mg	300mg
Sodium	Less than	2,400mg	2,400mg
Total Carbohydrate		300g	375g
Dietary Fiber		25g	30g

Calories per gram:
Fat 9 • Carbohydrate 4 • Protein 4

Here is a sample Nutrition Facts label, which the U.S. Food and Drug Administration (FDA) now requires on all packaged foods. Most people are familiar with the information about total calories and calories from fat given per serving. This information is helpful for people who count calories and monitor their daily percentage of calories from fat. Note also:

1 The serving size gives the amount of food (in grams) to which all other numbers on the label apply.

2 The % Daily Value is based on a diet of 2,000 calories and tells you what fraction of your total daily requirement will be met by a single serving of this food. In this example, four servings of this food would complete your total daily requirement for saturated fat. Any more saturated fat you take in that day would be excessive.

3 The Daily Values (total recommended amount in a day) for vitamins are based on the US Recommended Dietary Allowances (RDAs); these values prevent vitamin deficiency diseases.

4 If you have a 2,000- to 2,500-calorie diet, the Daily Values for total fat, saturated fat, cholesterol, sodium, carbohydrates, and dietary fiber are listed toward the bottom of the label. Amounts well above, or well below, these targets (on a regular basis) can cause health problems.

as those found in vegetable and fish oils, can reduce your level of LDL and increase your level of high-density lipoprotein cholesterol (HDL—the "good" cholesterol that is associated with lower rates of heart disease).

Regular exercise can also help you increase the amount of beneficial cholesterol in your blood and may give you a better cholesterol profile overall.

EXERCISE AND FITNESS

"That which is used develops. That which is not used wastes away."

HIPPOCRATES

Regular exercise protects against disease. It has more immediate benefits as well. It increases your endurance, helps your body more efficiently process the foods you eat, improves the quality of sleep, and can help reduce stress, depression, and anxiety.

People who get regular exercise feel better physically, but also report feeling more relaxed and able to handle stress. Exer-

cising releases hormones called endorphins in the brain, which have a calming effect on the body and make many people feel good. Exercise also improves your posture as your body loses fat and your muscle tone improves.

Even if you increase your food intake while increasing the amount you exercise (therefore not experiencing any weight loss), regular exercise will still benefit your health. And, if you are overweight, regular exercise that leads to weight loss has a double benefit.

How Exercise Protects Against Disease

Here are a few of the most important ways that regular exercise protects against disease:

Stronger heart Your heart becomes stronger. Like any other muscle, your heart muscle fibers get stronger with exercise and are able to pump more blood more efficiently throughout your body.

Better cholesterol levels The level of harmful LDL cholesterol is reduced and the level of beneficial HDL cholesterol is increased.

Determining Your Body Mass Index (BMI)

To estimate your body mass index (BMI), first identify your weight (to the nearest 10 pounds) in one of the columns across the top. Then move your finger down the column until you come to the row that represents your height. Inside the square where your weight and height meet is a number that is an estimate of your BMI. For example, if you weigh 160 pounds and are 5'7", your BMI is 25.

BMI INTERPRETATION

Underweight	Under 18.5
Normal	18.5–24
Overweight	25–29
Obese	30 and over

WEIGHT

HEIGHT	100	110	120	130	140	150	160	170	180	190	200	210	220	230	240	250
5'0"	20	21	23	25	27	29	31	33	35	37	39	41	43	45	47	49
5'1"	19	21	23	25	26	28	30	32	34	36	38	40	42	43	45	47
5'2"	18	20	22	24	26	27	29	31	33	35	37	38	40	42	44	46
5'3"	18	19	21	23	25	27	28	30	32	34	35	37	39	41	43	44
5'4"	17	19	21	22	24	26	27	29	31	33	34	36	38	39	41	43
5'5"	17	18	20	22	23	25	27	28	30	32	33	35	37	38	40	42
5'6"	16	18	19	21	23	24	26	27	29	31	32	34	36	37	39	40
5'7"	16	17	19	20	22	23	25	27	28	30	31	33	34	36	38	39
5'8"	15	17	18	20	21	23	24	26	27	29	30	32	33	35	36	38
5'9"	15	16	18	19	21	22	24	25	27	28	30	31	32	34	35	37
5'10"	14	16	17	19	20	22	23	24	26	27	29	30	32	33	34	36
5'11"	14	15	17	18	20	21	22	24	25	26	28	29	30	31	33	35
6'0"	14	15	16	18	19	20	22	23	24	26	27	28	30	31	33	34
6'1"	13	15	16	17	18	20	21	22	24	25	26	28	29	30	32	33
6'2"	13	14	15	17	18	19	21	22	23	24	26	27	28	30	31	32
6'3"	12	14	15	16	17	19	20	21	22	24	25	26	27	29	30	31
6'4"	12	13	15	16	17	18	19	21	22	23	24	26	27	28	29	30

Stronger lungs Your lungs become conditioned to taking in and using oxygen more efficiently so that, over time, you increase your breathing capacity.

Stronger bones and muscles Your joints become more flexible, and your muscles and bones strengthen. Building stronger bones is especially important for women after they reach menopause, when lower levels of estrogen can contribute to osteoporosis (see p.596).

Lower blood pressure Your blood pressure is lowered, which lowers your risk of heart disease, strokes, and other serious conditions.

Protection against cancer You may lower your risk of some types of cancer. Regular exercise may help prevent colon cancer, possibly by moving waste through the colon (large intestine) faster, reducing the time any cancer-causing substances spend in the colon.

Some scientists believe that exercise may also help reduce the risk of endometrial cancer and breast cancer, both of which are associated with increased estrogen levels. Because fat cells produce estrogen, it is possible that exercise may help reduce the risk of these cancers by lowering the amount of body fat.

Protection against diabetes You may well lower your risk of developing type 2 diabetes (see p.833), which is common in people over about age 40. At greatest risk are people who are even mildly overweight, those who have a family history of diabetes, people who do not exercise regularly, and Hispanics and Native Americans.

In type 2 diabetes, cells are resistant to the action of insulin, the hormone that helps the body use energy. Regular exercise helps muscle cells take up sugar from the bloodstream and use it for energy more efficiently.

Reduces appetite Although many people believe that exercise increases appetite, it some-

Major Muscle Groups and Everyday Activities in Which They Are Used

You may not realize it, but you use all your major muscle groups during the course of a normal day. Even moderate activity, such as brisk walking, carrying your groceries, or taking the stairs, has a beneficial impact on muscle groups.

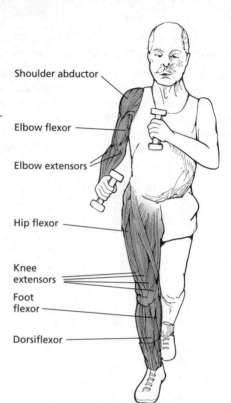

Stair climbing
Knee extensors
Hip extensors and flexors
Foot flexors
Dorsiflexors
Knee flexors and extensors
Hip flexors

Walking
Knee extensors
Hip extensors and flexors
Knee flexors and extensors
Dorsiflexors
Foot flexors

Getting up from a chair
Shoulder abductors
Elbow extensors
Knee extensors
Hip extensors and flexors
Dorsiflexors

Reaching
Shoulder abductors
Elbow extensors

Lifting or carrying
Elbow flexors
Shoulder abductors

Shoulder abductor
Elbow flexor
Elbow extensors
Hip flexor
Knee extensors
Foot flexor
Dorsiflexor

How Much Exercise Do I Need?

After you get started, work up to a minimum goal of 30 minutes of moderate activity every day. The 30 minutes does not have to be done all at once; it can be scattered throughout your day in the form of brisk walking (about 4 miles an hour), climbing stairs, and similar activities.

You do not need to jog, bike, swim, or perform more vigorous activities to meet this minimum, but the more intense and prolonged the exercise the better.

An exercise program that is optimal (rather than minimal) in its intensity level gets you to 55% to 85% of your maximal heart rate, a range commonly referred to as your "target heart rate" zone (see right).

If you are just starting to exercise, your numbers will be at the lower end of the range; you can progress to the higher end as your fitness level increases.

TARGET HEART RATE ZONE

To measure your heart rate, after exercising vigorously, locate your pulse in your wrist or neck and count the number of beats you feel during a 10-second period. Multiply that number by 6 to calculate your heart rate per minute. To determine your target heart rate zone:

1 Subtract your age from the number 220. The answer is your predicted maximum heart rate.

2 Multiply your predicted maximum heart rate (the answer to step 1) by .55. This number represents the low end of your heart rate range.

3 Multiply your predicted maximum heart rate (the answer to step 1) by .85. This number represents the high end of your heart rate range.

For example, if you are 40 years old, then your predicted maximum heart rate is 220 minus 40 (180). Therefore, the low end of the range for you is 180 x .55 (or 99 beats per minute) and the high end is 180 x .85 (or 153 beats per minute).

times decreases appetite, thereby having the additional benefit of helping you control your weight.

Getting Started

If you have not been active for a while, talk to your doctor before you begin an exercise program. When you start to exercise, begin slowly, getting just enough exercise to get your muscles and joints used to the increased activity. Then slowly increase the length and intensity of your workout over time.

To avoid injury and muscle strain, stretch and walk slowly for 5 or 10 minutes before you begin, using the flexibility exercises on p.55 before and after your workout. Build your exercise program gradually, starting with 20 minutes three times a week.

Brisk walking, swimming, or biking are good low-impact exercises to get you started, as is lifting light weights (see Strength Exercises, p.55; Strength Training for Seniors, p.1113). As you feel more fit, increase the benefits by

When Not to Exercise

Never exercise when you are ill. Too much activity can worsen your condition. In general, wait a couple of days to exercise if you have any of the following:

- Fever
- Sore throat
- Cough with phlegm (sputum)
- Painful urination
- Muscle and joint pain

exercising more vigorously, more often, and for a longer period of time.

Building Exercise Into Everyday Life

Many people find that the best way to increase the amount of exercise they get is to make activity a part of daily life. You can build exercise into your regular activities by:

- Walking up several flights of stairs (or as many as you can manage) instead of taking the elevator.

- Parking your car at the end of the parking lot so you have a short, healthy hike to and from your destination.

- Walking or riding your bike to the store, train station, or work.

- Taking a brisk, 20-minute walk during your lunch hour every day.

- Getting together with a friend to walk and talk, instead of sitting down for a cup of coffee.

- Shooting some baskets or throwing a disk with your children or a friend.

- Doing your own raking, mowing, and gardening.

Warm-Up and Cool-Down Exercises

No matter how physically fit you are, prepare your body for exercising by warming up your muscles and joints for at least 5 to 10 minutes; this helps prevent injury. The warm-up period also gets your blood moving and prepares you psychologically for exercise.

When you are done exercising, cool down your body by perform-

Warning Signs to Stop Exercising

Stop exercising and get help if you have any of the following symptoms:

- Chest pain or pressure
- Pain in the arms, neck, or jaw
- Light-headedness or dizziness
- Palpitations
- Nausea
- Blurred vision
- Breathlessness
- Faintness

ing the same movements. Never stop suddenly; taper your intensity level gradually and walk until your breathing rate returns to nearly normal. Cooling down after exercise prevents muscle cramps.

Follow these steps:

- Clasp your hands behind you and move your arms up and back so that you feel the upper part of your chest and shoulders stretching.

- To warm up your shoulders and arms, extend your arms straight out at the sides and make large arm circles. Circle both forward and backward several times.

- Loosen your knees and calves by gently placing one leg straight in front of the other, bending at the knee and being careful not to put too much pressure on the bent knee. This will stretch the calf muscles of the leg that is behind you.

- Stretch your hamstrings by standing straight and pulling one leg up toward your chest. Hold it and repeat with both legs several times.

■ Get your whole body moving by walking briskly before and after you exercise.

Types of Exercise

Exercise can be organized into three groups—aerobic, flexibility, and strength. Each provides different benefits. Most top athletes perform some of each type to balance their workout. You can easily incorporate all three types of exercise into a simple routine.

Aerobic exercises condition your heart and lungs by increasing your heart rate and breathing rate so that more oxygen goes to muscles. In addition to improving overall cardiovascular fitness, aerobic exercise also benefits your bones and muscles. Aerobic activities include jogging, brisk walking, biking, dancing, swimming, rowing, and stair-climbing.

Any time you exercise to a point where your heart rate rises above its resting level, your heart and lungs benefit. To achieve maximum benefit, do some aerobic exercise at least 5 days a week for at least 30 minutes a day, working hard enough to reach your target heart rate (see p.52).

Flexibility exercises stretch muscle groups and can help your body become more controlled and flexible. Flexibility exercises are helpful when warming up and cooling down after a workout. They help to stretch muscles that have been tightened during other forms of training or since your last workout. Flexibility exercises improve your muscles' ability to recover from exercise.

Aerobic Exercise

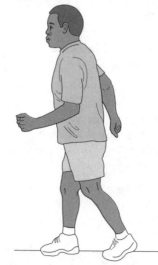

Aerobic exercise—such as brisk walking, jogging, biking, dancing, swimming, rowing, and stair-climbing—is one of the best forms of exercise because it conditions your heart and lungs and strengthens your bones and muscles. The term "aerobic" describes any form of moderately intense activity done for at least 12 minutes that uses oxygen to provide energy for the muscles. Brisk walking builds muscle, burns fat, and improves your overall cardiovascular fitness.

Done gently and slowly, flexibility exercises help prevent injury such as muscle strain.

Some people have difficulty staying flexible as they age. Maintaining flexibility can help you keep your strength and ability to perform daily tasks without injury. Yoga is one form of flexibility training. The simple stretches shown in the illustration on p.55 can be performed every day.

Strength exercises, also called resistance training, preserve bone density, increase muscle mass, and improve strength and

balance. Strength training involves working groups of muscles against some degree of resistance.

Strength exercises can be dynamic—such as weight lifting, in which the muscles actually change in length—or isometric, in which the muscles contract without shortening and are briefly tensed using one part of the body to resist the movement of another part.

As people get older, the amount of muscle begins to shrink. Muscle is regenerated by lifting weights (up to your maximum capacity—the maximum amount of weight you can lift eight times in a row) for 20 to 30 minutes three to four times a week.

Strength training is helpful for people of all ages, including seniors (see p.1113). Start by lifting heavy food cans and gradually increase the amount of weight you lift in ½-pound to 1-pound increments. Ankle and arm weights that permit extra weight to be added to them may be convenient. To give your muscles time to recover, allow 1 or 2 days of rest between each weight-training session.

Maintaining Fluids

Increase your intake of liquids both before and after exercising. At least 30 minutes before a workout, drink one or two glasses of water. Your body needs water to work properly, particularly in very hot weather.

You lose fluid through perspiration and through increased breathing. Drink another glass or two of water about a half hour after exercising; do not wait until you are thirsty.

Water is a good rehydration liquid; most people do not need sports drinks. Avoid caffeine-containing coffee, tea, and colas; caffeine acts as a diuretic (as does alcohol), increasing fluid loss by increasing urine formation.

The water you drink before and after a workout should be in addition to your daily intake of eight glasses of liquids.

Strength Exercises

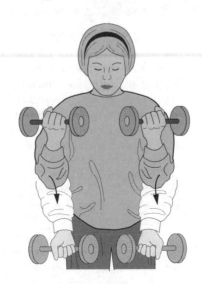

Hold a 1-pound hand weight (or soup can) in each hand. Stand with your back straight, knees slightly bent, and feet slightly apart. With your palms facing upward, hold the weights at thigh level. Lift the weights slowly up toward your chest. Lower them again down to thigh level. Do this with controlled, slow movements. When you can repeat this exercise 12 times, increase your weights by 1-pound increments.

Flexibility Exercises

Flexibility exercises help you warm up and cool down after a workout. Stretch gently, never pushing yourself to the point where you feel pain.

FOR TRICEPS

Sit or stand upright with your right arm behind your lower back, placed as far up your back as possible. Hold a rolled-up towel in your left hand, lift the left arm overhead, and bend your left elbow so that your left arm hangs down your back. Grasp the towel with your right hand. Work your hands together. Hold the stretch for 10 seconds, then relax. Reverse arm positions and repeat.

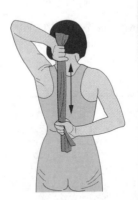

FOR CALF AND ACHILLES TENDON

Stand upright, slightly more than an arm's length from a wall. Place your right leg forward, keeping the left leg straight. Lean against the wall with your lower arms flat against the wall. Keep the heel of your left (back) foot down with the sole flat on the floor and the toes pointing forward. Hold the stretch for 10 seconds, then relax. Switch legs and repeat.

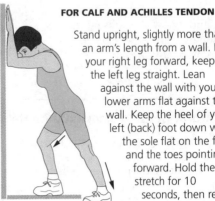

FOR LOWER BACK

Lie flat on your back. Bend both knees and slide your feet toward your buttocks. Grasp your thighs and pull your knees toward your chest, elevating your hips slightly. Hold the stretch for 30 seconds. Straighten your legs slowly, one at a time.

USING ADDICTIVE SUBSTANCES

Tobacco

Using tobacco is a life-threatening habit and the leading preventable cause of death in the United States. Yet 46 million Americans—1 of 4 adults—smoke. Nearly all of them started smoking before age 20. In addition, 6 million teenagers smoke, and smoking among adolescents is increasing. If you are a regular smoker, you lose about 5½ minutes of life expectancy for every cigarette you smoke.

There is no safe level of tobacco use. In both men and women, smoking cigarettes, pipes, or cigars is a cause of cardiovascular disease (heart attack and stroke), emphysema, chronic bronchitis, and cancers of the lung, larynx, mouth, esophagus, bladder, pancreas, and cervix. Lung cancer has long been the leading cause of cancer death in men, and it now also kills more women than any other cancer, including breast cancer.

Using smokeless tobacco in any form (including chewing tobacco or snuff) is also harmful and can lead to addiction. Like smoking, dipping or chewing has serious health effects, including cancers of the mouth, gum disease, loss of teeth, and heart problems.

Smoking cigarettes, cigars, or pipes jeopardizes the health of people close to you, including the fetus if you are pregnant.

Nonsmokers exposed to someone else's smoke (second-hand smoke) are at increased risk for the same diseases that affect smokers: lung cancer, coronary artery disease, and stroke.

The children of parents who smoke have more respiratory illnesses, such as bronchitis and asthma, than children of parents who do not smoke. Spouses of smokers have a higher risk of heart disease.

Using tobacco of any kind, in any way, and in any amount, is bad for your health. If you are a smoker, could you and the people close to you get lucky, and escape adverse health effects? Sure, anyone can get lucky. But do not count on it. If you use tobacco, you are gambling with your health and the health of those you love.

The odds are heavily against you. One of two smokers dies of a disease directly caused by the cigarette smoking, and each year tobacco is responsible for the deaths of more than 400,000 Americans.

WHAT HAPPENS WHEN YOU SMOKE?

Tobacco smoke contains more than 4,000 chemicals, many of which are known to be carcinogens (cancer-causing agents).

Three of these—tar, nicotine, and carbon monoxide—are especially dangerous. Tar is a mixture of hydrocarbons that becomes a sticky substance in the lungs and contains many cancer-causing substances.

Benefits of Quitting Smoking With Help

There are several supportive approaches (including nicotine replacement and taking the drug bupropion) available to help you quit smoking. You are more likely to be successful if you use one of these supportive approaches than if you do not.

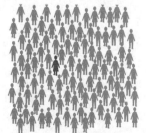

1 OF 100 SMOKERS WHO QUITS SMOKING WITHOUT AID OR COUNSELING WILL REMAIN A NON-SMOKER FOR 1 YEAR

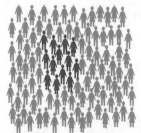

13 OF 100 SMOKERS WHO QUIT SMOKING USING ONLY THE NICOTINE PATCH WILL REMAIN NONSMOKERS FOR 1 YEAR

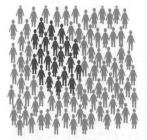

20 OF 100 SMOKERS WHO QUIT SMOKING USING ONLY THE DRUG BUPROPION WILL REMAIN NON-SMOKERS FOR 1 YEAR

Nicotine is an addictive chemical that, when absorbed through the lungs, affects the cardiovascular and nervous systems. A smoker smokes cigarettes to maintain a particular level of nicotine in the bloodstream.

Carbon monoxide robs the body of oxygen by decreasing the amount of oxygen that red blood cells can carry throughout the body.

There is no such thing as a safe cigarette, and that includes those that claim to deliver less tar and nicotine. People who switch to these "lighter" cigarettes eventually inhale longer and smoke more cigarettes to keep their level of nicotine up and prevent cravings for cigarettes. In the end, they spend more money on cigarettes, take the same amount of poison into their bodies, and run no less risk of disease.

DAMAGE AND EFFECTS

Damage to the respiratory system Toxic gases and particles of tar in tobacco smoke enter the lungs each time you inhale, damaging the lungs. Some of the damage can be repaired if you stop smoking, and some cannot.

Lung damage from smoking not only increases the risk of lung cancer, but also the risk of pneumonia, bronchitis, and emphysema. Smokers are also more susceptible to getting colds and the flu (influenza).

Damage to the cardiovascular system Smoking substantially increases your risk of cardiovascular disease, including stroke, heart attack, aortic aneurysms, and sudden death. Smoking cigarettes also increases the risk of peripheral vascular disease (poor circulation) and atherosclerosis

(hardening of the arteries) and lowers the level of high-density lipoprotein (HDL), the "good" cholesterol (see p.669).

Women who smoke and take oral contraceptives run a much greater risk of blood clots, heart attacks, and strokes than do non-smokers, especially after the age of 35.

Effects on the reproductive system Smoking during pregnancy greatly increases the chance a baby will be underweight (less than 5.5 pounds) at birth. A low birthweight baby is 40 times more likely to die during the first month of life than a baby of normal weight. Smoking slows the fetus's rate of growth in the uterus, probably because cigarette smoke in the mother's bloodstream crosses the placenta and introduces harmful chemicals into the fetus's blood.

Carbon monoxide reduces the amount of oxygen that can be carried in the blood of both the mother and the fetus; nicotine causes the fetus's blood vessels to constrict so that less oxygen and fewer nutrients reach it.

Smoking during pregnancy

has been linked to increased rates of miscarriage and stillbirth, as well as various bleeding problems. Smoking also increases the risk of infertility in both men and women.

Sudden infant death syndrome (SIDS) is two to four times more common in children of women who smoked while they were pregnant. Children of women who smoked during pregnancy also have a higher rate of brain damage, cerebral palsy, and behavioral disorders.

Damage to the musculoskeletal system Some studies have linked cigarette smoking to osteoporosis in women. This link may be due to some component of cigarette smoke itself, but it could also be due to the fact that women who smoke cigarettes tend to be thinner than non-smokers and tend to go through menopause earlier—both of which are risk factors for osteoporosis.

OTHER HEALTH RISKS

The skin of smokers wrinkles earlier and more severely than the skin of nonsmokers, no mat-

Alternative Medicine: Quitting Smoking

Many therapies, including acupuncture and herbal remedies, are offered to help smokers quit. None of these has been proven through scientific study to be effective. However, the health risks of continuing to smoke are so great that, if an alternative therapy helps you quit, it may be worthwhile. Discuss any alternative antismoking program you are considering with your physician before you undergo treatment. If an alternative method does not work, try one of the conventional smoking cessation methods (see p.59). Do not give up.

Preparing to Quit

You can quit smoking. In the United States today, there are more ex-smokers than smokers. All strategies to quit smoking recommend that a smoker establish a "quit date" and prepare for it in a way that minimizes the symptoms of nicotine withdrawal. Here are some recommendations for quitting:

■ Set a target date for quitting and make sure everyone knows about it. Friends and family can be an important source of support.

■ Before quitting, identify some activities that make you feel good, healthy, and energetic and plan to engage in them during the first few weeks of quitting. You will need to be distracted and rewarded during this time.

■ Start an exercise program. More people who exercise experience success than those who do not. This will help you avoid gaining weight and will improve your energy level.

■ Eat a healthy diet; snack on raw vegetables and drink eight glasses of water every day.

■ Avoid alcohol, coffee, and other caffeine-containing drinks, which can promote the desire for nicotine.

■ When you feel the urge to smoke, replace it with

several deep, slow breaths followed by a drink of water. You may need to do this frequently during the first week or two.

■ Avoid smoky environments.

■ Review any successful attempts at quitting in the past and identify factors that helped you succeed.

■ Make a list of all the reasons you want to quit (good health, better for family members, feel better). Every night before going to bed, repeat one of the reasons 10 times.

■ Recognize that withdrawal symptoms are temporary and usually last only 1 to 2 weeks.

■ Be aware that the first week will be your hardest because your body is still dependent on nicotine and the withdrawal symptoms are strongest.

■ Know that most relapses happen in the first 3 months after quitting, when situational triggers can occur, such as a stressful event or being with a friend who smokes.

■ Realize that most successful ex-smokers quit for good only after several attempts. If you slip and have a cigarette, make a decision to quit again immediately.

ter how much sun exposure they have had in their lives. Smokers are also at greater risk of developing stomach ulcers. Two leading causes of blindness in older adults—cataracts and macular degeneration—are more common in smokers.

BENEFITS OF QUITTING

Smokers often fear that they have smoked for so long that it is too late to derive benefit from stopping. Not so. It is true that the sooner in life a person quits smoking, the greater benefit he or she will gain. However, in most instances, no matter how long or

how heavily a person has smoked, quitting smoking reduces a smoker's risk of disease and increases life expectancy.

This is true even for smokers over the age of 65 and even for most smokers who have already developed a smoking-related disease. For example, smokers who stop smoking after suffering a heart attack reduce their chances of a future heart attack and of dying of heart disease by 25% to 50%.

Smokers who quit also avoid exposing their families to passive smoke and set a good example for their children, who are less

likely to smoke if their parents do not. Besides the health benefits, smokers who quit save money by not having to buy cigarettes and often feel a real sense of pride in their accomplishment.

OBSTACLES TO QUITTING

Most smokers already know that smoking is harmful to their health, and most smokers want to stop. Most have tried to do so at least once, but many of those who try to quit go back to smoking.

Quitting often takes several attempts because it is more than a matter of willpower. The majority of smokers are physically and

What Happens After I Quit?

Your body thanks you the minute you stop smoking cigarettes; the repair work begins immediately. If you smoke about 20 cigarettes a day, here is how your body begins the healing process.

- **After 2 hours** Nicotine begins to leave your system.

- **After 12 hours** The carbon monoxide has completely left your system. Your blood now carries oxygen more efficiently.

- **Within 1 week** Your senses of taste and smell sharpen. Your breath, hair, fingers, and teeth will be cleaner. Your circulation improves. All the nicotine will be gone from your system, along with the worst of the withdrawal symptoms.

- **Within 1 month** The cilia (the hairlike structures that line your airways) begin to recover and remove more mucus from your system. At first you will cough up mucus, which cleans your lungs and reduces the chance of infection. Soon you find yourself coughing less. Sinus congestion, fatigue, and shortness of breath will also decrease.

- **After 1 year** Your risk of having a heart attack or stroke is reduced and falls substantially over the first 2 to 4 years. The risk of lung cancer also falls, but more slowly.

psychologically dependent on cigarettes. Stopping any addictive drug can cause uncomfortable symptoms of drug withdrawal, and stopping nicotine is no different.

When a smoker quits, he or she can develop the following symptoms of nicotine withdrawal: cravings for a cigarette, irritability, anxiety, depression, inability to concentrate, impatience, anger, excessive hunger, and trouble sleeping. These withdrawal symptoms reach a peak 2 or 3 days after quitting and then wane gradually over a month or more.

Smokers also use cigarettes to handle anger, boredom, or frustration. When they quit they need to find alternative ways to cope with these situations. Certain events, such as finishing a meal

or having the first cup of morning coffee, become associated with lighting up a cigarette in the smoker's mind. In order to quit, a smoker must break these links.

People who smoke are also at higher risk of having symptoms of depression or problems abusing alcohol or other drugs. If not recognized and treated, these conditions can impede efforts to quit smoking. Many doctors recommend that smokers who are attempting to quit also give up alcohol temporarily because drinking can induce a return to smoking.

Fear of gaining weight is another issue that complicates the desire to quit smoking. Smokers who quit gain an average of 5 to 10 pounds. Partly, this is due to a decrease in the rate at which the body metabolizes

(processes) nutrients when nicotine is withdrawn. In addition, many people substitute food for cigarettes.

Starting a daily exercise program before you quit will minimize weight gain; ask your doctor for guidance. Overall, doctors agree that the weight gained does not pose nearly as serious a threat to health as smoking does.

SMOKING CESSATION METHODS

When you make a decision to quit smoking, you face two challenges: breaking the habit of smoking and overcoming your addiction to nicotine. Many people quit by themselves, some with the help of booklets that teach simple behavior-change strategies.

Groups that can help Many people find it easier to quit smoking if they join a group or participate in some organized program. Ask your doctor about groups in your area.

Another alternative is "Quitlines." These are programs available to every U.S. citizen over the telephone, organized by respected organizations such as the American Lung Association. You can talk to friendly and knowledgeable people over the phone, on toll-free numbers, who can provide you with free services including counseling and self-help kits. These programs have been proven successful: They double the chance that you will successfully quit. To find the number for a Quitline in your state, go to this Web site: http://www.smokefree.gov/usmap.html

While some people quit "cold turkey," others who have successfully quit smoking and not started again have found one of the following methods helpful in overcoming the initial withdrawal from nicotine. Ask your doctor for a recommendation on the methods that might work best for you.

Nicotine replacement therapy
A nicotine patch, nicotine gum, nicotine nasal spray, and a nico- tine inhaler all release nicotine into your bloodstream in amounts large enough to block the discomfort of withdrawal. In contrast to smoking, they pro- duce relatively constant blood levels of nicotine, and they do not contain any of the other toxic chemicals in tobacco.

Many smokers have quit by using these products, combined with support and encouragement from a smoking cessation group that teaches behavior modifica- tion techniques.

Statistically, using the nicotine patch or gum doubles your chances of quitting successfully. Less is known about the nasal spray or inhaler, which are

Coping with the Symptoms That Occur After Quitting Smoking

A number of frustrating symptoms can develop immediately after you quit smoking. If you are using the nicotine patch, gum, nasal spray, or inhaler, your withdrawal symptoms will be less intense than if you are not. Few people experi- ence all of the symptoms below, but most people experience some of them.

SYMPTOM	CAUSE	DURATION	RELIEF
Craving for cigarette	Body's craving for nicotine	Most intense during first week but can linger for months	Wait out the urge; distract your- self; take a brisk walk.
Irritability, impatience	Body's craving for nicotine	2 to 4 weeks	Exercise; take hot baths; use relax- ation techniques (see p.90); avoid caffeine.
Insomnia	Body's craving for nicotine temporarily reduces time spent in deep sleep	2 to 4 weeks	Avoid caffeine after 6 PM; use relaxation techniques (see p.90); exercise.
Fatigue	Body adjusting to lack of stimulation from nicotine	2 to 4 weeks	Take naps; do not push yourself.
Lack of concentration	Body adjusting to lack of stimulation from nicotine	A few weeks	Reduce workload; avoid stress.
Hunger	Craving for cigarettes may be confused with hunger pangs	Up to several weeks	Drink water or low-calorie drinks; eat low-calorie snacks.
Coughing, dry throat, nasal drip	Body ridding itself of mucus in lungs and airways	Several weeks	Drink plenty of fluids; use cough drops.
Constipation, gas	Intestinal movement decreases with lack of nicotine	1 to 2 weeks	Drink plenty of fluids; add fiber to diet; exercise.

newer products, but they appear to be about as effective as the patch and gum. Both the patch and the gum are available without a prescription and are safe for most people when used correctly. The nasal spray and inhaler require a doctor's prescription.

Never smoke or use snuff or chewing tobacco while using the patch or gum; this increases your risk of heart attack due to nicotine overdose. If you have heart disease or are pregnant or breast-feeding, talk to your doctor before starting nicotine replacement.

Nicotine patch The patch contains a fixed amount of nicotine that is released in doses and absorbed by your bloodstream throughout the day. On the day you plan to quit, you apply a nicotine patch to a hairless spot on your upper arm or torso. A typical patch is worn for 16 or 24 hours and replaced the next morning.

The patch is available in three strengths. Start with the highest dose unless you weigh less than 100 pounds or smoke less than half a pack a day. Most people should use the patch for 8 weeks. The major side effect is skin irritation at the site where the patch is worn. Do not use any tobacco products while wearing the patch.

Nicotine gum When nicotine gum is chewed, it releases nicotine that is absorbed through the lining of the mouth and passes into the bloodstream. The gum is available in two strengths. Chew the gum only long enough to release nicotine, producing a peppery taste, then place it between your gums and cheek to

allow the nicotine to be absorbed.

When the taste disappears, chew the gum again just enough to produce the distinctive taste, then push it back in the corner of your mouth. Each piece should be kept in the mouth for 30 minutes and then discarded. Keep in mind that it takes 20 minutes for the nicotine in the gum to be fully absorbed into the blood.

People using nicotine gum often chew too few pieces per day and for too few weeks to receive the gum's maximum benefits. Many doctors recommend a fixed schedule of at least one piece every 1 to 2 hours for 1 to 3 months. Some people develop side effects such as hiccups, upset stomach, a sore jaw, or a burning sensation in the mouth. Often these are the results of improper chewing technique.

Occasionally, nicotine gum users become dependent on the gum. To avoid this, do not use the gum for longer than 6 months and reduce your use gradually when you decide to quit. Never use any tobacco products while chewing nicotine gum.

Nicotine nasal spray and inhaler These methods of delivering nicotine to your bloodstream require a prescription from your doctor. The nicotine nasal spray is absorbed through the mucous membrane of your nose and into the bloodstream within 5 to 10 minutes. The nicotine in the inhaler is absorbed through your mouth, throat, and lungs and has its peak effect in 20 minutes.

Nicotine levels are maintained 1 to 2 hours, but there is a more dramatic rise in blood nicotine levels with the nasal spray than

with the patch, gum, or inhaler. This produces more rapid relief of withdrawal symptoms but it also poses greater potential for becoming dependent on the spray.

Side effects of the nasal spray include nose and throat irritation, watery eyes, sneezing, and coughing. Nicotine nasal spray is not recommended for people with asthma or chronic sinusitis. Side effects of the inhaler include coughing and mouth and throat irritation. Ask your doctor if one of these therapies might work for you.

Non-nicotine treatments In contrast to quitting aids that release nicotine into the bloodstream, the following therapies do not. Smokers who use these methods may also benefit from the support and encouragement of a smoking cessation group that teaches behavior modification techniques.

Bupropion is an antidepressant drug that is also an effective aid for smoking cessation. It is started 1 week before a smoker's planned "quit day" and continued for 8 to 12 weeks. Because the drug does not contain nicotine, it can be used in combination with nicotine replacement therapy.

Side effects include insomnia, agitation, anxiety, dry mouth, headache, and skin rash. Ask your doctor for information and a prescription if you want to try it.

Clonidine is a medicine that reduces the symptoms of withdrawal and can help double the chance that you will successfully quit. It is available in pill or patch form.

Nortriptyline is a medicine that helps fight depression, but for reasons that are unclear it helps smokers quit even when they do not suffer from depression. It is available in pill form.

Hypnosis (see p.394) is also popular among smokers who are trying to quit, although it has not been proven to be effective. While you are hypnotized, the therapist gives you suggestions to help you stop smoking. These might include reminders to help you relax when you get the urge to smoke and to feel good about the times you avoided the temptation to smoke.

Alcohol

Alcohol abuse is the second most common form of drug abuse in the United States, after tobacco addiction. Some people are more severely affected than others.

An estimated 9% of adult men and 4% of adult women have the most severe form of alcohol abuse known as alcohol dependence. These individuals have lost control of their drinking; they are unable to stop or cut down despite serious negative health consequences and the loss of valued activities or relationships.

Problem drinking is a milder disorder in which the use of alcohol leads to health problems or troubles at home, at work, at school, or with the law. Drinkers at risk are those who drink more than is considered safe—more than two drinks a day for men and more than one drink a day for women.

The cause of alcohol abuse or dependence is not fully understood, but a family history of addiction to alcohol places a person at higher risk. Children of parents who suffer from alcohol

Interaction of Alcohol with Commonly Used Medicines

Some medicines can cause problems when taken with alcohol. The problems are greatest when the dose of medication is high and you drink more than 1 to 2 drinks per day. Read the labels on prescription and over-the-counter drugs to determine if your drug will interact with alcohol. Some of the medicines that should be used cautiously with alcohol are listed below.

MEDICINE	INTERACTION OF ALCOHOL WITH MEDICINE
Ibuprofen	Increased risk of bleeding, especially in the digestive organs, due to alcohol's irritating effect on the stomach lining plus alcohol's effect on lowering the number of the blood-clotting cells called platelets.
Aspirin	Increased risk of bleeding; aspirin also enhances uptake of alcohol into the blood from the gastrointestinal tract, causing greater intoxication.
Acetaminophen	Increased risk of liver injury, since both acetaminophen and alcohol can be toxic to the liver.
Warfarin	Increased risk of bleeding, since alcohol increases the anticlotting effects of warfarin.
Anticonvulsants	Alcohol can either decrease or increase the effects of many anticonvulsant medicines.
Sedatives	Increased sedation and risk of losing consciousness from intoxication.
Metronidazole	Flushing, headache, nausea and vomiting, and sweating.
Oral hypoglycemic agents	Flushing, headache, nausea and vomiting, sweating, and unpredictable fluctuations in blood glucose levels.

abuse have a fourfold increased risk of the disorder.

Heavy drinking—more than two drinks a day for men and more than one drink a day for women—can seriously damage your liver, stomach, heart, brain, and nervous system.

Drinking also increases your risk of cancer of the mouth, throat, larynx (voice box), and

esophagus. Women who drink heavily are at higher risk of developing breast cancer and osteoporosis. In addition, people who drink heavily may not eat adequately, so they may develop vitamin and mineral deficiencies.

Although there are many risks to drinking alcohol, there also may be some benefits. Alcohol can be beneficial for adults who

Risk of Breast Cancer with Alcohol Consumption

A woman who consumes two to five drinks a day has an increased risk of breast cancer, whether she drinks wine, beer, or hard liquor. The increased risk caused by drinking moderate amounts of alcohol (one to two drinks a day) is about the same as the increased risk of having a first-degree relative with breast cancer. Alcohol may increase the levels of estrogen circulating in the blood. It has also been suggested that alcohol may act directly on breast tissue, causing it to be more susceptible to tumor growth.

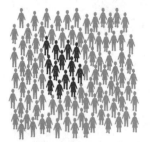

13 OF 100 WOMEN IN THE GENERAL POPULATION DEVELOP BREAST CANCER IN THEIR LIFETIME

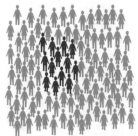

13 OF 100 WOMEN WHO HAVE ONE DRINK A DAY DEVELOP BREAST CANCER IN THEIR LIFETIME

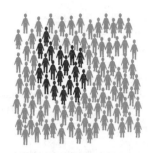

18 OF 100 WOMEN WHO HAVE TWO TO FIVE DRINKS A DAY DEVELOP BREAST CANCER IN THEIR LIFETIME

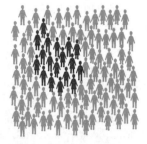

18 OF 100 WOMEN WHO HAVE A FAMILY HISTORY OF BREAST CANCER DEVELOP BREAST CANCER IN THEIR LIFETIME

are not at risk for alcohol dependence. Drinking 5 ounces of wine, 12 ounces of beer, or 1½ ounces of 80-proof distilled spirits daily appears to lower the risk of heart disease, stroke, and other circulatory diseases. There is evidence that a small amount of alcohol can boost levels of high-density lipoprotein (HDL), the beneficial cholesterol in your blood, as well as reduce the formation of plaque in blood vessels.

If too much alcohol is harmful but some is beneficial, how do you decide how much is too much? First, if you do not drink, do not start. The risks that come with drinking alcohol frequently outweigh the benefits. If you drink, do so in moderation—no more than one drink a day for women and no more than two drinks a day for men (see How

Much Alcohol in Your Drink, p.64, for drink equivalents).

There are no health benefits from binge drinking, intoxication, or chronic heavy alcohol use, only a significantly higher risk of death. Millions of people are dependent on alcohol and need help in quitting. For someone suffering from alcohol abuse, even one drink is too much.

People who should not drink include women who are trying to conceive or who are pregnant, people who plan to drive or operate equipment that requires attention or skill, and people using prescription or over-the-counter medicines that can cause drowsiness.

Alcohol can also alter the effectiveness and toxicity of medicines (see Interaction of Alcohol with Commonly Used Medicines, p.62). Some medicines increase

blood levels of alcohol or increase the adverse effects of alcohol on the brain.

ALCOHOL'S EFFECTS

Alcohol is a central nervous system depressant. It acts like a sedative or tranquilizer, slowing down your motor coordination and reaction time, as well as impairing judgment, memory, reasoning, and self-control. Paradoxically, alcohol disturbs sleep as its effects wear off; it is a major cause of insomnia.

Processing alcohol The size of your body, whether or not you have eaten recently, and the rate at which you drink also affect how your body processes alcohol. A large person has more blood circulating in his or her body than a smaller person, so alcohol concentration in larger people rises more slowly than in a smaller person, even if they drink identical amounts of alcohol.

Food slows the rate at which alcohol is absorbed into your bloodstream. It is ideal to have food in your stomach when you drink, or to drink only during meals. Drinking slowly is another way to reduce the rate at which alcohol is absorbed by your body. Having several nonalcoholic drinks between drinks of alcohol can also slow the effects of alcohol on your system.

Effect on women Drink for drink, women accumulate more alcohol in their bloodstream than men do. This is because women's bodies process alcohol differently than men's bodies do. Women have lower levels of the stomach enzyme that neutralizes alcohol before it moves into the bloodstream.

Women also tend to have a higher proportion of body fat, which does not absorb alcohol; this increases alcohol levels in the blood. Women also tend to weigh less than men, so drink for drink, there is more alcohol in a woman's bloodstream.

Driving There is no safe way to combine drinking and driving. As little as one drink can impair your ability to drive. To avoid driving after consuming alcohol, many adults find it helpful to establish a designated nondrinking driver, or to use public transportation. Your children should also understand that they should not drink and drive, and neither you nor your children should ever ride in a car with a driver who has been drinking.

Pregnancy There is no safe level of drinking during preg-

How Much Alcohol in Your Drink?

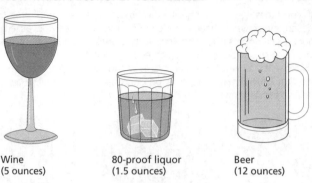

Wine
(5 ounces)

80-proof liquor
(1.5 ounces)

Beer
(12 ounces)

These three drinks have approximately the same amount of alcohol in them, despite the difference in serving size.

nancy. Women who are trying to get pregnant or who already are pregnant should not drink. During the first trimester, regular drinking—or even one period of heavy drinking—can damage the fetus. Women who drink alcohol heavily during pregnancy may give birth to babies with fetal alcohol syndrome, a group of birth defects that includes irreversible mental retardation.

Women who drink as few as one or two drinks a day while pregnant may give birth prematurely, and their children may have a low birthweight or neurological problems. Even occasional social drinking can increase the risk of miscarriage, particularly in the first trimester. If you are pregnant and have a problem with drinking, talk to your doctor immediately.

Teen drinking Each year more than 4 million children (age 14 to 17) in the United States have trouble at school, with their parents, and sometimes with the law because of the effects of drinking alcohol. Drinking impairs concentration, learning, and perfor-

mance at school and at home.

It also has a dramatic impact on personality and can bring on irritability, hostility, and aggression. A young person who drinks alcohol is also more likely to experiment with other drugs, and to run the risk of becoming addicted to them.

Teens who drink are also more likely to die by falling or drowning, and are more likely to drink and drive. Teach your children never to get into a car driven by a person who has been drinking; assure them that you will pick them up no matter what the hour.

Adults should also discuss with adolescents the dangers of binge drinking (consuming more than five drinks in a row). This is a serious problem among the 6 million full-time college students in the United States and has led to deaths from alcohol overdose.

Young men and women in this age group are also at risk of drinking-related injury, property damage, date rape, and unsafe sex while under the influence of alcohol.

SIGNS OF ALCOHOL ABUSE

Alcohol abuse and alcohol dependence are serious and progressive medical diseases. However, they both are treatable. If you think you or someone you care about has a problem with alcohol, learn more about the disease and ask your doctor for help. The earlier such problems are brought to the attention of a doctor, the easier the treatment will be.

Early symptoms of alcohol problems include drinking more than planned, continuing to drink alcohol despite the concerns of others, and frequent attempts to cut down or quit drinking. As alcohol abuse progresses, the individual develops a tolerance to alcohol. He or she must drink more alcohol to get the desired good feeling or to get intoxicated.

When a person becomes dependent on alcohol, he or she develops withdrawal symptoms such as headache, nausea and vomiting, anxiety, and fatigue.

As alcohol abuse worsens, the person becomes preoccupied with alcohol and can lose control. He or she may have blackouts, which are episodes in which a person completely forgets what occurred when he or she was drunk even though he or she was conscious at the time.

Finally, personality changes occur. Someone suffering from alcohol abuse can become more aggressive and his or her ability to function (hold a job or maintain relationships with friends and family) can seriously deteriorate. Heavy drinkers may experience tremors, panic attacks, confusion, hallucinations, and seizures.

How to Recognize a Drinking Problem

If you think you or someone you care about may have a drinking problem, answer the following questions "yes" or "no":

- Have you ever felt you should cut down on your drinking?
- Have you ever felt annoyed when people criticized your drinking?
- Have you ever felt bad or guilty about your drinking?
- Have you ever had a drink first thing in the morning to steady your nerves or to get rid of a hangover?

A person who answers "yes" to two or more of these questions may be dependent on alcohol. Talk to your doctor or call your local chapter of Alcoholics Anonymous (see p.1229).

People with alcohol problems frequently drink alone and say they use alcohol to help them sleep or deal with stress. People who drink excessively may also engage in risky sexual behavior or drive when they should not. They are also at higher risk for dependency on other drugs.

EFFECTS ON THE BODY

The effects of alcoholism on the body are devastating. Health consequences of heavy alcohol use include inflammation of the stomach (see Gastritis, p.752), inflammation of the liver (see Hepatitis, p.758), bleeding in the stomach and esophagus (see Esophageal Varices, p.751), impotence (see p.1092), permanent nerve and brain damage (numbness or tingling sensations, imbalance, inability to coordinate movements, forgetfulness, blackouts, or problems with short-term memory), and inflammation of the pancreas (see Pancreatitis, p.768).

Long-term use also can increase the risk and severity of pneumonia and tuberculosis; damage the heart, leading to heart failure; and cause cirrhosis of the liver, leading to liver failure.

TREATING ALCOHOLISM

A person who needs help for alcohol addiction may be the last to realize he or she has a problem. Even if the addicted person refuses treatment, family members can get help and support from Al Anon (see p.1229).

Many similar drug and alcohol rehabilitation programs offer counseling to family members, so that they can learn how to help the addicted person get the right kind of support and help. An important part of these programs is to make the individual drinker responsible for his or her behavior, and to help the family stop shielding the drinker from the consequences of drinking.

Treating alcohol abuse begins by helping the drinker understand that he or she has a problem and needs help. Once a drinker wants to stop, treatment can take place in an outpatient setting (such as regular appointments with a counselor) or in a hospital inpatient program (where the treatment is much more intensive).

Almost all treatment programs view alcohol dependence as a chronic, progressive disease, and most programs insist on complete abstinence from alcohol and other drugs.

Inpatient treatment usually begins with detoxification—supervised withdrawal from alcohol—usually with the help of medicine to ease the dangerous effects of withdrawal, including restlessness, agitation, hallucinations, delirium, and seizures. In its most severe form, alcohol withdrawal can be life-threatening.

Treatment for alcoholism also addresses the medical and psychological consequences of alcohol addiction. Health professionals counsel the person and family about the nature of addiction and help the person find positive alternatives to using alcohol. Health professionals also help the individual cope with any related problems, such as depression, job stress, legal consequences of drinking, or troubled personal relationships.

Maintaining sobriety—often called "recovery"—is a long-term process that can take many forms. Fellowship groups such as Alcoholics Anonymous are often very helpful.

Ongoing counseling and treatment with medicines can also play a role. Disulfiram may be prescribed for people who want to try a drug to help prevent them from drinking. Disulfiram disrupts the breakdown of alcohol in the liver so that the person will feel ill if he or she drinks alcohol.

Other drugs, such as naloxone, take away the pleasant feeling that comes with drinking alcohol, so there is less interest in drinking. Both drugs must be taken daily in order to work. In people who also are depressed, antidepressant drugs may be used in treatment.

Other Addicting Drugs

In addition to alcohol and tobacco, people can abuse or become addicted to illegal "street" drugs and to prescription drugs. While these drugs can make some people feel better for a brief period, with time the person begins to feel progressively worse if the drug is not in his or her body.

Dependence on the drug

Preventing Teen Drug Use

Your involvement in your child's life is a primary component of preventing drug use. Here are some additional suggestions for fostering a healthy start for children, who will almost assuredly be exposed to drugs at school and by contemporaries:

■ Talk to your child clearly and openly about drugs, but do it early, ideally between the ages of 10 and 12; do not wait until a problem exists.

■ Strongly discourage smoking. Besides the adverse health effects, studies show that young people who smoke are more likely to use alcohol and illicit drugs.

■ Be a role model yourself. Do not drink alcohol to excess, smoke cigarettes, or use other drugs. You are your child's role model.

■ Get your child involved in sports, exercise, and social activities. Fill up his or her spare time with healthy, challenging endeavors.

■ Monitor your child's whereabouts. Know where your teen is at all times and get to know the parents of your child's friends. If your children must be home alone after school, find adult supervision for them.

■ Make sure your child has a way to get home other than by being driven by someone who has been drinking.

■ Look for potential signs of drug use (aggressiveness, chronic or excessive anger, depression, rebellious behavior, or poor school performance).

■ Adopt and enforce standard rules of behavior, including no use of illegal drugs—ever. Tell teens they must abide by this rule no matter where they are—at home, at a friend's home, at school, or at a party—and no matter what the circumstances.

Illegal Drug Abuse

Illegal drugs of abuse can include drugs that are never used in medical treatment, such as LSD or PCP ("angel dust"), and drugs that have a medical use (such as barbiturates or morphine). Addiction to prescription drugs is discussed on p.1157. This chart shows some of the effects of some common drugs of abuse.

DRUG	EFFECTS	SIGNS OF USE	POSSIBLE EFFECTS OF LONG-TERM USE
Amphetamines	Stimulant; accelerates physical and mental states	Insomnia; shaking; weight loss	Violent behavior; paranoia
Barbiturates	Tranquilizer; causes profound drowsiness and lethargy	Decreased alertness; slurred speech; slowed thinking; problems with coordination	Anxiety; tremors; weakness; insomnia; double vision; coma or death from overdose
Cannabis (eg, marijuana and hashish)	Heightens perception; relaxes the body	Bloodshot eyes; dilated pupils; lack of coordination and energy; decreased concentration; memory problems; rapid heart rate	Lung damage; decreased sex drive and sperm count; menstrual disturbances
Cocaine	Stimulant; accelerates physical and mental states	Dilated pupils; rapid breathing; high blood pressure; agitation	Weight loss; lung damage; heart attack; stroke; seizures; sores in nasal passages and perforated nasal septum (see p.462) when snorted; burning of lips or throat when smoked
Hallucinogens (eg, LSD [lysergic acid diethylamide], mescaline, PCP [phencyclidine], or "designer drugs" such as MDMA [methylenedioxymethamphetamine])	Causes either terrifying or pleasant hallucinations	Dilated pupils; trembling, sweating, chills, and fever	Flashbacks; psychological problems; psychosis
Opiates (eg, heroin, opium, or morphine)	Produces euphoria; eases physical and mental pain	Pinpoint pupils when intoxicated; dilated pupils when going through withdrawal; weight loss; lethargy; sweating; slurred speech; mood swings	Risk of hepatitis and HIV if injected; absence of menstrual periods; decreased sex drive
Anabolic steroids (compounds derived from the male hormone testosterone)	Increases muscle strength and bulk; quickly improves performance in athletes	Acne; progressive baldness; personality disorders, including extreme aggression	Impotence; elevated blood pressure and cholesterol levels; heart irregularities
Solvents and aerosols (eg, glue fumes or cleaning fluids)	Causes giddiness, euphoria, hallucinations, and unconsciousness	Confusion; flushed face; bloodshot eyes; slurred speech; problems with coordination; sudden death from cardiac arrest	Damage to brain, liver, and kidneys

increases until it becomes a central part of a person's life. Like addiction to alcohol, addiction to other substances causes a gradual deterioration in the person's work, personal relationships, or both. Drugs offer only temporary solutions to underlying problems.

In addition to numerous mental health risks, drug abuse can have other serious consequences.

For example, sharing infected needles can lead to hepatitis or infection with HIV (the virus that causes AIDS).

There are no controls over the purity and strength of illegal drugs. They can be too pure or too strong, putting the user at risk of an inadvertent overdose, or they can be combined with poisonous substances. Since

street drugs are illegal, any person using them is breaking the law simply by possessing them.

If you or someone you care about is addicted to a drug, get help by calling your doctor or a drug counseling center. Treatment has many similarities to treatment of alcohol abuse (see Narcotics Anonymous, p.1229).

CONTRACEPTION AND SAFER SEX

Choosing an appropriate form of contraception and using it consistently can prevent pregnancy and sexually transmitted diseases (STDs). While there are many forms of birth control, there are only two that also prevent STDs: a male condom or a female condom.

Many methods of contraception involve drugs, such as hormones, or devices, such as a diaphragm. There are also "natural" methods for contraception that involve avoiding sexual relations during the time of each month when a woman is most likely to become pregnant.

Different forms of contraception have advantages and disadvantages, some of which are related to your current health.

If you are a man, your choices are limited to sterilization (vasectomy), which is permanent, or the male condom. Women have more contraception options, some of which require a doctor's prescription; others are available over the counter.

Ask yourself these questions as you review your contraceptive options:

Is the method easy to use and convenient? Contraception is effective only if it is used consistently. Ask yourself if you will remember to take a birth-control pill every day or how comfortable or diligent you will be in inserting a diaphragm or cervical cap every time you have intercourse. Forgetting even one time can lead to pregnancy. If you have sex infrequently, you may find it easier to use a condom, along with a spermicide or a diaphragm, than other forms of contraception.

If you prefer not to think about taking a pill every day, hormone implants or injections may be a better choice. Partners who choose natural family planning methods must be committed to rigorously monitoring changes in the woman's body and abstaining from sexual intercourse during fertile periods.

Does it protect against STDs? The male and female condoms are the only contraceptive methods that offer protection against STDs. If you are not in a mutually monogamous relationship (in which you and your partner are

having sex only with each other), use a latex or polyurethane male or female condom with a spermicide every time you have sex.

Is the method reliable? While sterilization (vasectomy for a man or tubal ligation for a woman) provides the most reliable protection against pregnancy, these surgical procedures permanently end your ability to reproduce. Other forms of contraception vary in their reliability, and all depend on using them properly and consistently. See p.69 for a chart of contraceptive methods and their effectiveness.

How expensive is the method? The birth-control pill, IUD (intrauterine device), and hormonal implants may be more expensive initially, but over time can be less expensive than other methods.

What method best suits your medical history? Ask your physician which contraception he or she would recommend, based on your overall medical history. For example, if someone in your family has had cancer of the ovary or endometrium, the birth-control pill

Reliability of Contraception

This chart shows the percentage of 18- to 44-year-old women who would not become pregnant (effectiveness rate) during the first year of using various methods of birth control. It is calculated by determining what percentage of women did not have an unintended pregnancy during the first year of using a particular form of contraception. The rates can be improved if you use your method consistently and reliably.

For the sake of comparison, if 100 typical women between ages 18 and 44 use no form of contraception for a year, 85 will become pregnant during that year (a 15% effectiveness rate).

METHOD	% EFFECTIVE
Hormone implants	99.9
Vasectomy	99.8
Hormone injections	99.6
Tubal ligation	99.5
IUD (intrauterine device)	98.0
Birth-control pill	97.0
Mini-pill	96.0
Male condom	88.0
Diaphragm	82.0
Natural family planning	81.0
Female condom	79.0
Cervical cap	73.0
Spermicides	70.0

may be recommended because it has been shown to reduce the risk of those cancers.

If you smoke and are over 35, you may be advised not to take birth-control pills because of the increased risk of blood clots. If you have had infections of the reproductive tract, or are at increased risk of infection, your doctor may discourage you from considering an IUD because it can increase your chances of infection. Your doctor can help you make the best choice.

Hormonal Contraceptives

Hormonal contraceptives work mainly by preventing the release of an egg from an ovary. To understand the role of both estrogen and progesterone, the two main sex hormones in contraceptive pills, see Health of Women (p.1039).

Contraceptives that incorporate hormones include pills, injections, and implants. Hormonal implants are popular because

they are reliable and convenient, with relatively few side effects. Both injections and implants can also reduce your risk of cancer of the endometrium.

Birth-control pills reduce your risk of cancer of the endometrium and cancer of the ovary while you take them (once you have been on them for 1 year) and for up to 18 years after you stop taking them. Hormonal contraceptives do not protect against STDs.

HORMONE INJECTIONS

In this type of contraception, a synthetic form of the female hormone progesterone is injected into a woman's buttocks or arm muscle every 3 months; it is highly effective.

Hormone injections reduce the likelihood of ovulation and change the consistency of the mucus covering the cervix (the opening to the uterus), preventing sperm from reaching the uterus and fallopian tubes, where the sperm can fertilize the egg.

The injections also reduce growth of the endometrium (the lining of the uterus), which reduces the chance that a fertilized egg will implant in the endometrium. The most common side effect of hormone injections is irregular bleeding and, after about 1 year, cessation of periods. Other side effects include weight gain.

HORMONE IMPLANTS

Hormone implants are soft matchsticklike capsules that are inserted by a physician just under the skin of a woman's upper arm. They release a constant but small dose of progestin (a synthetic version of the female hormone progesterone) to prevent ovulation (the monthly release of an egg by an ovary).

They also help prevent sperm from reaching the uterus by changing the consistency of the mucus that covers the cervix (the opening to the uterus).

The implants last 5 years. Side effects of hormone implants include spotting between periods, irregular periods, or no periods at all.

To insert the implants, your doctor will deaden an area of skin on your upper arm with a local anesthetic (see p.168). A single small incision is made and the six capsules are inserted in a fanlike pattern under the skin; the incision is so small that stitches are not needed. Small pieces of tape are used to close the incision.

Protection against pregnancy begins within 24 hours. Implants can be removed in a similar procedure.

BIRTH-CONTROL PILLS

Combined birth-control pills (also called oral contraceptives) contain estrogen and a synthetic form of progesterone, both female hormones. They work by interrupting the hormonal changes that cause a woman to ovulate (release an egg) and by causing the mucus in the cervix to change consistency, helping to block the passage of sperm into the uterus.

Aside from sterilization (see p.74), birth-control pills are the most effective way to prevent pregnancy. They do not affect your ability to become pregnant in the future.

Some oral contraceptives are packaged so that you take one

pill every day of the week for 21 days and then stop taking the pill for 7 days, when menstruation usually occurs. Others are packaged so that you take one pill every day of the week for 28 days but seven of the pills taken in a row are placebos. Menstruation occurs when you take the placebos.

If you forget to take a pill, take it as soon as you can, along with the pill for that day. If you forget to take two pills in a row, you must use another form of contraception in addition to taking the pills you missed.

Your doctor can tell you exactly how to take the missed pills and for how long you will require an additional form of birth control to prevent pregnancy. If you have difficulty remembering to take your pills, consider switching to hormone injections, implants, or another type of contraception.

There are several types of birth-control pills, each of which contains varying amounts of the two female hormones. Based on your medical history, your doctor can prescribe the best combination. Today's lower-dose birth-control pills contain less than half the estrogen of the pills that were prescribed 20 or more years ago and are therefore much safer.

However, doctors are unlikely to recommend the combined birth-control pill for women over 35 who smoke and for all women who have a history of diabetes, blood clots, high blood pressure, or breast or endometrial cancer. (Even though the birth-control pill protects against endometrial cancer, once a person has had endometrial cancer,

the estrogen in the pill may increase the chance of the cancer recurring.)

The side effects and risks of taking the pill are relatively minimal for women under 35. Some women have breakthrough bleeding or spotting between periods when they first start taking the pill; most women find that their periods become lighter and last fewer days.

Some women feel nauseous during the first few months on the pill while others feel a slight tenderness in their breasts. Switching to a pill with a lower dose of estrogen can reduce most of the side effects.

THE MINI-PILL

If you cannot take the combined birth-control pill, your doctor may recommend the mini-pill, so-called because it contains only progestin, a synthetic form of the female hormone progesterone. It is considered safer for women who have diabetes, a history of blood clots, high blood pressure, or other diseases that estrogen can complicate, and for women who smoke.

The mini-pill is slightly less effective than the combined pill, but it is an effective form of contraception if taken exactly as prescribed, which includes taking the pill at the same time every day.

The mini-pill works by preventing ovulation (release of an egg from an ovary), though not as effectively as the combined birth-control pill. It also thickens the mucus that covers the cervix (the opening to the uterus), thus preventing sperm from entering.

Ovulation is not always prevented with the mini-pill. You must rely on the protection offered by the thickened mucus on the cervix, so it is essential that you take your pill at the same time every day.

Because it contains no estrogen, the mini-pill inhibits the growth of the endometrium (the lining of the uterus into which a fertilized egg implants). This makes the endometrium less hospitable for implantation. The effect of the mini-pill on the endometrium can also cause your periods to be irregular or nonexistent. Instead, you may have a lot of spotting or breakthrough bleeding.

THE MORNING-AFTER PILL

Morning-after pills are taken within 72 hours of unprotected intercourse to prevent pregnancy. The most widely used pills contain estrogen and progesterone. Two pills are taken immediately and two are taken 12 hours later. They are about 80% effective, and work by preventing or delaying ovulation, inhibiting the sperm from reaching an egg, and interfering with implantation.

Morning-after pills are effective only when the first dose is taken within 72 hours of intercourse.

Barrier Methods

Barrier methods of contraception—such as the diaphragm, condom, and cervical cap—must always be used with spermicide jelly or cream, which contain chemicals that kill sperm before they can reach the uterus.

Even though they are called "barriers," the diaphragm and cervical cap used without spermicide

do not reliably block the passage of sperm. Their main function is to hold the spermicide in place over the cervix and kill any sperm trying to enter the uterus.

MALE CONDOM

The male condom is a thin latex or polyurethane sheath that is placed over the erect penis before intercourse. A condom prevents semen (and the sperm in semen) from being released into the vagina and the uterus, where sperm can reach a fallopian tube to fertilize an egg and cause pregnancy.

Latex or polyurethane condoms also prevent STDs (see p.889). Condoms made of materials such as lambskin do not protect against STDs because they are porous. When used correctly with a spermicide every time you have intercourse, the condom is highly effective. Some condoms

Spermicides

Spermicides are substances that kill sperm before they can fertilize an egg. They are available in many forms—including gels, creams, foams, suppositories, and films—and are placed in the vagina before sexual intercourse. Spermicides can be purchased at drugstores without a prescription.

The best way to use a spermicide is to combine it with a condom, diaphragm, or cervical cap. Alone, a spermicide is a poor method of preventing pregnancy. Also, you must read the directions on the spermicide packaging and use the product exactly as instructed; otherwise, it may not be effective. If you have intercourse more than once within a few hours, you must insert more spermicide.

Putting On and Taking Off a Male Condom

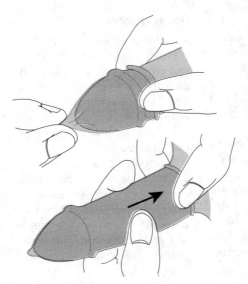

Pinch the top half inch of the condom to squeeze out air bubbles and leave a space for semen to collect. While still pinching the end of the condom, place it on the erect penis, unrolling it all the way down to the base. After ejaculation, hold the condom at its base to prevent it from slipping off the penis and immediately withdraw the penis from the vagina. The penis should be withdrawn right after ejaculation because once the penis becomes soft, the condom can slip off and accidentally deposit semen into the vagina.

How to Insert a Female Condom

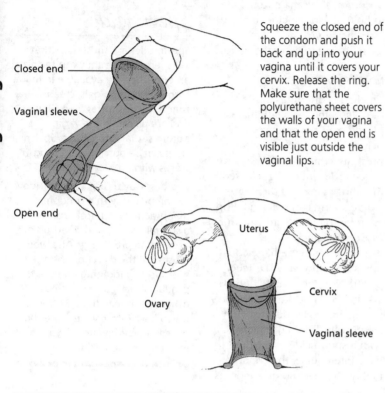

Closed end

Vaginal sleeve

Open end

Squeeze the closed end of the condom and push it back and up into your vagina until it covers your cervix. Release the ring. Make sure that the polyurethane sheet covers the walls of your vagina and that the open end is visible just outside the vaginal lips.

Uterus

Ovary

Cervix

Vaginal sleeve

are sold with a coating of spermicide on them.

To be effective, a condom must be put on before a man's genitals come into contact with a woman's genitals. After ejaculation, hold the base of the condom while the penis is withdrawn from the vagina to prevent the condom from pulling off and from emptying the semen into the vagina.

If the condom causes friction during intercourse, use a water-soluble lubricating jelly on the condom or in the vagina. Be sure the container of lubricating jelly contains the words "water soluble"; oil-based lubricants, such as petroleum jelly, can damage latex

and cause the condom to leak. Condoms can be purchased at drugstores without a prescription.

FEMALE CONDOM

The female condom, made of polyurethane, lines the vagina and prevents semen (which contains sperm) from being released into the vagina and the uterus, where sperm can reach a fallopian tube to fertilize an egg and cause pregnancy.

A portion of the female condom remains outside the vagina, where it helps protect against STDs (see p.889), such as genital warts and genital herpes, that can be spread to a woman's external genitals. The female condom is

lubricated and packaged with extra lubricant.

To be effective, the female condom must be inserted before a man's genitals come into contact with a woman's genitals. Female condoms can be purchased at drugstores without a prescription.

CERVICAL CAP

The cervical cap is a dome-shaped rubber cup that you fill with spermicide, insert into the vagina, and push up until it fits tightly over the cervix (the opening to the uterus). The cervical cap prevents sperm from entering the uterus, where they can reach a fallopian tube to fertilize an egg and cause pregnancy.

Your doctor must fit you for a cervical cap. To be effective, it is essential that the cap cover your cervix precisely; it is held over the cervix by suction.

It is best to insert the cervical cap about a half hour before intercourse (to be sure it is securely in place) and leave it in position for 8 hours afterward. It can be left in place for up to 48 hours after intercourse. To remove the cap, pull on the back edge of the rim and guide it out of your vagina.

The advantage of the cap is that it is less likely than the diaphragm to irritate the urethra, and can remain in the vagina longer. One disadvantage is that the cap probably does not protect very well against STDs.

DIAPHRAGM

A diaphragm resembles a rubber cup. Larger than the cervical cap, it covers your cervix (the opening to the uterus). To use the

Inserting and Removing a Cervical Cap

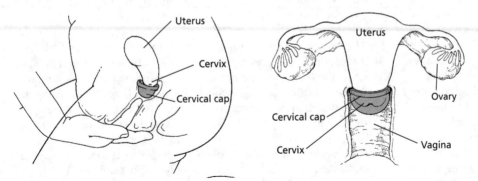

Uterus

Cervix

Cervical cap

Uterus

Ovary

Cervical cap

Cervix

Vagina

To insert a cervical cap, fill about a third of the cap with spermicidal jelly or cream. Push the cap into your vagina until it is positioned over the cervix, where it will make an airtight seal. To remove the cap, pull on the back edge of the rim and guide it out of your vagina.

Inserting and Removing a Diaphragm

INSERTION

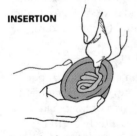

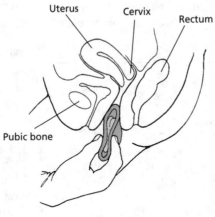

Uterus   Cervix

Rectum

2 Squeeze the rim together and insert the diaphragm into your vagina.

1 Apply about a teaspoon of spermicide to the center of the diaphragm; spread some around the rim.

Pubic bone

REMOVAL

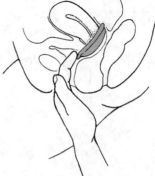

3 Using your finger, slide the back rim of the diaphragm past your cervix; make sure that the diaphragm covers your entire cervix.

4 After sexual intercourse, the diaphragm must be left in place for at least 6 hours. To remove it, place your finger over the top of the front rim and pull the diaphragm out of your vagina.

diaphragm, you apply a spermicide to the bowl-shaped area, insert it into your vagina, and push it up onto your cervix. It can be inserted several hours before intercourse and must stay in position at least 6 hours after intercourse.

The diaphragm itself does not prevent pregnancy. It is used to hold the spermicidal jelly or cream over the opening to the uterus, where it will kill sperm before they enter the uterus. The diaphragm requires a prescription and fitting by your doctor.

Other Contraceptive Methods

IUDS (INTRAUTERINE DEVICES)

An IUD is a T-shaped device made of plastic that your physician inserts into your uterus.

There are two types of IUDs. One gradually releases the female hormone progesterone into the body; the other is coated with copper.

The progesterone-containing IUD must be replaced every year. It works by thickening the mucus of the cervix (the opening to the uterus), which prevents sperm from reaching the uterus. It also kills the sperm as they try to get into the uterus and up the fallopian tubes, and produces changes in the endometrium (the lining of the uterus), inhibiting implantation of a fertilized egg.

An IUD coated with copper can remain in place for up to 10 years. It inhibits the fertilized egg from implanting in the endometrium.

To insert an IUD, your doctor first dilates (widens) your cervix. Uncommon complications related to insertion are injury to the wall of the uterus and the introduction of infection-causing bacteria into the uterus.

Once inserted, check monthly to ensure that you can feel the strings of your IUD, which hang down into your vagina. If you cannot feel the strings, call your doctor. The IUD may have moved out of the uterus during the mild contractions that occur with menstruation. Because it is only about 1 inch long by $\frac{1}{2}$ inch across, it can easily be lost in the toilet if it has become dislodged.

The most common side effects of the IUD are longer, heavier periods; spotting between periods; and menstrual pain. Using an IUD may increase your risk of pelvic inflammatory disease (see p.1077) and thereby increase the risk of infertility in the future.

STERILIZATION

Sterilization is surgery that permanently prevents reproduction in either a man or a woman; it is almost 100% effective. Sterilization for a woman is called tubal ligation; for a man, vasectomy.

While both procedures occasionally can be reversed, successful reversal is not common. If you are considering sterilization, you should view it as permanent.

Tubal ligation In tubal ligation, the fallopian tubes are either cut or clamped to prevent an egg released by an ovary from moving down the fallopian tube into the uterus. Tubal ligation is most often performed with the woman under general anesthesia (see p.168).

For the surgery, a laparoscope, a kind of endoscope (see

Position of IUD

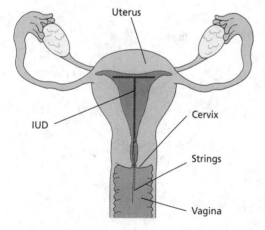

Uterus

IUD

Cervix

Strings

Vagina

An IUD (intrauterine device) is inserted by your doctor into your uterus. The strings of the IUD hang down through your cervix into your vagina. Feel for the strings every month after your period to ensure that the IUD is still in place. If you feel plastic (which is the IUD) pushing out through the cervix, see your doctor to have the position of the IUD checked.

Tubal Ligation: Female Sterilization

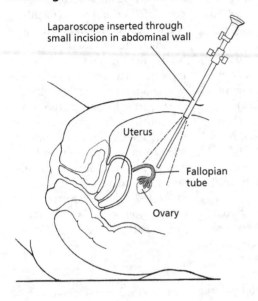

Laparoscope inserted through small incision in abdominal wall

Uterus

Fallopian tube

Ovary

VIEW THROUGH LAPAROSCOPE

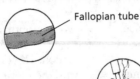

Fallopian tube

Burned

Cut and tied

Banded

Clamped

A tubal ligation interrupts an egg's passage from an ovary through the fallopian tube by cutting and tying, burning, banding, or clamping the fallopian tubes. Surgery is performed through two small incisions made just below the naval. A viewing instrument called a laparoscope is inserted through one incision; another instrument is inserted through a second incision to close off the fallopian tubes using one of the techniques shown.

p.142), is used to look inside the abdomen and pelvis. In the most common form of the procedure, two small incisions are made just below the navel, and the laparoscope is inserted through one of the incisions so the surgeon can see the fallopian tubes. A surgical instrument is inserted through the second incision to cut or clamp the fallopian tubes. The incisions are then stitched closed.

Tubal ligation can also be performed without a laparoscope, through a somewhat larger incision; this most often is done when a woman has had previous surgery in the area. Most women feel some abdominal discomfort for a few days after tubal ligation. The operation provides immediate protection against pregnancy; no other form of birth control is required.

Vasectomy In a vasectomy, the tubes (the vas deferens) that carry

Vasectomy: Male Sterilization

After administering a local anesthetic, the doctor performs a vasectomy as shown here.

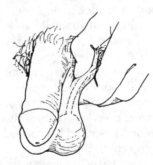

1 Doctor identifies position of vas deferens through touch.

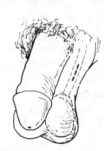

2 Skin incision is made over vas deferens.

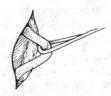

3 Vas deferens is pulled through incision.

4 Vas deferens is cut in two places.

5 Cut ends of vas deferens are tied off and incision is stitched closed.

sperm from the testicles to the penis are cut to prevent sperm from entering the semen, which is ejaculated during intercourse. (For a description of a man's reproductive system, see p.1086.)

Vasectomy can be performed in a doctor's office in about 20 minutes; it is simpler and safer than tubal ligation and requires only local anesthesia (see p.168).

The doctor first locates the vas deferens by feeling for it in the scrotum. The area is numbed and a small incision is made. The vas deferens is brought through the incision, cut, and the ends are either tied off or sealed with heat. The procedure is repeated with the other vas deferens and the incisions are stitched closed. Another type of vasectomy involves simply puncturing the skin instead of making an incision.

Two tests to confirm the absence of sperm in your semen are performed over a period of 8 weeks until the semen is sperm-free. You should use another form of birth control in the interim. A vasectomy does not affect a man's ability to achieve erection, have an orgasm, or ejaculate.

NATURAL METHODS

Effective natural family planning relies on completely avoiding sexual intercourse for at least 10 days per month—about a week before ovulation and several days afterward.

This method of birth control requires scrupulous attention to the signs of ovulation that occur throughout a woman's menstrual

cycle. It also requires the discipline not to have intercourse on risky days.

Every month, an egg is released by the ovary through ovulation. The egg then moves toward the uterus via the fallopian tubes, where fertilization occurs. An unfertilized egg can live from 12 to 24 hours; it is shed during menstruation if fertilization does not occur. Sperm can live up to 1 week in the fallopian tubes.

How do you tell when ovulation is likely to occur? There are several methods. In the cervical mucus method, you chart the consistency of your vaginal mucus (which is secreted by the cervix). The days surrounding ovulation are identified by the consistency of your mucus.

During the most fertile time, the mucus is slick, clear, and stretchy and feels like raw egg white. The mucus becomes cloudy and thick during safer times after ovulation. Some women cannot reliably use this method because they do not secret enough mucus to evaluate.

In the body temperature method, a woman takes her temperature every day (before she gets out of bed) with a special, highly sensitive thermometer, and charts each day's temperature on a monthly graph. Temperature rises slightly at the time of ovulation. You avoid intercourse for the days surrounding ovulation.

Particularly if your periods are regular, you can estimate when your next ovulation is likely to occur based on the pattern of previous ovulations. You then

avoid having unprotected intercourse for several days (ideally, a week) before the expected day of ovulation, and for at least 72 hours after the temperature rise indicates that you have ovulated.

Natural birth-control methods are the least reliable of the contraceptive methods because they require a high degree of commitment from both partners to be effective, and require very regular menstrual periods. If you are interested, ask your doctor for information on classes that teach these methods.

Safer Sex

You can greatly reduce your chance of acquiring STDs (see p.889), including HIV, by following these safer sex guidelines:

■ Engage in sexual intercourse only with a mutually monogamous partner—that is, one sex partner who has sex only with you.

■ Use a latex or polyurethane male condom or a female condom every time you have sex. In addition, use a spermicide that contains nonoxynol 9, which can help kill viruses.

■ For oral sex, use a latex or polyurethane male condom or a female condom.

■ For anal sex, use a latex or polyurethane male condom.

Semen, blood, and vaginal/cervical secretions can transmit HIV. Saliva may be capable of transmitting HIV but the transmission rate is extremely low. Sweat, tears, and urine do not transmit HIV.

MEDICAL CHECKUPS AND SCREENING TESTS

The complete annual physical once recommended has been replaced by periodic preventive examinations—health appraisals whose scope and frequency are tailored to your age, risk factors, and lifestyle.

Your behavior and habits strongly influence your risk of disease; sharing this information with your doctor is the best way to start appropriate preventive strategies.

Preventive physical examinations and screening tests are designed to identify diseases at an early stage, but the process is not perfect. No part of a physical examination and no screening test is perfectly accurate. Each can lead to "false negative" and "false positive" results. False negative test results can create a false sense of security, and false positive test results can create unnecessary fear and lead to additional tests.

Authoritative groups disagree about whether particular parts of the preventive physical examination or particular screening tests are worth doing. While almost all authorities agree on the value of certain tests (Pap smears, for example), there are differences of opinion concerning the value of other tests. Often, the differences of opinion are based on different judgments about how bad the consequences would be if a test result is falsely negative or positive.

The information on the following pages outlines what tests you should have regularly and how frequently they should be performed if you are at higher risk. These recommendations are strongly influenced by the US Preventive Services Task Force, a prestigious panel of experts who represent many medical disciplines. Your doctor can recommend a schedule that is tailored to your requirements.

Self-Examinations

You see the doctor only every so often, but you see yourself (if you have a bathroom mirror) every day. For that reason, it seems to make sense to examine yourself regularly.

Some physicians and medical organizations recommend that men and women perform certain examinations on themselves on a regular basis. The three most frequently recommended examinations are of the breasts, testicles, and skin.

Self-examinations are of unproven value. However, they are simple to do, and can identify a tumor at an early stage. The reason that some doctors do not recommend self-examination is that, in addition to being of unproven value, it has the potential for generating unnecessary apprehension. Most lumps turn out to be noncancerous, but it may take a few weeks before you know that.

Many physicians practicing at Harvard support self-examinations as a way to prevent disease. This is why you will find self-exams recommended elsewhere in this book. Talk to your own doctor about the value of self-examination as it relates to your particular medical needs and history.

Only you can make the judgment about whether you want to perform self-examinations. The three most common self-examinations are:

Breast self-exams are recommended by the American Cancer Society if you are a woman 20 or older. The American Cancer Society recommends that you examine your breasts every month, ideally at the end of your period, when your breasts are not tender or likely to be lumpy.

Performing this exam every month will acquaint you with the geography of your breasts and make it more likely that you will notice any unusual lump or swelling. To examine your breasts, follow the steps shown in the illustration on p.78. Talk to your doctor if you notice anything unusual.

Testicle self-exams are recommended by many doctors. To examine your testicles, follow the steps shown in the illustration on p.78. Choose an easy date to remember, like the first day of the month, to perform this examination.

Skin exams are best when performed by someone close to you (since you cannot see all parts of your own skin very well). The steps are described in the box Preventing Skin Cancer on p.548.

Most doctors agree that people who are at increased risk for developing the skin cancer melanoma (see p.543) should have their skin examined regularly by a doctor, supplemented by self-examination between doctor visits.

How to Examine Your Breasts

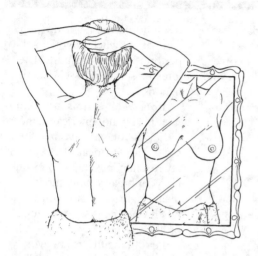 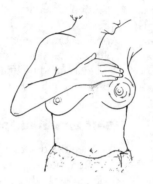 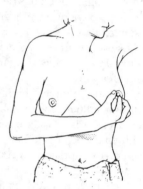

Examine your breasts every month several days after your period. Standing in front of a mirror with your arms hanging at your sides, look for any change in breast contour, such as a lump, swelling, puckering of the breast or nipple, prominent veins, or a difference in nipple color. Then, raise both arms over your head (left) and look for the same changes. Next, raise one arm (center), placing one hand behind your head. Press down gently on your breast with the middle three fingertips of your other hand, keeping your fingers straight. With small circular motions, spend at least 2 minutes feeling for hard lumps in every part of your breast, including your armpit. A hard lump of any size, even if it is not tender, should be brought to the attention of your doctor. Finally, squeeze each nipple gently (right) to check for discharge. Some women find that it is easier to feel for lumps in the bath or shower, when their skin is wet and soapy. Women with large breasts may find it easier to feel for lumps while lying down when doing the circular motions.

How to Examine Your Testicles

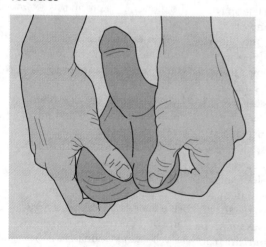

Examine your testicles during or after a shower, when the skin of your scrotum is relaxed. Use both hands to gently roll each testicle between your thumbs and fingers. Locate the tubelike structure at the back of each testicle (the epididymis) to become familiar with the way it feels. Feel the rest of your testicle for any lump, swelling, or tender area. Cancerous lumps are usually located on the sides, but can occur anywhere. If you feel any lump or have pain, tenderness, or swelling, see your doctor immediately.

79

Taking Charge of Your Health

HOME MEDICAL TESTS

Sophisticated and accurate home testing kits can be found in every pharmacy. Overall, about 300 home-test products have been approved by the U.S. Food and Drug Administration (FDA). FDA approval means a home test kit works and contains instructions written for consumers.

Home testing allows you to become more involved in your medical care, but should not replace regular visits to your doctor. Because your body changes from day to day, multiple measurements performed by you can add useful information to tests performed less frequently at your doctor's office.

The majority of the following kits are accurate and easy to use. However, all tests require that you follow the instructions carefully, including precise time intervals when directed.

Blood Cholesterol Test

You can test your total cholesterol at home with a simple blood test. This test is up to 97% accurate, but total cholesterol is only one of the measurements obtained on the cholesterol panel at your doctor's office.

Low-density lipoprotein (LDL) and high-density lipoprotein (HDL) readings (see p.669) are also important for some people. Current tests require several drops of blood. Because you need to poke your fingertip with a sharp lancet, some people find this test difficult to perform at home. Also, there is no evidence that tests performed at home reduce the risk of disease for most people.

Tests That Detect Blood in Bowel Movements

A fecal occult ("hidden") blood test can detect invisible amounts of blood in the bowel movement that are not apparent to the eye. You can obtain these home tests from your doctor or a pharmacy. If you follow the instructions carefully, the test is as reliable in your home as it is in your doctor's office.

In fact, because you can test more bowel movements, at different times, than is feasible for your doctor to test, the multiple tests you perform at home are more accurate than the single test your doctor performs in the office.

However, the test is not foolproof; it can give both falsely positive and falsely negative results. Follow these safeguards to make the test more accurate:

■ Do not use the test during your menstrual period or if you have hemorrhoids that are currently bleeding.

■ Certain foods (such as rare red meat, horseradish, cantaloupe, uncooked broccoli, cabbage, turnips, radishes, and cauliflower) should be avoided for 2 days before collecting a sample for testing because they can cause the test result to be abnormal or positive.

■ Certain medicines (such as aspirin and other nonsteroidal anti-inflammatory drugs and iron supplements) should be avoided for 2 days before collecting a sample for testing because they can cause the test result to be abnormal or positive.

■ Vitamin C pills or citrus fruits, which are high in vitamin C, should be avoided for 2 days

before collecting a sample for testing because they can cause the test result to be normal or negative when there actually is bleeding.

Your doctor will give you a set of three cards (each card will have two windows, labeled A and B), some wooden applicator sticks, and a special, foil-backed, return envelope. Use one of the wooden sticks to collect a small sample from one area of a bowel movement (or toilet paper used to wipe a bowel movement) and thinly smear it onto window A of one of the cards. Using the same wooden stick, get a second sample from a different area of the bowel movement and thinly smear it onto window B. Reseal the card.

Repeat this process, using the remaining two cards, the next two times you have a bowel movement. Then, in the special return envelope provided, send all three cards to your physician immediately. (You must use the envelope provided with your test; paper envelopes are not approved for this use by US postal regulations.)

At your doctor's office, a special developing solution will be added. If blood is present, the testing site of the card will turn blue.

TESTING TOILET WATER FOR BLOOD

An alternative to performing a fecal occult blood test is testing for blood in the toilet bowl water after a bowel movement. This test may be less accurate than testing the bowel movement directly. You can obtain a toilet water testing kit from your pharmacy. The kits contain sheets of special paper that you drop directly into the water of the

What Screening Tests Should Adults Have?

The recommended tests and examinations you should have are summarized here.

TEST	HOW OFTEN TEST SHOULD BE PERFORMED
Height and weight	Height: regularly in childhood, once in early adulthood, and every 10 years after age 50. Weight: regularly in childhood and every 1 to 3 years throughout adulthood.

VISION

Visual acuity	Every year after age 65.
For glaucoma	Every few years after age 50 if you are African-American or have a parent, brother, or sister with glaucoma; every few years after age 65.
Hearing	Every few years after age 21 if exposed to loud noises; every few years after age 65.
Blood pressure	Every doctor visit (or every 2 years) after age 18.

FOR HEART DISEASE RISK FACTORS

Cholesterol	Every 5 years after age 20 if a person has risk factors for atherosclerosis such as tobacco use, diabetes, family history of heart disease, high cholesterol, or high blood pressure. Every 1 to 3 years for men 35 and older, women 45 and older, until age 65.
Electrocardiogram (EKG)	Every 1 to 3 years after age 40 if you have coronary artery disease risk factors (see p.654) or if you are about to start a vigorous exercise program.

FOR DIABETES

Fasting blood sugar test	Every few years if you have had gestational diabetes (see p.930), are obese (see p.853), or have a parent, brother, or sister with diabetes.

FOR CERVICAL CANCER

Pap smear, plus HPV test as indicated (see p.1042)	Within 3 years of onset of sexual activity or age 21—whichever is first. Every 1 to 3 years thereafter.

FOR BREAST CANCER

Breast self-exam	Not of proven value as a screening test but recommended by some doctors because it is simple and has no expense.
Breast exam by physician	Every year after age 35 if mother or sister had breast cancer before menopause; every year after age 40. Every year after age 35 if mother or sister had breast cancer before menopause; every year after age 50.
Mammogram	Every 1 to 2 years for women aged 40 and older. Once for women between ages 35 and 40, if a parent or sibling has had breast cancer.

TEST	HOW OFTEN TEST SHOULD BE PERFORMED

FOR COLON CANCER

Testing stool for blood

Every 1 to 3 years after age 40 if you have a parent, brother, or sister with colorectal cancer (see p.791) or inflammatory bowel disease (see p.787). Every 1 to 3 years in all men and women age 50 and older.

Sigmoidoscopy (usually no need for sigmoidoscopy if colonoscopy performed)

Every 1 to 3 years after age 40 if you have a parent, brother, or sister with colorectal cancer (see p.791) or inflammatory bowel disease (see p.787).

Every 1 to 3 years after age 50 in all adults.

Colonoscopy

At least once after age 40 if you have more than one first-degree relative with colorectal cancer (see p.791) or have close relatives with familial polyposis (see p.129) or intestinal polyps (see p.790), or if you have had ulcerative colitis (see Inflammatory Bowel Disease, p.787) for more than 10 years, or have had intestinal polyps.

Every 10 years in all adults after age 50.

FOR PROSTATE CANCER

Rectal exam — Not of proven value as a screening test.

Prostate specific antigen (PSA) test — Not of proven value as a screening test.

FOR LUNG CANCER

Chest X-ray — Not of proven value as a screening test.

Low dose computerized tomography — Not of proven value as a screening test.

Sputum cytology — Not of proven value as a screening test.

FOR OSTEOPOROSIS

Bone density tests

Every 2 years in women over age 60, if she has risk factors for osteoporosis such as being thin and having thin bones, mother had osteoporosis, Asian or Caucasian, early menopause or ovaries surgically removed, diet low in calcium and vitamin D, physically inactive, smoking, or more than 2 alcoholic drinks a day.

Every 2 to 3 years in all women over age 65.

FOR HIV — Every few years if you have engaged in high risk behavior (see p.873)

FOR SYPHILIS — Every few years if you regularly engage in unprotected sexual intercourse, and during pregnancy if you are pregnant.

FOR THYROID DISEASE

Thyroid-stimulating hormone (TSH) blood test — Every few years after age 60 for women.

At What Age Do I Need Various Tests and Examinations?

This chart shows what tests and examinations you should have based on your age.

Birth to 20 years See Health of Infants and Children, p.945; Health of Adolescents, p.1021.

Ages 21 to 39 years

TEST	HOW OFTEN TEST SHOULD BE PERFORMED
Height and weight	Height once. Weight every 1 to 3 years.
Blood pressure	Every doctor visit (or every 2 years).
Cholesterol	Every 5 years after age 20 if a person has risk factors for atherosclerosis such as tobacco use, diabetes, family history of heart disease, high cholesterol, or high blood pressure. Every 1 to 3 years for men 35 and older.
For diabetes (fasting blood sugar)	Every few years if you have had gestational diabetes (see p.930), are obese (see p.853), or have a parent, brother, or sister with diabetes.
Pap smear, plus HPV test as indicated (see p.1042)	Within 3 years of onset of sexual activity or age 21—whichever is first. Every 1 to 3 years thereafter.
For HIV	Every few years if you have engaged in high risk behavior (see p.872)
Mammogram	Once for women between ages 35 and 40, if a parent or sibling has had breast cancer.
For syphilis	Every few years if you regularly engage in unprotected sexual intercourse, and during pregnancy if you are pregnant.

Ages 40 to 49 years

Same as for ages 21 to 39 years, except for the following:

TEST	FREQUENCY
Electrocardiogram (EKG)	Every 1 to 3 years after age 40 if you have coronary artery disease risk factors (see p.654) or if you are about to start a vigorous exercise program.
Mammogram	Every 1 to 2 years for women ages 40 and older. Once for women between ages 35 and 40, if a parent or sibling has had breast cancer.
Testing stool for blood	Every 1 to 3 years after age 40 if you have a parent, brother, or sister with colorectal cancer (see p.791) or inflammatory bowel disease (see p.787).
Sigmoidoscopy (usually no need for sigmoidoscopy if colonoscopy performed)	Every 1 to 3 years after age 40 if you have a parent, brother, or sister with colorectal cancer (see p.791) or inflammatory bowel disease (see p.787).
Colonoscopy	At least once after age 40 if you have more than one first-degree relative with colorectal cancer (see p.791) or have close relatives with familial polyposis (see p.129) or intestinal polyps (see p.790), or if you have had ulcerative colitis (see Inflammatory Bowel Disease, p.787) for more than 10 years or have had intestinal polyps.

Age 50 years and older
Same as for ages 21 to 39 years and 40 to 49 years, except for the following:

TEST	FREQUENCY
Height and weight	Height every 10 years. Weight every 1 to 3 years.
Visual acuity	Every year after age 65.
For glaucoma	Every few years after age 50 if you are African-American or have a parent, brother, or sister with glaucoma. Every few years after age 65 in all adults.

TEST	FREQUENCY
Hearing	Every few years if exposed to loud noises; every few years after age 65.
Mammogram	Every year until age 75.
For thyroid disease (thyroid-stimulating hormone [TSH] blood test)	Every few years after age 60 for women.

Benefits of Endoscopy for Colon Cancer

There is a strong association between the development of polyps in the colon and the development of colon or rectal cancer. Examination of the colon and rectum for polyps with a colonoscope or flexible sigmoidoscope, and removal of these polyps, has been shown to reduce your risk of colon cancer.

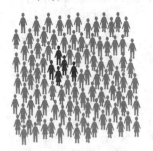

5 OF 100 PEOPLE IN THE GENERAL POPULATION WILL DEVELOP COLORECTAL CANCER IN THEIR LIFETIME

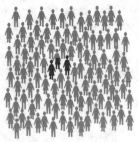

2.5 OF 100 PEOPLE WHO UNDERGO ROUTINE SCREEN-ING WITH ENDOSCOPY WILL DEVELOP COLORECTAL CANCER IN THEIR LIFETIME

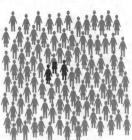

2.6 OF 100 PEOPLE IN THE GENERAL POPULATION WILL DIE OF COLORECTAL CANCER

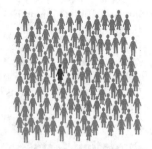

1 OF 100 PEOPLE WHO UNDERGO ROUTINE SCREEN-ING WITH ENDOSCOPY WILL DIE OF COLORECTAL CANCER

toilet bowl after you have had a bowel movement. The sheet turns blue if blood is detected.

Pregnancy Test

Home pregnancy tests are very accurate. They work by detecting the presence of the hormone human chorionic gonadotropin (HCG) in your urine. If you are pregnant, HCG is present in your urine by the first day of your missed period.

A pregnancy test is most accurate if the testing is done using the first urine of the morning because HCG accumulates overnight in urine stored in your bladder.

To perform the test, drop a small amount of urine into the well on the test disc. As the test begins to work, you will see a blush of color in the results window. Most tests use a plus sign (+) to indicate pregnancy, and a minus sign (-) to indicate that you are not pregnant. It is helpful if the test also has a control window that changes color to show the test is working.

If the test result is positive, you are probably pregnant; call your doctor and have a confirmation test. If the test result is negative, but you do not get your period within a week, consult your doctor. If the window remains colorless, call the test helpline.

Ovulation Tests

An ovulation test indicates when an egg is released from your ovary. You are most likely to become pregnant at this time. People trying to get pregnant can use this test so they can have sexual intercourse at the time of ovulation. The test senses a sub-

stance called luteinizing hormone (LH) in the urine. A sudden surge in LH triggers ovulation, which occurs within 36 hours.

To use the test, place a few drops of urine into the well on the test disc. After the specified time, watch for color changes in the control and results windows. The instructions will tell you if the test result is positive or negative. If the test result is negative, repeat it daily until the surge in LH occurs.

Another ovulation test measures the estrogen and progesterone levels in saliva to indicate when a woman is most fertile.

Hepatitis C Test

You can buy a kit at the drugstore that will test your blood for infection with the hepatitis C virus (see p.759). The kit consists of a lancet and special blotting paper. Prick your finger with the lancet and put a few drops of your blood on the paper provided. Mail it to the laboratory designated in the kit. You can keep your name anonymous.

The results will be mailed back to you in 4 to 10 business days. Let your doctor know if the result of the test is positive.

HIV Test

Many people would like to be tested for HIV, but some do not get tested because of inconvenience or concerns about privacy. You can order an anonymous HIV home test by mail or buy it in some pharmacies. Some companies have an 800 number you can call 24 hours a day that allows you to talk to counselors and order the test.

In 2004, a rapid HIV test that

uses a saliva sample instead of a blood sample was approved for use. Currently, it is approved for use only by a properly trained health professional, in a medical office setting. It is possible that it will someday be approved for home use.

If you order the home blood test by mail, it arrives in an unmarked package. If you pay for it by credit card, the bill is labeled only with the company's initials. When you receive the test, find the toll-free number and the unique code number of your test in the instructions. Call and register your number. The code number is needed to match your test with the results, which you will call for, later.

An automated voice will ask your age, sex, race, and zip code. You will be asked about your sexual history, intravenous drug use, blood transfusions, and sexual partners. If you do not want to answer a question, press the star ("*") key on your phone. If you want to speak to a counselor, press the operator ("0") key. Any information obtained is used to counsel you.

If your test result is positive, your zip code will allow the counselor to recommend an HIV specialist in your area.

To perform the test, you draw blood from your finger, drop the blood on the testing paper, and allow it to air-dry for 30 minutes. After the sample is dry, insert the specimen collection card in the foil-lined envelope provided, and mail it to the laboratory address.

To obtain the result, call the number listed in the instructions. You wait 7 days for the result of the standard test, or 3 days for the more expensive express version. You may hear a recorded message if your test result is negative. If your test result is positive, or if you have high-risk behaviors such as unsafe sexual practices or sharing needles, an experienced counselor will be available to speak with you.

Blood Sugar Test

Monitoring your blood glucose levels at home improves your ability to manage diabetes (see p.832). With proper instruction, glucose monitoring is easy to perform. By applying a single drop of blood to the test strip, you can immediately see if your blood sugar is under control. If it is not, you can adjust your diet, exercise, and medicine according to the plan you have established with your doctor.

Before you buy a blood glucose meter, ask your doctor or diabetes educator for a recommendation. They can also tell you about special meters that are available for people with vision or hearing impairment, tremors, or decreased manual dexterity.

Since treatment decisions will be based on your home test results, it is essential that your glucose meter provide an accurate reading. Periodically, check the blood glucose measured by your meter against the measurement taken in your doctor's office. Poor readings can occur if you are not familiar with the proper testing technique, if the strips are outdated, or if the

meter is dirty or has been stored at extreme temperatures.

You and your doctor will develop a specific schedule for measuring your blood sugar. If your blood glucose level is fluctuating or your medicine dose has been adjusted, or if you are not feeling well, you will need to check your blood sugar level more often than when your measurements are stable.

It is very important to keep a written record of your blood sugar readings and to bring them with you to your doctor. People who do not have diabetes do not need to check their blood glucose at home.

Blood Pressure Test

Home blood pressure monitors permit you to check your blood pressure or have a family member check it for you. Most pharmacies sell digital and manual machines. Both varieties have specially designed cuffs that you can slip over your arm without assistance.

Some of the digital models self-inflate; others require you to squeeze a hand pump. The manual cuffs are slightly more accurate, but require you to listen to heart sounds with a stethoscope while reading the blood pressure gauge.

The prices of digital and manual machines are comparable (the stethoscope is included with the manual cuff), but prices vary widely. Finger cuffs are also avail-

able, but they are not as accurate as cuffs that wrap around the arm.

Before using the cuff, take it to your doctor's office and compare simultaneous readings on the home and office machines. They should correlate closely.

Blood pressure naturally varies with your activities and the time of day. Do not worry if one recording is elevated; it is the average of many different measurements that matters. Check your blood pressure when you are relaxed. Your blood pressure reading can be up to 10 points higher when you are talking, and can also be elevated after you exercise or smoke cigarettes.

Urinary Tract Infection Test

A home test approved in 1998 permits you to test your urine when you have symptoms of a urinary tract infection (see p.804). The test is especially useful for women who have recurring urinary tract infections.

You collect a small amount of urine in a container and dip a strip of treated paper into the urine. A change in the color of the paper strip indicates a urinary tract infection.

Calling your doctor to describe your symptoms, along with the test result, may give the doctor enough information to prescribe antibiotics without examining you.

SAFETY AND PREVENTING INJURY

Unintended injuries are the leading cause of death in the United States for people ages 1 to 37 and the fourth leading cause of death for all ages. The largest number of these injuries occur in vehicle collisions. The other leading causes, in decreasing order, are falls, poisoning, and burns, all of which occur most often at home.

Home Safety

Falls Every year, 200,000 elderly people in the United States fracture their hips in a fall. Falls are also the leading cause of injury in infants. Look for ways to prevent falls in your home—whether ensuring a basement door has an out-of-reach safety lock to prevent a 2-year-old from falling down the stairs or securing throw rugs to the floor to prevent an elderly person from tripping and falling.

Also make sure that windows are closed and locked when children are in your house; screens cannot prevent children from falling out of windows. See p.1127 for steps you can take to prevent falls in older people.

Poisoning There were more than 1.8 million poisonings in U.S. homes in 1996. Children younger than age 6 are the most vulnerable. Substances that cause chemical burns, such as oven and toilet bowl cleaners, are particularly dangerous. Pesticides, alcoholic beverages, and antifreeze are dangerous as well.

Never mix cleaning products; mixing can produce potentially lethal gases. Medicines can also be poisonous. Store them in their original labeled containers away from the bedroom; do not leave them on a nightstand where they may be taken in the middle of the night accidentally.

For more information, read the recommendations for preventing poisoning on pp.963 and 990.

Fires You can cut your chances of dying in a home fire in half by having an operational smoke detector in your home. Install one on every floor of your home, including the basement, and install one in every bedroom. Test smoke detectors every month and install new batteries every 6 months.

Studies show that people have an average of 2 minutes to leave their homes during a fire; plan an escape route and practice it. Most fires start in the kitchen. Keep a small fire extinguisher near your cooking area. Also, have a home inspection of your electrical system to make sure it is in good working order.

Carbon monoxide poisoning Carbon monoxide is an odorless, colorless gas that can leak from faulty or improperly vented space heaters, furnaces, and clothes dryers. It can kill without warning. To guard against poisoning, clean flues and chimneys regularly and check them for leaks. Install a carbon monoxide detector in your home.

Radon Radon is a radioactive gas. If you live in an older building, ask your local public health department for a recommendation on having the radon level in your home checked to ensure

that radon is not endangering the health of family members.

The U.S. Environmental Protection Agency estimates that as many as 10% of all homes may have elevated levels of radon, which leaks through the foundations of older structures. Good ventilation, especially in the basement, reduces the risk.

Lead poisoning Lead poisoning poses a significant health risk to children and an occasional health risk to adults. Lead is a toxic substance in the environment that is either ingested or inhaled.

Ingested lead can come from elevated lead levels in your home water supply from pipes made of or soldered with lead. If you are concerned about the possibility of lead in your home, ask your local health department for suggestions on how to detect it.

Lead-based paint (outlawed in 1960, but still present in at least 30 million older homes in the United States) tastes sweet. Very young children can become poisoned by picking off and eating lead-based paint or putty from walls and other surfaces and by eating soil near contaminated houses.

Lead in the air can be inhaled into the lungs. This occurs when old paint is removed from buildings without the proper precautions. It formerly occurred when gasoline sold at gas stations contained lead, contributing to lead air pollution. Selling gasoline that contains lead is now against the law.

Lead poisoning can adversely affect many different organs of the body. In young children, it can affect the brain, creating serious learning, speech, coordination, and behavior problems. It can also cause anemia and kidney damage. For more discussion of lead poisoning, see Lead Poisoning: Dr Shannon's Advice (p.967).

Food Safety

About 7 million Americans have food-borne illnesses each year; 85% of food poisoning (see p.881) cases could be prevented with proper handling of food in the kitchen. Food poisoning is linked to at least 30 disease-causing bacteria—from *E coli* to salmonella—that cause abdominal cramps, nausea, vomiting, and diarrhea.

Although most cases of food poisoning are not grave, some occasionally produce serious medical conditions including kidney failure, stillbirth, and meningitis. The symptoms of food poisoning often do not appear until more than 24 hours after the bacteria have been ingested. Most disease-causing bacteria do not change the appearance, smell, or taste of food.

The United States has approved use of a drug spray that is expected to greatly reduce the infection of chickens with a variety of different dangerous bacteria. The spray consists of harmless bacteria that normally live in the intestines of chickens. By spraying newly hatched chickens, the harmless bacteria get into the intestines and prevent the harmful bacteria from growing.

SAFE FOOD PREPARATION

Follow these guidelines for safe food preparation:

Bacteria in the Kitchen

Potentially dangerous bacteria, including staphylococcus ("staph") and pseudomonas, can live on sponges, plastic scouring pads, and dish cloths. Touching them and then touching your own skin, or someone else's, can increase the risk of infections such as boils. Simply washing sponges and scouring pads in tap water does not eliminate the bacteria.

To be safe, once every week thoroughly rinse sponges and plastic scouring pads with tap water and then put them in a microwave oven at full power for 60 seconds. (Do not put metal scouring pads in the microwave.)

Shopping Look for "sell-by" and "use-by" dates on packaging. Purchase cold foods last and refrigerate immediately. Canned goods should be free of dents or bulging lids, which can indicate spoilage or contamination.

Storing Keep your refrigerator at 40°F and your freezer at 0°F.

Freeze fresh meat, fish, and poultry if you will not use it within 2 days. Do not let the juices from raw meat or fish drip onto other foods.

Preparation

■ Wash your hands before preparing food and after using the bathroom or changing diapers.

Safe Barbecuing

Many people enjoy the charred surface on meat caused by barbecuing. Unfortunately, that surface contains substances that cause cancer (carcinogens) in some animals. The potential carcinogens are more likely to be formed when the barbecue flames are high enough to sear the meat, or when you barbecue the meat for a long time.

Although it has not been proven that eating lots of barbecued meats causes cancer in humans, it is prudent to assume that it could, and to do what you can to reduce the risks. Here are some tips for safer barbecuing:

■ Precook meats in a microwave so that the inside is close to fully cooked before putting the meat on the barbecue. This reduces the amount of time the meat spends on the barbecue.

■ Grill fowl with its skin on, and remove the skin before eating. This will not only lower the fat content (because the fat is mainly in the skin) but will also lower the level of potential carcinogens.

■ Minimize grilling of fatty meat. Not only is too much saturated fat bad for you, but fat dripping off the meat causes flames to rise up and sear the meat.

■ Do not shut the lid on the barbecue. This increases the contact of potential carcinogens with the meat.

■ Cook foods thoroughly, using a meat thermometer to ensure that whole poultry is cooked to 180°F, roasts and steaks to 145°F, and ground meats to 160°F. Cook fish until it is opaque.

■ Eat cooked foods immediately.

■ Keep raw foods and cooked foods away from each other, and never use the same utensils on cooked meat that were used on raw meat.

■ Wash all spills from raw meat, fish, and poultry with hot soapy water.

■ Wash fruits and vegetables.

■ Do not use the same platter for raw and grilled meats.

■ Wash countertops, cutting boards, and all utensils in hot soapy water between preparation of food items.

■ Defrost foods only in the refrigerator or by microwaving.

Serving Never leave perishable food out of the refrigerator for more than 2 hours. Carry picnic foods and lunches in insulated containers.

Child Safety

If you have a baby, childproof your home. Install stairway gates to prevent falls, put plastic caps on all electrical outlets, and install safety locks on cabinets and windows. Put guards over windows to prevent falls (screens will not prevent a child from falling out a window) or keep windows closed and locked.

Never leave a child alone in the bathtub or near any pool of water, no matter how shallow. If you keep guns in your home,

keep them unloaded in a locked cabinet and store the key out of reach of children.

All children weighing 60 pounds or less should sit in an appropriately sized car seat that is secured by a safety belt to the back seat of your vehicle. Infants who weigh less that 20 pounds should be positioned with the infant seat facing the rear of the car in the back seat.

Children at play need to be monitored. If you have a swimming pool, install a fence around it with a gate, and keep the gate locked. Teach your children to swim and never leave them alone, even if they are competent swimmers.

Ensure that bicycles are in good working condition. When riding bicycles or motorcycles, skiing, snowboarding, skateboarding, or roller skating, you and your children should wear helmets—which greatly reduce the chance of head injury—and protective elbow, wrist, and knee pads.

Make sure your child knows and follows the rules and uses all the necessary equipment when participating in recreational activities. Set a good example.

Work Safety

Whether you have a desk job, drive a truck, or work in a factory, the government requires employers to provide you with a safe working environment.

Wherever you work, familiarize yourself with your employer's safety regulations and follow the standards set by the Occupational Safety and Health Act (OSHA). These standards are set

to protect workers from illness and injury caused by exposure to chemicals, dust, and physical hazards such as electricity.

Items such as respirators or eye or ear protection are sometimes required. A wide variety of protective equipment is available, but you must wear it consistently and correctly for it to be beneficial.

If you work at a computer, you can prevent repetitive strain injury by taking periodic breaks. Your desk should be of a height to permit your forearms to use a keyboard comfortably at an angle between 70 degrees and 90 degrees to your torso. Your computer screen should be at least an arm's distance away from your body.

Prevent neck and back strain by sitting in a chair that supports your lower back and that permits your feet to rest flat on the floor. Prevent eye strain by taking "blink breaks" (see p.422); look away from your monitor and completely blink your eyes.

If you use the telephone frequently, consider wearing a headset to avoid straining the muscles of your neck and shoulder from cradling the phone.

Car Safety

The majority of highway deaths are related to alcohol consumption. Never drink and drive, and never ride with a driver who has been drinking. Also, you should not drive while taking medicines that make you drowsy. In addition:

■ Obey speed limits and drive defensively.

- Make sure all passengers wear seat belts and that they stay in them. Using seat belts can reduce the risk of death by as much as 50% in a serious car crash.

- Position children in car seats or restraints appropriate for their age and weight. Never put a car seat in the front seat. The middle of the back seat is the safest location for a car seat.

- Never hold a baby or child on your lap in a moving vehicle. The child can turn into a human missile in a crash. If you are nursing a baby on a car trip, stop the car to nurse.

STRESS

If you are an average American, you probably describe your life as stressful. Stress has been defined as any circumstance that requires you to adapt. Today the term is loosely applied to virtually any event or situation that can evoke frustration, anger, or anxiety.

Stress can be physical, such as the stress of exercise or the stress of a debilitating disease, as well as situational or emotional, such as the stress of a high-pressure job or the emotional pain of divorce.

Many forms of stress can be positive. The stress triggered by exercise can be invigorating, as can the mental stress posed by a challenging athletic, school, or work assignment. Stress that motivates one person may frustrate another.

Scientists who study stress believe that situations that cause stress are more likely to be damaging if you cannot predict or control them, such as working in an environment where you have great responsibility but little control over how it is managed.

Stress is also more likely to have adverse effects if you lack social support or if you have personal, financial, or other pressing concerns.

FIGHT-OR-FLIGHT RESPONSE

Whatever its source, stress can trigger a hormonal reaction known as the fight-or-flight response. In this response, the brain sends signals to the adrenal glands that cause them to secrete the hormones epinephrine and norepinephrine. These hormones cause muscles to become tense, heart rate and blood pressure to increase, and breathing to accelerate.

The blood supply to your skin is increased, as is perspiration. Any person who faces a situation he or she finds stressful, such as public speaking, will recognize these features as the body's automatic response to the situation.

The fight-or-flight response originally evolved to prepare animals to respond to danger. It evolved as we did to prepare us to respond physically to a threat—to fight or to run. Today, however, most of us do not regularly face the same life-threatening situations that our ancestors did. The fight-or-flight response does not distinguish between a physical threat and the everyday stresses of life.

In some people, when the fight-or-flight response occurs repeatedly in the absence of a true emergency, it can increase the risk of stress-related medical problems.

It is important to find ways to control the harmful aspects of this response and neutralize the negative effects of modern stress on your health and well-being.

IMMUNIZATIONS AND TRAVEL HEALTH

In general, you need not be concerned about immunizations or special precautions with food and water if you travel to Australia, Canada, Scandinavia, New Zealand, or Western Europe.

For travel to other parts of the world, you need to receive appropriate immunizations before you go, bring pertinent health information and supplies with you, and be careful what you eat and drink. Read Immunizations for Travel (see p.94) for specific information.

Many cities in the United States have "travel clinics" that keep up with the latest recommendations, and that keep in stock fresh vaccines. Increasingly, travelers go to these travel clinics rather than to their doctor, to prepare for travel. A current list of travel clinics is updated on the

The Relaxation Response: Dr Benson's Advice

When the stress of modern life causes the fight-or-flight response, you can use the relaxation response to reduce and counteract the harmful effects. When you are under stress, your mind tells the heart to beat faster. In fact, your mind controls your heart rate and you can use your mind to voluntarily slow it down.

With practice and commitment, you may be able to use the relaxation response to achieve a decrease in stress, anxiety, compulsive worrying, and negative thoughts, and an increase in concentration and awareness, as well as greater self-confidence, enhanced performance, and improved sleep.

The relaxation response is a natural, physiological response; it can occur when you are not even aware of it. You can initiate this response through mental imaging techniques that involve focusing. Bring to mind, for example, a time when you were lying on a beach, fully relaxed, or the moments before you drift into sleep.

Two components are involved in eliciting the relaxation response:

1 A mental focusing device—such as focusing on your breathing or repeating a phrase, prayer, or sound to help you shift your mind from everyday thoughts and worries.

Warning Signs of Stress

These symptoms of stress should alert you to the need for change in your life. Many of these symptoms can be caused by depression, anxiety, or other medical disorders. See your physician if any of the following occur frequently:

PHYSICAL SYMPTOMS

Headache

Back pain

Indigestion

Tight neck and shoulders

Stomach pain

Racing heart

Sweaty palms

Restlessness

Sleep problems

Tiredness

Dizziness

Loss of appetite

Problem with sexual performance or enjoyment

Ringing in ears

CDC Web site (see Immunizations for Travel, p. 94) or by your state public health department.

Planning a Trip

If you are planning a trip, ask your doctor if any immunizations are needed. Discuss your travel plans with your physician at least 3 months before you leave; some immunizations must be given over a period of several weeks.

Because most Americans have received childhood immunizations against measles, mumps, rubella, diphtheria, pertussis, tetanus, and polio, you may not require further protection from these diseases.

If you receive your vaccines at a travel clinic, you will receive a small yellow booklet that lists all of the vaccines you have received. An official stamp is required for the yellow fever vaccine. You can fill in your name,

address, list of medical problems, medicines, allergies, prescription for eyeglasses, and other information in the spaces provided. Keep the yellow booklet with your passport at all times (even after you get home so you will be able to find it for future trips).

If you are not receiving assistance from a travel clinic, copy and complete the form on p.1246 to take with you.

2 A passive attitude toward distracting thoughts, which means not worrying about how well you are doing (or about the laundry or a business report), but gently directing your mind back to your focus when you notice yourself being distracted.

The relaxation response must be learned and practiced, ideally at least once a day. Follow these steps. It may take several attempts before you begin to feel the effects. Once you have mastered the art of the relaxation response, you will be able to use it at your desk, before a speech, or during any other event that is stressful for you.

Step 1 Pick a focus phrase, image, or prayer. You may also choose to focus on your breathing.

Step 2 Find a quiet place and sit calmly in a comfortable position.

Step 3 Close your eyes.

Step 4 Relax all of your muscles.

Step 5 Breathe slowly and naturally; as you do, repeat your focus word or phrase as you exhale.

Step 6 Assume a passive attitude. Do not worry about how well you are doing. When other thoughts come to mind, simply return to the repetition.

Step 7 Continue for 10 to 20 minutes.

Step 8 Practice the technique once or twice daily.

HERBERT BENSON, MD
BETH ISRAEL DEACONESS MEDICAL CENTER
HARVARD MEDICAL SCHOOL

BEHAVIORAL SYMPTOMS

Increase in smoking
Grinding teeth
Bossiness
Increase in use of alcohol
Compulsive gum chewing
Compulsive eating
Criticizing others
Inability to get things done

EMOTIONAL SYMPTOMS

Crying
Overwhelming sense of pressure
Nervousness; anxiety
Anger
Feeling that there is no meaning to life
Loneliness
Edginess; feeling of being ready to explode
Unhappiness for no reason
Feeling powerless to change things
Being easily upset

COGNITIVE SYMPTOMS

Trouble thinking clearly
Inability to make decisions
Forgetfulness
Thoughts of running away
Lack of creativity
Constant worry
Memory loss
Loss of sense of humor

Be Prepared for Illness or Injury

Planning ahead can make a difference in the quality of your trip if you become ill or need medical help in another country. You may have to go to a major city in an undeveloped country if you need medical or dental care. Take these steps:

■ Be sure your medical insurance will cover you when you travel out of the country; not all insurance policies do.

■ Injury is the most common cause of hospitalization and death in healthy travelers. Avoid activities that will increase risk, such as driving on unfamiliar roads at night; never drink and drive. As a pedestrian, be aware that traffic may run opposite to the direction you are used to. If you use a bicycle, motorbike, or motorcycle, be sure to wear a helmet.

■ In the United States, mosquitoes are a nuisance but only rarely transmit infections. In many tropical regions of the world, mosquitoes can carry malaria, dengue, yellow fever, Japanese encephalitis, and many other serious infections. Take a good insect repellent and use it.

■ Needles and syringes (even the disposable ones) are often reused in many parts of the world, frequently without being sterilized. Do not get a tattoo or body

PREVENTING INFECTION

An infectious disease is, by nature, transmissible—that is, it can be passed by a person, animal, insect, or by something in the environment, such as food or water.

When treatment is available for an infection, it is important to get treated. However, preventing transmission is essential because some common infections cannot be treated. This chart gives some examples of infectious diseases. For more information on infections, see p.863.

DISEASE	CAUSES	WAYS TO AVOID TRANSMITTING INFECTION	WAYS TO AVOID ACQUIRING INFECTION
Common cold (see p.460)	Many viruses	Cover your mouth and nose when you cough or sneeze. Wash hands regularly (cold viruses can live on hands).	Wash hands regularly (cold viruses can live on hands).
Strep throat (see p.467)	Streptococcus bacteria	Cover your mouth and nose when you cough or sneeze. Wash hands regularly (bacteria can live on hands).	Wash hands regularly. Avoid close contact with people who have strep throat.
Sexually transmitted diseases (STDs) (see p.889)	Many different microorganisms	Use a latex or polyurethane condom every time you have sexual intercourse. See Safer Sex, p.76.	Use a latex or polyurethane condom every time you have sexual intercourse. See Safer Sex, p.76.
Body lice; scabies (see p.549)	Insects; mites	Wash clothes and bed sheets. Infected person and close contacts should be treated with a lotion containing the prescription medicine lindane.	Do not sleep in the same bed or share towels or linens with infested people until their infestation is gone. Otherwise, use lotion containing the prescription medicine lindane or permethrin.
Chickenpox (see p.948)	Varicella-zoster virus	Keep away from anyone who has not had chickenpox until 5 days after your blisters appeared. Be especially careful to avoid pregnant women.	If you have not been vaccinated and have never had chickenpox, avoid being in the same room as a person with active infection. Particularly, avoid contact with the skin blisters. Also avoid contact with skin blisters of a person with shingles.
Flu (see p.875)	Influenza virus	Cover your mouth and nose when you cough or sneeze. Wash hands regularly (flu virus can live on hands).	Avoid sharing a closed space with a person who has influenza. Wash hands regularly (flu virus can live on hands).
Pneumonia (see p.496)	Many different microorganisms	Cover your mouth and nose when you cough or sneeze. Wash your hands frequently.	Avoid the air near an infected person who is coughing. Wash your hands after contact with an infected person.
AIDS (see p.872)	Human immunodeficiency virus	Use a latex or polyurethane condom every time you have sexual intercourse. If you use intravenous drugs, never share needles. See Safer Sex, p.76.	Use a latex or polyurethane condom every time you have sexual intercourse. If you use intravenous drugs, never share needles. See Safer Sex, p.76.

DISEASE	CAUSES	WAYS TO AVOID TRANSMITTING INFECTION	WAYS TO AVOID ACQUIRING INFECTION
Hepatitis (see p.758)	Several viruses	Wash your hands after using the bathroom. Use a latex or polyurethane condom every time you have sexual intercourse. If you use intravenous drugs, never share needles. If you have hepatitis, do not prepare food for others.	Use a latex or polyurethane condom every time you have sexual intercourse. If you use intravenous drugs, never share needles. If you live with someone who has hepatitis, he or she should not prepare food for others.
Food poisoning (see p.881)	*E coli* and salmonella organisms	Wash hands after using the bathroom and before preparing food. Follow safe food handling instructions on p.87.	See Food Safety (p.87).

Good Hygiene Prevents Infections

You can avoid acquiring or transmitting many infections by following the guidelines below. Other important measures include vaccination against infectious diseases and practicing safer sex (see p.77).

■ Cover your mouth and nose with a tissue when you sneeze or cough.

■ Stay away from people who have a respiratory infection such as a cold. If you shake hands often, wash your hands often. Infections can be transmitted by shaking hands with an infected person and then touching your eyes, mouth, or nose, which allows the infectious organisms to enter the body through the mucous membranes.

■ Wash your hands with soap and water before preparing food and after using the bathroom.

■ Wash and bandage all cuts. Any serious cut or animal or human bite should be examined by a doctor.

■ Wear gloves when working with soil, and get a tetanus shot every 10 years.

■ Do not pick at healing wounds or blemishes or squeeze pimples.

How Are Infections Transmitted?

Different infections can be transmitted in the following ways:

■ Sexual contact

■ Eating contaminated food or drinking contaminated water

■ Blood transfusion with contaminated blood (although this is rare in industrialized countries)

■ Coughing or sneezing

■ Contact with infectious organisms that can live in water, in soil, or in some animals

■ Animal bites

■ Skin-to-skin contact

■ Touching infected person and then touching your eyes, nose, or mouth

■ Through broken skin, such as a cut

■ Insect bites, such as ticks and mosquitoes

■ Needles, such as those used in tattooing and for drug use

piercing unless you are absolutely sure needles have been handled safely.

■ If you have not obtained the small yellow booklet at a traveler's clinic, copy and complete the form on p.1246. This form includes dates for immunizations; any long-term health conditions; your physician's name, address, and phone number; a list of all medicines you take (both generic and brand names) and their doses; a copy of your vision correction prescription; and the name and number of a relative to notify in an emergency. Pack your medicines and medical record in a bag that you do not check, and keep it with you as you travel.

■ The nonprofit International Association for Medical Assistance to Travelers (see p.1237) provides a world directory of English-speaking physicians to its members.

■ A small first-aid kit can be useful when traveling to a foreign country. Include painkillers (aspirin or acetaminophen), a

Immunizations for Travel

A list of common travel immunizations is presented here. Other vaccines are recommended under special circumstances. The U.S. Centers for Disease Control and Prevention (CDC) can provide you with the most recent information on immunization requirements for the countries on your itinerary. The recommendations change frequently. To check the most updated information, go to the CDC Web site: http://www.cdc.gov/travel.

IMMUNIZATION	WHEN REQUIRED/RECOMMENDED	DETAILS
Cholera	Not officially required by any country.	There is no longer a vaccine licensed for use in the United States.
Diphtheria	Recommended for anyone not fully immunized as a child.	Most Americans receive vaccine as children. Booster is recommended every 10 years.
Immune serum globulin	Recommended for travelers who have not been immunized against hepatitis A for travel to areas other than Australia, Canada, New Zealand, Scandinavia, or Western Europe.	Can protect against hepatitis A for up to 3 months.
Hepatitis A	Recommended for travelers visiting areas other than Australia, Canada, New Zealand, Scandinavia, or Western Europe.	First dose protects at least 1 year; second dose at least a decade.
Hepatitis B	Recommended for travelers to most of Africa, Asia, India, the former Soviet Union, the Middle East, and to some of South and Central America. Check with your doctor, a travel clinic, or the CDC.	Second dose is given 1 month after first dose; third dose is given 6 months after first dose.
Japanese encephalitis virus	Recommended for travelers to rural areas for prolonged periods in China, Japan, Korea, and eastern areas of Russia.	Three doses given over 30 days.

thermometer, antiseptic cream, bandages, alcohol wipes, insect repellent, sunscreen, antacids, laxatives, and a decongestant.

Food and Water Precautions

The availability of a safe food and water supply is something

More Health Advice for Travelers

For more health information related to travel, see:

- Traveler's diarrhea, p.780
- Jet lag, p.385
- Travelers' Health Information, p.1236

IMMUNIZATION	WHEN REQUIRED/RECOMMENDED	DETAILS
Measles	Recommended for anyone who did not receive two doses as a child and who has not had measles.	Most Americans receive two doses of the vaccine as children.
Meningitis (meningococcal)	Required for travelers to Ethiopia (in some seasons). Recommended for those traveling to sub-Saharan Africa and other countries with the potential for an epidemic. Check with the CDC.	Protection lasts at least 3 years.
Polio	Full vaccine series is recommended for anyone not immunized as a child. Most of the world's poliovirus transmission takes place in Afghanistan, India, Niger, Nigeria, and Pakistan.	Most Americans receive the vaccine as children.
Rabies	Not required for travel anywhere. Recommended for travelers with considerable exposure to wild or domestic animals in most parts of the world except Western Europe and North America.	Three injections over 3 to 4 weeks (several different vaccines available).
Tetanus	Full vaccine series is recommended for anyone not immunized as a child. A booster shot is needed every 10 years.	Most Americans receive the vaccine as children. A booster shot is needed every 10 years.
Typhoid	Recommended for those traveling to Asia, Africa, Central and South America, and the Indian subcontinent, particularly to those planning on visiting small cities, villages, or rural areas.	Oral vaccine gives protection for about 5 years; injection gives protection for about 2 years. Protection level is moderate, and booster doses can be given if necessary.
Yellow fever	Required for entry to some countries. Recommended for travel to sub-Saharan Africa and tropical South America.	Vaccine is effective for 10 years.

most Americans take for granted. It is easy to forget that many nonindustrialized countries do not have similar standards of hygiene. If you have any doubt about the safety of food and water, take these precautions:

■ Do not use ice.

■ Drink only bottled drinks—such as soft drinks or bottled water that have secure caps (indi-cating they have not been refilled with local water). Be aware that some fruit juices may be made with impure local water.

■ Boil all water before drinking or drink only bottled water; use bottled or boiled water to brush your teeth.

■ Do not eat uncooked vegetables, including lettuce; do not eat fruit you have not peeled yourself.

■ Do not eat partially cooked or raw shellfish or undercooked meat.

■ Do not consume dairy prod-ucts (milk may not be pasteur-ized).

■ In general, steaming hot, well-cooked foods are safe, since heat kills most of the microbes that can make you sick.

How Your Body Works

HOW YOU READ AND REMEMBER

1 Signals from the eye travel to the primary visual cortex in the occipital lobe and then to several other regions of the brain used to interpret visual stimuli, allowing the brain to see the shapes of the letters.

2 For the letters to be recognized as words and language, and for the words to be understood, another part of the brain (the Wernicke area) and nearby structures are used.

3 The hippocampus, deep inside the brain, is required for storing memories of recent experiences. It participates in the process of storing long-term memories. Long-term memories are stored in the cerebral cortex, in ways that are not well understood.

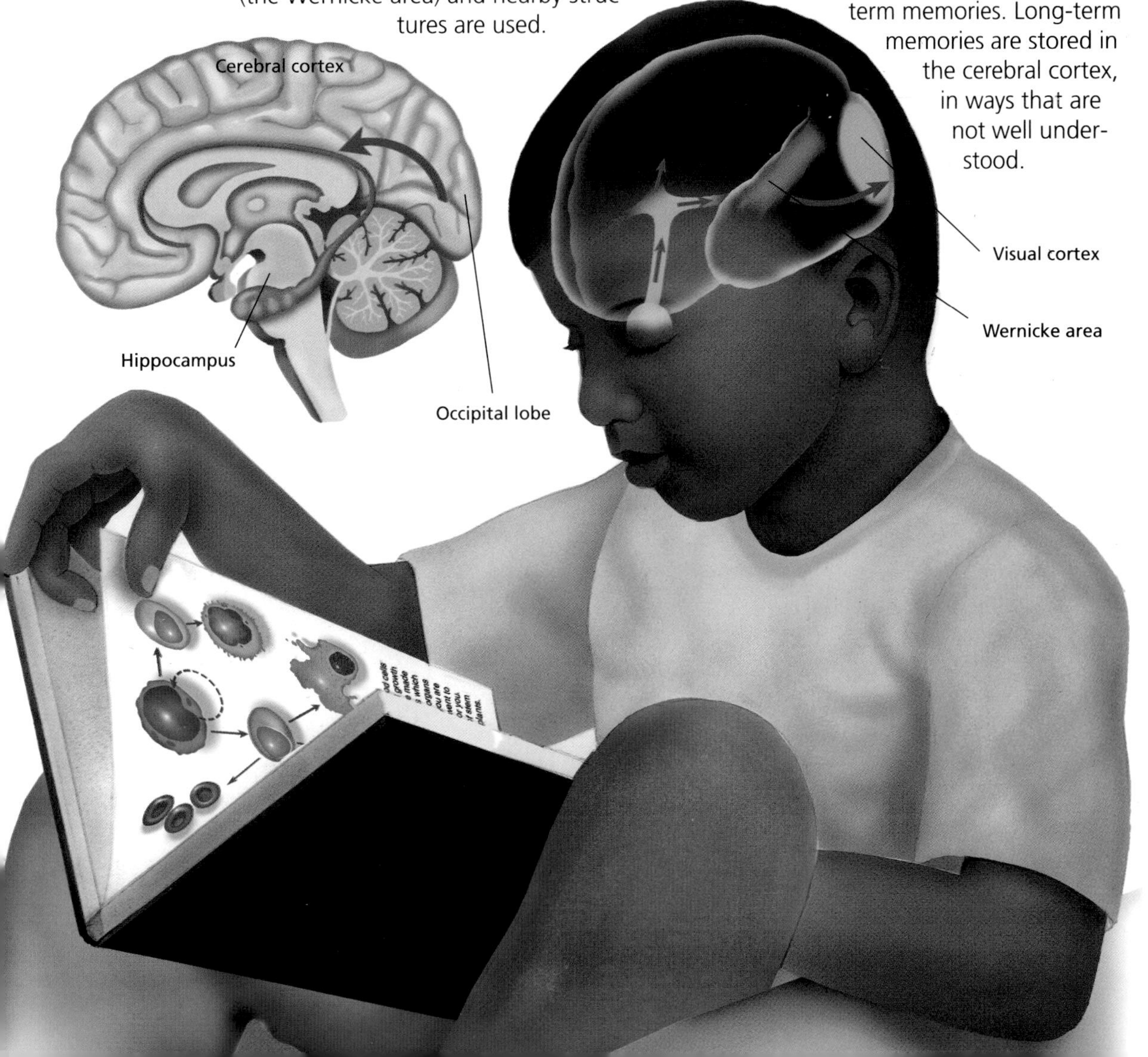

Cerebral cortex

Hippocampus

Occipital lobe

Visual cortex

Wernicke area

HOW YOU SPEAK AND UNDERSTAND SPEECH

1 The woman on the right is using many regions of her brain and other parts of her body to speak. Speaking requires that she breathe air out past her vocal cords, creating sound. Her tongue shapes the sounds as they pass up from the vocal cords, transforming the sounds into words. Breathing out and moving the tongue are both controlled by muscles under the brain's direction, including an important part of the frontal lobe called the Broca area.

2 The woman on the left is listening and comprehending her friend's speech. Hearing, interpreting sounds as speech, and understanding what the words mean requires her to use a part of the left temporal and parietal lobes called the Wernicke area.

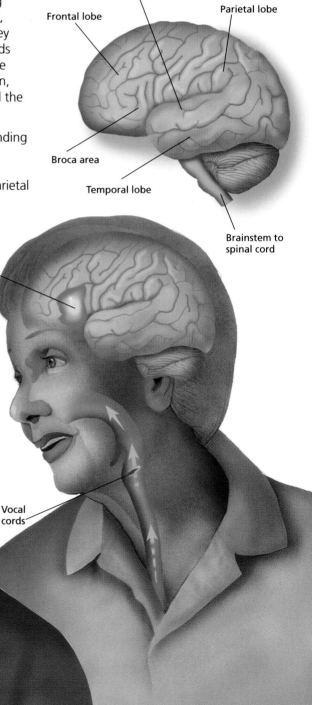

Wernicke area

Frontal lobe

Parietal lobe

Broca area

Temporal lobe

Brainstem to spinal cord

Wernicke area

Broca area

Vocal cords

HOW YOU RECOGNIZE OBJECTS

1 The parietal and temporal lobes are essential for recognizing and naming objects. As the boy prepares to make his next chess move, his parietal and temporal lobes are activated.

2 The right brain is important in recognizing your position in space, such as distinguishing between right and left or remembering how to get home; in recognizing objects, such as the chess pieces; and in recognizing sounds, such as the sound of the chess piece hitting the board (along with other physical sensations). The boy can recognize the type of chess piece he is holding, even without looking at it, by touch.

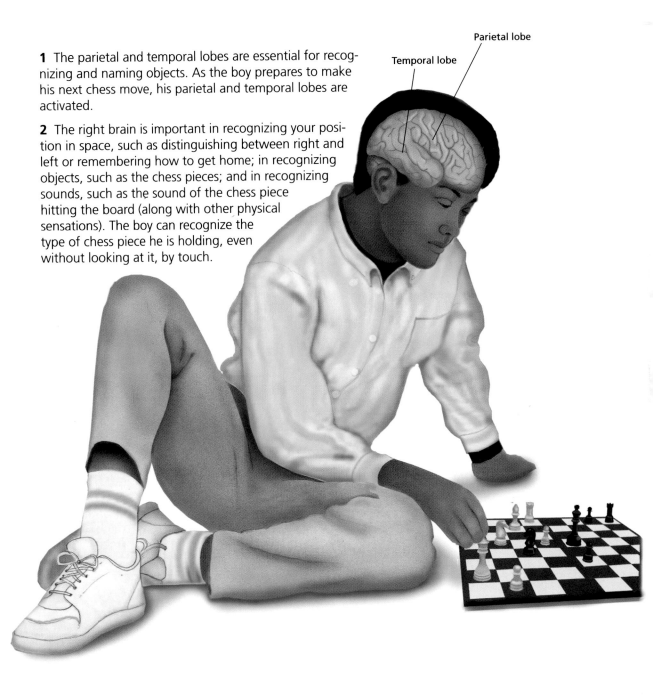

Parietal lobe

Temporal lobe

HOW YOU SEE

The girl's six eye muscles (inset) move her eyes in a coordinated way.

1 Light waves from the bird and the tree branch travel to the girl's eyes through the cornea, anterior (front) chamber, pupil, and lens, where the waves are focused.

2 The light waves land on the retina where, as with a camera, the image of the bird is upside down.

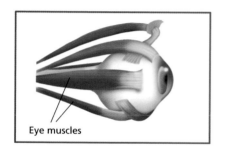

Eye muscles

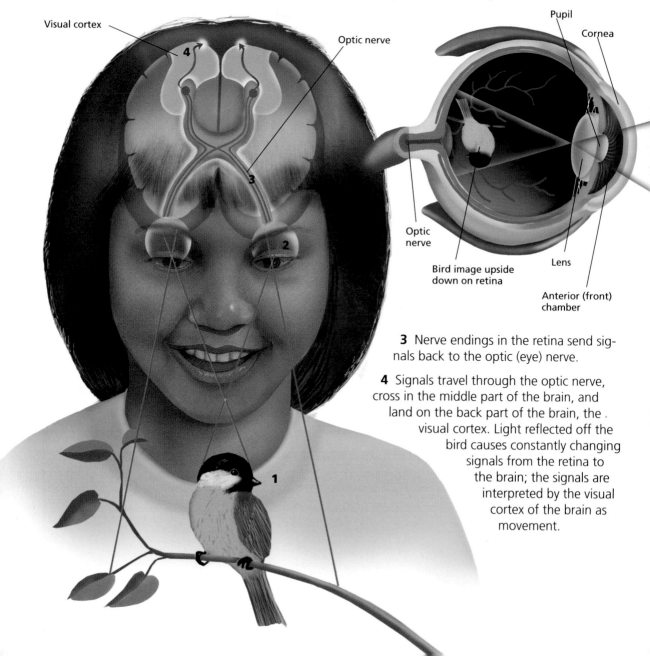

Visual cortex

Optic nerve

Pupil

Cornea

Optic nerve

Bird image upside down on retina

Lens

Anterior (front) chamber

3 Nerve endings in the retina send signals back to the optic (eye) nerve.

4 Signals travel through the optic nerve, cross in the middle part of the brain, and land on the back part of the brain, the visual cortex. Light reflected off the bird causes constantly changing signals from the retina to the brain; the signals are interpreted by the visual cortex of the brain as movement.

HOW YOU HEAR

6
Hearing center
in temporal lobe

1 Sound waves are created by the telephone.

2 Waves travel down the ear canal and bounce against the eardrum.

3 The eardrum vibrates and transmits the vibrations to the tiny bones in the middle ear.

4 The bones send the vibrations to the cochlea, a snail-shaped organ in the inner ear, where they move in a circle.

5 The tiny hairs of the cochlea vibrate, creating signals in the auditory (hearing) nerve.

6 The signals are carried by the auditory nerve to the hearing center in the temporal lobe of the brain, where sounds are interpreted. Here, the sounds are recognized as a human voice as heard through a tele-phone.

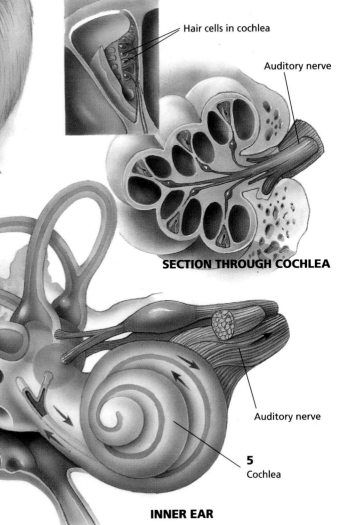

Hair cells in cochlea

Auditory nerve

SECTION THROUGH COCHLEA

4
Bones in middle ear

Ear canal

Auditory nerve

2
Sound waves

3
Eardrum

5
Cochlea

OUTER EAR

MIDDLE EAR

INNER EAR

HOW YOU FEEL PAIN

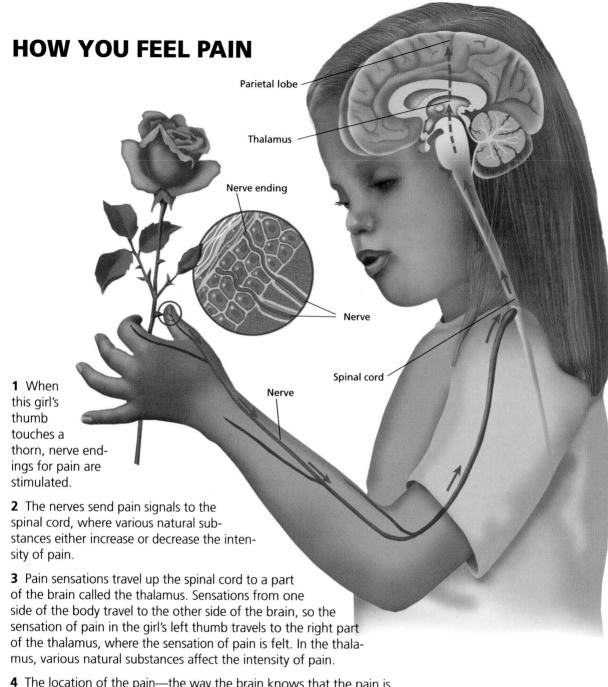

Parietal lobe

Thalamus

Nerve ending

Nerve

Spinal cord

Nerve

1 When this girl's thumb touches a thorn, nerve endings for pain are stimulated.

2 The nerves send pain signals to the spinal cord, where various natural substances either increase or decrease the intensity of pain.

3 Pain sensations travel up the spinal cord to a part of the brain called the thalamus. Sensations from one side of the body travel to the other side of the brain, so the sensation of pain in the girl's left thumb travels to the right part of the thalamus, where the sensation of pain is felt. In the thalamus, various natural substances affect the intensity of pain.

4 The location of the pain—the way the brain knows that the pain is occurring in the girl's left thumb—is determined when pain signals travel from the thalamus to the right parietal lobe. Pain signals also travel to other parts of the brain, including the frontal lobes.

5 Internal pain (such as that of a heart attack) travels the same route to and up the spinal cord as pain from the skin's surface. Therefore, pain from inside the body is often sensed as coming from the body's surface. It tends to feel more like burning or aching and is less sharp than pain from the skin.

HOW YOU SMELL AND TASTE

1 Molecules from the coffee evaporate, hang in the air above the cup, and enter the woman's nostrils when she breathes.

2 The coffee molecules attach to certain olfactory (smell) receptor cells that send signals to the olfactory (smelling) nerve.

3 The olfactory nerve carries the signals to the smell centers in the brain; the woman recognizes the sensation as the smell of coffee.

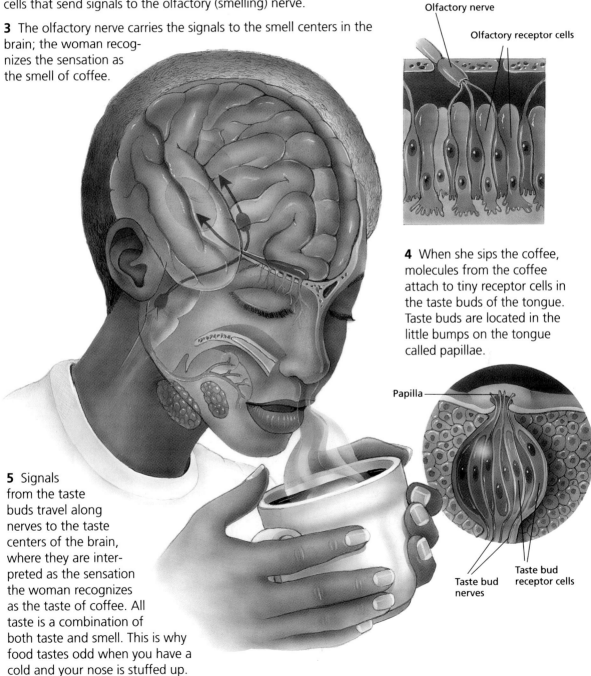

Olfactory nerve

Olfactory receptor cells

4 When she sips the coffee, molecules from the coffee attach to tiny receptor cells in the taste buds of the tongue. Taste buds are located in the little bumps on the tongue called papillae.

Papilla

Taste bud nerves

Taste bud receptor cells

5 Signals from the taste buds travel along nerves to the taste centers of the brain, where they are interpreted as the sensation the woman recognizes as the taste of coffee. All taste is a combination of both taste and smell. This is why food tastes odd when you have a cold and your nose is stuffed up.

HOW YOU MOVE

1 The boy's arm is cocked and he is ready to throw. To throw the ball, the boy must first see where he wants to throw it, using his eyes and visual cortex, and must feel where his body is in space using the balance centers in his ears and brain.

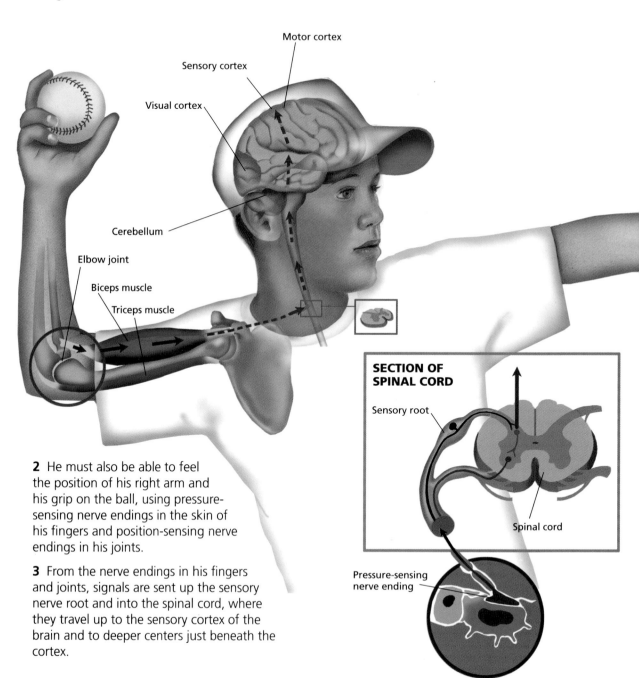

Motor cortex

Sensory cortex

Visual cortex

Cerebellum

Elbow joint

Biceps muscle

Triceps muscle

SECTION OF SPINAL CORD

Sensory root

Spinal cord

2 He must also be able to feel the position of his right arm and his grip on the ball, using pressure-sensing nerve endings in the skin of his fingers and position-sensing nerve endings in his joints.

3 From the nerve endings in his fingers and joints, signals are sent up the sensory nerve root and into the spinal cord, where they travel up to the sensory cortex of the brain and to deeper centers just beneath the cortex.

Pressure-sensing nerve ending

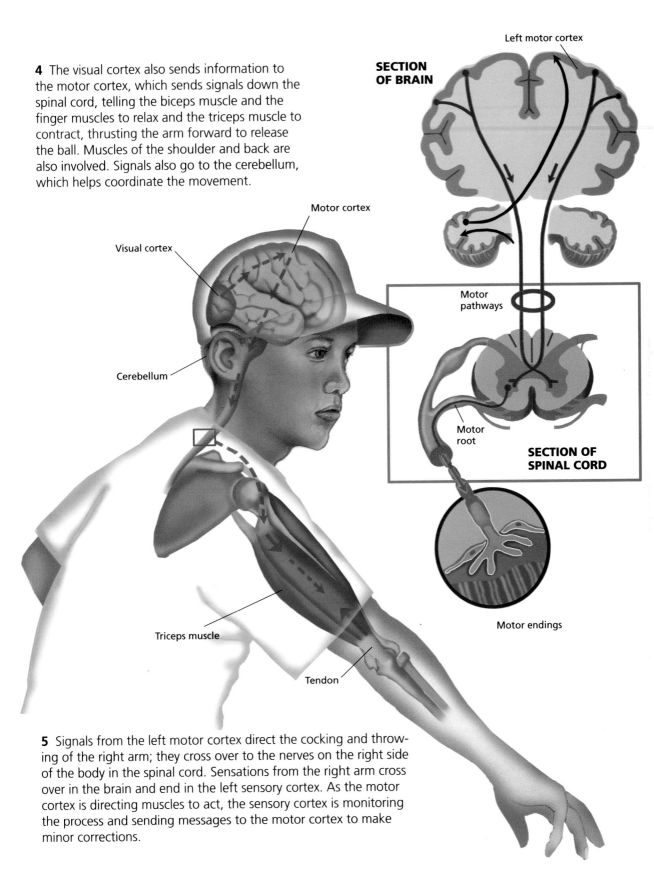

4 The visual cortex also sends information to the motor cortex, which sends signals down the spinal cord, telling the biceps muscle and the finger muscles to relax and the triceps muscle to contract, thrusting the arm forward to release the ball. Muscles of the shoulder and back are also involved. Signals also go to the cerebellum, which helps coordinate the movement.

SECTION OF BRAIN

Left motor cortex

Motor cortex

Visual cortex

Cerebellum

Motor pathways

Motor root

SECTION OF SPINAL CORD

Motor endings

Triceps muscle

Tendon

5 Signals from the left motor cortex direct the cocking and throwing of the right arm; they cross over to the nerves on the right side of the body in the spinal cord. Sensations from the right arm cross over in the brain and end in the left sensory cortex. As the motor cortex is directing muscles to act, the sensory cortex is monitoring the process and sending messages to the motor cortex to make minor corrections.

YOUR VITAL FUNCTIONS AND THE AUTONOMIC NERVOUS SYSTEM

Your body's vital functions are controlled by the autonomic nervous system, which starts in the hypothalamus in the center of the brain. The autonomic nervous system sends nerves out to all parts of the body to direct various functions and has other nerves coming in from all parts of the body carrying messages to the brain. The system is divided into sympathetic (green) and parasympathetic (blue) nerves, which work together.

THE SYMPATHETIC NERVES

The sympathetic nerves carry signals to all parts of the body to prepare it for physical action—the fight-or-flight response.

BLOOD PRESSURE AND HEART RATE

When you exercise, arterioles in your heart, lungs, and muscles widen, and blood flow greatly increases.

The hypothalamus directs the sympathetic nerves to decrease blood flow to the skin, stomach, and intestines, so that more blood is available to the heart, lungs, and muscles.

Sympathetic nerves to the adrenal glands stimulate them to make more of the hormone epinephrine (adrenaline).

Messages from the sympathetic nerves to the heart, along with epinephrine in the blood, cause the heart to pump more rapidly and forcefully. Parasympathetic nerves (see right) stand by to moderate these effects.

Sympathetic nerves and epinephrine in the blood widen bronchial tubes (airways), so you can move more air in and out of your lungs.

CONTROLLING BODY TEMPERATURE

A temperature control center, also in the hypothalamus, keeps the temperature of your blood within the right range. When you exercise, contraction of the muscles generates heat, which causes body temperature to rise. As it rises, the hypothalamus sends signals down the nerves to increase sweating and blood flow to the skin, which causes body heat to be lost to the surrounding air.

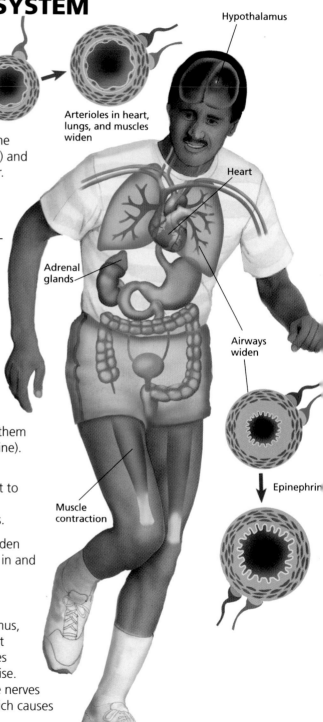

Arterioles in heart, lungs, and muscles widen

Hypothalamus

Heart

Adrenal glands

Airways widen

Muscle contraction

Epinephrine

THE PARASYMPATHETIC NERVES

The parasympathetic nerves maintain a balance with the function of the sympathetic nerves by sending signals to all parts of the body that quiet the body after exercise.

The parasympathetic nerves send signals to the heart's pacemaker, the sinoatrial node, to slow down the heart. When exercise begins again, the resting parasympathetic signals are withdrawn as the sympathetic nerves and epinephrine signal the heart to pump more rapidly and forcefully.

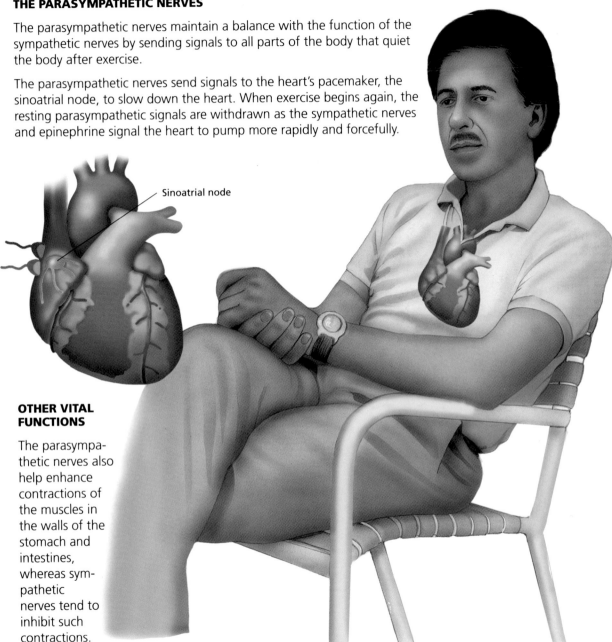

Sinoatrial node

OTHER VITAL FUNCTIONS

The parasympathetic nerves also help enhance contractions of the muscles in the walls of the stomach and intestines, whereas sympathetic nerves tend to inhibit such contractions.

Working together, the parasympathetic and sympathetic nerves:

- Encourage the elimination of urine and intestinal waste by stimulating muscles in the wall of the bladder and intestines

- Cause erection of the penis and clitoris during sexual arousal

- Cause the lacrimal glands in the eyes to form tears

HOW YOU CIRCULATE BLOOD

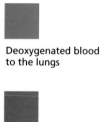

Deoxygenated blood
to the lungs

Oxygenated blood
to the body

From all parts of the body, deoxygenated blood (purple) flows into the heart—first to the right atrium (**1**), then to the right ventricle (**2**), pulmonary artery (**3**), and lungs (**4**).

In the lungs, blood fills up with oxygen and unloads carbon dioxide.

Oxygenated blood (red) enters the pulmonary veins (**5**) and then the left atrium (**6**) and left ventricle (**7**), which pumps blood through the aorta (**8**) to all parts of the body.

Blood that passes through the intestines (**9**) picks up nutrients and liquids that have been digested and absorbed.

Blood from the intestine travels to the liver (**10**), which removes toxic substances and makes them harmless, and also adds essential proteins (such as clotting factors) to the blood.

In the kidneys (**11**), blood unloads excess fluids, acids, and minerals.

In the spleen (**12**), blood unloads old, exhausted blood cells, which are then broken down.

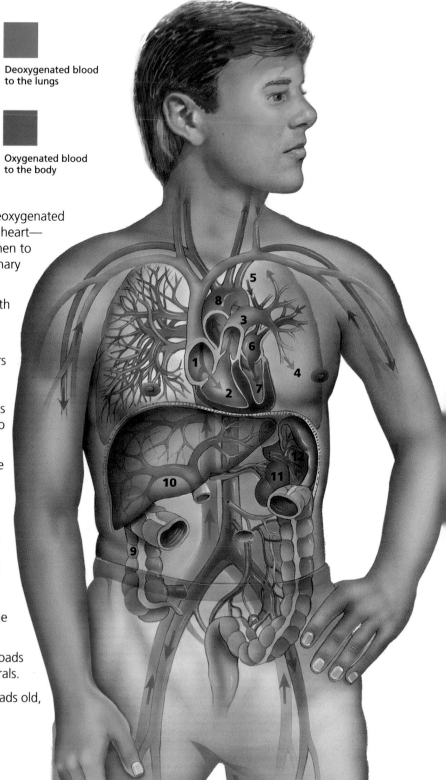

HOW YOU MAKE BLOOD

Your blood includes liquid (plasma) and blood cells. The amount of blood is controlled by the kidneys. The liver produces most of the proteins in the plasma. The bone marrow produces blood cells. Oxygen-carrying red blood cells are by far the most numerous—they make up nearly half the blood.

Blood cells are born and mature in the marrow of certain bones, including the breastbone, pelvis, ribs, spinal vertebrae, and the long bones of the legs (the femur and tibia). When blood cells reach maturity, they enter blood vessels in the bone marrow and travel via the blood throughout your body. Lymphocytes enter the lymph nodes, thymus, and spleen, mature further, and then re-enter the blood.

All mature blood cells develop originally from primitive cells called stem cells. Main stem cells (also called multipotential stem cells) can produce lymphoid stem cells, which make white blood cells (lymphocytes). Main stem cells also produce myeloid stem cells, which make red blood cells and other white blood cells, including megakaryocytes (which make platelets). Main stem cells also make more main stem cells (dotted line). In between the stem cells and the fully mature cells are less mature cells (not shown).

The growth and maturation of blood cells is stimulated by substances called growth factors, some of which are made in the marrow; additional growth factors are hormones made in other organs that travel to the marrow in the blood. Growth factors can be given as medicines to stimulate the production of different blood cells. You can also get transfusions of stem cells during a bone marrow transplant.

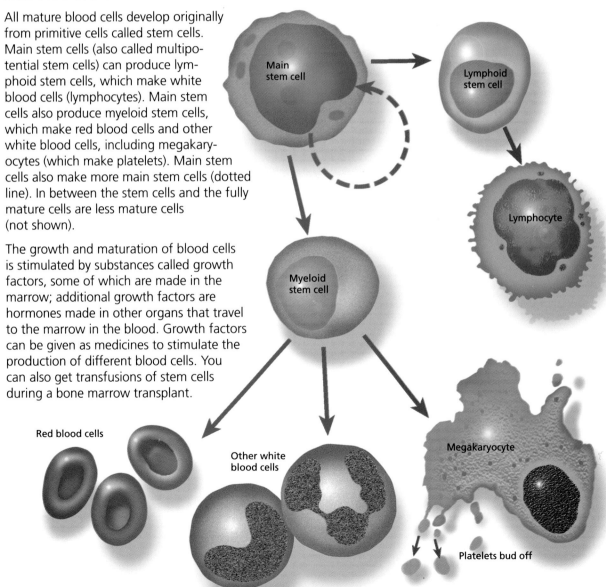

Main stem cell

Lymphoid stem cell

Lymphocyte

Myeloid stem cell

Red blood cells

Other white blood cells

Megakaryocyte

Platelets bud off

HOW YOU BREATHE

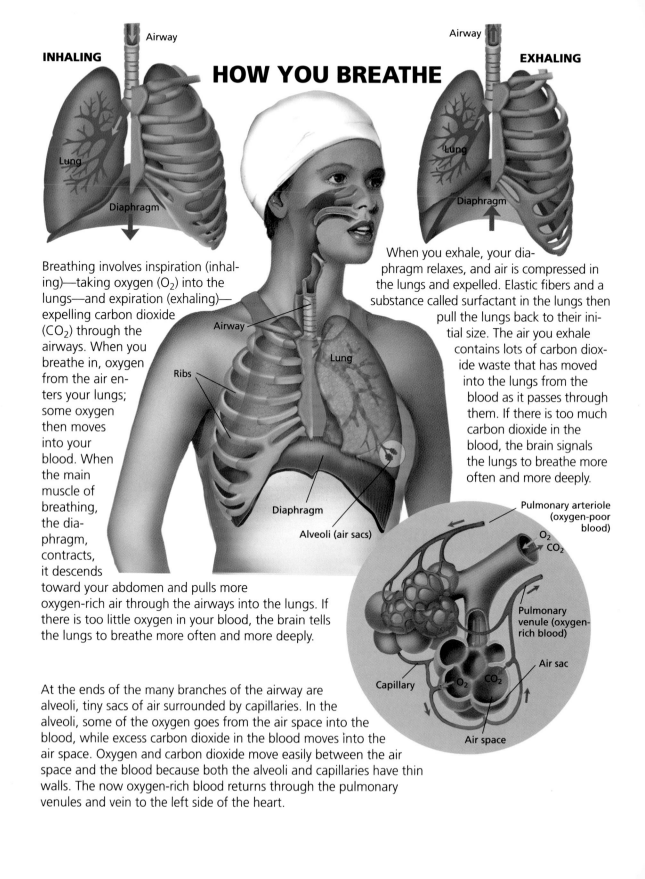

INHALING

Airway

Lung

Diaphragm

EXHALING

Airway

Lung

Diaphragm

Breathing involves inspiration (inhaling)—taking oxygen (O_2) into the lungs—and expiration (exhaling)—expelling carbon dioxide (CO_2) through the airways. When you breathe in, oxygen from the air enters your lungs; some oxygen then moves into your blood. When the main muscle of breathing, the diaphragm, contracts, it descends toward your abdomen and pulls more oxygen-rich air through the airways into the lungs. If there is too little oxygen in your blood, the brain tells the lungs to breathe more often and more deeply.

When you exhale, your diaphragm relaxes, and air is compressed in the lungs and expelled. Elastic fibers and a substance called surfactant in the lungs then pull the lungs back to their initial size. The air you exhale contains lots of carbon dioxide waste that has moved into the lungs from the blood as it passes through them. If there is too much carbon dioxide in the blood, the brain signals the lungs to breathe more often and more deeply.

Airway

Lung

Ribs

Diaphragm

Alveoli (air sacs)

Pulmonary arteriole (oxygen-poor blood)

O_2
CO_2

Pulmonary venule (oxygen-rich blood)

Air sac

Capillary

O_2 CO_2

Air space

At the ends of the many branches of the airway are alveoli, tiny sacs of air surrounded by capillaries. In the alveoli, some of the oxygen goes from the air space into the blood, while excess carbon dioxide in the blood moves into the air space. Oxygen and carbon dioxide move easily between the air space and the blood because both the alveoli and capillaries have thin walls. The now oxygen-rich blood returns through the pulmonary venules and vein to the left side of the heart.

HOW HORMONES WORK

1 The boy is having a cut on his arm treated and the antiseptic on the cotton ball makes the cut sting. The boy's brain recognizes stress and causes the hypothalamus to increase the production of corticotropin-releasing hormone (CRH).

2 CRH travels from the hypothalamus into the pituitary gland through the portal vessels.

3 In response, the pituitary gland increases production of adrenocorticotropic hormone (ACTH), which is released into the blood and carried to the adrenal glands.

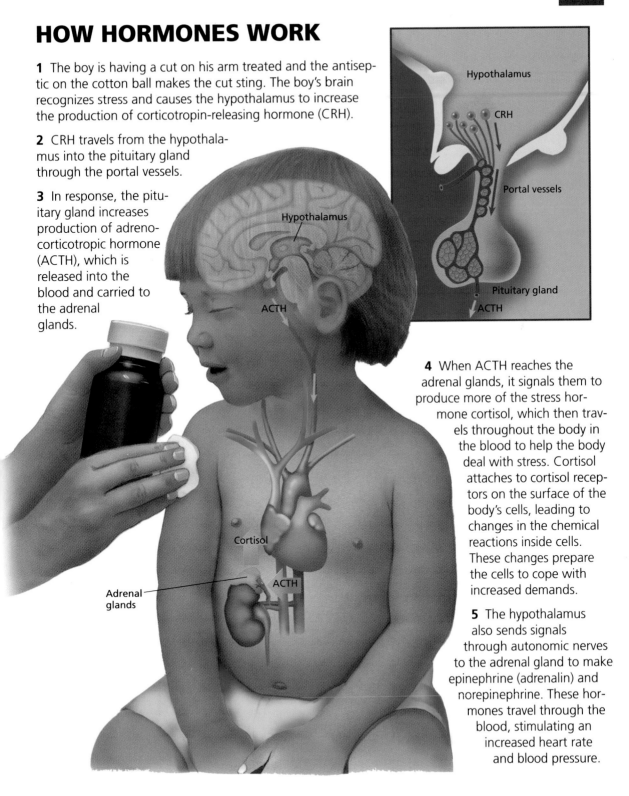

Hypothalamus

CRH

Portal vessels

Pituitary gland

ACTH

Hypothalamus

ACTH

Cortisol

Adrenal glands

ACTH

4 When ACTH reaches the adrenal glands, it signals them to produce more of the stress hormone cortisol, which then travels throughout the body in the blood to help the body deal with stress. Cortisol attaches to cortisol receptors on the surface of the body's cells, leading to changes in the chemical reactions inside cells. These changes prepare the cells to cope with increased demands.

5 The hypothalamus also sends signals through autonomic nerves to the adrenal gland to make epinephrine (adrenalin) and norepinephrine. These hormones travel through the blood, stimulating an increased heart rate and blood pressure.

HOW YOU DIGEST

1 When the amount of sugar in the blood, or fat inside fat cells, gets low, the appetite center in the brain receives signals that create the sensation of hunger.

2 The process of digestion begins in the mouth. Digestion involves breaking down food into countless molecules that are tiny enough to be absorbed by the body. The teeth grind food into small pieces, and enzymes in saliva chemically break the small pieces into even smaller pieces.

3 Food is swallowed down the esophagus into the stomach.

4 In the stomach, food is digested further by stomach acid.

5 Food reaches the small intestine where it is digested further by enzymes made in the pancreas and small intestine into tiny sugar, fat, and protein molecules. The sugar, fat, and protein molecules are absorbed through the wall of the small intestine.

6 The contents of the digestive tract reach the large intestine about 5 or 6 hours after leaving the stomach. The large intestine primarily absorbs water and electrolyte ions.

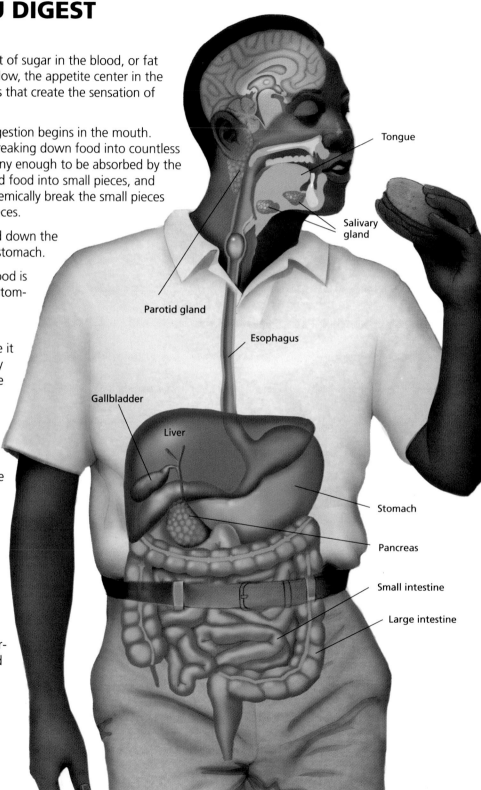

Tongue

Salivary gland

Parotid gland

Esophagus

Gallbladder

Liver

Stomach

Pancreas

Small intestine

Large intestine

THE PROCESS OF DIGESTION

1 The wall of the stomach consists of an outer layer, three layers of muscle (which create the churning action that breaks up food and mixes it with secretions), and an inner lining that produces digestive enzymes.

2 The stomach lining (gastric mucosa) forms a layer of pits. In the pits are cells that produce hydrochloric acid and the enzyme pepsin. A layer of mucus over the lining prevents the stomach from digesting itself.

3 Food is converted to a milky liquid, chyme, which is forced into the small intestine.

4 Bile is produced in the liver, stored in the gallbladder, and flows into the intestine where, with lipase from the pancreas, it digests fats. The pancreas also produces the hormones insulin and glucagon, which affect the level of sugar in the blood.

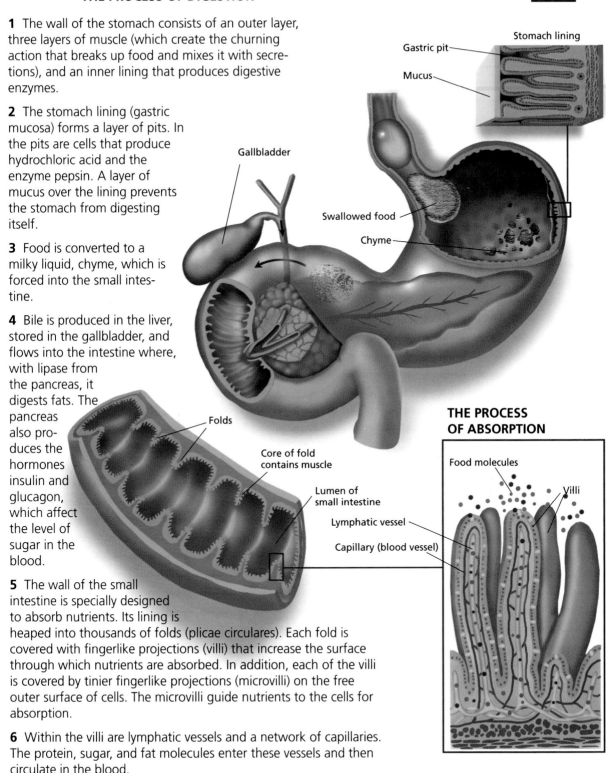

Stomach lining

Gastric pit

Mucus

Gallbladder

Swallowed food

Chyme

Folds

Core of fold contains muscle

Lumen of small intestine

Lymphatic vessel

Capillary (blood vessel)

THE PROCESS OF ABSORPTION

Food molecules

Villi

5 The wall of the small intestine is specially designed to absorb nutrients. Its lining is heaped into thousands of folds (plicae circulares). Each fold is covered with fingerlike projections (villi) that increase the surface through which nutrients are absorbed. In addition, each of the villi is covered by tinier fingerlike projections (microvilli) on the free outer surface of cells. The microvilli guide nutrients to the cells for absorption.

6 Within the villi are lymphatic vessels and a network of capillaries. The protein, sugar, and fat molecules enter these vessels and then circulate in the blood.

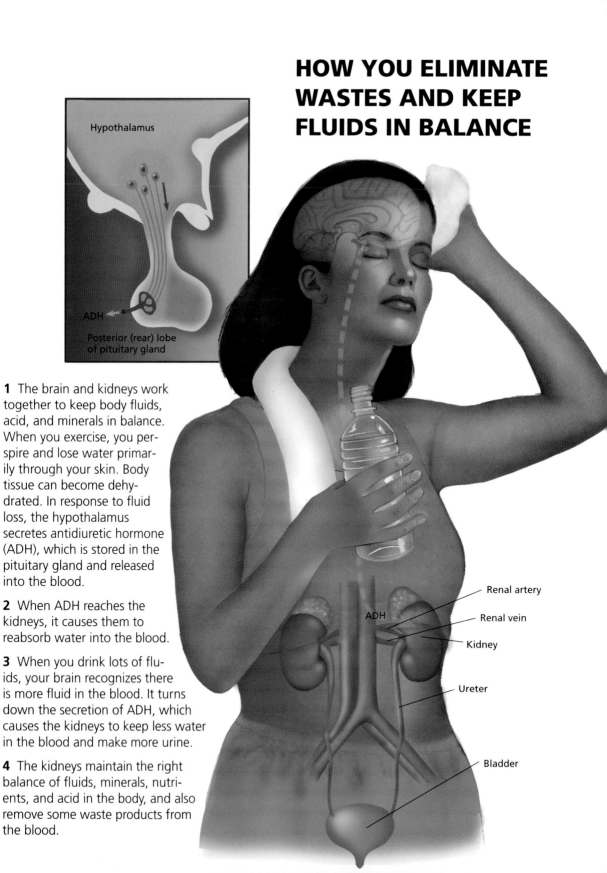

HOW YOU ELIMINATE WASTES AND KEEP FLUIDS IN BALANCE

Hypothalamus

ADH

Posterior (rear) lobe
of pituitary gland

1 The brain and kidneys work together to keep body fluids, acid, and minerals in balance. When you exercise, you perspire and lose water primarily through your skin. Body tissue can become dehydrated. In response to fluid loss, the hypothalamus secretes antidiuretic hormone (ADH), which is stored in the pituitary gland and released into the blood.

2 When ADH reaches the kidneys, it causes them to reabsorb water into the blood.

3 When you drink lots of fluids, your brain recognizes there is more fluid in the blood. It turns down the secretion of ADH, which causes the kidneys to keep less water in the blood and make more urine.

4 The kidneys maintain the right balance of fluids, minerals, nutrients, and acid in the body, and also remove some waste products from the blood.

ADH

Renal artery

Renal vein

Kidney

Ureter

Bladder

HOW YOUR KIDNEYS WORK

Nephron

Arteriole
and venule

Artery

Vein

Ureter

The job of the kidneys is to keep the right amounts of water, minerals, nutrients, and acid in the body, and to remove any waste products, such as urea (a substance created by the metabolism of proteins). Your kidneys maintain the balance by first filtering most of these substances out of the blood, and then taking back into the blood just what your body needs. The rest is excreted in urine.

The initial filtering is performed by a million tiny units (glomeruli). Blood pressure forces fluid through tufts of tiny capillaries in each glomerulus into a long tubule (nephron). The nephron empties into a larger tube called the collecting tubule, which carries urine to the center of the kidney. From there, the urine travels through the ureter into the bladder.

Beginning of nephron

Glomerulus

NEPHRON

Tubule

Arteriole

Venule

Capillaries

Collecting tubule
to ureter

The cells forming the wall of each nephron have proteins that pump minerals, acid, and nutrients out of the tubule and into capillaries that run alongside each tubule. The minerals, acid, and nutrients re-enter the bloodstream and travel throughout the body. Just enough of each is taken back into the body to keep the supply in balance.

For example, when you do not have enough water in your body, the hypothalamus in the brain makes antidiuretic hormone (ADH). ADH makes the wall of the tubule leak more, so water flows more easily out of the tubule and back into the blood.

The kidneys make the hormones renin and erythropoietin. Renin increases blood pressure when the kidneys sense that blood pressure or the mineral sodium is too low. Erythropoietin stimulates the production of red blood cells.

HOW YOU REPRODUCE

1 Hormones released from the pituitary gland and carried by the blood initiate sperm production in the testicles. Testosterone produced by the testicles helps sperm mature.

2 Sperm travel to the epididymis, the vas deferens, and then up the vas deferens to mix with semen.

3 The prostate gland and the seminal vesicles produce semen, a thick liquid that nourishes sperm.

4 At the time of male orgasm, sperm are ejaculated from the ejaculatory duct into the urethra, where they travel through the penis.

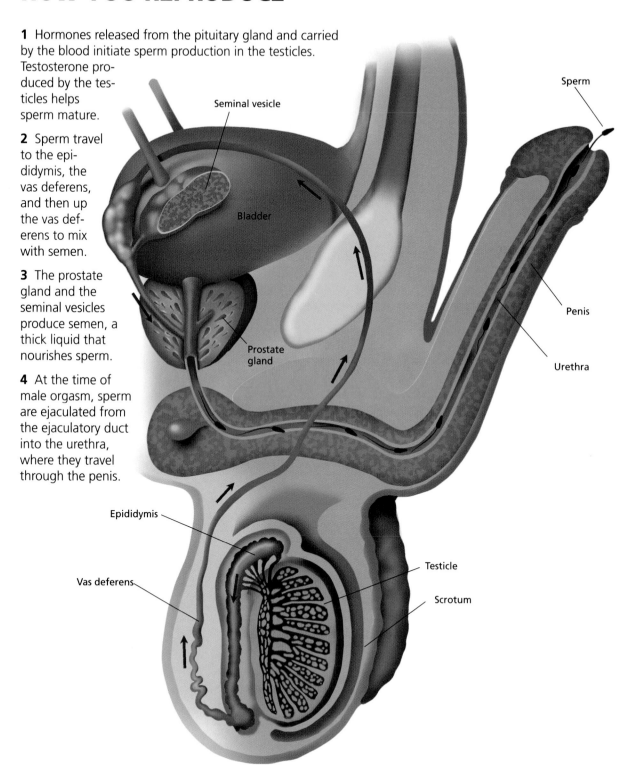

Seminal vesicle

Bladder

Prostate gland

Sperm

Penis

Urethra

Epididymis

Vas deferens

Testicle

Scrotum

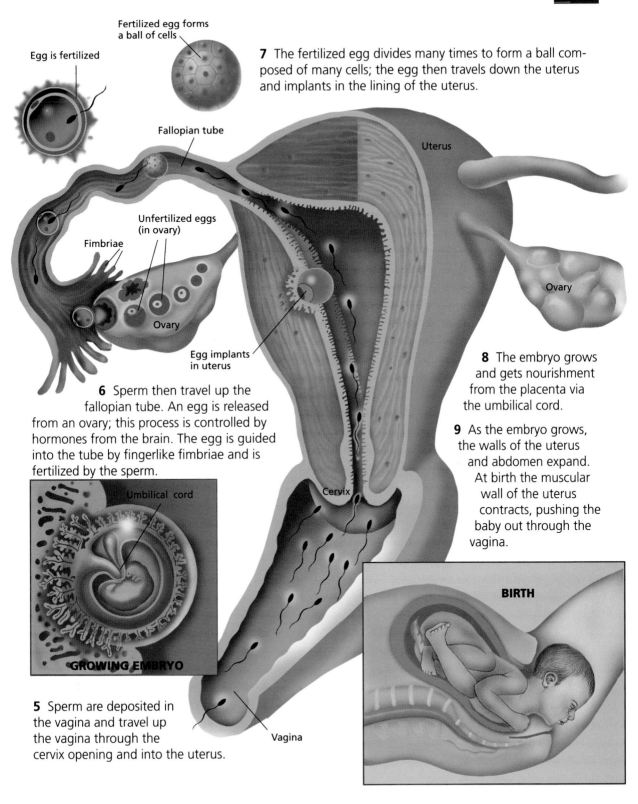

Fertilized egg forms
a ball of cells

Egg is fertilized

7 The fertilized egg divides many times to form a ball composed of many cells; the egg then travels down the uterus and implants in the lining of the uterus.

Fallopian tube

Uterus

Unfertilized eggs
(in ovary)

Fimbriae

Ovary

Ovary

Egg implants
in uterus

8 The embryo grows and gets nourishment from the placenta via the umbilical cord.

6 Sperm then travel up the fallopian tube. An egg is released from an ovary; this process is controlled by hormones from the brain. The egg is guided into the tube by fingerlike fimbriae and is fertilized by the sperm.

9 As the embryo grows, the walls of the uterus and abdomen expand. At birth the muscular wall of the uterus contracts, pushing the baby out through the vagina.

Umbilical cord

Cervix

BIRTH

GROWING EMBRYO

5 Sperm are deposited in the vagina and travel up the vagina through the cervix opening and into the uterus.

Vagina

HOW YOU FIGHT BACTERIAL INFECTIONS

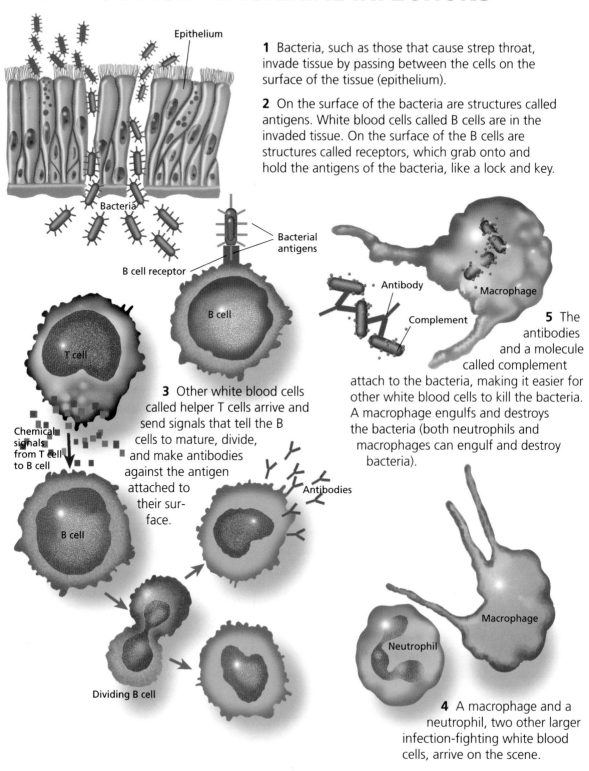

Epithelium

1 Bacteria, such as those that cause strep throat, invade tissue by passing between the cells on the surface of the tissue (epithelium).

2 On the surface of the bacteria are structures called antigens. White blood cells called B cells are in the invaded tissue. On the surface of the B cells are structures called receptors, which grab onto and hold the antigens of the bacteria, like a lock and key.

Bacteria

Bacterial antigens

B cell receptor

B cell

T cell

Antibody

Complement

Macrophage

5 The antibodies and a molecule called complement attach to the bacteria, making it easier for other white blood cells to kill the bacteria. A macrophage engulfs and destroys the bacteria (both neutrophils and macrophages can engulf and destroy bacteria).

Chemical signals from T cell to B cell

3 Other white blood cells called helper T cells arrive and send signals that tell the B cells to mature, divide, and make antibodies against the antigen attached to their surface.

Antibodies

B cell

Dividing B cell

Macrophage

Neutrophil

4 A macrophage and a neutrophil, two other larger infection-fighting white blood cells, arrive on the scene.

HOW YOU FIGHT VIRAL INFECTIONS

1 A virus is a coil of genetic material (nucleic acid) surrounded by a coat of protein. Viruses cannot survive and reproduce until they get inside a cell. B cells make antibodies that attack viruses floating temporarily in the blood (just as B cells do with bacteria). Some viruses escape being destroyed by antibodies and enter cells. Killer (cytotoxic) T cells attack the infected cells. Here, a virus attaches itself to a cell by having one or more of the molecules on its outer surface fit (like a key into a lock) onto projections on the outer surface of the cell.

2 After it attaches itself to the cell, the virus is pulled inside the cell.

3 After the virus is inside the cell, it unwraps its coat of protein. Pieces of the protein travel to the cell's surface. The virus's genetic material inside the cell either remains dormant or reproduces itself.

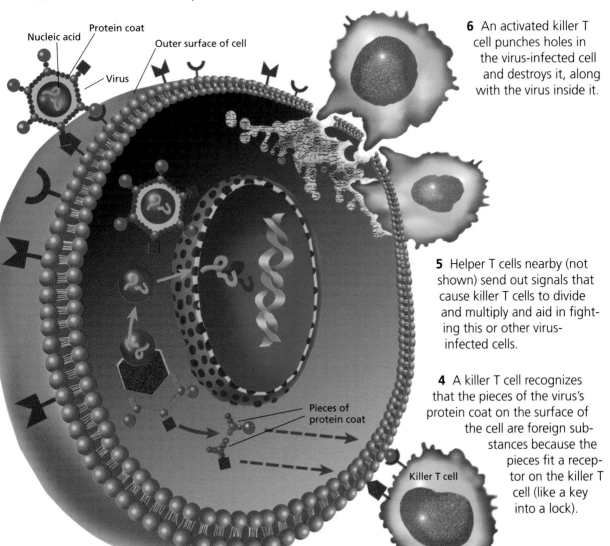

Nucleic acid
Protein coat
Outer surface of cell
Virus
Pieces of protein coat
Killer T cell

6 An activated killer T cell punches holes in the virus-infected cell and destroys it, along with the virus inside it.

5 Helper T cells nearby (not shown) send out signals that cause killer T cells to divide and multiply and aid in fighting this or other virus-infected cells.

4 A killer T cell recognizes that the pieces of the virus's protein coat on the surface of the cell are foreign substances because the pieces fit a receptor on the killer T cell (like a key into a lock).

HOW YOU HEAL INJURIES

1 How will the body heal this cut to the finger? Blood vessels that are cut prevent major loss of blood by sealing the holes in their walls with platelets. Proteins in the blood form a clot; white blood cells move out of the injured blood vessels and travel to the injured tissue. They engulf and remove dirt, dead cells, bacteria, and other foreign material in the wound.

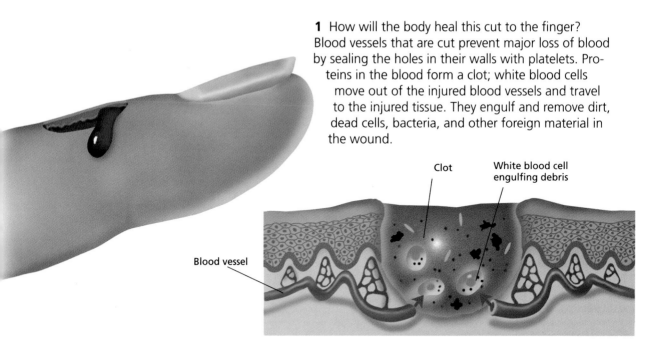

Clot

White blood cell engulfing debris

Blood vessel

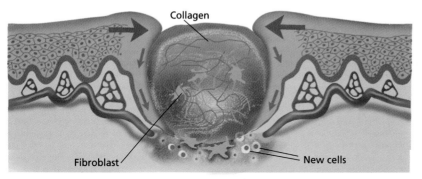

Collagen

Fibroblast

New cells

2 Within 24 hours, the top layer of skin cells at the edge of the wound begin to multiply and move across the wound.

At the same time, another type of cell, called a fibroblast, moves into the injury and lays down a thread of a fiber called collagen that adds strength to the new skin.

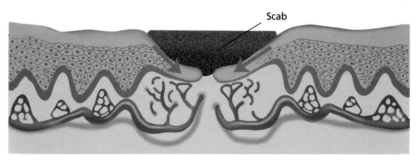

Scab

3 A scab, which is a mix of collagen and clotted blood, forms to create a temporary roof to protect the cells underneath as they complete the process of healing.

Diagnosing Disease

YOU AND YOUR DOCTOR

To make the most of the partnership with your doctor, be honest with him or her about any disturbing symptoms and any problems you are having following medical advice. If you find it difficult to discuss health-related topics that you feel are embarrassing or sensitive, remember that doctors are accustomed to discussing very personal issues with those in their care. Any information that can help your physician protect your health or treat a medical condition, such as incontinence or sexual problems, is worth raising during your office appointment.

When you have a new symptom, your doctor will try to make a diagnosis, a systematic process used to determine what disease or disorder could be causing the symptoms you are experiencing.

The diagnostic process begins well before a physical examination and often even before you speak. Your doctor will note your general appearance when he or she first sees you. Some illnesses cause characteristic abnormalities that can be seen immediately.

For example, bulging eyes could indicate an overactive thyroid gland, sunken cheeks and a very thin appearance could indicate cancer, a face with little expressiveness could indicate Parkinson disease, or an apathetic

attitude could indicate depression.

To make a diagnosis, the doctor always needs to ask you questions, often needs to perform a physical examination, and sometimes needs to order laboratory tests. At each step of the way, your physician is trying to solve a puzzle: "What is wrong with you?"

The questions he or she asks follow a logical order, based on how you have answered the previous question. From the beginning, your physician is keeping a mental list of illnesses that could explain your symptoms. Your answers to each question make certain illnesses more likely and others less so.

Your doctor's goal is to rule out the unlikely illnesses, leaving one as highly likely. Usually, this requires that parts of a physical examination be performed. Often, a few pertinent tests are needed (based on what you have said during the medical history) to help the doctor be even more certain about the diagnosis.

The Medical History

You might be surprised to learn that, despite all of the sophisticated tests that are available today, many doctors still consider the medical history to be the single most important part of making a diagnosis. Obviously, your

doctor will ask you about the symptoms for which you are seeking medical care. He or she may also ask about previous illnesses, tests, or treatments you have had.

Your doctor may want to discuss your work, home and family life, and relationships. Who you are and what is happening in your life can affect how you respond to illness. For example, if you injure a part of your body that is critically important in your work, you are likely to be much more concerned about even a minor injury than another person would be. The amount of stress in your life can also affect your health. Finally, the amount of family and social support you have can be crucially important as you cope with a chronic (ongoing) illness. For these reasons and many more, your doctor needs to know about you and your life.

You may be asked about things that seem unnecessarily personal or irrelevant: Do you use any illegal drugs? Do you drink alcohol and, if so, how much? Do you use any alternative medicine? Do you engage in any sexual practices that could endanger your health? Each of these practices can affect your health.

For example, even if you have

not used illegal drugs for many years, back when you did use them, you could have been exposed to diseases—such as the human immunodeficiency virus (HIV)—that can lie dormant in the body for years but become medical problems later in life.

Questions about race or nationality may be asked because some diseases are much more (or less) common in people of certain races or from certain parts of the world. For example, sickle cell anemia is more common in blacks and some cancers are more common in people from Southeast Asia. You may also be asked about illnesses in members of your extended family because many diseases run in families.

During the medical history, your doctor will ask you to describe your symptoms. It is vital that you not hold back any information; all of it is useful. If your doctor uses medical words you do not understand, do not be reluctant to ask for clarification.

DESCRIBING YOUR SYMPTOMS

When you describe a new symptom, your doctor will ask you questions to help determine the cause. Think about the answers to the following questions in advance (keep a journal if you find it helpful):

■ Approximately when did the symptom start (what day and what time)?

■ What were you doing when it started?

■ How severe was it at the start and how has it changed over time?

■ Did it start suddenly or gradually, and did it get worse over time?

■ Does anything regularly make the symptom better?

■ Does anything regularly make it worse?

■ Have you tried any treatments (such as over-the-counter medicines, medications you had in your medicine cabinet, or home remedies)? Have any of them helped?

■ Besides the main symptom, are there any other symptoms that seem to be connected to the main symptom, getting better when it gets better or worse when it gets worse?

■ Is anyone else in your family or workplace having the same problem?

■ Have you received treatment for this problem or for a similar problem before?

■ How is this problem affecting

Medical Instruments: When You Visit Your Doctor

Your physician may use several instruments during the examination. The most common are:

■ **Stethoscope** This instrument amplifies sounds and is used mainly to listen to the sounds made by the heart, arteries, lungs, and organs in the abdomen. Sometimes the doctor will ask you to say letters (like "A" or "E") so that he or she can hear how the letters sound coming through the tissue of your lungs.

■ **Ophthalmoscope** This instrument lets the doctor look inside your eyes, starting with the outermost part (the cornea), then going deeper into the eye through the lens, and finally to the retina.

■ **Otoscope** This instrument helps your physician look inside your ears, nose, and mouth. It may include a device for blowing air into your ear canal to see how easily the tympanic membrane—your eardrum—moves.

■ **Tongue depressor** This wooden instrument is used to press down your tongue so that the doctor can better see the back of your throat. The view is even better if you say "Ahhh."

■ **Reflex hammer** This little rubber hammer lets the doctor test your reflexes. The most commonly tested reflexes are at the knees, ankles, and forearms.

■ **Vaginal speculum** This metal or plastic instrument is placed inside the vagina to allow the doctor to see the walls of the vagina and the cervix. It also permits your doctor to perform a Pap smear (p.1067) and to take cultures (p.159).

■ **Tuning fork** This metal fork vibrates when it is struck. Your doctor uses it to test your ability to hear the tone it gives off, and to feel the vibrations it creates.

The Physical Examination: Dr Taylor's Advice

Q I've always wondered why my doctor taps on various parts of my body during a physical examination. Can you tell me?

A This decidedly low-tech diagnostic technique is called percussion. It is an extremely valuable part of the physical exam. In percussion, your doctor places a finger from one hand over a part of your body and taps with the other hand, listening to the resonance of the sound. The sound tells your doctor a great deal about the area being tapped. For example, a healthy lung that is filled with air produces a clear hollow sound; when part of the lung is filled with fluid, which can occur in pneumonia, it causes a dull sound over that part.

Q What are doctors feeling for when they push on my abdomen?

A They are feeling for enlargement of the organs, particularly the liver, spleen, and kidneys. They also are feeling for any unusual lumps that could indicate cysts or cancer. Abnormalities of large blood vessels can sometimes be felt by the doctor as abnormal pulsations. Finally, they are feeling for areas of tenderness that could indicate a medical problem.

WILLIAM C. TAYLOR, MD
BETH ISRAEL DEACONESS MEDICAL CENTER
HARVARD MEDICAL SCHOOL

---

your family life, job, finances, and emotions?

The Physical Examination

After taking your medical history, your doctor usually performs a physical examination. It may be a complete examination, such as the one you have during your first visit with a new doctor or for a general checkup. More often, only a part of the complete examination is necessary, based on the reason for your visit.

Sometimes, it may seem the doctor is examining parts of your body that do not relate to your symptoms. This is because a symptom in one part of the body could be caused by a condition that affects another part. For example, if you have difficulty breathing, the doctor is likely to examine not only your lungs but also your feet. This is because

difficulty breathing can be caused by heart failure, and heart failure can cause a buildup of fluid in the legs and feet.

Some parts of the physical examination, such as a rectal examination, can be uncomfortable. By relaxing, you can alleviate some of the discomfort. Take slow, deep breaths to relax any tension in your muscles. Other portions of the physical examination can be painful, particularly if you are seeing the doctor because something hurts, and the doctor is pushing on that something. Some amount of pain is unavoidable. The doctor will be as gentle as possible while trying to locate the source of your pain.

The physical examination is obviously an intimate experience, particularly when it involves examining your sex organs. Your doctor is a professional who is trained to perform this examination, and usually does so many

times every day. Remembering this can help reduce any embarrassment you may feel.

After the Examination

After you are dressed you will again sit down and talk with your doctor. During this time he or she will explain what was found during the physical examination and what is suggested as a next step. If more tests are recommended, your physician should explain what those tests are, who will perform them, and how the results might help make an accurate diagnosis.

Make sure you understand how long it will take to get the results of the tests, and how you will be informed (for instance, by mail or phone). If your doctor has already made a diagnosis and wants to discuss treatment options, he or she should carefully explain each option and dis-

When Should You Call Your Doctor?

It can be difficult to decide when to call your physician. You generally do not need to see a doctor about a minor condition, such as a common cold, that will go away on its own. On the other hand, you should not wait too long before seeing a doctor about a problem that could be serious. The symptom charts (see p.171) in this book can help you decide if a phone call is appropriate.

If you are not feeling well but are uncertain about what to do, it is always best to phone your physician. In most medical offices, someone other than the doctor answers the phone and takes messages. In some offices, a nurse or a physician's assistant will be the first person to answer a call. These health professionals are trained to know when the problem requires the doctor's attention and how urgent the situation is.

Most physicians are not available to take phone calls except in cases of emergencies. Many doctors set aside hours during which they take phone calls; others talk to their patients using electronic mail. The better you and your doctor know each other, the easier it is for him or her to know when you need to be examined.

there to answer them. If you feel it is necessary, ask for a longer-than-normal appointment or schedule a follow-up phone call. In some situations, your physician may recommend that you speak to a nurse on staff about your questions.

Diagnostic Tests

After your medical history and physical examination are complete, your doctor may order diagnostic tests (see p.153) to help determine the cause of your symptoms or the state of a chronic (ongoing) illness. Alternately, the tests may simply be screening tests (see p.80) to identify any problems early.

Some tests, such as those performed on blood or urine, can be done immediately, right in the office. Others, such as x-rays or other imaging tests (see p.135), may require that you go to another office or building. Still others may have to be scheduled for another day. Some of the tests may be completed immediately by your doctor's office staff; in that case, you will be asked to wait a few minutes until the doctor has seen the test results. More often, the results of the tests may take a day or more.

If your physician recommends a treatment or procedure that you question, do not feel embarrassed about obtaining a second opinion before proceeding. A good doctor will respect your wishes, discuss the pros and cons of getting a second opinion, and may be able to refer you to other doctors from whom you can obtain other opinions.

cuss procedures, effectiveness, side effects, and costs.

Primary care doctors are trained to care for most medical problems without referring you to a specialist. However, if your physician wants you to see a specialist, he or she should explain why this step is necessary and what the specialist can offer. If seeing a specialist is not recommended but you think it might be helpful, discuss this with your doctor also.

Make sure you understand everything your physician says. Ask your doctor to repeat or re-explain anything you do not understand; medical terminology is easy to misunderstand. For example, a tumor does not always mean life-threatening cancer; some tumors are benign (noncancerous). If you feel over-

whelmed by the news your doctor gives you, ask if you may make another appointment or telephone to discuss it further.

If you have trouble remembering everything your doctor says, take a pen and paper or tape recorder to your appointment. Some people, especially elderly adults, find it helpful to bring along a friend or family member as an extra set of ears. Friends and family can provide valuable information, and doctors are often grateful to have them in the room to help answer questions if needed.

Because your time with the doctor is limited, it is a good idea to write down a list of important questions before your appointment. Do not worry that your doctor will find your questions silly or unrelated; he or she is

How Often Should You Have a Checkup?

While an annual complete physical examination is no longer considered necessary for everyone, you should see your doctor for a checkup as often as he or she recommends. For example, it may be important to check your blood pressure once a year, but not necessary for you to undergo a complete physical examination.

Your doctor may also want to schedule certain screening procedures (see p.80), such as a mammogram or rectal examination, on a regular basis. Screening examinations can detect disease long before you notice any signs of trouble, giving you the best possible chance to control or cure the condition before it becomes life-threatening. Your doctor is also a good source of information for the correct way to perform self-examinations (see p.78), such as those for the breasts, testicles, and skin. These can also increase your chances of finding disease early.

If you have a sudden new illness, or if you have a chronic (ongoing) illness, your doctor will want to see you regularly, sometimes more often than once a year. These return visits are very important to be certain the condition is improving or being kept under control.

PREPARING FOR YOUR FIRST VISIT WITH A PRIMARY CARE DOCTOR

Your primary care doctor is the doctor responsible for knowing about all of your health problems, and for organizing your care when specialists are needed. Many people think that a doctor they are seeing for the first time should be able to determine what is wrong with them just by asking a few questions, performing a physical examination, and ordering some tests. It is not always that simple. Often what is most important for a new doctor is knowing the result of a test done by a previous physician.

Before you visit a new primary care doctor, gather your medical records to take with you or have them sent by your former doctor to your new physician. In most states, you must sign a written authorization to allow one doctor to send your records to another.

If you cannot obtain the records, do your best to complete the personal health record on p.1246; it summarizes the information that is usually most important. At a minimum, bring a list of all medicines you are taking, including any nonprescription drugs. If you find it easier, take all your pill bottles with you to the doctor's office.

If you are seeing a doctor who practices with your primary care doctor (such as when your physician is on vacation), it is not necessary for you to gather records.

The new doctor should have access to all of your records.

Likewise, when your primary care doctor refers you to a specialist, it should be your primary care doctor's responsibility to be sure that the specialist has all the information that is needed; it is the specialist's responsibility to communicate the results of your visit to your primary care doctor.

HELPING YOUR DOCTOR TREAT A CHRONIC CONDITION

If you have a chronic (ongoing) condition, the partnership with your doctor is even more important. Your physician's challenge is to determine whether you are having any complications from the condition or from its treatment.

When you see your doctor, he or she will ask you whether you have had symptoms that could indicate complications. These symptoms vary greatly, depending on the chronic condition you have, and the medicines used to treat it. Part of your role is to understand which symptoms are significant so that if any develop you can contact your doctor immediately.

You may be asked to keep a written record of symptoms or the results of tests you do at home—from taking your weight to testing your blood for sugar. Taking an active role in your treatment will ensure the best possible outcome.

UNDERSTANDING GENETICS

You have about 20,000 to 25,000 genes, and the state of your health is linked to the information in them.

Advances in medicine, including the identification of genes that can cause disease and the use of genes to treat disease, make your genetic profile increasingly important.

What Are Genes?

Your genes provide a blueprint for your life. They help determine everything from the color of your skin and hair to your susceptibility and resistance to disease.

Most of your genes are located in the nucleus of each body cell, but some are found in the energy-producing mitochondria within each cell. You inherit half of the genes in the nucleus of your cells (and all of the mitochondrial genes) from your mother and half from your father at the moment of conception—when egg meets sperm.

After conception, the one-celled organism, and its full set of genes, divides again and again. As the cells differentiate into various organs and body parts, every cell carries your genetic blueprint.

In the cells of your body, your genes are carried on 23 pairs of chromosomes—22 pairs, plus a pair of sex chromosomes (XX for females and XY for males). Eggs and sperm each carry half the number of chromosomes so that there will be a full set when they unite to form a fertilized egg. Sperm bear an X or a Y chromosome, which determines the sex of the baby.

One chromosome of each of your pairs was inherited from your father, the other from your mother. Each chromosome is actually a long, coiled double strand (the double helix) of DNA and is composed of 50 million to 250 million tiny molecules known as nucleotide bases.

These nucleotide bases (adenine, cytosine, guanine, and thymine) are arranged like beads on two parallel strings. Just as letters (when they are arranged in a certain order) spell words, bases (when they are arranged in a certain order) can convey information. A stretch of several thousand of these DNA "words" put together in a "sentence" is called a gene.

How Do Genes Work?

Genes control your body's growth and function primarily by providing a code or program that enables cells to make proteins they need to carry out certain jobs.

For example, one gene "sentence" might contain instructions for making the protein insulin, which is required for sugar to be

How You Inherit Genes

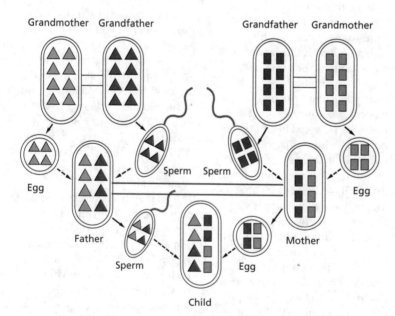

Half of your genes come from each parent. Each of your parents received half of their genes from each of their parents. Consequently, you inherit one quarter of your genes from each grandparent.

A Gene at Work

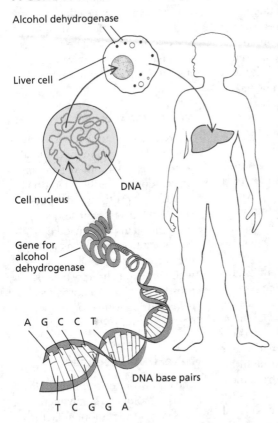

The language of our genes is written in units of DNA called bases. The order of the four bases—adenine, thymine, cytosine, and guanine—determines the structure of a gene's protein. Although all genes are contained in a 6-foot strand of DNA in every cell, specific genes are activated only in cells that require the protein it encodes. For example, the gene for alcohol dehydrogenase, which is required to break down alcohol, is turned on primarily in the liver cells.

helpful results, allowing us to adapt to changes in the environment and to survive as a species.

However, a harmful mutation of a gene can give very different instructions to a cell, with the result that not enough of a protein is made, the wrong protein is made, or some other error occurs. Such changes might seem small, but they can cause serious diseases. Sickle cell anemia (see p.721), for example, is caused by a mutation in a single gene.

GENE MUTATIONS

There are two main types of gene mutations—acquired mutations and hereditary mutations.

An acquired mutation is one that arises in a single body cell. This type of coding error is not passed on to your children, but it is transmitted during cell division to all descendants of that cell.

Abnormal cells developing from an acquired mutation may be destroyed by your immune system, may die on their own, or may continue to grow and spread, forming cancer.

A hereditary mutation may have occurred many generations ago, been passed down to you from a parent, and thus is found in all your cells. It can also be passed on to your children through your sperm or egg.

However, because sperm and egg cells contain only half of your DNA, a mutated gene will not necessarily show up in any of your offspring.

Whether or not a hereditary mutation will cause problems in the next generation depends on the half of the genes inherited from your mother as well as on

used by cells for energy. Another gene might tell a cell how and when to make hemoglobin, a blood protein that carries oxygen in the bloodstream.

Not all genes are "turned on" at the same time. Most function only when they are needed to direct a certain process.

Sometimes the DNA coding in a particular gene is altered; this is called a mutation. A mutation can represent a large change or an alteration of only a single nucleotide.

The mutation of genes is the cause of natural variation among animal and plant species over hundreds of thousands of years— a cornerstone of Charles Darwin's theory of evolution.

Genetic mutation can have

the half inherited from your father. For instance, one gene from your mother codes for blue eyes, while the other gene of that pair from your father codes for brown eyes. The various mutations or changed forms of these genes that control for your eye color are called alleles.

DOMINANT VS RECESSIVE ALLELES

Alleles are either dominant or recessive. The traits carried by a dominant allele usually override those carried by a recessive allele, and are more powerfully expressed—that is, apparent in the person.

For example, if you inherit one gene for brown eye color (a dominant allele) and one for blue eye color (a recessive allele), you will have brown eyes, because the dominant allele overrode the recessive allele.

Recessive alleles are expressed only when there is no dominant allele present; for example, if you inherited two genes for blue eye color, your eyes will be blue.

When a person inherits two alleles that are the same, whether they are both dominant or both recessive, the person is said to be homozygous for that trait. If the two alleles are different (one dominant and one recessive), the person is said to be heterozygous.

If a disease or trait is carried by a dominant allele, a heterozygous person will most likely develop that condition, because the dominant allele will override the other one.

However, if a disease or trait is carried on a recessive allele, a heterozygous person may not demonstrate the condition, be-

cause the normal dominant allele will be expressed. In that case, a heterozygous person is considered a carrier of the condition, because, although the condition may not affect the carrier, the person can pass the mutated gene on to offspring.

DISEASES CARRIED ON NONSEX AND SEX CHROMOSOMES

Many disorders are carried from one generation to the next by a single dominant or recessive gene on an autosome (a nonsex chromosome). They are called autosomal dominant or autosomal recessive disorders.

Other diseases and traits are on the sex chromosomes (the X and Y chromosomes). Males have one X chromosome (from their mother) and one Y chromosome (from their father); females have two X chromosomes (one from their mother and one from their father).

The sex chromosome-related diseases are called X-linked, because they are caused by a gene carried on the X sex chromosome. These X-linked diseases are usually found in males because males have only one X chromosome, since their second sex chromosome is the Y chromosome.

Thus, whatever mutated, unhealthy genes are on a male's single X chromosome will be expressed, since there is no non-mutated, healthy gene on a second X chromosome to oppose it.

In the same way, females, because they have two X chromosomes, can be carriers of unhealthy, mutated genes. That is, they can pass one of a pair on to their children, but their normal

gene on their other X chromosome keeps them healthy.

Females are affected themselves only if the mutated gene is dominant, or if they have inherited two copies of a recessive mutation.

MULTIFACTORIAL CONDITIONS

There are also multifactorial conditions. They require that several genes plus environmental factors be present before the condition or trait is expressed in the person. Some diseases arise not from problems in individual genes but from problems with the chromosome itself, such as when an extra chromosome is present, or part of a chromosome is lost during formation of the egg or sperm.

Inherited Diseases

The ethnic or geographic origin of your biological family members can be an important factor in your risk for some inheritable diseases, because certain genetic mutations are more common in some groups of people.

For example, people of Ashkenazi Jewish descent are more likely to carry genes for Tay-Sachs disease (see p.129) and a type of breast cancer caused by the BRCA1 gene mutation. Blacks of African descent are more likely to carry genes for sickle cell anemia (see p.721). People of Chinese descent are more likely to carry genes for thalassemia (see p.723). Many other ethnic groups have been linked to specific inheritable diseases.

Some common gene muta-

Examples of Genetic Disorders

More than 4,000 diseases are known to be inheritable, but the responsible genes have been identified for only a fraction of those. The following are examples of genetic disorders, some of which are inheritable diseases:

DISEASE OR DISORDER	SYMPTOMS, DESCRIPTION, AND/OR EFFECT
Acute intermittent porphyria	Severe abdominal pain and sometimes nervous system problems
Adult polycystic kidney disease	Numerous cysts in kidneys and eventual kidney failure
Albinism	Absence of pigment in skin, hair, and eyes
Alkaptonuria	Degenerative disease of the spine and joints
BRCA1 and BRCA2 breast cancer	Inheritable forms of breast cancer
Cystic fibrosis	Chronic lung and digestive system disorder
Down syndrome	Mental retardation and physical problems
Duchenne muscular dystrophy	Muscle wasting
Fragile X syndrome	Mental retardation
Gaucher disease	Spleen problems and bone pain
Hemophilia	Deficiency of blood-clotting factors leading to severe bleeding
Huntington disease	Nervous system degeneration with memory loss
Klinefelter syndrome	Disproportionately long legs and arms, small testicles, and male infertility
Marfan syndrome	Disease of connective tissues, causing problems in skeletal and cardiovascular systems
Neurofibromatosis	Numerous soft tumors and patches of pigmented skin
Phenylketonuria	Mental retardation
Polyposis of the colon	Numerous polyps (which can become cancerous) in large intestine
Sickle cell anemia	Misshapen red blood cells, severe anemia, painful clotting, and tissue damage
Tay-Sachs disease	Degenerative and fatal neurological disease
Thalassemia	Deficiency of hemoglobin, leading to anemia or death

tions allowed populations to survive in the past, even though these same genetic defects have produced diseases. For example, ancestors of present-day cystic fibrosis carriers survived cholera epidemics in Northern Europe and sickle cell carriers survived malaria in Africa because their genetic defects protected them.

Compiling a Family Medical History

Your first step in exploring your genetic profile is to gather a family health history. Start with your own health history, using the personal health record on p.1246. Then compile a similar list for each family member, including your parents, children, grandchil-

dren, brothers, sisters, aunts, uncles, cousins, grandparents, and great-grandparents.

For deceased relatives, include the age at death and cause of death. Also include information about relatives who were stillborn or died very young.

If you or your doctor are seriously concerned about the possibility you could have a genetic

Human Genome Project

The Human Genome Project has been a remarkable international effort to identify the structure of the human genome, which includes every human gene. The huge effort was supported by both public and private funds. In April 2003, the public agencies funding the Human Genome Project in the United States announced that over 99% of human DNA had been accurately and definitively sequenced.

This endeavor will have tremendous implications for health and science in the next few decades. The project has provided scientists with a "parts list." Knowing the structure of every human gene will make it much easier for scientists to identify genes involved in particular diseases, to develop screening tests that identify people at risk for certain diseases and diagnose others, to determine which drugs are likely to be most potent and least toxic in a given individual, and to design treatments that promote health and cure disease. Already, scientists are using the results of the project to create genetic "fingerprints" of patients with cancer to determine the best treatment for that patient, and to give improved information about prognosis. Scientists and ethicists are currently debating all the ethical issues raised by the Human Genome Project.

disease, you may need to do some detective work.

Ask relatives what they recall about deceased family members. Call the doctors or hospitals that cared for deceased relatives and ask for information. Call the state health department and request copies of death certificates, which usually note the age and cause of death. Even old family photos can sometimes help your doctor track a genetic disorder through generations.

Create a family tree that shows how your family members are related to one another. Note also information about ethnic and geographic origin. Apparently minor pieces of information may provide important clues for your doctor. You may also be referred to a genetic counselor or physician geneticist for a more focused examination of you or your family history.

Genetic Counseling

A genetic counselor can help you understand your genetic profile and help you make decisions about genetic testing. He or she is trained to translate complex scientific concepts into language you can understand and to help you use this information to make decisions about childbearing and other health issues.

If you are interested in genetic counseling, ask your doctor for a referral or call one of the organizations listed in the Appendix under Genetic Diseases/Testing (see p.1233) or Birth Defects (see p.1230).

Your genetic counselor will work with you and your doctor to gather medical records and your family's medical history. With that information, he or she will prepare a family pedigree that tracks possible inherited dis-

eases through several generations.

Even before any genetic testing is done, a family pedigree can often reveal much about the risks you or your offspring might face from a genetic disorder. Many people are relieved to find that they have greatly overestimated their risk for a genetic disorder.

Next, your counselor will explain inheritable diseases and the particular disorders that might affect your family. This typically begins with the basic principles of genetics: how genes work and how genetic disorders can be passed from one generation to the next.

You will also discuss the medical implications of the gene in question. Questions you might ask include: what risk the gene poses, whether it is a dominant or recessive gene (see Gene Mutations, p.127) and how this relates to your developing manifestations of the disease, whether the disease will develop in everyone who has the gene, and whether the disease is likely to develop in all your children or only in some of them.

Your counselor can also supply medical information about the disease in question, including treatment options, and can refer you to medical specialists.

The counselor will explain the genetic tests available and will describe how the tests are performed, what they can and cannot reveal, and how accurate they are. He or she will help you consider the psychological implications of having the test, and may ask if you are certain you want to know the results.

Who Should Consider Genetic Counseling or Testing?

While there are not always easy answers to the questions that genetic counseling and testing can reveal, a counselor can help you understand your options, support your decisions, and prepare you for the future.

Doctors recommend that people in the following situations consider genetic counseling or testing or that they receive educational brochures on hereditary disorders (which are available in many different languages):

■ Adults (and parents of children) who are carriers of, or at an increased risk for, genetic diseases, chromosomal disorders, birth defects, or hereditary psychiatric diseases.

■ Parents of newborns who have tested positively in state-mandated newborn screening (which tests for a number of treatable diseases such as phenylketonuria) shortly after birth.

■ Couples who are planning to have a child and who have a family history of, or an increased risk for, genetic disorders or birth anomalies.

■ Women who are pregnant and will be older than 35 years at the time of delivery or men who will be older than 40 years at conception. Older women have an increased risk for having a fetus with an extra chromosome, which occurs in Down syndrome. Older men have an increased risk of spontaneous mutations in their sperm, leading to autosomal dominant disorders such as very short stature.

■ Couples in which one or both partners have a genetic disorder.

■ Couples in which one or both partners are known carriers of a genetic disorder.

■ Adults with a family history of multiple cancers appearing in one family member or a single type of cancer occurring in multiple family members.

■ Individuals or couples who have had several miscarriages or babies who died in infancy.

■ Couples who are closely related by blood (such as first cousins).

■ Pregnant women taking medicine for a chronic medical condition, such as a seizure disorder or lupus, that could possibly cause genetic damage to the fetus.

■ Pregnant women who have smoked tobacco or used alcohol, prescription medicines, or street drugs during pregnancy.

■ Couples in which either partner has been exposed to chemicals, radiation, or other agents that could cause genetic damage.

■ All pregnant women, regardless of known risk level, should have screening tests for alpha fetoprotein, human chorionic gonadotropin, and estriol (see Prenatal Testing and Genetic Disorders, p.917). Tests may reveal problems and indicate a need for further testing.

Initially, many people want to have genetic testing but, on further reflection, change their minds.

There are many issues to consider:

■ If you are pregnant already, do you want to know if your fetus has inherited or acquired a genetic disorder? Will this information be useful to you in deciding whether to continue the pregnancy or in planning for the child's birth and care?

■ Will prenatal diagnosis provide you welcome reassurance or heightened anxiety?

■ If you are not pregnant, will knowing about genetic disorders that your children could inherit influence your family planning? If you decide to have children regardless of the outcome of testing, such information could help you be better prepared for a child with health problems. You might also consider other reproductive options or adoption if

you consider the risk of having an affected child to be too high.

■ Do you want to know about a disease that might affect you in the near or distant future? Ask yourself how such knowledge could affect the way you live your life today, and how it could affect family planning, marriage, career, and financial decisions.

■ Do you want to know about a disease that might affect you later in life only if there are steps you can take to help prevent it or lessen its severity?

■ How will having the test affect other family members? In some cases, the test can also reveal information about their genetic profiles, information they might choose not to know. Consider how the information could affect family relationships if some people are found to be affected and others are not.

■ Are you concerned about privacy? Ask the counselor who else might see your test results and why (see Ethical and Social Issues, p.134).

If you decide to be tested, your counselor will arrange for the tests, explain the results, and help you make decisions about your future, based on the information. He or she may suggest you attend a support group, schedule a visit with a specialist who can closely monitor your health, or recommend options for pregnancy.

In all cases, your genetic counselor is there to provide information, support, and resources, not to push you toward one decision or another.

Genetic Testing

A genetic test can be simple; for instance, some tests can be performed on a small sample of blood. In other cases, the test is more complex. In amniocentesis (see p.917), for example, a small amount of the amniotic fluid that bathes the fetus is withdrawn from the uterus. In chorionic villus sampling (see p.918), a tiny piece of tissue from the placenta is removed for testing.

Genetic tests can be highly accurate if done by a professional laboratory that has experience in these techniques, but errors in testing and interpretation are possible. Your doctor can refer you to a facility that has experience in the type of test you need.

There are three basic types of genetic tests: biochemical tests, chromosome analysis, and DNA analysis.

Biochemical tests Biochemical tests are used to diagnose certain genetic disorders that cause an imbalance of a protein the body needs to function. The test measures the protein (not the DNA that makes the protein). An example is Tay-Sachs disease, in which a genetic mutation leads to an absence of the enzyme hexosaminidase A.

Biochemical tests usually involve chemically examining a sample of blood, urine, amniotic fluid, or amniotic cells for the presence or absence of a protein or related substance, which indicates the presence of the genetic defect. A tiny sample of tissue is sometimes needed to perform the analysis.

Biochemical tests are also used to diagnose phenylketonuria (see p.983) and cystic fibrosis (see p.1003). Some biochemical tests are performed on all newborns.

Chromosome analysis Chromosome analysis is used to diagnose abnormalities in the number and structure of the chromosomes themselves, rather than looking for a mutation of a specific gene on one of the chromosomes. It is commonly used to diagnose abnormalities in fetuses.

One of the most common of

these disorders is the presence of an extra chromosome, which can cause Down syndrome. Cells are obtained from a blood sample or, in the case of a fetus, through amniocentesis or chorionic villus sampling. The frozen cells are placed on a slide, stained so the chromosomes stand out, and examined under a powerful microscope.

DNA analysis DNA analysis is used primarily to identify genetic disorders that can be caused by a single gene, such as Huntington disease or cystic fibrosis. As in chromosome analysis, the DNA is usually obtained from blood or from fetal cells.

DNA analysis uses a variety of techniques to search for mutated genes. When scientists go looking for the DNA "fingerprint" of a particular gene in your DNA, they have to know what to look for. They might know the complete structure of the gene or only part of the structure. Sometimes they do not know the structure of the gene but know the structure of a "marker" piece of DNA that is located very close to the gene, on the same chromosome. If you have that marker, you have a high likelihood of having the gene in question.

The search usually uses a "probe," which is a small piece of nucleic acid that is the same as a part of the gene or the marker that lies near the gene. Because that probe has the same structure as a part of the gene, it will bind to the gene (if you have the gene). Once the probe finds its target, it gives off radiation that can be seen on photographic film.

In cases where a mutation is

Gene Therapy

Gene therapy, an exciting approach to treating disease, is still in the experimental stages. The premise is that a healthy, functioning gene is inserted into cells to do the job that a defective gene has failed to do. The new gene is carried into the body by a variety of means. It may be piggybacked onto a harmless virus that spreads among the body's cells or carried on a fat globule. Once it reaches its target cells, the new gene settles in and directs the cell to make the missing protein or do another job, such as suppressing another gene. Some introduced genes seem to set up permanent residence, while others need to be replenished periodically.

Numerous clinical trials are underway to test the effectiveness of gene therapy in inherited diseases such as cystic fibrosis. Cancer therapy trials are exploring the use of genes to do such things as trigger the immune system to attack cancer cells or make cancer cells more likely to respond to treatment. Heart specialists are using gene therapy to encourage the heart to grow new blood vessels, a kind of biological bypass that could help those with heart disease avoid surgery.

While these treatments could theoretically cure people, those whose disorders are caused by defective genes could still pass on the mutation to their children. However, it may someday also be possible to prevent offspring from having problems by inserting healthy genes into embryos to replace defective genes.

How Gene Therapy May Work

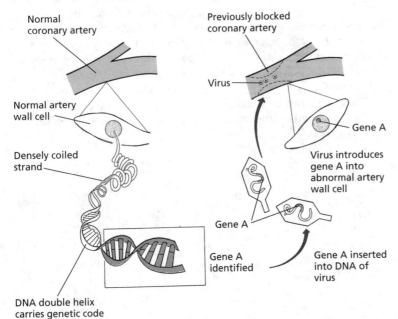

Normal coronary artery

Normal artery wall cell

Densely coiled strand

DNA double helix carries genetic code

Previously blocked coronary artery

Virus

Gene A

Virus introduces gene A into abnormal artery wall cell

Gene A

Gene A identified

Gene A inserted into DNA of virus

In gene therapy, a specific gene (here, gene A) that inhibits the recurrence of blockages in the coronary artery would be inserted into the DNA of a virus. The virus would carry that gene into the nucleus of the target cells in the diseased vessel wall. The cell could then make many copies of a specific protein that prevents further blockages.

known to be carried in a family (but its exact nature or location on the chromosome is not known), linkage analysis may be used. Because the exact mutation is not known, it is necessary to have DNA samples from affected and unaffected family members for comparison.

In some cases, finding a mutation means that the person will definitely get the disease. This is the case in testing for Huntington disease. In other situations, however, the presence of a mutation means only that the person is more likely to develop the disease. Also, testing negatively for one known mutation does not always mean that the person will never get the disease. There can be other, unknown mutations involved.

Ethical and Social Issues

The Human Genome Project, and the work that preceded it, has led to the identification of a growing number of genes that cause disease (see p. 130). Tests have been developed that can determine who carries a mutated gene and who does not. Deciding whether or not to have genetic testing involves deeply personal choices. However, it also raises ethical and social questions.

One of the most pressing issues is the confidentiality of genetic information. Who will have access to your test results? Discrimination based on your genetic profile is a real possibility.

Might you be denied a job because a potential employer knows that you are likely to develop breast cancer and could drive up insurance costs? Could you be denied insurance for the same reason? Will genetic profiles be considered pre-existing conditions by insurance companies and used to deny coverage?

Could you be denied admittance to a professional school if it is known that you are going to develop Huntington disease? Would an adoption agency deny you a child?

These scenarios may sound far-fetched, but they are increasingly common. Many cases of genetic discrimination have already occurred. You have some protection under federal law with the Americans with Disabilities Act, a federal law called the Health Insurance Portability and Accountability Act (HIPAA), and under some state laws, but how far these protections extend is not yet clear.

Consequently, many people who have genetic testing elect to keep their results private and decide to pay for tests themselves rather than reveal their condition to their insurance company and others who have access to their records.

Another question to consider is stigmatization by peers based on your genetic profile. How will family members feel about relatives who test negative or positive for a genetic mutation?

Should children be tested? Many doctors believe children should not be tested for medical disorders that occur later in life, but that they should wait until they are old enough to make the decision to be tested themselves.

GUIDE TO IMAGING

Electrocardiogram

An electrocardiogram (ECG), formerly abbreviated EKG, is a test that records the electrical current that naturally runs through the heart muscle. In order to pump blood through the chambers of the heart, the heart muscle must contract (squeeze) in a coordinated manner.

A specialized area of the heart—the sinoatrial node—acts as a natural pacemaker by maintaining a regular beat and producing electrical impulses that tell the heart muscle when to contract. The contraction itself produces an electrical signal that can be recorded on the ECG graph (see below).

Your doctor examines the graph for abnormal electrical currents. An ECG can detect a new or old injury to the heart (such as from a heart attack), abnormal heart rhythms, thickening or thinning of the heart muscle wall, inflammation of the tissue covering the heart (the pericardium), and many other conditions.

Getting an ECG is painless. A recording called a resting ECG is made while you lie still on an examining table. An exercise stress test is an ECG performed while you exert yourself physically.

Several electrodes—small, round, metal sensors that pick up electrical signals—are placed at specific sites on your chest, arms, and legs. The electrodes are attached to the skin with suction cups or stickers; they do not pierce your skin and they do not transmit any electricity into your body.

The electrodes detect the electrical signals generated by your heart and send this information through wires to a recording machine. The recording machine produces a graph of the electrical impulses from several heartbeats on a long sheet of paper.

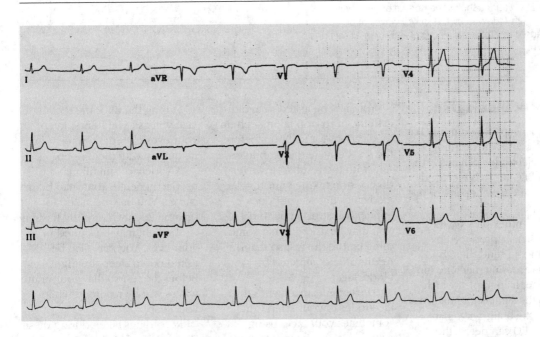

ELECTROCARDIOGRAM OF A HEALTHY HEART

This electrocardiogram shows 12 different views returned from 12 electrodes (labeled I, II, III, aVR, aVL, aVF, and V1 through V6) graphing the electrical current from different parts of a healthy heart. Differences in the direction and shape of the waves alert your doctor to problems with the heart's blood supply or rhythm. The unlabeled graph at the bottom is called a rhythm strip. It helps your doctor see your heart rhythm.

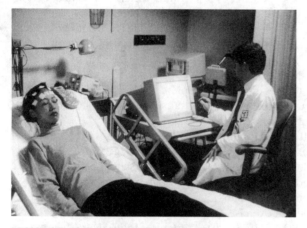

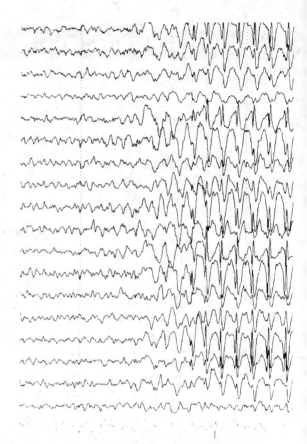

RECORDING AN ELECTROENCEPHALOGRAM OF A PERSON HAVING AN ABSENCE SEIZURE

For an electroencephalogram (EEG), electrodes are placed on the head to record brain waves from different parts of the brain. The EEG at right shows the normal brain waves of sleep on the left followed by the spiked waves of an absence seizure, caused by abnormal electrical activity in all sections of the brain.

Electroencephalogram

An electroencephalogram (EEG) is similar to an electrocardiogram. Through electrodes placed on the scalp, an EEG records electrical activity from different parts of the brain.

The electrodes pick up the electrical signals produced by your brain and send them by wire to a recording machine (an electroencephalograph), which amplifies the signals and makes a tracing of the brain-wave patterns. An EEG can detect the abnormalities in brain waves present in a variety of disorders, including epilepsy and sleep disorders. An EEG cannot diagnose psychiatric disorders.

You may be asked to avoid caffeine or to stop taking certain medications for 24 hours before the test because they can interfere with the results. However, do not stop taking your regular medicines unless your doctor explicitly instructs you to do so. You may be asked to eat something before the test so that the results are not affected by low blood sugar.

The technician attaches the electrodes to your scalp (and sometimes your face) using paste, suction, or tape. In some cases, tiny needle electrodes that slip under the skin of the scalp are used; these cause only minor discomfort. Your hair does not need to be cut for this test.

During the EEG, the technician will ask you to first keep your eyes closed, then to sit or lie quietly with them open.

A variety of stimuli may be used to generate abnormal brain waves. You may be asked to breathe deeply. A rapidly flashing strobe light may be shined in your eyes. You may also be asked not to sleep the night before the test so that your brain waves will be recorded while you sleep.

Recordings taken during these instructions show your doctor how your brain responds to various stimuli and may indicate abnormalities.

Nuclear Medicine (Radionuclide Scanning) and Single Photon Emission Computed Tomography

Nuclear medicine scans (also known as radionuclide scans) are made by injecting a substance containing a tiny amount of radioactivity into a blood vessel and taking a picture with a sophisticated camera of where the substance goes. This basic method is used with different forms of radiation to obtain pictures of various parts of the body.

The radioactive substances, referred to as radionuclides or radioisotopes, are either injected into the body or swallowed. The substance used depends on what part of the body is being examined.

For example, to examine your thyroid gland, your doctor uses radioactive iodine, which naturally collects in the thyroid. Other substances collect in the lungs, bones, liver, or other body parts.

For some procedures, you may have to wait several hours for the radionuclides to travel to and be concentrated in the designated organ. Then, a camera is positioned near your body so it can detect the gamma rays given off by the radionuclides. Areas of disease can give off abnormal amounts of radiation.

For example, an infection in a bone can cause the bone to take up more of the radionuclides, which the camera detects and records as an abnormally high level of gamma rays. Radionuclides may also concentrate in tumors, making them stand out.

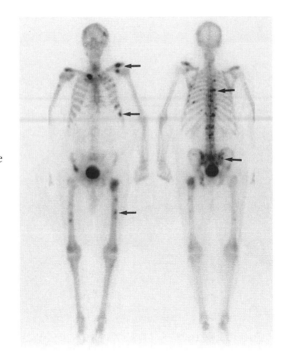

ABNORMAL BONE SCAN

Black spots in both skeletons (arrows) are areas of increased radioisotope uptake. These are areas where cancer has spread to the bones.

SINGLE PHOTON EMISSION COMPUTED TOMOGRAPHY OF NORMAL HEART AND ABNORMAL HEART

The normal scan just below shows a cross-sectional view through the heart. The heart muscle takes up the radioisotope that has been injected and appears as a series of brightly colored rings. The abnormal scan of the heart (bottom) shows interruption of the colored rings, indicating areas of the heart that are deprived of blood.

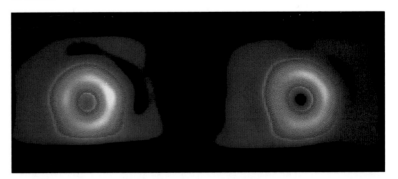

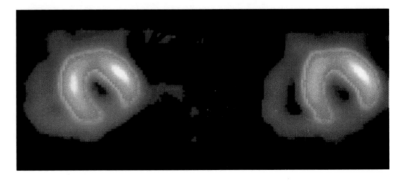

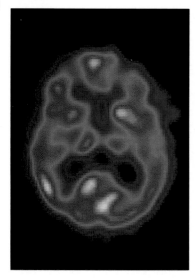 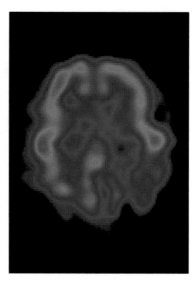

**SINGLE PHOTON EMISSION COMPUTED TOMOGRAPHY
OF NORMAL BRAIN AND BRAIN OF PERSON WITH ALZHEIMER DISEASE**

The scan at left shows a section of a normal brain. Blood flow (orange) and brain metabolism (pink) are evenly distributed throughout the brain. At right, the scan shows a section of a brain from a person who had Alzheimer disease. There is decreased blood flow (orange) and brain metabolism (pink).

In other cases, a lower level of radiation than expected suggests the tissue is unhealthy or not functioning. For example, an area of the heart that has died in a heart attack may show decreased radioactivity with certain radionuclides.

Most radionuclide scans also use a computer to enhance the image. In this technique, known as single photon emission computed tomography (SPECT), the camera circles around you, taking readings of the gamma rays from many angles. The computer uses this information to build an even more detailed and precise picture. Positron emission tomography scanning is another type of radionuclide scan.

Radionuclide scanning is a safe procedure that causes no discomfort. Your exposure to radiation is less from radionuclide scanning than from an x-ray and there is no risk of allergic reaction.

**SINGLE PHOTON EMISSION COMPUTED TOMOGRAPHY OF BRAIN
BEFORE AND DURING A SEIZURE**

These two scans show normal brain activity (left) and brain activity during a seizure (right). The scan showing normal brain activity has color evenly distributed on both sides of the brain. The scan showing the seizure indicates uneven brain activity (arrows).

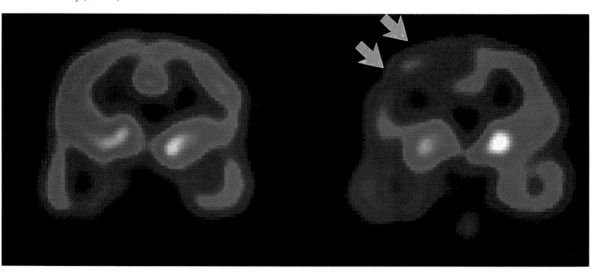

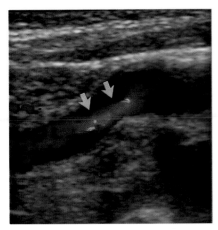

ULTRASOUND OF CAROTID ARTERY

This ultrasound shows a carotid artery blockage caused by plaque. Normal blood flow (far left) is deep red. Abnormal flow or blockage (arrows) is indicated by yellow, orange, and blue.

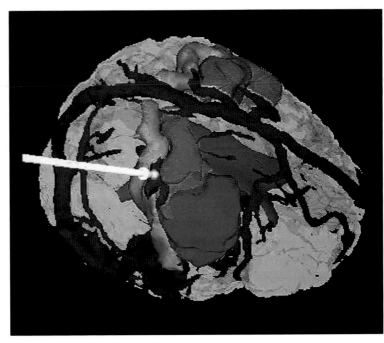

FUNCTIONAL MAGNETIC RESONANCE IMAGING OF BRAIN

This image shows the head of a woman with a brain tumor (green). During the taking of this image, she was asked to move her left hand so that doctors could view the part of the brain that functioned as she moved it (causing the area to show up as red, highlighted by the white pointer). Taking functional magnetic resonance images before surgery helps surgeons identify essential brain tissue and enables them to avoid removing it during surgery. Veins are shown in dark blue.

Doppler Ultrasound

Doppler ultrasound examines the flow of blood through blood vessels. It can identify possible blockages in the veins and arteries where blood flow looks abnormal. Like conventional ultrasound, Doppler ultrasound uses a handheld instrument to send sound waves into your body and receive their echoes.

Doppler ultrasound can make pictures of blood flowing by using the Doppler effect. Just as the pitch of a fire engine siren changes as the distance between you and it changes—seeming to rise as it moves closer to you and fall as it moves away—sound waves reflected back by blood also change. The Doppler ultrasound machine detects those changes and translates the sound-wave data into a picture of the moving blood.

Doppler ultrasound is useful for detecting the turbulence in narrowed blood vessels that is

known as "noisy" blood flow, which translates into changes in color in the ultrasound picture.

The turbulence suggests the presence of a blockage of the blood vessel. Decreases in blood flow caused by the blockage can also be measured.

Functional Magnetic Resonance Imaging

Standard magnetic resonance imaging (MRI) can provide a very detailed view of the shape of structures inside your body. However, it cannot tell doctors how well those structures are

functioning. Just like positron emission tomography scans (see next page), functional MRI reveals information about metabolism—that is, how well an organ or parts of an organ are working.

Functional MRI works like standard MRI, but goes further, detecting minute changes in the amount of oxygen found in blood vessels. These changes in oxygen levels indicate which parts of the organ are functioning. In the brain, for example, an area toward the back of the head "lights up" during a functional MRI of your eyes.

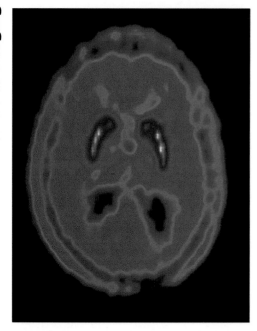
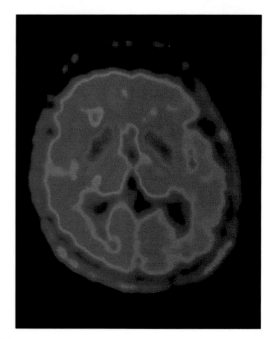

**POSITRON EMISSION TOMOGRAPHY OF NORMAL BRAIN
AND BRAIN OF A PERSON WITH PARKINSON DISEASE**

In a healthy person's brain (left) there are normal amounts of the brain neuro-transmitter dopamine (yellow and red) deep in the part of the brain called the basal ganglia. In a person with Parkinson disease (right) there are deficient amounts of dopamine.

Positron Emission Tomography

Doctors can use positron emission tomography (PET) scanning to look at more than the shape and structure of an organ. By looking at the chemical and metabolic (functional) activity of tissues, particularly in the brain, PET scanning can evaluate how well an organ is working and can detect nonfunctioning areas that may look normal on a regular scan.

Like nuclear medicine procedures, PET requires the use of very small amounts of radioactive substances called radioisotopes. The radioisotope is attached to a host substance such as glucose or a hormone that is actively used by the tissues to be imaged by

the PET scan. The isotope/host substance combination is injected into the bloodstream, travels to the part of the body to be imaged, and concentrates in the tissues that are most biologically active.

The scan is named for the positron particles produced by the radioisotope that collide with other particles and give off gamma rays. A large ring of detectors around your head or body picks up the gamma rays. A computer then translates the information into a picture detailing the structure as well as areas of high and low activity through changes in color.

Initially, PET scanning was used for research, primarily to study brain or heart function. Increasingly, PET scanning is

being used in major medical centers to diagnose and treat diseases. Some applications involve distinguishing cancer from benign lesions, cardiac exercise testing, and identifying sources of hidden infection. It has been widely used to map brain function after strokes or in the study of diseased brain states.

Because the amount of radioactivity used is very small, there is little risk associated with PET scanning. It is a painless procedure. Some doctors believe that PET scanning will be replaced by functional magnetic resonance imaging (see previous page), a less complicated procedure that does not require the injection of a radioactive substance into the body.

Magnetic Resonance Imaging in the Operating Room

Another specialized use of magnetic resonance imaging (MRI) occurs in the operating room. During surgery, doctors can use a "real-time" (how a body part looks at that moment) MRI to obtain a very close and detailed look at the region being operated on.

While performing brain surgery, for example, physicians can use MRI to locate part of a brain tumor that otherwise would be invisible to the eye.

Using MRI in the operating room allows the surgeon to identify with greater accuracy the sections of healthy tissue that, before MRI, may have been removed on the chance that they contained cancerous cells.

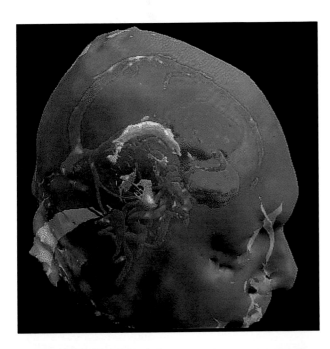

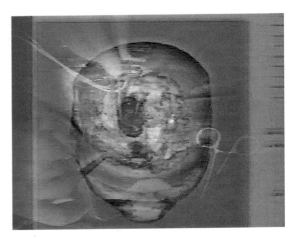

WHAT MAGNETIC RESONANCE IMAGING SHOWS

In the operating room on a monitor, a video of the patient's brain is superimposed on the magnetic resonance imaging (MRI) picture (above). Instead of looking directly down onto brain tissue, where the color of the tumor is hard to distinguish from the surrounding normal brain, the surgeon can see the tumor (green) much more clearly. In this photograph, surgical instruments can also be seen.

MAGNETIC RESONANCE IMAGING OF DIFFERENT BRAIN TUMORS

At top left, magnetic resonance imaging makes it possible to see inside the brain with extraordinary clarity. In this person, arteries (red), fluid-filled ventricles (light blue), and a large brain tumor (green) are evident. At lower left, the veins (darker blue), ventricles (light blue), and a large tumor (green) of a different person are seen.

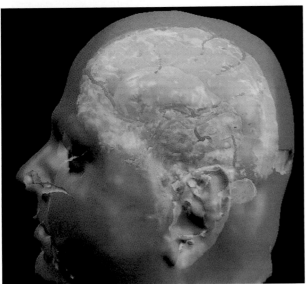

Endoscopy

Endoscopy is a general term for the examination of the inside of your body with an endoscope. An endoscope is a thin flexible tube with a camera at its tip that is inserted into the body; it permits the doctor to look directly at internal organs.

Most endoscopes carry a light that illuminates the area being examined, a viewer that reflects images back up the scope, and a lens that enlarges the image. Sometimes the image is sent to a monitor above the doctor.

Some endoscopes have tiny compartments for the passage of instruments that are used to collect samples of tissue for a biopsy or to perform an operation. For example, tiny scissors can be attached to the end of an endoscope to remove a polyp.

Endoscopes are most commonly used to look at the gastrointestinal tract, such as the esophagus, stomach, or the uppermost part of the small intestine. To view these structures, the endoscope is inserted through your mouth.

If the rectum or lower colon is to be examined, the procedure is called proctoscopy or sigmoidoscopy, and the endoscope is inserted through the anus. Colonoscopy is used to examine the entire colon; in this procedure, a longer endoscope is inserted through the anus. Although these procedures may cause some discomfort, they are not usually painful.

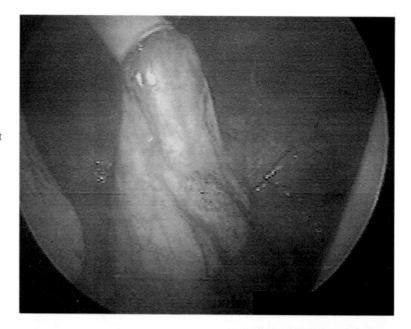

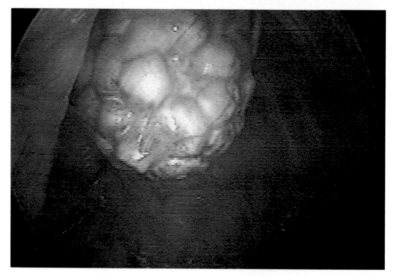

LAPAROSCOPIC CHOLECYSTECTOMY (GALLBLADDER REMOVAL)

A laparoscopic gallbladder removal can be performed using only a few small incisions in the abdomen. At top, the gallbladder is cut away from the liver and pulled up toward the abdominal wall with a surgical tool. At bottom, many gallstones (packed inside the gallbladder) are evident as the gallbladder is pulled by suction toward the incision in the navel, to be removed from the body.

Endoscopes are also used to look at many other parts of the body, including the sinuses, lungs, abdomen, pelvis, bladder, and joints. In a technique called laparoscopy, the doctor uses the endoscope to directly view the abdominal organs.

After using a local anesthetic to numb the skin and underlying tissue, one or more incisions the size of a buttonhole are made in the skin of the abdomen. The endoscope is passed into the abdominal space to look at the organs or help perform surgery.

During laryngoscopy, the doctor uses a thin endoscope to look farther down your throat to visualize the larynx and vocal cords. A bronchoscope is used to view the large airways of the lung. Tumors or areas of infection can be seen and biopsies of abnormal lung tissue can be taken.

Endoscopes are increasingly used to perform surgery. For example, the gallbladder can be removed using an endoscope.

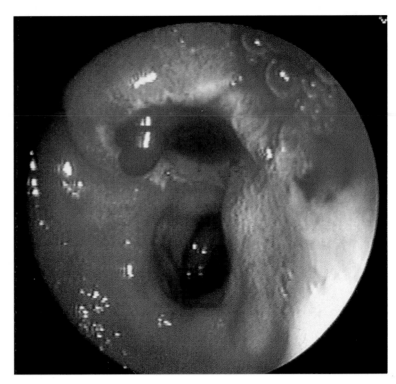

BLEEDING ULCER

This view through a gastroscope, looking down into the duodenum (the first part of the small intestine), shows a bleeding ulcer. A drop of blood is about to drip down at top. The lower opening is the passage into the rest of the small intestine.

NORMAL KNEE AND KNEE WITH DISEASED CARTILAGE

At left, an arthroscope placed inside a healthy knee joint shows the smooth cartilage surface of the femur and tibia, the two main bones that meet in the knee. The cartilage of the diseased knee at right has been severely damaged by arthritis and is worn away and irregular.

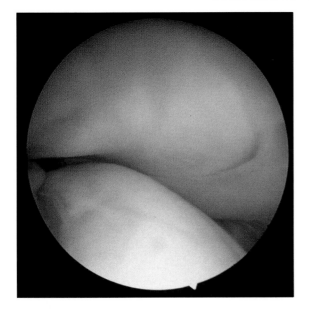

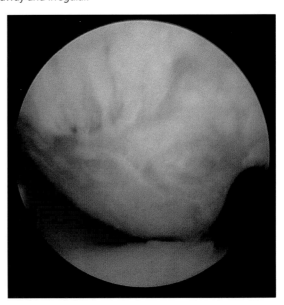

Microscopic Tests

The microscope, developed in the 17th century, remains an essential diagnostic tool. Your physician can look at body fluids, such as urine, under the micro-scope to detect signs of infection, bleeding, or other abnormalities.

Cells scraped from the surface of the body can be examined microscopically for signs of cancer. This is called a cytology examination, and the most famil-iar example is a Pap smear.

A tissue biopsy can be examined under the microscope to look for various abnormalities, including cancer.

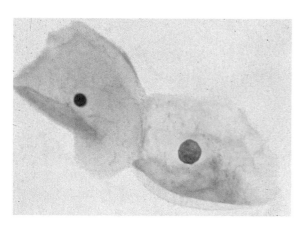
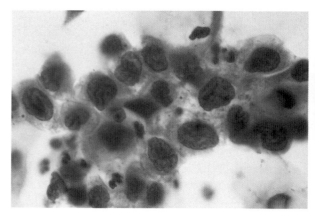

MICROSCOPIC VIEWS OF NORMAL AND ABNORMAL CERVICAL CELLS

During a Pap smear, cells are brushed off the surface of the cervix, placed on a slide, and examined under a microscope. The two cells above left are normal cells from the outer portion of the cervix. The dark circles in the middle of the cells are the nuclei of the cells and contain DNA. The view above right is of cancerous cells taken from an abnormal Pap smear. The cancer cells are much smaller than the normal cells and have abnormally shaped nuclei.

MICROSCOPIC VIEW OF SKIN CANCER CELLS

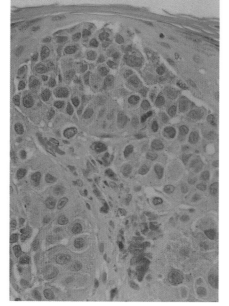

In a skin biopsy, a tiny piece of tissue is removed for examination under a micro-scope. Chemicals are used to preserve and stain the tissue. The sample at left, from a skin biopsy of a person with malignant melanoma, shows some of the cells that contain melanin, the brown pigment that gives this cancer its name. Almost all the larger, purple-colored, variably shaped cells in the picture are cancerous.

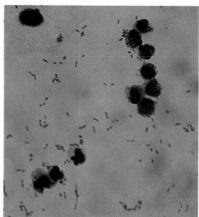

MICROSCOPIC VIEW OF INFECTED URINE

Many small, rod-shaped bacteria are apparent in the urine of a woman with a urinary tract infection. The large, dark purple cells are the infection-fighting white cells.

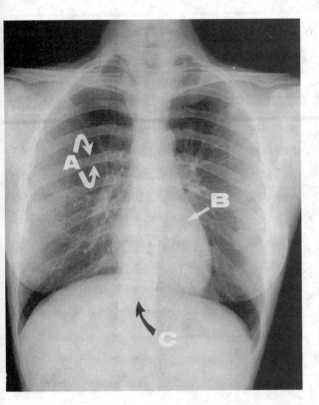

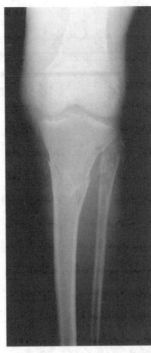

NORMAL CHEST X-RAY

In the normal chest x-ray at far left, the ribs are visible; one rib is marked with arrows (A). The lungs appear black because they contain air. The heart (B) and the spine (C) can also be seen.

X-RAY OF A BROKEN LEG

The x-ray at left shows two fractured bones below the knee. The fracture in the large bone (the tibia) is easier to see.

Conventional X-Rays

Doctors have used x-rays to help diagnose disease for more than 100 years. In 1895, Wilhelm Roentgen, a German professor, found that he could produce a picture of his bones by placing his hand in the path of x-rays, with a photographic film behind his hand.

The x-rays Roentgen used were produced by natural radioactive substances in the environment; today x-rays are produced and controlled by machines.

An x-ray beam is produced by a machine that is positioned near your body. The beam travels through your body and strikes a photographic plate placed on the other side. Dense structures, such as bone, absorb a lot of the beam, and block the x-rays from reaching the photographic plate. This results in a white area on the film.

Hollow body parts, such as the lungs, allow most of the x-rays to pass through and strike the photographic plate, resulting in a dark area of film. Soft tissues such as skin and muscles, which are more dense than air but less dense than bone, show up as shades of gray.

Although x-ray images have traditionally been captured on photographic film, the images are increasingly being made using digital technology and stored in computers.

X-rays help doctors detect many problems, including lung cancer, breast cancer (through mammography), skull fractures, pneumonia, broken bones, and dental problems.

To take an x-ray picture, you lie on an examining table or stand in front of a photographic plate. You may be given a lead apron to wear over the parts of your body that are not being examined to protect them from radiation.

The technician will make sure the machine is directed at the part of the body being examined and may step out of the room. He or she will ask you to hold your breath for a few seconds (to avoid body motion caused by breathing, which can blur the image) and then turn on the x-ray machine.

The beam passes through your body in a fraction of a second and causes no discomfort. X-ray pictures of the same body part may be taken from several angles. Usually, x-rays are used

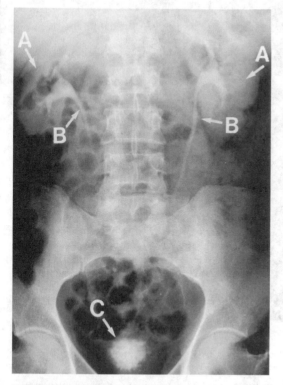

NORMAL INTRAVENOUS PYELOGRAM

In an intravenous pyelogram, a dye that shows up on x-rays is injected into the blood, and travels to highlight the kidneys (A), which are visible on both sides, as are the ureters (B). The dye also is seen collecting in the bladder (C).

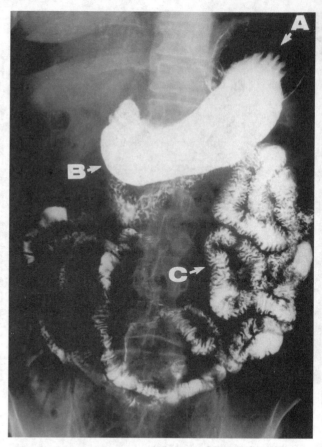

NORMAL UPPER GASTROINTESTINAL TRACT X-RAY

The upper part of the stomach (A) is filled with air and appears black. Swallowed barium, which shows up white on x-rays, reveals the lower part of the stomach (B). The small intestine (C) is clearly outlined.

to make images or photographs of one moment in time. However, a film or video camera can record action by using a constant beam of x-rays over a period of time to record multiple pictures in a series.

Another type of x-ray uses a contrast medium (dye) to better visualize parts of the body. The dye is a dense chemical that absorbs x-rays (as bone does), and therefore creates a white image on the film. In some cases, the dye is used to fill a space that

normally has only air in it, thereby revealing the shape of that space.

For example, a regular x-ray of your stomach cannot reveal much about the shape or lining of the stomach. If you drink the contrast medium, however, your stomach appears highlighted in white.

The contrast medium may also be given in an enema to reveal the shape of the large intestine. It can also be injected into the bloodstream to indicate the

shape or function of an organ or to look for areas of infection or bleeding or for a tumor.

One example of conventional x-ray imaging is pyelography, in which an iodine-containing contrast agent is injected into a vein and photographed as it reaches the kidneys, revealing the shape of the kidneys (particularly the inner part where urine collects) and the tubes (ureters) through which urine flows out of the kidneys.

Angiography

An angiogram is an x-ray picture of your veins or arteries that uses a contrast medium (usually iodine dye) to define the outlines of the blood vessel. The contrast helps show any blockages or unusual widening in the blood vessels.

Angiograms are complex procedures because the dye must be injected directly into the blood vessel being evaluated. The doctor uses a local anesthetic to numb an area of your skin and then guides a catheter (a plastic tube) through the skin and into a blood vessel near the skin, often an artery in the arm or leg.

The catheter is guided farther into the system of arteries until it reaches the target, such as the arteries of the heart, kidneys, or lungs. X-rays are taken while the catheter is being positioned so the catheter can be directed to the correct blood vessel.

Once the catheter is in posi-

tion, the contrast medium is injected. The movement of the contrast medium through the blood vessels is recorded by a camera or on a series of films.

Most people feel a sensation of warmth when the contrast medium is injected. As in any invasive procedure, there is a small risk of complications. Some people develop an allergic reaction to the contrast medium.

Allergy to Iodine in Contrast Medium

Some people have an allergic reaction to the iodine in the contrast medium (dye) injected during some imaging procedures. An allergic reaction to iodine can cause a rash, swelling of the face or throat, headache, abdominal pain, and vomiting.

People who have a higher risk of having an allergic reaction to the dye include those who have asthma or who have had a previous allergic reaction to more than one type of food or medicine.

If you think you may have an allergy to iodine, tell your doctor and radiologist. They can use a different type of contrast for the test or give you medicines beforehand to help prevent a reaction.

MAGNETIC RESONANCE ANGIOGRAPHY

Like magnetic resonance imaging (MRI), magnetic resonance angiography (MRA) uses a strong magnetic field and radio waves to produce images of internal organs. Unlike MRI, MRA shows blood vessels clearly. Unlike a conventional angiogram, it does not require the use of a needle and catheter or dye, or exposure to radiation. It is especially useful in investigating narrowing of arteries and aneurysms in the head and for viewing arteries in the abdomen and legs.

Before MRA was available, an x-ray angiogram was required in order to take pictures of the blood vessels. An angiogram still provides a more accurate picture of some blood vessels than current types of MRA.

MRA is painless. You lie still on a table in the center of a tube-shaped machine, which makes a thumping sound as it obtains the images. You should not have MRA if you have certain types of metal implants or devices, such as a brain aneurysm clip or a pacemaker. Tell your radiologist if you have any metal inside your body.

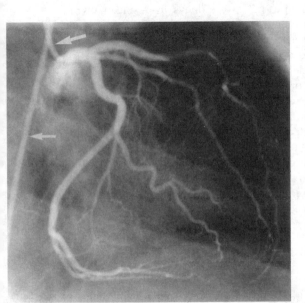

NORMAL CORONARY ANGIOGRAM

The straight white line at left (bottom arrow) is a catheter inside the aorta, the body's largest artery. X-ray dye is being injected from the tip of the catheter (top arrow) into the coronary arteries, which are the curved white lines. These arteries carry blood to the heart muscle.

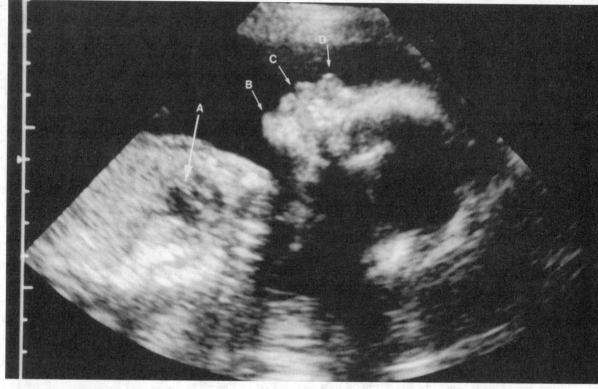

ULTRASOUND OF A FETUS

This ultrasound shows the head and chest of a fetus in profile. The heart (A) is visible in the chest. The chin (B), lips (C), and nose (D) can also be seen.

Conventional Ultrasound

Ultrasound uses sound waves instead of radiation to create pictures of internal body structures. It is similar to marine sonar, which sends out sound waves to detect objects in the ocean.

During an ultrasound examination, a handheld instrument transmits painless sound waves toward a part of your body. Some of the waves bounce off tissues and echo back to the surface, where the same instrument picks up their echo. A computer then transforms the sound waves into a picture that is displayed on a monitor.

Ultrasound is very useful for looking at fluid-filled organs, such as the gallbladder. However it is not very useful for examining parts of the body surrounded by bone (such as the brain) because sound waves do not pass through bone.

Ultrasound was originally used to visualize a fetus in the uterus. Today it is also used to look for cysts, tumors, and other abnormalities of organs such as the kidneys, liver, spleen, thyroid gland, breasts, bladder, testicles, ovaries, and eyes. In echocardiography, it is also used to examine the chambers of the heart.

An ultrasound examination takes from 15 to 30 minutes. You lie down or sit and a jelly is spread on the instrument to help it make good contact with your skin. The technician then slides the instrument to a variety of locations on your skin while viewing the image on the screen.

Computed Tomography

A computed tomography (CT) scan uses x-rays to obtain pictures of your body. But instead of passing a single, wide x-ray beam through your body to a flat sheet of x-ray film (and obtaining a simple picture like a chest x-ray), CT scanning sends numerous, very narrow x-ray beams through your body.

The beams are collected by a camera that rotates around you and the information is sent to a computer that combines the images to produce cross-sectional pictures of the body—as though a slice had been made through it. Like conventional x-rays, the beams are absorbed by some organs and tissues and easily pass through others.

For a CT scan, you lie still on a table that slides into a cylindrical scanner. The scanner rotates around you, taking pictures in one plane of the body from numerous angles. The table is then moved slightly and pictures are taken of the next "slice" of the body. In some machines, the table moves continuously; in others, it starts and stops. The scanner never touches you, but it can be noisy.

Some people feel claustrophobic inside the cylinder; your doctor can give you a sedative before the scan to lessen this feeling. For some CT scans, you are first injected with a contrast medium to make your blood vessels show up more clearly on the pictures. These contrast substances may cause a feeling of warmth when they are injected.

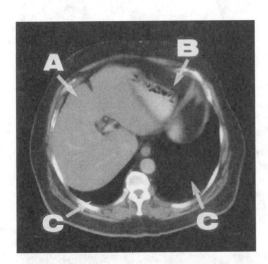

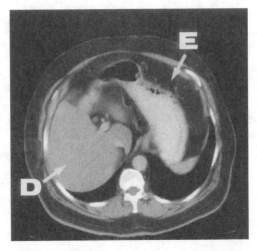

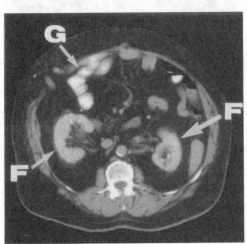

COMPUTED TOMOGRAPHY OF UPPER, MIDDLE, AND LOWER ABDOMEN

The cross-sectional slice (above left) from a computed tomography (CT) scan of the abdomen shows the liver as gray (A). The stomach (B) appears both black (air) and white (due to barium that was previously swallowed). The lungs (C) appear black because they contain air. The spine is the bright white area toward the bottom.

The slice above is taken slightly lower. The liver (D) and more of the stomach (E) are visible.

The slice at left is taken still lower in the abdomen. It shows the kidneys (F). Loops of small intestines toward the top of the image (G) are white because of barium that was swallowed previously (not as part of the CT scan).

HAVING A COMPUTED TOMOGRAPHY SCAN

For a computed tomography scan, you are positioned inside the scanner, which is like a large tunnel.

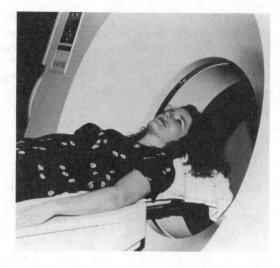

Some people are allergic to the contrast medium.

The pictures produced by a CT scan are more detailed than those of a conventional x-ray. In addition to showing a cross-section of the body, the images can be combined by the computer to produce a three-dimensional picture of internal organs.

CT scanning was originally used to look at the brain. Today it is used to help doctors investigate a wide variety of conditions, including tumors, aneurysms, organ damage, and infections.

Radiation Exposure

A rem is a unit of radiation used to measure the amount of damage to your body's tissue caused by radiation exposure. It stands for roentgen equivalents man (or mammal). The units shown below are given in millirems (mrem); 1,000 mrem are equivalent to 1 rem.

The average annual exposure to radiation in the United States is about 360 mrem. About 310 mrem come from natural sources; only about 50 mrem per year come from medical sources.

By way of comparison, the exposure limit for nuclear power plant workers is 5,000 mrem per year. Your doctor regulates your exposure to radiation by recommending only those medical tests whose potential diagnostic and treatment benefits outweigh the risks of exposure to radiation.

RADIATION FROM NATURAL SOURCES	DOSAGE IN MREM
Cosmic radiation in Denver, Colo	50 per year
Average U.S. terrestrial radiation	28 per year
Average U.S. cosmic radiation	27 per year
Cosmic radiation at sea level	26 per year
Natural gas in the home	9 per year
Sitting close to a TV	6 per year
Radiation in drinking water	5 per year
Pocket watch with radium dial	5 per year
Airplane trip	0.5 per hour

RADIATION FROM MEDICAL SOURCES	SINGLE EXPOSURE IN MREM
Computed tomography of head and body	1,100
Lower gastrointestinal tract series	405
Upper gastrointestinal tract series	245
Hip x-ray	83
Pelvic x-ray	44
Cervical (neck area) spine x-ray	22
Head and/or neck x-ray	20
Dental x-ray	10
Chest x-ray	8
Arm or leg x-ray	1

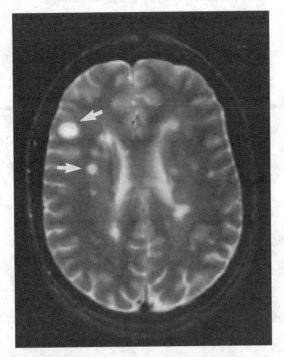

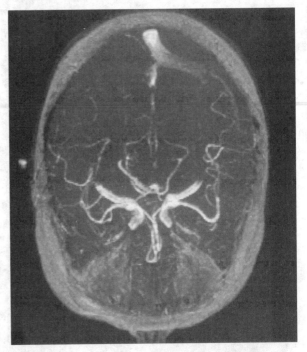

MAGNETIC RESONANCE IMAGING OF ABNORMAL BRAIN

On this scan of a person with multiple sclerosis, the bright white dots (arrows point to the largest ones) indicate areas damaged by multiple sclerosis.

MAGNETIC RESONANCE ANGIOGRAM OF NORMAL BRAIN

This view, taken looking down from the top of the head into the brain, shows blood flow through blood vessels (white), achieved without injecting x-ray dye. The blood vessels of the entire brain are visible.

Magnetic Resonance Imaging

Magnetic resonance imaging (MRI) does not use radiation to look inside the body. Instead, it uses a very large magnet, a radio-wave transmitter, and a computer to construct detailed pictures.

During an MRI scan, you lie on a table that slides into a machine that contains a large magnet and a radio-wave transmitter. Exposing your tissues to the magnetic field and to pulses of radio waves causes your tissues to emit signals that are detected by the machine that surrounds you. The information is then sent to the computer, which forms an image from the signals.

Tissues that have a high water content and a large number of hydrogen atoms, such as fat, show up as light images. Tissues that have less water and fewer hydrogen atoms, such as bone, appear darker. Sometimes, a contrast medium is injected into the blood to enhance the images.

Like CT scanning, MRI can show the insides of organs much better than conventional x-rays. People who have certain types of metal implants inside the body, such as a brain aneurysm clip or a pacemaker, cannot have an MRI because the strong magnetic field can dislodge the device.

Surgical clips and orthopedic metal implants are usually considered safe, but you should let the radiologist know if you have any metal inside your body.

Although MRI is painless, some people find the MRI cylinder makes them claustrophobic; it is also noisy. Many facilities provide headphones so you can listen to music to block the noise. Also, some MRI machines are more open; most of your body is not inside the cylinder and only the body part being scanned is covered by an arch containing the equipment.

MRI can provide pictures of body parts that are surrounded by bone, so it is particularly useful for viewing the brain and spinal cord. It is also commonly used to look at joints. A related technique, magnetic resonance angiography, may be used when detailed pictures of blood vessels are required.

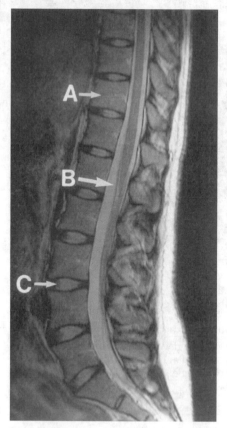

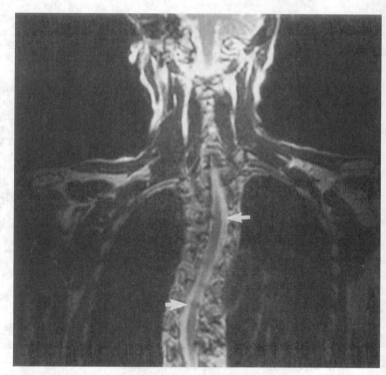

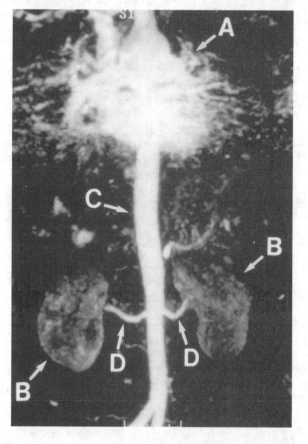

MAGNETIC RESONANCE IMAGING OF NORMAL SPINE

The magnetic resonance imaging scan above shows the structures of the spine, including bony vertebrae (A), spinal cord (B), and spongy disks (C) that lie between the vertebrae.

MAGNETIC RESONANCE IMAGING OF ABNORMAL SPINE

The scan above right shows the curved spine and spinal cord (arrows) of a person with scoliosis. When viewed from the front or back, the spine is normally straight.

MAGNETIC RESONANCE ARTERIOGRAPHY OF CHEST AND ABDOMEN

In the image at right, the heart (A) is seen at the top and the kidneys (B) are outlined on either side of the aorta (C), the largest artery in the body. The arteries supplying the kidneys (D) are clearly visible.

DIAGNOSTIC TESTS

Years ago, a doctor made a diagnosis on little more than the person's description of symptoms and the doctor's own observations. Today, a dizzying array of tests provides much more information.

The most commonly used tests are blood and urine analyses, which can reveal how well many of the organs and systems of the body are functioning. Many physicians start the diagnostic process with these and other less expensive and less invasive tests. More complex tests, such as imaging tests (see p.135), are performed only if necessary.

When your doctor suggests you have a test, you should understand why and exactly what is involved in having it. Some questions to ask your physician:

- Why was the test suggested?

- What will it show?

- What do I need to do to prepare for it?

- How will it feel?

- How long will it take?

- How will I feel afterward?

- Who will perform it?

- Does it have any risks?

- When will I learn the results?

- How might the results affect future treatment plans?

- How much will it cost?

Blood Tests

Your blood carries nourishing substances your body needs (such as oxygen and nutrients

How to Locate Tests in This Book

The descriptions of many common diagnostic tests are listed here; many more are described in Diseases and Disorders (see p.5). The most direct route to find the test you are interested in is through the Index (see p.1251). To find further information, look up the name of the test in the Index and note the page numbers on which it appears.

from food) and wastes that are eliminated by the liver, lungs, or kidneys. It also carries medicines to the parts of the body where they are needed.

Blood is composed of several types of blood cells as well as a salt-water fluid called plasma (see Blood Disorders, p.709). The following blood tests can reveal the presence of abnormal blood cells and can measure substances that are present in the blood's fluid.

ALANINE AMINOTRANSFERASE (ALT)

ALT is an enzyme normally found primarily in liver tissue. If the liver is injured, ALT spills into the blood. Elevated levels of ALT in the blood can indicate acute liver damage.

ALBUMIN

Albumin is a protein made by the liver and essential for normal body function. The levels of albumin in blood help your doctor diagnose liver and kidney disease. When people are seriously ill, from a temporary or ongoing illness, their albumin levels often fall.

ALCOHOL

Measuring the level of alcohol in the blood can determine if a person is legally drunk.

ALKALINE PHOSPHATASE

Alkaline phosphatase is an enzyme found in both liver and bone. When the liver is affected by disease, alkaline phosphatase enters the bloodstream. Elevated levels can indicate liver cancer, inflammation, hepatitis, gallstones, and bone disease. This test is usually done as part of liver function tests.

ALPHA FETOPROTEIN (AFP)

AFP is a protein produced by a fetus. High levels of AFP in a pregnant woman can indicate birth defects such as spina bifida and anencephaly (absence of the brain and/or spinal cord) in the fetus. High levels can also occur in people who have cancer of the liver or testicle, or who have hepatitis.

AMYLASE

Amylase is an enzyme produced by the pancreas. It aids in the digestion of starch molecules.

High blood levels of amylase may indicate a disease of the pancreas such as pancreatitis. This test is usually done at the same time as the lipase test (see p.156), another test for disease of the pancreas.

ANTINEUTROPHIL CYTOPLASMIC ANTIBODY (ANCA)

ANCAs are antibodies produced by various autoimmune conditions and aid in the diagnosis of those conditions. There are two types of ANCAs. The cANCA antibodies are quite specific for an unusual disorder, Wegener granulomatosis. pANCA antibodies are seen in conditions such as nephritis and colitis.

ANTINUCLEAR ANTIBODY (ANA)

ANAs are produced by the body when the immune system mistakenly recognizes the nuclei of some of its own cells as foreign. ANAs are found in the blood of people with autoimmune diseases such as lupus and rheumatoid arthritis. They are detected by looking at a blood sample using an ultraviolet microscope.

ARTERIAL BLOOD GAS (ABG)

This test measures the levels in the blood of the gases oxygen and carbon dioxide as well as the acid level in the arteries. The test can identify various problems involving the lungs, heart, and kidneys.

ASPARTATE AMINOTRANSFERASE (AST)

AST is an enzyme normally found primarily in liver and heart tissue. If the liver or heart is injured, AST spills into the blood, raising the blood level above normal.

BETA HUMAN CHORIONIC GONADOTROPIN (BETA HCG)

Beta hCG is a hormone produced when a fertilized egg implants in the uterus. It stimulates the body to secrete the hormones estrogen and progesterone, both of which help to maintain pregnancy. Beta hCG can be detected in a pregnant woman's blood and urine to verify pregnancy. The blood test is slightly more accurate, but urine tests are used more often because samples are easier to obtain.

BILIRUBIN

Bilirubin is the orange-colored pigment produced when the liver metabolizes the hemoglobin in red blood cells. Bilirubin collects in the liver, is excreted in bowel movements, and colors the stool. When liver disease causes bilirubin to accumulate abnormally, it causes jaundice (yellowing of the skin and whites of the eyes). Testing for bilirubin can point to liver disease, bile duct obstruction, and some forms of anemia.

BLOOD UREA NITROGEN (BUN)

Urea nitrogen is a waste product that is usually filtered out of the blood as it passes through the kidneys. An abnormal BUN level can indicate that the kidneys are not working properly. It can also show the degree to which a person is dehydrated.

CALCIUM

Calcium is a naturally occurring mineral that is stored in bones. It plays a role in many body functions, including the heartbeat and the transmission of messages along nerves. Abnormal levels of calcium can indicate kidney disease, vitamin D deficiency, parathyroid gland problems, or bone cancer.

CARBAMAZEPINE

Carbamazepine is an anticonvulsant drug used to treat seizure disorders and bipolar disorder. To avoid toxicity, close monitoring of its concentration in the blood is necessary.

CARCINOEMBRYONIC ANTIGEN (CEA)

Levels of the protein CEA are elevated in cancers of the digestive system and are monitored during cancer treatment. High CEA levels may also be found in people who have hepatitis or smoke heavily.

COMPLEMENT

Complement is the name of a group of blood proteins that help the body destroy foreign substances and microorganisms. In some active inflammatory diseases (such as lupus), levels are low; in others, levels are high.

COMPLETE BLOOD CELL COUNT (CBC)

A complete blood cell count is one of the most common laboratory tests. It measures the number of several blood components, including red blood cells, different types of white blood cells, and platelets. It also measures the size of red blood cells. Abnormal findings can indicate anemia, infection, and other conditions.

CORTISOL

Cortisol is a hormone secreted by the adrenal glands. It helps regulate the immune system. Abnormal levels can indicate a hormonal problem such as Cushing syndrome or Addison disease.

C-REACTIVE PROTEIN

These proteins are usually produced within 24 to 48 hours of the onset of inflammation. Testing for C-reactive protein does not point to a specific disease, but can indicate underlying inflammation. C-reactive proteins may be produced with disorders such as rheumatic fever, arthritis, coronary artery disease, and other conditions.

CREATINE KINASE (CK)

This enzyme is found mainly in the heart and other muscles. When the heart or other muscle tissue is injured, CK spills into the blood, raising the blood level of the enzyme. Measuring the levels of CK (particularly a form called "MB") is often used to diagnose a heart attack. The levels may also be elevated in various muscle diseases.

CREATININE

Creatinine is a waste product that is normally filtered out of the blood by the kidneys. Measuring the amount of creatinine in the blood over time reveals how well the kidneys are working.

FERRITIN

Ferritin is a protein that aids in the body's ability to store iron. Measuring the amount of ferritin in the blood indicates how much iron is stored in the body. This test is used to help diagnose iron deficiency and iron overload.

FOLATE (FOLIC ACID)

Folate is a term for a group of vitamins (including folic acid) that is essential for many body functions. A deficiency of folate, which is more common during pregnancy, can cause anemia, abnormal fetal growth, graying hair, diarrhea, and other conditions. Folate deficiency may also contribute to atherosclerosis.

FOLLICLE-STIMULATING HORMONE (FSH)

This hormone is produced by the pituitary gland; it triggers the growth of sperm in males and the development of eggs in females. Measuring FSH level can help diagnose fertility problems and the onset of menopause.

GLUCOSE

Glucose (blood sugar) is a breakdown product of food that is absorbed into the blood from the intestines and then used as energy for cells. Testing the level of glucose can indicate abnormally high glucose levels (which occur in diabetes) or abnormally low levels (which occur in overtreatment of diabetes and other rare conditions).

GLUCOSE TOLERANCE

This test measures the amount of glucose in the blood at different times over a period of several hours following a sugary meal. You eat a special diet for several days before the test and then drink a solution with a set amount of glucose in it. The test is most often used to diagnose diabetes.

HEMATOCRIT

This test indicates how much of total blood volume is composed of red blood cells. It can be used to diagnose different types of anemia. This test is done as part of a complete blood cell count.

HEMOGLOBIN

Hemoglobin is a substance found in red blood cells. It carries oxygen from the lungs to the rest of the body and carbon dioxide back to the lungs, where it is exhaled. A hemoglobin test can indicate if you are anemic.

HEMOGLOBIN ELECTROPHORESIS

This test detects the presence of an abnormal form of hemoglobin, which occurs in genetic blood diseases such as sickle cell anemia.

IRON

This common metal is an essential part of hemoglobin, the oxygen-carrying substance in red blood cells. A lack of iron due to poor diet, poor absorption, or chronic bleeding can cause iron deficiency anemia. An iron test determines how much iron is in the blood.

IRON BINDING CAPACITY

This test measures the levels of the protein transferrin, which carries iron from the bloodstream into the bone marrow, where it is incorporated into new blood cells. It is usually used to help diagnose the cause of anemia.

LACTATE DEHYDROGENASE (LDH)

LDH is an enzyme normally found in tissues of the heart, liver, lungs, and kidneys. When one of those organs is damaged, LDH is released into the bloodstream. This test is commonly used to help diagnose a heart attack, liver disease, or diseases that cause red blood cells to be destroyed.

LEAD

Lead is a common metal that is normally found only in very low amounts in the body; it can be toxic at higher levels. Children and adults can develop lead poisoning by eating or inhaling lead from paint chips, drinking water from lead pipes, or by eating from lead-glazed pottery, as well as other means. Lead poisoning can cause learning disabilities and severe physical symptoms.

LIPASE

Lipase is an enzyme produced by the pancreas; it helps the body break down fats. When present in the blood in high amounts, it can indicate pancreatitis. This test is usually done at the same time as the amylase test (see p.153).

LUTEINIZING HORMONE (LH)

LH is produced by the pituitary gland. It stimulates the secretion of other hormones by the ovaries and testicles, triggering ovulation and sperm production. Testing blood levels of LH can help evaluate fertility problems or the cause of absent menstrual periods. It also helps monitor therapies being used to induce ovulation.

PARATHYROID HORMONE

Parathyroid hormone is produced by the parathyroid glands, which are small structures situated near the thyroid gland. This hormone regulates the level of calcium and phosphate in the body. Testing the blood for parathyroid hormone can indicate overactive or underactive parathyroid glands.

PARTIAL THROMBOPLASTIN TIME (PTT)

This test is one measure of how well your blood is clotting. It can detect low levels of different blood substances that help blood clot. The test is performed before surgery to monitor people on blood-thinning medicines and to diagnose diseases such as hemophilia.

PHENOBARBITAL

Phenobarbital is a drug used to control seizures; it is also used as a sedative. The level of phenobarbital in the blood is measured to ensure that the dosage is high enough to control seizures but not so high that it will cause a toxic reaction. In people who are unconscious for unknown reasons, the level is often tested to determine if an overdose has been taken.

PHENYTOIN

Phenytoin is an anticonvulsant used primarily to treat seizure disorders. The phenytoin blood level is measured to ensure that the dosage is high enough to control seizures but not so high that it will cause a toxic reaction.

PHOSPHATE

Phosphates play a role in the storage and use of energy and other critical body functions. Phosphate levels are often measured to help diagnose bone and kidney conditions and abnormalities of parathyroid hormone.

PLATELET COUNT

Platelets are small, disk-shaped cell fragments that play a role in blood clotting. This test evaluates the amount of platelets in a blood sample. Both low and high levels, which can alter normal blood clotting, occur in several diseases.

POTASSIUM

Potassium is a mineral needed for proper muscle function, nerve impulse conduction, and other functions in the body. A severe imbalance in potassium levels can cause an irregular heartbeat. Low potassium levels are usually caused by diuretic drugs rather than by an underlying disease. Testing for potassium levels is often done to evaluate the amount in the blood of people taking diuretic drugs.

PROLACTIN

Prolactin is a hormone produced by the pituitary gland. It acts with estrogen and other hormones to produce breast milk and to prepare the breasts for nursing. Elevated blood levels are caused by pituitary gland tumors and can lead to leakage of milk from the breasts in non-nursing women, and breast swelling and impotence in men.

PROSTATE-SPECIFIC ANTIGEN (PSA)

PSA is a protein produced by the prostate gland. Many men with prostate cancer have elevated PSA levels, but many men with noncancerous prostate conditions also have high PSA levels. In men who are being treated for prostate cancer, a falling PSA level is an indication that the treatment is working.

PROTHROMBIN TIME (PT)

PT is one measure of the blood's ability to clot, and indicates the blood level of several essential blood-clotting factors. The test is often done before surgery to diagnose liver disease and to monitor people taking blood-thinning medicine.

RADIOALLERGOSORBENT (RAST)

In certain allergic conditions, the immune system produces an unusually large amount of immunoglobulin E (IgE) antibodies against an allergen (such as ragweed, cat dander, or certain foods). RAST tests detect the presence of IgE against specific antigens in the blood, and thus indicate what you are allergic to.

RETICULOCYTE COUNT

A reticulocyte is an immature red blood cell normally present in very low quantities. A larger-than-normal number of reticulocytes may indicate that the body is trying to combat anemia or restore blood volume after excessive bleeding.

RHEUMATOID FACTOR

Rheumatoid factor is a protein that the immune system produces, usually in people who have rheumatoid arthritis. Testing for rheumatoid factor is often done to help diagnose rheumatoid arthritis. Rheumatoid factor may also be found in people who have other diseases.

RH-FACTOR COMPATIBILITY

Rh factor is an antigen found in the blood of about 85% of all people; these people are said to be Rh positive. The rest of the population is Rh negative. Rh testing is done as a part of the process of determining your blood type, so that you receive a blood transfusion only from someone with the same Rh status. Rh factor is also tested in all pregnant women because the fetus can be damaged if its cells are Rh positive and its mother's cells are Rh negative.

SEDIMENTATION RATE

This test determines the rate at which red blood cells settle to the bottom of a test tube. The rate is elevated in various infections, inflammatory diseases, and cancers.

SERUM PROTEIN ELECTROPHORESIS

This test is used to screen the blood for abnormally high levels of several proteins, particularly immunoglobulins and related molecules. It is most often used to help diagnose the blood cell disease multiple myeloma.

SODIUM

The mineral sodium is important in maintaining the body's water balance and also plays a role in muscle contraction and nerve impulse transmission. The body normally keeps sodium levels under tight control, but sodium levels can become abnormally high or low in various diseases.

THEOPHYLLINE

Theophylline is a drug used to treat asthma. It can cause abnormal heart rhythms or seizures in higher concentrations, so the levels of the drug in the bloodstream must be carefully monitored.

THYROID-STIMULATING HORMONE (TSH)

TSH is produced by the pituitary gland and helps regulate the production of triiodothyronine and thyroxine by the thyroid gland. When thyroid hormones are too low or too high, TSH signals the thyroid to increase or decrease production. The TSH test is usually used to diagnose hyperthyroidism or hypothyroidism.

THYROXINE (T_4)

The T_4 hormone, produced by the thyroid gland, helps regulate growth and development as well as control metabolism and body temperature. Elevated levels indicate hyperthyroidism; reduced levels indicate hypothyroidism.

TOXIC SCREEN

A toxic screen tests the blood for the presence of potentially poisonous substances, such as narcotics, tranquilizers, antidepressants, antipsychotic medicines, alcohol, amphetamines, and hallucinogens. It is usually done in an emergency setting to investigate symptoms such as coma, confusion, irrational behavior, or heart irregularities.

TRICYCLIC LEVEL

Tricyclic antidepressants (also called heterocyclics) are commonly used to treat depression. Because elevated levels can cause heart damage, the blood levels of these drugs must be periodically monitored.

TRIGLYCERIDES

Triglycerides are fats that travel in the bloodstream and can contribute to cardiac disease and other conditions. Triglyceride levels are often checked when cholesterol levels are tested to determine your risk for developing heart disease.

TRIIODOTHYRONINE (T₃)

The T_3 hormone, produced by the thyroid gland, helps regulate growth and development as well as control metabolism and body temperature. Elevated levels indicate hyperthyroidism; reduced levels indicate hypothyroidism.

URIC ACID

Uric acid is a waste product that is normally excreted by the kidneys. High blood levels of uric acid usually occur with the inflammatory condition gout, and can also occur with leukemia and severe kidney damage.

VITAMIN B₁₂

Low levels of vitamin B_{12} can be caused by an inadequate intake of the vitamin in the diet (such as in vegetarians) or by conditions in which the intestines and stomach are unable to absorb the vitamin. Low levels of vitamin B_{12} cause anemia and neurological and other conditions.

WHITE BLOOD CELL COUNT

White blood cells help the body fight infections. The test is part of a complete blood cell count, and is often done when infection is suspected. Leukemia also causes elevated numbers of white blood cells. Certain drug reactions and diseases can cause low numbers of white blood cells.

WHITE BLOOD CELL DIFFERENTIAL CELL COUNT

The body produces different types of white blood cells. This test reveals the relative percentages of each type in the blood, which can help determine the kind of infection (such as bacterial versus viral) you might have.

Urine Tests

As blood circulates through your body, it picks up many waste substances. To rid itself of waste products, blood passes through the kidneys, which filter out substances that are not needed and expel them in urine. For a more complete description, see How You Eliminate Wastes and Keep Fluids in Balance (p.114).

Testing urine for the high or low levels of various chemicals can reveal many things about how your body is functioning.

A test sample is easily obtained by urinating into a container. Some urine tests are done in the doctor's office with chemically treated paper. Others are performed in an outside laboratory. (See also Common Tests for Kidney and Urinary Tract Disorders, p.805.)

BETA HUMAN CHORIONIC GONADOTROPIN (BETA HCG)

Beta hCG is a hormone produced soon after a fertilized egg implants in the uterus. Beta hCG can be detected in both a woman's urine and blood. The urine test is used in the doctor's office and also in home test kits.

BLOOD

Blood is not usually found in the urine. Testing for blood in urine is usually performed as part of a complete urinalysis. Its presence can indicate kidney stones, urinary tract infection, tumors of the urinary tract, or other problems.

CALCIUM

Calcium is important in maintaining several metabolic functions in the body. Abnormal levels can occur in various diseases, including disorders of the parathyroid glands. Elevated levels often occur in people who form calcium-containing kidney stones.

CASTS

Casts are tubular-shaped clumps of material or cells formed in the kidney tubules and excreted in the urine. Some kinds of casts (such as red blood cell casts) indicate disease, whereas others are normal.

CATECHOLAMINES

Catecholamines, which include epinephrine and norepinephrine, are secreted by the adrenal glands. Their levels are measured in people who have high blood pressure to determine if the condition is being caused by a tumor called a pheochromocytoma. This tumor often occurs in the adrenal gland and produces high levels of catecholamines.

CREATININE

This substance is eliminated from the body by the kidneys. The amount of creatinine excreted in the urine can tell doctors whether kidneys are functioning properly.

GLUCOSE

When glucose (blood sugar) levels are elevated in the blood, such as in diabetes, glucose is excreted in the urine. Urine sugar tests are a simple way of suspecting diabetes and of monitoring how well controlled diabetes is.

5-HYDROXYINDOLEACETIC ACID (5-HIAA)

5-HIAA is a normal byproduct of the body's metabolic processes. Its level in urine may be elevated in people with carcinoid cell tumors. These unusual tumors cause high levels of 5-HIAA in both blood and urine.

LEUKOCYTE ESTERASE

This enzyme is found in some white blood cells. When it is detected in urine, it indicates that there are white blood cells in the urine due to inflammation, which can be caused by a bacterial infection.

METANEPHRINES

Metanephrines may be present in high levels in people with the tumor pheochromocytoma (see Catecholamines, p.158).

NITRITES

The bacteria that cause urinary infections cause substances called nitrites to appear in the urine. Elevated urine nitrite levels can indicate the presence of a urinary infection.

PROTEIN

Proteins are not usually found in urine because they are large molecules that normally stay in the blood and are not passed into the urine. If the kidneys' filtering system is damaged, proteins may pass through and be detected in the urine.

RED BLOOD CELLS

Red blood cells are not normally found in the urine and can indicate an abnormality of the urinary tract such as an infection, a tumor, or nephritis.

SPECIFIC GRAVITY

This test measures the concentration of particles in the urine and is used to gauge how well a person is hydrated and how well the kidneys are functioning in keeping body fluid at the right levels.

URIC ACID

Uric acid is a component of the genetic material DNA. Abnormally high levels of uric acid can indicate gout, kidney failure, or other conditions. People with recurring uric acid–containing kidney stones often have high levels of uric acid in their urine.

WHITE BLOOD CELLS

When white blood cells are found in the urine, it usually indicates an infection of the kidneys or bladder.

Cytology (Cell) Tests

Cytology tests involve looking at cells under a microscope for abnormal shapes that indicate the cells are turning or have turned cancerous.

A Pap smear is an example of a cytology test. In a Pap smear, a sample of cells is taken from a woman's cervix and smeared onto a slide. When examined under a microscope, the cells are ranked according to one of five classes, ranging from normal through clearly cancerous (see p.1071).

Because a cytology test can identify cell changes at their earliest stages, it is a useful tool in diagnosing cancer at a stage when it is most easily treated, as well as identifying precancerous cell changes that should be monitored.

Tests for Blood in Bowel Movements

Many conditions can cause bleeding in the gastrointestinal tract. Sometimes the bleeding is apparent, such as when a person vomits blood or passes bright red blood in a bowel movement. Sometimes, however, the bleeding is not obvious, and a test of the bowel movements is needed to detect it.

For a stool sample, you will be asked to defecate and then transfer a small amount of the stool, using a small wooden spatula, to a container or a special card. (See also Tests That Detect Blood in Bowel Movements, p.79.) Alternatively, your doctor may take a stool sample during a rectal examination.

Microbiology Tests

Several common types of microbiology tests are described here:

CULTURES

Cultures are used to identify microorganisms such as bacteria that are causing disease. To perform a culture, a cotton swab or similar device is used to collect possibly infected material from such areas as the throat or vagina. The sample is sent to a laboratory, where it is smeared on top of or poked into a nutrient gel or fluid. Different bacteria grow in different nutrient gels.

When a few invisible bacteria multiply on the nutrient gel, they form colonies of millions of bacteria that are visible to the eye. These bacterial colonies can then be tested by chemical techniques and by microscopic examination to determine what kind of bacteria they are. Cultures take a day or more to grow and be analyzed.

STAINS

One important way of identifying the kind of bacteria causing an infection is to stain the wall of the bacterium. The most commonly used stain is called the Gram stain, which turns some bacteria a violet-blue (gram-positive bacteria) or pink (gram-negative bacteria).

Along with the shape of a bacterium, the stain helps indicate the kind of bacterium present. The results of a stain can be known in a few minutes.

ANTIBACTERIAL SENSITIVITY

After a disease-causing bacterium has been identified in the laboratory, it may be subjected to an antibacterial sensitivity test to see which antibiotic will be effective in killing it.

The most common method is to place several paper disks, each soaked in different antibiotics, on top of a nutrient gel on which the bacteria are growing. The degree to which bacteria do not grow near each disk indicates how sensitive the bacteria are to each antibiotic.

MICROSCOPIC OBSERVATION

Many disease-causing microorganisms can be identified under the microscope, with or without any special stains. Some, such as viruses, are too small to be seen with the kind of light microscope found in a doctor's office, although they can be seen with the much more powerful electron microscope.

Looking at samples of blood, phlegm (sputum), urine, feces, pus, and other secretions, laboratory technicians can identify many types of bacteria, fungi, protozoa, and worms.

ANTIBODIES

When a foreign infectious agent or substance (such as an allergen like ragweed pollen) enters the body, the immune system recognizes parts (called antigens) of the agent or substance as foreign, and produces antibodies specifically designed to attach to and help destroy the intruder. A blood test for these antibodies can reveal the type of foreign infectious agent or substance that has entered the body.

Autoantibodies, which are antibodies that the immune system has mistakenly produced against its own tissues, can occur in autoimmune diseases (see p.870) and are also detectable.

ANTIGENS

An antigen is a part of a natural or foreign agent or substance that can be recognized by the immune system. If it is foreign, its presence triggers the immune system to try to attack it. In some cases, antigen tests can provide a more accurate diagnosis than antibody tests. They are most commonly used to detect specific infectious agents, such as hepatitis B and Legionnaires disease.

NUCLEIC ACIDS

Every cell in the body and every kind of infectious agent (except prions) contains nucleic acids. The nucleic acids of an infectious agent are like a fingerprint that identifies the agent.

Tests that measure the type and the amount of nucleic acids are increasingly used to diagnose infectious diseases, and to monitor the effects of treatment.

The most commonly used test for nucleic acid is called the polymerase chain reaction (PCR). It can detect a very small amount of foreign nucleic acid, such as from a virus, in human tissues. It can find the proverbial needle in a haystack. The technique finds and then amplifies the nucleic acid. Once the amount is amplified, the structure of the nucleic acid can be determined.

Nucleic acid testing can also be used to detect unusual human nucleic acids such as cancer-causing genes. This technique is rapidly improving the accuracy of determining whether cancer has spread to various parts of the body. The process is called cancer staging and leads to improved choice of treatment and more accurate information about prognosis (outlook).

TOXINS

Some microorganisms that invade the body produce toxins, or poisons, that are responsible for damaging the body. The toxins can often be detected by performing tests on body fluids. Examples include the toxin that causes toxic shock syndrome and the toxin that causes the *Clostridium difficile* infection in the intestine.

OTHER MICROBIOLOGY TESTS
DARK-FIELD EXAMINATION FOR SYPHILIS

Treponema pallidum, the bacterium that causes syphilis, is not easily seen using a standard microscope. One way to identify it is to examine a specimen under a special dark-field microscope, in which organisms are made to glow against a dark background.

FECAL LEUKOCYTES

Fecal leukocytes are white blood cells in a stool sample. They are found in some kinds of infections that cause diarrhea, but not in all kinds.

SKIN FUNGUS

In many cases, a skin fungus can be readily seen, scraped off, and sent to a laboratory for analysis. At other times, the fungus may not be easily seen with the naked eye. In such cases, shining a special ultraviolet light on it may make it visible.

STOOL EXAMINATION FOR OVA (EGGS) AND PARASITES

A stool sample can be examined under a microscope for parasites and their eggs. This test can uncover various protozoa and worms that cause infections of the digestive system.

THICK BLOOD SMEAR FOR RED BLOOD CELL PARASITES

This microscopic inspection of a blood sample is used to detect the parasites that cause diseases such as malaria and babesiosis.

Biopsies

A biopsy is a sample of tissue that is taken from the body and examined under the microscope. Biopsies are performed during surgery, during endoscopy (see p.142), and by passing needles deep into parts of the body, often with the needle guided by a diagnostic imaging technique (see p.135).

Biopsies are used to diagnose many different conditions. The most common reason for a biopsy is a suspicion of cancer or the presence of precancerous cells. Biopsies can also be used to diagnose cirrhosis of the liver, kidney inflammation, bone infections, and other conditions.

Taps

In addition to blood, your body contains other reservoirs of body fluids. Some reservoirs are normal (such as the spinal fluid that bathes the brain and spinal cord) and some are abnormal (such as collections of fluid at the bottom of the lung called pleural effusions or collections of fluid in the abdomen called ascites).

The fluid is usually withdrawn from the body by means of a needle inserted through the skin and into the cavity containing the fluid. Once the fluid is removed, it is analyzed using chemical and microbiology tests.

A lumbar puncture (also known as a spinal tap) is one of the most common taps. You lie on your side with your legs drawn up. A local anesthetic is used to deaden the skin and a needle is inserted between two vertebrae in the lower back and then into the spinal canal. A small amount of cerebrospinal fluid is withdrawn for analysis.

Other taps withdraw fluid from the abdomen (paracentesis), uterus (amniocentesis), joints (arthrocentesis), pleural cavity of the lungs (thoracentesis), the cavity around the heart (pericardicentesis), and the eardrum (tympanocentesis).

Bone Density Tests

With age, some people (primarily women) develop abnormally porous bones, a condition known as osteoporosis. Osteoporosis weakens bone structure, causing bone to lose mass and strength.

Bone density tests can reveal how much mineral loss and bone thinning has occurred. Several tests may be used to gauge bone density, but the most reliable is dual energy x-ray absorptiometry (DXA). In DXA, you lie on a table while an imager similar to a standard x-ray machine (but which delivers a lower dose of radiation) passes over your body. The degree to which the radiation is absorbed by the bones determines their density.

Manometry

Manometry is used to measure the amount of pressure in a particular part of the body. It is used most often to measure increased pressure at the bottom of the esophagus, where it passes into the stomach.

Another form of manometry, tympanometry, is used to estimate the amount of pressure needed to move the eardrum (when there is a middle ear infection, more pressure is required to move the eardrum). A manometer may also be used during a lumbar puncture to evaluate the pressure in the spinal canal.

Electrical Studies

Your body depends on electrical energy to perform many functions, such as heartbeat and muscle contractions. This energy can be detected on the outside of the body through electrodes placed on the skin. Abnormal readings are used to help diagnose conditions such as coronary artery disease or epilepsy.

Two common electrical studies are an electrocardiogram (see p.135) and electroencephalogram (see p.136).

Some of the electrical studies doctors use to evaluate disorders of the brain and nerves are described below:

EVOKED POTENTIALS

These tests monitor how the brain reacts to various stimuli. Electrodes are positioned on the person's scalp and the brain is stimulated with light, noise, or touch. The brain's electrical responses can indicate disorders such as multiple sclerosis or epilepsy.

ELECTRONYSTAGMOGRAPHY

Electrodes measure the movement of eye muscles. Abnormal eye movements (called nystagmus) may occur without provocation or during a caloric test, in which water of various temperatures is squirted into the ear canal.

ELECTROMYOGRAPHY

An electromyogram measures the electrical activity in muscle. A thin needle with a recording electrode is inserted into the muscle. Electrical impulses created while you contract and relax the muscle are then measured. Electromyography can be used to diagnose disorders such as muscular dystrophy.

NERVE CONDUCTION STUDY

This test uses skin electrodes to study the functioning of a particular nerve. A mild electrical impulse is sent into the nerve, and the electrodes record the time it takes for the impulse to travel the length of the nerve. It is often used to diagnose carpal tunnel syndrome, in which a pinching of the median nerve in the wrist delays the electrical impulse.

Skin Tests

Skin tests are used to diagnose a wide range of conditions, ranging from allergies to infections such as tuberculosis. Common procedures include injecting a substance just below the skin surface or taping a small patch that has been soaked in the agent to the skin surface.

To test for allergies, a small amount of each possible allergen is placed on the skin or injected into it; if a reaction develops, the person is allergic to that substance.

To test for tuberculosis exposure, a small amount of dead tuberculosis bacteria (known as a purified protein derivative) is injected under the skin. The injection site is later examined for a reaction.

Sometimes skin testing is performed to see if a person's immune system is underactive, which can occur in serious infections or cancers.

Chromosome Tests

Chromosome analysis involves extracting the chromosomes from some of your cells and examining them under a microscope to see if they are normal in number and structure.

The most common chromosomal disorder is Down syndrome, which is caused by an extra chromosome. Instead of two copies of chromosome number 21, there are three. Fetal chromosomes are obtained either through amniocentesis (see p.917) or chorionic villus sampling (see p.918), which provides a sample of the placental tissue. See also Understanding Genetics, p.126.

GOING TO THE HOSPITAL

It is likely that you will need to be hospitalized some time during your life—for a diagnostic test or surgery, to help you recover from a disease or accident, or during labor and delivery of a baby.

Today, due to technological advances, many conditions that in the past were treated with long hospital stays are treated on an outpatient basis or require only a brief hospital stay.

Financial incentives to shorten hospital stays have also resulted in increased availability of home health services such as visiting nurses, physical therapists, and home health aids.

Before You Enter the Hospital

You will be admitted to a hospital only with a doctor's authorization. The doctor must be on the admitting hospital's staff and he or she must have privileges to admit patients to that hospital.

Hospitals have the right to decide which doctors they will appoint to their staffs. Appointment to the medical staff of the most highly rated hospitals is sought by many doctors, but granted only to some. In considering whether to appoint a doctor to its staff, the hospital judges the quality of the doctor's training and certification by professional societies, as well as the doctor's past performance at other hospitals (taking into consideration factors such as malpractice suits).

Some doctors can admit patients to more than one hospital. In choosing a primary care physician, or in working with your primary care physician to pick a specialist, you may want to consider the hospital with which that physician is affiliated. What is its reputation? Is it conveniently located? Are there other factors that matter (such as whether it is affiliated with a particular religion)?

An admission to the hospital can be either an emergency admission or an elective admission. An elective admission is scheduled for some future time. A physical examination and diagnostic tests are often arranged in the days prior to a scheduled elective admission. For emergency admissions, this information is obtained in the hospital emergency or admitting department.

Particularly when an elective admission for a surgical procedure has been recommended, some people seek (or their insurance companies require) a second opinion as to whether surgery is necessary or whether the proper surgical procedure has been planned.

When the second opinion differs from the first, it does not mean that the second opinion is correct or incorrect. Two knowledgeable doctors may simply disagree; different doctors have different ways of approaching a problem. A second opinion can give you more confidence about the initial recommendation or it can guide you toward another form of treatment.

HAVING AN ADVOCATE

It can be useful to bring a relative or friend with you to your doctor visits before hospitalization and to accompany you during some parts of your hospitalization.

Someone who is well versed in your medical condition and who knows your wishes may be particularly helpful. This person can take notes during discussions with your doctor, surgeons, and other specialists and can be nearby when procedures are performed. He or she can also be with you in the hospital and relay your needs to the doctors and nurses.

PLANNING YOUR HOSPITALIZATION

If your primary care doctor recommends a procedure by a specialist, you can meet with and interview the physician who will perform it. It is appropriate to ask how often the specialist has performed the procedure, what percentage of his or her patients have had complications, and if he or she is board certified (see p.18).

Ask if he or she will perform the procedure alone or if a doctor in training will be present or participate. You should be open to a trainee participating in your care or surgery for two reasons. First, the senior doctor closely supervises the trainees. Second, the very best physicians and surgeons often work in hospitals that have active training programs; if you want these senior physicians to be in charge of your care, you may have to accept the involvement of trainees.

In preparation for hospitalization, many doctors suggest getting plenty of rest, eating well, exercising moderately, avoiding stress, and limiting alcohol.

If you use tobacco, the period before hospitalization is an excellent time to quit (see p.60). For some procedures, including any surgery that involves general anesthesia, quitting ahead of time is particularly important.

Choosing a Hospital

Your primary care physician will help you consider which hospital is best-equipped for the procedure you will have. When looking at your hospital choices, there are several factors to consider. One is the hospital staff's experience with the procedure you will have. If it is a highly complex procedure (such as a bone marrow transplant), your doctor may refer you to a hospital whose staff has expertise in that area.

Another factor is the rating of the hospital by the accreditation authorities. You can obtain information from organizations that inspect and accredit hospitals. The Joint Commission on Accreditation of Healthcare Organizations (JCAHO) (see p.21) inspects about 18,000 facilities regularly. Ask your librarian about local hospital ratings.

TYPES OF ACUTE-CARE HOSPITALS

Acute care hospitals are designed to care for people with serious conditions, rather than to provide long-term rehabilitation or care.

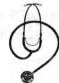

Hospitalization: Questions to Ask Your Doctor

Here are some questions to ask your doctor before you are hospitalized:

- Is there anything I can do in the weeks before hospitalization to prepare?

- How long will I be in the hospital if all goes well?

- What kinds of complications might develop from the hospitalization itself or from the specific treatments I will get in the hospital?

- What can I expect after surgery? Will I need to stay in bed or will I be out of bed and moving around shortly afterward?

- What sorts of monitors or other equipment will be used?

- How likely is it that I will require a blood transfusion during surgery? Should I donate my own blood (see p.711) several weeks before surgery?

- How long will it take until I can resume normal activities?

- After I am discharged, will I need the services of a visiting nurse, home health aid, or physical therapist? Will family members need to help care for me?

There are several kinds of acute-care hospitals:

Community hospitals These facilities serve the more common medical needs of the community, focusing on patient care rather than research. Some community hospitals take care of complex medical problems; others provide care mainly for straightforward problems. A big advantage of many community hospitals is that they are located close to where you (and visiting family members and friends) live.

Specialty centers These hospitals are geared toward treating specific types of diseases (such as cancer or orthopedic problems) or specific groups (such as children).

Academic medical centers These institutions often include the care of people with the most complex medical problems. They also train doctors and other health professionals and conduct medical research. They are usually affiliated with medical schools. Academic medical centers are often the most highly respected hospitals in their communities and invariably rank at the top of the lists of the nation's leading hospitals. At academic medical centers, doctors in training (such as interns, residents, and fellows) are likely to play a direct role in your care.

Teaching hospitals All academic medical centers and many community hospitals train doctors. They include medical students (who do not yet have their doctor-of-medicine degree) and interns, residents, and fellows (who have their degree but are getting additional training). In general, teaching hospitals in a community are highly respected for the care they provide because they attract a talented medical staff and, through teaching, keep the staff up-to-date.

Public hospitals These hospitals are owned by the federal or local government and usually provide care regardless of ability to pay. Many of these hospitals offer excellent care and many are also teaching hospitals. Public hospitals are often part of academic medical centers.

TYPES OF CHRONIC (LONG-TERM) CARE FACILITIES

Patients are frequently discharged from an acute care hospital to a chronic care facility, where they remain 24 hours a day. Chronic care facilities are very different from each other in many respects.

Rehabilitation hospitals These are institutions where patients are sent to receive the care that is necessary to improve their level of function. For example, they may need many weeks or months of physical therapy to recover their strength or their ability to walk or talk. They may need continued treatment of an injury or a surgical wound. People are admitted to rehabilitation hospitals when it is judged that the care they will receive there

will improve their level of function.

Nursing homes Nursing homes provide ongoing care with activities of daily living, such as meals or bathing, when people cannot manage at home. Unlike rehabilitation hospitals, there is often no expectation that the care will improve their level of function. Although most people prefer to remain at home when they need care and there is increasing use of home care instead of nursing home care, home care is not practical for many people. This is particularly true when family and friends are not nearby and not able to assist with various tasks.

Hospices Hospices provide care to people who have terminal illnesses. Some hospices are institutions in which the dying person remains 24 hours a day. However, there are many hospice programs that can bring necessary support services into a person's home or into a nursing home. For more information, see p.1141.

What to Expect in the Hospital

Many hospitals offer a booklet detailing what you can bring to the hospital and what to expect when you are admitted. Call the admissions office to have this information mailed to you.

Hospital Specialty Units

Many hospitals have the following units, which provide specialized care:

Intensive care unit (ICU) An ICU is a section of a hospital that provides care for those who can benefit from intensive medical care, but is not designed to care for people who are in the last stages of a fatal illness. ICUs bring together several key elements: intensive nursing care, physicians with specialized training, and special equipment (such as a respirator, which is a machine that takes over breathing for people who cannot breathe on their own). There is usually one nurse for every one or two patients so that each person is monitored closely and problems can be responded to quickly.

Many hospitals have both a surgical intensive care unit (for those who require intensive nursing care after surgery) and a medical intensive care unit (for nonsurgical intensive care). Some hospitals have a neurological intensive care unit to care for people with severe brain disorders or after brain surgery. ICUs provide little privacy and may have limited visiting hours.

Coronary care unit (CCU) This is a kind of ICU that is designed to care specifically for people who have had a heart attack or who have another serious heart condition (such as a heart rhythm disturbance) that could be life-threatening.

Neonatal intensive care unit (NICU) This kind of ICU is designed to provide intensive care for seriously ill newborns, including premature babies.

WHAT TO BRING WITH YOU

Particularly if you are scheduled for an elective admission to the hospital, here are the things you should bring with you:

Forms Bring whatever information you have about your health insurance. At a minimum, this means the card that identifies your insurance plan and your personal number. Also bring some form of identification such as a driver's license. Do not forget to bring a list of the medicines you are currently taking (if you can, bring the actual medicines so the physicians can review dosage instructions). The doctors at the hospital will also want to know if you are allergic to any medicines. Finally, bring along a copy of any appropriate legal documents such as a living will or health care proxy (see p.1243).

Personal items Bring whatever will make you feel comfortable. Most people bring toiletries, reading material, photographs, a small amount of cash, a list of phone numbers, robe, slippers, and pajamas (if you do not want to wear a hospital gown). Some hospitals provide lockers where your possessions can be stored securely, but it is generally wisest to avoid bringing valuables with you. Thefts occur even in hospitals.

PREADMISSION TESTS

Until recently, required tests were performed after you were admitted to the hospital. It is now more likely that any tests you need (such as blood work or x-rays) will be done before you are admitted. The type of procedure you will be having, along with the state of your general health, will guide your physician and anesthesiologist in determining what tests you will need.

EXPLAINING RISKS AND BENEFITS (INFORMED CONSENT)

When your doctor recommends particular treatments, including surgery or experimental medical treatments, you will be asked to give "informed consent." Your physician or another health professional working with the doctor will explain the risks and benefits of the treatment; he or she may also provide a written description of the risks and benefits.

Think about how you would like the information concerning your procedure to be explained to you. Do you want as much detail as possible, just a general overview, or something in between? Do you want an advocate, such as a family member or friend, to be with you when the procedure is explained? If a specialist has recommended the treatment, you may want to talk to your primary care physician before deciding; it may be easier for you to talk to your own doctor than one you just met.

Arrange for the discussion to occur at a time that allows your advocate to be present. Feel free to ask questions or seek clarification of any points before signing the document.

For an elective hospitalization, it is reasonable to ask the hospital if you can obtain informed consent forms several days before you are admitted so that you can read the forms when you are less anxious and rushed. If, after considering the risks and benefits, you decide to go ahead with the treatment, you will be asked to sign a document indicating when you have given your informed consent.

If you are undergoing emergency treatment, there will be times when immediate treatment (and an immediate decision from you) is needed.

STANDARDS OF CARE

Doctors, nurses, and other health care providers are expected to perform their duties according to professional standards set by the hospital and professional organizations.

If you feel that any aspect of the care you are receiving is not in accordance with standards, contact the hospital's patient representative for help. Minor problems can usually be resolved by talking things over. Doctors and nurses have professional certifying bodies (such as the board of registration in medicine) that have ways of resolving problems.

Most hospitals follow a Patient's Bill of Rights such as the one first developed at Boston's Beth Israel Hospital (see Your Rights When You Are Hospitalized: Dr Rabkin's Advice, p.167). These guidelines help ensure that patients are treated with respect and consideration, that they are fully informed of the consequences of treatment, and that their privacy is respected.

Your hospital may give you a copy of similar guidelines when you are admitted. You may also be protected by laws or regulations in your state that affect hospital care. You can ask the hospital's admitting office for this information.

Your Rights When You Are Hospitalized:
Dr Rabkin's Advice

In 1972, when I served as President of Boston's Beth Israel Hospital (now Beth Israel Deaconess Medical Center), we were the first in the nation to put into writing a clear statement by a provider of care on the rights of hospitalized patients.

This was followed a few months later by nationwide distribution of a similar statement by the American Hospital Association, leading over time to the adoption of this approach by many hospitals throughout the nation.

Here is an outline of what we share with all our patients, both those admitted to the hospital and those who are outpatients:

1 You have the right to receive the best care medically indicated for your problem regardless of your race, color, religion, national origin, or the source of payment for your care.

2 You have the right to be treated respectfully by others, and to be addressed by your proper name and without undue familiarity.

3 You have the right to privacy. You may expect to talk with your doctor, nurse, other health worker, or an administrative officer in private, and know that the information you supply will not be overheard or given to others without your permission.

4 You have the right to seek and receive all the information necessary for you to understand your medical situation. You have the right to know the name of the doctor who is responsible for your care and the right to talk with that doctor and any others who give you care. You are entitled to know fully about the planned course of diagnosis and treatment (including explanation of each day's procedures and tests), and the prognosis or medical outlook for your future.

5 You have the right to know when students are to perform specific examinations or treatments that pertain to your care, and the right to refuse to participate, without prejudice to the attention we give you.

6 You have the right to full explanation of any research study in which you may be asked to partici-

pate. No research study is ever carried out on any patient without his or her informed consent. If you are asked to participate in a study, you have the right to refuse to participate; you will still receive the best care the medical center can provide.

7 You have the right to leave the hospital even if your doctors advise against it, unless you have certain infectious diseases that may influence the health of others, or if you are incapable of maintaining your own safety, as defined by law.

8 By Massachusetts law, you have the right of access to your medical record. As a general rule, we do not recommend that you review your medical record in the midst of a hospital stay because, while you are an inpatient, your medical record is incomplete; it serves more as a worksheet for your physicians and nurses than as a clear-cut listing of the pertinent medical facts of your case. During your hospitalization, we urge you to direct questions to your physicians and your primary nurse, but if you still wish to see your record, you have the right to do so.

9 You have the right to inquire about the possibility of financial aid to help you in the understanding and payment of hospital bills and the right to receive information and assistance in securing such aid.

10 We believe you are entitled to know whether any facilities recommended for your use are businesses in which those making such recommendations have a significant financial interest, such as nursing homes, pharmacies, or laboratories.

11 You have the right not to be exposed to the smoking of others.

12 You have the right to take part in decisions relating to your health care. Should you become unable to communicate your health care wishes, or simply if you so desire, you may appoint an agent to make those decisions for you by completing a health care proxy.

MITCHELL T. RABKIN, MD
BETH ISRAEL DEACONESS MEDICAL CENTER
HARVARD MEDICAL SCHOOL

Preparing Children for the Hospital

Being admitted to the hospital is not easy for anyone, but it can be particularly difficult for a child. Parents can do many things to help children prepare, starting by familiarizing them with the hospital setting and medical procedures. Find out if the hospital offers a preadmission tour geared to children, where your child can meet with nurses, see rooms, and look at the various machines and other hospital equipment. Read your child a book about going to the hospital and reassure him or her that you will be there.

Explain medical procedures as honestly and completely as possible, and be sure to answer (or have the doctor answer) any questions your child might have. Remember that children have vivid imaginations; they may be worried about things that would never occur to you. For example, sometimes children worry that they will run out of blood and die if their blood is repeatedly tested, so they may need to be told that their bodies are constantly making more blood.

For young children, it can help to play out scenarios with dolls. For example, for a child awaiting surgery, it may be helpful to put a doll to "sleep" with anesthesia and have the doll wake up later wearing a bandage.

Ask if you may stay overnight in your child's room. If you are not permitted to do so, explain to your son or daughter exactly when you have to leave and when you will be back. Do not lie to the child or try to slip quietly out of the room after your child has fallen asleep.

If one of your children is frequently hospitalized, look into programs for your other children, who might feel neglected or guilty. Some specialized hospitals have counselors to help children understand these feelings.

Anesthesia

Before surgery, and before many other procedures, you will be given some form of anesthesia. Anesthesia consists of drugs that block the sensation of pain in a part of your body or that make you unconscious, preventing your awareness of pain.

If you are being admitted to a hospital or outpatient clinic for surgery, you will meet with the anesthesiologist beforehand to discuss your medical history and decide on the best form of anesthesia. For surgical procedures that will be performed in your doctor's office, your physician will discuss anesthesia with you.

It is important to be accurate and complete in answering the questions about your medical history and lifestyle; any omissions could have serious health consequences. In general, the discussion will cover your health history, your use of tobacco and alcohol, current medicines, allergies, dental devices, and previous reactions to anesthesia.

You should be informed about the risks and benefits of the anesthesia that is planned; the doctor should also explain when the effects will wear off and how you will feel after surgery. Do not hesitate to ask questions, including clarification of what you have already been told. For outpatient procedures, you will want to ask if you should arrange for someone to drive you home.

GENERAL ANESTHESIA

General anesthesia induces loss of consciousness and is used for most major surgery. The anesthetic medicine causes a deep "sleep" and reduces the motion of your muscles.

The anesthesiologist first inserts an intravenous (IV) line in a vein and administers medicines that relax your muscles and make you unconscious. After you are unconscious, you may have a tube placed in your windpipe to deliver oxygen as well as anesthetic gases to your lungs.

While you are unconscious, the anesthesiologist will closely monitor many functions—including your breathing rate, pulse, blood pressure, and body temperature—and keep them in the correct range.

When the operation is over, the anesthesiologist will stop or change the drugs you are taking, to allow you to gradually wake up from anesthesia.

LOCAL ANESTHESIA

Local anesthesia is usually much less complex than general anesthesia. It stops sensation only in the area being treated and can be administered as an injection, spray, or ointment. Local anesthesia wears off over time; feeling slowly returns to the anesthetized area of the body.

Hospital Emergency Departments

It is sometimes difficult to know whether or not you should go to an emergency department. If you think you are dealing with a sudden, life-threatening emergency (such as a heart attack), first call 911 and then your primary care doctor. The symptom charts (see p.171) in this book can help you decide if your symptoms are a medical emergency.

If you are concerned, but do not think you are dealing with a life-threatening emergency, you should always call your primary care doctor first. Emergency departments can be hectic places. They are set up to deal with unplanned, life-threatening situations, and the staff must decide who needs care the most.

If your problem is not as severe as other problems in the emergency department, you may have to wait a long time to be helped. The emergency department is not the place to be treated for minor health problems; call your primary care doctor instead.

needle. The tube is left in place and the needle withdrawn. The anesthesiologist then injects anesthetic drugs prior to and during the operation. Epidural anesthesia is often used during childbirth.

In spinal anesthesia, drugs are injected directly into the spinal fluid that surrounds the spinal cord. This method acts faster than an epidural and produces a more complete, temporary numbness and temporary paralysis.

However, unlike an epidural, the drugs cannot be adjusted during the operation. Sedatives may be given before and during both epidural and spinal anesthesia to help you relax.

Sedatives are sometimes given with local anesthesia to help you relax and reduce your awareness of sensations such as pulling or pressure.

REGIONAL ANESTHESIA

Regional anesthesia stops sensation in an entire region of your body, such as an arm or leg. Unlike general anesthesia, you are not put into an unconscious state.

Regional anesthesia can be used to block all sensation from the waist down. One of the most common regional anesthetics is an epidural. The anesthesiologist inserts a thin plastic catheter (tube) into the space that surrounds the spinal cord (the epidural space), using a

PATIENT-CONTROLLED PAINKILLERS

When you awaken after many types of surgery, or if you have a nonsurgical condition that causes constant pain, you will need pain medicine—often a narcotic drug. Traditionally, narcotics were given by hospital staff as tablets or through an intravenous (IV) line, at a time determined by a doctor and administered by a

Regional Anesthesia

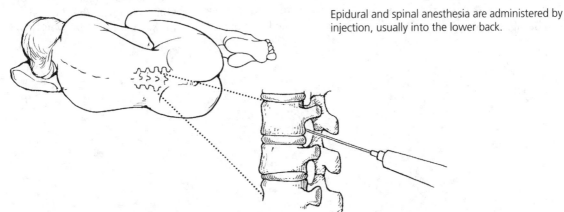

Epidural and spinal anesthesia are administered by injection, usually into the lower back.

nurse; the patient had no direct control.

In recent years, a new approach called patient-controlled analgesia (PCA) has been developed. PCA is delivered via an IV line attached to a small pump that you control to adjust the amount of narcotic delivered. When you feel the pain coming back or becoming too unpleasant, you push a button and get some more relief. A regulator controls the maximum amount of medicine that you can administer.

While some people were concerned that patients might overuse or misuse this pain-relief technique, studies show that people who use PCA often actually require less pain medicine than if they had been placed on a schedule determined by a doctor.

The Cost of Hospitalization

Charges for medical care are complicated. You will receive separate bills from the hospital and from your doctor, as well as from other doctors (such as specialists). If you have insurance, your insurance company will pay part of the bills, but you may have to pay some portion.

Since even the leftover portion can be significant, ask in advance what your insurance will cover and what portion you will be liable for. Before you enter the hospital, read your insurance policy and talk to your doctors and the hospital about fees. Call or write your insurance company or talk to your employee benefits manager to find out what will be covered (see Paying for Your Health Care, p.21).

The portion for which you are billed (after your insurance pays its portion) is limited under certain circumstances in some states. For example, doctors who participate in Medicare (see p.27) may not be permitted to charge you for the difference between what they usually charge and what Medicare permits them to charge.

If you do not have health insurance, you may be able to obtain help paying your bills. Many states have a "free care" pool or another mechanism whereby the hospital receives money as reimbursement for caring for uninsured people, depending on their incomes. Ask the hospital's financial office for information.

If you file a claim and your insurer refuses to pay for some or all charges, do not drop the matter. Ask questions, write letters, and enlist the help of your doctor, the hospital, or your employee benefits office. If the discrepancy is significant, consider hiring a private advocate who will review your bill and negotiate with the insurance company on your behalf.

Advance Directives

There is always a possibility that at some time during your hospitalization you will not be able to speak for yourself or direct your medical care. To ensure that you get the kind of care you want under such circumstances, prepare an advance directive (see p.1142) such as a living will, health care proxy, or durable power of attorney. Different states have different legal requirements for these documents; ask your doctor which mechanism is best for you.

If you are hospitalized for a serious condition, and there is a chance you might die, your advance directive should consider if you want to donate any of your healthy organs to a living person who desperately needs them or if you want to will your body to a medical school (see p.1143).

Many people find comfort in the possibility that they will be able to help another human being after they die.

Symptom Charts

HOW TO USE THE SYMPTOM CHARTS

The charts in this chapter can help you become an active participant in the diagnostic process and a true partner, with your physician, in your health care.

The charts are not intended to replace your physician, but rather to help you make a decision about when to call your doctor. They are only guidelines, and are not a substitute for medical advice, which can be properly given only by your doctor in relation to specific facts.

In some charts, you will be advised to wait to see if your symptoms subside on their own. Use your best judgment in all cases; if your symptoms worsen or concern you, call your physician promptly.

Each symptom chart will lead you through a series of questions that suggest possible diagnoses and provide page references to other parts of the book where you can find additional information about the condition.

Organization

The symptom charts are organized into four categories:

■ General symptoms (these charts generally apply to everyone)

■ Women's symptoms

■ Men's symptoms

■ Symptoms of infants and children

Finding the Right Chart

First, identify the symptom. Decide if the symptom is general or specific to age or gender. For example, if your infant is vomiting, assume that the Vomiting in Infants chart would offer a better path to a possible diagnosis than the chart that applies to all ages.

Next, find your symptom and the page number for the appropriate chart in the Index (see p.1250).

How to Use the Charts

Each chart has a symptom title followed by a brief description of the symptom or other introductory information. Use the title and description to confirm that you have located the appropriate chart for your symptom.

Begin by answering the first question. It is important to start at the top left of the chart and work your way down to the bottom right. The order of questions is important in leading you to the appropriate possible diagnosis.

Each symptom chart is divided into the following sections:

SYMPTOMS

This section contains questions that require a "yes" or a "no" answer. For a "yes" answer, follow the arrow to the right to another question or to Taking Action. For a "no" answer, follow the arrow down to the next question. Continue to answer the questions, following the arrows,

until you reach the Taking Action section of the chart.

TAKING ACTION

Recommendations include:

■ **EMERGENCY!** Call 911 or go immediately to a hospital emergency department.

■ **Call your doctor now** Telephone your doctor and be prepared to describe your symptoms, when they started, under what conditions you became aware of them, and what you have done in the way of self-treatment.

■ **Call your doctor** or **See your doctor** Call the doctor when convenient or make an appointment to see your doctor soon. Be prepared to describe your symptoms, when they started, under what conditions you became aware of them, and what you have done in the way of self-treatment.

In some situations, you will be advised to wait a period of days or weeks, to see if your symptoms subside, before calling your doctor. Again, use your best judgment and always phone your physician promptly if your symptoms concern you.

MORE INFORMATION

After you have taken the action indicated, review the entries listed in the More Information section. The page references will guide you to more detailed information.

ANXIETY

Anxiety includes feelings of fear, dread, or danger. Anxiety can be a vague or intense feeling caused by physical or psychological conditions. The frequency of anxiety can range from a one-time event to recurring episodes.

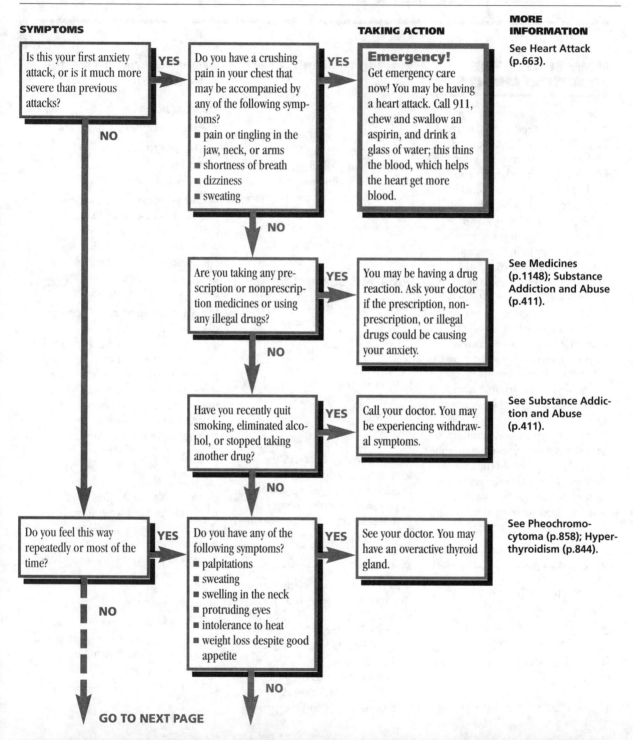

SYMPTOMS

Is this your first anxiety attack, or is it much more severe than previous attacks?

YES → Do you have a crushing pain in your chest that may be accompanied by any of the following symptoms?
- pain or tingling in the jaw, neck, or arms
- shortness of breath
- dizziness
- sweating

NO

TAKING ACTION

YES → **Emergency!** Get emergency care now! You may be having a heart attack. Call 911, chew and swallow an aspirin, and drink a glass of water; this thins the blood, which helps the heart get more blood.

NO

Are you taking any prescription or nonprescription medicines or using any illegal drugs?

YES → You may be having a drug reaction. Ask your doctor if the prescription, nonprescription, or illegal drugs could be causing your anxiety.

NO

Have you recently quit smoking, eliminated alcohol, or stopped taking another drug?

YES → Call your doctor. You may be experiencing withdrawal symptoms.

NO

Do you feel this way repeatedly or most of the time?

YES → Do you have any of the following symptoms?
- palpitations
- sweating
- swelling in the neck
- protruding eyes
- intolerance to heat
- weight loss despite good appetite

NO

YES → See your doctor. You may have an overactive thyroid gland.

NO

GO TO NEXT PAGE

MORE INFORMATION

See Heart Attack (p.663).

See Medicines (p.1148); Substance Addiction and Abuse (p.411).

See Substance Addiction and Abuse (p.411).

See Pheochromocytoma (p.858); Hyperthyroidism (p.844).

**CONTINUED FROM
PREVIOUS PAGE**

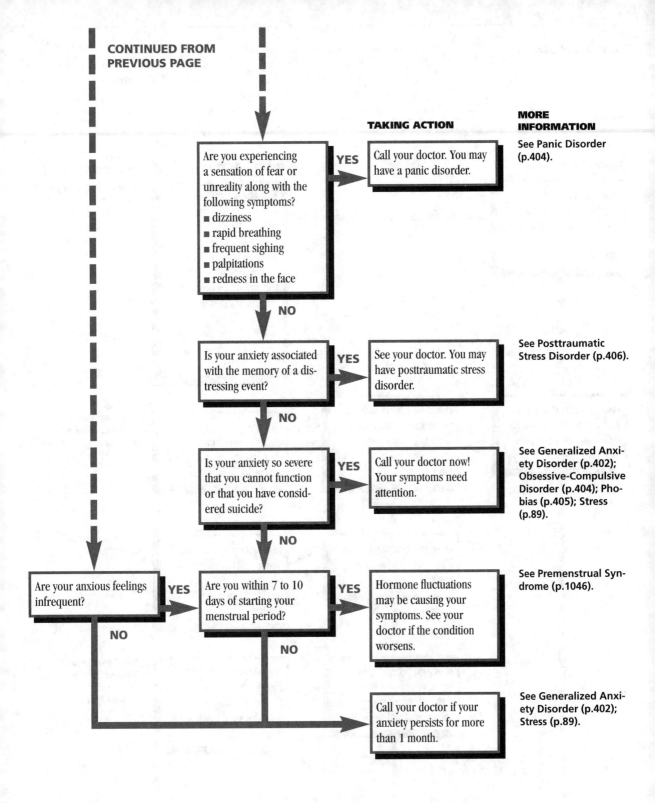

TAKING ACTION

Are you experiencing a sensation of fear or unreality along with the following symptoms?
- dizziness
- rapid breathing
- frequent sighing
- palpitations
- redness in the face

YES → Call your doctor. You may have a panic disorder.

See Panic Disorder (p.404).

NO

Is your anxiety associated with the memory of a distressing event?

YES → See your doctor. You may have posttraumatic stress disorder.

See Posttraumatic Stress Disorder (p.406).

NO

Is your anxiety so severe that you cannot function or that you have considered suicide?

YES → Call your doctor now! Your symptoms need attention.

See Generalized Anxiety Disorder (p.402); Obsessive-Compulsive Disorder (p.404); Phobias (p.405); Stress (p.89).

NO

Are your anxious feelings infrequent?

YES → Are you within 7 to 10 days of starting your menstrual period?

YES → Hormone fluctuations may be causing your symptoms. See your doctor if the condition worsens.

See Premenstrual Syndrome (p.1046).

NO

NO

Call your doctor if your anxiety persists for more than 1 month.

See Generalized Anxiety Disorder (p.402); Stress (p.89).

DEPRESSION

Depression causes feelings of sadness, hopelessness, or despair. For most people, depression is a passing mood.

For others, it is a debilitating illness with physical as well as emotional symptoms.

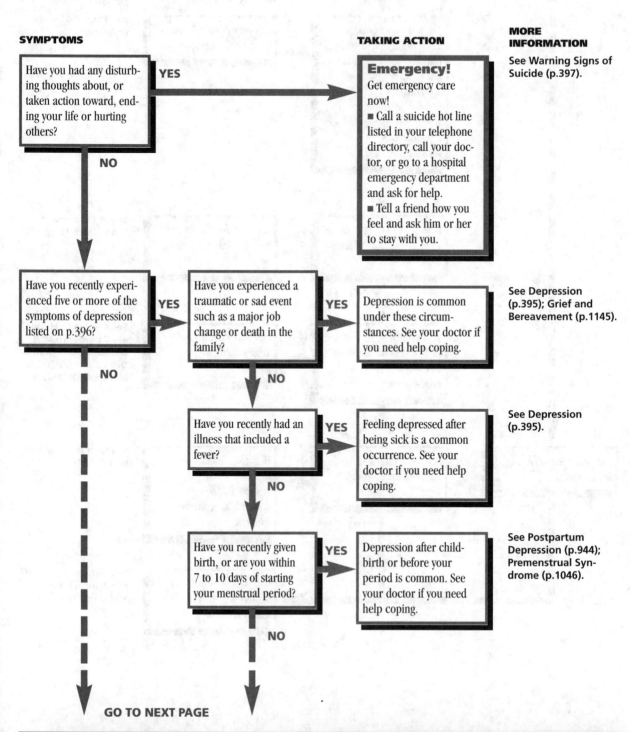

SYMPTOMS

Have you had any disturbing thoughts about, or taken action toward, ending your life or hurting others?

YES →

NO ↓

Have you recently experienced five or more of the symptoms of depression listed on p.396?

YES →

NO ↓

Have you experienced a traumatic or sad event such as a major job change or death in the family?

YES →

NO ↓

Have you recently had an illness that included a fever?

YES →

NO ↓

Have you recently given birth, or are you within 7 to 10 days of starting your menstrual period?

YES →

NO ↓

TAKING ACTION

Emergency!
Get emergency care now!
■ Call a suicide hot line listed in your telephone directory, call your doctor, or go to a hospital emergency department and ask for help.
■ Tell a friend how you feel and ask him or her to stay with you.

Depression is common under these circumstances. See your doctor if you need help coping.

Feeling depressed after being sick is a common occurrence. See your doctor if you need help coping.

Depression after childbirth or before your period is common. See your doctor if you need help coping.

MORE INFORMATION

See Warning Signs of Suicide (p.397).

See Depression (p.395); Grief and Bereavement (p.1145).

See Depression (p.395).

See Postpartum Depression (p.944); Premenstrual Syndrome (p.1046).

GO TO NEXT PAGE

TAKING ACTION

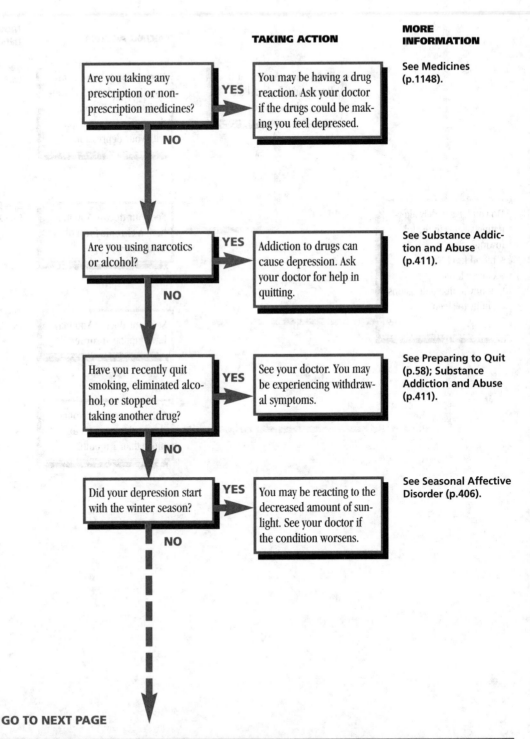

Are you taking any prescription or non-prescription medicines?

YES → You may be having a drug reaction. Ask your doctor if the drugs could be making you feel depressed.

See Medicines (p.1148).

NO

Are you using narcotics or alcohol?

YES → Addiction to drugs can cause depression. Ask your doctor for help in quitting.

See Substance Addiction and Abuse (p.411).

NO

Have you recently quit smoking, eliminated alcohol, or stopped taking another drug?

YES → See your doctor. You may be experiencing withdrawal symptoms.

See Preparing to Quit (p.58); Substance Addiction and Abuse (p.411).

NO

Did your depression start with the winter season?

YES → You may be reacting to the decreased amount of sunlight. See your doctor if the condition worsens.

See Seasonal Affective Disorder (p.406).

NO

GO TO NEXT PAGE

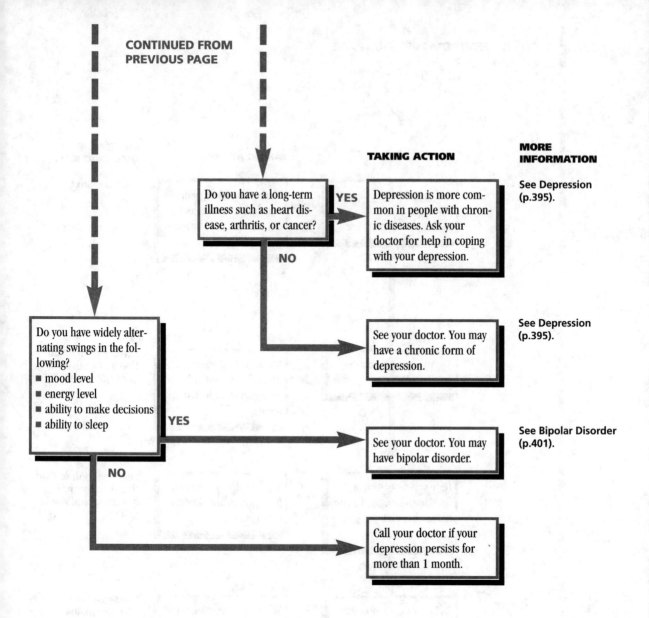

CONTINUED FROM PREVIOUS PAGE

TAKING ACTION

MORE INFORMATION

Do you have a long-term illness such as heart disease, arthritis, or cancer?

YES → Depression is more common in people with chronic diseases. Ask your doctor for help in coping with your depression.

See Depression (p.395).

NO

Do you have widely alternating swings in the following?
- mood level
- energy level
- ability to make decisions
- ability to sleep

See your doctor. You may have a chronic form of depression.

See Depression (p.395).

YES → See your doctor. You may have bipolar disorder.

See Bipolar Disorder (p.401).

NO → Call your doctor if your depression persists for more than 1 month.

DIZZINESS

Dizziness is a spinning sensation and/or a feeling of light-headedness or unsteadiness. Dizziness is a symptom of many medical conditions.

When it occurs after a head injury or is accompanied by paralysis, difficulty breathing, or impaired vision, it is an emergency.

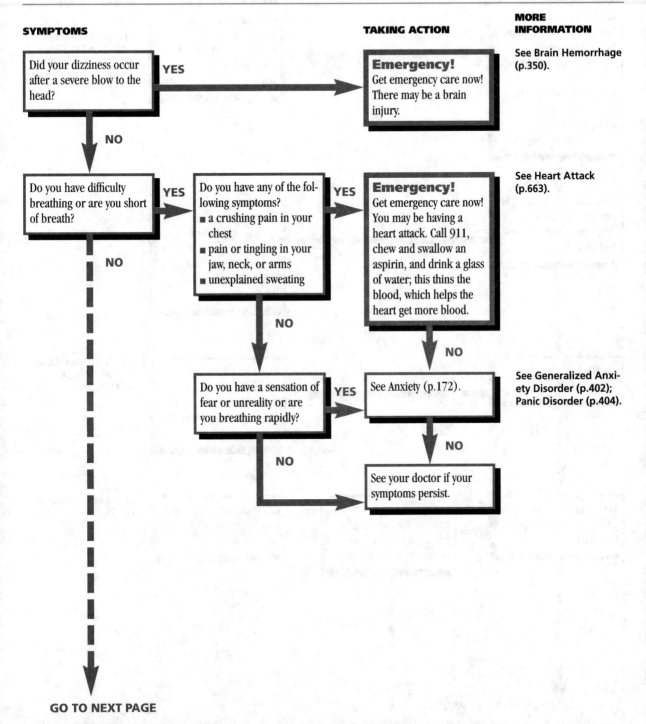

SYMPTOMS

TAKING ACTION

MORE INFORMATION

Did your dizziness occur after a severe blow to the head?

YES →

Emergency!
Get emergency care now! There may be a brain injury.

See Brain Hemorrhage (p.350).

NO ↓

Do you have difficulty breathing or are you short of breath?

YES →

Do you have any of the following symptoms?
- a crushing pain in your chest
- pain or tingling in your jaw, neck, or arms
- unexplained sweating

YES →

Emergency!
Get emergency care now! You may be having a heart attack. Call 911, chew and swallow an aspirin, and drink a glass of water; this thins the blood, which helps the heart get more blood.

See Heart Attack (p.663).

NO ↓ (from difficulty breathing)

NO ↓ (from symptoms)

NO ↓ (from Emergency)

Do you have a sensation of fear or unreality or are you breathing rapidly?

YES →

See Anxiety (p.172).

See Generalized Anxiety Disorder (p.402); Panic Disorder (p.404).

NO ↓

NO ↓

See your doctor if your symptoms persist.

GO TO NEXT PAGE

CONTINUED FROM PREVIOUS PAGE

SYMPTOMS		TAKING ACTION	MORE INFORMATION
Do you have any of the following symptoms? ■ paralysis on one side of your face ■ numbness or tingling in your arms or legs ■ slurred speech ■ blurred or double vision	YES →	**Emergency!** Get emergency care now! You may have a brain or nerve disorder.	See Stroke (p.342); Transient Ischemic Attack (p.342); Multiple Sclerosis (p.368); Vision Loss or Impairment (p.204).
NO ↓			
Are you taking any prescription or nonprescription medicines?	YES →	You may be having a drug reaction. Call your doctor. Ask if your prescription or nonprescription drugs could be causing your dizziness.	See Medicines (p.1148).
NO ↓			
Are you using narcotics or alcohol?	YES →	Dizziness can be caused by drinking too much alcohol or using narcotic drugs. Ask your doctor for help.	See Substance Addiction and Abuse (p.411).
NO ↓			
Is your dizziness accompanied by nausea and/or vomiting?	YES → Does your dizziness recur and is it accompanied by ringing in your ears or a decreased ability to hear? YES →	Call your doctor now. You may have a serious inner ear disorder.	See Ménière Disease (p.456).
NO ↓	NO ↓		

GO TO NEXT PAGE

CONTINUED FROM PREVIOUS PAGE

Has your dizziness lasted from a few hours to a few days?

YES → Call your doctor. You may have a mild inner ear disorder.

See Labyrinthitis (p.456).

NO ↓

Have you been in a car, boat, or airplane within the last 12 hours?

YES → Your condition is probably temporary motion sickness. Call your doctor if your symptoms persist for more than 3 days.

NO ↓

See your doctor if your symptoms persist for more than 3 days.

Has the dizziness lasted at least several weeks, and do you have hearing loss in one ear and/or pain, numbness, or tingling of the face?

YES → See your doctor. You may have nerve damage or a blockage in your ear. See Hearing Loss (p.187).

See Acoustic Neuroma (p.449); Unblocking Earwax (p.451); Hearing Loss (p.451).

NO ↓

Is your dizziness accompanied by headaches?

YES → Did you experience dizziness immediately before a headache?

YES → Call your doctor. You may have a migraine headache.

See Migraine Headache (p.355).

NO ↓

NO ↓

GO TO NEXT PAGE

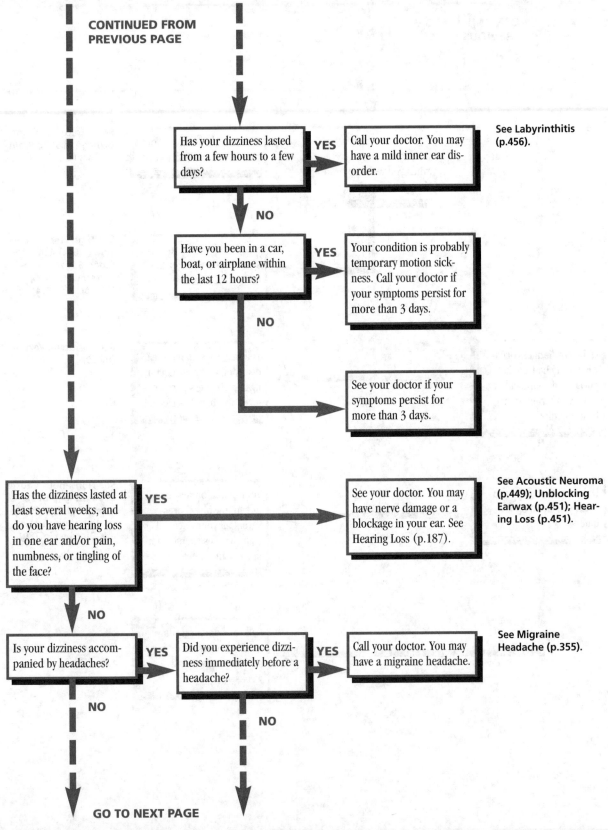

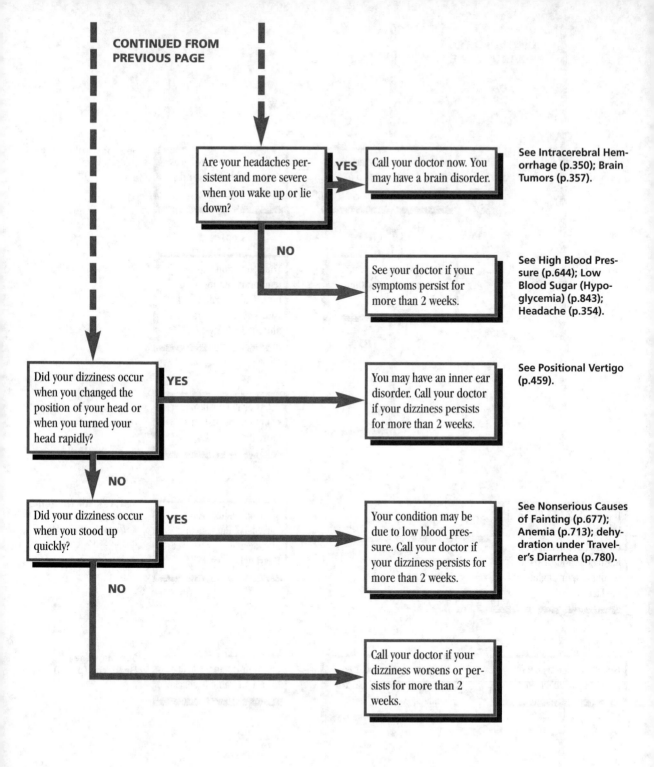

CONTINUED FROM
PREVIOUS PAGE

Are your headaches persistent and more severe when you wake up or lie down?

YES → Call your doctor now. You may have a brain disorder.

See Intracerebral Hemorrhage (p.350); Brain Tumors (p.357).

NO

See your doctor if your symptoms persist for more than 2 weeks.

See High Blood Pressure (p.644); Low Blood Sugar (Hypoglycemia) (p.843); Headache (p.354).

Did your dizziness occur when you changed the position of your head or when you turned your head rapidly?

YES → You may have an inner ear disorder. Call your doctor if your dizziness persists for more than 2 weeks.

See Positional Vertigo (p.459).

NO

Did your dizziness occur when you stood up quickly?

YES → Your condition may be due to low blood pressure. Call your doctor if your dizziness persists for more than 2 weeks.

See Nonserious Causes of Fainting (p.677); Anemia (p.713); dehydration under Traveler's Diarrhea (p.780).

NO

Call your doctor if your dizziness worsens or persists for more than 2 weeks.

DROWSINESS

Drowsiness is difficulty waking up or remaining awake. Short-term drowsiness can be caused by lifestyle factors such as not getting enough sleep. Long-term drowsiness may have a physiological or psychological basis.

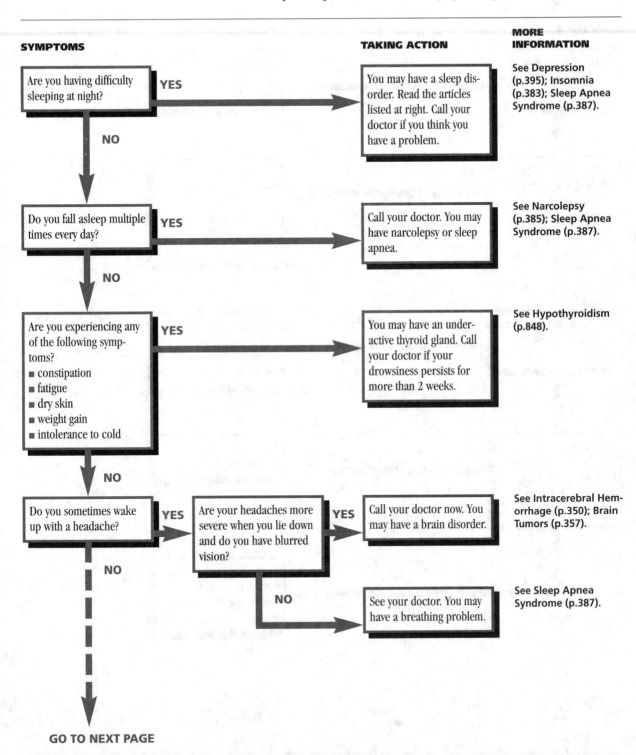

SYMPTOMS

TAKING ACTION

MORE INFORMATION

Are you having difficulty sleeping at night?

YES → You may have a sleep disorder. Read the articles listed at right. Call your doctor if you think you have a problem.

See Depression (p.395); Insomnia (p.383); Sleep Apnea Syndrome (p.387).

NO ↓

Do you fall asleep multiple times every day?

YES → Call your doctor. You may have narcolepsy or sleep apnea.

See Narcolepsy (p.385); Sleep Apnea Syndrome (p.387).

NO ↓

Are you experiencing any of the following symptoms?
- constipation
- fatigue
- dry skin
- weight gain
- intolerance to cold

YES → You may have an underactive thyroid gland. Call your doctor if your drowsiness persists for more than 2 weeks.

See Hypothyroidism (p.848).

NO ↓

Do you sometimes wake up with a headache?

YES → Are your headaches more severe when you lie down and do you have blurred vision?

YES → Call your doctor now. You may have a brain disorder.

See Intracerebral Hemorrhage (p.350); Brain Tumors (p.357).

NO → See your doctor. You may have a breathing problem.

See Sleep Apnea Syndrome (p.387).

NO ↓

GO TO NEXT PAGE

CONTINUED FROM PREVIOUS PAGE

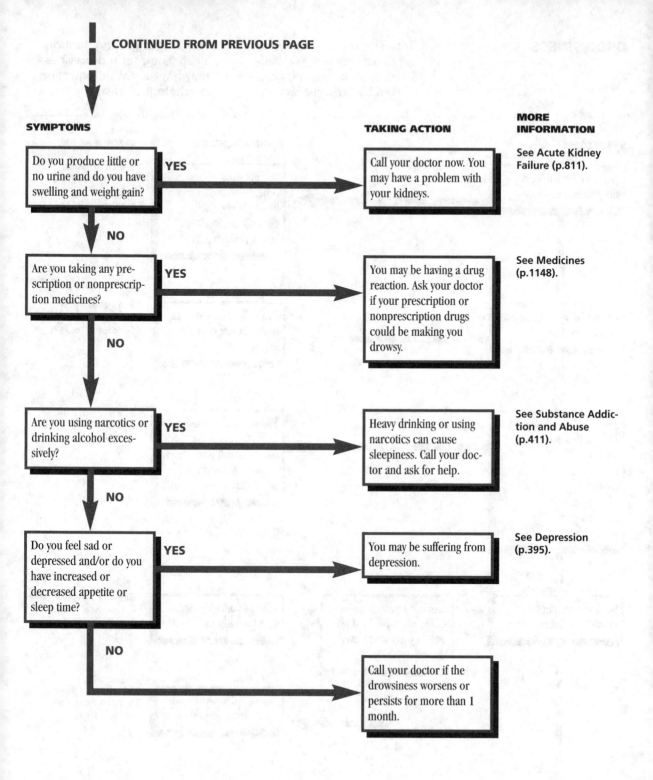

SYMPTOMS

TAKING ACTION

Do you produce little or no urine and do you have swelling and weight gain?

YES → Call your doctor now. You may have a problem with your kidneys.

See Acute Kidney Failure (p.811).

NO ↓

Are you taking any prescription or nonprescription medicines?

YES → You may be having a drug reaction. Ask your doctor if your prescription or nonprescription drugs could be making you drowsy.

See Medicines (p.1148).

NO ↓

Are you using narcotics or drinking alcohol excessively?

YES → Heavy drinking or using narcotics can cause sleepiness. Call your doctor and ask for help.

See Substance Addiction and Abuse (p.411).

NO ↓

Do you feel sad or depressed and/or do you have increased or decreased appetite or sleep time?

YES → You may be suffering from depression.

See Depression (p.395).

NO ↓

Call your doctor if the drowsiness worsens or persists for more than 1 month.

HEADACHE

Headaches can be caused by a variety of factors, such as muscle tension or drinking too much alcohol. Headaches can also occur with common illnesses such as the flu. Severe headaches that are accompanied by confusion or high fever can indicate a serious health condition and require your doctor's immediate attention.

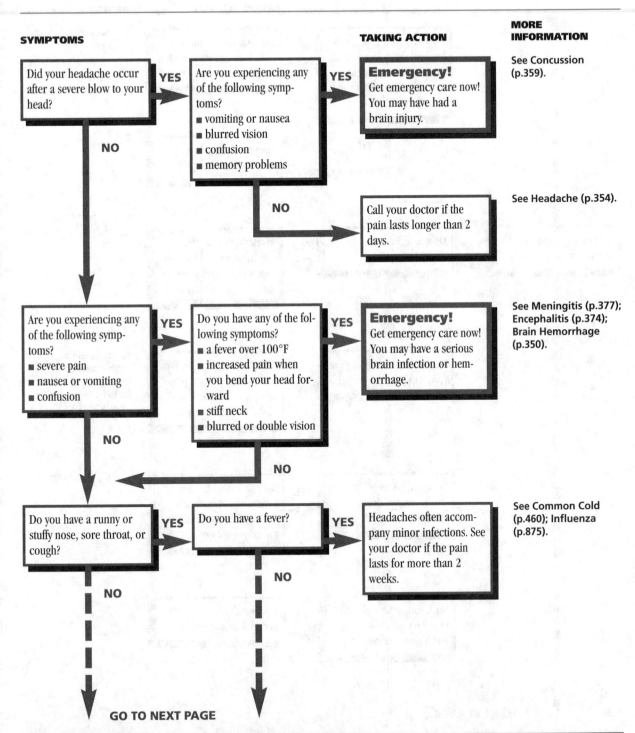

SYMPTOMS

Did your headache occur after a severe blow to your head?

YES → Are you experiencing any of the following symptoms?
- vomiting or nausea
- blurred vision
- confusion
- memory problems

YES → **Emergency!** Get emergency care now! You may have had a brain injury.

MORE INFORMATION
See Concussion (p.359).

NO → Call your doctor if the pain lasts longer than 2 days.

See Headache (p.354).

TAKING ACTION

Are you experiencing any of the following symptoms?
- severe pain
- nausea or vomiting
- confusion

YES → Do you have any of the following symptoms?
- a fever over 100°F
- increased pain when you bend your head forward
- stiff neck
- blurred or double vision

YES → **Emergency!** Get emergency care now! You may have a serious brain infection or hemorrhage.

See Meningitis (p.377); Encephalitis (p.374); Brain Hemorrhage (p.350).

NO

Do you have a runny or stuffy nose, sore throat, or cough?

YES → Do you have a fever?

YES → Headaches often accompany minor infections. See your doctor if the pain lasts for more than 2 weeks.

See Common Cold (p.460); Influenza (p.875).

NO → **GO TO NEXT PAGE**

CONTINUED FROM PREVIOUS PAGE

TAKING ACTION

MORE INFORMATION

See Sinusitis (p.464).

Do you have a green, yellow, or rust-colored nasal discharge and increasing pain when you bend your head forward?

YES → You may have a sinus infection. Call your doctor if your symptoms persist.

NO → See your doctor if your symptoms persist.

Are you experiencing nausea or vomiting?

YES → Do you feel confused or dizzy?

YES → **Emergency!** Get fresh air and emergency care now! You may be breathing toxic air.

See Poisonous Fumes (p.1213).

NO

NO

Do you have throbbing eye pain with blurred vision?

YES → Call your doctor now. You may have increased pressure in your eyes or high blood pressure.

See Glaucoma (p.435); High Blood Pressure (p.644); Brain Tumors (p.357); Migraine Headache (p.355).

NO

Have you recently consumed a great deal of alcohol?

YES → Nausea, vomiting, and headache are common effects of excessive alcohol consumption.

See Alcohol (p.62).

NO

Have you just traveled to or exercised at an unusually high elevation?

YES → Your headache may be due to a lack of oxygen.

NO

GO TO NEXT PAGE

TAKING ACTION

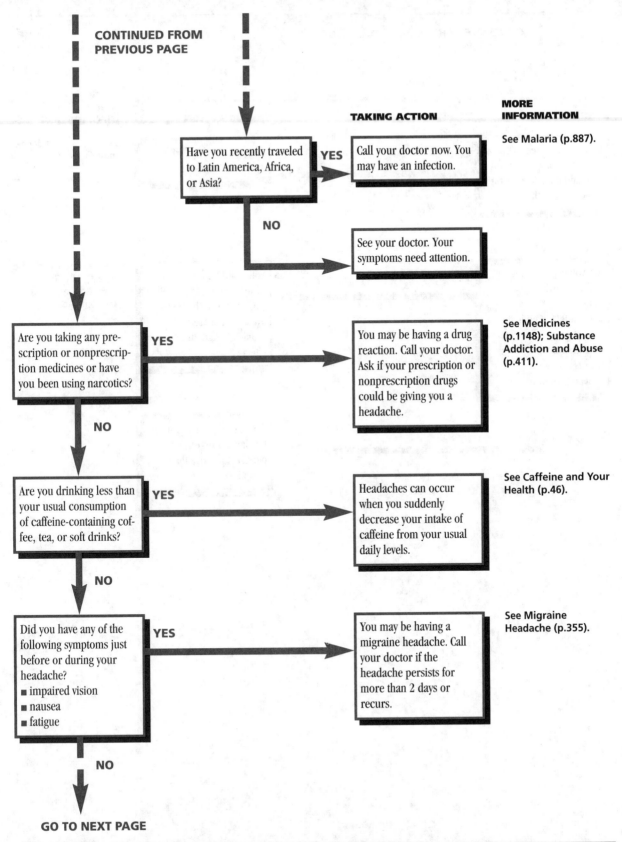

Have you recently traveled to Latin America, Africa, or Asia?

YES → Call your doctor now. You may have an infection.

See Malaria (p.887).

NO → See your doctor. Your symptoms need attention.

Are you taking any prescription or nonprescription medicines or have you been using narcotics?

YES → You may be having a drug reaction. Call your doctor. Ask if your prescription or nonprescription drugs could be giving you a headache.

See Medicines (p.1148); Substance Addiction and Abuse (p.411).

NO

Are you drinking less than your usual consumption of caffeine-containing coffee, tea, or soft drinks?

YES → Headaches can occur when you suddenly decrease your intake of caffeine from your usual daily levels.

See Caffeine and Your Health (p.46).

NO

Did you have any of the following symptoms just before or during your headache?
- impaired vision
- nausea
- fatigue

YES → You may be having a migraine headache. Call your doctor if the headache persists for more than 2 days or recurs.

See Migraine Headache (p.355).

NO

GO TO NEXT PAGE

CONTINUED FROM PREVIOUS PAGE

SYMPTOMS

TAKING ACTION

Do attacks of headaches tend to recur over several days and then go away for weeks or months?

YES →

See your doctor if your symptoms worsen.

See Cluster Headache (p.354).

NO ↓

Are you experiencing any of the following symptoms?
- a bandlike pain in the front or back of your head or neck
- stress
- sleep problems

YES →

Your pain may be caused by tension or stress. Call your doctor if the treatments suggested in the articles at right are not effective.

See Tension Headache (p.354); The Relaxation Response: Dr Benson's Advice (p.90).

NO →

Call your doctor if your headache worsens or persists for more than 1 week.

HEARING LOSS

Hearing loss can be a complete loss of hearing or a diminished ability to hear.

Hearing loss accompanied by ear pain, pressure, or a discharge is usually a symptom of infection. When it is accompanied by dizziness, loss of balance, nausea, or vomiting, it can indicate a disorder of the nerves or bones, and requires your doctor's attention.

SYMPTOMS

TAKING ACTION

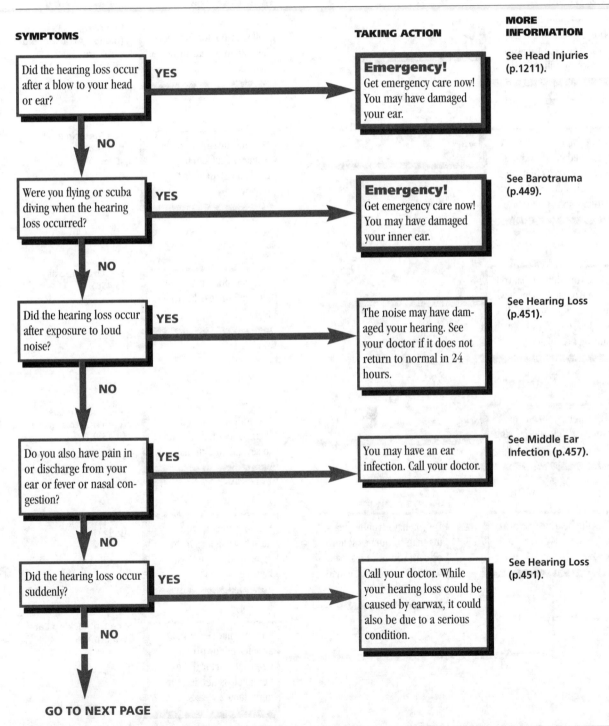

Did the hearing loss occur after a blow to your head or ear? — **YES** →

Emergency! Get emergency care now! You may have damaged your ear.

See Head Injuries (p.1211).

NO ↓

Were you flying or scuba diving when the hearing loss occurred? — **YES** →

Emergency! Get emergency care now! You may have damaged your inner ear.

See Barotrauma (p.449).

NO ↓

Did the hearing loss occur after exposure to loud noise? — **YES** →

The noise may have damaged your hearing. See your doctor if it does not return to normal in 24 hours.

See Hearing Loss (p.451).

NO ↓

Do you also have pain in or discharge from your ear or fever or nasal congestion? — **YES** →

You may have an ear infection. Call your doctor.

See Middle Ear Infection (p.457).

NO ↓

Did the hearing loss occur suddenly? — **YES** →

Call your doctor. While your hearing loss could be caused by earwax, it could also be due to a serious condition.

See Hearing Loss (p.451).

NO ↓

GO TO NEXT PAGE

CONTINUED FROM PREVIOUS PAGE

SYMPTOMS

TAKING ACTION

Do you also have dizziness, vertigo, or nausea or are you vomiting?

YES →

Call your doctor. You may have an inner ear or nerve disorder.

See Ménière Disease (p.456); Acoustic Neuroma (p.449).

NO ↓

Have you been taking any new medicines over the past few weeks, particularly high doses of aspirin, antibiotics, or diuretics?

YES →

You may be experiencing a side effect from the medicine. Call your doctor.

See Medicines (p.1148).

NO ↓

Have you noticed that you have trouble hearing low-frequency sounds, or that the hearing loss worsened during pregnancy?

YES →

See your doctor. You may have middle ear hearing loss.

See Otosclerosis (p.458).

NO ↓

Are you over 40 and do you have difficulty hearing low-frequency sounds?

YES →

See your doctor. Your hearing loss may be due to several conditions.

See Hearing Loss (p.451); Otosclerosis (p.458).

NO ↓

Has the hearing loss progressed slowly over the years?

YES →

Do you have trouble hearing high-frequency sounds or have you been exposed to loud noise for extended periods of time?

YES →

See your doctor. You may have hearing loss from aging or damage to your hearing.

See Hearing Loss (p.451).

NO ↓

NO →

You may have earwax or another minor problem. Call your doctor if the hearing loss persists for more than 2 weeks.

See Unblocking Earwax (p.451).

RINGING IN THE EARS

Ringing in the ears is noise that you can hear when there is no sound in the environment. It can be a whistling, hissing, whooshing, or pulsing noise. Usually there is no serious medical condition. When ringing in the ears occurs with other symptoms, however, it can indicate serious problems.

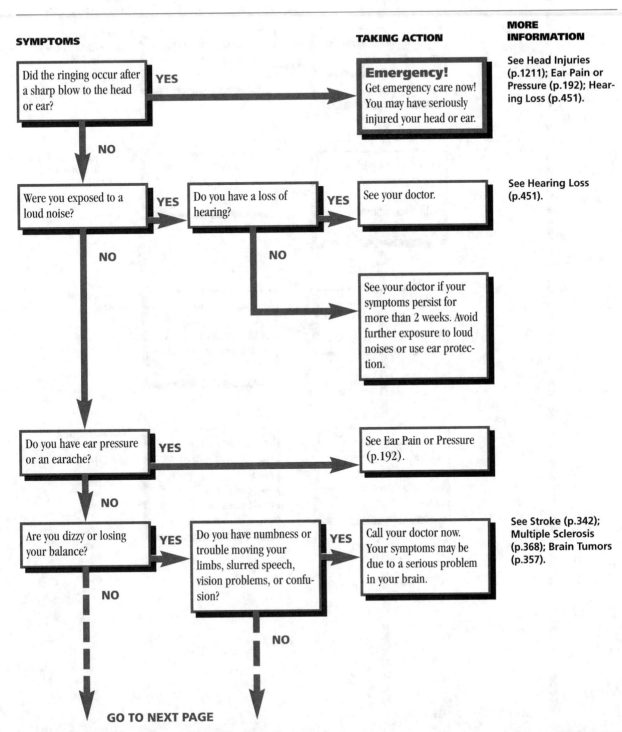

SYMPTOMS

TAKING ACTION

MORE INFORMATION

Did the ringing occur after a sharp blow to the head or ear?

YES

Emergency!
Get emergency care now! You may have seriously injured your head or ear.

See Head Injuries (p.1211); Ear Pain or Pressure (p.192); Hearing Loss (p.451).

NO

Were you exposed to a loud noise?

YES

Do you have a loss of hearing?

YES

See your doctor.

See Hearing Loss (p.451).

NO

NO

See your doctor if your symptoms persist for more than 2 weeks. Avoid further exposure to loud noises or use ear protection.

Do you have ear pressure or an earache?

YES

See Ear Pain or Pressure (p.192).

NO

Are you dizzy or losing your balance?

YES

Do you have numbness or trouble moving your limbs, slurred speech, vision problems, or confusion?

YES

Call your doctor now. Your symptoms may be due to a serious problem in your brain.

See Stroke (p.342); Multiple Sclerosis (p.368); Brain Tumors (p.357).

NO

NO

GO TO NEXT PAGE

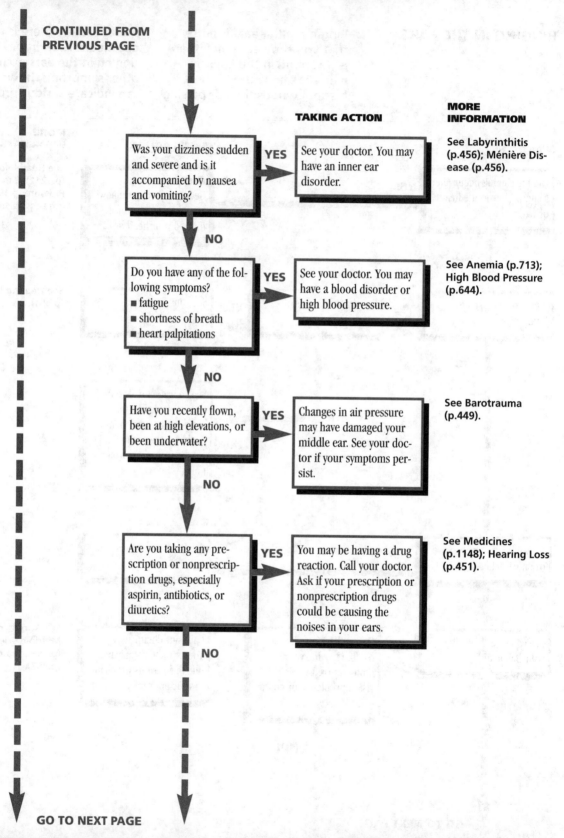

TAKING ACTION

**MORE
INFORMATION**

Was your dizziness sudden and severe and is it accompanied by nausea and vomiting?

YES → See your doctor. You may have an inner ear disorder.

See Labyrinthitis (p.456); Ménière Disease (p.456).

NO ↓

Do you have any of the following symptoms?
- fatigue
- shortness of breath
- heart palpitations

YES → See your doctor. You may have a blood disorder or high blood pressure.

See Anemia (p.713); High Blood Pressure (p.644).

NO ↓

Have you recently flown, been at high elevations, or been underwater?

YES → Changes in air pressure may have damaged your middle ear. See your doctor if your symptoms persist.

See Barotrauma (p.449).

NO ↓

Are you taking any prescription or nonprescription drugs, especially aspirin, antibiotics, or diuretics?

YES → You may be having a drug reaction. Call your doctor. Ask if your prescription or nonprescription drugs could be causing the noises in your ears.

See Medicines (p.1148); Hearing Loss (p.451).

NO ↓

GO TO NEXT PAGE

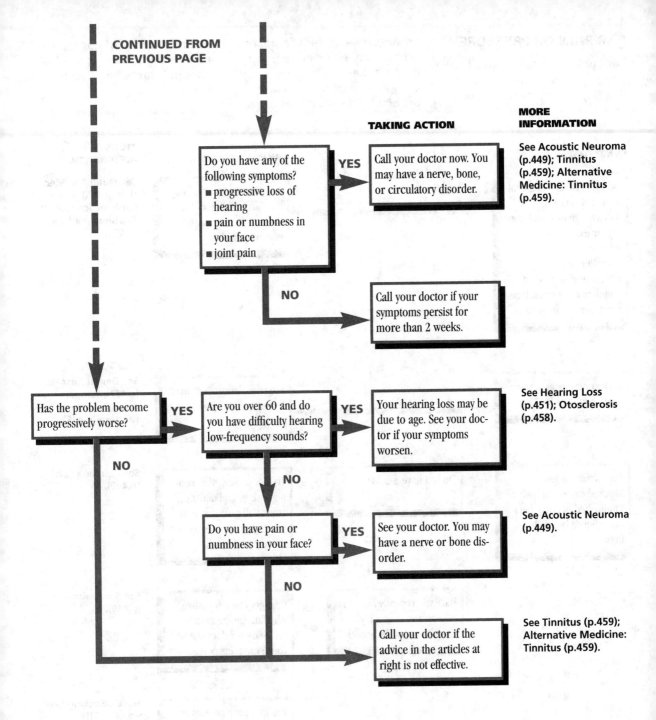

TAKING ACTION

Do you have any of the following symptoms?
- progressive loss of hearing
- pain or numbness in your face
- joint pain

YES → Call your doctor now. You may have a nerve, bone, or circulatory disorder.

See Acoustic Neuroma (p.449); Tinnitus (p.459); Alternative Medicine: Tinnitus (p.459).

NO → Call your doctor if your symptoms persist for more than 2 weeks.

Has the problem become progressively worse?

YES → Are you over 60 and do you have difficulty hearing low-frequency sounds?

YES → Your hearing loss may be due to age. See your doctor if your symptoms worsen.

See Hearing Loss (p.451); Otosclerosis (p.458).

NO

NO ↓

Do you have pain or numbness in your face?

YES → See your doctor. You may have a nerve or bone disorder.

See Acoustic Neuroma (p.449).

NO

Call your doctor if the advice in the articles at right is not effective.

See Tinnitus (p.459); Alternative Medicine: Tinnitus (p.459).

EAR PAIN OR PRESSURE

Ear pain or pressure includes any pain, tenderness, aching, throbbing, or pressure in or around the ear. Most earaches accompany colds or allergies. An earache also may be caused by earwax or a jaw problem. Ear infections are a common cause of ear pain in infants and children; see Ear Pain in Infants and Children, p.310.

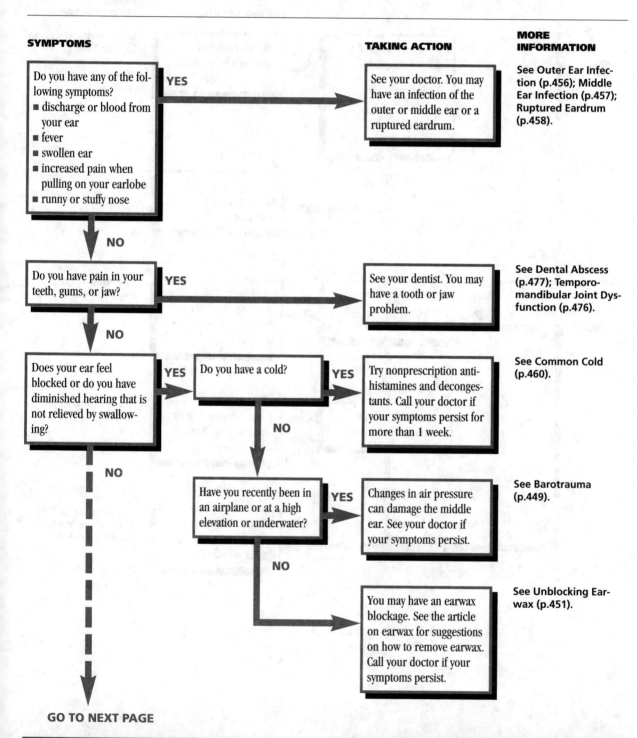

SYMPTOMS

TAKING ACTION

MORE INFORMATION

Do you have any of the following symptoms?
- discharge or blood from your ear
- fever
- swollen ear
- increased pain when pulling on your earlobe
- runny or stuffy nose

YES → See your doctor. You may have an infection of the outer or middle ear or a ruptured eardrum.

See Outer Ear Infection (p.456); Middle Ear Infection (p.457); Ruptured Eardrum (p.458).

NO ↓

Do you have pain in your teeth, gums, or jaw?

YES → See your dentist. You may have a tooth or jaw problem.

See Dental Abscess (p.477); Temporomandibular Joint Dysfunction (p.476).

NO ↓

Does your ear feel blocked or do you have diminished hearing that is not relieved by swallowing?

YES → Do you have a cold?

YES → Try nonprescription antihistamines and decongestants. Call your doctor if your symptoms persist for more than 1 week.

See Common Cold (p.460).

NO ↓

Have you recently been in an airplane or at a high elevation or underwater?

YES → Changes in air pressure can damage the middle ear. See your doctor if your symptoms persist.

See Barotrauma (p.449).

NO ↓

You may have an earwax blockage. See the article on earwax for suggestions on how to remove earwax. Call your doctor if your symptoms persist.

See Unblocking Earwax (p.451).

NO ↓

GO TO NEXT PAGE

SYMPTOMS

TAKING ACTION

MORE INFORMATION

Are you feeling pressure in your ear, rather than pain?

YES →

Do you have a cold or allergy?

YES →

You probably have a blocked eustachian tube. Take fluids and decongestants.

See Common Cold (p.460); Allergic Rhinitis (Hay Fever) (p.462).

NO ↓

Have you flown or scuba dived recently?

YES →

You may have mild barotrauma. See your doctor if your symptoms persist for more than 1 week.

See Barotrauma (p.449).

NO ↓

You may have an earwax blockage. See the article on earwax for suggestions on how to remove earwax. Call your doctor if your symptoms persist for more than 1 week.

Unblocking Earwax (p.451).

NO ↓

Have you recently had a blow to your ear or head?

YES →

See your doctor immediately. You may have damaged your ear.

NO ↓

Is the pain worse when you chew or yawn?

YES →

See your dentist. You may have a problem with your jaw.

See Temporomandibular Joint Dysfunction (p.476).

NO ↓

Have you flown or gone scuba diving recently?

YES →

See your doctor immediately. You may have barotrauma.

See Barotrauma (p.449).

NO ↓

See your doctor if your symptoms persist for more than 2 weeks.

TOOTH PAIN

Mild or severe pain in one or more teeth, or in the gums, can be caused by tooth decay, a tooth abscess, or gum disease. These common conditions require the attention of your dentist. When accompanied by pain in the face, neck, or chest, or by breathing difficulties, tooth pain may be part of a more complex and potentially serious medical condition.

SYMPTOMS

TAKING ACTION

MORE INFORMATION

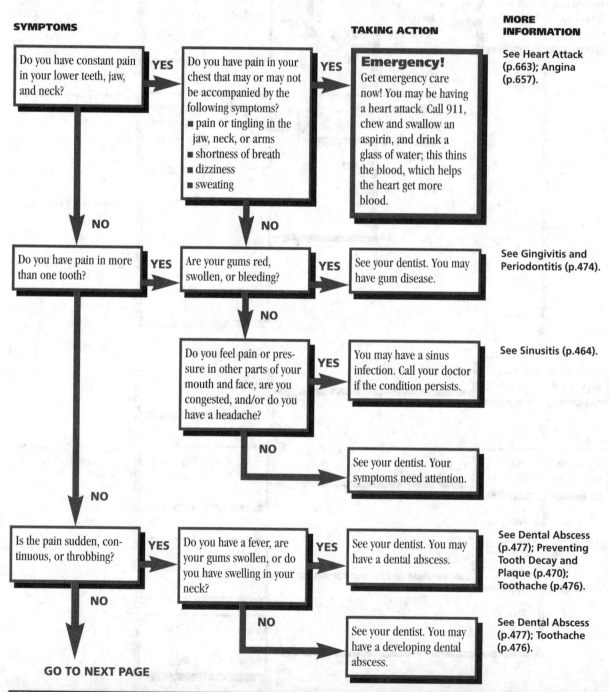

Do you have constant pain in your lower teeth, jaw, and neck?

YES → Do you have pain in your chest that may or may not be accompanied by the following symptoms?
■ pain or tingling in the jaw, neck, or arms
■ shortness of breath
■ dizziness
■ sweating

YES → **Emergency!** Get emergency care now! You may be having a heart attack. Call 911, chew and swallow an aspirin, and drink a glass of water; this thins the blood, which helps the heart get more blood.

See Heart Attack (p.663); Angina (p.657).

NO ↓   **NO** ↓

Do you have pain in more than one tooth?

YES → Are your gums red, swollen, or bleeding?

YES → See your dentist. You may have gum disease.

See Gingivitis and Periodontitis (p.474).

NO ↓

Do you feel pain or pressure in other parts of your mouth and face, are you congested, and/or do you have a headache?

YES → You may have a sinus infection. Call your doctor if the condition persists.

See Sinusitis (p.464).

NO ↓

See your dentist. Your symptoms need attention.

NO ↓

Is the pain sudden, continuous, or throbbing?

YES → Do you have a fever, are your gums swollen, or do you have swelling in your neck?

YES → See your dentist. You may have a dental abscess.

See Dental Abscess (p.477); Preventing Tooth Decay and Plaque (p.470); Toothache (p.476).

NO ↓

See your dentist. You may have a developing dental abscess.

See Dental Abscess (p.477); Toothache (p.476).

NO ↓

GO TO NEXT PAGE

Does your tooth hurt when you chew or bite down on it?

YES →

Has your dentist recently put a filling in one of your teeth?

YES →

Your filling may be uneven. Call your dentist if the condition persists.

See Toothache (p.476).

NO

See your dentist. You may have a developing dental abscess.

See Dental Abscess (p.477); Toothache (p.476).

NO

Do you have pain in your jaw accompanied by clicking sounds and headaches?

YES →

See your dentist. You may have a problem in your jaw joint.

See Temporo-mandibular Joint Dysfunction (p.476).

NO

Does your tooth hurt when you eat hot, cold, or sweet substances?

YES →

See your dentist. You may have a cavity or a broken filling.

See Preventing Tooth Decay and Plaque (p.470); Sensitive Teeth and Gums (p.476).

NO

Your symptoms do not need immediate attention. Call your dentist if your symptoms persist for more than a week or worsen.

SWOLLEN GLANDS

Swollen glands in the neck, armpit, or groin are usually caused by infections such as the flu and are usually temporary. Glands that stay swollen for more than 2 months can indicate a more serious health condition and require your doctor's attention.

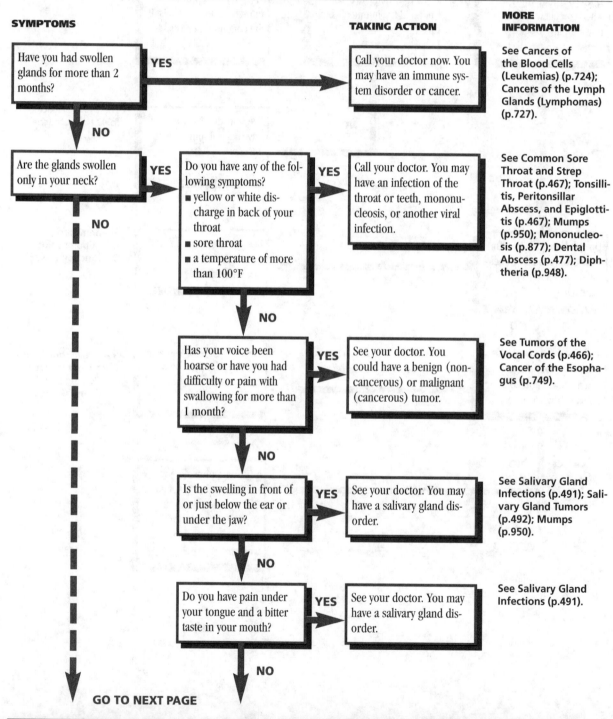

SYMPTOMS

TAKING ACTION

MORE INFORMATION

Have you had swollen glands for more than 2 months?

YES → Call your doctor now. You may have an immune system disorder or cancer.

See Cancers of the Blood Cells (Leukemias) (p.724); Cancers of the Lymph Glands (Lymphomas) (p.727).

NO ↓

Are the glands swollen only in your neck?

YES → Do you have any of the following symptoms?
- yellow or white discharge in back of your throat
- sore throat
- a temperature of more than 100°F

YES → Call your doctor. You may have an infection of the throat or teeth, mononucleosis, or another viral infection.

See Common Sore Throat and Strep Throat (p.467); Tonsillitis, Peritonsillar Abscess, and Epiglottitis (p.467); Mumps (p.950); Mononucleosis (p.877); Dental Abscess (p.477); Diphtheria (p.948).

NO ↓

Has your voice been hoarse or have you had difficulty or pain with swallowing for more than 1 month?

YES → See your doctor. You could have a benign (noncancerous) or malignant (cancerous) tumor.

See Tumors of the Vocal Cords (p.466); Cancer of the Esophagus (p.749).

NO ↓

Is the swelling in front of or just below the ear or under the jaw?

YES → See your doctor. You may have a salivary gland disorder.

See Salivary Gland Infections (p.491); Salivary Gland Tumors (p.492); Mumps (p.950).

NO ↓

Do you have pain under your tongue and a bitter taste in your mouth?

YES → See your doctor. You may have a salivary gland disorder.

See Salivary Gland Infections (p.491).

NO ↓

GO TO NEXT PAGE

**CONTINUED FROM
PREVIOUS PAGE**

TAKING ACTION

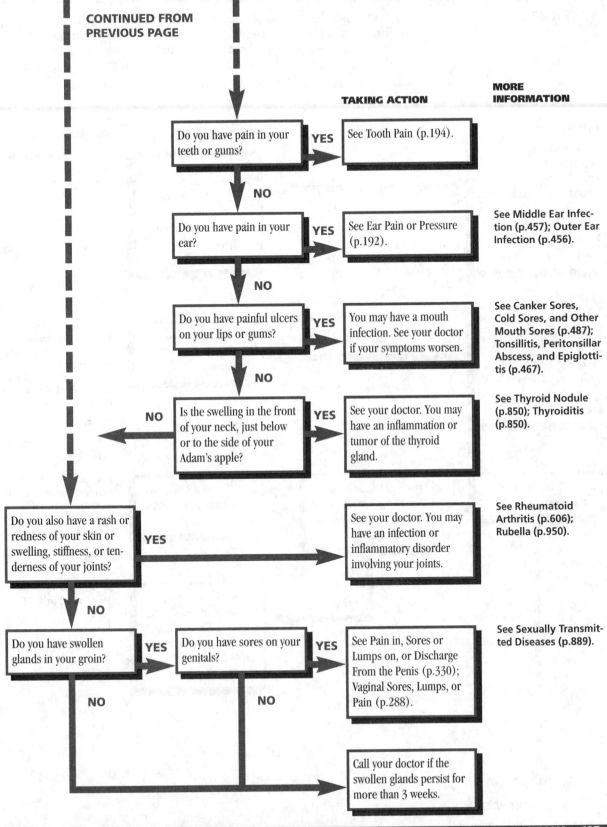

Do you have pain in your teeth or gums? — **YES** → See Tooth Pain (p.194).

NO

Do you have pain in your ear? — **YES** → See Ear Pain or Pressure (p.192).

See Middle Ear Infection (p.457); Outer Ear Infection (p.456).

NO

Do you have painful ulcers on your lips or gums? — **YES** → You may have a mouth infection. See your doctor if your symptoms worsen.

See Canker Sores, Cold Sores, and Other Mouth Sores (p.487); Tonsillitis, Peritonsillar Abscess, and Epiglottitis (p.467).

NO

NO ← Is the swelling in the front of your neck, just below or to the side of your Adam's apple? — **YES** → See your doctor. You may have an inflammation or tumor of the thyroid gland.

See Thyroid Nodule (p.850); Thyroiditis (p.850).

Do you also have a rash or redness of your skin or swelling, stiffness, or tenderness of your joints? — **YES** → See your doctor. You may have an infection or inflammatory disorder involving your joints.

See Rheumatoid Arthritis (p.606); Rubella (p.950).

NO

Do you have swollen glands in your groin? — **YES** → Do you have sores on your genitals? — **YES** → See Pain in, Sores or Lumps on, or Discharge From the Penis (p.330); Vaginal Sores, Lumps, or Pain (p.288).

See Sexually Transmitted Diseases (p.889).

NO   **NO**

Call your doctor if the swollen glands persist for more than 3 weeks.

SORE THROAT

Pain, soreness, rawness, burning, or discomfort in the throat are symptoms of many different viral and bacterial infections and can occur in people of all ages. Sore throats also accompany many childhood illnesses. For information on sore throat in children, see p.1018.

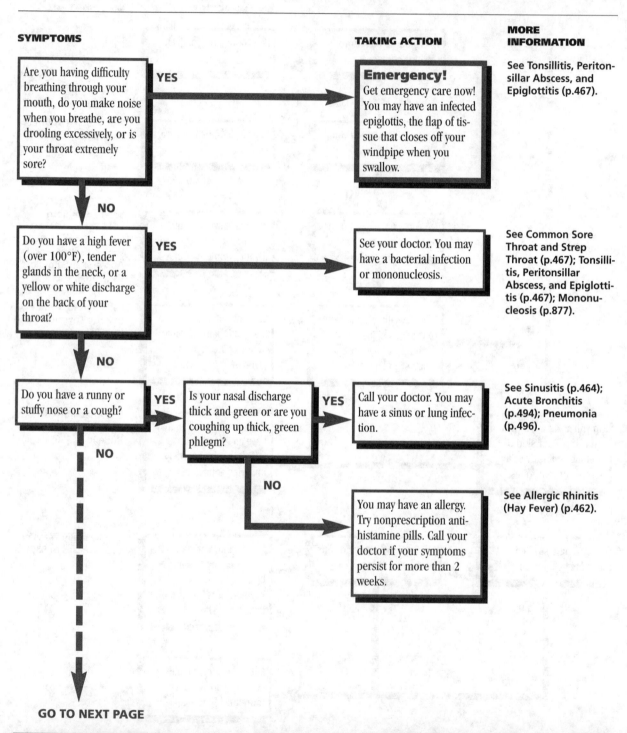

SYMPTOMS

TAKING ACTION

MORE INFORMATION

Are you having difficulty breathing through your mouth, do you make noise when you breathe, are you drooling excessively, or is your throat extremely sore?

YES

Emergency!
Get emergency care now! You may have an infected epiglottis, the flap of tissue that closes off your windpipe when you swallow.

See Tonsillitis, Peritonsillar Abscess, and Epiglottitis (p.467).

NO

Do you have a high fever (over 100°F), tender glands in the neck, or a yellow or white discharge on the back of your throat?

YES

See your doctor. You may have a bacterial infection or mononucleosis.

See Common Sore Throat and Strep Throat (p.467); Tonsillitis, Peritonsillar Abscess, and Epiglottitis (p.467); Mononucleosis (p.877).

NO

Do you have a runny or stuffy nose or a cough?

YES

Is your nasal discharge thick and green or are you coughing up thick, green phlegm?

YES

Call your doctor. You may have a sinus or lung infection.

See Sinusitis (p.464); Acute Bronchitis (p.494); Pneumonia (p.496).

NO

NO

You may have an allergy. Try nonprescription antihistamine pills. Call your doctor if your symptoms persist for more than 2 weeks.

See Allergic Rhinitis (Hay Fever) (p.462).

GO TO NEXT PAGE

CONTINUED FROM PREVIOUS PAGE

SYMPTOMS   **TAKING ACTION**   **MORE INFORMATION**

Is your voice hoarse?   **YES** →   Your vocal cords may be inflamed.   See Laryngitis (p.466).

NO ↓

Does your sore throat feel acidic or is it accompanied by heartburn?   **YES** →   You may have an irritation of the throat caused by stomach acid. Try antacids. Call your doctor if your sore throat persists for 2 weeks despite treatment.   See Inflammation of the Esophagus (p.747).

NO ↓

Has your throat been sore for more than 2 weeks?   **YES** →   See your doctor. You probably have only a minor infection, but it could be something more serious.   See Tumors of the Vocal Cords (p.466); Cancer of the Esophagus (p.749).

NO ↓

You probably have a viral throat infection. See your doctor if your sore throat persists for 2 weeks.

EYE PAIN OR PROBLEMS WITH THE EYELID

Eye irritation, itching, or redness is often caused by a common cold or allergies. Symptoms that last more than 2 days or are accompanied by a severe headache, discharge from the eye, excessive tear production, loss of vision, facial swelling, or weak facial muscles may indicate a serious condition that requires your doctor's attention.

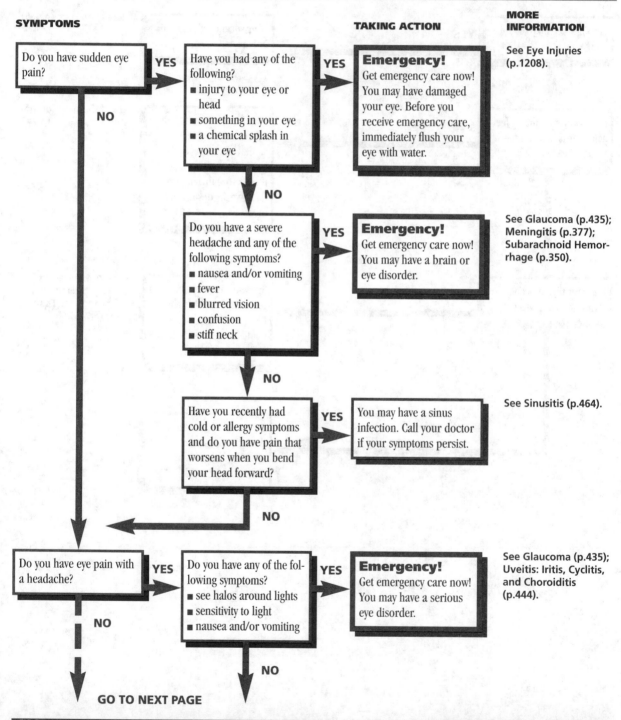

SYMPTOMS

TAKING ACTION

MORE INFORMATION

Do you have sudden eye pain? → **YES** → Have you had any of the following?
- injury to your eye or head
- something in your eye
- a chemical splash in your eye

→ **YES** → **Emergency!** Get emergency care now! You may have damaged your eye. Before you receive emergency care, immediately flush your eye with water.

See Eye Injuries (p.1208).

NO ↓

Do you have a severe headache and any of the following symptoms?
- nausea and/or vomiting
- fever
- blurred vision
- confusion
- stiff neck

→ **YES** → **Emergency!** Get emergency care now! You may have a brain or eye disorder.

See Glaucoma (p.435); Meningitis (p.377); Subarachnoid Hemorrhage (p.350).

NO ↓

Have you recently had cold or allergy symptoms and do you have pain that worsens when you bend your head forward?

→ **YES** → You may have a sinus infection. Call your doctor if your symptoms persist.

See Sinusitis (p.464).

NO

Do you have eye pain with a headache? → **YES** → Do you have any of the following symptoms?
- see halos around lights
- sensitivity to light
- nausea and/or vomiting

→ **YES** → **Emergency!** Get emergency care now! You may have a serious eye disorder.

See Glaucoma (p.435); Uveitis: Iritis, Cyclitis, and Choroiditis (p.444).

NO ↓ **GO TO NEXT PAGE**

NO ↓

200 GENERAL SYMPTOMS EYE PAIN OR PROBLEMS WITH THE EYELID

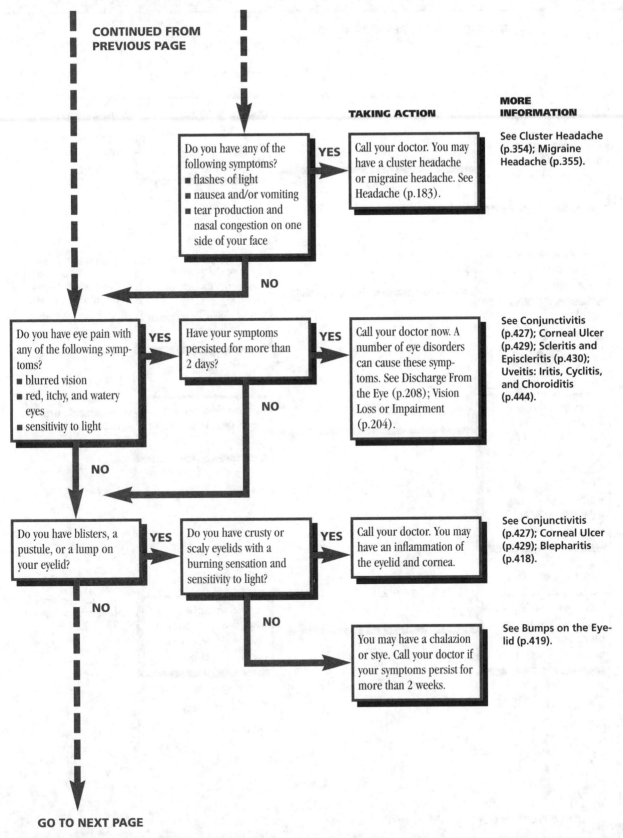

CONTINUED FROM
PREVIOUS PAGE

TAKING ACTION

MORE
INFORMATION

Do you have any of the
following symptoms?
- flashes of light
- nausea and/or vomiting
- tear production and
  nasal congestion on one
  side of your face

YES → Call your doctor. You may
have a cluster headache
or migraine headache. See
Headache (p.183).

See Cluster Headache
(p.354); Migraine
Headache (p.355).

NO

Do you have eye pain with
any of the following symptoms?
- blurred vision
- red, itchy, and watery
  eyes
- sensitivity to light

YES → Have your symptoms
persisted for more than
2 days?

YES → Call your doctor now. A
number of eye disorders
can cause these symp-
toms. See Discharge From
the Eye (p.208); Vision
Loss or Impairment
(p.204).

See Conjunctivitis
(p.427); Corneal Ulcer
(p.429); Scleritis and
Episcleritis (p.430);
Uveitis: Iritis, Cyclitis,
and Choroiditis
(p.444).

NO

NO

Do you have blisters, a
pustule, or a lump on
your eyelid?

YES → Do you have crusty or
scaly eyelids with a
burning sensation and
sensitivity to light?

YES → Call your doctor. You may
have an inflammation of
the eyelid and cornea.

See Conjunctivitis
(p.427); Corneal Ulcer
(p.429); Blepharitis
(p.418).

NO

NO → You may have a chalazion
or stye. Call your doctor if
your symptoms persist for
more than 2 weeks.

See Bumps on the Eye-
lid (p.419).

GO TO NEXT PAGE

CONTINUED FROM PREVIOUS PAGE

SYMPTOMS

TAKING ACTION

MORE INFORMATION

Do you have watery eyes or a yellow, crusty discharge in one or both eyes?

YES → See Discharge From the Eye (p.208).

See Conjunctivitis (p.427).

NO ↓

Do you have bulging eyes and eye pain?

YES → Call your doctor now. Your condition may be due to a growth, an inflammation, or a thyroid disorder.

See Brain Tumors (p.357); Tumors of the Eye (p.443); Hyperthyroidism (p.844).

NO ↓

Do you have drooping eyelids and any of the following symptoms?
■ weakness in your face, arms, or legs
■ ear pain
■ difficulty swallowing
■ difficulty breathing
■ watery eyes

YES → Call your doctor now. You may have a nerve or muscle disorder.

See Bell Palsy (p.373); Myasthenia Gravis (p.377); Stroke (p.342).

NO ↓

Do you suddenly have a red, bloody patch in the white of your eye but no worsening of your vision?

YES → You may have injured the blood vessels in your eye. This should heal slowly over 1 to 2 weeks.

See Subconjunctival Hemorrhage (p.429).

NO ↓

GO TO NEXT PAGE

CONTINUED FROM PREVIOUS PAGE

SYMPTOMS

TAKING ACTION

MORE
INFORMATION

Do you have dry eyes?

YES

NO

Do you have poor night vision that may be accompanied by any of the following symptoms?
- loss of appetite
- diarrhea
- yellow or foul-smelling stools
- weakness

YES

Call your doctor. You may have a malabsorption disorder.

See Malabsorption (p.775).

NO

Do you have a dry mouth, dry skin, and joint pain?

YES

Call your doctor. You may have an autoimmune disorder.

See Rheumatoid Arthritis (p.606); Sjøgren Syndrome (p.898).

NO

Call your doctor if your symptoms persist for more than 2 weeks or worsen.

VISION LOSS OR IMPAIRMENT

Any sudden change in vision or a complete loss of vision requires your doctor's attention. Blurred vision is not uncommon, especially with age; it usually comes on gradually and is caused by a focusing problem that can be corrected with glasses, contact lenses, or (in the case of cataracts) surgery.

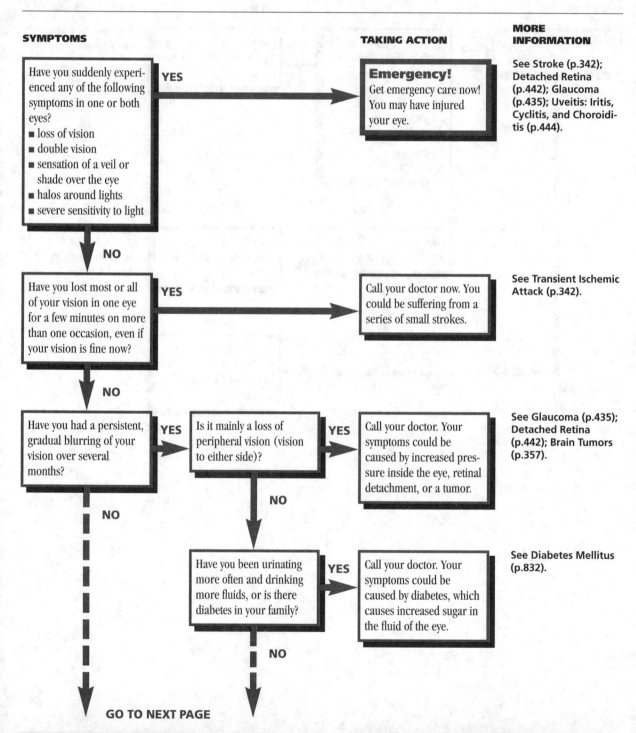

SYMPTOMS

Have you suddenly experienced any of the following symptoms in one or both eyes?
- loss of vision
- double vision
- sensation of a veil or shade over the eye
- halos around lights
- severe sensitivity to light

YES →

TAKING ACTION

Emergency!
Get emergency care now! You may have injured your eye.

MORE INFORMATION

See Stroke (p.342); Detached Retina (p.442); Glaucoma (p.435); Uveitis: Iritis, Cyclitis, and Choroiditis (p.444).

NO ↓

Have you lost most or all of your vision in one eye for a few minutes on more than one occasion, even if your vision is fine now?

YES →

Call your doctor now. You could be suffering from a series of small strokes.

See Transient Ischemic Attack (p.342).

NO ↓

Have you had a persistent, gradual blurring of your vision over several months?

YES →

Is it mainly a loss of peripheral vision (vision to either side)?

YES →

Call your doctor. Your symptoms could be caused by increased pressure inside the eye, retinal detachment, or a tumor.

See Glaucoma (p.435); Detached Retina (p.442); Brain Tumors (p.357).

NO ↓

Have you been urinating more often and drinking more fluids, or is there diabetes in your family?

YES →

Call your doctor. Your symptoms could be caused by diabetes, which causes increased sugar in the fluid of the eye.

See Diabetes Mellitus (p.832).

NO ↓

GO TO NEXT PAGE

TAKING ACTION

Are you experiencing any of the following symptoms?
- blurred vision when viewing near or far objects
- worsening blurred vision, especially in bright light
- difficulty driving at night
- difficulty perceiving colors

YES → Call your doctor. Your condition may be due to a cataract, or you may need glasses.

See Cataracts (p.430); Presbyopia (p.425); Focusing Problems (p.420).

NO ↓

Has your vision become gradually blurred since you began taking any new prescription or nonprescription medicine?

YES → Call your doctor. You may be having a drug reaction.

See Medicines (p.1148).

NO → Call an eye doctor. You may need corrective lenses or a change in your lenses.

See Focusing Problems (p.420).

Do you have any of the following symptoms?
- discharge from the eye
- itching
- swollen eyelids
- sensitivity to light

YES → You may have an eye inflammation. Call your doctor if your symptoms persist for more than 2 days.

See Conjunctivitis (p.427); Eye Pain or Problems with the Eyelid (p.200); Discharge From the Eye (p.208).

NO ↓

GO TO NEXT PAGE

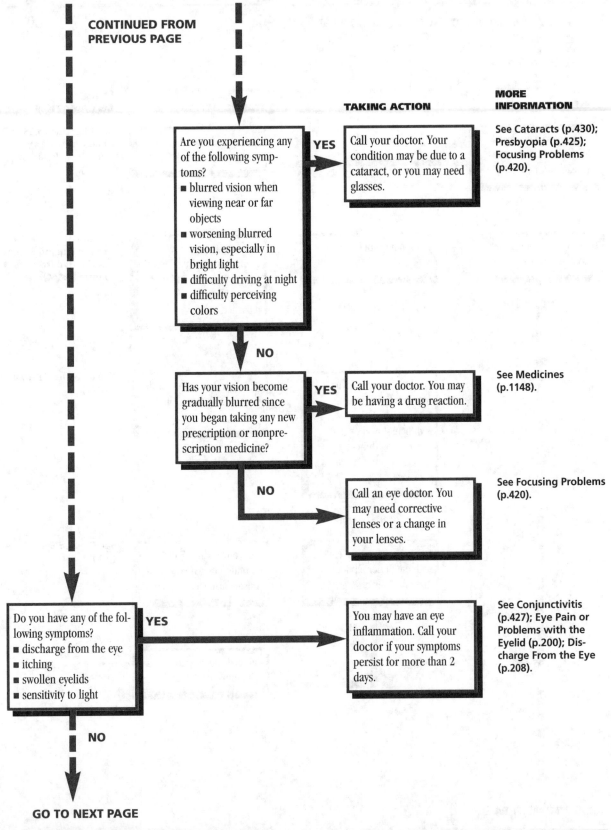

CONTINUED FROM PREVIOUS PAGE

SYMPTOMS

TAKING ACTION

Do you have a headache with flashes of light and nausea and/or vomiting?

YES →

Call your doctor. You may have a migraine.

See Migraine (p.355); Headache (p.354); Nausea or Vomiting (p.254).

NO ↓

Do you have double vision?

YES →

Do you have bulging eyes?

YES →

Call your doctor now. Your condition may be due to a growth, inflammation, or a thyroid disorder.

See Tumors of the Eye (p.443); Bulging Eyes (p.427); Hyperthyroidism (p.844).

NO ↓ (double vision)

NO ↓ (bulging eyes)

Do you have any of the following symptoms?
- drooping eyelids
- difficulty swallowing
- breathing difficulty
- weakness in your arms or legs

YES →

Call your doctor now. You may have a muscle disorder.

See Myasthenia Gravis (p.377).

NO ↓

Do you have a problem with depth perception, or are your eyes crossed?

YES →

Call your doctor. Your condition may be due to a muscle disorder.

See Crossed Eyes (p.445).

NO ↓

Call your doctor. Your symptoms need attention.

GO TO NEXT PAGE

CONTINUED FROM PREVIOUS PAGE

SYMPTOMS

TAKING ACTION

Do you have poor night vision that may or may not be accompanied by the following symptoms?
- dry eyes
- loss of appetite
- diarrhea or yellow or foul-smelling stools
- weakness

YES ▶

Call your doctor. You may have a malabsorption disorder.

See Malabsorption (p.775).

NO ▶

Call your doctor if your symptoms persist for more than 2 weeks or worsen.

DISCHARGE FROM THE EYE

Discharge from the eye can range from watery eyes (due to excessive tears) to a thick, yellow discharge. Watery eyes are often caused by a common cold or allergies. Symptoms that are accompanied by eye pain, loss of vision, facial swelling, or muscle weakness in the face can indicate a serious condition that requires your doctor's attention.

SYMPTOMS　　　　　　　　　　　　**TAKING ACTION**　　　**MORE INFORMATION**

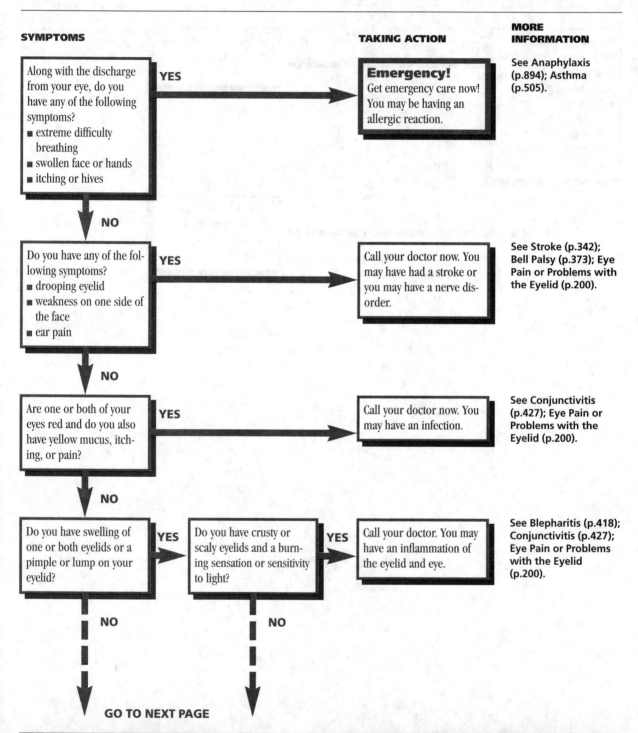

Along with the discharge from your eye, do you have any of the following symptoms?
- extreme difficulty breathing
- swollen face or hands
- itching or hives

YES →

Emergency! Get emergency care now! You may be having an allergic reaction.

See Anaphylaxis (p.894); Asthma (p.505).

NO ↓

Do you have any of the following symptoms?
- drooping eyelid
- weakness on one side of the face
- ear pain

YES →

Call your doctor now. You may have had a stroke or you may have a nerve disorder.

See Stroke (p.342); Bell Palsy (p.373); Eye Pain or Problems with the Eyelid (p.200).

NO ↓

Are one or both of your eyes red and do you also have yellow mucus, itching, or pain?

YES →

Call your doctor now. You may have an infection.

See Conjunctivitis (p.427); Eye Pain or Problems with the Eyelid (p.200).

NO ↓

Do you have swelling of one or both eyelids or a pimple or lump on your eyelid?

YES →

Do you have crusty or scaly eyelids and a burning sensation or sensitivity to light?

YES →

Call your doctor. You may have an inflammation of the eyelid and eye.

See Blepharitis (p.418); Conjunctivitis (p.427); Eye Pain or Problems with the Eyelid (p.200).

NO ↓　　　　　　**NO** ↓

GO TO NEXT PAGE

TAKING ACTION

**MORE
INFORMATION**

Do you have a painful pimple on your eyelid? **YES** → You may have a stye. Place warm compresses on the eyelid.

See Bumps on the Eyelid (p.419).

NO

Do you have a blister on your eyelid? **YES** → Call your doctor. You may have a herpes virus infection.

NO

Do you have a red, watery eye and a headache on the same side of the head as the affected eye? **YES** → You may have a migraine or cluster headache. Take pain medication and call your doctor if your symptoms persist.

See Migraine Headache (p.355); Cluster Headache (p.354); Sinusitis (p.464).

NO

Do you have a runny or stuffy nose, cough, or sore throat? **YES** → You probably have a cold.

See Common Cold (p.460); Allergic Rhinitis (Hay Fever) (p.462).

NO

Do you have a watery eye with any of the following symptoms?
- eye pain
- blurred or spotted vision
- sensitivity to light

YES → Call your doctor now. A number of eye disorders may cause your symptoms.

See Corneal Ulcer (p.429); Uveitis: Iritis, Cyclitis, and Choroiditis (p.444); Scleritis and Episcleritis (p.430); Eye Pain or Problems with the Eyelid (p.200); Vision Loss or Impairment (p.204).

NO → Call your doctor if your symptoms worsen or persist for more than 1 month.

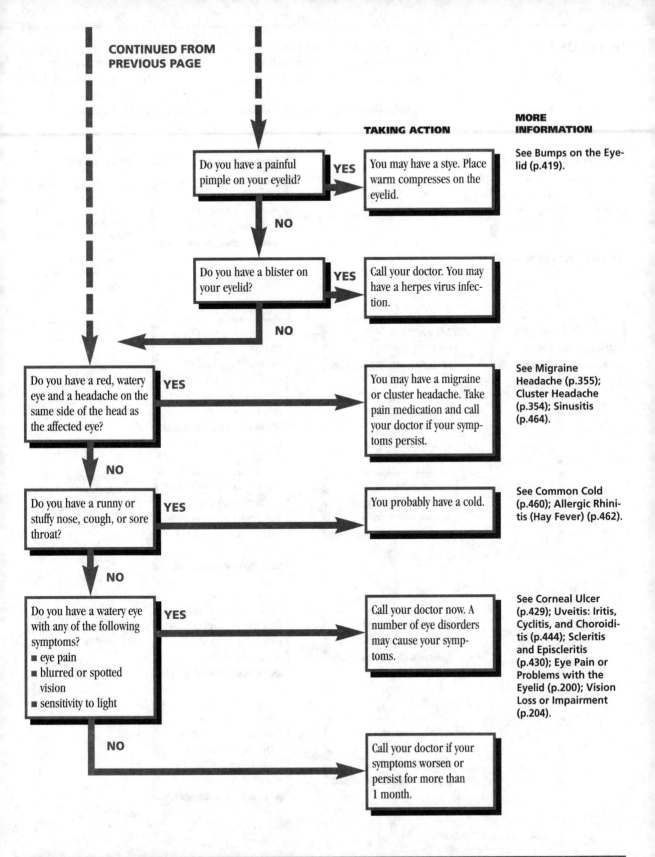

HAIR LOSS

Hair loss can be sudden or gradual loss or thinning of hair on your head or on other parts of the body. A gradual loss or thinning of hair without any accompanying symptoms is common. However, hair loss that is accompanied by general ill health requires your doctor's attention.

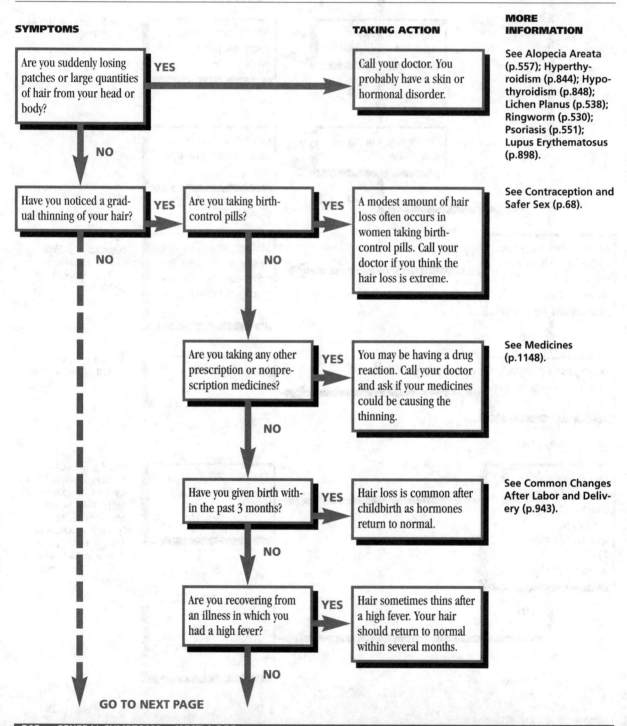

SYMPTOMS

TAKING ACTION

MORE INFORMATION

Are you suddenly losing patches or large quantities of hair from your head or body?

YES → Call your doctor. You probably have a skin or hormonal disorder.

See Alopecia Areata (p.557); Hyperthyroidism (p.844); Hypothyroidism (p.848); Lichen Planus (p.538); Ringworm (p.530); Psoriasis (p.551); Lupus Erythematosus (p.898).

NO

Have you noticed a gradual thinning of your hair?

YES → Are you taking birth-control pills?

YES → A modest amount of hair loss often occurs in women taking birth-control pills. Call your doctor if you think the hair loss is extreme.

See Contraception and Safer Sex (p.68).

NO

Are you taking any other prescription or nonprescription medicines?

YES → You may be having a drug reaction. Call your doctor and ask if your medicines could be causing the thinning.

See Medicines (p.1148).

NO

Have you given birth within the past 3 months?

YES → Hair loss is common after childbirth as hormones return to normal.

See Common Changes After Labor and Delivery (p.943).

NO

Are you recovering from an illness in which you had a high fever?

YES → Hair sometimes thins after a high fever. Your hair should return to normal within several months.

NO

GO TO NEXT PAGE

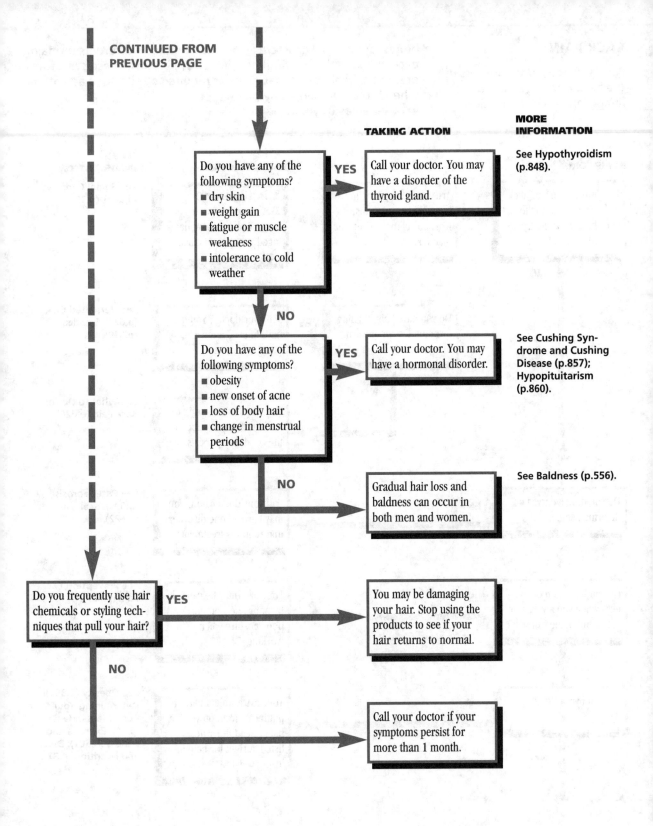

TAKING ACTION

MORE INFORMATION

Do you have any of the following symptoms?
- dry skin
- weight gain
- fatigue or muscle weakness
- intolerance to cold weather

YES → Call your doctor. You may have a disorder of the thyroid gland.

See Hypothyroidism (p.848).

NO

Do you have any of the following symptoms?
- obesity
- new onset of acne
- loss of body hair
- change in menstrual periods

YES → Call your doctor. You may have a hormonal disorder.

See Cushing Syndrome and Cushing Disease (p.857); Hypopituitarism (p.860).

NO → Gradual hair loss and baldness can occur in both men and women.

See Baldness (p.556).

Do you frequently use hair chemicals or styling techniques that pull your hair?

YES → You may be damaging your hair. Stop using the products to see if your hair returns to normal.

NO → Call your doctor if your symptoms persist for more than 1 month.

BACK PAIN

Pain, stiffness, or tenderness in the back is usually caused by minor injury to the muscles, bones, or nerves. Persistent back pain, numbness, tingling, or muscle weakness, especially when it is accompanied by pain in other areas of your body, may indicate disorders of major body systems. These symptoms require your doctor's attention.

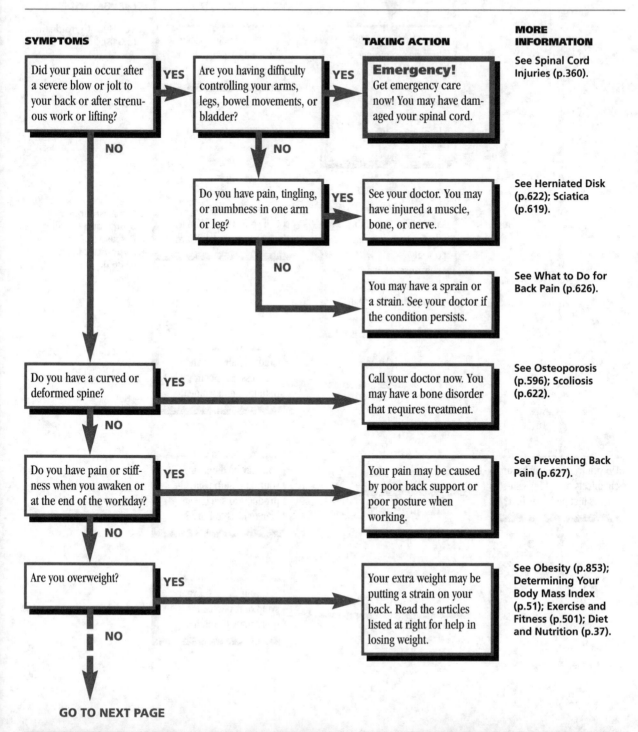

SYMPTOMS

TAKING ACTION

MORE INFORMATION

Did your pain occur after a severe blow or jolt to your back or after strenuous work or lifting?

YES → Are you having difficulty controlling your arms, legs, bowel movements, or bladder?

YES → **Emergency!** Get emergency care now! You may have damaged your spinal cord.

See Spinal Cord Injuries (p.360).

NO ↓

NO ↓

Do you have pain, tingling, or numbness in one arm or leg?

YES → See your doctor. You may have injured a muscle, bone, or nerve.

See Herniated Disk (p.622); Sciatica (p.619).

NO ↓

You may have a sprain or a strain. See your doctor if the condition persists.

See What to Do for Back Pain (p.626).

Do you have a curved or deformed spine?

YES → Call your doctor now. You may have a bone disorder that requires treatment.

See Osteoporosis (p.596); Scoliosis (p.622).

NO ↓

Do you have pain or stiffness when you awaken or at the end of the workday?

YES → Your pain may be caused by poor back support or poor posture when working.

See Preventing Back Pain (p.627).

NO ↓

Are you overweight?

YES → Your extra weight may be putting a strain on your back. Read the articles listed at right for help in losing weight.

See Obesity (p.853); Determining Your Body Mass Index (p.51); Exercise and Fitness (p.501); Diet and Nutrition (p.37).

NO ↓

GO TO NEXT PAGE

CONTINUED FROM PREVIOUS PAGE

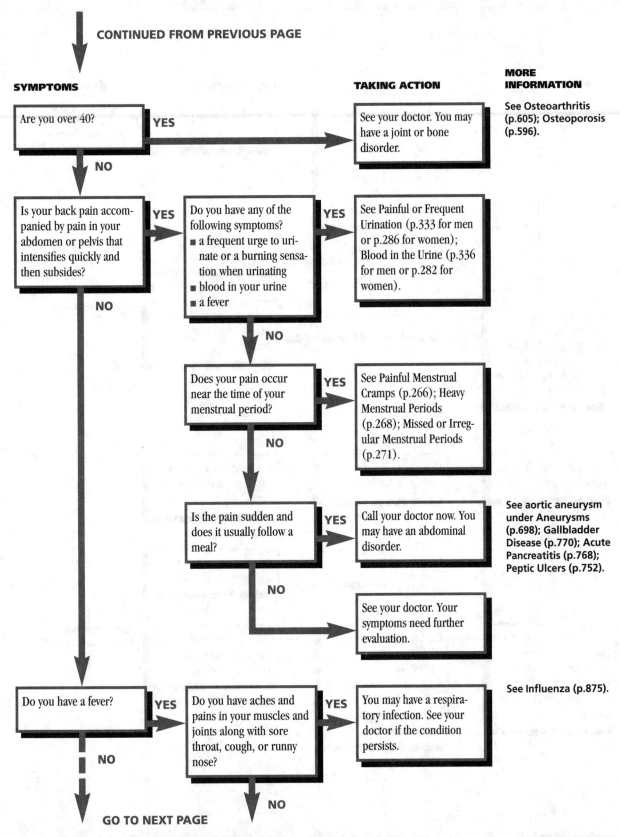

SYMPTOMS

TAKING ACTION

**MORE
INFORMATION**

Are you over 40?

YES

See your doctor. You may have a joint or bone disorder.

See Osteoarthritis (p.605); Osteoporosis (p.596).

NO

Is your back pain accompanied by pain in your abdomen or pelvis that intensifies quickly and then subsides?

YES

Do you have any of the following symptoms?
■ a frequent urge to urinate or a burning sensation when urinating
■ blood in your urine
■ a fever

YES

See Painful or Frequent Urination (p.333 for men or p.286 for women); Blood in the Urine (p.336 for men or p.282 for women).

NO

NO

Does your pain occur near the time of your menstrual period?

YES

See Painful Menstrual Cramps (p.266); Heavy Menstrual Periods (p.268); Missed or Irregular Menstrual Periods (p.271).

NO

Is the pain sudden and does it usually follow a meal?

YES

Call your doctor now. You may have an abdominal disorder.

See aortic aneurysm under Aneurysms (p.698); Gallbladder Disease (p.770); Acute Pancreatitis (p.768); Peptic Ulcers (p.752).

NO

See your doctor. Your symptoms need further evaluation.

Do you have a fever?

YES

Do you have aches and pains in your muscles and joints along with sore throat, cough, or runny nose?

YES

You may have a respiratory infection. See your doctor if the condition persists.

See Influenza (p.875).

NO

NO

GO TO NEXT PAGE

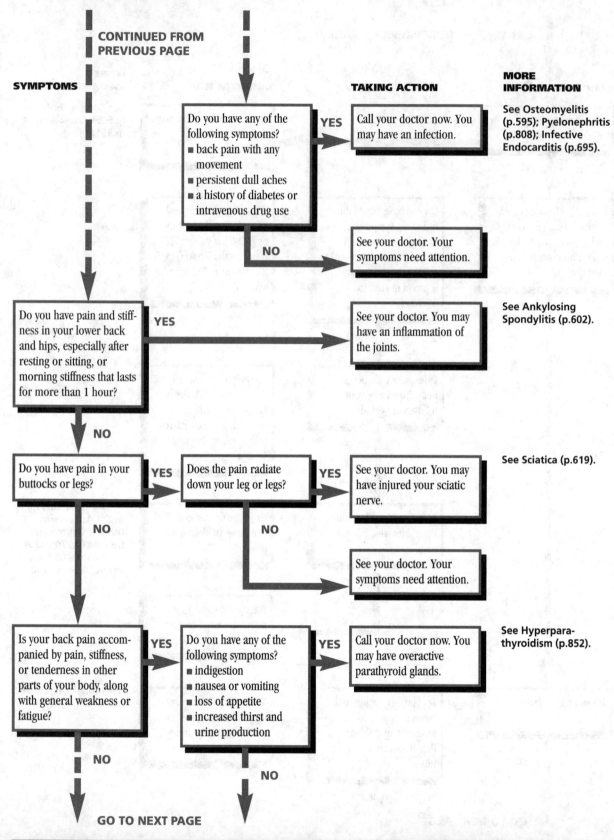

CONTINUED FROM
PREVIOUS PAGE

SYMPTOMS

TAKING ACTION

**MORE
INFORMATION**

Do you have any of the following symptoms?
- back pain with any movement
- persistent dull aches
- a history of diabetes or intravenous drug use

YES → Call your doctor now. You may have an infection.

See Osteomyelitis (p.595); Pyelonephritis (p.808); Infective Endocarditis (p.695).

NO → See your doctor. Your symptoms need attention.

Do you have pain and stiffness in your lower back and hips, especially after resting or sitting, or morning stiffness that lasts for more than 1 hour?

YES → See your doctor. You may have an inflammation of the joints.

See Ankylosing Spondylitis (p.602).

NO ↓

Do you have pain in your buttocks or legs?

YES → Does the pain radiate down your leg or legs?

YES → See your doctor. You may have injured your sciatic nerve.

See Sciatica (p.619).

NO ↓

NO → See your doctor. Your symptoms need attention.

Is your back pain accompanied by pain, stiffness, or tenderness in other parts of your body, along with general weakness or fatigue?

YES → Do you have any of the following symptoms?
- indigestion
- nausea or vomiting
- loss of appetite
- increased thirst and urine production

YES → Call your doctor now. You may have overactive parathyroid glands.

See Hyperparathyroidism (p.852).

NO ↓

NO ↓

GO TO NEXT PAGE

CONTINUED FROM PREVIOUS PAGE

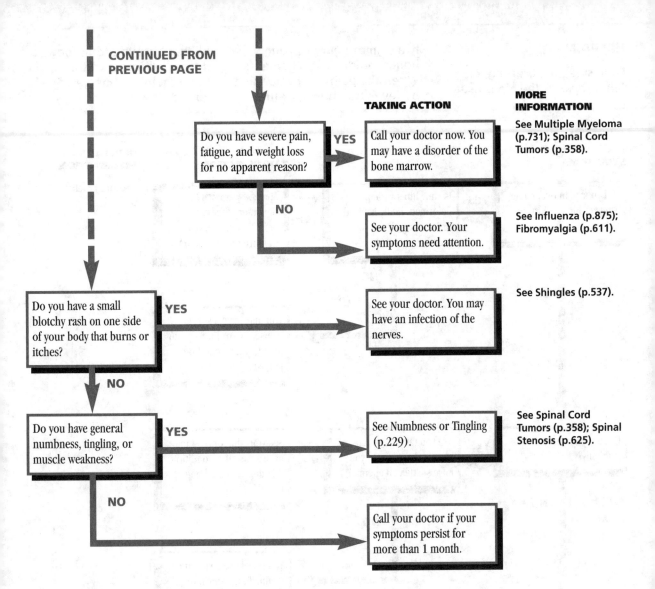

TAKING ACTION

Do you have severe pain, fatigue, and weight loss for no apparent reason?

YES → Call your doctor now. You may have a disorder of the bone marrow.

See Multiple Myeloma (p.731); Spinal Cord Tumors (p.358).

NO → See your doctor. Your symptoms need attention.

See Influenza (p.875); Fibromyalgia (p.611).

Do you have a small blotchy rash on one side of your body that burns or itches?

YES → See your doctor. You may have an infection of the nerves.

See Shingles (p.537).

NO

Do you have general numbness, tingling, or muscle weakness?

YES → See Numbness or Tingling (p.229).

See Spinal Cord Tumors (p.358); Spinal Stenosis (p.625).

NO → Call your doctor if your symptoms persist for more than 1 month.

HIP PAIN

Pain, swelling, bruising, or tenderness of the hip is usually a sign of injury to your bones, tendons, or ligaments. When the pain is accompanied by fever, numbness, or tingling, your symptoms may be due to a disorder of the bones, joints, or nerves. See your doctor.

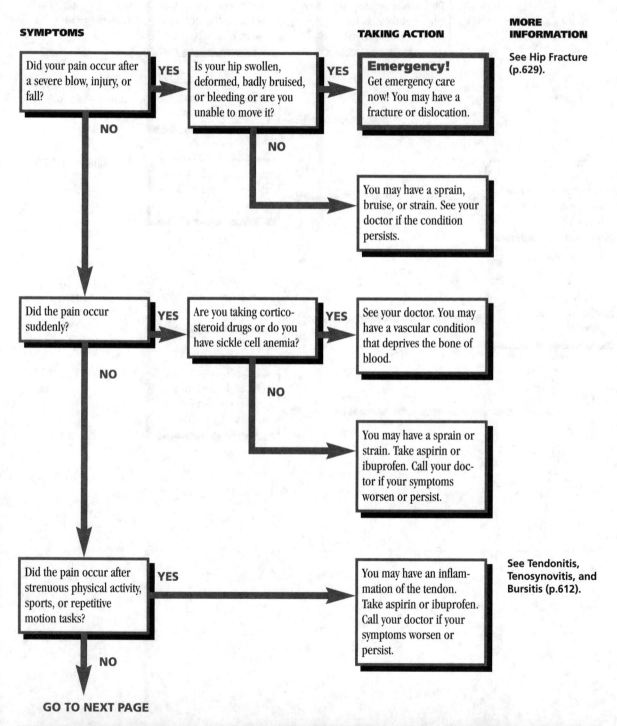

SYMPTOMS

Did your pain occur after a severe blow, injury, or fall?

YES →

Is your hip swollen, deformed, badly bruised, or bleeding or are you unable to move it?

YES →

NO

TAKING ACTION

Emergency! Get emergency care now! You may have a fracture or dislocation.

You may have a sprain, bruise, or strain. See your doctor if the condition persists.

NO

Did the pain occur suddenly?

YES →

Are you taking corticosteroid drugs or do you have sickle cell anemia?

YES →

NO

See your doctor. You may have a vascular condition that deprives the bone of blood.

You may have a sprain or strain. Take aspirin or ibuprofen. Call your doctor if your symptoms worsen or persist.

NO

Did the pain occur after strenuous physical activity, sports, or repetitive motion tasks?

YES →

You may have an inflammation of the tendon. Take aspirin or ibuprofen. Call your doctor if your symptoms worsen or persist.

NO

GO TO NEXT PAGE

MORE INFORMATION

See Hip Fracture (p.629).

See Tendonitis, Tenosynovitis, and Bursitis (p.612).

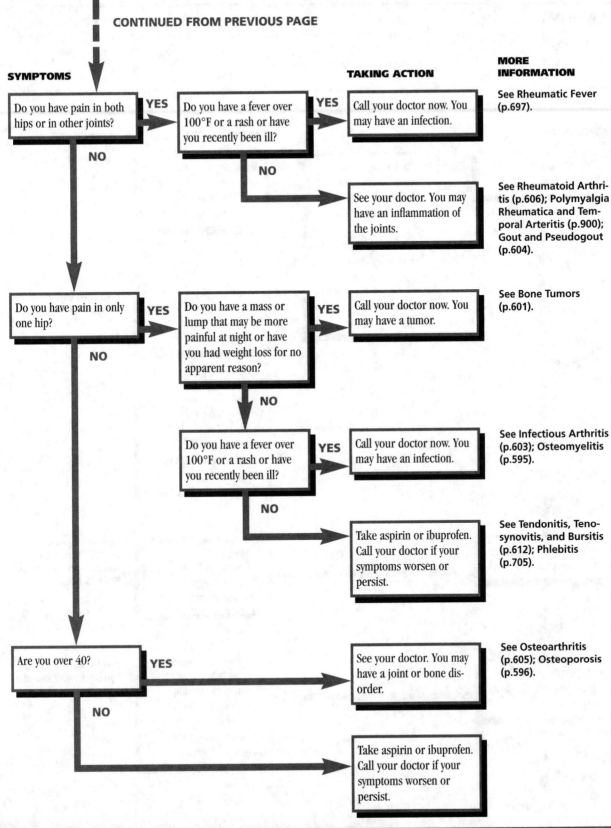

SYMPTOMS

Do you have pain in both hips or in other joints?

YES

Do you have a fever over 100°F or a rash or have you recently been ill?

YES

NO

NO

Do you have pain in only one hip?

YES

Do you have a mass or lump that may be more painful at night or have you had weight loss for no apparent reason?

YES

NO

NO

Do you have a fever over 100°F or a rash or have you recently been ill?

YES

NO

Are you over 40?

YES

NO

TAKING ACTION

Call your doctor now. You may have an infection.

See your doctor. You may have an inflammation of the joints.

Call your doctor now. You may have a tumor.

Call your doctor now. You may have an infection.

Take aspirin or ibuprofen. Call your doctor if your symptoms worsen or persist.

See your doctor. You may have a joint or bone disorder.

Take aspirin or ibuprofen. Call your doctor if your symptoms worsen or persist.

MORE INFORMATION

See Rheumatic Fever (p.697).

See Rheumatoid Arthritis (p.606); Polymyalgia Rheumatica and Temporal Arteritis (p.900); Gout and Pseudogout (p.604).

See Bone Tumors (p.601).

See Infectious Arthritis (p.603); Osteomyelitis (p.595).

See Tendonitis, Tenosynovitis, and Bursitis (p.612); Phlebitis (p.705).

See Osteoarthritis (p.605); Osteoporosis (p.596).

KNEE PAIN

Pain, swelling, bruising, or tenderness of the knee is usually a sign that you have injured your bones, tendons, or ligaments. When accompanied by fever, numbness, or tingling, your symptoms may be due to a disorder of the bones, joints, or nerves. See your doctor.

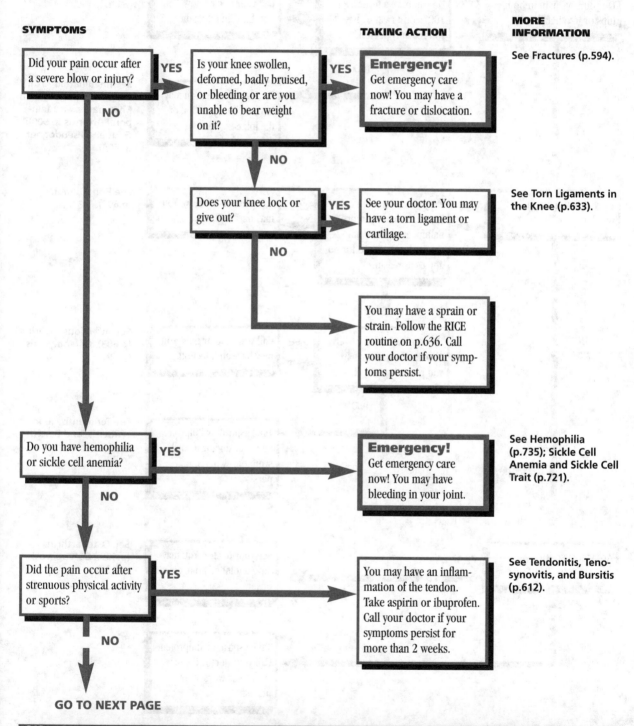

SYMPTOMS

TAKING ACTION

MORE INFORMATION

Did your pain occur after a severe blow or injury? — **YES** →

Is your knee swollen, deformed, badly bruised, or bleeding or are you unable to bear weight on it? — **YES** →

Emergency! Get emergency care now! You may have a fracture or dislocation.

See Fractures (p.594).

NO ↓

Does your knee lock or give out? — **YES** →

See your doctor. You may have a torn ligament or cartilage.

See Torn Ligaments in the Knee (p.633).

NO ↓

You may have a sprain or strain. Follow the RICE routine on p.636. Call your doctor if your symptoms persist.

NO ↓

Do you have hemophilia or sickle cell anemia? — **YES** →

Emergency! Get emergency care now! You may have bleeding in your joint.

See Hemophilia (p.735); Sickle Cell Anemia and Sickle Cell Trait (p.721).

NO ↓

Did the pain occur after strenuous physical activity or sports? — **YES** →

You may have an inflammation of the tendon. Take aspirin or ibuprofen. Call your doctor if your symptoms persist for more than 2 weeks.

See Tendonitis, Tenosynovitis, and Bursitis (p.612).

NO ↓

GO TO NEXT PAGE

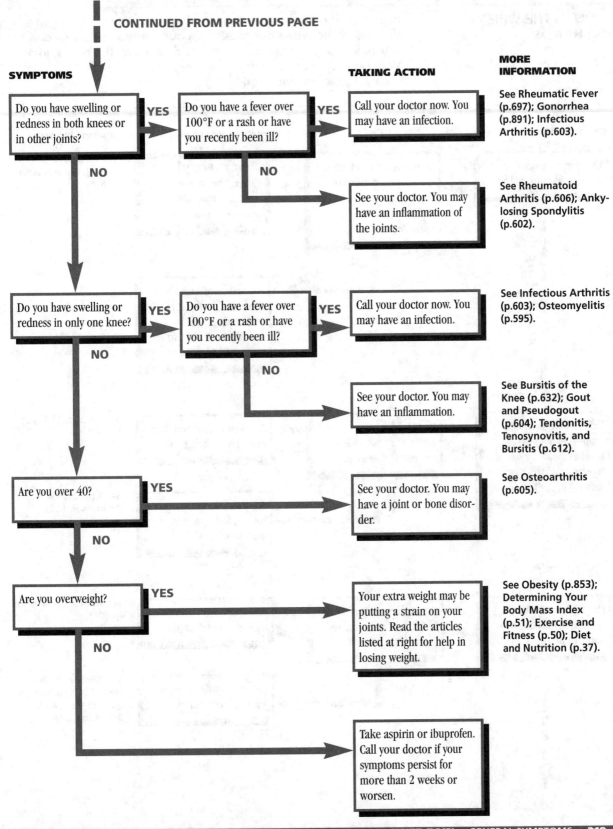

SYMPTOMS

TAKING ACTION

Do you have swelling or redness in both knees or in other joints?

YES → Do you have a fever over 100°F or a rash or have you recently been ill?

YES → Call your doctor now. You may have an infection.

See Rheumatic Fever (p.697); Gonorrhea (p.891); Infectious Arthritis (p.603).

NO

NO → See your doctor. You may have an inflammation of the joints.

See Rheumatoid Arthritis (p.606); Anky-losing Spondylitis (p.602).

Do you have swelling or redness in only one knee?

YES → Do you have a fever over 100°F or a rash or have you recently been ill?

YES → Call your doctor now. You may have an infection.

See Infectious Arthritis (p.603); Osteomyelitis (p.595).

NO

NO → See your doctor. You may have an inflammation.

See Bursitis of the Knee (p.632); Gout and Pseudogout (p.604); Tendonitis, Tenosynovitis, and Bursitis (p.612).

Are you over 40?

YES → See your doctor. You may have a joint or bone disorder.

See Osteoarthritis (p.605).

NO

Are you overweight?

YES → Your extra weight may be putting a strain on your joints. Read the articles listed at right for help in losing weight.

See Obesity (p.853); Determining Your Body Mass Index (p.51); Exercise and Fitness (p.50); Diet and Nutrition (p.37).

NO

Take aspirin or ibuprofen. Call your doctor if your symptoms persist for more than 2 weeks or worsen.

PAIN IN THE WRISTS OR HANDS

Pain, swelling, bruising, or tenderness of the wrists or hands is usually a sign of injury to your bones, tendons, or ligaments. When accompanied by fever, numbness, or tingling, your symptoms may be due to a disorder of the bones, joints, or nerves.

SYMPTOMS

TAKING ACTION

MORE INFORMATION

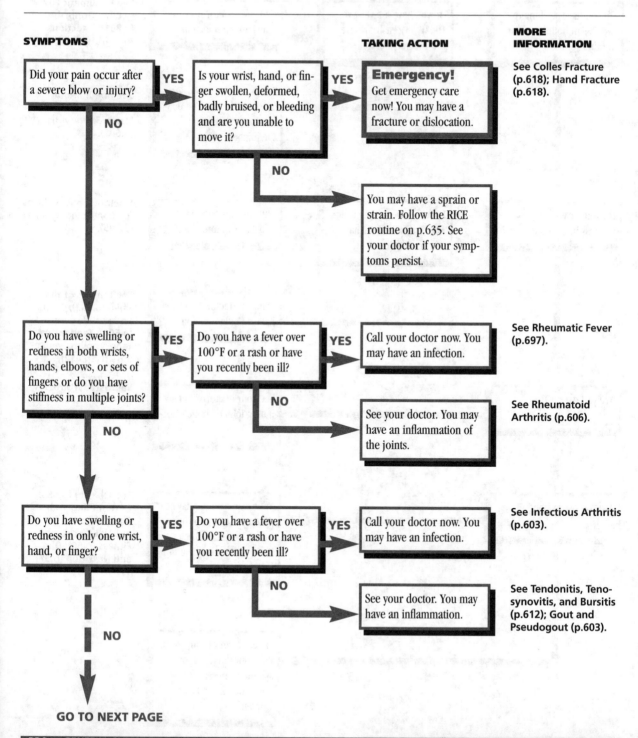

Did your pain occur after a severe blow or injury?

YES → Is your wrist, hand, or finger swollen, deformed, badly bruised, or bleeding and are you unable to move it?

YES → **Emergency!** Get emergency care now! You may have a fracture or dislocation.

See Colles Fracture (p.618); Hand Fracture (p.618).

NO → You may have a sprain or strain. Follow the RICE routine on p.635. See your doctor if your symptoms persist.

NO

Do you have swelling or redness in both wrists, hands, elbows, or sets of fingers or do you have stiffness in multiple joints?

YES → Do you have a fever over 100°F or a rash or have you recently been ill?

YES → Call your doctor now. You may have an infection.

See Rheumatic Fever (p.697).

NO → See your doctor. You may have an inflammation of the joints.

See Rheumatoid Arthritis (p.606).

NO

Do you have swelling or redness in only one wrist, hand, or finger?

YES → Do you have a fever over 100°F or a rash or have you recently been ill?

YES → Call your doctor now. You may have an infection.

See Infectious Arthritis (p.603).

NO → See your doctor. You may have an inflammation.

See Tendonitis, Tenosynovitis, and Bursitis (p.612); Gout and Pseudogout (p.603).

NO

GO TO NEXT PAGE

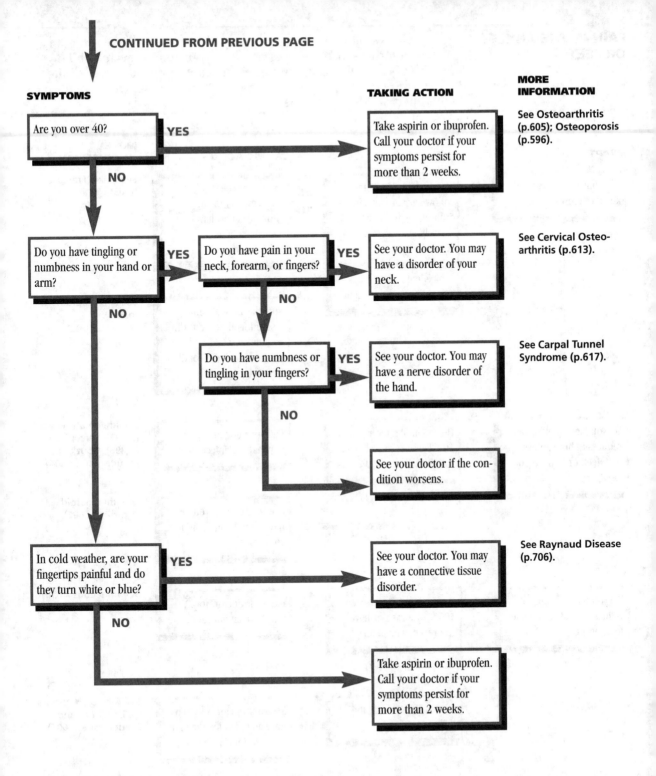

SYMPTOMS

TAKING ACTION

Are you over 40?

YES → Take aspirin or ibuprofen. Call your doctor if your symptoms persist for more than 2 weeks.

See Osteoarthritis (p.605); Osteoporosis (p.596).

NO ↓

Do you have tingling or numbness in your hand or arm?

YES → Do you have pain in your neck, forearm, or fingers?

YES → See your doctor. You may have a disorder of your neck.

See Cervical Osteo-arthritis (p.613).

NO ↓

Do you have numbness or tingling in your fingers?

YES → See your doctor. You may have a nerve disorder of the hand.

See Carpal Tunnel Syndrome (p.617).

NO ↓

See your doctor if the condition worsens.

NO ↓

In cold weather, are your fingertips painful and do they turn white or blue?

YES → See your doctor. You may have a connective tissue disorder.

See Raynaud Disease (p.706).

NO ↓

Take aspirin or ibuprofen. Call your doctor if your symptoms persist for more than 2 weeks.

PAIN IN THE ANKLES OR FEET

Pain, swelling, bruising, or tenderness of the ankles or feet is usually a sign of injury to the bones, tendons, or ligaments. When accompanied by fever, numbness, or tingling, your symptoms may be caused by a disorder of the bones, joints, or nerves.

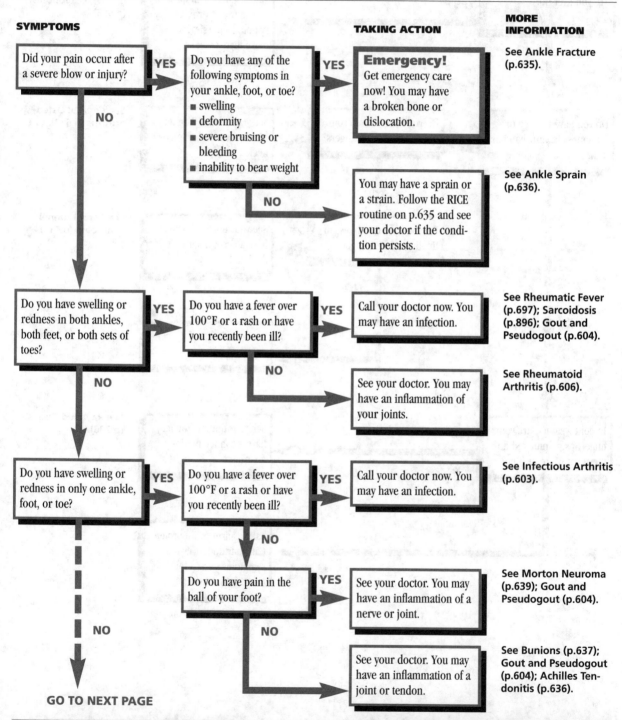

SYMPTOMS

Did your pain occur after a severe blow or injury? — **YES** → Do you have any of the following symptoms in your ankle, foot, or toe?
- swelling
- deformity
- severe bruising or bleeding
- inability to bear weight

— **YES** →

TAKING ACTION

Emergency! Get emergency care now! You may have a broken bone or dislocation.

MORE INFORMATION

See Ankle Fracture (p.635).

NO → You may have a sprain or a strain. Follow the RICE routine on p.635 and see your doctor if the condition persists.

See Ankle Sprain (p.636).

Do you have swelling or redness in both ankles, both feet, or both sets of toes? — **YES** → Do you have a fever over 100°F or a rash or have you recently been ill? — **YES** → Call your doctor now. You may have an infection.

See Rheumatic Fever (p.697); Sarcoidosis (p.896); Gout and Pseudogout (p.604).

NO → See your doctor. You may have an inflammation of your joints.

See Rheumatoid Arthritis (p.606).

Do you have swelling or redness in only one ankle, foot, or toe? — **YES** → Do you have a fever over 100°F or a rash or have you recently been ill? — **YES** → Call your doctor now. You may have an infection.

See Infectious Arthritis (p.603).

NO → Do you have pain in the ball of your foot? — **YES** → See your doctor. You may have an inflammation of a nerve or joint.

See Morton Neuroma (p.639); Gout and Pseudogout (p.604).

NO → See your doctor. You may have an inflammation of a joint or tendon.

See Bunions (p.637); Gout and Pseudogout (p.604); Achilles Tendonitis (p.636).

NO → **GO TO NEXT PAGE**

TAKING ACTION

MORE INFORMATION

Are you over 40? — **YES** → See your doctor. You may have a joint or bone disorder. — See Osteoarthritis (p.605).

NO ↓

Are you overweight? — **YES** → Your extra weight may be putting a strain on your joints. Read the articles listed at right for help in losing weight. — See Obesity (p.853); Determining Your Body Mass Index (p.51); Exercise and Fitness (p.50); Diet and Nutrition (p.37).

NO ↓

Do you have a tough, raised patch of skin on the bottom of your foot or toes? — **YES** → **Is the area painful when you apply pressure?** — **YES** → You may have a plantar wart. See your doctor if the condition worsens. — See Warts (p.541).

NO ↓

Are your toes in a clenched or clawlike position? — **YES** → You may have a foot deformity. See your doctor if the condition worsens. — See Hammer Toe (p.639).

NO ↓

See your doctor if the condition worsens. — See Bunions (p.637); Corns and Calluses (p.555).

NO ↓ (from "Do you have a tough, raised patch...")

Do you have pain in your sole or heel, especially when you walk or run? — **YES** → See your doctor. You may have a circulatory or ligament problem. — See Atherosclerosis (p.653); Plantar Fasciitis (p.640); Peripheral Vascular Disease (p.701).

NO ↓

Do you have numbness or tingling in your feet that moves up your legs? — **YES** → See Numbness or Tingling (p.229). — See Peripheral Neuropathy (p.379).

NO ↓

Call your doctor if your symptoms persist for more than 1 month.

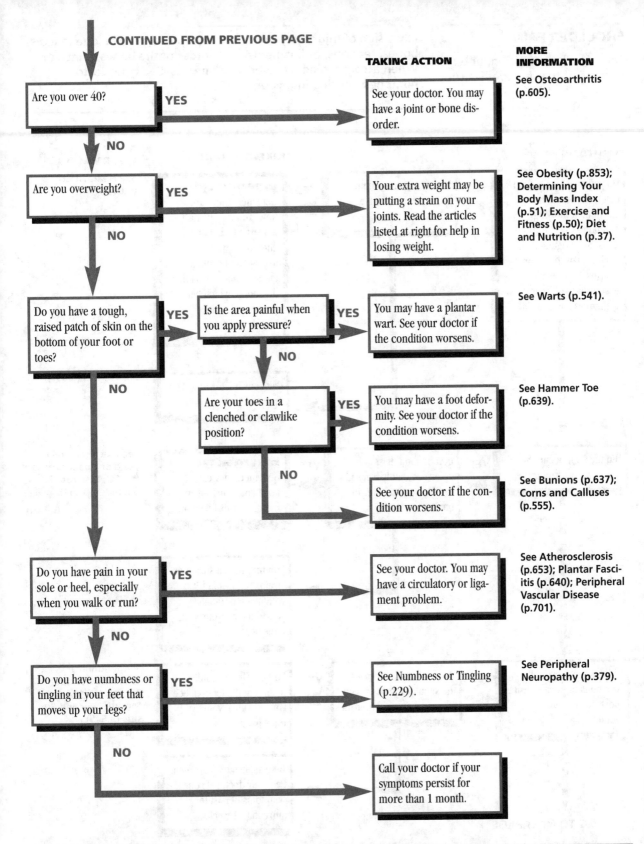

SHOULDER PAIN

Pain, swelling, bruising, or tenderness of the shoulder is usually a sign of injury to your bones, tendons, or ligaments. When accompanied by fever, numbness, or tingling, your symptoms may be due to a disorder of the bones, joints, or nerves. See your doctor.

SYMPTOMS

TAKING ACTION

MORE INFORMATION

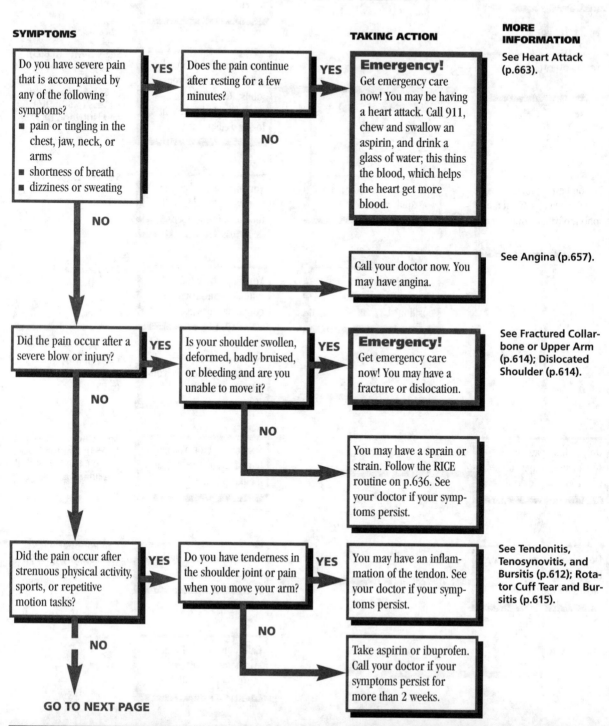

Do you have severe pain that is accompanied by any of the following symptoms?
- pain or tingling in the chest, jaw, neck, or arms
- shortness of breath
- dizziness or sweating

YES → Does the pain continue after resting for a few minutes?

YES → **Emergency!** Get emergency care now! You may be having a heart attack. Call 911, chew and swallow an aspirin, and drink a glass of water; this thins the blood, which helps the heart get more blood.

See Heart Attack (p.663).

NO → Call your doctor now. You may have angina.

See Angina (p.657).

NO

Did the pain occur after a severe blow or injury?

YES → Is your shoulder swollen, deformed, badly bruised, or bleeding and are you unable to move it?

YES → **Emergency!** Get emergency care now! You may have a fracture or dislocation.

See Fractured Collarbone or Upper Arm (p.614); Dislocated Shoulder (p.614).

NO → You may have a sprain or strain. Follow the RICE routine on p.636. See your doctor if your symptoms persist.

NO

Did the pain occur after strenuous physical activity, sports, or repetitive motion tasks?

YES → Do you have tenderness in the shoulder joint or pain when you move your arm?

YES → You may have an inflammation of the tendon. See your doctor if your symptoms persist.

See Tendonitis, Tenosynovitis, and Bursitis (p.612); Rotator Cuff Tear and Bursitis (p.615).

NO → Take aspirin or ibuprofen. Call your doctor if your symptoms persist for more than 2 weeks.

NO

GO TO NEXT PAGE

CONTINUED FROM PREVIOUS PAGE

SYMPTOMS

TAKING ACTION

**MORE
INFORMATION**

Has your shoulder pain become more severe recently, possibly causing sleep difficulties?

YES → See your doctor. You may have an inflammation that is complicated by adhesions.

See Frozen Shoulder (p.615).

NO ↓

Do you have swelling or redness in both shoulders or in other joints?

YES → Do you have a fever over 100°F or a rash or have you recently been ill?

YES → Call your doctor now. You may have an infection.

See Rheumatic Fever (p.697).

NO → See your doctor. You may have an inflammation of the joints.

See Rheumatoid Arthritis (p.606).

NO ↓

Do you have swelling or redness in only one shoulder?

YES → Do you have a fever over 100°F or a rash or have you recently been ill?

YES → Call your doctor now. You may have an infection.

See Infectious Arthritis (p.603); Osteomyelitis (p.596).

NO → See your doctor. You may have an inflammation.

See Tendonitis, Tenosynovitis, and Bursitis (p.612); Gout and Pseudogout (p.604).

NO ↓

Are you over 40?

YES → Take aspirin or ibuprofen. Call your doctor if your symptoms persist for more than 2 weeks.

See Osteoarthritis (p.605); Osteoporosis (p.596).

NO ↓

Do you have tingling or numbness in your neck, hand, or arm?

YES → See your doctor. You may have a disorder of your neck.

See Cervical Osteo-arthritis (p.613).

NO ↓

Take aspirin or ibuprofen. Call your doctor if your symptoms persist for more than 2 weeks.

NECK PAIN

Neck pain is any pain, stiffness, swelling, lumps, or spasms in your neck. Neck pain and stiffness often occur as a result of muscle strain. However, neck pain accompanied by other symptoms requires medical evaluation. If you have swollen glands, see the chart on p.867.

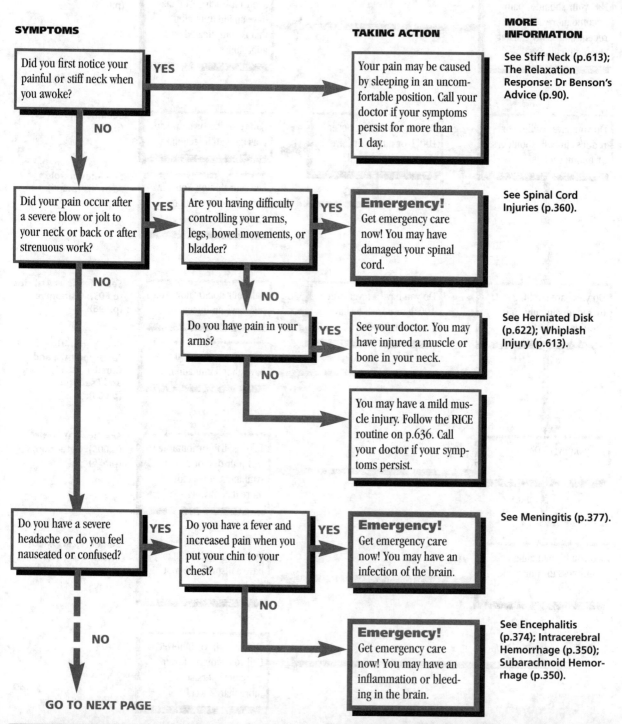

SYMPTOMS

TAKING ACTION

MORE INFORMATION

Did you first notice your painful or stiff neck when you awoke?

YES → Your pain may be caused by sleeping in an uncomfortable position. Call your doctor if your symptoms persist for more than 1 day.

See Stiff Neck (p.613); The Relaxation Response: Dr Benson's Advice (p.90).

NO ↓

Did your pain occur after a severe blow or jolt to your neck or back or after strenuous work?

YES → Are you having difficulty controlling your arms, legs, bowel movements, or bladder?

YES → **Emergency!** Get emergency care now! You may have damaged your spinal cord.

See Spinal Cord Injuries (p.360).

NO ↓

Do you have pain in your arms?

YES → See your doctor. You may have injured a muscle or bone in your neck.

See Herniated Disk (p.622); Whiplash Injury (p.613).

NO ↓

You may have a mild muscle injury. Follow the RICE routine on p.636. Call your doctor if your symptoms persist.

NO ↓

Do you have a severe headache or do you feel nauseated or confused?

YES → Do you have a fever and increased pain when you put your chin to your chest?

YES → **Emergency!** Get emergency care now! You may have an infection of the brain.

See Meningitis (p.377).

NO ↓

Emergency! Get emergency care now! You may have an inflammation or bleeding in the brain.

See Encephalitis (p.374); Intracerebral Hemorrhage (p.350); Subarachnoid Hemorrhage (p.350).

NO ↓

GO TO NEXT PAGE

CONTINUED FROM PREVIOUS PAGE

SYMPTOMS

TAKING ACTION

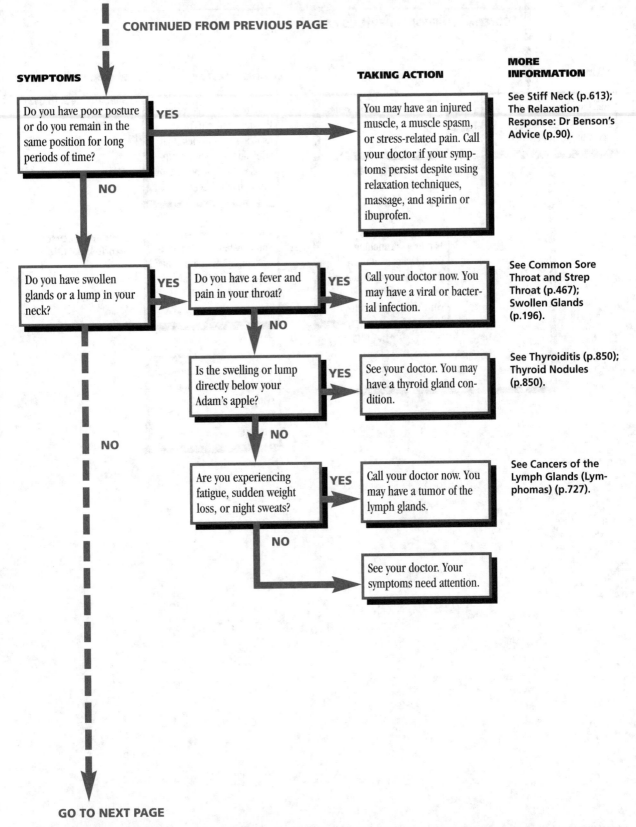

Do you have poor posture or do you remain in the same position for long periods of time?

YES

You may have an injured muscle, a muscle spasm, or stress-related pain. Call your doctor if your symptoms persist despite using relaxation techniques, massage, and aspirin or ibuprofen.

See Stiff Neck (p.613); The Relaxation Response: Dr Benson's Advice (p.90).

NO

Do you have swollen glands or a lump in your neck?

YES

Do you have a fever and pain in your throat?

YES

Call your doctor now. You may have a viral or bacterial infection.

See Common Sore Throat and Strep Throat (p.467); Swollen Glands (p.196).

NO

Is the swelling or lump directly below your Adam's apple?

YES

See your doctor. You may have a thyroid gland condition.

See Thyroiditis (p.850); Thyroid Nodules (p.850).

NO

NO

Are you experiencing fatigue, sudden weight loss, or night sweats?

YES

Call your doctor now. You may have a tumor of the lymph glands.

See Cancers of the Lymph Glands (Lymphomas) (p.727).

NO

See your doctor. Your symptoms need attention.

GO TO NEXT PAGE

SYMPTOMS

TAKING ACTION

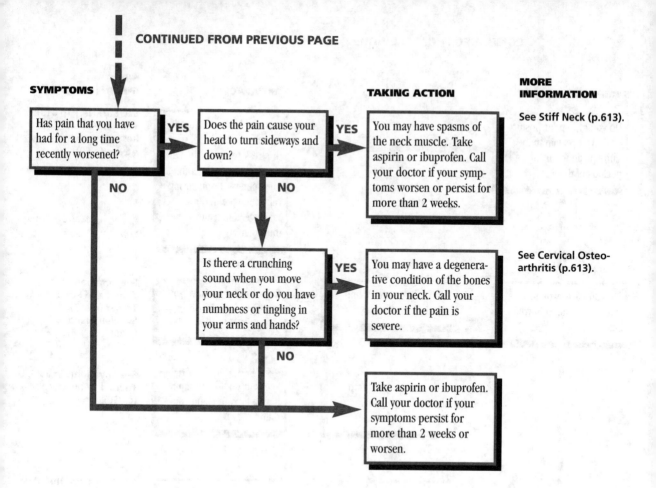

Has pain that you have had for a long time recently worsened?

YES

Does the pain cause your head to turn sideways and down?

YES

You may have spasms of the neck muscle. Take aspirin or ibuprofen. Call your doctor if your symptoms worsen or persist for more than 2 weeks.

See Stiff Neck (p.613).

NO

NO

Is there a crunching sound when you move your neck or do you have numbness or tingling in your arms and hands?

YES

You may have a degenerative condition of the bones in your neck. Call your doctor if the pain is severe.

See Cervical Osteo-arthritis (p.613).

NO

Take aspirin or ibuprofen. Call your doctor if your symptoms persist for more than 2 weeks or worsen.

NUMBNESS OR TINGLING

Numbness or tingling causes little or no feeling of the skin or a prickly sensation. Numbness or tingling is a symptom of many conditions. When accompanied by paralysis, however, either symptom can be an emergency.

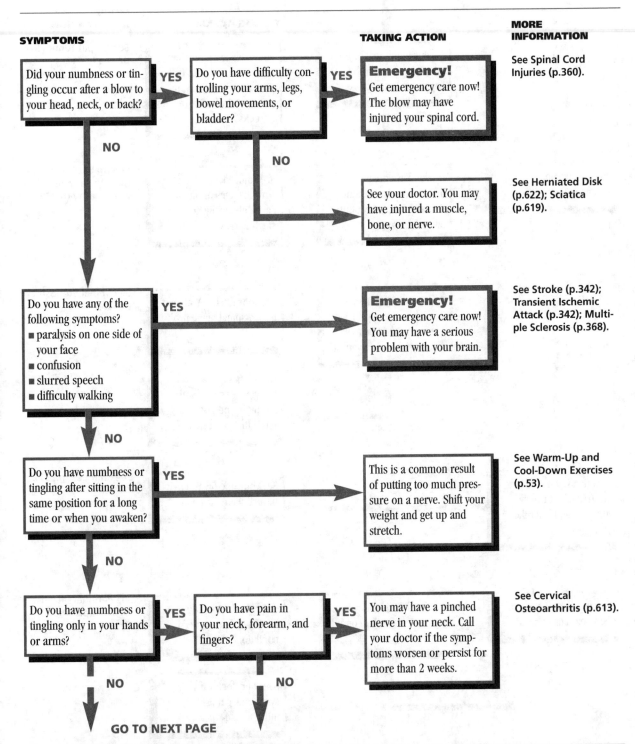

SYMPTOMS

TAKING ACTION

MORE INFORMATION

Did your numbness or tingling occur after a blow to your head, neck, or back?

YES → Do you have difficulty controlling your arms, legs, bowel movements, or bladder?

YES → **Emergency!** Get emergency care now! The blow may have injured your spinal cord.

See Spinal Cord Injuries (p.360).

NO

See your doctor. You may have injured a muscle, bone, or nerve.

See Herniated Disk (p.622); Sciatica (p.619).

NO

Do you have any of the following symptoms?
- paralysis on one side of your face
- confusion
- slurred speech
- difficulty walking

YES → **Emergency!** Get emergency care now! You may have a serious problem with your brain.

See Stroke (p.342); Transient Ischemic Attack (p.342); Multiple Sclerosis (p.368).

NO

Do you have numbness or tingling after sitting in the same position for a long time or when you awaken?

YES → This is a common result of putting too much pressure on a nerve. Shift your weight and get up and stretch.

See Warm-Up and Cool-Down Exercises (p.53).

NO

Do you have numbness or tingling only in your hands or arms?

YES → Do you have pain in your neck, forearm, and fingers?

YES → You may have a pinched nerve in your neck. Call your doctor if the symptoms worsen or persist for more than 2 weeks.

See Cervical Osteoarthritis (p.613).

NO

NO

GO TO NEXT PAGE

CONTINUED FROM PREVIOUS PAGE

TAKING ACTION

Is your numbness or tingling associated with repetitive motion tasks?

YES → You may have a pinched nerve in your hand. Call your doctor if the symptoms persist for more than 2 weeks.

See Carpal Tunnel Syndrome (p.617).

NO

Do you have numbness or tingling in your feet?

YES → Do you have greatly increased urine production and frequency of urination?

YES → See your doctor. You may have diabetes or another cause of damage to the small nerves.

See Diabetes Mellitus (p.832); Peripheral Neuropathy (p.379).

NO

NO

Does your numbness or tingling occur in your legs when you stand or walk and improve when you sit?

YES → See your doctor. You may have a spinal nerve problem.

See Spinal Stenosis (p.625).

NO → See your doctor if your symptoms persist for more than 2 weeks.

Do you have tingling in one area of your body with a small, blisterlike rash?

YES → See your doctor. You may have a nerve infection.

See Shingles (p.537).

NO

Have you had tingling for many years or months?

YES → Do any close blood relatives have a similar condition?

YES → See your doctor. You may have an inherited nerve condition.

See Peripheral Neuropathy (p.379).

NO

NO → See your doctor if your symptoms persist for more than 4 weeks.

NAIL PROBLEMS

Fingernail and toenail problems are usually caused by inflammation of the skin around the nail or by an infection. A persistently painful and inflamed fingernail or toenail requires your doctor's attention.

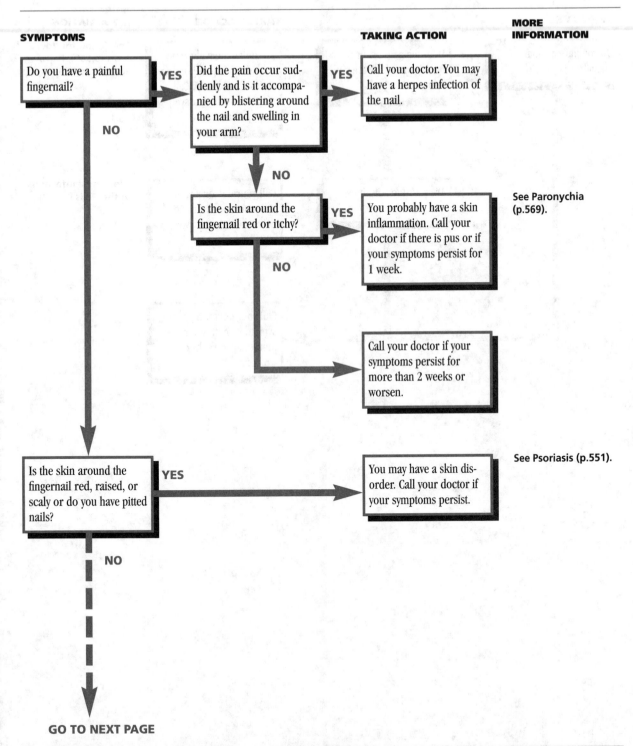

SYMPTOMS

Do you have a painful fingernail?

YES → Did the pain occur suddenly and is it accompanied by blistering around the nail and swelling in your arm?

NO

Is the skin around the fingernail red or itchy?

NO

YES → Is the skin around the fingernail red, raised, or scaly or do you have pitted nails?

NO

TAKING ACTION

YES → Call your doctor. You may have a herpes infection of the nail.

YES → You probably have a skin inflammation. Call your doctor if there is pus or if your symptoms persist for 1 week.

Call your doctor if your symptoms persist for more than 2 weeks or worsen.

YES → You may have a skin disorder. Call your doctor if your symptoms persist.

MORE INFORMATION

See Paronychia (p.569).

See Psoriasis (p.551).

GO TO NEXT PAGE

CONTINUED FROM PREVIOUS PAGE

SYMPTOMS

TAKING ACTION

Do you have a painful toenail?

YES → Does the pain occur on the big toe where the nail touches the skin?

YES → Trimming the nail properly and wearing well-fitting shoes should help. Call your doctor if your symptoms persist.

See Caring for Your Nails (p.569); Ingrown Toenails (p.560).

NO

NO

Are your toenails thick and yellow?

YES → Call your doctor if your symptoms persist or you do not like the way your nails look.

See Fungal Infections of the Nails (p.560).

NO

Call your doctor if your symptoms persist for more than 2 weeks or worsen.

COUGH

Coughing is a symptom of many conditions, the most common of which is respiratory infection. Coughing up blood, coughing accompanied by shortness of breath, or long-term coughing with a fever can indicate a condition that requires your doctor's attention.

SYMPTOMS

TAKING ACTION

MORE INFORMATION

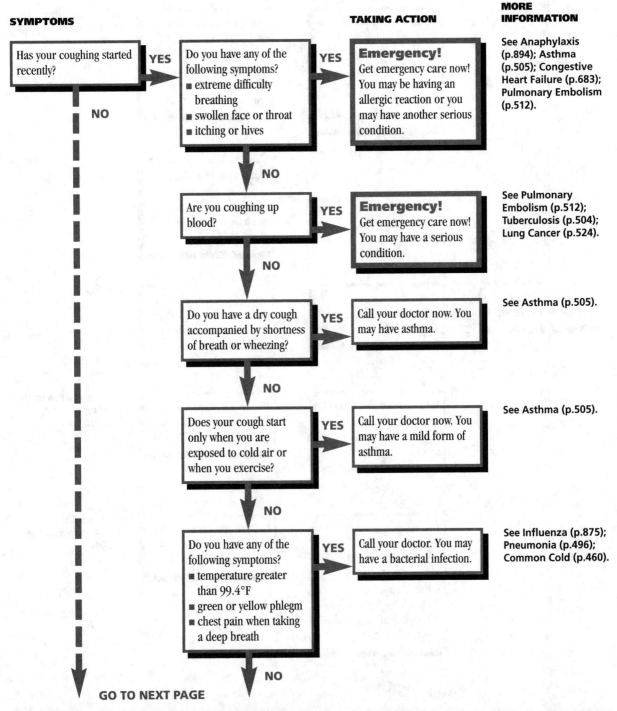

Has your coughing started recently?

YES → Do you have any of the following symptoms?
- extreme difficulty breathing
- swollen face or throat
- itching or hives

YES → **Emergency!** Get emergency care now! You may be having an allergic reaction or you may have another serious condition.

See Anaphylaxis (p.894); Asthma (p.505); Congestive Heart Failure (p.683); Pulmonary Embolism (p.512).

NO ↓

Are you coughing up blood?

YES → **Emergency!** Get emergency care now! You may have a serious condition.

See Pulmonary Embolism (p.512); Tuberculosis (p.504); Lung Cancer (p.524).

NO ↓

Do you have a dry cough accompanied by shortness of breath or wheezing?

YES → Call your doctor now. You may have asthma.

See Asthma (p.505).

NO ↓

Does your cough start only when you are exposed to cold air or when you exercise?

YES → Call your doctor now. You may have a mild form of asthma.

See Asthma (p.505).

NO ↓

Do you have any of the following symptoms?
- temperature greater than 99.4°F
- green or yellow phlegm
- chest pain when taking a deep breath

YES → Call your doctor. You may have a bacterial infection.

See Influenza (p.875); Pneumonia (p.496); Common Cold (p.460).

NO ↓

NO (left path)

GO TO NEXT PAGE

CONTINUED FROM
PREVIOUS PAGE

TAKING ACTION

Do you have any of the following symptoms?
- runny nose
- sore throat
- minimal phlegm with your cough
- weak, run-down feeling

YES → You may have an upper respiratory infection. Call your doctor if your symptoms persist for more than 14 days or if you have a temperature over 101°F.

See Acute Bronchitis (p.494); Common Cold (p.460).

NO → Call your doctor if your symptoms persist for more than 14 days or if you have a temperature over 101°F.

Do you have a chronic cough and do you smoke? **YES** → Do you have minimal phlegm and a hoarse voice? **YES** → Your coughing is probably due to smoking. Ask your doctor for help in quitting smoking.

See Tobacco (p.56).

NO

NO → Have you had shortness of breath for at least 3 months when you are active? **YES** → Call your doctor. You may have chronic obstructive pulmonary disease.

See Chronic Bronchitis and Emphysema (p.517).

NO → Do you have any of the following symptoms?
- coughing up blood
- pains in your chest
- loss of appetite
- unexplained weight loss (more than 10 pounds over 6 months)

YES → Call your doctor now. You may have a lung tumor or tuberculosis.

See Lung Cancer (p.524); Tuberculosis (p.504).

NO

GO TO NEXT PAGE

SYMPTOMS

TAKING ACTION

Do you have a chronic cough?

YES →

Do you have any of the following symptoms?
- fever
- night sweats
- weight loss
- history of tuberculosis
- exposure to someone with tuberculosis

YES →

Call your doctor now. You may have tuberculosis.

See Tuberculosis (p.504).

NO ↓

NO ↓

Do you have any of the following symptoms?
- history of heart disease
- a cough that is worse when lying down
- swollen legs

YES →

Call your doctor now. You may have congestive heart failure.

See Congestive Heart Failure (p.683).

NO ↓

Does your cough occur only when you are exposed to cold air or when you exercise?

YES →

Call your doctor. You may have a mild form of asthma.

See Asthma (p.505).

NO ↓

Are you taking angiotensin-converting enzyme (ACE) inhibitors for high blood pressure?

YES →

You may be having a side effect from the ACE inhibitor. Ask your doctor if your medicines could be causing your cough.

See Medicines (p.1148).

NO ↓

Are you exposed to smoky conditions or polluted air?

YES →

Your cough may be due to secondhand smoke or pollution.

See Tobacco (p.56).

NO ↓

Call your doctor if your symptoms worsen or persist for more than 1 month.

SHORTNESS OF BREATH

Labored, rapid breathing, or an inability to get air in or out of the lungs characterizes shortness of breath. It almost always indicates a condition that requires your doctor's attention. When accompanied by chest pain or swelling of the face or abdomen, immediate treatment is required.

SYMPTOMS

TAKING ACTION

MORE INFORMATION

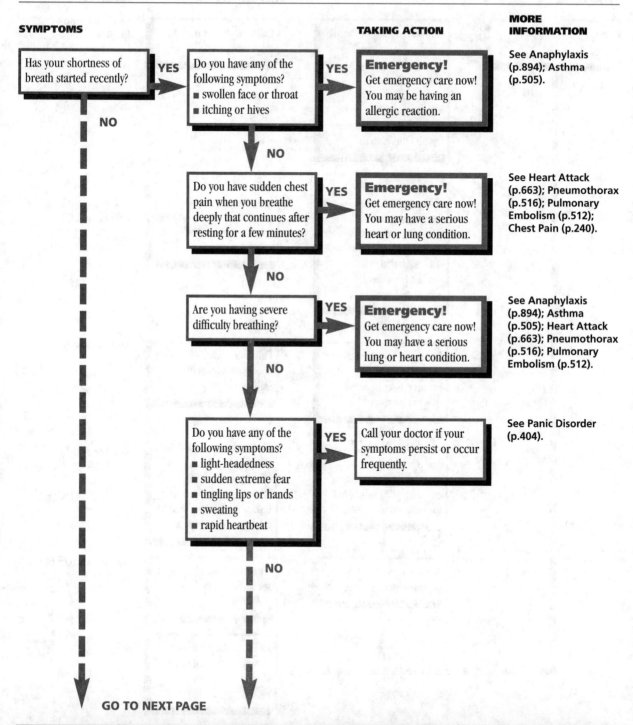

Has your shortness of breath started recently?

YES →

Do you have any of the following symptoms?
- swollen face or throat
- itching or hives

YES →

Emergency!
Get emergency care now! You may be having an allergic reaction.

See Anaphylaxis (p.894); Asthma (p.505).

NO ↓

Do you have sudden chest pain when you breathe deeply that continues after resting for a few minutes?

YES →

Emergency!
Get emergency care now! You may have a serious heart or lung condition.

See Heart Attack (p.663); Pneumothorax (p.516); Pulmonary Embolism (p.512); Chest Pain (p.240).

NO ↓

Are you having severe difficulty breathing?

YES →

Emergency!
Get emergency care now! You may have a serious lung or heart condition.

See Anaphylaxis (p.894); Asthma (p.505); Heart Attack (p.663); Pneumothorax (p.516); Pulmonary Embolism (p.512).

NO ↓

Do you have any of the following symptoms?
- light-headedness
- sudden extreme fear
- tingling lips or hands
- sweating
- rapid heartbeat

YES →

Call your doctor if your symptoms persist or occur frequently.

See Panic Disorder (p.404).

NO ↓

GO TO NEXT PAGE

CONTINUED FROM
PREVIOUS PAGE

TAKING ACTION

MORE
INFORMATION

See Influenza (p.875);
Pneumonia (p.496);
Common Cold (p.460).

Do you have any of the following symptoms?
- temperature more than 99.4°F
- green or yellow phlegm
- chest pain with breathing

YES → Call your doctor. You may have a bacterial infection.

NO → Call your doctor. Your symptoms need attention.

Do you have chronic shortness of breath, with or without a cough?

YES →

Do you have any of the following symptoms?
- fever
- night sweats
- loss of appetite
- weight loss
- coughing up blood
- history of tuberculosis

YES → Call your doctor now. You may have a lung tumor, a lung abscess, or tuberculosis.

See Lung Cancer
(p.524); Tuberculosis
(p.504).

NO →

NO →

Do you have any of the following symptoms?
- shortness of breath or a cough that is worse when lying down
- swollen legs
- history of heart disease

YES → Call your doctor now. You may have congestive heart failure.

See Congestive Heart
Failure (p.683).

NO →

GO TO NEXT PAGE

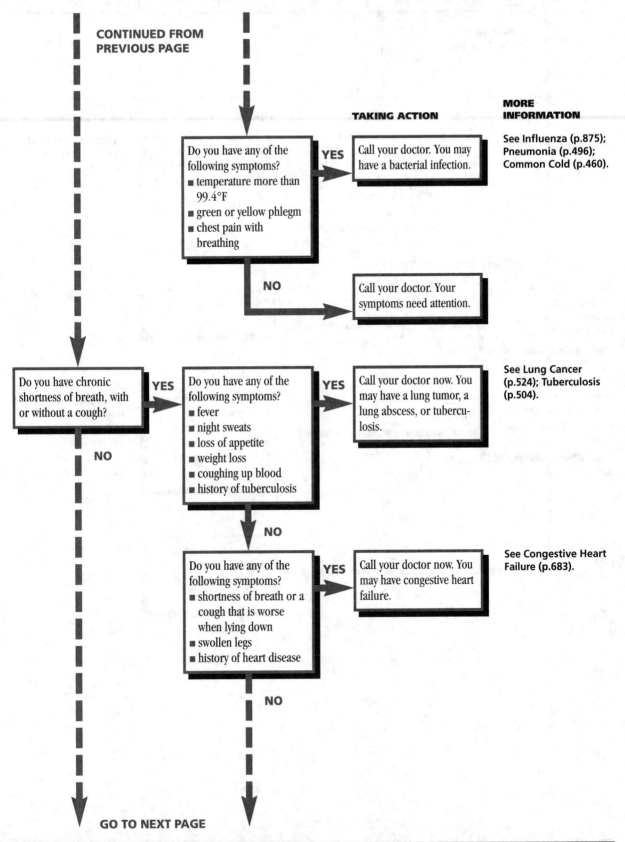

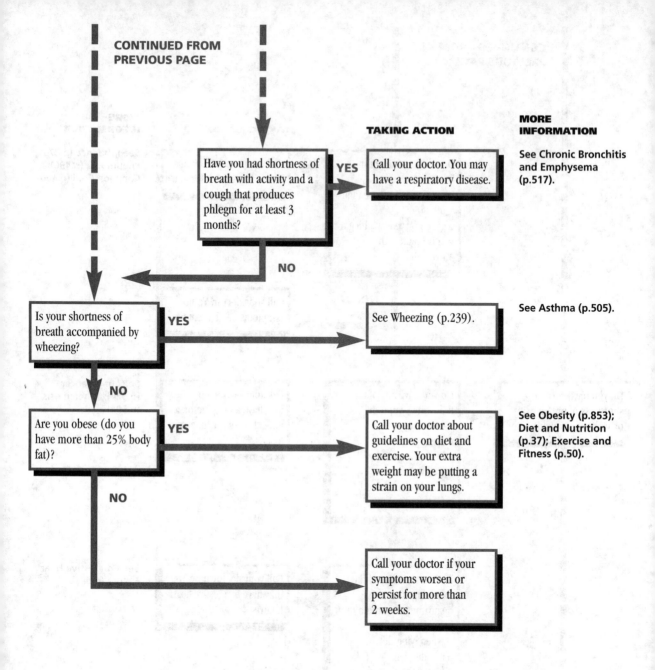

CONTINUED FROM
PREVIOUS PAGE

TAKING ACTION

**MORE
INFORMATION**

Have you had shortness of breath with activity and a cough that produces phlegm for at least 3 months?

YES ▶ Call your doctor. You may have a respiratory disease.

**See Chronic Bronchitis
and Emphysema
(p.517).**

NO

Is your shortness of breath accompanied by wheezing?

YES ▶ See Wheezing (p.239).

See Asthma (p.505).

NO

Are you obese (do you have more than 25% body fat)?

YES ▶ Call your doctor about guidelines on diet and exercise. Your extra weight may be putting a strain on your lungs.

**See Obesity (p.853);
Diet and Nutrition
(p.37); Exercise and
Fitness (p.50).**

NO

Call your doctor if your symptoms worsen or persist for more than 2 weeks.

WHEEZING

Wheezing is unusually noisy or labored breathing. It can range from mild breathing discomfort to a life-threatening restriction of air flow. Breathing problems require your doctor's attention. Bronchiolitis (see p.969) and croup (see p.1002) can cause wheezing in infants and young children. Rapid and shallow breathing accompanies bronchiolitis. Hoarseness and a barking cough indicate croup. Talk to your child's doctor if either condition persists.

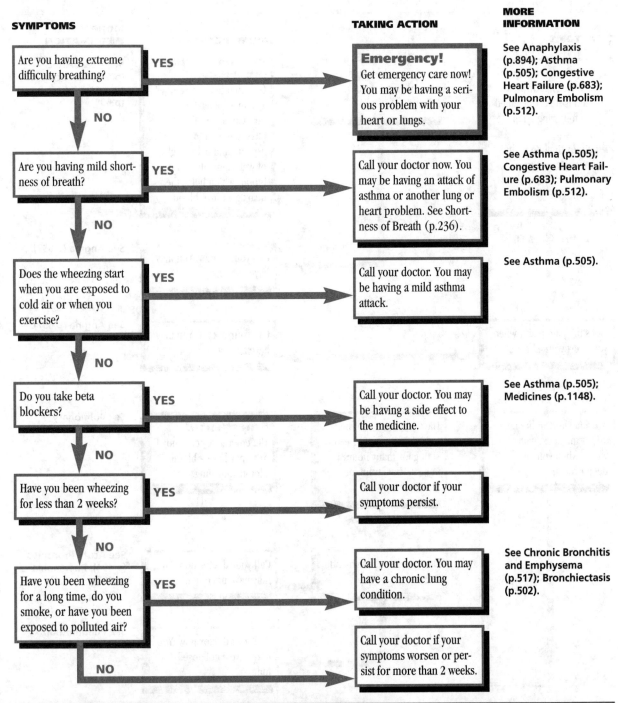

SYMPTOMS

TAKING ACTION

MORE INFORMATION

Are you having extreme difficulty breathing? — **YES** →

Emergency! Get emergency care now! You may be having a serious problem with your heart or lungs.

See Anaphylaxis (p.894); Asthma (p.505); Congestive Heart Failure (p.683); Pulmonary Embolism (p.512).

NO ↓

Are you having mild shortness of breath? — **YES** →

Call your doctor now. You may be having an attack of asthma or another lung or heart problem. See Shortness of Breath (p.236).

See Asthma (p.505); Congestive Heart Failure (p.683); Pulmonary Embolism (p.512).

NO ↓

Does the wheezing start when you are exposed to cold air or when you exercise? — **YES** →

Call your doctor. You may be having a mild asthma attack.

See Asthma (p.505).

NO ↓

Do you take beta blockers? — **YES** →

Call your doctor. You may be having a side effect to the medicine.

See Asthma (p.505); Medicines (p.1148).

NO ↓

Have you been wheezing for less than 2 weeks? — **YES** →

Call your doctor if your symptoms persist.

NO ↓

Have you been wheezing for a long time, do you smoke, or have you been exposed to polluted air? — **YES** →

Call your doctor. You may have a chronic lung condition.

See Chronic Bronchitis and Emphysema (p.517); Bronchiectasis (p.502).

NO →

Call your doctor if your symptoms worsen or persist for more than 2 weeks.

CHEST PAIN

Any pain below the neck and above the abdomen is considered chest pain. Chest pain can be caused by many conditions that range in severity from mildly inconvenient to life-threatening. Heart and lung conditions are the most serious causes. Very often, the most ominous chest pain causes a discomfort that is not perceived as a pain but rather as a fullness, pressure, constriction, or tearing sensation. Chest pains caused by disorders of the digestive system, muscles, bones, or nerves are also common but are usually less serious.

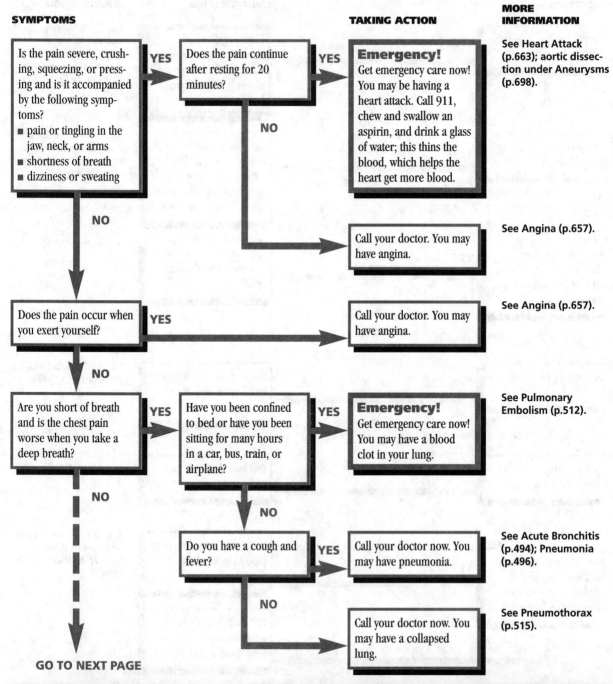

SYMPTOMS

Is the pain severe, crushing, squeezing, or pressing and is it accompanied by the following symptoms?
- pain or tingling in the jaw, neck, or arms
- shortness of breath
- dizziness or sweating

YES → Does the pain continue after resting for 20 minutes?

YES → **TAKING ACTION**

Emergency!
Get emergency care now! You may be having a heart attack. Call 911, chew and swallow an aspirin, and drink a glass of water; this thins the blood, which helps the heart get more blood.

MORE INFORMATION

See Heart Attack (p.663); aortic dissection under Aneurysms (p.698).

NO → Call your doctor. You may have angina.

See Angina (p.657).

NO → Does the pain occur when you exert yourself?

YES → Call your doctor. You may have angina.

See Angina (p.657).

NO → Are you short of breath and is the chest pain worse when you take a deep breath?

YES → Have you been confined to bed or have you been sitting for many hours in a car, bus, train, or airplane?

YES → **Emergency!**
Get emergency care now! You may have a blood clot in your lung.

See Pulmonary Embolism (p.512).

NO → Do you have a cough and fever?

YES → Call your doctor now. You may have pneumonia.

See Acute Bronchitis (p.494); Pneumonia (p.496).

NO → Call your doctor now. You may have a collapsed lung.

See Pneumothorax (p.515).

NO → **GO TO NEXT PAGE**

CONTINUED FROM PREVIOUS PAGE

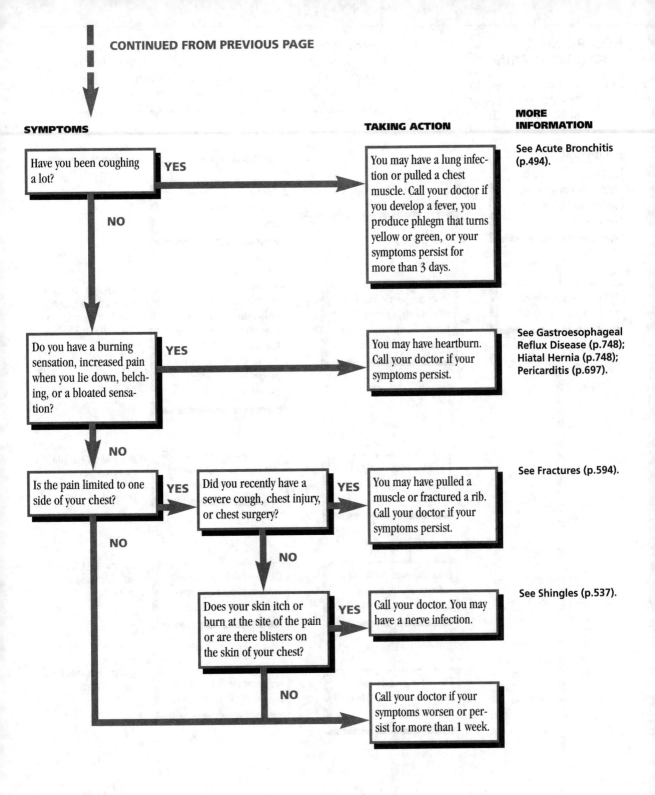

SYMPTOMS

TAKING ACTION

Have you been coughing a lot?

YES

You may have a lung infection or pulled a chest muscle. Call your doctor if you develop a fever, you produce phlegm that turns yellow or green, or your symptoms persist for more than 3 days.

See Acute Bronchitis (p.494).

NO

Do you have a burning sensation, increased pain when you lie down, belching, or a bloated sensation?

YES

You may have heartburn. Call your doctor if your symptoms persist.

See Gastroesophageal Reflux Disease (p.748); Hiatal Hernia (p.748); Pericarditis (p.697).

NO

Is the pain limited to one side of your chest?

YES

Did you recently have a severe cough, chest injury, or chest surgery?

YES

You may have pulled a muscle or fractured a rib. Call your doctor if your symptoms persist.

See Fractures (p.594).

NO

NO

Does your skin itch or burn at the site of the pain or are there blisters on the skin of your chest?

YES

Call your doctor. You may have a nerve infection.

See Shingles (p.537).

NO

Call your doctor if your symptoms worsen or persist for more than 1 week.

RECURRING ABDOMINAL PAIN

Recurring abdominal pain is pain in the abdomen (below the chest but above the groin) that you have had repeatedly over months or years. Recurring abdominal pain is caused by many conditions, from mild to life-threatening. If you have abdominal pain you have never had before, or severe abdominal pain, see Severe or Sudden Abdominal Pain (p.245).

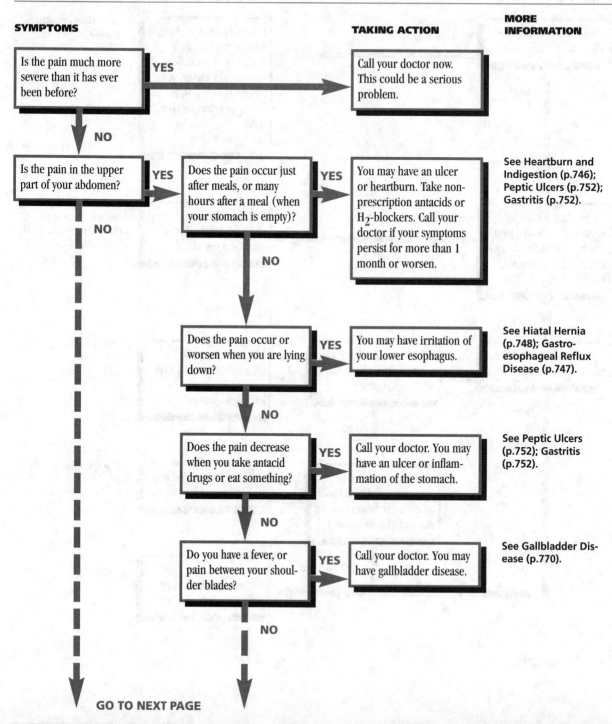

SYMPTOMS

TAKING ACTION

MORE INFORMATION

Is the pain much more severe than it has ever been before? — **YES** → Call your doctor now. This could be a serious problem.

NO ↓

Is the pain in the upper part of your abdomen? — **YES** → Does the pain occur just after meals, or many hours after a meal (when your stomach is empty)? — **YES** → You may have an ulcer or heartburn. Take non-prescription antacids or H$_2$-blockers. Call your doctor if your symptoms persist for more than 1 month or worsen.

See Heartburn and Indigestion (p.746); Peptic Ulcers (p.752); Gastritis (p.752).

NO (under "Is the pain in the upper part of your abdomen?")

NO ↓ (under "Does the pain occur just after meals...")

Does the pain occur or worsen when you are lying down? — **YES** → You may have irritation of your lower esophagus.

See Hiatal Hernia (p.748); Gastroesophageal Reflux Disease (p.747).

NO ↓

Does the pain decrease when you take antacid drugs or eat something? — **YES** → Call your doctor. You may have an ulcer or inflammation of the stomach.

See Peptic Ulcers (p.752); Gastritis (p.752).

NO ↓

Do you have a fever, or pain between your shoulder blades? — **YES** → Call your doctor. You may have gallbladder disease.

See Gallbladder Disease (p.770).

NO ↓

GO TO NEXT PAGE

CONTINUED FROM PREVIOUS PAGE

TAKING ACTION

Have you lost your appetite, and have you had an unexplained weight loss of more than 10 pounds over the past 6 months?

YES → Call your doctor now. You may have a serious condition.

See Cancer of the Pancreas (p.770); Stomach Cancer (p.756); Liver Cancer (p.766); Chronic Pancreatitis (p.769); Malabsorption (p.775).

NO ↓

Are you tired and do you have black or tarlike stools?

YES → Call your doctor now. You may have a bleeding ulcer.

See Peptic Ulcers (p.752).

NO ↓

Call your doctor. Your symptoms need attention.

Is the pain in the lower part of your abdomen?

YES → Do you have diarrhea that contains blood or mucus?

YES → Call your doctor. You may have an inflammation of the large intestine.

See Inflammatory Bowel Disease (p.787); Viral Gastroenteritis (p.778); Diverticulosis and Diverticulitis (p.783).

NO ↓ (left)

NO ↓

Do you have diarrhea, fever, and pain in your abdomen?

YES → Call your doctor. You may have an inflammation of the large intestine.

See Diverticulosis and Diverticulitis (p.783).

NO ↓

Do you have alternating bouts of diarrhea and constipation along with bloating?

YES → You may have a disorder of the small or large intestine. Call your doctor if your symptoms persist.

See Irritable Bowel Syndrome (p.789).

NO ↓

GO TO NEXT PAGE

CONTINUED FROM PREVIOUS PAGE

TAKING ACTION

MORE INFORMATION

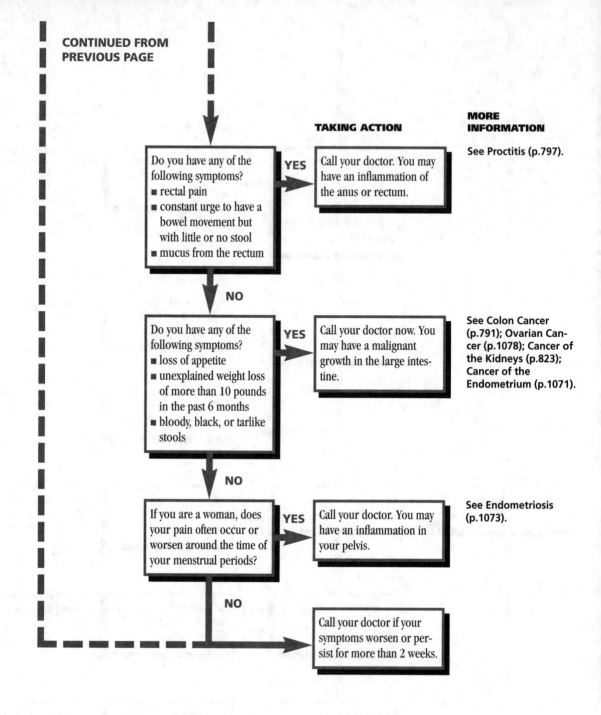

See Proctitis (p.797).

Do you have any of the following symptoms?
- rectal pain
- constant urge to have a bowel movement but with little or no stool
- mucus from the rectum

YES → Call your doctor. You may have an inflammation of the anus or rectum.

NO

Do you have any of the following symptoms?
- loss of appetite
- unexplained weight loss of more than 10 pounds in the past 6 months
- bloody, black, or tarlike stools

YES → Call your doctor now. You may have a malignant growth in the large intestine.

See Colon Cancer (p.791); Ovarian Cancer (p.1078); Cancer of the Kidneys (p.823); Cancer of the Endometrium (p.1071).

NO

If you are a woman, does your pain often occur or worsen around the time of your menstrual periods?

YES → Call your doctor. You may have an inflammation in your pelvis.

See Endometriosis (p.1073).

NO

Call your doctor if your symptoms worsen or persist for more than 2 weeks.

SEVERE OR SUDDEN ABDOMINAL PAIN

Suddenly feeling pain in your abdomen (below the chest but above the groin) is often not serious. However, if the pain is severe, it can indicate a life-threatening condition.

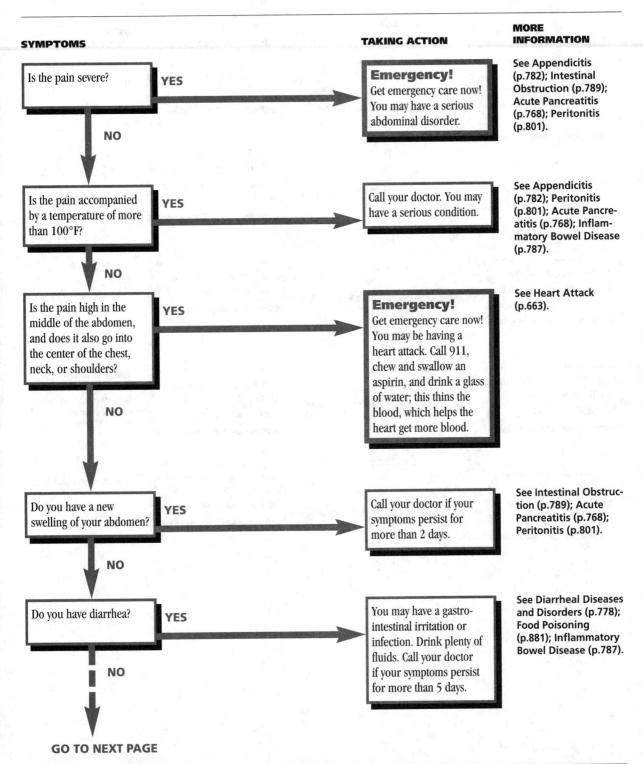

SYMPTOMS

Is the pain severe? — YES →

Emergency!
Get emergency care now! You may have a serious abdominal disorder.

See **Appendicitis (p.782); Intestinal Obstruction (p.789); Acute Pancreatitis (p.768); Peritonitis (p.801).**

NO ↓

Is the pain accompanied by a temperature of more than 100°F? — YES →

Call your doctor. You may have a serious condition.

See **Appendicitis (p.782); Peritonitis (p.801); Acute Pancreatitis (p.768); Inflammatory Bowel Disease (p.787).**

NO ↓

Is the pain high in the middle of the abdomen, and does it also go into the center of the chest, neck, or shoulders? — YES →

Emergency!
Get emergency care now! You may be having a heart attack. Call 911, chew and swallow an aspirin, and drink a glass of water; this thins the blood, which helps the heart get more blood.

See **Heart Attack (p.663).**

NO ↓

Do you have a new swelling of your abdomen? — YES →

Call your doctor if your symptoms persist for more than 2 days.

See **Intestinal Obstruction (p.789); Acute Pancreatitis (p.768); Peritonitis (p.801).**

NO ↓

Do you have diarrhea? — YES →

You may have a gastrointestinal irritation or infection. Drink plenty of fluids. Call your doctor if your symptoms persist for more than 5 days.

See **Diarrheal Diseases and Disorders (p.778); Food Poisoning (p.881); Inflammatory Bowel Disease (p.787).**

NO ↓

GO TO NEXT PAGE

CONTINUED FROM PREVIOUS PAGE

SYMPTOMS			TAKING ACTION	MORE INFORMATION
Do you have a frequent urge to urinate, or does urinating cause a burning sensation?	YES → Do you also have pain in your groin?	YES →	Call your doctor. You may have a kidney stone.	See Kidney Stones (p.818).
		NO →	Call your doctor. You may have a urinary tract infection.	See Cystitis (p.804); Pyelonephritis (p.808).
NO ↓				
Do you have pain in your shoulder blades and nausea, bloating, or belching?	YES →		Call your doctor now. You may have gallstones.	See Gallbladder Disease (p.770).
NO ↓				
Do you have heartburn, an acid taste, or a growling stomach?	YES →		You may have mild indigestion. Call your doctor if your symptoms persist.	See Heartburn and Indigestion (p.746); Gastroesophageal Reflux Disease (p.747); Hiatal Hernia (p.748).
NO ↓				
Does your skin blister, itch, or burn at the site of the pain?	YES →		Call your doctor. You may have a nerve infection.	See Shingles (p.537).
NO ↓				

GO TO NEXT PAGE

CONTINUED FROM PREVIOUS PAGE

SYMPTOMS

TAKING ACTION

Are you a woman? — **YES** → Have you missed a menstrual period? — **YES** → Call your doctor now. You may have a pregnancy developing outside the uterus.

See Ectopic Pregnancy (p.929).

NO ↓

Have you had a heavy or painful menstrual period? — **YES** → Call your doctor. You may have a gynecological problem.

See Painful Periods (p.1045); Ovarian Cysts (p.1080); Ovarian Cancer (p.1078).

NO

Are you a man, and does the pain spread to your genitals? — **YES** → Is the pain severe and is there a lump, redness, and swelling in your genital area? — **YES** → **Emergency!** Get emergency care now! Your testicle may be twisted.

See Torsion of the Testicle (p.1089).

NO ↓

Is the pain a dull ache and do you have a lump that comes and goes in your lower abdomen? — **YES** → Call your doctor now. You may have a hernia.

See Hernias (p.800).

NO

Call your doctor if your symptoms worsen or persist for more than 2 weeks.

CONSTIPATION

Constipation—infrequent, painful, dry, hard, or uncomfortable bowel movements— can be caused by a low-fiber diet, inadequate water intake, lack of exercise, disorders of the intestines, inflammation of the anus or rectum, hormonal changes, and medicines.

SYMPTOMS

TAKING ACTION

MORE INFORMATION

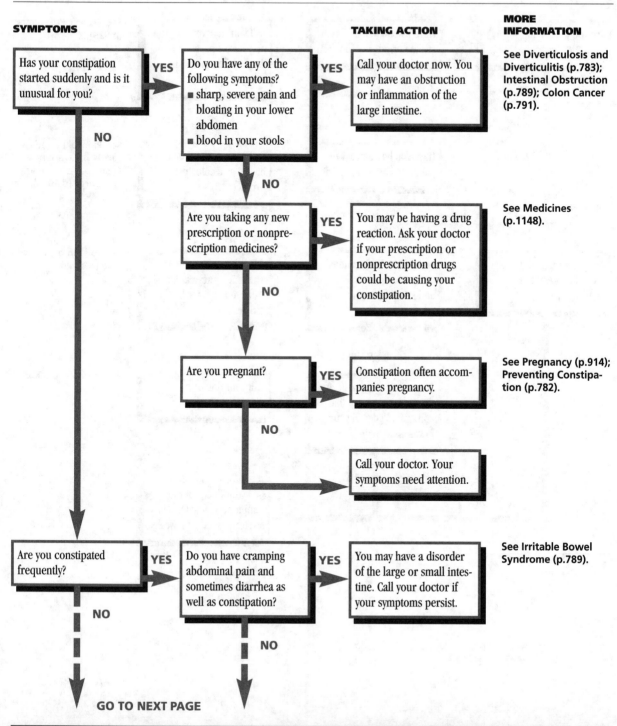

Has your constipation started suddenly and is it unusual for you?

YES → Do you have any of the following symptoms?
- sharp, severe pain and bloating in your lower abdomen
- blood in your stools

YES → Call your doctor now. You may have an obstruction or inflammation of the large intestine.

See Diverticulosis and Diverticulitis (p.783); Intestinal Obstruction (p.789); Colon Cancer (p.791).

NO

Are you taking any new prescription or nonprescription medicines?

YES → You may be having a drug reaction. Ask your doctor if your prescription or nonprescription drugs could be causing your constipation.

See Medicines (p.1148).

NO

Are you pregnant?

YES → Constipation often accompanies pregnancy.

See Pregnancy (p.914); Preventing Constipation (p.782).

NO

Call your doctor. Your symptoms need attention.

Are you constipated frequently?

YES → Do you have cramping abdominal pain and sometimes diarrhea as well as constipation?

YES → You may have a disorder of the large or small intestine. Call your doctor if your symptoms persist.

See Irritable Bowel Syndrome (p.789).

NO

NO

GO TO NEXT PAGE

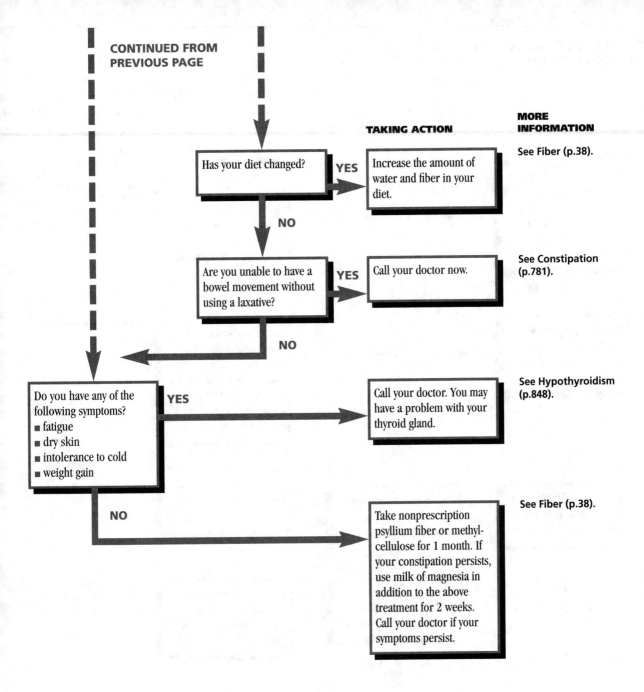

CONTINUED FROM PREVIOUS PAGE

Has your diet changed? — **YES** → Increase the amount of water and fiber in your diet.

See Fiber (p.38).

NO

Are you unable to have a bowel movement without using a laxative? — **YES** → Call your doctor now.

See Constipation (p.781).

NO

Do you have any of the following symptoms?
- fatigue
- dry skin
- intolerance to cold
- weight gain

YES → Call your doctor. You may have a problem with your thyroid gland.

See Hypothyroidism (p.848).

NO → Take nonprescription psyllium fiber or methyl-cellulose for 1 month. If your constipation persists, use milk of magnesia in addition to the above treatment for 2 weeks. Call your doctor if your symptoms persist.

See Fiber (p.38).

BELCHING, GROWLING STOMACH, OR GAS

Belching and having a growling stomach or gas are common conditions often related to foods you have eaten and eating habits. However, if accompanied by pain in the chest or a change in bowel habits, they may indicate a condition that requires your doctor's attention.

SYMPTOMS

TAKING ACTION

**MORE
INFORMATION**

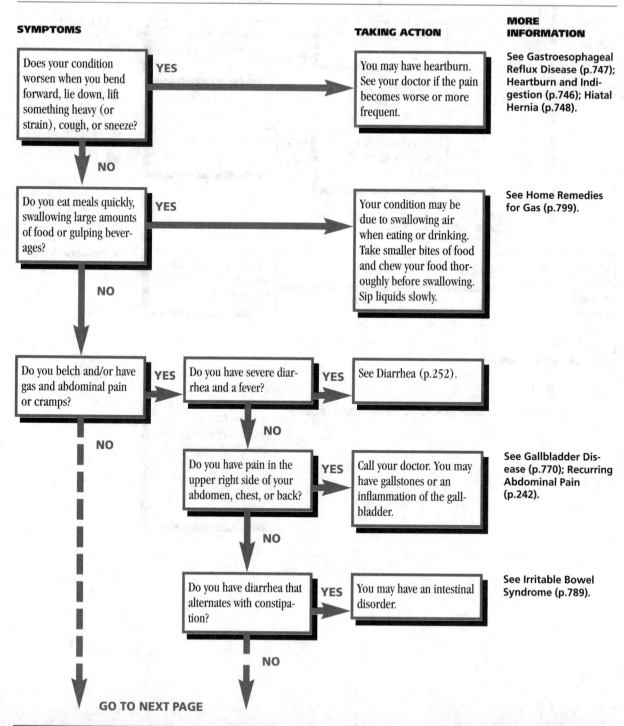

Does your condition worsen when you bend forward, lie down, lift something heavy (or strain), cough, or sneeze?

YES → You may have heartburn. See your doctor if the pain becomes worse or more frequent.

See Gastroesophageal Reflux Disease (p.747); Heartburn and Indigestion (p.746); Hiatal Hernia (p.748).

NO ↓

Do you eat meals quickly, swallowing large amounts of food or gulping beverages?

YES → Your condition may be due to swallowing air when eating or drinking. Take smaller bites of food and chew your food thoroughly before swallowing. Sip liquids slowly.

See Home Remedies for Gas (p.799).

NO ↓

Do you belch and/or have gas and abdominal pain or cramps?

YES → Do you have severe diarrhea and a fever?

YES → See Diarrhea (p.252).

NO ↓

Do you have pain in the upper right side of your abdomen, chest, or back?

YES → Call your doctor. You may have gallstones or an inflammation of the gallbladder.

See Gallbladder Disease (p.770); Recurring Abdominal Pain (p.242).

NO ↓

Do you have diarrhea that alternates with constipation?

YES → You may have an intestinal disorder.

See Irritable Bowel Syndrome (p.789).

NO ↓

NO ↓

GO TO NEXT PAGE

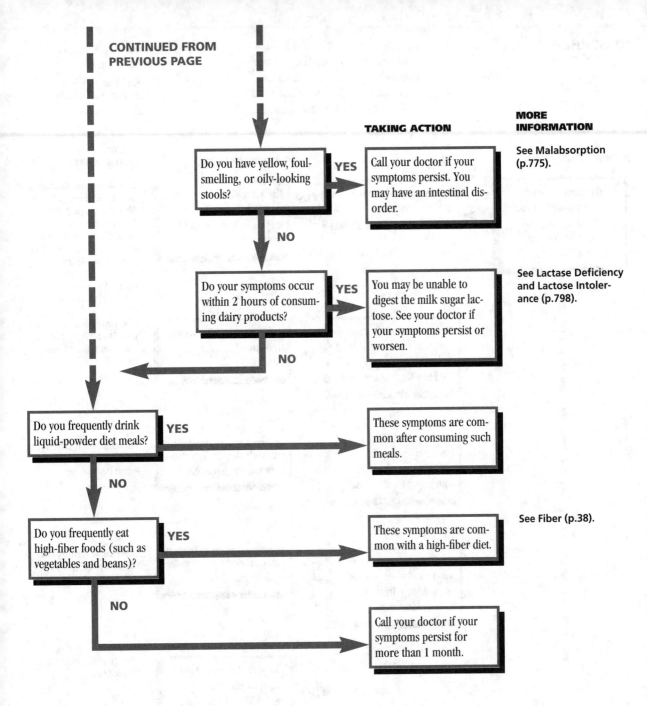

TAKING ACTION

Do you have yellow, foul-smelling, or oily-looking stools?

YES → Call your doctor if your symptoms persist. You may have an intestinal disorder.

See Malabsorption (p.775).

NO

Do your symptoms occur within 2 hours of consuming dairy products?

YES → You may be unable to digest the milk sugar lactose. See your doctor if your symptoms persist or worsen.

See Lactase Deficiency and Lactose Intolerance (p.798).

NO

Do you frequently drink liquid-powder diet meals?

YES → These symptoms are common after consuming such meals.

NO

Do you frequently eat high-fiber foods (such as vegetables and beans)?

YES → These symptoms are common with a high-fiber diet.

See Fiber (p.38).

NO

Call your doctor if your symptoms persist for more than 1 month.

DIARRHEA

Loose, watery bowel movements are a symptom of many intestinal disorders and can also be caused by what you eat. When diarrhea is fre- quent or accompanied by abdominal pain or fever, it may indicate a condition that requires your doctor's attention.

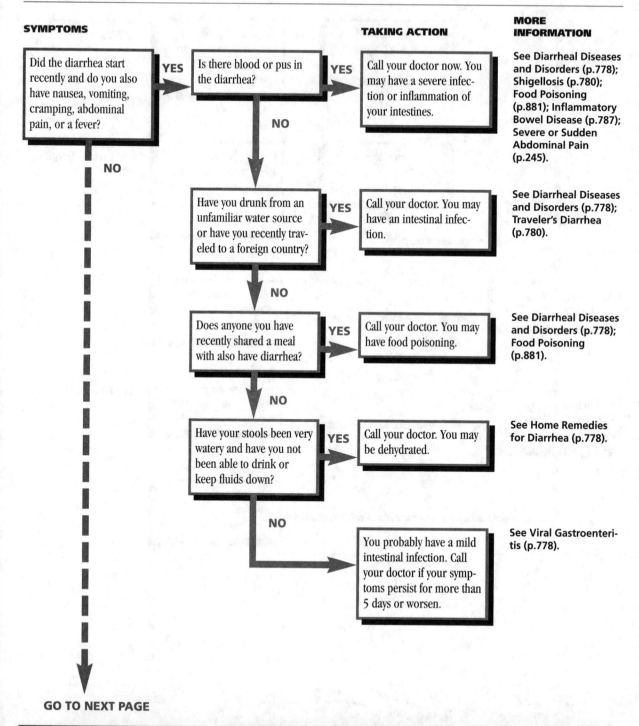

SYMPTOMS

Did the diarrhea start recently and do you also have nausea, vomiting, cramping, abdominal pain, or a fever?

YES → Is there blood or pus in the diarrhea?

YES → Call your doctor now. You may have a severe infection or inflammation of your intestines.

NO ↓

Have you drunk from an unfamiliar water source or have you recently traveled to a foreign country?

YES → Call your doctor. You may have an intestinal infection.

NO ↓

Does anyone you have recently shared a meal with also have diarrhea?

YES → Call your doctor. You may have food poisoning.

NO ↓

Have your stools been very watery and have you not been able to drink or keep fluids down?

YES → Call your doctor. You may be dehydrated.

NO ↓

You probably have a mild intestinal infection. Call your doctor if your symptoms persist for more than 5 days or worsen.

NO ↓ (from first question)

TAKING ACTION

MORE INFORMATION

See Diarrheal Diseases and Disorders (p.778); Shigellosis (p.780); Food Poisoning (p.881); Inflammatory Bowel Disease (p.787); Severe or Sudden Abdominal Pain (p.245).

See Diarrheal Diseases and Disorders (p.778); Traveler's Diarrhea (p.780).

See Diarrheal Diseases and Disorders (p.778); Food Poisoning (p.881).

See Home Remedies for Diarrhea (p.778).

See Viral Gastroenteritis (p.778).

GO TO NEXT PAGE

CONTINUED FROM PREVIOUS PAGE

SYMPTOMS   **TAKING ACTION**   **MORE INFORMATION**

Are you taking any new prescription or nonprescription medicines?

YES →

Call your doctor. Your medicine may be causing your diarrhea.

See Medicines (p.1148).

NO ↓

Are you also belching and having gas?

YES →

You may be reacting to a specific food or beverage.

See Home Remedies for Gas (p.799).

NO ↓

Is your diarrhea a recurring problem, one that you have had for many months or even years?

YES →

Do you have any of the following symptoms?
- abdominal pain that subsides after the diarrhea
- bloody diarrhea
- fever

YES →

Call your doctor. You may have an intestinal disorder. See Recurring Abdominal Pain (p.242); Rectal Bleeding (p.256).

See Inflammatory Bowel Disease (p.787); Diarrheal Diseases and Disorders (p.778).

NO ↓

Do you have foul-smelling or oily-looking stools?

YES →

Call your doctor. You may have an intestinal disorder.

See Malabsorption (p.775); Celiac Disease (p.774).

NO ↓

Is your diarrhea accompanied by cramping pain in different parts of your abdomen and intermittent bouts of constipation?

YES →

Eat more fruits and vegetables and take nonprescription psyllium husk fiber or methylcellulose every day. Call your doctor if your symptoms persist.

See Irritable Bowel Syndrome (p.789).

NO ↓

Eat more fruits and vegetables and take nonprescription psyllium husk fiber or methylcellulose every day. Call your doctor if your symptoms persist.

See Fiber (p.38).

NAUSEA OR VOMITING

Nausea and vomiting accompany many disorders. When brought on by injury, or accompanied by severe abdominal pain or headache, nausea or vomiting may indicate a serious condition that requires your doctor's attention.

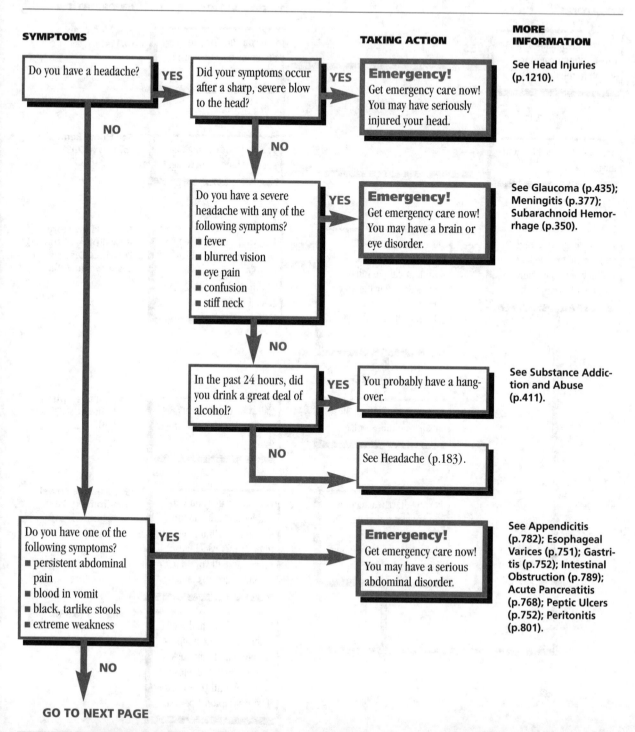

SYMPTOMS

Do you have a headache?

YES → Did your symptoms occur after a sharp, severe blow to the head?

NO ↓

TAKING ACTION

YES → **Emergency!** Get emergency care now! You may have seriously injured your head.

NO ↓

Do you have a severe headache with any of the following symptoms?
- fever
- blurred vision
- eye pain
- confusion
- stiff neck

YES → **Emergency!** Get emergency care now! You may have a brain or eye disorder.

NO ↓

In the past 24 hours, did you drink a great deal of alcohol?

YES → You probably have a hangover.

NO → See Headache (p.183).

Do you have one of the following symptoms?
- persistent abdominal pain
- blood in vomit
- black, tarlike stools
- extreme weakness

YES → **Emergency!** Get emergency care now! You may have a serious abdominal disorder.

NO ↓

GO TO NEXT PAGE

MORE INFORMATION

See Head Injuries (p.1210).

See Glaucoma (p.435); Meningitis (p.377); Subarachnoid Hemorrhage (p.350).

See Substance Addiction and Abuse (p.411).

See Appendicitis (p.782); Esophageal Varices (p.751); Gastritis (p.752); Intestinal Obstruction (p.789); Acute Pancreatitis (p.768); Peptic Ulcers (p.752); Peritonitis (p.801).

CONTINUED FROM PREVIOUS PAGE

SYMPTOMS

TAKING ACTION

Do you have abdominal cramps and fever or diarrhea?

YES → You may have a gastrointestinal irritation or infection. Call your doctor if your symptoms persist for more than 3 days.

See Diarrheal Diseases and Disorders (p.778); Food Poisoning (p.881); Gastritis (p.752).

NO ↓

Are you dizzy?

YES → See Dizziness (p.177).

NO ↓

Are you taking any new prescription or nonprescription medicines?

YES → Call your doctor. Your medicines could be causing your symptoms.

See Medicines (p.1148).

NO ↓

Do you drink an excessive amount of alcohol?

YES → Your symptoms are probably due to alcohol abuse. Call your doctor for help with your problem.

See Substance Addiction and Abuse (p.411).

NO ↓

Are you in the first 6 months of pregnancy?

YES → This is a common occurrence.

See Morning Sickness (p.926).

NO ↓

Call your doctor if you vomit more than three times or if the nausea persists for more than 5 days. You could have a serious problem.

See Brain Tumors (p.357).

RECTAL BLEEDING

Rectal bleeding includes red blood from the anus or obvious blood in the stools, both of which may be noticed in the toilet or on toilet tissue after a bowel movement. Rectal bleeding, especially when accompanied by a change in bowel habits, requires your doctor's attention.

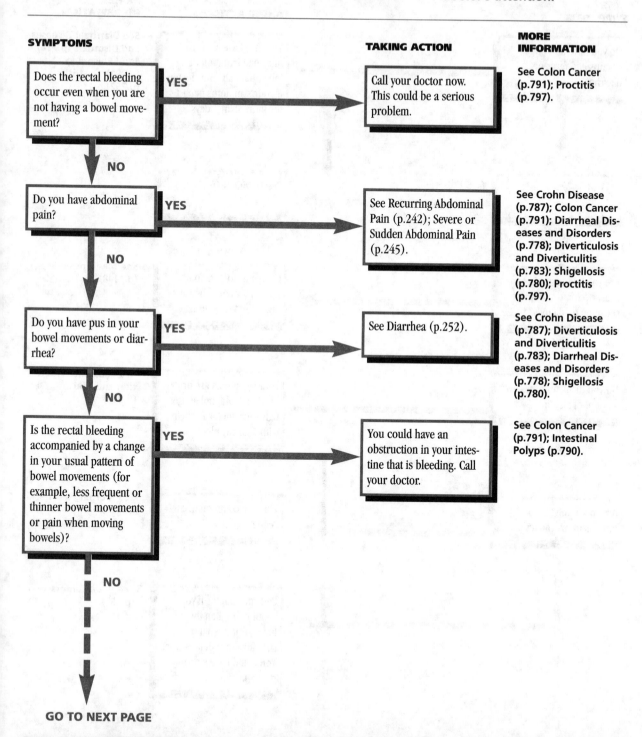

SYMPTOMS

Does the rectal bleeding occur even when you are not having a bowel movement?

YES

NO

Do you have abdominal pain?

YES

NO

Do you have pus in your bowel movements or diarrhea?

YES

NO

Is the rectal bleeding accompanied by a change in your usual pattern of bowel movements (for example, less frequent or thinner bowel movements or pain when moving bowels)?

YES

NO

GO TO NEXT PAGE

TAKING ACTION

Call your doctor now. This could be a serious problem.

See Recurring Abdominal Pain (p.242); Severe or Sudden Abdominal Pain (p.245).

See Diarrhea (p.252).

You could have an obstruction in your intestine that is bleeding. Call your doctor.

MORE INFORMATION

See Colon Cancer (p.791); Proctitis (p.797).

See Crohn Disease (p.787); Colon Cancer (p.791); Diarrheal Diseases and Disorders (p.778); Diverticulosis and Diverticulitis (p.783); Shigellosis (p.780); Proctitis (p.797).

See Crohn Disease (p.787); Diverticulosis and Diverticulitis (p.783); Diarrheal Diseases and Disorders (p.778); Shigellosis (p.780).

See Colon Cancer (p.791); Intestinal Polyps (p.790).

CONTINUED FROM PREVIOUS PAGE

SYMPTOMS

TAKING ACTION

Do you have rectal pain or itching?

YES → See Rectal Pain or Itching (p.258).

See Anal Fissure and Fistula (p.794); Hemorrhoids (p.795); Colon Cancer (p.791).

NO ↓

Do you have infrequent bowel movements with hard, dry stools?

YES → See Constipation (p.248).

See Constipation (p.781); Colon Cancer (p.791).

NO ↓

Are you over 45, or do you have a close relative (such as a parent, sibling, or child) who has developed colon polyps or colon cancer?

YES → Call your doctor. Your symptoms need attention.

See Colon Cancer (p.791).

NO →

Call your doctor if your symptoms worsen or persist for more than 1 week. There could be a serious problem.

RECTAL PAIN OR ITCHING

Rectal pain or itching usually is not serious when it accompanies occasional difficulty having a bowel movement. However, long-term rectal pain, especially when accompanied by bleeding or a change in bowel movements, requires your doctor's attention.

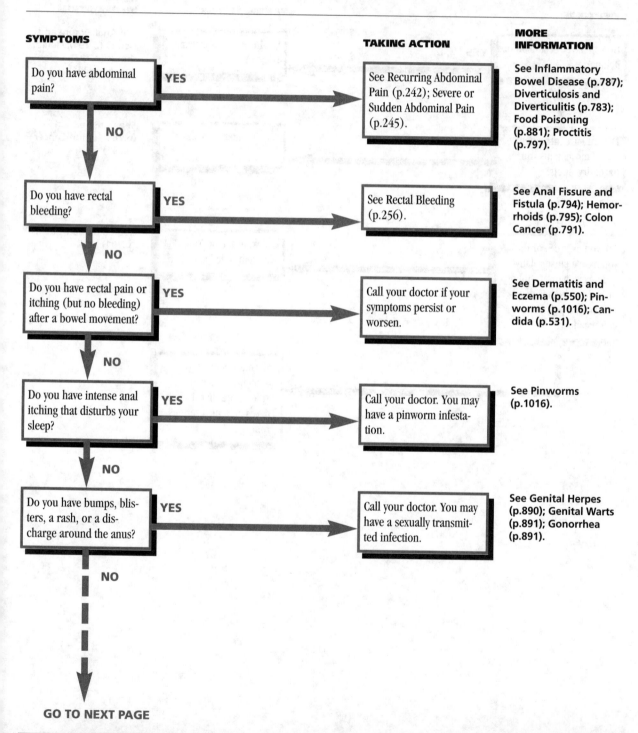

SYMPTOMS

Do you have abdominal pain?

YES →

See Recurring Abdominal Pain (p.242); Severe or Sudden Abdominal Pain (p.245).

NO ↓

Do you have rectal bleeding?

YES →

See Rectal Bleeding (p.256).

NO ↓

Do you have rectal pain or itching (but no bleeding) after a bowel movement?

YES →

Call your doctor if your symptoms persist or worsen.

NO ↓

Do you have intense anal itching that disturbs your sleep?

YES →

Call your doctor. You may have a pinworm infestation.

NO ↓

Do you have bumps, blisters, a rash, or a discharge around the anus?

YES →

Call your doctor. You may have a sexually transmitted infection.

NO ↓

GO TO NEXT PAGE

TAKING ACTION

MORE INFORMATION

See Inflammatory Bowel Disease (p.787); Diverticulosis and Diverticulitis (p.783); Food Poisoning (p.881); Proctitis (p.797).

See Anal Fissure and Fistula (p.794); Hemorrhoids (p.795); Colon Cancer (p.791).

See Dermatitis and Eczema (p.550); Pinworms (p.1016); Candida (p.531).

See Pinworms (p.1016).

See Genital Herpes (p.890); Genital Warts (p.891); Gonorrhea (p.891).

CONTINUED FROM PREVIOUS PAGE

SYMPTOMS

TAKING ACTION

MORE INFORMATION

Do you have infrequent bowel movements with hard, dry stools?

YES

See Constipation (p.248).

See Constipation (p.781).

NO

Your symptoms may be due to a tear in the anus or hemorrhoids. Take nonprescription psyllium husk fiber and stool-softening medicine, and apply nonprescription hydrocortisone cream once a day. Call your doctor if your symptoms persist for more than 2 weeks or worsen.

See Anal Fissure and Fistula (p.794); Hemorrhoids (p.795).

UNEXPLAINED WEIGHT GAIN

In most people, the explanation for weight gain is simple—you are taking in more calories than you burn with exercise. When weight gain is accompanied by swelling or difficulty breathing, however, it may indicate a condition that requires your doctor's attention.

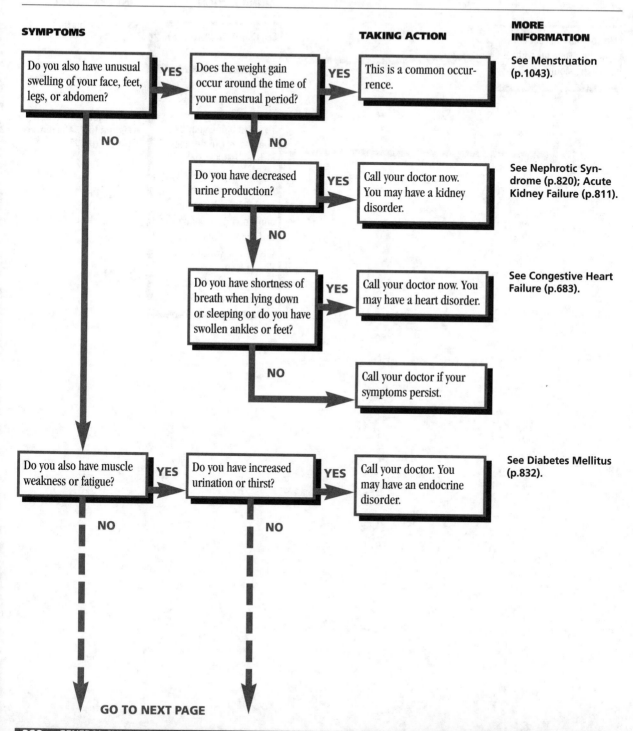

SYMPTOMS

TAKING ACTION

MORE INFORMATION

Do you also have unusual swelling of your face, feet, legs, or abdomen?

YES → Does the weight gain occur around the time of your menstrual period?

YES → This is a common occurrence.

See Menstruation (p.1043).

NO

Do you have decreased urine production?

YES → Call your doctor now. You may have a kidney disorder.

See Nephrotic Syndrome (p.820); Acute Kidney Failure (p.811).

NO

Do you have shortness of breath when lying down or sleeping or do you have swollen ankles or feet?

YES → Call your doctor now. You may have a heart disorder.

See Congestive Heart Failure (p.683).

NO → Call your doctor if your symptoms persist.

Do you also have muscle weakness or fatigue?

YES → Do you have increased urination or thirst?

YES → Call your doctor. You may have an endocrine disorder.

See Diabetes Mellitus (p.832).

NO

NO

GO TO NEXT PAGE

CONTINUED FROM PREVIOUS PAGE

TAKING ACTION

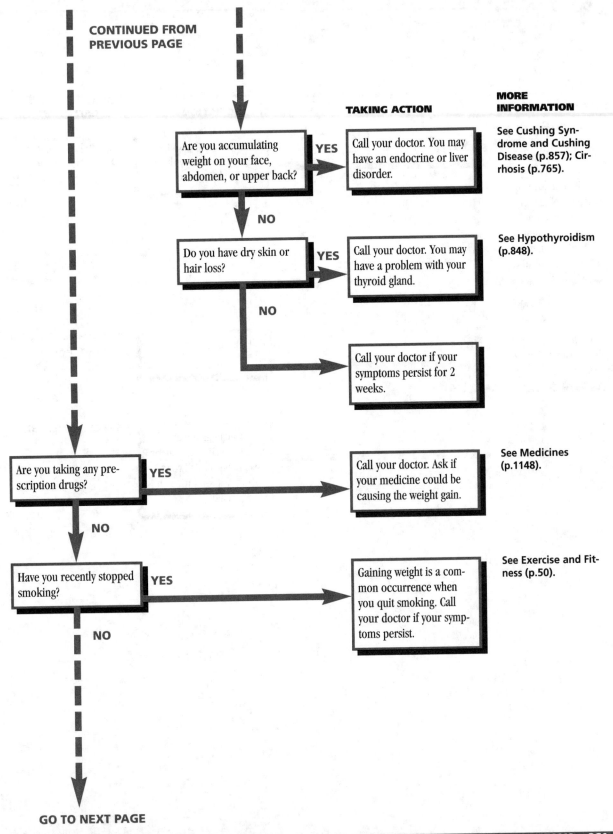

Are you accumulating weight on your face, abdomen, or upper back?

YES → Call your doctor. You may have an endocrine or liver disorder.

See Cushing Syndrome and Cushing Disease (p.857); Cirrhosis (p.765).

NO ↓

Do you have dry skin or hair loss?

YES → Call your doctor. You may have a problem with your thyroid gland.

See Hypothyroidism (p.848).

NO ↓

Call your doctor if your symptoms persist for 2 weeks.

Are you taking any prescription drugs?

YES → Call your doctor. Ask if your medicine could be causing the weight gain.

See Medicines (p.1148).

NO ↓

Have you recently stopped smoking?

YES → Gaining weight is a common occurrence when you quit smoking. Call your doctor if your symptoms persist.

See Exercise and Fitness (p.50).

NO ↓

GO TO NEXT PAGE

CONTINUED FROM PREVIOUS PAGE

SYMPTOMS

TAKING ACTION

Have you recently experienced any of the following?
- death of a loved one
- change of career
- traumatic event
- change in eating or sleeping patterns
- feeling sad or low

YES → Call your doctor. Your weight gain may be due to emotional pressure.

See Generalized Anxiety Disorder (p.402); Depression (p.395).

NO ↓

Does your weight gain occur with a change in seasons?

YES → Call your doctor.

See Seasonal Affective Disorder (p.406).

NO ↓

Your weight gain may be genetic, environmental, or psychological. Call your doctor. Ask for advice on losing weight.

See Obesity (p.853).

UNEXPLAINED WEIGHT LOSS

Weight loss that occurs when you expend more energy than you take in from food is common. When you lose more than 5% of your usual body weight, or more than 10 pounds, without trying to lose weight, see your doctor. If you have unintended weight loss of a lesser degree that is accompanied by persistent pain, difficulty breathing, or bleeding, it can indicate a condition that requires your doctor's attention.

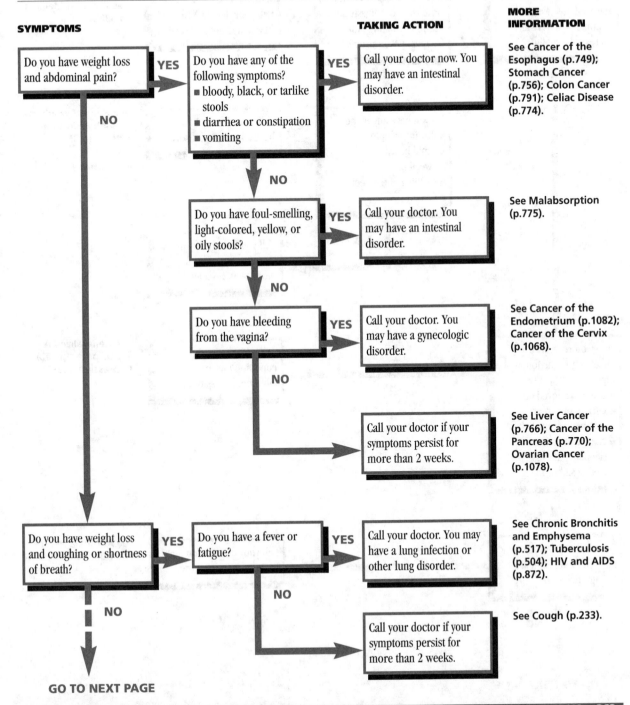

SYMPTOMS

TAKING ACTION

MORE INFORMATION

Do you have weight loss and abdominal pain? — **YES** → Do you have any of the following symptoms?
- bloody, black, or tarlike stools
- diarrhea or constipation
- vomiting

YES → Call your doctor now. You may have an intestinal disorder.

See Cancer of the Esophagus (p.749); Stomach Cancer (p.756); Colon Cancer (p.791); Celiac Disease (p.774).

NO ↓

Do you have foul-smelling, light-colored, yellow, or oily stools? — **YES** → Call your doctor. You may have an intestinal disorder.

See Malabsorption (p.775).

NO ↓

Do you have bleeding from the vagina? — **YES** → Call your doctor. You may have a gynecologic disorder.

See Cancer of the Endometrium (p.1082); Cancer of the Cervix (p.1068).

NO ↓

Call your doctor if your symptoms persist for more than 2 weeks.

See Liver Cancer (p.766); Cancer of the Pancreas (p.770); Ovarian Cancer (p.1078).

NO ↓

Do you have weight loss and coughing or shortness of breath? — **YES** → Do you have a fever or fatigue? — **YES** → Call your doctor. You may have a lung infection or other lung disorder.

See Chronic Bronchitis and Emphysema (p.517); Tuberculosis (p.504); HIV and AIDS (p.872).

NO ↓

Call your doctor if your symptoms persist for more than 2 weeks.

See Cough (p.233).

NO ↓

GO TO NEXT PAGE

CONTINUED FROM PREVIOUS PAGE

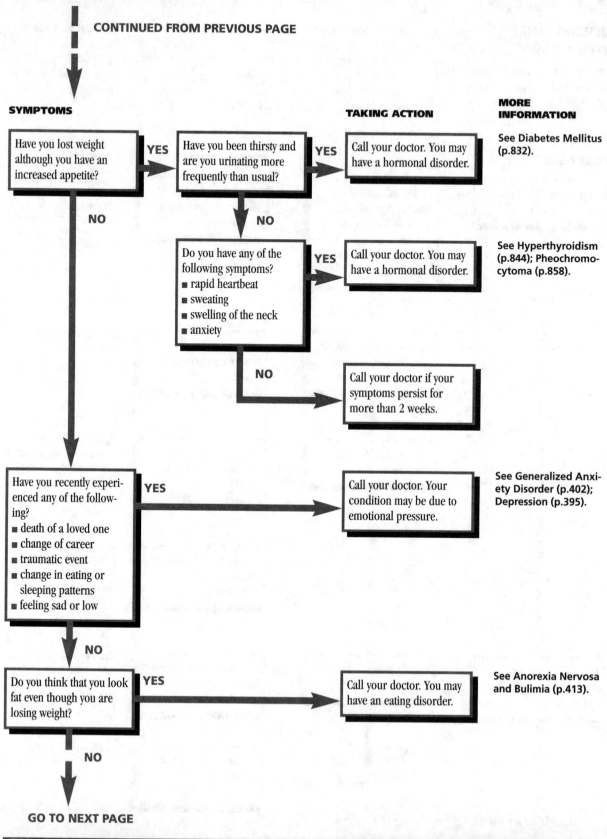

SYMPTOMS

TAKING ACTION

MORE INFORMATION

Have you lost weight although you have an increased appetite?

YES → Have you been thirsty and are you urinating more frequently than usual?

YES → Call your doctor. You may have a hormonal disorder.

See Diabetes Mellitus (p.832).

NO ↓

NO ↓

Do you have any of the following symptoms?
■ rapid heartbeat
■ sweating
■ swelling of the neck
■ anxiety

YES → Call your doctor. You may have a hormonal disorder.

See Hyperthyroidism (p.844); Pheochromo-cytoma (p.858).

NO ↓

Call your doctor if your symptoms persist for more than 2 weeks.

Have you recently experienced any of the following?
■ death of a loved one
■ change of career
■ traumatic event
■ change in eating or sleeping patterns
■ feeling sad or low

YES → Call your doctor. Your condition may be due to emotional pressure.

See Generalized Anxiety Disorder (p.402); Depression (p.395).

NO ↓

Do you think that you look fat even though you are losing weight?

YES → Call your doctor. You may have an eating disorder.

See Anorexia Nervosa and Bulimia (p.413).

NO ↓

GO TO NEXT PAGE

CONTINUED FROM PREVIOUS PAGE

SYMPTOMS

TAKING ACTION

Do you feel extremely weak and lack energy?

YES →

Call your doctor. You may have a serious condition.

See Cancer (p.738); Anemia (p.713).

NO

Are you taking any prescription drugs?

YES →

Call your doctor. Ask if your medicine could be causing your symptoms.

See Medicines (p.1148).

NO

Have you lost more than 10% of your body weight in the past 4 to 6 months?

YES →

Call your doctor now. A number of chronic conditions could be causing your symptoms.

See Cancer (p.738); HIV and AIDS (p.872).

NO

Call your doctor if your weight loss continues for another 2 weeks or if you lose 5% of your usual body weight or 10 pounds.

PAINFUL MENSTRUAL CRAMPS

Most women experience cramping pain, usually in the abdomen, around the time of their periods at some point in their lives. In addition to pain in the lower abdomen, pain may occur in the hips, lower back, or thighs. Menstrual cramps are common and usually not a cause for concern.

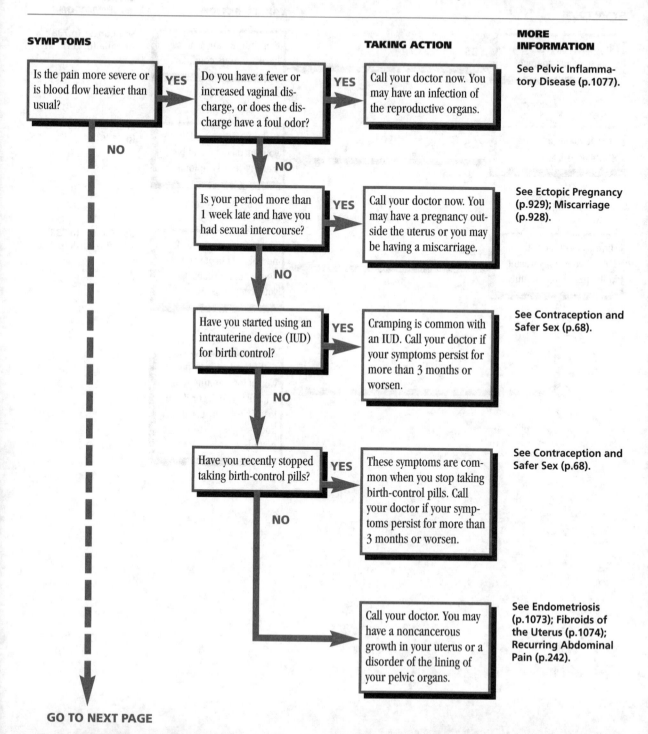

SYMPTOMS

Is the pain more severe or is blood flow heavier than usual?

YES → Do you have a fever or increased vaginal discharge, or does the discharge have a foul odor?

NO

Is your period more than 1 week late and have you had sexual intercourse?

NO

Have you started using an intrauterine device (IUD) for birth control?

NO

Have you recently stopped taking birth-control pills?

NO

TAKING ACTION

YES → Call your doctor now. You may have an infection of the reproductive organs.

YES → Call your doctor now. You may have a pregnancy outside the uterus or you may be having a miscarriage.

YES → Cramping is common with an IUD. Call your doctor if your symptoms persist for more than 3 months or worsen.

YES → These symptoms are common when you stop taking birth-control pills. Call your doctor if your symptoms persist for more than 3 months or worsen.

Call your doctor. You may have a noncancerous growth in your uterus or a disorder of the lining of your pelvic organs.

MORE INFORMATION

See Pelvic Inflammatory Disease (p.1077).

See Ectopic Pregnancy (p.929); Miscarriage (p.928).

See Contraception and Safer Sex (p.68).

See Contraception and Safer Sex (p.68).

See Endometriosis (p.1073); Fibroids of the Uterus (p.1074); Recurring Abdominal Pain (p.242).

GO TO NEXT PAGE

CONTINUED FROM PREVIOUS PAGE

SYMPTOMS

TAKING ACTION

MORE INFORMATION

Did you start menstruating within the past 2 years?

YES

NO

These symptoms are common at the start of menstruation. Call your doctor if your symptoms worsen.

See Menstruation (p.1043); Home Remedies for Premenstrual Symptoms and Cramps (p.1046).

Call your doctor if your symptoms worsen.

See Painful Periods (p.1045); Polycystic Ovary Syndrome (p.1081).

HEAVY MENSTRUAL PERIODS

Heavy periods are those in which the amount of blood or the duration of the flow is greater than usual. A menstrual period is considered heavy if bleeding requires you to change a sanitary napkin or tampon more than once an hour for more than 6 hours, if your period lasts longer than 7 days, or if there is a significant increase in the volume or length of flow.

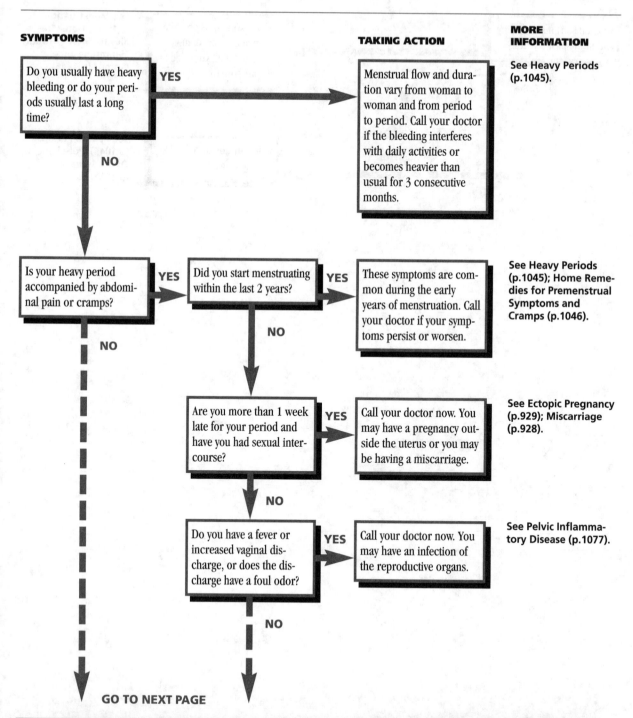

SYMPTOMS

Do you usually have heavy bleeding or do your periods usually last a long time?

— YES →

NO ↓

Is your heavy period accompanied by abdominal pain or cramps?

— YES →

NO ↓ (dashed)

Did you start menstruating within the last 2 years?

— YES →

NO ↓

Are you more than 1 week late for your period and have you had sexual intercourse?

— YES →

NO ↓

Do you have a fever or increased vaginal discharge, or does the discharge have a foul odor?

— YES →

NO ↓

GO TO NEXT PAGE

TAKING ACTION

Menstrual flow and duration vary from woman to woman and from period to period. Call your doctor if the bleeding interferes with daily activities or becomes heavier than usual for 3 consecutive months.

These symptoms are common during the early years of menstruation. Call your doctor if your symptoms persist or worsen.

Call your doctor now. You may have a pregnancy outside the uterus or you may be having a miscarriage.

Call your doctor now. You may have an infection of the reproductive organs.

MORE INFORMATION

See Heavy Periods (p.1045).

See Heavy Periods (p.1045); Home Remedies for Premenstrual Symptoms and Cramps (p.1046).

See Ectopic Pregnancy (p.929); Miscarriage (p.928).

See Pelvic Inflammatory Disease (p.1077).

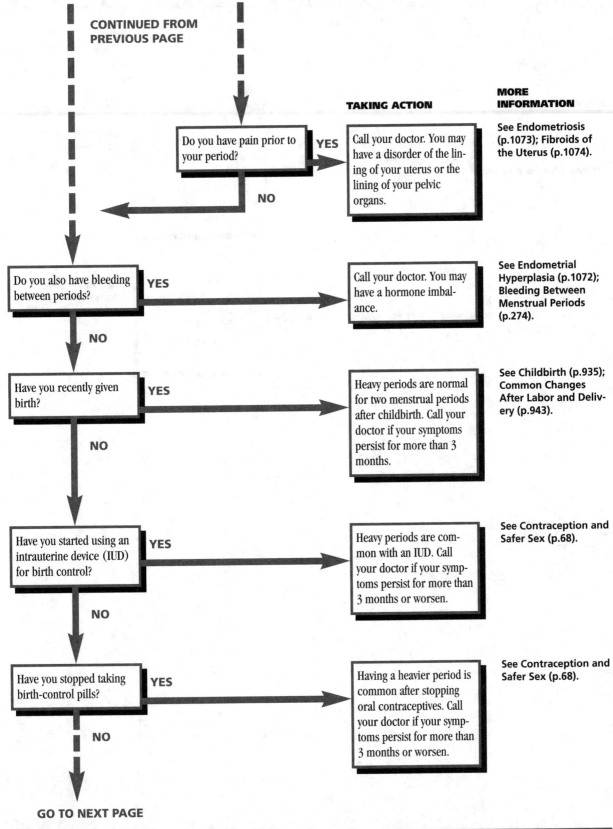

CONTINUED FROM PREVIOUS PAGE

TAKING ACTION

MORE INFORMATION

Do you have pain prior to your period? **YES**

Call your doctor. You may have a disorder of the lining of your uterus or the lining of your pelvic organs.

See Endometriosis (p.1073); Fibroids of the Uterus (p.1074).

NO

Do you also have bleeding between periods? **YES**

Call your doctor. You may have a hormone imbalance.

See Endometrial Hyperplasia (p.1072); Bleeding Between Menstrual Periods (p.274).

NO

Have you recently given birth? **YES**

Heavy periods are normal for two menstrual periods after childbirth. Call your doctor if your symptoms persist for more than 3 months.

See Childbirth (p.935); Common Changes After Labor and Delivery (p.943).

NO

Have you started using an intrauterine device (IUD) for birth control? **YES**

Heavy periods are common with an IUD. Call your doctor if your symptoms persist for more than 3 months or worsen.

See Contraception and Safer Sex (p.68).

NO

Have you stopped taking birth-control pills? **YES**

Having a heavier period is common after stopping oral contraceptives. Call your doctor if your symptoms persist for more than 3 months or worsen.

See Contraception and Safer Sex (p.68).

NO

GO TO NEXT PAGE

CONTINUED FROM PREVIOUS PAGE

SYMPTOMS

TAKING ACTION

Are you over 40?

YES

Heavy periods sometimes occur in the years before menopause. Call your doctor if your symptoms persist or interfere with daily activities.

See Menopause (p.1047).

NO

A number of conditions can cause these symptoms. Call your doctor if your symptoms persist or worsen.

See Heavy Periods (p.1045); Fibroids of the Uterus (p.1074).

MISSED OR IRREGULAR MENSTRUAL PERIODS

Most women experience absent, short, or irregular periods at some point in their lives. A wide range of conditions can cause these symptoms, including pregnancy, stress, weight loss, lifestyle changes, hormone imbalance, infection, tumors, or the approach of menopause.

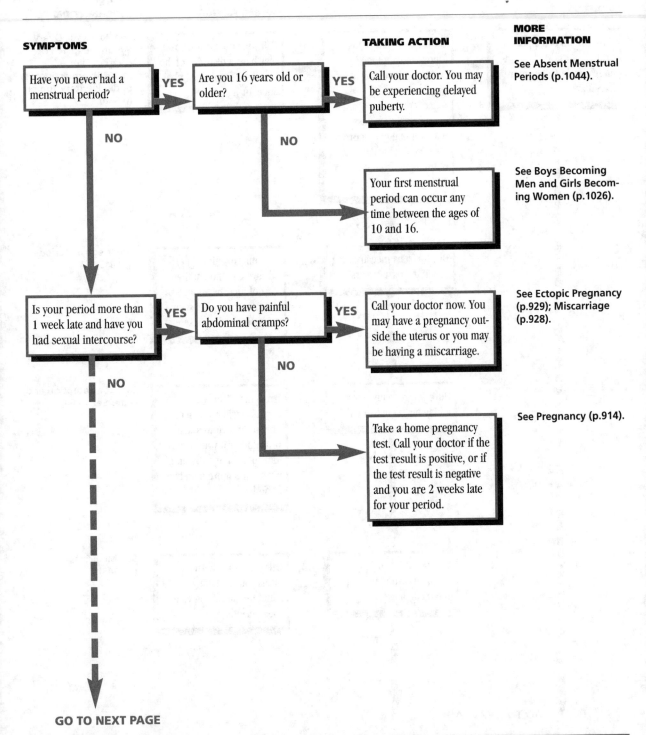

SYMPTOMS

Have you never had a menstrual period?

YES → Are you 16 years old or older?

YES → **TAKING ACTION**

Call your doctor. You may be experiencing delayed puberty.

MORE INFORMATION

See Absent Menstrual Periods (p.1044).

NO

Your first menstrual period can occur any time between the ages of 10 and 16.

See Boys Becoming Men and Girls Becoming Women (p.1026).

NO

Is your period more than 1 week late and have you had sexual intercourse?

YES → Do you have painful abdominal cramps?

YES → Call your doctor now. You may have a pregnancy outside the uterus or you may be having a miscarriage.

See Ectopic Pregnancy (p.929); Miscarriage (p.928).

NO

Take a home pregnancy test. Call your doctor if the test result is positive, or if the test result is negative and you are 2 weeks late for your period.

See Pregnancy (p.914).

NO

GO TO NEXT PAGE

SYMPTOMS

TAKING ACTION

MORE INFORMATION

Have you missed a period, or are your periods shorter, less frequent, or more irregular?

YES →

Do you have any of the following symptoms?
- unexplained weight gain or loss
- deeper voice
- abnormal hairiness
- abdominal pain more severe than usual
- discharge from the nipples

YES →

Call your doctor now. You may have a disorder of the ovaries, a hormone imbalance, or a tumor.

See Polycystic Ovary Syndrome (p.1081); Ovarian Cancer (p.1078); prolactinoma under Pituitary Tumors (p.860).

NO ↓

NO ↓

Did you start menstruating within the past 2 years?

YES →

Irregular or missed periods are common at the start of menstruation. Call your doctor if your symptoms persist or worsen.

See Irregular Periods (p.1045).

NO ↓

Have you recently started taking birth-control pills?

YES →

Irregular periods are common when you start oral contraceptives. Call your doctor if your symptoms persist or worsen, or if you miss more than two periods.

See Contraception and Safer Sex (p.68).

NO ↓

Are you taking any prescription or nonprescription medicines?

YES →

Call your doctor. The drugs you are taking could be interfering with your periods.

See Medicines (p.1148).

NO ↓

GO TO NEXT PAGE

TAKING ACTION

MORE
INFORMATION

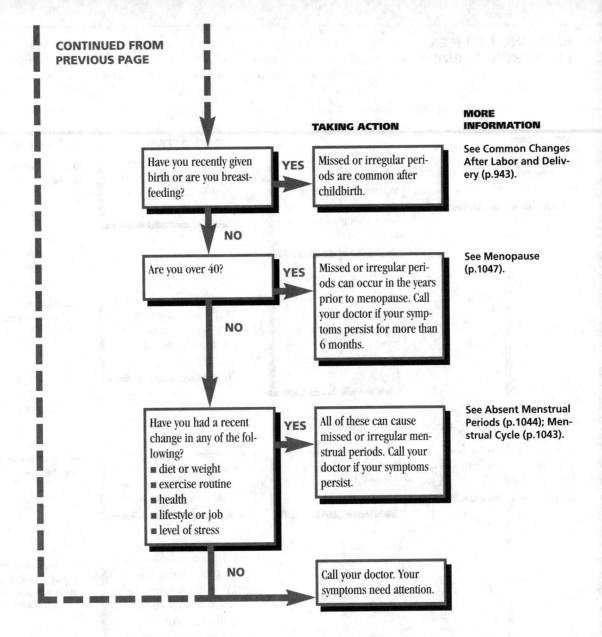

Have you recently given birth or are you breast-feeding?

YES → Missed or irregular periods are common after childbirth.

See Common Changes After Labor and Delivery (p.943).

NO ↓

Are you over 40?

YES → Missed or irregular periods can occur in the years prior to menopause. Call your doctor if your symptoms persist for more than 6 months.

See Menopause (p.1047).

NO ↓

Have you had a recent change in any of the following?
- diet or weight
- exercise routine
- health
- lifestyle or job
- level of stress

YES → All of these can cause missed or irregular menstrual periods. Call your doctor if your symptoms persist.

See Absent Menstrual Periods (p.1044); Menstrual Cycle (p.1043).

NO → Call your doctor. Your symptoms need attention.

BLEEDING BETWEEN MENSTRUAL PERIODS

It is not unusual for women to experience breakthrough bleeding or spotting between periods. The causes of bleed-ing between periods or during pregnancy range from normal fluctuations in body chemistry to life-threatening conditions.

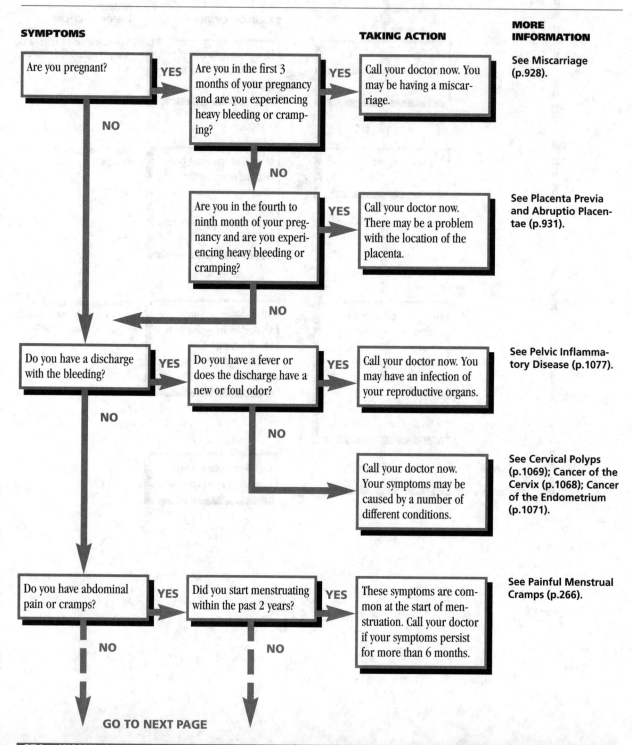

SYMPTOMS

TAKING ACTION

MORE INFORMATION

Are you pregnant?

YES → Are you in the first 3 months of your pregnancy and are you experiencing heavy bleeding or cramping?

YES → Call your doctor now. You may be having a miscarriage.

See Miscarriage (p.928).

NO

NO ↓

Are you in the fourth to ninth month of your pregnancy and are you experiencing heavy bleeding or cramping?

YES → Call your doctor now. There may be a problem with the location of the placenta.

See Placenta Previa and Abruptio Placentae (p.931).

NO

Do you have a discharge with the bleeding?

YES → Do you have a fever or does the discharge have a new or foul odor?

YES → Call your doctor now. You may have an infection of your reproductive organs.

See Pelvic Inflammatory Disease (p.1077).

NO

NO ↓

Call your doctor now. Your symptoms may be caused by a number of different conditions.

See Cervical Polyps (p.1069); Cancer of the Cervix (p.1068); Cancer of the Endometrium (p.1071).

Do you have abdominal pain or cramps?

YES → Did you start menstruating within the past 2 years?

YES → These symptoms are common at the start of menstruation. Call your doctor if your symptoms persist for more than 6 months.

See Painful Menstrual Cramps (p.266).

NO

NO

GO TO NEXT PAGE

CONTINUED FROM PREVIOUS PAGE

	TAKING ACTION	MORE INFORMATION
Have you started using an intrauterine device (IUD) for birth control? YES →	Bleeding between periods is common when using an IUD. Call your doctor if your symptoms persist for more than 6 months or worsen.	See Contraception and Safer Sex (p.68).
NO ↓ Did you miss or are you more than 1 week late for your last period and could you be pregnant? YES →	Call your doctor now. You may have a pregnancy outside the uterus or you may be having a miscarriage.	See Ectopic Pregnancy (p.929); Miscarriage (p.928).
NO →	Many women experience breakthrough bleeding between menstrual cycles. Call your doctor if your symptoms persist.	See Irregular Periods (p.1045).
Do you usually have heavy periods or was your last period especially heavy? YES →	Call your doctor. You may have a high estrogen level. See Heavy Menstrual Periods (p.268).	See Endometrial Hyperplasia (p.1072).
NO ↓		

GO TO NEXT PAGE

CONTINUED FROM PREVIOUS PAGE

SYMPTOMS

TAKING ACTION

Are you taking any pre-scription or nonprescrip-tion medicines?

YES → Are you taking birth-control pills?

YES → Bleeding between periods can occur when taking birth-control pills. Call your doctor if your symp-toms worsen.

See Contraception and Safer Sex (p.68).

NO

NO

You may be having a side effect of a medicine. Ask your doctor if any of the drugs you are taking could be interfering with your periods.

See Medicines (p.1148).

Are you over 40?

YES → Bleeding between periods can occur in the years preceding menopause. Call your doctor if your symptoms persist or worsen.

See Menopause (p.1047).

NO

Call your doctor. Your symptoms need attention.

See Cervical Polyps (p.1071); Cancer of the Cervix (p.1068); Cancer of the Endometrium (p.1071).

BLEEDING AFTER MENOPAUSE

Vaginal bleeding after menopause may be light or heavy and often is one of the normal effects of menopause and fluctuating hormone levels. However, more serious disorders also can cause bleeding after menopause.

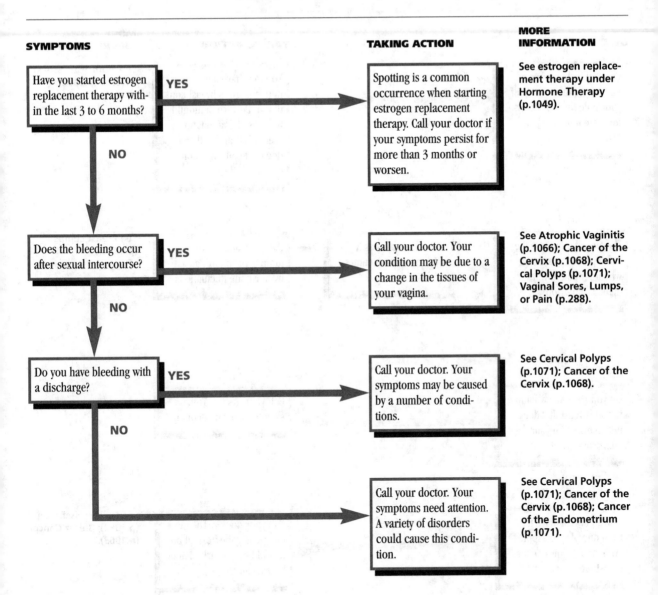

SYMPTOMS

TAKING ACTION

MORE INFORMATION

Have you started estrogen replacement therapy within the last 3 to 6 months?

YES → Spotting is a common occurrence when starting estrogen replacement therapy. Call your doctor if your symptoms persist for more than 3 months or worsen.

See estrogen replacement therapy under Hormone Therapy (p.1049).

NO

Does the bleeding occur after sexual intercourse?

YES → Call your doctor. Your condition may be due to a change in the tissues of your vagina.

See Atrophic Vaginitis (p.1066); Cancer of the Cervix (p.1068); Cervical Polyps (p.1071); Vaginal Sores, Lumps, or Pain (p.288).

NO

Do you have bleeding with a discharge?

YES → Call your doctor. Your symptoms may be caused by a number of conditions.

See Cervical Polyps (p.1071); Cancer of the Cervix (p.1068).

NO → Call your doctor. Your symptoms need attention. A variety of disorders could cause this condition.

See Cervical Polyps (p.1071); Cancer of the Cervix (p.1068); Cancer of the Endometrium (p.1071).

BREAST LUMP

Touch alone cannot distinguish a malignant (cancerous) lump from a benign (noncancerous) one. Most breasts are lumpy to some degree. However, there are certain signs to look for and bring to the attention of your doctor.

SYMPTOMS

TAKING ACTION

MORE INFORMATION

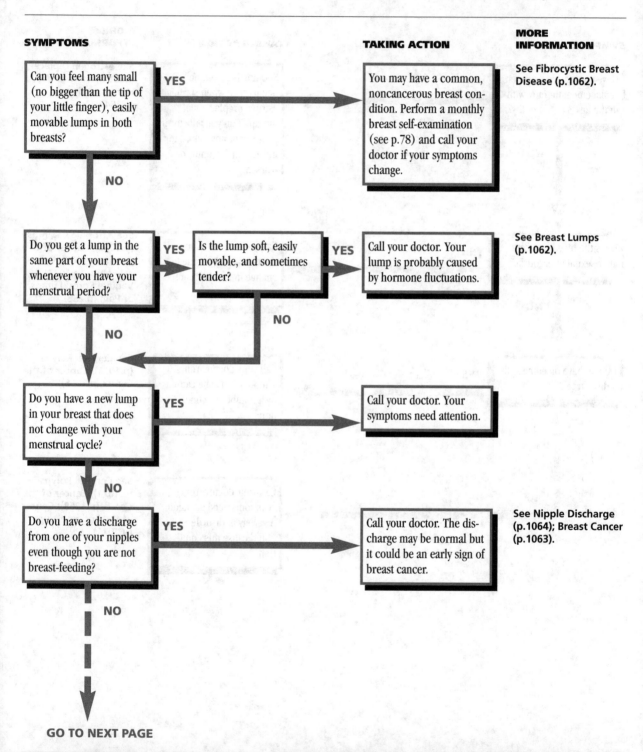

Can you feel many small (no bigger than the tip of your little finger), easily movable lumps in both breasts?

YES → You may have a common, noncancerous breast condition. Perform a monthly breast self-examination (see p.78) and call your doctor if your symptoms change.

See Fibrocystic Breast Disease (p.1062).

NO ↓

Do you get a lump in the same part of your breast whenever you have your menstrual period?

YES → Is the lump soft, easily movable, and sometimes tender?

YES → Call your doctor. Your lump is probably caused by hormone fluctuations.

See Breast Lumps (p.1062).

NO

NO ↓

Do you have a new lump in your breast that does not change with your menstrual cycle?

YES → Call your doctor. Your symptoms need attention.

NO ↓

Do you have a discharge from one of your nipples even though you are not breast-feeding?

YES → Call your doctor. The discharge may be normal but it could be an early sign of breast cancer.

See Nipple Discharge (p.1064); Breast Cancer (p.1063).

NO ↓

GO TO NEXT PAGE

CONTINUED FROM PREVIOUS PAGE

SYMPTOMS

TAKING ACTION

When you lift your hands above your head and look at your breasts in a mirror, is there an indentation in the contour of the breast?

YES →

Call your doctor. This could be an early sign of breast cancer.

See Breast Cancer (p.1063).

NO ↓

Has the skin of your breast become dimpled, like the surface of an orange?

YES →

Call your doctor. This could be an early sign of breast cancer.

See Breast Cancer (p.1063).

NO ↓

Has the nipple of one breast become retracted (pulled inside the breast tissue)?

YES →

Call your doctor. This could be an early sign of breast cancer.

See Breast Cancer (p.1063).

NO →

Call your doctor. Your symptoms need attention.

BREAST PAIN

Pain, soreness, or tenderness in one or both breasts often precedes or accompanies menstrual periods but can also occur during pregnancy, breast-feeding, and menopause. Consult your doctor if you have breast pain that is accompanied by a breast lump or nipple discharge.

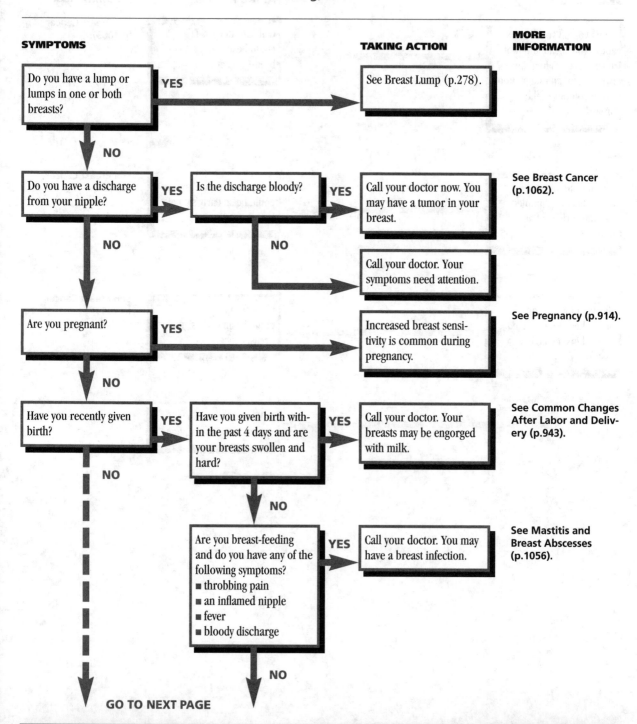

SYMPTOMS

TAKING ACTION

MORE INFORMATION

Do you have a lump or lumps in one or both breasts? — **YES** → See Breast Lump (p.278).

NO

Do you have a discharge from your nipple? — **YES** → Is the discharge bloody? — **YES** → Call your doctor now. You may have a tumor in your breast. — **See Breast Cancer (p.1062).**

NO (discharge bloody) → Call your doctor. Your symptoms need attention.

NO (discharge from nipple)

Are you pregnant? — **YES** → Increased breast sensitivity is common during pregnancy. — **See Pregnancy (p.914).**

NO

Have you recently given birth? — **YES** → Have you given birth within the past 4 days and are your breasts swollen and hard? — **YES** → Call your doctor. Your breasts may be engorged with milk. — **See Common Changes After Labor and Delivery (p.943).**

NO

Are you breast-feeding and do you have any of the following symptoms?
- throbbing pain
- an inflamed nipple
- fever
- bloody discharge

— **YES** → Call your doctor. You may have a breast infection. — **See Mastitis and Breast Abscesses (p.1056).**

NO

GO TO NEXT PAGE

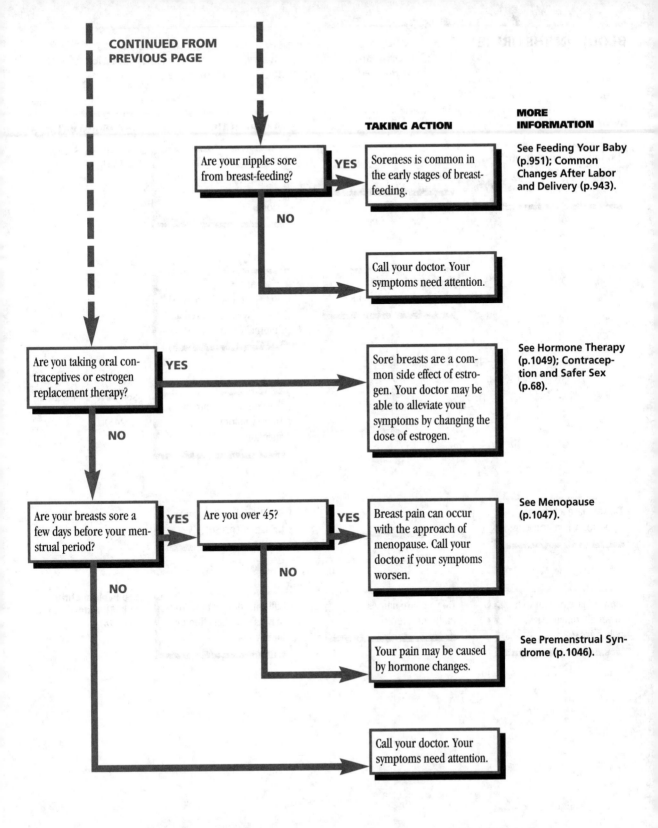

TAKING ACTION

Are your nipples sore from breast-feeding?

YES → Soreness is common in the early stages of breast-feeding.

See Feeding Your Baby (p.951); Common Changes After Labor and Delivery (p.943).

NO

Call your doctor. Your symptoms need attention.

Are you taking oral contraceptives or estrogen replacement therapy?

YES → Sore breasts are a common side effect of estrogen. Your doctor may be able to alleviate your symptoms by changing the dose of estrogen.

See Hormone Therapy (p.1049); Contraception and Safer Sex (p.68).

NO

Are your breasts sore a few days before your menstrual period?

YES → Are you over 45?

YES → Breast pain can occur with the approach of menopause. Call your doctor if your symptoms worsen.

See Menopause (p.1047).

NO

Your pain may be caused by hormone changes.

See Premenstrual Syndrome (p.1046).

NO

Call your doctor. Your symptoms need attention.

BLOOD IN THE URINE

Blood in urine can appear cloudy, pink, or red. Some food colorings (both natural and artificial) and medicines can change the color of your urine.

SYMPTOMS

TAKING ACTION

MORE INFORMATION

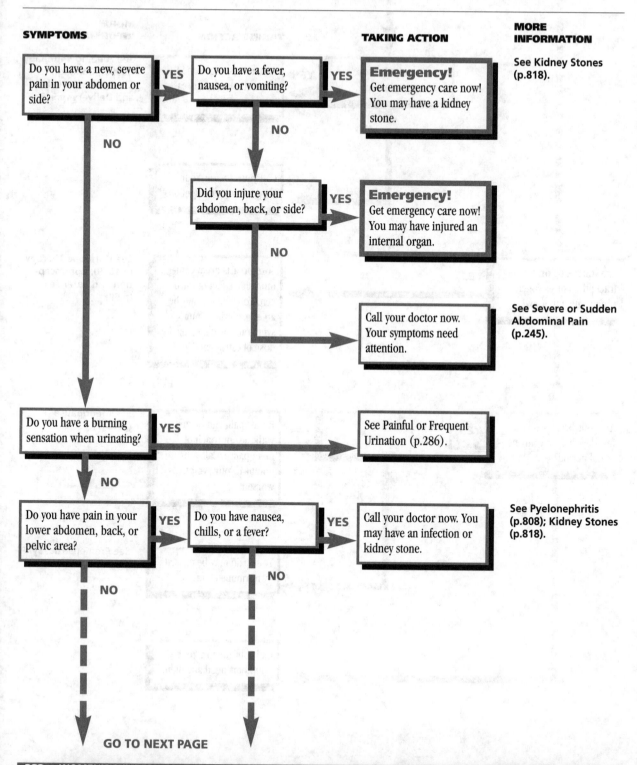

Do you have a new, severe pain in your abdomen or side?

YES → Do you have a fever, nausea, or vomiting?

YES → **Emergency!** Get emergency care now! You may have a kidney stone.

See Kidney Stones (p.818).

NO

NO → Did you injure your abdomen, back, or side?

YES → **Emergency!** Get emergency care now! You may have injured an internal organ.

NO → Call your doctor now. Your symptoms need attention.

See Severe or Sudden Abdominal Pain (p.245).

Do you have a burning sensation when urinating?

YES → See Painful or Frequent Urination (p.286).

NO

Do you have pain in your lower abdomen, back, or pelvic area?

YES → Do you have nausea, chills, or a fever?

YES → Call your doctor now. You may have an infection or kidney stone.

See Pyelonephritis (p.808); Kidney Stones (p.818).

NO

NO

GO TO NEXT PAGE

**CONTINUED FROM
PREVIOUS PAGE**

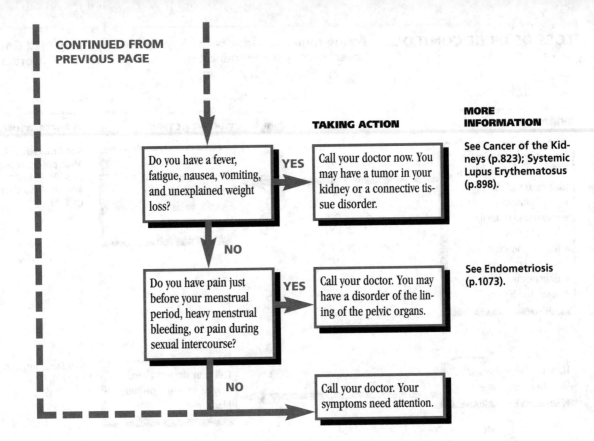

TAKING ACTION

**MORE
INFORMATION**

Do you have a fever, fatigue, nausea, vomiting, and unexplained weight loss?

YES → Call your doctor now. You may have a tumor in your kidney or a connective tissue disorder.

See Cancer of the Kidneys (p.823); Systemic Lupus Erythematosus (p.898).

NO ↓

Do you have pain just before your menstrual period, heavy menstrual bleeding, or pain during sexual intercourse?

YES → Call your doctor. You may have a disorder of the lining of the pelvic organs.

See Endometriosis (p.1073).

NO →

Call your doctor. Your symptoms need attention.

LOSS OF URINE CONTROL

Losing control of urine is called urinary incontinence. It can be caused by conditions related to aging, medicines, or a serious medical disorder.

SYMPTOMS

TAKING ACTION

MORE INFORMATION

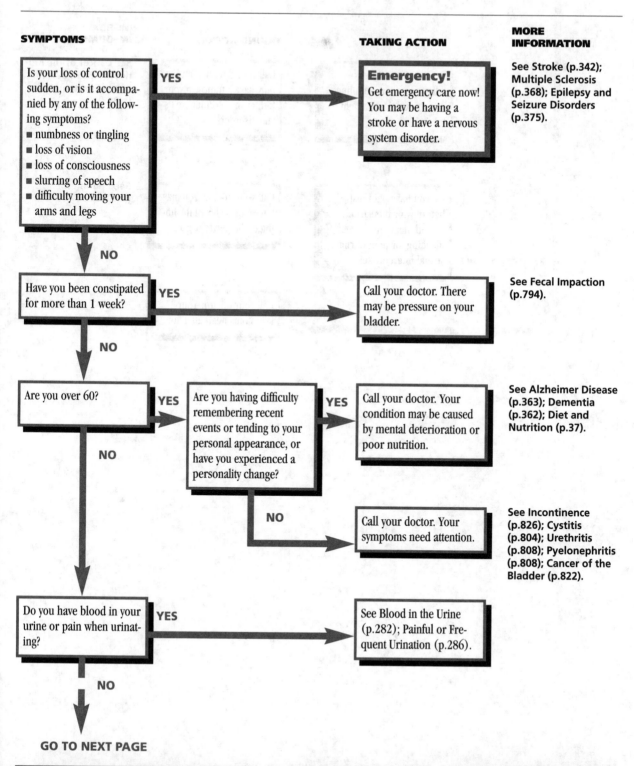

Is your loss of control sudden, or is it accompanied by any of the following symptoms?
- numbness or tingling
- loss of vision
- loss of consciousness
- slurring of speech
- difficulty moving your arms and legs

YES →

Emergency! Get emergency care now! You may be having a stroke or have a nervous system disorder.

See Stroke (p.342); Multiple Sclerosis (p.368); Epilepsy and Seizure Disorders (p.375).

NO ↓

Have you been constipated for more than 1 week?

YES →

Call your doctor. There may be pressure on your bladder.

See Fecal Impaction (p.794).

NO ↓

Are you over 60?

YES →

Are you having difficulty remembering recent events or tending to your personal appearance, or have you experienced a personality change?

YES →

Call your doctor. Your condition may be caused by mental deterioration or poor nutrition.

See Alzheimer Disease (p.363); Dementia (p.362); Diet and Nutrition (p.37).

NO ↓

Call your doctor. Your symptoms need attention.

See Incontinence (p.826); Cystitis (p.804); Urethritis (p.808); Pyelonephritis (p.808); Cancer of the Bladder (p.822).

NO ↓

Do you have blood in your urine or pain when urinating?

YES →

See Blood in the Urine (p.282); Painful or Frequent Urination (p.286).

NO ↓

GO TO NEXT PAGE

CONTINUED FROM PREVIOUS PAGE

SYMPTOMS

TAKING ACTION

Are you taking any prescription or nonprescription medicines?

YES

Call your doctor. Your incontinence may be a side effect of your medicine.

See Medicines (p.1148).

NO

Do you have a small leakage of urine when you cough, sneeze, laugh, or run?

YES

Your loss of control may be due to sudden pressure on the abdomen. Try doing Kegel exercises to strengthen pelvic muscles. Call your doctor if your symptoms persist.

See stress incontinence under Incontinence (p.826); Kegel Exercises for Pelvic Floor Muscles (p.1051).

NO

Call your doctor. Your symptoms need attention.

See Incontinence (p.826).

PAINFUL OR FREQUENT URINATION

Pain during or just after urinating, difficulty urinating, or changes in frequency or volume of urination can be caused by infections, hormone changes, metabolic disorders, tumors, medicines, or merely an excessive consumption of liquids.

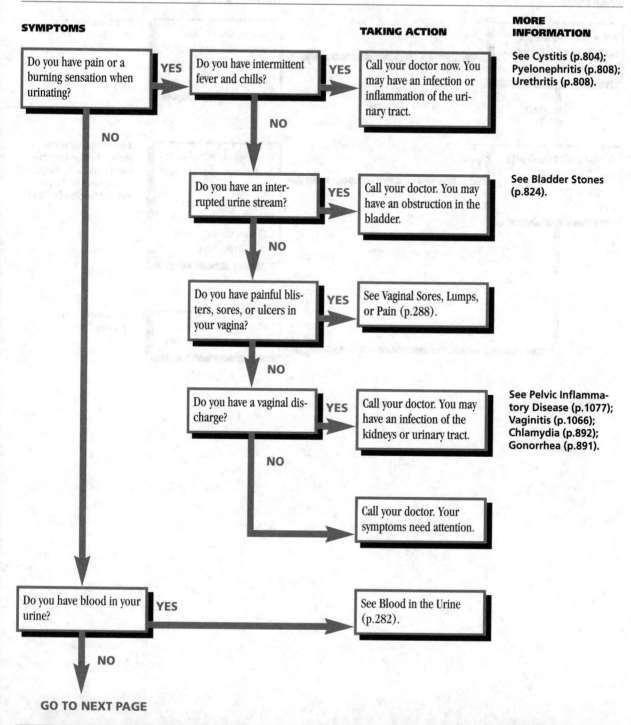

SYMPTOMS

Do you have pain or a burning sensation when urinating?

YES → Do you have intermittent fever and chills?

YES → **TAKING ACTION**

Call your doctor now. You may have an infection or inflammation of the urinary tract.

MORE INFORMATION

See Cystitis (p.804); Pyelonephritis (p.808); Urethritis (p.808).

NO ↓

Do you have an interrupted urine stream?

YES → Call your doctor. You may have an obstruction in the bladder.

See Bladder Stones (p.824).

NO ↓

Do you have painful blisters, sores, or ulcers in your vagina?

YES → See Vaginal Sores, Lumps, or Pain (p.288).

NO ↓

Do you have a vaginal discharge?

YES → Call your doctor. You may have an infection of the kidneys or urinary tract.

See Pelvic Inflammatory Disease (p.1077); Vaginitis (p.1066); Chlamydia (p.892); Gonorrhea (p.891).

NO ↓

Call your doctor. Your symptoms need attention.

NO (from first question) ↓

Do you have blood in your urine?

YES → See Blood in the Urine (p.282).

NO ↓

GO TO NEXT PAGE

CONTINUED FROM PREVIOUS PAGE

SYMPTOMS

TAKING ACTION

MORE INFORMATION

Do you urinate frequently or has your frequency of urination increased?

YES → Are you pregnant?

YES → Frequent urination is common during pregnancy.

See Pregnancy (p.914).

NO

NO

Do you have any of the following symptoms?
- increased thirst and appetite
- genital itching
- fatigue
- weight loss

YES → Call your doctor. You may have increased sugar in your blood and urine.

See Diabetes Mellitus (p.832).

NO

Are you taking any diuretic drugs?

YES → Increased urination is one of the effects of diuretic drugs.

See loop diuretic under Common Drug Classes (p.1160).

NO

Do you drink large amounts of alcoholic beverages or caffeine-containing drinks such as coffee, tea, or soft drinks?

YES → Increased urination is a common effect of caffeine and alcohol.

NO

Do you lose control of your urine?

YES → See Loss of Urine Control (p.284).

See Incontinence (p.826).

NO

Call your doctor if your symptoms worsen or persist for more than 2 weeks.

VAGINAL SORES, LUMPS, OR PAIN

Sores and lumps in the vagina can be caused by a sexually transmitted disease. See your doctor now so any disease can be diagnosed and, if necessary, you and all sexual partners can be treated. Vaginal pain that is accompanied by discharge, bleeding, or painful urination, or that occurs during intercourse, may indicate a disorder of the vagina or other reproductive organs, or a urinary tract infection. These conditions also require your doctor's attention.

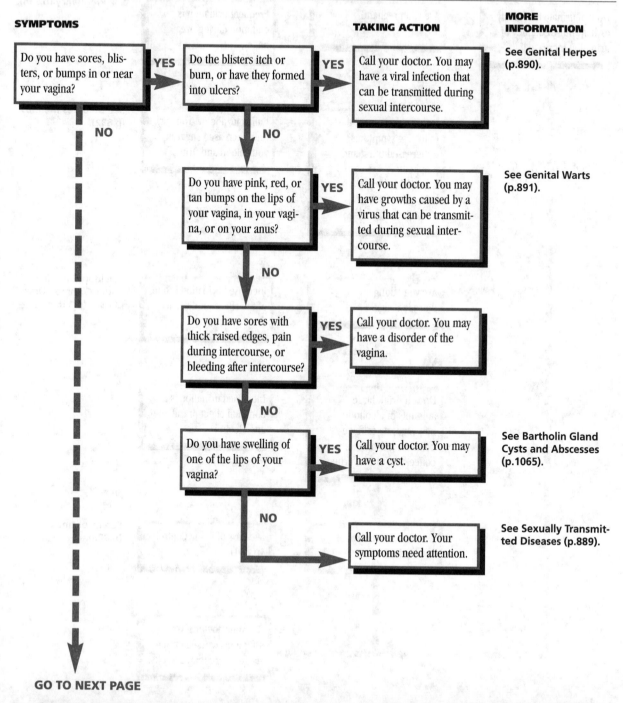

SYMPTOMS

TAKING ACTION

MORE INFORMATION

Do you have sores, blisters, or bumps in or near your vagina?

YES → Do the blisters itch or burn, or have they formed into ulcers?

YES → Call your doctor. You may have a viral infection that can be transmitted during sexual intercourse.

See Genital Herpes (p.890).

NO

Do you have pink, red, or tan bumps on the lips of your vagina, in your vagina, or on your anus?

YES → Call your doctor. You may have growths caused by a virus that can be transmitted during sexual intercourse.

See Genital Warts (p.891).

NO

Do you have sores with thick raised edges, pain during intercourse, or bleeding after intercourse?

YES → Call your doctor. You may have a disorder of the vagina.

NO

Do you have swelling of one of the lips of your vagina?

YES → Call your doctor. You may have a cyst.

See Bartholin Gland Cysts and Abscesses (p.1065).

NO

Call your doctor. Your symptoms need attention.

See Sexually Transmitted Diseases (p.889).

GO TO NEXT PAGE

SYMPTOMS

TAKING ACTION

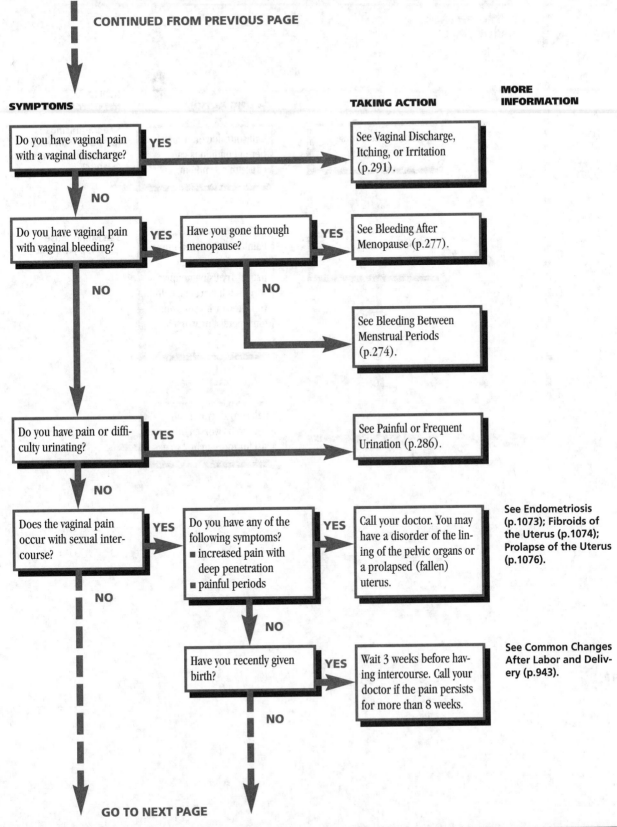

Do you have vaginal pain with a vaginal discharge? **YES** → See Vaginal Discharge, Itching, or Irritation (p.291).

NO

Do you have vaginal pain with vaginal bleeding? **YES** → Have you gone through menopause? **YES** → See Bleeding After Menopause (p.277).

NO

See Bleeding Between Menstrual Periods (p.274).

NO

Do you have pain or difficulty urinating? **YES** → See Painful or Frequent Urination (p.286).

NO

Does the vaginal pain occur with sexual intercourse? **YES** → Do you have any of the following symptoms?
■ increased pain with deep penetration
■ painful periods
YES → Call your doctor. You may have a disorder of the lining of the pelvic organs or a prolapsed (fallen) uterus.

See Endometriosis (p.1073); Fibroids of the Uterus (p.1074); Prolapse of the Uterus (p.1076).

NO

NO

Have you recently given birth? **YES** → Wait 3 weeks before having intercourse. Call your doctor if the pain persists for more than 8 weeks.

See Common Changes After Labor and Delivery (p.943).

NO

GO TO NEXT PAGE

**CONTINUED FROM
PREVIOUS PAGE**

TAKING ACTION

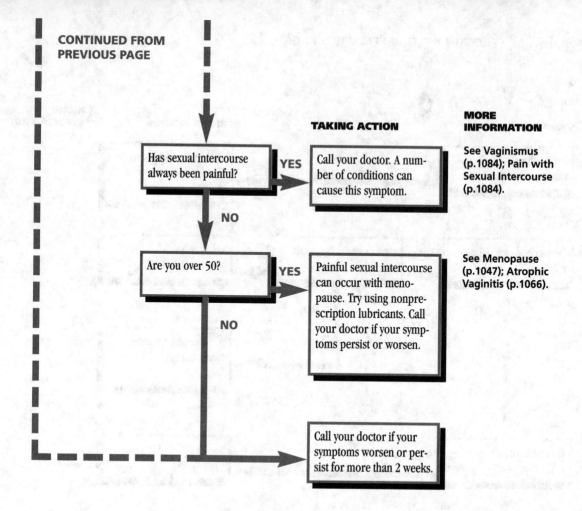

Has sexual intercourse always been painful?

YES → Call your doctor. A number of conditions can cause this symptom.

See Vaginismus (p.1084); Pain with Sexual Intercourse (p.1084).

NO

Are you over 50?

YES → Painful sexual intercourse can occur with menopause. Try using nonprescription lubricants. Call your doctor if your symptoms persist or worsen.

See Menopause (p.1047); Atrophic Vaginitis (p.1066).

NO

Call your doctor if your symptoms worsen or persist for more than 2 weeks.

VAGINAL DISCHARGE, ITCHING, OR IRRITATION

The amount and consistency of vaginal discharge change during the menstrual cycle. Significant changes in volume, color, consistency, or odor indicate that you should see your doctor.

SYMPTOMS

TAKING ACTION

MORE INFORMATION

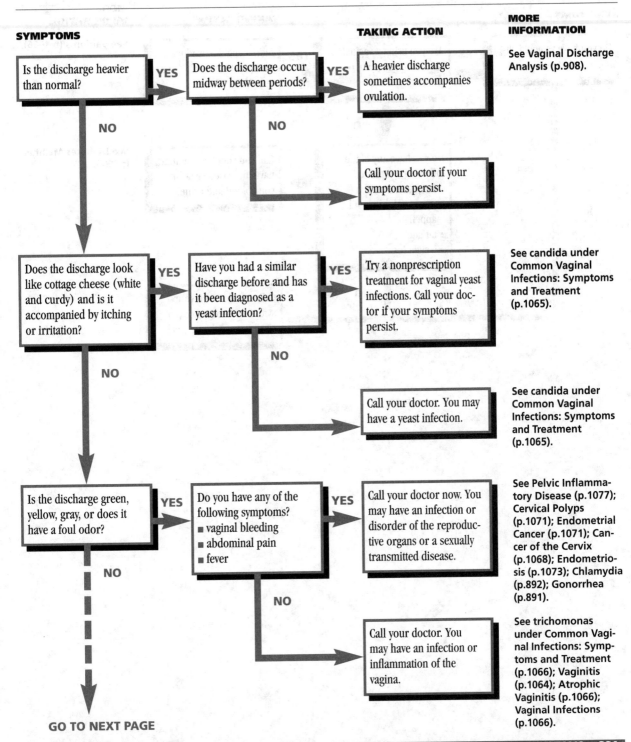

Is the discharge heavier than normal? **YES** → Does the discharge occur midway between periods? **YES** → A heavier discharge sometimes accompanies ovulation.

See Vaginal Discharge Analysis (p.908).

NO ↓ **NO** ↓

Call your doctor if your symptoms persist.

Does the discharge look like cottage cheese (white and curdy) and is it accompanied by itching or irritation? **YES** → Have you had a similar discharge before and has it been diagnosed as a yeast infection? **YES** → Try a nonprescription treatment for vaginal yeast infections. Call your doctor if your symptoms persist.

See candida under Common Vaginal Infections: Symptoms and Treatment (p.1065).

NO ↓ **NO** ↓

Call your doctor. You may have a yeast infection.

See candida under Common Vaginal Infections: Symptoms and Treatment (p.1065).

Is the discharge green, yellow, gray, or does it have a foul odor? **YES** → Do you have any of the following symptoms?
■ vaginal bleeding
■ abdominal pain
■ fever
YES → Call your doctor now. You may have an infection or disorder of the reproductive organs or a sexually transmitted disease.

See Pelvic Inflammatory Disease (p.1077); Cervical Polyps (p.1071); Endometrial Cancer (p.1071); Cancer of the Cervix (p.1068); Endometriosis (p.1073); Chlamydia (p.892); Gonorrhea (p.891).

NO ↓ **NO** ↓

Call your doctor. You may have an infection or inflammation of the vagina.

See trichomonas under Common Vaginal Infections: Symptoms and Treatment (p.1066); Vaginitis (p.1064); Atrophic Vaginitis (p.1066); Vaginal Infections (p.1066).

GO TO NEXT PAGE

CONTINUED FROM PREVIOUS PAGE

SYMPTOMS | **TAKING ACTION** | **MORE INFORMATION**

Do you have vaginal itching or irritation?

YES → Are you using a vaginal spray, cream, foam, or douche?

YES → Stop using the product and see if your symptoms subside.

See Vaginitis (p.1066).

NO → Do you have any of the following symptoms?

- frequent urination
- increased thirst and appetite
- fatigue
- weight loss

YES → Call your doctor. You may have increased sugar in your blood and urine.

See Diabetes Mellitus (p.832).

NO → Call your doctor if your symptoms worsen or persist for more than 2 weeks.

CRYING IN INFANTS

Changes in the pattern, sound, or duration of your baby's crying can occur for no apparent reason. All infants cry and for many common reasons, including hunger, a wet diaper, gas, and the need to be held. Crying that may be due to illness or injury, or crying that is inconsolable, requires your doctor's attention.

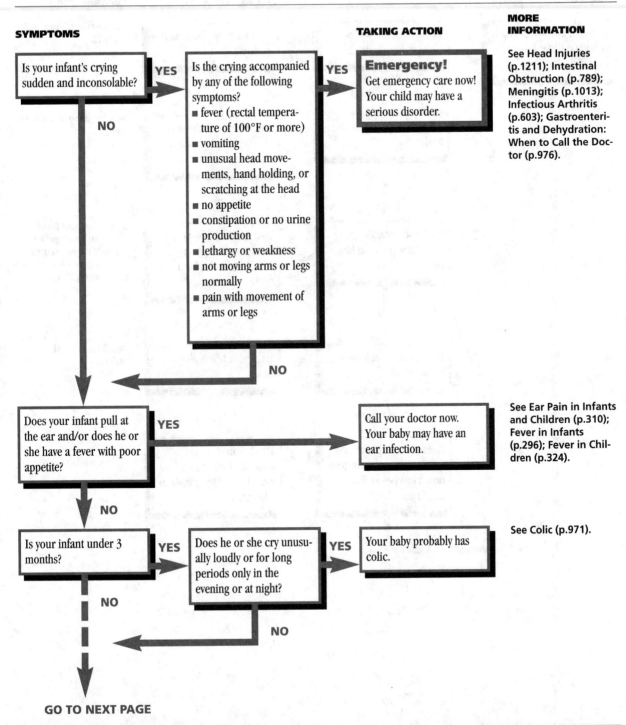

Is your infant's crying sudden and inconsolable?

YES → Is the crying accompanied by any of the following symptoms?

- fever (rectal temperature of 100°F or more)
- vomiting
- unusual head movements, hand holding, or scratching at the head
- no appetite
- constipation or no urine production
- lethargy or weakness
- not moving arms or legs normally
- pain with movement of arms or legs

YES → **Emergency!** Get emergency care now! Your child may have a serious disorder.

See Head Injuries (p.1211); Intestinal Obstruction (p.789); Meningitis (p.1013); Infectious Arthritis (p.603); Gastroenteritis and Dehydration: When to Call the Doctor (p.976).

NO

Does your infant pull at the ear and/or does he or she have a fever with poor appetite?

YES → Call your doctor now. Your baby may have an ear infection.

See Ear Pain in Infants and Children (p.310); Fever in Infants (p.296); Fever in Children (p.324).

NO

Is your infant under 3 months?

YES → Does he or she cry unusually loudly or for long periods only in the evening or at night?

YES → Your baby probably has colic.

See Colic (p.971).

NO

NO

GO TO NEXT PAGE

CONTINUED FROM PREVIOUS PAGE

SYMPTOMS

TAKING ACTION

Is your infant not feeding as usual or does he or she seem sick?

YES →

Does his or her crying stop after feeding?

YES →

Your baby may be hungry or thirsty.

See Feeding Your Baby (p.951).

NO ↓

Does the crying start after feeding?

YES →

Your baby probably has gas. Try burping your infant more often.

See Feeding Your Baby (p.951).

NO ↓

Does your infant's crying stop when you hold him or her?

YES →

Your baby may be bored, lonely, or want attention. Hold him or her for a while.

See The Child Development Touchpoints Model: Dr Brazelton's Advice on Child Development (p.954).

NO ↓

Does your infant have diaper rash?

YES →

Treat your baby's diaper rash.

See Diaper Rash (p.973).

NO ↓

Does the crying start and do his or her arms or legs twitch just before your child falls asleep?

YES →

This is common. Hold your child securely or wrap him or her snugly in a blanket.

NO ←

NO (from first symptom, down left side)

GO TO NEXT PAGE

CONTINUED FROM PREVIOUS PAGE

SYMPTOMS

TAKING ACTION

Is there a great deal of stress in your home?

YES

Your infant may be reacting to your anxiety. Try to modify your home environment.

See The Child Development Touchpoints Model: Dr Brazelton's Advice (p.954).

NO

Is your infant crying and salivating more than usual?

YES

He or she is probably getting a new tooth.

See Teething (p.964).

NO

Call your doctor if your infant's symptoms worsen or persist for more than 1 week.

FEVER IN INFANTS

Your infant's temperature can fluctuate with the time of day or activity level. A fever is a rectal temperature of 100.4°F or above. Generally, a high fever in an infant under age 1 is 104°F or above. However, call your doctor if your infant is less than 3 months and has any fever, even a low one. Call your doctor if your infant is between 3 and 12 months and has a fever over 101°F.

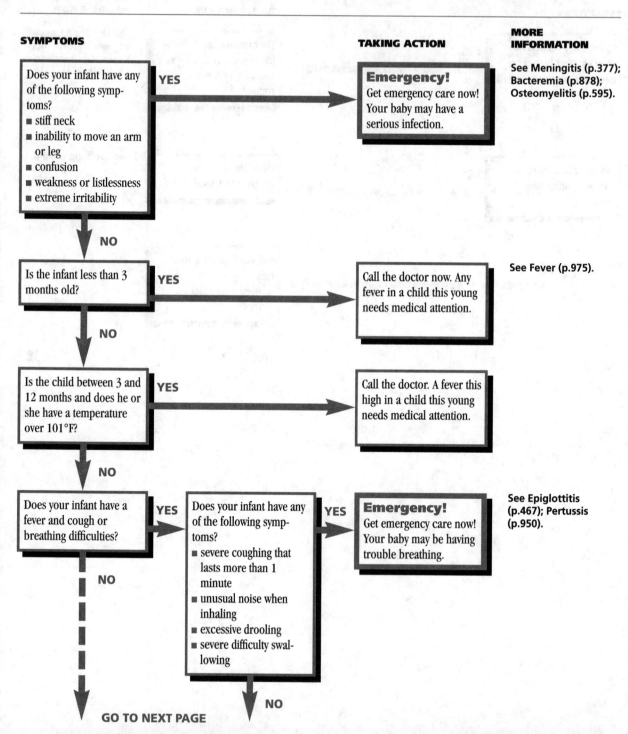

SYMPTOMS

Does your infant have any of the following symptoms?
- stiff neck
- inability to move an arm or leg
- confusion
- weakness or listlessness
- extreme irritability

YES →

TAKING ACTION

Emergency!
Get emergency care now! Your baby may have a serious infection.

MORE INFORMATION

See Meningitis (p.377); Bacteremia (p.878); Osteomyelitis (p.595).

NO ↓

Is the infant less than 3 months old?

YES →

Call the doctor now. Any fever in a child this young needs medical attention.

See Fever (p.975).

NO ↓

Is the child between 3 and 12 months and does he or she have a temperature over 101°F?

YES →

Call the doctor. A fever this high in a child this young needs medical attention.

NO ↓

Does your infant have a fever and cough or breathing difficulties?

YES →

Does your infant have any of the following symptoms?
- severe coughing that lasts more than 1 minute
- unusual noise when inhaling
- excessive drooling
- severe difficulty swallowing

YES →

Emergency!
Get emergency care now! Your baby may be having trouble breathing.

See Epiglottitis (p.467); Pertussis (p.950).

NO ↓

GO TO NEXT PAGE

NO ↓

**CONTINUED FROM
PREVIOUS PAGE**

TAKING ACTION

Does your infant have a noisy, barking cough, especially at night?

YES

Call the doctor now. Your infant may have an infection of the vocal cords and large breathing tubes.

See Croup (p.1002).

NO

Call the doctor now. Your baby may have an infection.

See Coughing in Infants and Children (p.307); Shortness of Breath in Infants and Children (p.312).

Does your infant have a fever with unusual or jerking movements of the arms, legs, or face or periods of listlessness?

YES

Call the doctor now. A sudden, high fever can cause seizures.

See Febrile Seizure (p.1007).

NO

Does your infant have a fever with a rash?

YES

Your baby may have an infection.

See Rash in Infants and Children (p.304).

NO

Does your infant have a fever with diarrhea or vomiting?

YES

Call the doctor now. Your baby may have an infection.

See Gastroenteritis (p.976); Diarrhea in Infants (p.299); and Vomiting in Infants (p.301).

NO

GO TO NEXT PAGE

CONTINUED FROM PREVIOUS PAGE

SYMPTOMS

TAKING ACTION

Does your infant have a fever with a runny nose or coldlike symptoms?

YES →

Your baby may have an infection.

See Colds (p.1000); respiratory syncytial virus under Bronchiolitis (p.969).

NO ↓

Does your infant have a fever, and is he or she pulling at the ear and crying?

YES →

Call the doctor now. Your baby may have an ear infection.

See Ear Pain in Infants and Children (p.310).

NO ↓

Has your infant recently been immunized?

YES →

A fever sometimes occurs after immunization. See the doctor if your child's symptoms persist.

See Childhood Immunization Schedule (p.947).

NO ↓

Is your infant wrapped tightly or wearing heavy clothing or is it hot in your home?

YES →

A baby's temperature can be affected by clothing and air temperature. Remove some layers of clothing from your child and give him or her fluids.

See Gastroenteritis and Dehydration: When to Call the Doctor (p.976).

NO ↓

Call your doctor if your child's fever persists for more than 2 to 3 days, or rises to a high level.

DIARRHEA IN INFANTS

Loose, watery, or more frequent bowel movements indicate diarrhea. Gastrointestinal infections or changes in diet are common causes of diarrhea in an infant. When accompanied by persistent abdominal pain or vomiting, diarrhea may require a doctor's attention.

SYMPTOMS

TAKING ACTION

MORE INFORMATION

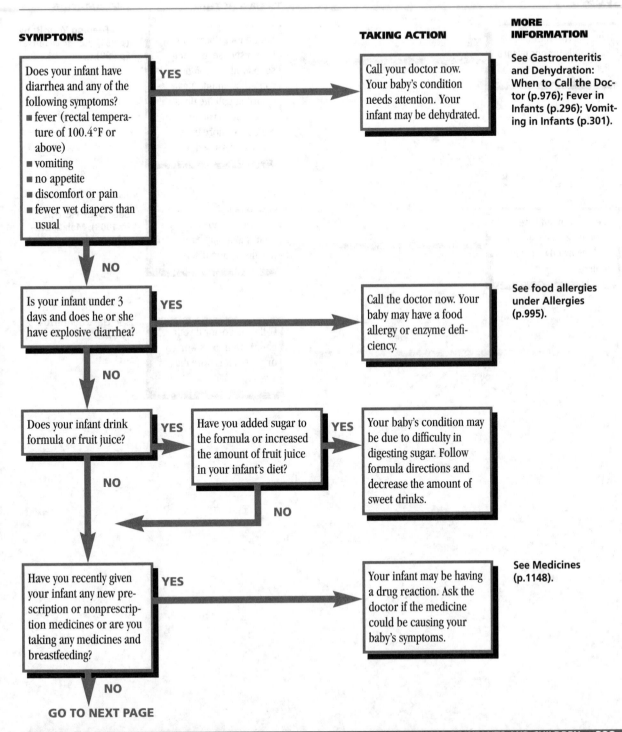

Does your infant have diarrhea and any of the following symptoms?
- fever (rectal temperature of 100.4°F or above)
- vomiting
- no appetite
- discomfort or pain
- fewer wet diapers than usual

YES → Call your doctor now. Your baby's condition needs attention. Your infant may be dehydrated.

See Gastroenteritis and Dehydration: When to Call the Doctor (p.976); Fever in Infants (p.296); Vomiting in Infants (p.301).

NO ↓

Is your infant under 3 days and does he or she have explosive diarrhea?

YES → Call the doctor now. Your baby may have a food allergy or enzyme deficiency.

See food allergies under Allergies (p.995).

NO ↓

Does your infant drink formula or fruit juice?

YES → Have you added sugar to the formula or increased the amount of fruit juice in your infant's diet?

YES → Your baby's condition may be due to difficulty in digesting sugar. Follow formula directions and decrease the amount of sweet drinks.

NO ←

NO ↓

Have you recently given your infant any new prescription or nonprescription medicines or are you taking any medicines and breastfeeding?

YES → Your infant may be having a drug reaction. Ask the doctor if the medicine could be causing your baby's symptoms.

See Medicines (p.1148).

NO ↓

GO TO NEXT PAGE

CONTINUED FROM PREVIOUS PAGE

SYMPTOMS

TAKING ACTION

Have you just introduced solid foods to your infant's diet?

YES

Your baby's diarrhea may be a response to eating solid foods or could be caused by an intestinal disorder. Call the doctor if your child's symptoms persist for more than 1 week or worsen.

See Feeding Your Baby (p.951); Celiac Disease (p.999).

NO

Does your infant have chronic diarrhea and foul-smelling or oily looking stools?

YES

Call your doctor now. Your infant may have a malabsorption disorder.

See Cystic Fibrosis (p.1003); Malabsorption syndrome (p.775).

NO

Call your doctor if your child's symptoms worsen or persist for more than 1 week.

See Gastroenteritis (p.976).

VOMITING IN INFANTS

Emptying of stomach contents through the mouth (spitting up) is common in infants.

However, vomiting that is more frequent or more forceful than is typical for your child, or that is accompanied by fever, reluctance to nurse, constipation, or diarrhea, may require your doctor's attention.

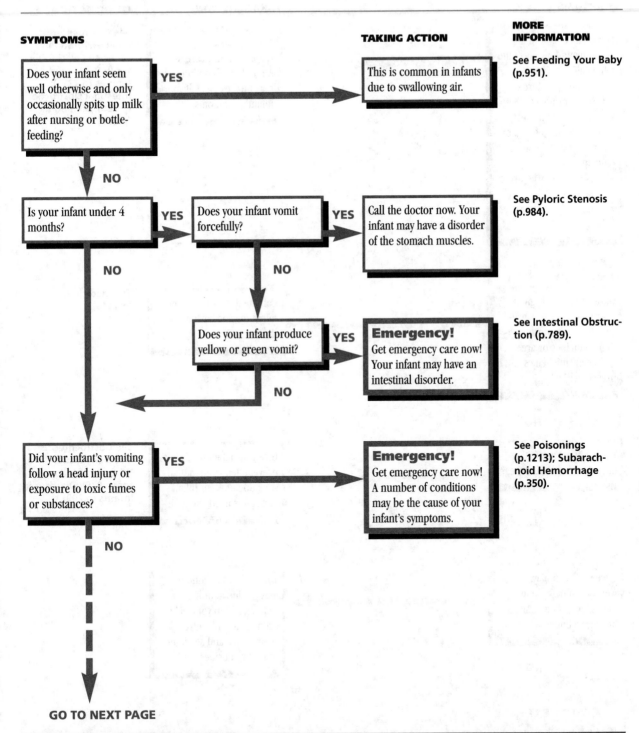

SYMPTOMS

TAKING ACTION

MORE INFORMATION

Does your infant seem well otherwise and only occasionally spits up milk after nursing or bottle-feeding?

YES → This is common in infants due to swallowing air.

See Feeding Your Baby (p.951).

NO ↓

Is your infant under 4 months?

YES → Does your infant vomit forcefully?

YES → Call the doctor now. Your infant may have a disorder of the stomach muscles.

See Pyloric Stenosis (p.984).

NO ↓

NO ↓

Does your infant produce yellow or green vomit?

YES → **Emergency!** Get emergency care now! Your infant may have an intestinal disorder.

See Intestinal Obstruction (p.789).

NO ←

Did your infant's vomiting follow a head injury or exposure to toxic fumes or substances?

YES → **Emergency!** Get emergency care now! A number of conditions may be the cause of your infant's symptoms.

See Poisonings (p.1213); Subarachnoid Hemorrhage (p.350).

NO ↓

GO TO NEXT PAGE

CONTINUED FROM PREVIOUS PAGE

SYMPTOMS

TAKING ACTION

Is your infant's vomiting accompanied by any of the following?
- fever (temperature of 100.4°F or above)
- unusual head movements, hand holding, or scratching at the head
- no appetite
- constipation or no urine production
- lethargy

YES →

Emergency!
Get emergency care now! A number of conditions may be the cause of your infant's symptoms.

See Gastroenteritis and Dehydration: When to Call the Doctor (p.976); Head Injuries (p.1211); Intestinal Obstruction (p.789); Meningitis (p.377).

NO ↓

Have you recently given your infant any new prescription or nonprescription medicines or are you taking any medicines and breast-feeding?

YES →

Call the doctor now. Your infant may be having a drug reaction.

See Medicines (p.1148).

NO ↓

Is your infant's vomiting accompanied by diarrhea?

YES →

Give your infant fluids to prevent dehydration. Call your doctor. Your infant's symptoms need attention.

See Gastroenteritis and Dehydration: When to Call the Doctor (p.976); Diarrhea in Infants (p.299).

NO ↓

Have you been playing with or bouncing your infant, or has he or she been traveling?

YES →

Your infant's condition may be due to motion sickness. Keep your baby calm for a while, give clear fluids, and see if the vomiting subsides.

NO ↓

GO TO NEXT PAGE

CONTINUED FROM PREVIOUS PAGE

SYMPTOMS

TAKING ACTION

Have you just introduced solid foods to your infant's diet?

YES

NO

It is common for infants to spit up their first solid foods, but your baby may also have an intestinal problem. Call your doctor if your infant's symptoms persist for more than 1 week or your infant appears to be ill.

See Feeding Your Baby (p.951); Celiac Disease (p.999).

Call your doctor if your infant's symptoms worsen or persist for more than 2 weeks.

See food allergy under Allergies (p.995).

RASH IN INFANTS AND CHILDREN

Rashes are very common. Blisters, bumps, or scaly patches can indicate a variety of minor skin conditions, including diaper rash. When accompanied by a fever, they may require your doctor's attention.

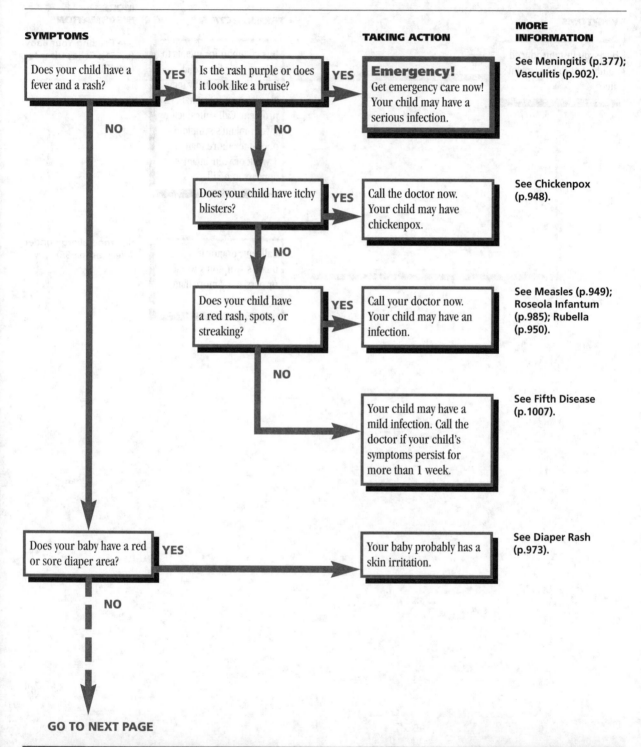

SYMPTOMS

TAKING ACTION

MORE INFORMATION

Does your child have a fever and a rash? — **YES** → Is the rash purple or does it look like a bruise? — **YES** →

Emergency!
Get emergency care now! Your child may have a serious infection.

See Meningitis (p.377); Vasculitis (p.902).

NO

Does your child have itchy blisters? — **YES** →

Call the doctor now. Your child may have chickenpox.

See Chickenpox (p.948).

NO

Does your child have a red rash, spots, or streaking? — **YES** →

Call your doctor now. Your child may have an infection.

See Measles (p.949); Roseola Infantum (p.985); Rubella (p.950).

NO

Your child may have a mild infection. Call the doctor if your child's symptoms persist for more than 1 week.

See Fifth Disease (p.1007).

Does your baby have a red or sore diaper area? — **YES** →

Your baby probably has a skin irritation.

See Diaper Rash (p.973).

NO

GO TO NEXT PAGE

CONTINUED FROM PREVIOUS PAGE

SYMPTOMS	TAKING ACTION	MORE INFORMATION
Does your child have scaly or crusty patches on the scalp, hands, or feet or in skin folds? **YES** →	Your child may have a skin irritation, allergy, or infestation. Call your doctor if your child's symptoms worsen or persist.	See Cradle Cap (p.972); Infantile Eczema (p.568); Scabies (p.550).
NO ↓		
Does your child have pus-filled blisters? **YES** →	Call your doctor. Your child may have a bacterial skin infection.	See Impetigo (p.531).
NO ↓		
Does your child have raised red bumps that may or may not itch or hurt? **YES** →	Call your doctor now. Your child may have an allergy or an infection.	See Hives (p.536); Impetigo (p.531).
NO ↓		
Does your child have clear blisters and slight redness in one spot, and is this area painful? **YES** →	Call your doctor. The child may have an infection.	See Shingles (p.537).
NO ↓		
Does your child complain of pain or stiffness in his or her joints? **YES** →	Call your doctor. Your child may have an inflammatory disorder.	See Lupus Erythematosus (p.898); Juvenile Rheumatoid Arthritis (p.1010).
NO ↓		
	Call your doctor if your child's symptoms worsen or persist for more than 2 weeks.	

CONSTIPATION IN INFANTS AND CHILDREN

Infrequent, painful, dry, hard, or uncomfortable bowel movements indicate constipation. Common causes of constipation in children include a low-fiber diet, inadequate water intake, lack of exercise, and anxiety. When constipation occurs in an infant, or is accompanied by abdominal pain in a child of any age, it requires your doctor's attention.

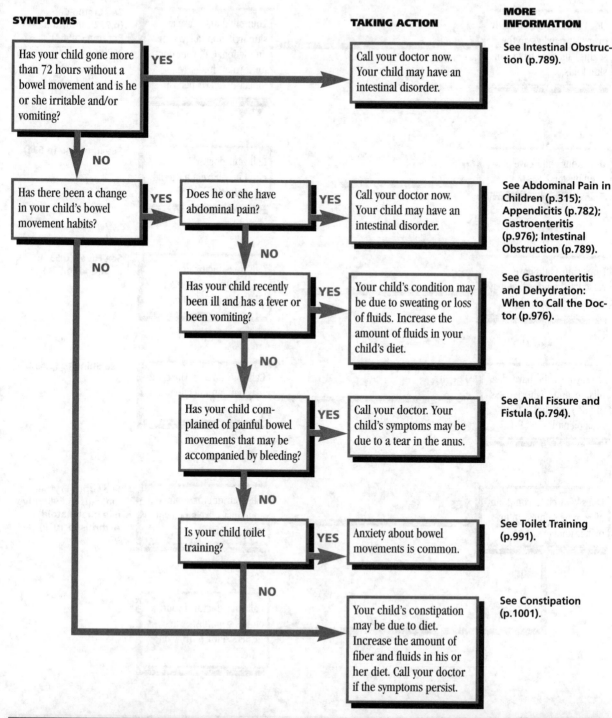

SYMPTOMS

TAKING ACTION

MORE INFORMATION

Has your child gone more than 72 hours without a bowel movement and is he or she irritable and/or vomiting?

YES → Call your doctor now. Your child may have an intestinal disorder.

See Intestinal Obstruction (p.789).

NO

Has there been a change in your child's bowel movement habits?

YES → Does he or she have abdominal pain?

YES → Call your doctor now. Your child may have an intestinal disorder.

See Abdominal Pain in Children (p.315); Appendicitis (p.782); Gastroenteritis (p.976); Intestinal Obstruction (p.789).

NO

Has your child recently been ill and has a fever or been vomiting?

YES → Your child's condition may be due to sweating or loss of fluids. Increase the amount of fluids in your child's diet.

See Gastroenteritis and Dehydration: When to Call the Doctor (p.976).

NO

Has your child complained of painful bowel movements that may be accompanied by bleeding?

YES → Call your doctor. Your child's symptoms may be due to a tear in the anus.

See Anal Fissure and Fistula (p.794).

NO

Is your child toilet training?

YES → Anxiety about bowel movements is common.

See Toilet Training (p.991).

NO

Your child's constipation may be due to diet. Increase the amount of fiber and fluids in his or her diet. Call your doctor if the symptoms persist.

See Constipation (p.1001).

COUGHING IN INFANTS AND CHILDREN

A dry cough, a cough that produces phlegm (sputum), or coughing that is short-term or long-term can be cause for concern. Coughing is often due to a respiratory infection. When coughing is accompanied by shortness of breath or a rectal temperature of 100.4°F or above in a child, or if coughing occurs in an infant, a doctor's attention is required.

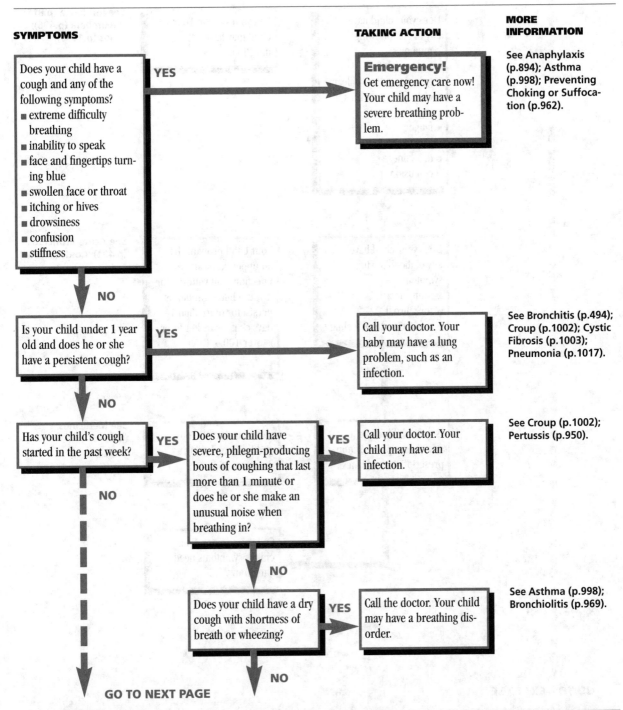

SYMPTOMS

Does your child have a cough and any of the following symptoms?
- extreme difficulty breathing
- inability to speak
- face and fingertips turning blue
- swollen face or throat
- itching or hives
- drowsiness
- confusion
- stiffness

YES →

NO ↓

Is your child under 1 year old and does he or she have a persistent cough?

YES →

NO ↓

Has your child's cough started in the past week?

YES →

NO ↓

Does your child have severe, phlegm-producing bouts of coughing that last more than 1 minute or does he or she make an unusual noise when breathing in?

YES →

NO ↓

Does your child have a dry cough with shortness of breath or wheezing?

YES →

NO ↓

GO TO NEXT PAGE

TAKING ACTION

Emergency!
Get emergency care now! Your child may have a severe breathing problem.

Call your doctor. Your baby may have a lung problem, such as an infection.

Call your doctor. Your child may have an infection.

Call the doctor. Your child may have a breathing disorder.

MORE INFORMATION

See Anaphylaxis (p.894); Asthma (p.998); Preventing Choking or Suffocation (p.962).

See Bronchitis (p.494); Croup (p.1002); Cystic Fibrosis (p.1003); Pneumonia (p.1017).

See Croup (p.1002); Pertussis (p.950).

See Asthma (p.998); Bronchiolitis (p.969).

**CONTINUED FROM
PREVIOUS PAGE**

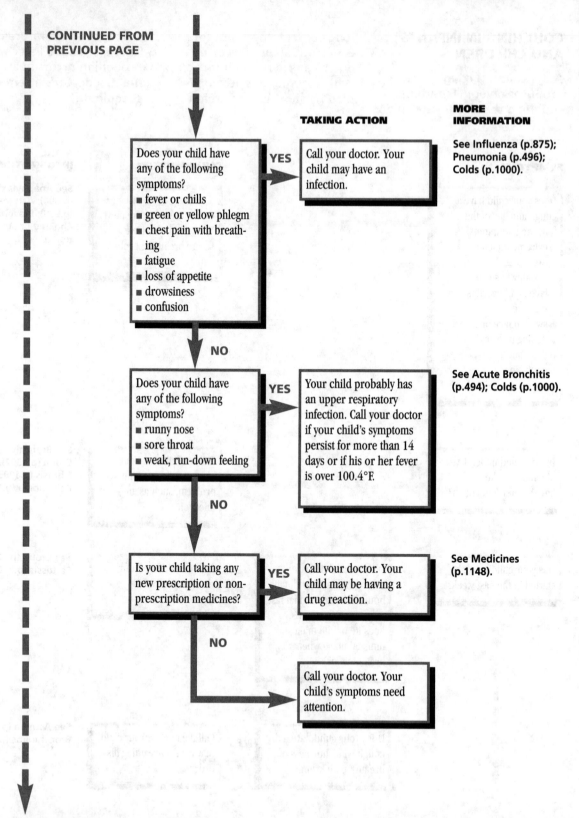

TAKING ACTION

**MORE
INFORMATION**

Does your child have
any of the following
symptoms?
- fever or chills
- green or yellow phlegm
- chest pain with breath-
  ing
- fatigue
- loss of appetite
- drowsiness
- confusion

YES → Call your doctor. Your
child may have an
infection.

**See Influenza (p.875);
Pneumonia (p.496);
Colds (p.1000).**

NO

Does your child have
any of the following
symptoms?
- runny nose
- sore throat
- weak, run-down feeling

YES → Your child probably has
an upper respiratory
infection. Call your doctor
if your child's symptoms
persist for more than 14
days or if his or her fever
is over 100.4°F.

**See Acute Bronchitis
(p.494); Colds (p.1000).**

NO

Is your child taking any
new prescription or non-
prescription medicines?

YES → Call your doctor. Your
child may be having a
drug reaction.

**See Medicines
(p.1148).**

NO

Call your doctor. Your
child's symptoms need
attention.

GO TO NEXT PAGE

CONTINUED FROM PREVIOUS PAGE

SYMPTOMS

TAKING ACTION

Has your child had a cough for many weeks?

YES →

Does your child constantly have a runny or stuffy nose or bad breath or does he or she persistently breathe through his or her mouth?

YES →

Call your doctor. Several conditions could be causing your child's symptoms.

See enlarged adenoids under Enlarged Adenoids (p.1006); Allergies (p.995); Sinusitis (p.464).

NO

NO

Is your child exposed to secondhand smoke from smokers or polluted air?

YES →

Your child's symptoms may be due to the effects of secondhand smoke or polluted air. You should try to quit smoking.

See Tobacco (p.56).

NO

Call your doctor if your child's symptoms persist for more than 1 week.

EAR PAIN IN INFANTS AND CHILDREN

Pain, tenderness, throbbing, ringing, or a blockage in the ear can occur frequently in children 3 months to 3 years. The pain usually indicates an infection or, less commonly, injury to the ear. Diminished hearing may be caused by a blockage of earwax or fluid behind the eardrum.

SYMPTOMS

TAKING ACTION

MORE INFORMATION

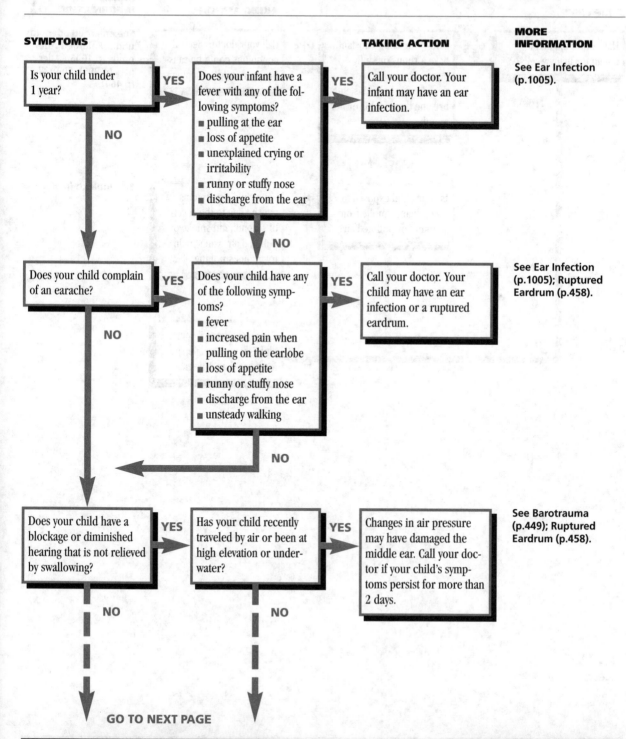

Is your child under 1 year?

YES → Does your infant have a fever with any of the following symptoms?
- pulling at the ear
- loss of appetite
- unexplained crying or irritability
- runny or stuffy nose
- discharge from the ear

YES → Call your doctor. Your infant may have an ear infection.

See Ear Infection (p.1005).

NO

NO

Does your child complain of an earache?

YES → Does your child have any of the following symptoms?
- fever
- increased pain when pulling on the earlobe
- loss of appetite
- runny or stuffy nose
- discharge from the ear
- unsteady walking

YES → Call your doctor. Your child may have an ear infection or a ruptured eardrum.

See Ear Infection (p.1005); Ruptured Eardrum (p.458).

NO

NO

Does your child have a blockage or diminished hearing that is not relieved by swallowing?

YES → Has your child recently traveled by air or been at high elevation or underwater?

YES → Changes in air pressure may have damaged the middle ear. Call your doctor if your child's symptoms persist for more than 2 days.

See Barotrauma (p.449); Ruptured Eardrum (p.458).

NO

NO

GO TO NEXT PAGE

CONTINUED FROM PREVIOUS PAGE

TAKING ACTION

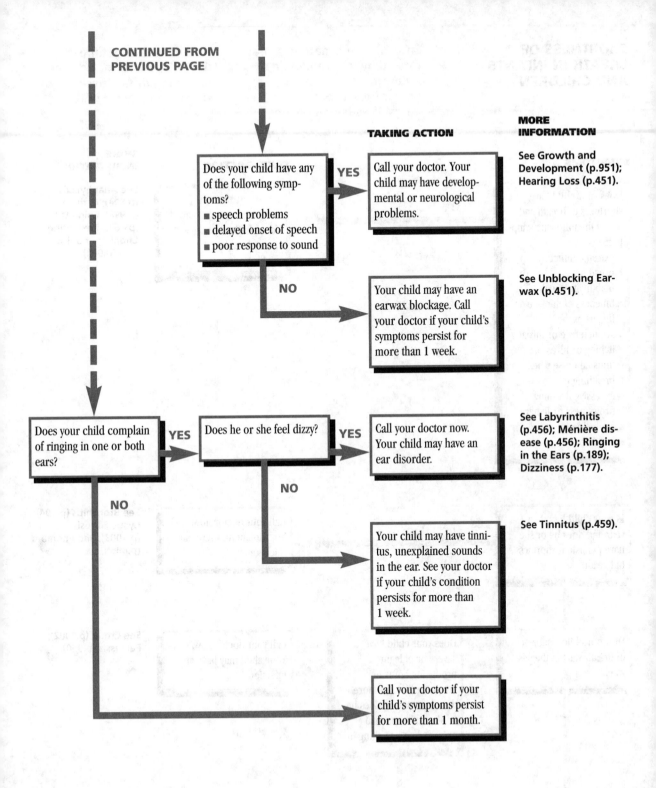

Does your child have any of the following symptoms?
- speech problems
- delayed onset of speech
- poor response to sound

YES → Call your doctor. Your child may have developmental or neurological problems.

See Growth and Development (p.951); Hearing Loss (p.451).

NO → Your child may have an earwax blockage. Call your doctor if your child's symptoms persist for more than 1 week.

See Unblocking Earwax (p.451).

Does your child complain of ringing in one or both ears?

YES → Does he or she feel dizzy?

YES → Call your doctor now. Your child may have an ear disorder.

See Labyrinthitis (p.456); Ménière disease (p.456); Ringing in the Ears (p.189); Dizziness (p.177).

NO → Your child may have tinnitus, unexplained sounds in the ear. See your doctor if your child's condition persists for more than 1 week.

See Tinnitus (p.459).

NO → Call your doctor if your child's symptoms persist for more than 1 month.

SHORTNESS OF BREATH IN INFANTS AND CHILDREN

Shortness of breath is characterized by labored, rapid breathing or an inability to get air into or out of the lungs. It usually indicates a condition that requires a doctor's attention. Extreme breathing difficulties may call for emergency treatment.

SYMPTOMS

TAKING ACTION

MORE INFORMATION

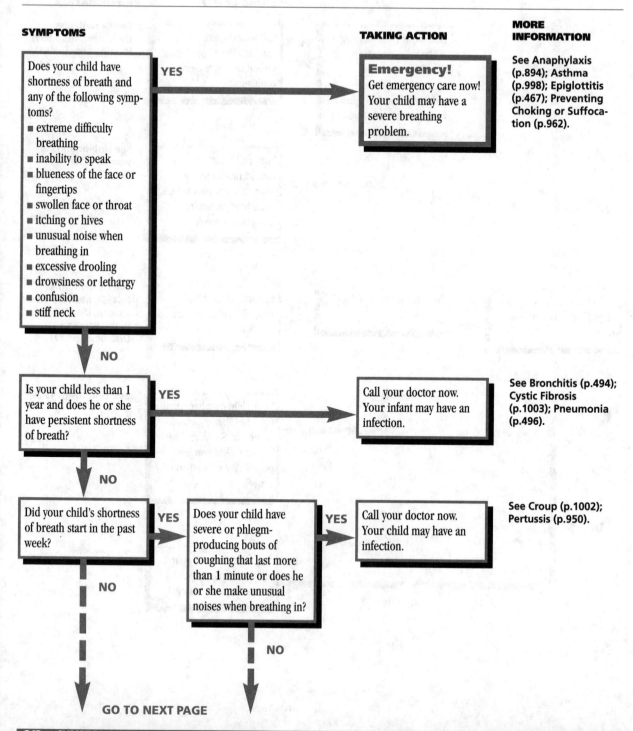

Does your child have shortness of breath and any of the following symptoms?
- extreme difficulty breathing
- inability to speak
- blueness of the face or fingertips
- swollen face or throat
- itching or hives
- unusual noise when breathing in
- excessive drooling
- drowsiness or lethargy
- confusion
- stiff neck

YES

Emergency!
Get emergency care now! Your child may have a severe breathing problem.

See Anaphylaxis (p.894); Asthma (p.998); Epiglottitis (p.467); Preventing Choking or Suffocation (p.962).

NO

Is your child less than 1 year and does he or she have persistent shortness of breath?

YES

Call your doctor now. Your infant may have an infection.

See Bronchitis (p.494); Cystic Fibrosis (p.1003); Pneumonia (p.496).

NO

Did your child's shortness of breath start in the past week?

YES

Does your child have severe or phlegm-producing bouts of coughing that last more than 1 minute or does he or she make unusual noises when breathing in?

YES

Call your doctor now. Your child may have an infection.

See Croup (p.1002); Pertussis (p.950).

NO

NO

GO TO NEXT PAGE

CONTINUED FROM
PREVIOUS PAGE

TAKING ACTION

Does your child have a dry cough or wheezing?

YES → Call your doctor now. Your child may have a breathing disorder.

See Asthma (p.998); Bronchiolitis (p.969).

NO

Does your child have any of the following symptoms?
■ fever or chills
■ green or yellow sputum
■ chest pain with breathing
■ fatigue
■ loss of appetite
■ drowsiness
■ confusion

YES → See your doctor. Your child may have a bacterial infection.

See Influenza (p.875); Pneumonia (p.496); Colds (p.1000).

NO

Is your child taking any prescription or nonprescription medicines?

YES → Call your doctor now. Your child may be having a drug reaction.

See Medicines (p.1148).

NO

Does your child have any of the following symptoms?
■ light-headedness
■ fear
■ anxiety
■ tingling lips or hands

YES → Call your doctor if your child's symptoms persist or if they occur frequently.

See Panic Disorder (p.404).

NO → Call your doctor if the symptoms persist for more than 1 week.

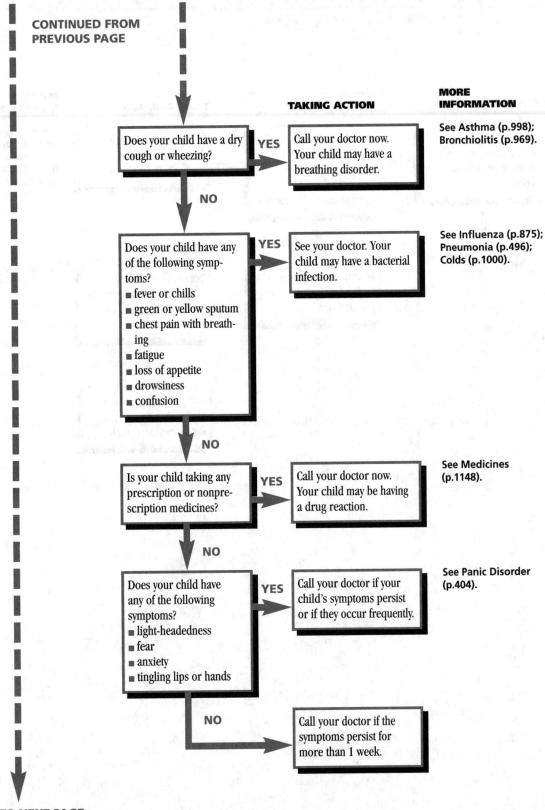

GO TO NEXT PAGE

CONTINUED FROM PREVIOUS PAGE

SYMPTOMS
TAKING ACTION
MORE INFORMATION
Has your child had shortness of breath or breathing problems for many weeks?
YES
Does he or she have a persistent runny or stuffy nose or bad breath and constantly breathe through his or her mouth?
YES
Call your doctor. A number of conditions can cause these symptoms.
See enlarged adenoids under Enlarged Tonsils and Adenoids (p.1006); Allergies (p.995); Sinusitis (p.464).
NO
NO
Is your child exposed to smoke from smokers or polluted air?
YES
Your child's symptoms may be due to the effect of secondhand smoke or polluted air.
See Smoking Cessation Methods (p.59).
NO
Call your doctor if your child's symptoms persist for more than 1 week.

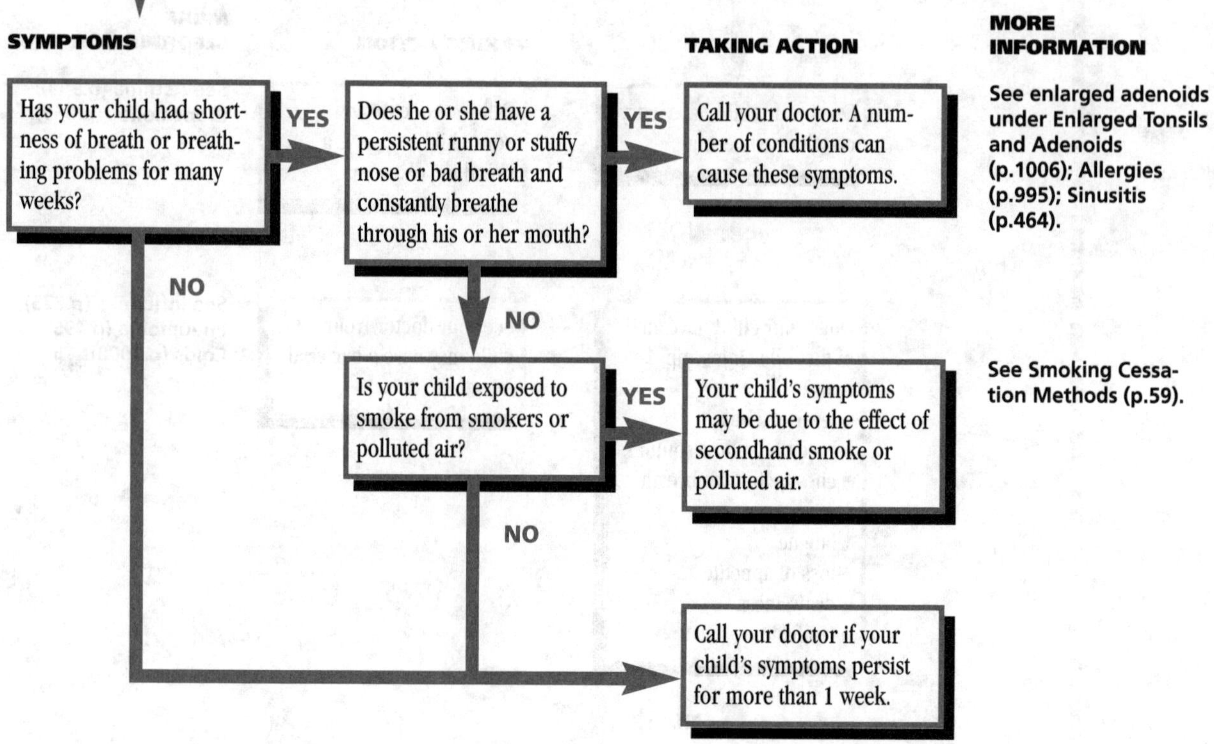

ABDOMINAL PAIN IN CHILDREN

Abdominal pain is pain in the region between the bottom of the rib cage and the groin. It is common in children. When it persists for more than 3 hours, is accompanied by recurrent vomiting or constipation, or occurs in an infant, abdominal pain may require your doctor's attention.

SYMPTOMS

TAKING ACTION

MORE INFORMATION

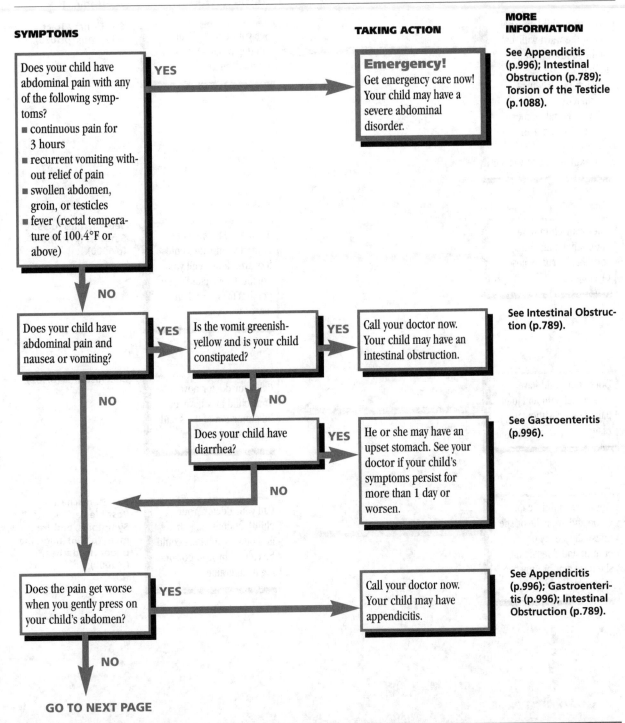

Does your child have abdominal pain with any of the following symptoms?
- continuous pain for 3 hours
- recurrent vomiting without relief of pain
- swollen abdomen, groin, or testicles
- fever (rectal temperature of 100.4°F or above)

YES →

Emergency!
Get emergency care now! Your child may have a severe abdominal disorder.

See Appendicitis (p.996); Intestinal Obstruction (p.789); Torsion of the Testicle (p.1088).

NO ↓

Does your child have abdominal pain and nausea or vomiting?

YES → Is the vomit greenish-yellow and is your child constipated?

YES → Call your doctor now. Your child may have an intestinal obstruction.

See Intestinal Obstruction (p.789).

NO ↓

Does your child have diarrhea?

YES → He or she may have an upset stomach. See your doctor if your child's symptoms persist for more than 1 day or worsen.

See Gastroenteritis (p.996).

NO ←

NO ↓

Does the pain get worse when you gently press on your child's abdomen?

YES → Call your doctor now. Your child may have appendicitis.

See Appendicitis (p.996); Gastroenteritis (p.996); Intestinal Obstruction (p.789).

NO ↓

GO TO NEXT PAGE

SYMPTOMS

TAKING ACTION

MORE INFORMATION

Does your child have pain below the waist with any of the following symptoms?
- painful or frequent urination
- fever (rectal temperature of 100.4°F or above)
- unexplained bed-wetting

YES →

See your doctor. Your child may have a urinary tract infection.

See Urinary Tract Infections (p.1020).

NO ↓

Does your child have abdominal pain and a sore throat, runny nose, or cough?

YES →

Abdominal pain sometimes accompanies cold-like symptoms. Call your doctor if your child's pain persists for more than 1 day or worsens.

See Allergies (p.995); Sinusitis (p.464); Colds (p.1000).

NO ↓

Does your child have abdominal pain and joint pain with or without a rash?

YES →

Call your doctor now. Your child may have an inflammation of the small blood vessels.

See Vasculitis (p.902).

NO ↓

Does your child's pain come and go, is he or she unusually sleepy or cranky, and does he or she have a poor appetite or headaches?

YES →

Call your doctor. Your child's abdominal pain and other symptoms could be caused by lead poisoning or migraines.

See Stomachache: Possible Causes, Symptoms, and Treatment (p.996); migraine under Headaches (p.1009).

NO ↓

GO TO NEXT PAGE

CONTINUED FROM PREVIOUS PAGE

SYMPTOMS

TAKING ACTION

Does your child's pain come and go, and usually occur after drinking milk?

YES

Call your doctor. Your child may have an allergy to dairy products.

See Lactose Intolerance (p.1012).

NO

Your child may have an upset stomach. Call your doctor if your child's pain lasts for more than 2 or 3 days or worsens.

See Gastroenteritis (p.996).

BED-WETTING AND TOILET TRAINING

Problems with bowel and bladder control can occur at any age. The age at which children become toilet trained varies, but it usually occurs between 2 and 5 years. Accidents during and after toilet training are common. However, frequent bladder- and bowel-control problems after toilet training may indicate a physical or psychological condition that requires your doctor's attention.

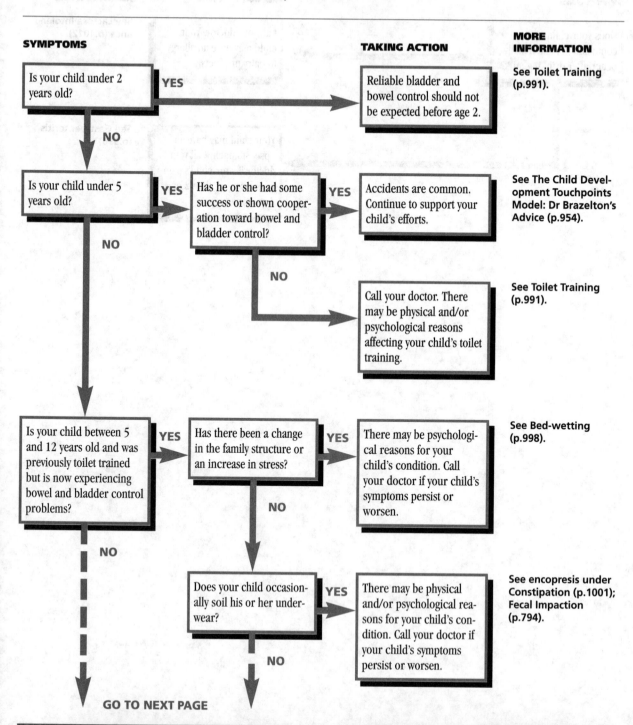

SYMPTOMS

Is your child under 2 years old?

YES → Reliable bladder and bowel control should not be expected before age 2.

MORE INFORMATION
See Toilet Training (p.991).

NO

Is your child under 5 years old?

YES → Has he or she had some success or shown cooperation toward bowel and bladder control?

YES → **TAKING ACTION** Accidents are common. Continue to support your child's efforts.

See The Child Development Touchpoints Model: Dr Brazelton's Advice (p.954).

NO

NO → Call your doctor. There may be physical and/or psychological reasons affecting your child's toilet training.

See Toilet Training (p.991).

Is your child between 5 and 12 years old and was previously toilet trained but is now experiencing bowel and bladder control problems?

YES → Has there been a change in the family structure or an increase in stress?

YES → There may be psychological reasons for your child's condition. Call your doctor if your child's symptoms persist or worsen.

See Bed-wetting (p.998).

NO

NO → Does your child occasionally soil his or her underwear?

YES → There may be physical and/or psychological reasons for your child's condition. Call your doctor if your child's symptoms persist or worsen.

See encopresis under Constipation (p.1001); Fecal Impaction (p.794).

NO

GO TO NEXT PAGE

CONTINUED FROM
PREVIOUS PAGE

TAKING ACTION

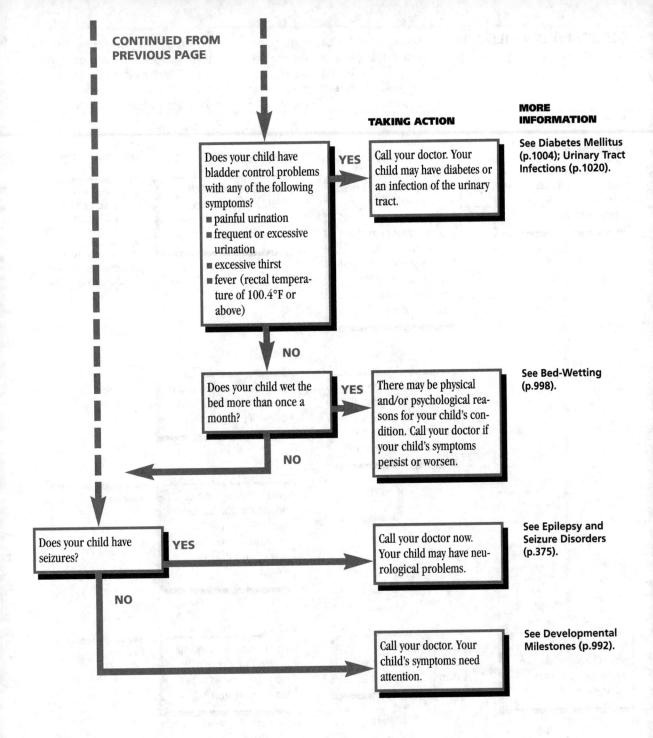

Does your child have bladder control problems with any of the following symptoms?
- painful urination
- frequent or excessive urination
- excessive thirst
- fever (rectal temperature of 100.4°F or above)

YES → Call your doctor. Your child may have diabetes or an infection of the urinary tract.

See Diabetes Mellitus (p.1004); Urinary Tract Infections (p.1020).

NO

Does your child wet the bed more than once a month?

YES → There may be physical and/or psychological reasons for your child's condition. Call your doctor if your child's symptoms persist or worsen.

See Bed-Wetting (p.998).

NO

Does your child have seizures?

YES → Call your doctor now. Your child may have neurological problems.

See Epilepsy and Seizure Disorders (p.375).

NO

Call your doctor. Your child's symptoms need attention.

See Developmental Milestones (p.992).

DIARRHEA IN CHILDREN

Diarrhea is loose, watery, or more frequent bowel movements. Gastrointestinal infections and anxiety are common causes of diarrhea in children.

When accompanied by persistent abdominal pain or vomiting, diarrhea may indicate a condition that requires a doctor's attention.

SYMPTOMS

TAKING ACTION

MORE INFORMATION

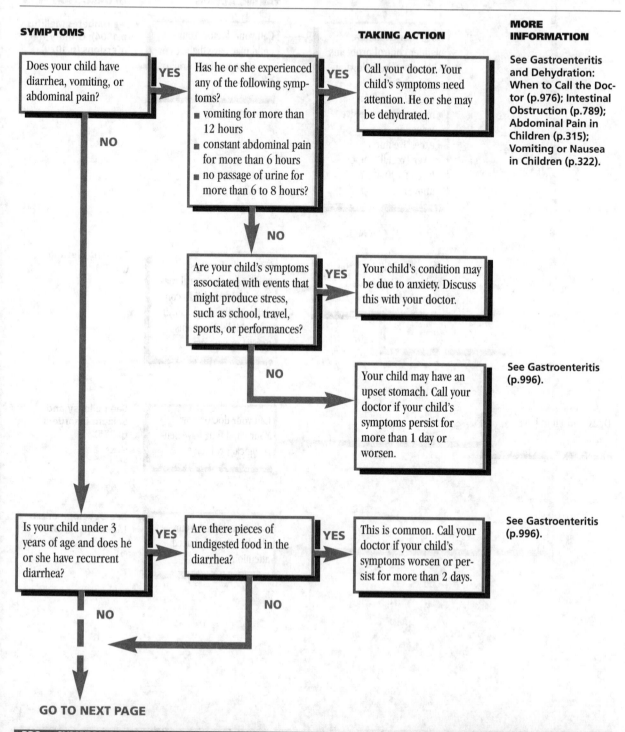

Does your child have diarrhea, vomiting, or abdominal pain?

YES

Has he or she experienced any of the following symptoms?
- vomiting for more than 12 hours
- constant abdominal pain for more than 6 hours
- no passage of urine for more than 6 to 8 hours?

YES

Call your doctor. Your child's symptoms need attention. He or she may be dehydrated.

See Gastroenteritis and Dehydration: When to Call the Doctor (p.976); Intestinal Obstruction (p.789); Abdominal Pain in Children (p.315); Vomiting or Nausea in Children (p.322).

NO

NO

Are your child's symptoms associated with events that might produce stress, such as school, travel, sports, or performances?

YES

Your child's condition may be due to anxiety. Discuss this with your doctor.

NO

Your child may have an upset stomach. Call your doctor if your child's symptoms persist for more than 1 day or worsen.

See Gastroenteritis (p.996).

Is your child under 3 years of age and does he or she have recurrent diarrhea?

YES

Are there pieces of undigested food in the diarrhea?

YES

This is common. Call your doctor if your child's symptoms worsen or persist for more than 2 days.

See Gastroenteritis (p.996).

NO

NO

GO TO NEXT PAGE

CONTINUED FROM PREVIOUS PAGE

SYMPTOMS

TAKING ACTION

MORE INFORMATION

Did your child's diarrhea follow constipation or is it associated with toilet training or anxiety?

YES →

This is a common occurrence. Call your doctor if your child's symptoms persist for more than 1 week.

See Toilet Training (p.991); encopresis under Constipation (p.1001).

NO ↓

Have you given your child any new prescription or nonprescription medicines?

YES →

Your child may be having a drug reaction. Ask your doctor if the medicine could be causing the diarrhea.

See Medicines (p.1148).

NO ↓

See your doctor if your child's symptoms worsen or persist for more than 2 days.

VOMITING OR NAUSEA IN CHILDREN

Nausea and vomiting are common in children and can occur with many disorders. Nausea and vomiting that occur after an injury, or that are accompanied by severe abdominal pain or headache, require a doctor's attention.

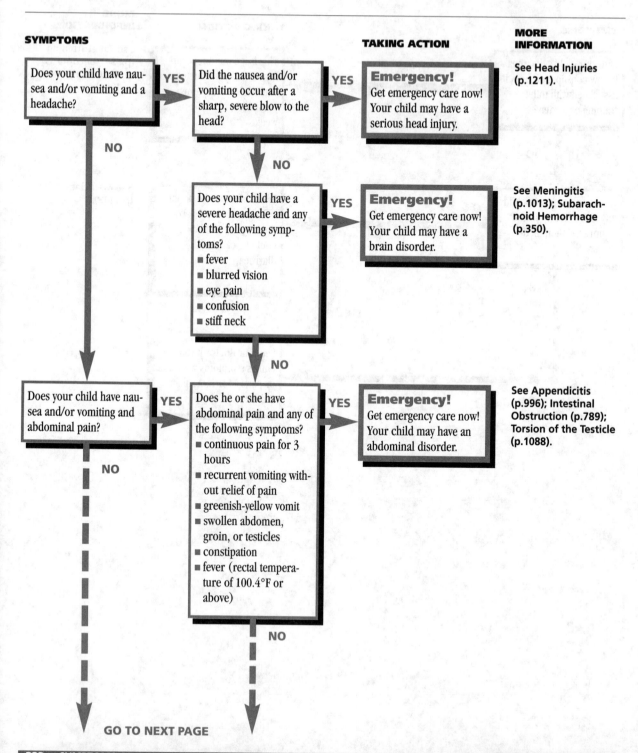

SYMPTOMS

Does your child have nausea and/or vomiting and a headache?

YES → Did the nausea and/or vomiting occur after a sharp, severe blow to the head?

YES →

NO ↓

Does your child have a severe headache and any of the following symptoms?
- fever
- blurred vision
- eye pain
- confusion
- stiff neck

YES →

NO ↓

Does your child have nausea and/or vomiting and abdominal pain?

YES → Does he or she have abdominal pain and any of the following symptoms?
- continuous pain for 3 hours
- recurrent vomiting without relief of pain
- greenish-yellow vomit
- swollen abdomen, groin, or testicles
- constipation
- fever (rectal temperature of 100.4°F or above)

YES →

NO ↓

NO ↓

GO TO NEXT PAGE

TAKING ACTION

Emergency!
Get emergency care now! Your child may have a serious head injury.

Emergency!
Get emergency care now! Your child may have a brain disorder.

Emergency!
Get emergency care now! Your child may have an abdominal disorder.

MORE INFORMATION

See Head Injuries (p.1211).

See Meningitis (p.1013); Subarachnoid Hemorrhage (p.350).

See Appendicitis (p.996); Intestinal Obstruction (p.789); Torsion of the Testicle (p.1088).

CONTINUED FROM PREVIOUS PAGE

TAKING ACTION

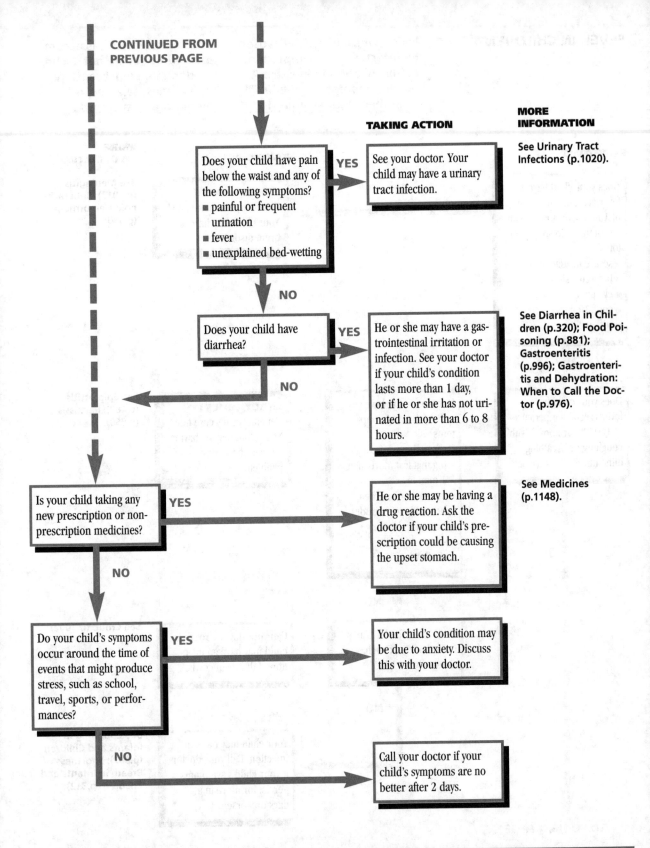

Does your child have pain below the waist and any of the following symptoms?
- painful or frequent urination
- fever
- unexplained bed-wetting

YES → See your doctor. Your child may have a urinary tract infection.

See Urinary Tract Infections (p.1020).

NO

Does your child have diarrhea?

YES → He or she may have a gastrointestinal irritation or infection. See your doctor if your child's condition lasts more than 1 day, or if he or she has not urinated in more than 6 to 8 hours.

See Diarrhea in Children (p.320); Food Poisoning (p.881); Gastroenteritis (p.996); Gastroenteritis and Dehydration: When to Call the Doctor (p.976).

NO

Is your child taking any new prescription or non-prescription medicines?

YES → He or she may be having a drug reaction. Ask the doctor if your child's prescription could be causing the upset stomach.

See Medicines (p.1148).

NO

Do your child's symptoms occur around the time of events that might produce stress, such as school, travel, sports, or performances?

YES → Your child's condition may be due to anxiety. Discuss this with your doctor.

NO → Call your doctor if your child's symptoms are no better after 2 days.

FEVER IN CHILDREN

Fever, which is usually caused by infection, is a symptom of many childhood illnesses. A rectal temperature of 100.4°F or higher requires your doc-tor's attention if it is accompanied by severe headache, abdominal pain, breathing difficulties, seizures, recurrent vomiting, or stiff neck.

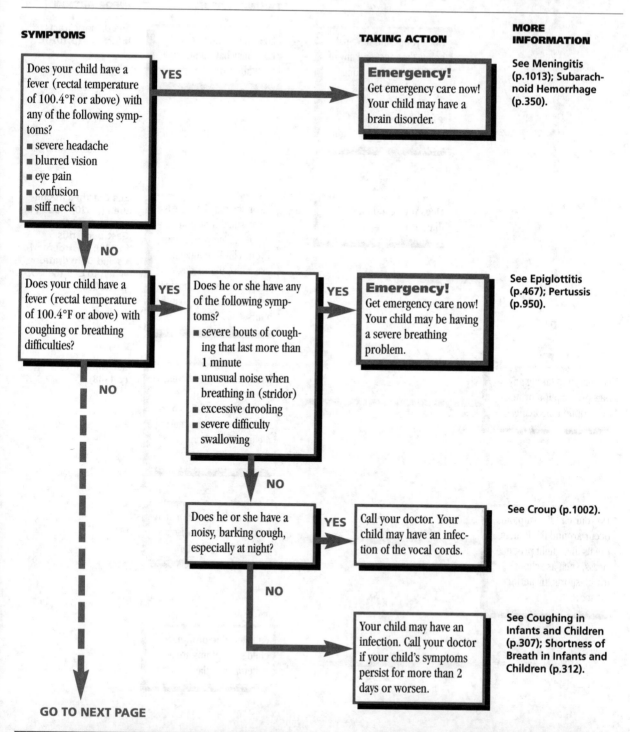

SYMPTOMS

Does your child have a fever (rectal temperature of 100.4°F or above) with any of the following symptoms?
- severe headache
- blurred vision
- eye pain
- confusion
- stiff neck

YES

NO

Does your child have a fever (rectal temperature of 100.4°F or above) with coughing or breathing difficulties?

YES

NO

Does he or she have any of the following symptoms?
- severe bouts of coughing that last more than 1 minute
- unusual noise when breathing in (stridor)
- excessive drooling
- severe difficulty swallowing

YES

NO

Does he or she have a noisy, barking cough, especially at night?

YES

NO

TAKING ACTION

Emergency!
Get emergency care now! Your child may have a brain disorder.

Emergency!
Get emergency care now! Your child may be having a severe breathing problem.

Call your doctor. Your child may have an infection of the vocal cords.

Your child may have an infection. Call your doctor if your child's symptoms persist for more than 2 days or worsen.

MORE INFORMATION

See Meningitis (p.1013); Subarachnoid Hemorrhage (p.350).

See Epiglottitis (p.467); Pertussis (p.950).

See Croup (p.1002).

See Coughing in Infants and Children (p.307); Shortness of Breath in Infants and Children (p.312).

GO TO NEXT PAGE

CONTINUED FROM PREVIOUS PAGE

SYMPTOMS

TAKING ACTION

Does your child have a fever (rectal temperature of 100.4°F or above) with abdominal pain?

YES →

Has he or she had any of the following symptoms?
- continuous pain for 3 hours
- recurrent vomiting without relief from pain
- greenish-yellow vomit
- swollen abdomen, groin, or testicles
- constipation

YES →

Emergency!
Get emergency care now! Your child may have an abdominal disorder.

See Appendicitis (p.996); Intestinal Obstruction (p.789); Torsion of the Testicle (p.1088).

NO ↓ (from first box)

NO ↓ (from symptoms box)

Does your child have pain below the waist with any of the following symptoms?
- painful urination
- frequent urination
- unexplained bed-wetting

YES →

See the doctor. Your child may have a urinary tract infection.

See Urinary Tract Infections (p.1020).

NO ↓

Does your child have diarrhea?

YES →

Your child may have a gastrointestinal irritation or infection. Call your doctor if your child's symptoms persist for more than 2 days.

See Food Poisoning (p.881); Gastroenteritis (p.996); Gastroenteritis and Dehydration: When to Call the Doctor (p.976).

NO ↓

Call your doctor if your child's condition worsens.

See Abdominal Pain in Children (p.315).

GO TO NEXT PAGE

CONTINUED FROM PREVIOUS PAGE

SYMPTOMS

TAKING ACTION

Does your child have a fever (rectal temperature of 100.4°F or above) with unusual or jerking movements of the arms, legs, or face, or periods of listlessness?

YES →

Call your doctor now. A sudden, high fever can cause seizures.

See Febrile Seizure (p.1007).

NO ↓

Does your child have a fever (rectal temperature of 100.4°F or above) with a rash?

YES →

Your child may have an infection.

See Rash in Infants and Children (p.304).

NO ↓

Does your child have a fever (rectal temperature of 100.4°F or above) and a runny nose or coldlike symptoms?

YES →

Your child may have an infection. Call your doctor if your child's symptoms worsen.

See Colds (p.1000); respiratory syncytial virus under Bronchiolitis (p.969).

NO ↓

Does your child have a fever (rectal temperature of 100.4°F or above) and swelling between the ear and jaw?

YES →

Call your doctor now. Your child may have an infection.

See Mumps (p.950).

NO ↓

GO TO NEXT PAGE

SYMPTOMS

TAKING ACTION

Does your child have a fever (rectal temperature of 100.4°F or above) with a sore throat?

YES →

Your child may have an infection. Call your doctor if your child's symptoms persist or worsen.

See Sore Throat (p.1018).

NO ↓

Does your child have a fever (rectal temperature of 100.4°F or above) and is he or she pulling on his or her ear and crying?

YES →

Your child may have an ear infection. Call your doctor if your child's symptoms persist or worsen.

See Ear Pain in Infants and Children (p.310).

NO ↓

Has your child recently been immunized?

YES →

A fever sometimes occurs after immunization. Call your doctor if your child's symptoms persist for more than 2 to 3 days or worsen.

See Childhood Immunization Schedule (p.947).

NO ↓

Has your child been playing in hot weather or in a hot environment?

YES →

A child's temperature can be affected by exercise in heat. Remove some of his or her clothing and give fluids.

See dehydration under Gastroenteritis and Dehydration: When to Call the Doctor (p.976).

NO ↓

Call your doctor if your child's symptoms persist for more than 3 days or worsen.

IRRITABLE OR ILL CHILD

General and unexplained irritability, crying, or behavior change can sometimes indicate illness. Your child may be unaware or unable to articulate his or her symptoms without your help.

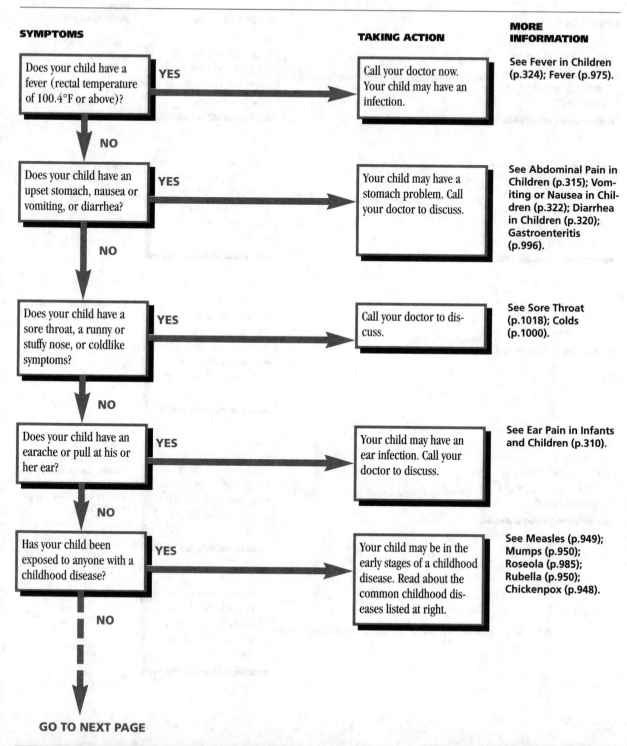

SYMPTOMS

Does your child have a fever (rectal temperature of 100.4°F or above)?

YES →

NO ↓

Does your child have an upset stomach, nausea or vomiting, or diarrhea?

YES →

NO ↓

Does your child have a sore throat, a runny or stuffy nose, or coldlike symptoms?

YES →

NO ↓

Does your child have an earache or pull at his or her ear?

YES →

NO ↓

Has your child been exposed to anyone with a childhood disease?

YES →

NO ↓

GO TO NEXT PAGE

TAKING ACTION

Call your doctor now. Your child may have an infection.

Your child may have a stomach problem. Call your doctor to discuss.

Call your doctor to discuss.

Your child may have an ear infection. Call your doctor to discuss.

Your child may be in the early stages of a childhood disease. Read about the common childhood diseases listed at right.

MORE INFORMATION

See Fever in Children (p.324); Fever (p.975).

See Abdominal Pain in Children (p.315); Vomiting or Nausea in Children (p.322); Diarrhea in Children (p.320); Gastroenteritis (p.996).

See Sore Throat (p.1018); Colds (p.1000).

See Ear Pain in Infants and Children (p.310).

See Measles (p.949); Mumps (p.950); Roseola (p.985); Rubella (p.950); Chickenpox (p.948).

CONTINUED FROM PREVIOUS PAGE

SYMPTOMS

TAKING ACTION

Are there any events that might cause your child stress, such as school, travel, sports, or performances?

YES → Your child's condition may be due to anxiety. Discuss this with your doctor.

NO ↓

Is your child very restless or unable to pay attention?

YES → Is he or she like this most of the time?

YES → Call your doctor. Your child may have an attention disorder.

See attention deficit hyperactivity disorder under Learning Disabilities (p.1012).

NO ↓

NO ↓

Call your doctor if your child's symptoms persist for more than 1 week or worsen.

PAIN IN, SORES OR LUMPS ON, OR DISCHARGE FROM THE PENIS

Sores or lumps on the penis, or a discharge from the penis, are often caused by a sexually transmitted disease. See your doctor now so that your condition can be diagnosed and so you and all of your sexual partners can be treated.

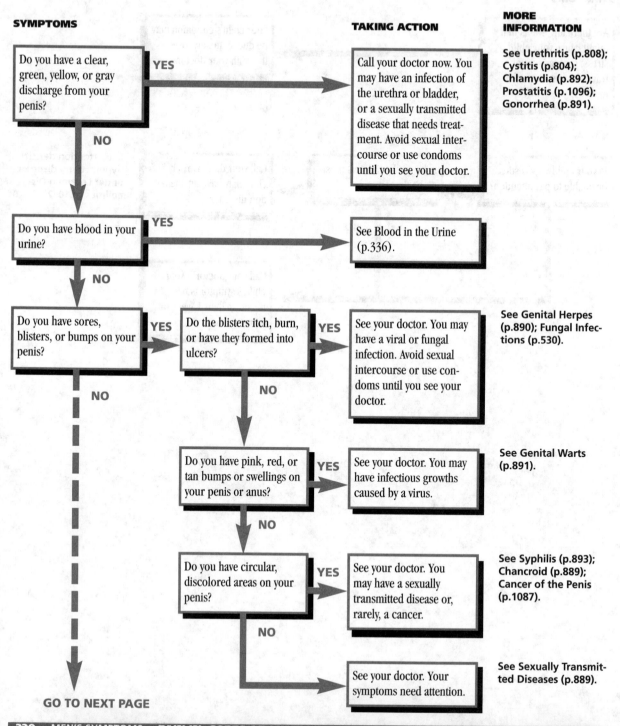

SYMPTOMS

Do you have a clear, green, yellow, or gray discharge from your penis?

YES → Call your doctor now. You may have an infection of the urethra or bladder, or a sexually transmitted disease that needs treatment. Avoid sexual intercourse or use condoms until you see your doctor.

NO ↓

Do you have blood in your urine?

YES → See Blood in the Urine (p.336).

NO ↓

Do you have sores, blisters, or bumps on your penis?

YES → Do the blisters itch, burn, or have they formed into ulcers?

YES → See your doctor. You may have a viral or fungal infection. Avoid sexual intercourse or use condoms until you see your doctor.

NO ↓

Do you have pink, red, or tan bumps or swellings on your penis or anus?

YES → See your doctor. You may have infectious growths caused by a virus.

NO ↓

Do you have circular, discolored areas on your penis?

YES → See your doctor. You may have a sexually transmitted disease or, rarely, a cancer.

NO ↓

See your doctor. Your symptoms need attention.

NO ↓

GO TO NEXT PAGE

TAKING ACTION

MORE INFORMATION

See Urethritis (p.808); Cystitis (p.804); Chlamydia (p.892); Prostatitis (p.1096); Gonorrhea (p.891).

See Genital Herpes (p.890); Fungal Infections (p.530).

See Genital Warts (p.891).

See Syphilis (p.893); Chancroid (p.889); Cancer of the Penis (p.1087).

See Sexually Transmitted Diseases (p.889).

CONTINUED FROM PREVIOUS PAGE

SYMPTOMS

TAKING ACTION

Do you have redness and swelling on the tip of your penis?

YES →

See your doctor. You may have balanitis.

See Balanitis (p.1088).

↓ **NO**

Do you have pain or a burning sensation when you urinate?

YES →

See Painful or Frequent Urination (p.333).

↓ **NO**

Do you have pain during or after sexual intercourse?

YES →

Your pain may be due to friction from your partner or an allergic reaction to a latex condom or diaphragm.

See Contraception and Safe Sex (p.68); Atrophic Vaginitis (p.1066).

NO

Call your doctor if your symptoms persist for more than 2 weeks or worsen.

LOSS OF URINE CONTROL

Losing control of your urine is called urinary incontinence. It can be caused by aging, serious disorders, or some medicines. Talk to your doctor to rule out any serious problem.

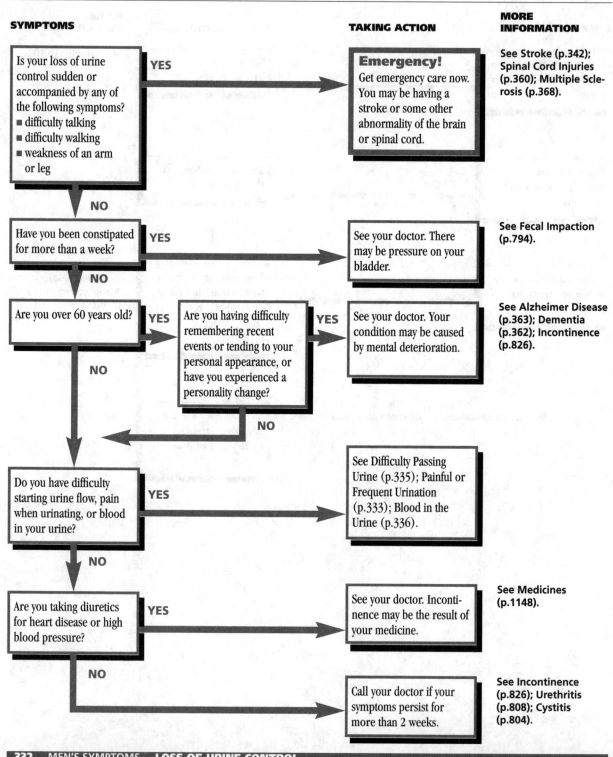

SYMPTOMS

Is your loss of urine control sudden or accompanied by any of the following symptoms?
- difficulty talking
- difficulty walking
- weakness of an arm or leg

YES →

NO ↓

Have you been constipated for more than a week?

YES →

NO ↓

Are you over 60 years old?

YES →

Are you having difficulty remembering recent events or tending to your personal appearance, or have you experienced a personality change?

YES →

NO ↓ (Are you over 60)

NO → (personality change)

Do you have difficulty starting urine flow, pain when urinating, or blood in your urine?

YES →

NO ↓

Are you taking diuretics for heart disease or high blood pressure?

YES →

NO ↓

TAKING ACTION

Emergency!
Get emergency care now. You may be having a stroke or some other abnormality of the brain or spinal cord.

See your doctor. There may be pressure on your bladder.

See your doctor. Your condition may be caused by mental deterioration.

See Difficulty Passing Urine (p.335); Painful or Frequent Urination (p.333); Blood in the Urine (p.336).

See your doctor. Incontinence may be the result of your medicine.

Call your doctor if your symptoms persist for more than 2 weeks.

MORE INFORMATION

See Stroke (p.342); Spinal Cord Injuries (p.360); Multiple Sclerosis (p.368).

See Fecal Impaction (p.794).

See Alzheimer Disease (p.363); Dementia (p.362); Incontinence (p.826).

See Medicines (p.1148).

See Incontinence (p.826); Urethritis (p.808); Cystitis (p.804).

PAINFUL OR FREQUENT URINATION

Pain before, during, or after urinating can be caused by infection. Frequent urination can be caused by infection, diabetes, diuretic medicines, or simply by high intake of liquids.

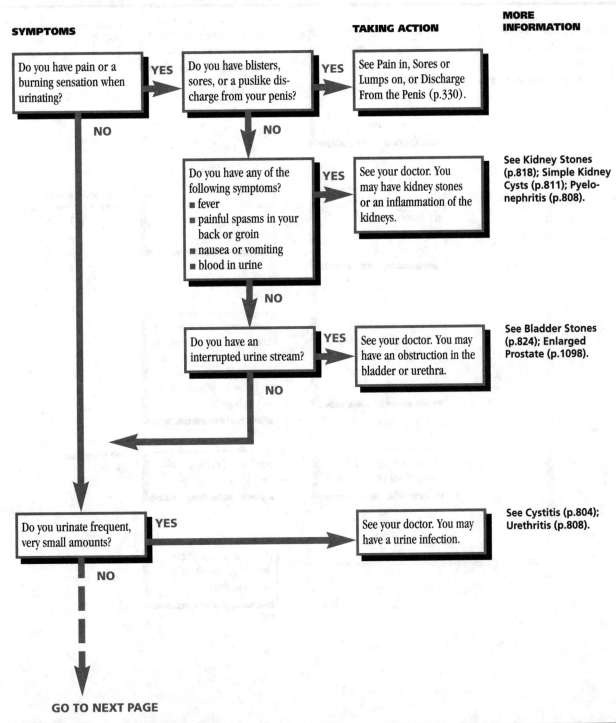

SYMPTOMS

TAKING ACTION

MORE INFORMATION

Do you have pain or a burning sensation when urinating?

YES →

Do you have blisters, sores, or a puslike discharge from your penis?

YES →

See Pain in, Sores or Lumps on, or Discharge From the Penis (p.330).

NO

Do you have any of the following symptoms?
- fever
- painful spasms in your back or groin
- nausea or vomiting
- blood in urine

YES →

See your doctor. You may have kidney stones or an inflammation of the kidneys.

See Kidney Stones (p.818); Simple Kidney Cysts (p.811); Pyelonephritis (p.808).

NO

Do you have an interrupted urine stream?

YES →

See your doctor. You may have an obstruction in the bladder or urethra.

See Bladder Stones (p.824); Enlarged Prostate (p.1098).

NO

Do you urinate frequent, very small amounts?

YES →

See your doctor. You may have a urine infection.

See Cystitis (p.804); Urethritis (p.808).

NO

GO TO NEXT PAGE

CONTINUED FROM PREVIOUS PAGE

SYMPTOMS

TAKING ACTION

Do you urinate frequently or has your frequency increased?

YES →

Do you have any of the following symptoms?
- increased thirst and appetite
- fatigue
- weight loss
- blurred vision

YES →

See your doctor. You may have diabetes mellitus.

See Diabetes Mellitus (p.832).

NO

NO ↓

Do you take any diuretic medicines for heart disease or high blood pressure?

YES →

Frequent urination is common when taking diuretic drugs.

See loop diuretic under Common Drug Classes (p.1160).

NO ↓

Do you drink a lot of coffee, tea, soft drinks, or alcoholic beverages or excessive amounts of other fluids?

YES →

Frequent urination is a common effect of drinking beverages containing caffeine or alcohol or of drinking large amounts of any liquid.

NO ↓

Do you wet yourself or lose control of your urine?

YES →

See Loss of Urine Control (p.332).

See Incontinence (p.826).

NO ↓

Call your doctor if your symptoms persist for 2 weeks or worsen.

DIFFICULTY PASSING URINE

Very little urine production, the inability to start urine flow, or difficulty producing urine or starting urine flow can indicate problems with the kidneys or prostate gland. These symptoms always require your doctor's attention.

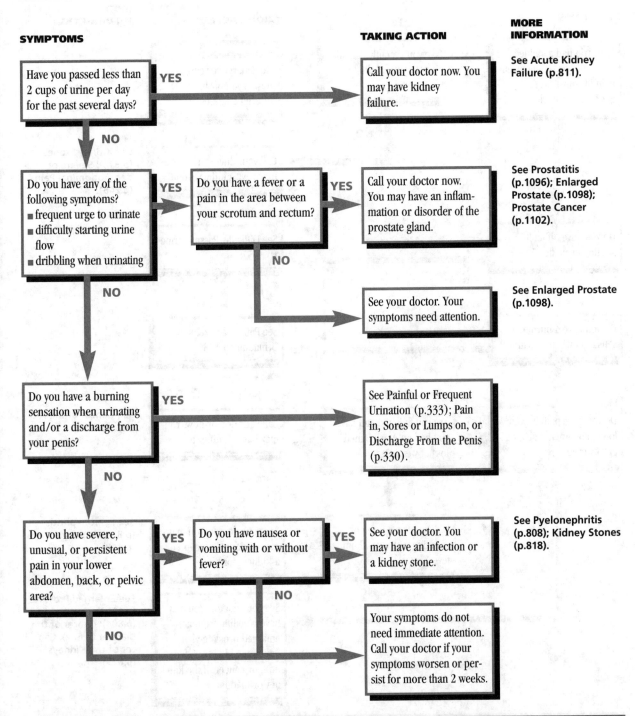

SYMPTOMS

TAKING ACTION

MORE INFORMATION

Have you passed less than 2 cups of urine per day for the past several days?

YES → Call your doctor now. You may have kidney failure.

See Acute Kidney Failure (p.811).

NO ↓

Do you have any of the following symptoms?
- frequent urge to urinate
- difficulty starting urine flow
- dribbling when urinating

YES → Do you have a fever or a pain in the area between your scrotum and rectum?

YES → Call your doctor now. You may have an inflammation or disorder of the prostate gland.

See Prostatitis (p.1096); Enlarged Prostate (p.1098); Prostate Cancer (p.1102).

NO ↓

See your doctor. Your symptoms need attention.

See Enlarged Prostate (p.1098).

NO ↓

Do you have a burning sensation when urinating and/or a discharge from your penis?

YES → See Painful or Frequent Urination (p.333); Pain in, Sores or Lumps on, or Discharge From the Penis (p.330).

NO ↓

Do you have severe, unusual, or persistent pain in your lower abdomen, back, or pelvic area?

YES → Do you have nausea or vomiting with or without fever?

YES → See your doctor. You may have an infection or a kidney stone.

See Pyelonephritis (p.808); Kidney Stones (p.818).

NO ↓

Your symptoms do not need immediate attention. Call your doctor if your symptoms worsen or persist for more than 2 weeks.

NO →

BLOOD IN THE URINE

Urine that contains blood can appear cloudy, smoky, pink, or red. Blood in the urine can be caused by infection, inflammation, or a tumor in the urinary tract. However, food colorings, some foods, and some medicines can also change the color of your urine. Your doctor will want to test a sample of your urine to make a diagnosis.

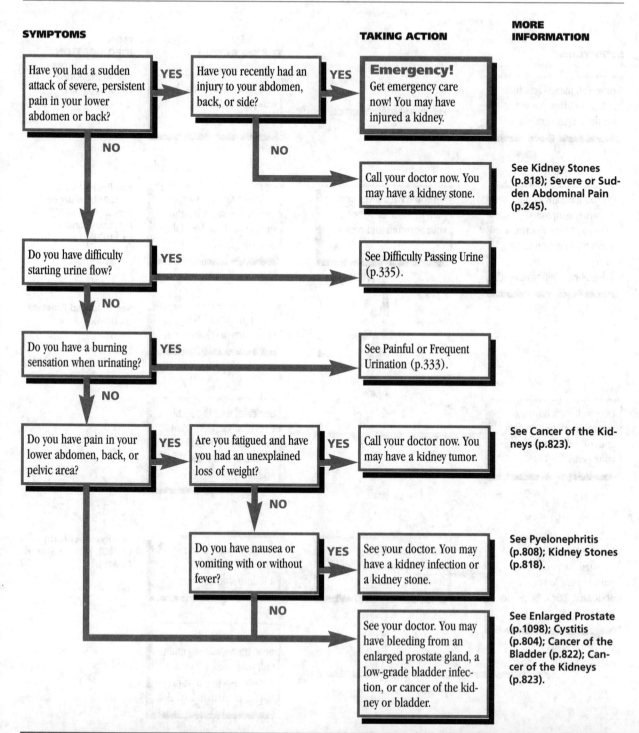

SYMPTOMS

TAKING ACTION

MORE INFORMATION

Have you had a sudden attack of severe, persistent pain in your lower abdomen or back?

YES → Have you recently had an injury to your abdomen, back, or side?

YES → **Emergency!** Get emergency care now! You may have injured a kidney.

NO → Call your doctor now. You may have a kidney stone.

See Kidney Stones (p.818); Severe or Sudden Abdominal Pain (p.245).

NO ↓

Do you have difficulty starting urine flow?

YES → See Difficulty Passing Urine (p.335).

NO ↓

Do you have a burning sensation when urinating?

YES → See Painful or Frequent Urination (p.333).

NO ↓

Do you have pain in your lower abdomen, back, or pelvic area?

YES → Are you fatigued and have you had an unexplained loss of weight?

YES → Call your doctor now. You may have a kidney tumor.

See Cancer of the Kidneys (p.823).

NO ↓

Do you have nausea or vomiting with or without fever?

YES → See your doctor. You may have a kidney infection or a kidney stone.

See Pyelonephritis (p.808); Kidney Stones (p.818).

NO →

See your doctor. You may have bleeding from an enlarged prostate gland, a low-grade bladder infection, or cancer of the kidney or bladder.

See Enlarged Prostate (p.1098); Cystitis (p.804); Cancer of the Bladder (p.822); Cancer of the Kidneys (p.823).

Brain and Nervous System

The brain is the most remarkable organ in the body. It organizes a large number of very mechanical functions, such as movement and the pumping heart, but it is also the organ responsible for speech, thought, memory, emotion, pleasure, pain, dreams, and creativity. Human beings share many organs in common with other animals, but the organ that makes us human is our brain.

Central nervous system Together, the brain and the spinal cord are called the central nervous system. The central nervous system is in direct, two-way communication with all the body's nerves, which as a group are called the peripheral nervous system.

Like any organ, the nervous system is made up of billions of cells, called neurons, that perform the main functions of the brain. Neurons are special cells that usually have a fiber called an axon. An axon can be several feet long; it sends information. Neurons also contain very short fibers (dendrites); they receive information.

Neurons rapidly communicate commands from the brain to the body (such as instructing the muscles of your arms to reach out and hug a friend) and from the body to the brain (such as pulling your hand away when you touch a hot object).

The brain and spinal cord are as soft as gelatin, and quite vulnerable. Both the brain and spinal cord are bathed in a layer of nourishing and cushioning fluid called cerebrospinal fluid. Thin layers of tissue called the meninges encase the cerebrospinal fluid around the brain.

Doctors Who Treat the Brain

Primary care doctors are often the first to identify medical conditions of the brain and nervous system. For many common problems, such as headaches, no specialist is necessary.

Neurologists are doctors who specialize in diagnosing and treating conditions of the brain and nervous system, but who do not perform surgery. Neurosurgeons perform surgery on the brain and other parts of the nervous system. Oncologists (cancer specialists) help care for people with brain cancer.

Other specialists may be called for expertise when a medical condition involving the brain and nervous system involves their area of special knowledge. For example, infectious disease specialists may help treat brain infections, and cardiologists may assist when blood clots from the heart have caused a stroke.

A neurologic examination usually starts by the doctor evaluating your mental state by asking simple questions that reveal your perception of time and place. He or she then performs a physical examination that tests muscle strength (from the muscles of your face to the muscles of your legs), various sensations (such as your capacity to hear, see, smell, or feel light touch or a pinprick), coordination and balance, ability to speak, and reflexes (you may be familiar with having your knee jerk reflex checked by having your knee tapped with a rubber hammer).

If disease of the central nervous system is suspected, the doctor may check the Babinski reflex, in which a metal object such as a key is dragged across the outer portion of the sole of your foot while the movement of your toes in response is noted.

Central Nervous System

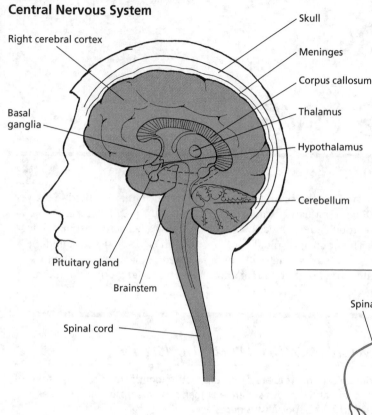

Right cerebral cortex

Basal ganglia

Pituitary gland

Brainstem

Spinal cord

Skull

Meninges

Corpus callosum

Thalamus

Hypothalamus

Cerebellum

The central nervous system consists of the brain and spinal cord. The meninges, three thin layers of tissue, encase the brain and are protected by the skull bones. Most messages from the brain start (and many end) in the cerebral cortex, the seat of thought, language, vision, and hearing. At the core of the brain lie the thalamus (involved in receiving and processing many sensations), hypothalamus (part of the limbic system), pituitary gland (which makes several hormones), and brainstem (which controls many vital functions such as blood pressure and body temperature). The cerebellum is essential in coordinating movement and may play a role in thinking.

Each of the 31 spinal nerves has two roots. The dorsal root carries sensations such as touch, pain, heat, or cold into the spinal cord, where they travel to the brain. The ventral root carries messages from the brain to the muscles that direct movement.

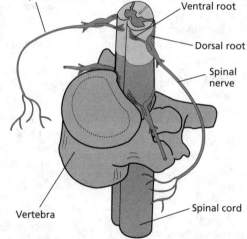

Spinal nerve

Ventral root

Dorsal root

Spinal nerve

Vertebra

Spinal cord

Inflammation of the meninges is called meningitis.

The brain is ultimately protected by the bones of the skull, while the spinal cord is protected by the bones of the back (vertebrae). The spinal cord runs through a canal down the center of the vertebrae, surrounded by a halo of hard bone.

Peripheral nervous system The nerves that extend from the brain

(cranial nerves) and spinal cord (spinal nerves) make up the peripheral nervous system. This system is composed of a second set of neurons that, like the neurons of the central nervous system, also have long axons and short dendrites. These neurons relay information to and from the central nervous system.

For example, when you reach out to shake a hand, certain neurons in the brain send messages

through the long axons that travel down through the spinal cord. Somewhere in your neck, the tips of the axons from the brain neurons send a message to the dendrites of the peripheral neurons. The peripheral neuron axons carry the message to your arm and tell the arm muscles what action to take.

In a similar manner, sensations from the body are relayed by the peripheral neurons to the central

Peripheral Nervous System

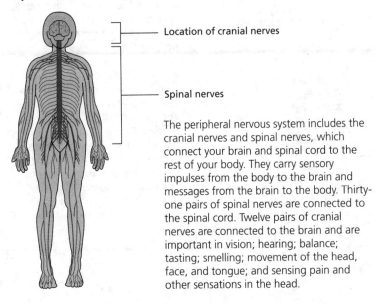

Location of cranial nerves

Spinal nerves

The peripheral nervous system includes the cranial nerves and spinal nerves, which connect your brain and spinal cord to the rest of your body. They carry sensory impulses from the body to the brain and messages from the brain to the body. Thirty-one pairs of spinal nerves are connected to the spinal cord. Twelve pairs of cranial nerves are connected to the brain and are important in vision; hearing; balance; tasting; smelling; movement of the head, face, and tongue; and sensing pain and other sensations in the head.

nervous system neurons. The brain then takes all of these messages and organizes them to interpret the experience.

For example, the feeling of sipping an icy drink presents itself to the brain as a number of separate sensory signals: the temperature of the fluid, the textures of the fluid and ice, the shape and feeling of the glass—even the glass's condensation. Your thalamus weaves together these threads of sensory signals so that the cerebrum can identify the experience as "icy drink."

Autonomic nervous system The autonomic (automatic) nervous system controls important body functions like heart rate, body temperature, and blood pressure. It is divided into two nerve pathways: the sympathetic and parasympathetic.

The sympathetic division takes over during stressful situa-

tions such as fear, anxiety, anger, and even exercise. It primes the body for quick action—heartbeat increases, muscles contract, blood vessels open up to allow increased blood flow to carry more oxygen to the muscles, and pupils dilate to make vision keener. Without this defensive mechanism, called the fight-or-flight response, we might not be able to move quickly enough to avoid danger, such as an oncoming car.

This response was particularly valuable when humans faced physical threats such as wild animals. Today's threats more commonly take the shape of emotional and psychological stresses, such as frustration, anger, and worry.

The parasympathetic division takes over during nonstressful times to maintain normal organ function. For example, once the body is stimulated to action by

the sympathetic division, the parasympathetic division helps return it to normal—heart rate slows down, diameter of blood vessels becomes smaller, and pupils constrict.

How the nervous system works
The neurons of the central and peripheral nervous systems are something like electrical wires—the long, signal-carrying axons are often covered by a protective sheath called myelin.

The axons of one neuron communicate with other neurons by sending chemical signals (see Neurotransmitters: Neurons Talking to Neurons, p.341). This is how messages are relayed from the brain neurons to all the specific neurons that tell the muscles what to do.

Of course, it is not this simple. Even moving an arm, let alone having a creative idea, is a highly complex process that requires the coordinated involvement of many thousands of neurons in different parts of the nervous system.

The brain has different areas that serve specific functions. The cerebrum, or cerebral cortex, is an extensively folded mass of tissue that covers the top and sides of the brain. It is divided into two hemispheres, commonly called the left brain and the right brain. Each hemisphere is divided into lobes in charge of different functions. For example, the frontal lobes generate voluntary movement, such as picking up a pen. The left frontal lobe directs movement on the right side of the body; and the right frontal lobe directs movement on the left side of the body.

Within the temporal lobes are the auditory (hearing) areas and the olfactory (sense of smell)

Functions of the Brain

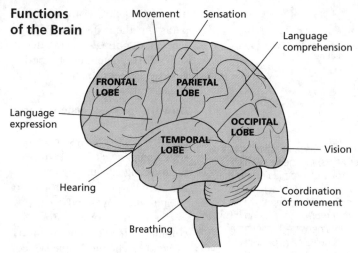

Movement
Sensation
Language comprehension
FRONTAL LOBE
PARIETAL LOBE
OCCIPITAL LOBE
Language expression
TEMPORAL LOBE
Vision
Hearing
Coordination of movement
Breathing

Each hemisphere, or half, of the cortex of the brain is divided into four specialized lobes: the frontal lobe, parietal lobe, temporal lobe, and occipital lobe. In general, the frontal lobe controls movement, planning, and language expression. The parietal lobe interprets sensation. The occipital lobe perceives and interprets vision. The temporal lobe is involved in hearing, long-term memory, behavior, and understanding and expressing language. Memory and behavior are located deep within the temporal and frontal lobes (not shown).

The Seat of Emotion: The Limbic System and Nearby Parts of the Brain

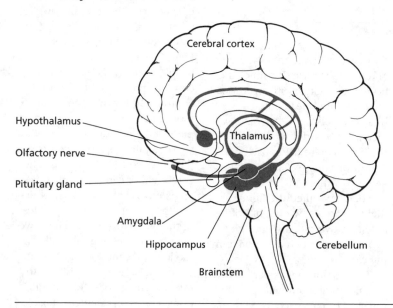

Cerebral cortex
Hypothalamus
Olfactory nerve
Pituitary gland
Thalamus
Amygdala
Hippocampus
Cerebellum
Brainstem

The parts of the limbic system are shown here. Feelings of pleasure, relaxation, fear, aggression, and rage arise from the hypothalamus. It coordinates the flight-or-fight response and triggers sexual arousal by stimulating the nearby pituitary gland to produce hormones. The hypothalamus also regulates appetite, thirst, and body temperature. The olfactory nerves connect the nasal passages directly to the hippocampus and amygdala. Since these structures coordinate memory storage and recall, their direct connection to our sense of smell may explain how an odor can so powerfully evoke a memory of long ago.

areas. The parietal lobes perceive and interpret sensations from the skin. The occipital lobes receive and interpret visual stimuli. Several different parts of the cerebrum control your understanding of language and your ability to express yourself through language. In most people, the language areas

are in the left hemisphere.

Lying between the cerebrum and the deeper parts of the brain is the limbic system, which controls instinctual behavior, emotions, and sexual function. It also is important in memory.

Deep within the brain are the hypothalamus, thalamus, and

brainstem (which includes the medulla, pons, and midbrain). The components of the brainstem govern basic life functions such as heart rate, breathing, and balance.

The hypothalamus sits on top of the brainstem and controls hormones (see p.829) as well as the basic urges to eat, drink,

How Nerve Cells Communicate

BRAIN TISSUE

NEUROTRANSMISSION

The brain's basic unit of processing information is the neuron (left). Neurons communicate with one another by generating an electrical impulse that travels down an axon (the long, fiberlike part of the nerve) to the axon terminal (the end of the axon). At the axon terminal (right), this electrical signal causes substances called neurotransmitters to be released from tiny pores. The neurotransmitters from the first neuron spill into the synapse (the space between neurons) and attach to receptors on the surface of a dendrite of the second neuron, activating the second neuron to generate an electrical impulse that travels down the axon.

Neurotransmitters: Neurons Talking to Neurons

The brain can do nothing and perceive nothing unless thousands of its neurons (nerve cells) communicate in a coordinated fashion with thousands of other neurons. Communicating requires certain neurons to "turn on" and to send a message to another neuron or group of neurons. Often, the message must travel a long distance. The final neuron in the circuit must receive the message and command another cell (such as a muscle) to perform a function or, in the brain, interpret the information.

Messages are transmitted by an intricate set of chemical signals. A neuron sends an electrical signal down its long axon. The tips of the axon then release little sacs of chemicals called neurotransmitters. Norepinephrine, serotonin, and dopamine are common neurotransmitters.

Neurons communicate with each other at a junction called a synapse, where the tip of one axon sits next to the tips of dendrites from another neuron. The neurotransmitters released by the axon float through the fluid-filled space to the tips of the dendrites of the next neuron. The neurotransmitter then attaches

to a receptor on the tip of a dendrite, the way a key fits into a lock. This causes the second neuron to pass an electrical signal down its axon, passing the message from the first neuron to the second neuron.

Many illnesses are related to problems with neurotransmitters and their receptors. If there are not enough neurotransmitters, the signal cannot be passed. If there is a problem with the receptors, the second neuron cannot receive the signal or may not be able to turn off the signal. Problems with neurotransmitters can cause diseases affecting strength, coordination of muscles, mood (such as depression), thought (such as schizophrenia), or speech.

To treat these diseases, medicines are used to correct the levels of neurotransmitter or the problem with the receptor. Antidepressant drugs increase norepinephrine and serotonin signals; antipsychotic drugs block receptors for dopamine. Further investigation of the actions of neurotransmitters should lead to the development of more effective treatments and to a better understanding of psychiatric disorders in general.

reproduce, and flee in the face of danger. The thalamus rests on the hypothalamus and works in tandem with the cerebrum to process, and sometimes suppress, sensory information.

Sitting at the base of the brain, the cerebellum stores and exe- cutes common conscious and unconscious muscular move- ments. While the cerebrum might decide that it is time for you to reset your watch, it is the cere- bellum that recalls and coordi- nates the millions of learned and programmed movements required for you to accomplish this task. The cerebellum is important for the smooth coordi- nation of movement, and it has recently been recognized as important for thinking and rea- soning, as well.

STROKE

There are two general categories of stroke, each of which has a different cause.

Ischemic strokes occur when there is an interruption in the flow of blood to the brain, almost always due to a clot blocking a blood vessel. About 80% of strokes fall into this category.

The remaining 20% are brain hemorrhages, which occur when a blood vessel in the brain rup- tures.

A stroke, or brain attack, occurs when the blood flow to the brain is disrupted because a vessel supplying it has either rup- tured or is blocked. Deprived of blood and oxygen (a condition called ischemia), brain cells and brain tissue die, and are not replaced. As a result, the parts of the body once controlled by those cells can lose their ability to function.

Approximately 500,000 Ameri- cans have strokes each year, and about one third die within several months. About 10% of those who survive a stroke return home to their previous level of activity, about 50% return home but require some assistance, and about 40% require institutionaliza- tion and constant help in daily liv- ing. A stroke can cause a loss of function that is often permanent.

Sometimes the loss of function is temporary, lasting less than 24 hours. These temporary spells are called transient ischemic attacks and they can warn of an impend- ing stroke.

Transient Ischemic Attack

A transient ischemic attack (TIA) results from a temporary inter- ruption in blood flow to the brain. A TIA can occur when small pieces of debris (emboli) such as blood clots, cholesterol deposits, or other foreign matter travel through the blood and temporarily lodge in the small blood vessels in the brain. When the debris interrupts the flow of blood to brain tissue, the tissue temporarily stops functioning until the debris dissolves.

The emboli that cause a TIA most frequently result from atherosclerosis (see p.653), a dis- ease that develops when plaque, a buildup of fatty deposits, forms inside the large arteries that sup-

Living with a Transient Ischemic Attack

It happened the first time on Labor Day. I started to feel a little light- headed. I really noticed something was going on while I was talking to my brother on the phone. He was talking about his son, Frank. Frank is my godson, and I know him really well. But in the middle of his story about Frank and his car, I asked him, "Who is Frank?" I just could not understand what he was talking about. Then I lost feeling in my left arm and had this numbness that went up my arm to my left shoulder. I did not know what had happened but I did not call the doctor because I thought maybe it was related to a shoulder injury I had. I went to the doctor a couple of days later. He thought it was nothing, but sent me to an orthopedist. The orthopedist thought I had had a stroke. Finally, I was seen in the emergency room and met a neurologist who told me it was a TIA, not really a stroke. I started on treatment and have not had any more TIAs since then.

Arthur K., 62 years old

Arteries Supplying Blood to the Brain

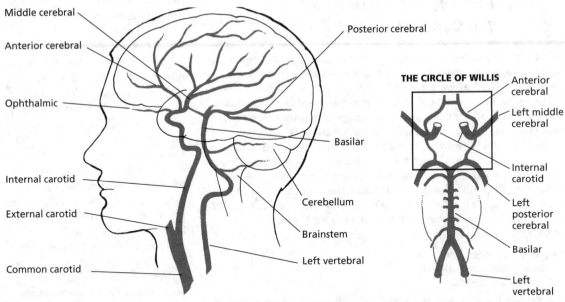

Middle cerebral

Anterior cerebral

Ophthalmic

Internal carotid

External carotid

Common carotid

Posterior cerebral

Basilar

Cerebellum

Brainstem

Left vertebral

THE CIRCLE OF WILLIS

Anterior cerebral

Left middle cerebral

Internal carotid

Left posterior cerebral

Basilar

Left vertebral

The carotid and vertebral arteries (left) run up the neck. The carotid arteries supply the front and middle of the brain with blood. The vertebral and basilar arteries supply the back of the cerebral cortex, cerebellum, and brainstem with blood. The vertebral arteries join at the back of the head to become the basilar artery. The blood supply from the carotid and basilar arteries forms the circle of Willis (right), which provides other routes for blood flow if a major vessel is blocked.

Types of Stroke

BRAIN HEMORRHAGE

Blood

Brain

Intracerebral Hemorrhage

ISCHEMIC STROKES

Embolic Stroke

Blood clot

Blood supply cut off

Brain

Thrombotic Stroke

Blood clot in narrowed vessel

Plaque (buildup that occurs in atherosclerosis)

Brain hemorrhages, such as an intracerebral hemorrhage (left), are caused by a rupture of a blood vessel in the brain. The subsequent accumulation of blood compresses both the brain tissue and other blood vessels that nourish brain tissue. Ischemic strokes, [such as an embolic stroke (top right) or a thrombotic stroke (bottom right)], are caused by an interruption in blood flow to the brain. In an embolic stroke, a clot forms elsewhere in the body and travels through the circulatory system to the brain. It lodges in a small vessel and cuts off the supply of blood. In a thrombotic stroke, a vessel in the brain is progressively narrowed by a buildup of plaque. A clot eventually forms at the site of the narrowing, cutting off the blood supply.

Preventing Strokes: Dr Samuels' Advice

Strokes are preventable, yet strokes are unfortunately very common. As a neurologist, nearly every day I see people who have suffered from a stroke. Yesterday, they were happy, healthy people, and today they cannot talk, or cannot understand, or cannot move one side of their body. Too often, they had experienced the symptoms of a transient ischemic attack (TIA) but had not contacted their doctor about it. Sometimes, they had been told they were at risk for a stroke and advised to take a medicine to reduce the risk, but they chose not to. The medicine often is simple—one pill a day—and quite safe, if properly monitored by the doctor, but they chose not to take it. And now there is nothing that they or I can do. It is a very sad situation. If you or a loved one may have had TIAs, or has an irregular heart rhythm, talk to the doctor. If medicine is prescribed, think twice about refusing to take it.

MARTIN A. SAMUELS, MD
BRIGHAM AND WOMEN'S HOSPITAL
HARVARD MEDICAL SCHOOL

ply the brain. Emboli can also originate from clots in the heart or from debris on heart valves.

TIAs are different from strokes in that they are brief and temporary. Symptoms usually develop abruptly, last a few hours, and go away in less than 24 hours. Essentially, blood flow is restored quickly enough so that brain tissue is not permanently damaged.

TIAs serve as a warning that a person could have a stroke in the future. Almost half of people who have had an ischemic stroke (see p.345) had at least one TIA some months before their stroke. But not all people who have TIAs will have a stroke. TIAs are more likely to occur in people with high blood pressure, certain types of heart disease, and diabetes; people who smoke; or people who are of an advanced age.

SYMPTOMS

The symptoms vary widely depending on the portion of the brain affected. TIAs may cause weakness, numbness, or paralysis of the face, arm, or leg; dizziness, loss of balance, or loss of coordination; sudden blurring or loss of vision in one or both eyes; and loss of one half of the visual field in one or both eyes. See your doctor immediately if you have any of these symptoms.

TREATMENT OPTIONS

Your doctor will first check for other conditions that can mimic a TIA or stroke, including migraine, seizures, low blood sugar, low blood pressure, brain tumor, irregular heart rhythms, and labyrinthitis (see p.456).

If you have recurring TIAs with symptoms that are always the same, it suggests recurring blockage of the same artery. If the symptoms vary from one TIA to the next, emboli may be blocking different arteries each time.

Your physician will use a stethoscope to listen for bruits, which are noises heard when blood flow in the arteries is impaired. To aid in diagnosis, you may need to have one of several radiology tests, such as computed tomography (see p.149), magnetic resonance imaging (see p.151), ultrasound (see p.148), magnetic resonance angiography (see p.147), or conventional angiography (see p.147). These tests can identify blockages in your neck and brain. Further tests may be necessary to evaluate your heart.

You may be hospitalized if you see your doctor while you are having a TIA. He or she may give you a fast-acting, blood-thinning medicine (heparin) to try to keep the clot that is blocking the flow of blood to your brain from getting bigger or to keep the clot from coming back if it has started to dissolve naturally.

Since TIAs usually resolve on their own, treatment aims to prevent another TIA or a stroke (see Preventing Stroke, p.346). Your doctor will help you improve control of any risk factors such as high blood pressure or diabetes. He or she will also discuss with you ways to stop smoking.

Anticoagulants, most commonly aspirin, may be prescribed to thin the blood and reduce the chance of clotting. Carotid endarterectomy (see p.345), which is surgery to remove plaque from the large arteries leading from the neck to the brain, may be recommended if you have had a TIA and have a significant blockage (more than 70%) in a carotid artery.

Cerebral Angiography

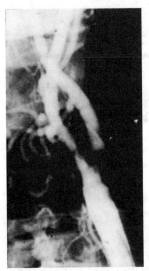

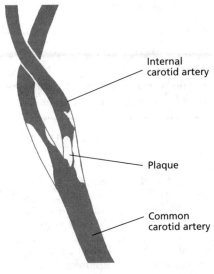

Internal carotid artery

Plaque

Common carotid artery

The angiogram (left) shows a narrowing of the internal carotid artery. The buildup of plaque (right) that caused the narrowing is also evident.

Ischemic Stroke

Ischemic stroke occurs when there is a blockage in one of the arteries that supplies blood to the brain. If the blockage lasts longer than about 2 hours, the part of the brain nourished by the artery dies. The symptoms depend on the part of the brain that has been affected.

There are two types of ischemic strokes: thrombotic and embolic. Thrombotic stroke occurs when an atherosclerotic plaque (see p.343) in a brain artery becomes large enough to block the blood supply to brain tissue. What happens during a thrombotic stroke is similar to what happens during a heart attack (see p.663).

Embolic stroke is the result of a blockage in an artery by a

Carotid Endarterectomy

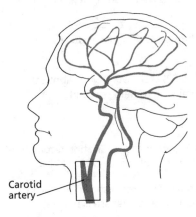

Carotid artery

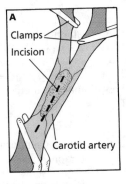

A
Clamps
Incision
Carotid artery

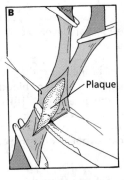

B
Plaque

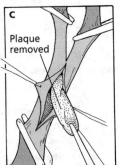

C
Plaque removed

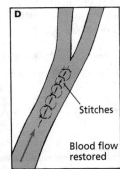

D
Stitches
Blood flow restored

In a carotid endarterectomy, which removes the lining of a carotid artery narrowed by atherosclerosis, the surgeon clamps off the carotid artery and makes an incision (A). The blocked area is exposed to reveal the plaque buildup of atherosclerosis (B). The plaque is scraped away and removed, along with any blood clot that has formed (C). The incision is stitched closed, and blood flows more freely to the brain (D).

Preventing Stroke

Many strokes can be prevented by eliminating or reducing risk factors. The factors that contribute to your risk of having a stroke, and what you can do to reduce that risk, are outlined below. In addition, research indicates that drinking one to two alcoholic drinks per day may cut the risk of stroke in half. Drinking more than this amount increases your risk of stroke.

RISK FACTORS	HOW YOU CAN REDUCE YOUR RISK
Untreated high blood pressure (see p.644) is the leading cause of stroke in the United States. High blood pressure damages vessel walls, encouraging scarring, plaque buildup, and atherosclerosis (see p.653).	Have your blood pressure checked at least every 2 years (more often if you have high blood pressure in your family). If your blood pressure is high, reducing your diastolic blood pressure by just a little can cut your risk of stroke nearly in half.
Atrial fibrillation (see p.673) is a common heart rhythm disturbance in which the upper chambers of the heart quiver erratically, allowing blood to form small clots that can cause a stroke if a clot travels to the brain.	The blood-thinning prescription drug warfarin or aspirin can greatly decrease the risk of stroke. Ask your doctor about warfarin.
Atherosclerosis (see p.653) and elevated cholesterol levels (see p.669) can contribute to stroke in several ways.	Have your cholesterol levels checked, eat a low-fat diet, and exercise regularly.
Your risk of stroke is very high for 3 to 6 months after a transient ischemic attack (TIA) (see p.342).	If you have the warning signs of a TIA, your physician can give you treatments that reduce the chance of a stroke.
People who have heart failure can develop clots in their heart from slower blood flow.	Blood-thinning drugs or aspirin may reduce your stroke risk.
Smoking makes blood more prone to clotting, raises blood pressure, and damages the lining of blood vessels. The more you smoke, the greater your risk of stroke.	Quit smoking (see p.59). Ask your doctor about the many strategies available to help you quit.
Diabetes (see p.832) increases your risk of stroke.	Follow your doctor's dietary and medication recommendations for lowering your blood sugar.
Obesity increases the risk of stroke as much as twofold. You are considered obese if you weigh at least 20% more than you should (see p.853).	Discuss with your doctor how to lose weight through a sensible diet (see p.37) and exercise (see p.50) program.
Blood clots can develop on mechanical heart valves if the blood is not made thin enough with the anticoagulant warfarin.	If you have mechanical heart valves, you should be taking warfarin, and your doctor should do blood tests regularly to make sure the dose is correct.
Low levels of vitamin E in your diet.	Although unproven, a diet rich in foods containing vitamin E (see p.42) may reduce the severity of a stroke.

Atrial Fibrillation and Ischemic Stroke

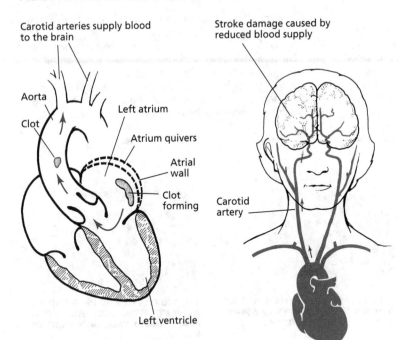

During atrial fibrillation (left), the atria (the upper chambers of the heart) quiver rapidly and ineffectively. Instead of being efficiently pumped out of the atria, some blood remains in the atria. Blood that has pooled along the walls of the left atrium can form clots, which break loose and travel through the left ventricle to the aorta and then into the circulation. The clot travels to an artery, such as the carotid artery, that supplies blood to the brain (right), obstructing blood flow and causing an ischemic stroke.

clot or plaque fragment that is formed elsewhere in the body, often in the heart, and travels in the blood until it lodges in a small blood vessel in the brain.

Embolic strokes are like transient ischemic attacks (TIAs) (see p.342), except that the blockage of the artery is more complete, leading to death of a part of the brain and a prolonged and often permanent loss of some function.

Embolic strokes and TIAs are often a complication of atrial fibrillation (see p.673), a condition in which the heart beats rapidly and irregularly. The fluttering motion allows blood to pool in the heart and form clots that can travel to the brain.

Ischemic stroke is more prevalent among people with high blood pressure (see p.644), some types of heart disease (see p.652), diabetes (see p.832), and advanced age. Cigarette smoking, high cholesterol (see p.669), heavy alcohol consumption, obesity (see p.853), and a family history of stroke increase your risk.

SYMPTOMS

The symptoms of ischemic stroke vary, depending on the size of the blockage, the region of the brain affected, and how quickly the blockage of the artery developed. Stroke is a medical emergency. It is critical to recognize the symptoms of stroke and get immediate medical help by phoning 911 or your local emergency service.

The longer a stroke remains untreated, the greater the damage. Within the first 4 to 6 hours, treatment can be administered that may restore blood flow and prevent permanent damage to the brain.

WARNING SIGNS OF STROKE

Here are the warning signs of stroke:

■ Sudden weakness in an arm, hand, or leg on one side of the body

■ Sudden numbness on one side of the face or body

■ Sudden dimness or loss of vision, particularly in only one eye

■ Sudden difficulty speaking or sudden inability to understand what someone is saying

■ Sudden dizziness or loss of balance

■ Sudden, excruciating headache

It is the suddenness of the onset of these symptoms that typifies stroke; gradual development of some of these symptoms may be an indication of other nervous system conditions, such as a brain tumor (see p.357) or Parkinson disease (see p.371).

Benefits and Risks of Blood Thinners for Stroke

If you have atrial fibrillation and have had an ischemic stroke from an embolism, the use of blood-thinning medicine (such as aspirin or an anticoagulant drug) is often advised to protect you against another stroke. Blood-thinning medicines reduce your risk of having another ischemic stroke but increase your risk of major bleeding, which can cause either temporary or permanent damage.

If major bleeding occurs in the stomach or intestines (as is often the case) or other areas of the body (such as a joint), it usually can be treated successfully. If bleeding occurs in the brain (see Brain Hemorrhage, p.350), it can cause severe brain damage, just as an ischemic stroke can. However, the risk of having another ischemic stroke from not taking blood thinners is much greater than the risk of a brain hemorrhage from taking blood thinners.

NO MEDICINE

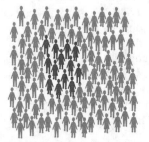

13 OF 100 PEOPLE WHO HAVE HAD AN ISCHEMIC STROKE AND TAKE NO MEDICINE WILL HAVE ANOTHER STROKE

ASPIRIN

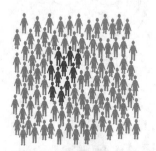

10 OF 100 PEOPLE WHO HAVE HAD AN ISCHEMIC STROKE AND TAKE ASPIRIN WILL HAVE ANOTHER STROKE

ANTICOAGULANTS

4 OF 100 PEOPLE WHO HAVE HAD AN ISCHEMIC STROKE AND TAKE ANTI-COAGULANTS WILL HAVE ANOTHER STROKE

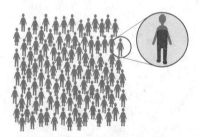

0.7 OF 100 PEOPLE WHO HAVE HAD AN ISCHEMIC STROKE AND TAKE NO MEDICINE WILL HAVE AN EPISODE OF MAJOR BLEEDING

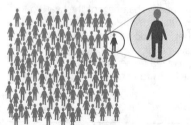

0.9 OF 100 PEOPLE WHO HAVE HAD AN ISCHEMIC STROKE AND TAKE ASPIRIN WILL HAVE AN EPISODE OF MAJOR BLEEDING

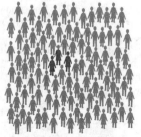

2.8 OF 100 PEOPLE WHO HAVE HAD AN ISCHEMIC STROKE AND TAKE ANTICOAGULANTS WILL HAVE AN EPISODE OF MAJOR BLEEDING

TREATMENT OPTIONS

The person's symptoms and results of a physical examination in the first hours after a stroke provide doctors with clues about the type and location of the stroke. Often, diagnostic tests are ordered, including computed tomography (see p.149) and magnetic resonance imaging (see p.151). These tests can usually distinguish an ischemic stroke from a brain hemorrhage (see p.350) and can identify the area of the brain affected.

Magnetic resonance angiography (see p.147) or conventional angiography (see p.147) can identify the precise blood vessel inside the brain that is blocked.

A person with a severe stroke requires hospitalization in the intensive care unit to monitor the brain, heart, and other body functions. Depending on the extent of the damage, life-support measures may be necessary to supply oxygen, nutrients, and medicines. A feeding tube may be required for people who have lost their ability to eat.

Medicines or, in severe cases, emergency surgery may be required if the stroke has caused brain swelling. The medicines or surgery are necessary to relieve

Benefits and Risks of Thrombolytic Drugs for Stroke

Intravenous treatment with thrombolytic drugs to break up blood clots, if given within the first 3 hours of having an ischemic stroke, increases your risk of death in the first few days and first 6 months, but lowers your risk of dying or living in an impaired dependent state over the next 6 months. Despite the early risks, most physicians recommend that the drug be given to prevent the longer-term risk.

WITH TREATMENT

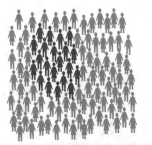

21 OF 100 PEOPLE WHO HAVE HAD A STROKE AND TAKE THROMBOLYTIC DRUGS WILL DIE WITHIN A FEW DAYS

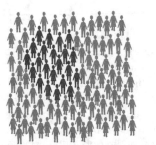

22 OF 100 PEOPLE WHO HAVE HAD A STROKE AND TAKE THROMBOLYTIC DRUGS WILL DIE WITHIN 6 MONTHS

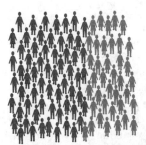

62 OF 100 PEOPLE WHO HAVE HAD A STROKE AND TAKE THROMBOLYTIC DRUGS WILL DIE OR BE LIVING IN AN IMPAIRED, DEPENDENT STATE WITHIN THE FOLLOWING 6 MONTHS

WITHOUT TREATMENT

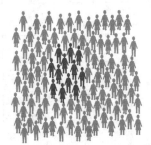

12 OF 100 PEOPLE WHO HAVE HAD A STROKE AND DO NOT TAKE THROMBOLYTIC DRUGS WILL DIE WITHIN A FEW DAYS

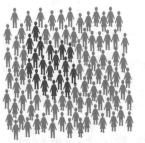

18 OF 100 PEOPLE WHO HAVE HAD A STROKE AND DO NOT TAKE THROMBOLYTIC DRUGS WILL DIE WITHIN 6 MONTHS

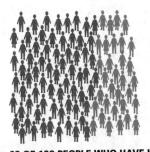

68 OF 100 PEOPLE WHO HAVE HAD A STROKE AND DO NOT TAKE THROMBOLYTIC DRUGS WILL DIE OR BE LIVING IN AN IMPAIRED, DEPENDENT STATE WITHIN THE FOLLOWING 6 MONTHS

pressure as the swollen brain tissue crushes other brain tissue or vessels. More minor strokes result in less brain damage and require less monitoring. Sometimes, people with minor strokes can be cared for at home without being hospitalized.

If you have had an ischemic stroke, you may be given a fast-acting, blood-thinning medicine (heparin) to try to keep the clot that is blocking the flow of blood to your brain from getting bigger or to keep it from coming back if it has started to dissolve naturally.

If you have had an ischemic stroke and are seen by a physician within the narrow 3-hour window, you will probably receive thrombolytic therapy, a treatment that rapidly dissolves blood clots. In some people, particularly people with bleeding conditions, this potent therapy cannot be used. When thrombolytic therapy is properly used, results are superior to previous treatments in reducing the risk of disability and death. Stroke experts are now conducting pilot programs to make the public aware of stroke symptoms so that people with symptoms of a possible stroke go to an emergency room as soon as possible.

Particularly in the case of an embolic stroke, the doctor will try to identify the site where the clot formed. Echocardiography (see p.665) may be used to look for clots in the heart and to see if the heart is pumping weakly, which could contribute to the development of clots in its chambers.

A portable device called a Holter monitor records the heart rate and identifies heart irregularities such as atrial fibrillation (see p.673) that could cause clot formations. Ultrasound may be used

How Thrombolytic Drugs Break Up Clots

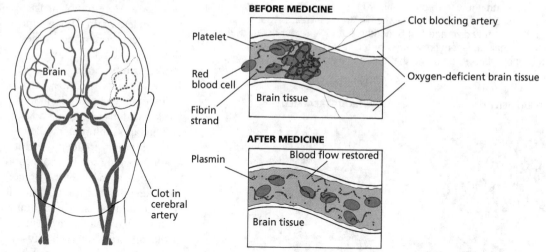

A blood clot (left and top right), which contains platelets and red blood cells trapped in fibrin strands, may form on plaque in a brain artery or, more commonly, travel to the brain from another part of the body. Unless the clot is dissolved promptly, brain tissue will die because of lack of blood and oxygen. Recombinant tissue-plasminogen activator breaks up the clot and restores blood flow (bottom right) by helping generate the enzyme plasmin, which digests the fibrin strands. To be most effective, it should be injected into the bloodstream within 3 hours of the stroke.

to identify narrowing of blood vessels in the brain, as well as plaque in the carotid artery or in the arteries leading from the heart to the carotid artery, another common source of clots.

An operation called a carotid endarterectomy (see p.345) removes plaque deposits from one of the major arteries leading to the brain. Most often it is performed after a TIA or stroke to prevent a recurrence, especially if a carotid artery is narrowed by 80% or more.

BRAIN HEMORRHAGE

A brain hemorrhage, also called a hemorrhagic stroke or cerebral hemorrhage, is the rupture of a small blood vessel in the brain. Brain damage occurs because of lack of blood and oxygen to the

tissues, as well as a buildup of pressure from the bleeding.

This type of stroke is more likely to occur in a person with high blood pressure, which weakens vessel walls. An abnormality called an arteriovenous malformation (see Intracerebral and Subarachnoid Hemorrhages, right) can also cause a brain hemorrhage.

Although every stroke is serious, brain hemorrhages are often devastating because they can affect younger people and are more likely to cause death. High blood pressure is the leading cause of a brain hemorrhage, but other risk factors include cocaine use, alcohol abuse, head injury, diabetes (see p.832), and bleeding disorders.

Brain hemorrhage can occur in either of two places. When bleeding takes place inside the

brain, the stroke is called an intracerebral hemorrhage. When a vessel on the surface of the brain bursts, it is called a subarachnoid hemorrhage, a subdural hemorrhage, or an epidural hemorrhage, depending on the location of the pool of blood.

Intracerebral and Subarachnoid Hemorrhages

An intracerebral hemorrhage occurs inside the brain. This type of stroke often occurs when people are awake and sometimes when they are under stress. Usually, the person's first symptoms are a sudden, severe headache or sudden vomiting, or even unconsciousness. These symptoms develop over several minutes.

Other neurological symptoms

follow shortly, such as weakness or difficulty speaking. When bleeding has occurred in the cerebellum—where movement and balance are coordinated—the person may experience abrupt dizziness and loss of balance that affects walking or standing.

In a subarachnoid hemorrhage, a blood vessel bursts on the surface of the brain. The surface of the brain is covered by three thin membranes called meninges (see p.378). The outside membrane adheres to the skull and the innermost membrane adheres to the brain. Between the layers is the subarachnoid space, which is normally filled with fluid.

In a subarachnoid hemorrhage, blood leaks into this space. Damage can be more extensive than in an intracerebral hemorrhage because blood accumulates between the brain and the skull and presses on a large area of the surface of the brain.

Subarachnoid hemorrhages are caused by abnormally shaped, weak-walled arteries in the brain—either an aneurysm or an arteriovenous malformation.

Aneurysms are small, balloon-like structures that stick out of the wall of a small artery. Some people are born with a tendency to form aneurysms. High blood pressure probably increases the tendency of aneurysms to form and surely increases the risk that they will rupture.

Arteriovenous malformations are unusual tangles of thin-walled arteries and veins that create a little sac filled with blood. The malformations bleed easily. Men are more likely to have arteriovenous malformations than

women, and it is not unusual for families to have several affected members.

As many as half of all arteriovenous malformations leak blood intermittently into the subarachnoid space. Even without rupturing, arteriovenous malformations can cause symptoms (mainly headaches and seizures) by pressing on brain tissue. The symptoms usually occur between the ages of 10 and 30.

While surgical treatment of arteriovenous malformations is often successful, it is also technically difficult because the malformations often are located in vital areas of the brain. Moderate-sized arteriovenous malformations that cause no symptoms and are discovered incidentally through other tests are best left alone. People who have seizures but have no other symptoms are usually treated with anticonvulsant drugs.

About 45% of people with a subarachnoid hemorrhage have severe headache as the first major symptom. People often describe the headache as "exploding" or "bursting." About half lose consciousness. Other early symptoms include a stiff neck, nausea and vomiting, mental impairment, or seizures.

More than half of people who survive this type of stroke have significant neurological damage, including partial paralysis, weakness, or numbness. Vision and speech problems may also occur. The ultimate recovery depends on how soon and what kind of treatment is given.

TREATMENT OPTIONS

Treatment is guided by the location and extent of the hemor-

rhage, which can be detected by computed tomography (see p.149). The internal bleeding has usually stopped by the time the affected person arrives at the hospital.

For an intracerebral hemorrhage, there is often little that can be done. If the hemorrhage has produced a large pool of blood that is putting pressure on the brain, surgery may be required to remove the pool of blood.

If the brain hemorrhage is caused by a ruptured aneurysm, surgery often is attempted; the skull is opened and the surgeon clips off the aneurysm. If this is not possible because the aneurysm is located deep inside the brain, where it is difficult to reach, doctors can sometimes thread a catheter through the circulation and into the blood vessel that has the aneurysm and try to seal the aneurysm from the inside.

If the person has high blood pressure, medicine will be given to bring it under control. In addition, supportive care to manage breathing, feeding, and the ingestion of fluids may be necessary. Angiograms (see p.147) are performed to locate the source of bleeding and to identify any additional aneurysms that are likely to rupture.

Survival and recovery depend on the size, location, and cause of the bleeding. Approximately 75% of people with a hemorrhage related to high blood pressure die. In survivors, major improvement can result when the blood is reabsorbed by the brain, allowing the brain tissue to resume its normal function.

Chances of a full recovery are best for those who regain consciousness and survive for 6 months with no recurrence.

Epidural Hemorrhage

Epidural (also called extradural) hemorrhage usually results from a head injury that causes a blood vessel in the outer surface of the dura mater (the outermost of three membrane layers that cover the brain) to rupture. Blood then leaks between the dura mater and the skull to form a pool of clotted blood (hematoma) that presses on the brain.

Because the blood vessel that bursts is usually an artery, a substantial amount of blood leaks into the narrow space between the brain and skull, increasing the pressure on the brain as more blood collects.

SYMPTOMS

Symptoms occur within minutes to a few hours after the injury, and may include sudden severe headache, nausea, dizziness, vomiting, confusion, and increasing drowsiness. If untreated, an epidural hemorrhage may lead to permanent brain damage, and even death. Immediate diagnosis and prompt treatment are essential.

TREATMENT OPTIONS

Doctors may use skull x-rays to identify a skull injury and computed tomography (see p.149) to locate the hemorrhage. If diagnostic tests confirm an epidural hemorrhage, surgery is necessary to stop the bleeding and remove the clot.

Most people make a complete recovery if surgery is performed promptly, although a period of convalescence may be required.

Adults regain most of the function they will have within about 6 months. Children tend to heal faster from head injuries and make steady improvement.

Subdural Hemorrhage

Subdural hemorrhage occurs when injury causes a blood vessel to rupture underneath the dura mater (the outermost of the three membranes that cover the brain). As in an epidural hemorrhage (see p.352), the slowly leaking blood forms a clotted pool (hematoma) between the surface of the brain and the dura mater, compressing the brain tissue as it gets larger.

In a subdural hemorrhage, the leaking usually originates from a vein and proceeds slowly, so symptoms may take days or weeks to develop. (In an epidural hemorrhage, the leaking originates from an artery, so symptoms develop rapidly.)

While a subdural hemorrhage can be caused by an obvious severe head injury, it also can occur after an apparently minor injury, such as a bumped head. Infants and elderly people are most prone to subdural hemorrhage.

SYMPTOMS

Symptoms, including drowsiness, confusion, partial paralysis on one side of the body, imbalance, nausea, seizures, and persistent or fluctuating headaches, may begin gradually or intermittently, but eventually they worsen over a period of hours or weeks. If the subdural hemorrhage is not diagnosed and treated promptly, death may result.

TREATMENT OPTIONS

If you or a member of your family has the symptoms of a subdural hemorrhage, see a physician immediately (especially if you have had a head injury).

To diagnose the condition, doctors use computed tomography (see p.149) or magnetic resonance imaging (see p.151). Some small hematomas are gradually absorbed by your body and do not require surgery. Often however, it is necessary for a brain surgeon to drill a small hole into your skull and drain the hematoma, thereby relieving the pressure on the brain.

Larger hematomas and those that are made up of clotted blood may be removed by cutting out a section of the skull. Brain swelling may be controlled with corticosteroid drugs (see p.895).

During the recovery period, you may experience amnesia, anxiety, and headache for the first 6 months. Your ability to concentrate may be temporarily impaired.

STROKE REHABILITATION

A number of rehabilitation specialists can help the stroke survivor recover the greatest possible function. Leading the team is a physiatrist, a physician who specializes in physical medicine and rehabilitation. Depending on the needs of the individual, other team members may include physical therapists, occupational therapists, speech therapists, social workers, and psychologists. Therapy is focused on making the most of the person's capabilities for self-care, mobility, and reestablishing recreational and vocational pursuits.

Rehabilitation usually begins in the hospital. At this stage, some people with stroke are unable to breathe, eat, or drink unassisted. Therapy usually begins with range-of-motion exercises performed by a physical therapist, nurse, or family member, who does most of the work by moving the person's limbs; this helps keep circulation flowing, prevents bedsores (see p.1123), and maintains muscle tone.

Later, the individual will be able to take a more active role in exercise. After leaving the hospital, rehabilitation may continue at a nursing home or outpatient clinic, or at home with the help of family members and visiting professionals.

A home environment with a supportive and healthy partner and/or family is important in the rehabilitation process. Stroke survivors going home to a positive environment are more likely to become independent and productive. It is sometimes necessary to adapt the home with such architectural modifications as ramps, railings, and grab bars (see p.1122 for other assistive devices) near the tub and toilet.

Language Difficulties After Stroke

Speech or language disorders occur in up to 40% of people who have had a stroke. Those with a speech or language disorder should first have a hearing

evaluation to ensure that the difficulty in communication stems from damage to the language center in the brain and not a hearing problem.

It is important to remember that people with speech disorders do not necessarily have an intellectual deficit. They may be able to think as well as they did before the stroke but have difficulty expressing these thoughts, which can be extremely frustrating for the person who has had a stroke.

Speech-language pathologists or speech therapists help the person who has had a stroke improve his or her capacity to produce and understand speech.

Aphasia, the partial or total loss of the ability to use language, is common after a stroke, especially if any part of the brain where language is processed has been damaged.

Aphasia takes several different forms. Some people have trouble talking but can easily understand what others are saying; some people can talk easily but cannot understand when others speak.

Some people who have had a stroke recover quickly on their own or with therapy, while others continue to have trouble speaking or finding the words to say, or have problems with reading, writing, or math.

People with dysarthria may be able to understand speech and to form proper words in their mind, but they cannot control their mouth to articulate. Speech may be slow or slurred, and one side of the face may droop due to

muscle paralysis. Drooling may also occur. Dysarthria is caused by an injury to the brain centers that control the tongue, palate, and lips.

Emotional Impact of Stroke

Many people need psychological help to cope with the consequences of a stroke. Sudden emotional changes such as an increased tendency to laugh or cry inappropriately or get angry easily are common. Many people recovering from a stroke also experience sexual problems. Counseling or psychotherapy can play an important role in rehabilitation.

Depression (see p.395) often sets in after a stroke; up to two thirds of people report feeling sad for months afterward, and about 25% experience major depression. Untreated depression can undermine efforts at rehabilitation and worsen speech and language. Several factors may contribute to the depression: a normal reaction to the losses caused by the stroke, injury to certain parts of the brain, or a side effect of prescribed medicine.

Support and encouragement from family and friends can help motivate a depressed stroke survivor to participate in a rehabilitation program. To alleviate severe depression, however, psychotherapy or antidepressant medicines may also be necessary.

HEADACHE

Tension Headache

The pain of a tension headache is one of the most common symptoms human beings experience. Doctors do not know what causes tension headaches. Many people experience tension headaches only intermittently; others have them almost daily or two or more times weekly.

Tension headaches usually develop during middle age, and continue off and on for several years. They affect men and women equally.

SYMPTOMS

The typical sensation is one of steady tightness or pressure, often like a band tightening around the head. The headache often starts late in the day and may continue for minutes, days, months, or even years. The pain may be barely noticeable or severe, or fall somewhere in between. Its intensity may wax and wane. The discomfort can make falling asleep difficult but usually is not intense enough to wake you from sleep.

TREATMENT OPTIONS

To pinpoint the cause of your headaches, it is useful to keep a headache diary, noting the pattern and events that trigger the headache. Your physician may look for other potential sources for your head pain by performing vision tests or examining your sinuses. You will not need diagnostic tests such as skull x-rays or computed tomography (see p.149) if your symptoms indicate that you are suffering from tension headaches.

There is no cure for tension headaches, but the pain can be relieved with over-the-counter painkillers such as aspirin, acetaminophen, or ibuprofen. Tension headaches occur more often in people who are depressed or anxious, so stress management or treatment for depression can help.

Some people have found relief by taking a heterocyclic antidepressant (see p.400), even when they do not have depression. Tension headaches also respond to massage, hot or cold showers, relaxation, proper diet, rest, and exercise.

When a Headache Signals Danger

The vast majority of headaches are not a sign of any serious brain condition. On occasion, however, a headache can be a warning sign of an underlying disorder or serious medical condition that requires immediate medical attention. Call your physician or go to a hospital emergency department immediately if you notice any of the following symptoms:

- The worst headache of your life

- Headaches after age 50 (especially if you usually do not get headaches or the pain is different than you usually have)

- Headache accompanied by a fever, stiff neck, and/or rash

- A different kind of headache in people with human immuno-deficiency virus or cancer

- Headache with numbness or weakness of a limb or visual changes (if such a headache has never happened before)

- Headache that develops after a head injury

- Abrupt, severe headache that reaches its peak within 5 minutes

- Persistent headache that worsens after exertion, coughing, or sudden movement

Cluster Headache

Cluster headaches are among the most severe of all headaches; they cause intense penetrating pain in and around one eye.

Most people with cluster headaches have them episodically—a cluster of one to three headaches a day over a period of weeks or months, alternating with headache-free periods.

About 20% of people have the chronic form, in which daily bouts continue for a year or longer before remission sets in. Chronic headaches are less easily treated by drug therapy than episodic cluster headaches.

There is no known cause or cure for cluster headaches, which can be a lifelong disorder. Although they are excruciatingly painful, there is no permanent harm or link to other diseases. However, intense pain around one eye may also suggest acute glaucoma (see p.435), a condition that requires immediate medical attention.

Cluster headaches predominantly affect men, with the first attack usually striking during adolescence or the early 20s. For people who get cluster headaches, smoking cigarettes and drinking alcohol can trigger attacks during cluster periods but not during remissions.

SYMPTOMS

The typical cluster headache starts suddenly, usually 2 to 3 hours after the person falls asleep. The pain is an intense, steady, burning, penetrating sensation, usually behind one eye but occasionally in the cheek, near the ear, or at some other adjacent site. The affected eye may be teary and bloodshot, the eyelid droopy, the nostril initially stuffy and then runny, and the cheek flushed and swollen.

During a single bout, all symptoms occur on either the left or the right side, never both at once. Most people find that the same side is always affected. After an hour or two, the pain and other symptoms usually recede, sometime as suddenly as they started, only to recur at the same time day after day.

TREATMENT OPTIONS

Pain medicines such as aspirin, ibuprofen, and acetaminophen are not effective against cluster headaches, mainly because they take effect too slowly. Indomethacin, a painkiller and anti-inflammatory drug, is often very effective.

For cluster headaches that occur primarily at night, inhaling oxygen supplied by a tank through a mask for 15 minutes often provides relief. The drug ergotamine, which can be used to prevent attacks as well as relieve pain, is taken as an inhaled spray, oral tablet, or rectal suppository. Other medicines include antihistamines, corticosteroids (see p.895), lithium, or calcium channel blockers.

Migraine Headache

Migraine headaches produce a constellation of symptoms. Characterized by a throbbing pain that starts on one side of the head and may spread, a migraine attack is usually preceded and accompanied by other symptoms (see p.356).

On occasion, the only symptoms of migraine are the symptoms of the aura: the headache itself never materializes.

The physiologic causes are yet to be fully understood. An old theory was that the aura results from an initial narrowing of the arteries that supply blood to the brain, and the headache results from a subsequent widening of these same arteries.

Newer research suggests that abnormalities of the neurotransmitter serotonin (see p.341) or the serotonin receptors on brain cells may be responsible for migraine.

Migraine headaches are more common in women and tend to run in families. The frequency of attacks varies from a few in a lifetime to several per week. A first attack usually occurs after puberty but before age 40. For most people, the intensity and frequency of migraine headaches subside with age. This pattern in women suggests that estrogen, the female hormone, may play a role. However, migraines affect children as well as adults.

Migraines can strike at any time, but onset is common during periods of relaxation after a stressful day. Other triggers include menstruation, fatigue, excessive or insufficient sleep, changes in weather, and exposure to bright light, loud noises, or strong odors.

There are also many dietary triggers, the most common being alcohol (especially red wine),

Alternative Medicine: Migraine

Biofeedback, acupuncture, and relaxation techniques are effective in treating migraines in some people. In some studies, magnesium supplements (approximately 20 millimoles a day) reduced the frequency of migraines. Taking a high dose (400 milligrams) of vitamin B$_2$ (riboflavin) daily also seems to reduce the frequency of migraine attacks.

peanuts, chocolate, aged cheese, the artificial sweetener aspartame, caffeine (in excess or during withdrawal), and fermented foods.

PHASES OF MIGRAINE

There are five well-defined phases of a classic migraine attack: prodrome, aura, headache, termination, and postdrome. You may experience more than one phase, although not necessarily all of them.

Prodrome phase The prodrome phase occurs hours to days before the headache. During this time, about 60% of migraine sufferers experience symptoms. The symptoms can be psychological (such as depression or extreme happiness), neurological (such as enhanced smell or heightened sensitivity to light), or constitutional (such as fatigue, loss of appetite, or increased thirst).

Some people also experience gastrointestinal symptoms such as nausea, constipation, or diarrhea. Although symptoms in the prodrome vary widely, each person usually has his or her own specific set of symptoms that signal a migraine.

Aura phase The aura phase immediately precedes or accompanies an attack. About 20% of migraine sufferers experience neurologic symptoms (the aura), usually developing over 5 to 20 minutes and lasting less than an hour. Migraines with visual disturbances are called classic migraines. The most common aura is flashing lights in a herringbone pattern. Some people see bright lights in other geometric patterns, or half of their visual field is blank.

Others may experience diffi-

culty speaking, weakness on one side of the body, or numbness or tingling in a hand or arm or on one side of the face. The most prevalent form of migraine (common migraine) occurs without an aura. Common migraines typically last longer and occur more often than classic migraines.

Headache phase The typical migraine headache is throbbing, with pain starting on one side of the head and then spreading to both sides. Jabs and jolts of sharp, shooting pain in various areas of the head are common. The onset is gradual, with the pain increasing in intensity for the first 30 minutes to 2 hours, then leveling off and slowly subsiding. The average duration of the headache phase is a day, but it can last for up to 3 days.

In 90% of people, the headache is accompanied by nausea, vomiting, or loss of appetite. Other accompanying symptoms include blurred vision, nasal stuffiness, diarrhea, neck stiffness, memory impairment, and difficulty concentrating.

Termination phase In this phase, pain relief occurs. The pain gradually decreases in intensity over a period of several hours, leaving most people with fatigue and irritability. In many people, vomiting or falling asleep signals the end of an attack.

Postdrome phase The postdrome phase is the period after the pain subsides. During this phase, some sufferers feel drained or irritable, while others are refreshed or euphoric. Some residual symptoms may persist after the pain is gone.

There are several unusual forms of migraine. In familial hemi-

plegic migraine, the aura involves paralysis on one side of the body; the affected person usually has a family member with the same symptoms.

Some people have a migraine aura (such as changes in vision) without headache; this type of migraine is more common in midlife or later. In ophthalmoplegic migraine, the aura includes partial paralysis of the eyes. The most severe form of migraine involves a stroke that occurs in association with the migraine.

TREATMENT OPTIONS

There is no diagnostic test for migraine; the diagnosis is based on your symptoms. In the unusual episodes of migraine that involve temporary loss of brain function (such as partial loss of vision in one eye), other possible diagnoses, such as transient ischemic attack (see p.342), may lead your doctor to order tests.

Although there is no cure for migraine, treatment can reduce frequency, decrease severity, or abort headaches in the prodrome or aura phase. If you think you have migraines, or you experience frequent, disruptive headaches, see your doctor to discuss treatment strategies.

There are two things you can do: prevent or reduce the number of the attacks and cut them short when they occur.

Preventing migraines Try to avoid situations that trigger migraine attacks, such as particular lights, sounds, or odors; changes in humidity or barometric pressure; alcohol; stress; estrogen therapy (30% of women have increased attacks when taking birth-control pills); alterations in eating habits; or eating certain foods (particularly chocolate or foods with nitrate preservatives).

Keep a diary of your headaches, recording what you were doing and the sensations you were having at the time.

Certain prescription medicines can reduce the number of migraine attacks: beta blockers, heterocyclic antidepressants (see p.400), calcium channel blockers, valproic acid, and methysergide (rarely used because of side effects).

There is also evidence that one aspirin every day (not just when you get a headache) can reduce the number of migraine attacks.

Cutting migraine attacks short
As soon as you recognize the signs of a migraine, minimize sensory stimuli. You will probably naturally seek out a dark, quiet room and lie down. Nonprescription pain medicines containing a combination of aspirin, acetaminophen, and caffeine (proved to be effective in treating migraine headaches) are sometimes all that are needed.

Nonsteroidal anti-inflammatory drugs (NSAIDs), including those available without a prescription, work by reducing the inflammation of the cerebral blood vessels. Because pills tend to be absorbed more slowly during migraine attacks, some people prefer to take their medicines in faster-acting forms such as injections, nasal sprays, or suppositories.

Some of the most effective NSAIDs include indomethacin given as a rectal suppository and ketorolac, which is injected under a doctor's supervision.

Ergotamine may also stop a migraine. It can be taken as a pill, injection, suppository, or nasal spray. It is usually taken with an antinausea drug since it may also cause or worsen nausea.

Injections of dihydroergotamine, an ergotamine derivative with few side effects, have been particularly effective for migraines associated with menstrual periods. Because ergotamine (and related drugs) may constrict blood vessels throughout the body, many people with diseases that narrow blood vessels, such as coronary artery disease (see p.652), should not use it. It also is generally not used by

people with high blood pressure, kidney disease, or liver disease, or by pregnant women.

A relatively new group of drugs called triptans—including sumatriptan, rizatriptan, zolmitriptan, and naratriptan—act at a receptor for the neurotransmitter serotonin (see p.341) and can relieve both headache and nausea. They can be taken as pills, injections, or nasal sprays. The first dose is often given under a doctor's supervision to watch for serious side effects.

People with heart disease (particularly related to angina; see p.657), or people who have had heart attacks or who have risk factors for heart attack should generally avoid triptans. If you have high blood pressure that is not under control, triptans could make it worse. Compared to ergotamine, sumatriptan works faster but its effects are not as long-lasting.

Butorphanol, a rapidly acting opiate analgesic, is available by prescription as a nasal spray. Your doctor will monitor the use of butorphanol closely because it is a narcotic and can be addicting.

CANCER

Brain Tumors

A brain tumor is any growth of abnormal cells in the brain or skull. Brain tumors can be malignant (cancerous and likely to spread) or benign (unlikely to spread). Brain tumors of any kind are serious because a growing tumor in the brain does not have to grow too large before it compresses and damages other structures in the brain.

There are two categories of cancerous brain tumor: primary and secondary. Primary tumors start in brain tissue. Secondary brain tumors are cancers that start in another organ, most commonly the lung or breast, and metastasize (spread) to the brain. Secondary brain tumors are more common than primary tumors and occur in 25% of people who have cancer elsewhere in the body.

Brain tumors affect both genders and can occur at any age, although secondary tumors are more common later in life, when all cancers are more likely to develop.

SYMPTOMS

Some brain tumors are discovered when they are still small when they cause a seizure or hemorrhage. Most produce no symptoms until they grow large enough to compress neighboring brain tissue and cause an impairment such as weakness of an arm or leg or difficulty speaking.

Sometimes the only symptom of a brain tumor is a headache, caused by an increase in the pressure inside the skull. A headache in someone who has not tended to have headaches may be the first symptom. On rare occasions, an unexplained change in personality may be the first sign of a brain tumor.

TREATMENT OPTIONS

If untreated, brain tumors can lead to permanent brain damage, and many types are fatal despite the best efforts at treatment. For benign and some malignant tumors, early discovery and treatment offer the best chance of recovery.

To look for a brain tumor, your physician will perform a variety of tests, including computed tomography (see p.149) or magnetic resonance imaging (see p.153), which take pictures of the brain and determine the size and location of any tumors. Since secondary brain tumors develop from cancers in other organs, you may also have radiology tests of other parts of your body.

If surgery is planned, cerebral angiography (see p.147) may also be required to further evaluate the size and site of the tumor. Depending on what your doctor finds, you may be referred to a neurologist, oncologist, or neurosurgeon (see Doctors Who Treat the Brain, p.337).

Surgery to remove some benign and malignant tumors can be successful. However, if the entire tumor cannot be cut out because it is attached to vital brain structures, recurrence is likely. Even when the tumor cannot be completely removed or is incurable, it is sometimes possible to remove a portion of it in order to reduce pressure and relieve symptoms. Computer-assisted surgery (see What Magnetic Resonance Imaging Shows, p.141) has increased the ability of surgeons to remove tumors deep inside the brain that were previously impossible to reach.

Radiation therapy (see p.741) or chemotherapy (see p.741) may also be used. Corticosteroid drugs (see p.895) may be given to reduce the swelling of brain tissue, and anticonvulsant drugs can control seizures related to tumor growth.

Studies are being done to see whether cancer-fighting drugs or radioactive disks placed directly into a tumor are more effective. If the cancer has spread throughout the body, or if a malignancy cannot be cured with surgery and drugs, efforts are directed at relieving symptoms and providing comfort.

Spinal Cord Tumors

Spinal cord tumors are masses of abnormal cells that can grow in the spinal cord itself, between its protective sheaths, or on the surface of the sheath that covers the spinal cord. Benign (unlikely to spread) tumors are more common than malignant (cancerous and likely to spread) tumors.

Most spinal cord tumors are primary (originating in the spine itself), although some start as cancer elsewhere in the body and metastasize (spread) to the spine; these are called secondary tumors. Benign tumors can occur more often in certain families. However, in most cases, the cause of the tumor is unknown.

SYMPTOMS

The most prominent symptom is back pain that worsens as the growing tumor presses against the spinal cord. Other symptoms of spinal cord tumor vary, depending on which part of the spinal cord is affected and whether or not nerves are compressed.

In general, symptoms can include numbness, tingling, or cold sensations in your body; progressive muscle weakness in any arm or leg; and loss of bowel or bladder control.

TREATMENT OPTIONS

If you experience any of these symptoms, your physician will check for other medical conditions that can cause similar symptoms and may refer you to a neurologist (a physician who specializes in disorders of the brain and nervous system). He or she may perform a variety of diagnostic tests, including computed tomography (see p.149) or magnetic resonance imaging (see p.151).

Surgery to remove tumors outside the spinal cord is usually successful, but other tumors may not be able to be removed without significant damage to the spinal cord itself. In these cases, you may receive radiation therapy (see p.741) to retard further growth of the tumor. Surgical removal of parts of the surrounding vertebrae (the bony sections that make up the spine) can also relieve pain and other symptoms by reducing pressure on the spinal nerves.

Corticosteroid drugs (see p.895) may be prescribed to reduce spinal cord swelling. You may need physical therapy to regain muscle strength and control after surgery or radiation therapy.

INJURIES

Concussion

A concussion is a momentary loss of consciousness and brain function that occurs after a blow to the head; unconsciousness may last for seconds, minutes, or hours but recovery occurs within a day. There is no detectable damage to brain structures.

Researchers are not clear as to the nature of the injury in concussion. In most concussions, the damage is mild and may be of little consequence. However, in others there may be a major disruption of brain function.

Doctors grade cerebral concussions on a scale from 1 to 3. A grade 1 concussion usually is not accompanied by loss of consciousness. People with a grade 2 concussion usually lose consciousness for less than 5 minutes; grade 3 concussions typically cause unconsciousness for more than 5 minutes and may produce memory loss for more than 24 hours.

SYMPTOMS

The symptoms of concussion can include headache, nausea or vomiting, and loss of memory. Some symptoms require immediate medical attention. If you feel confused or drowsy, act irrationally, become more and more fatigued, have difficulty speaking clearly, have numbness or paralysis in one part of your body, or notice that one pupil is larger than the other, call your doctor immediately.

During the year after a concussion, some people experience postconcussion syndrome. Symptoms may not appear for hours, days, or even weeks and can include dizziness, headache, fatigue, and insomnia. You may experience a decrease in creativity or motivation—symptoms that may be mistaken for depression.

A typical feature of postconcussion syndrome is a reduced tolerance for alcohol. Personality changes also may occur, and people may become more assertive and less diplomatic than before.

TREATMENT OPTIONS

In diagnosing concussion, your doctor will first rule out a brain hemorrhage (see p.350) and spine injuries. He or she may take x-rays or a computed tomography (see p.149) scan of your head. No treatment for the concussion itself is necessary since symptoms usually go away on their own.

Your physician may recommend that you have someone at home with you for a day or two to watch for any other symptoms that may develop. You will be advised to rest and avoid strenuous activity for several days.

Your doctor may recommend acetaminophen or prescribe a more potent painkiller for headache. You should avoid aspirin and other nonsteroidal anti-inflammatory drugs such as ibuprofen, naproxen, and indomethacin because they can promote bleeding.

Recovery from postconcussion syndrome may come suddenly after a long period of little progress. Recovery typically takes longer in older people and in those who have had a previous head injury. There is no treatment for postconcussion syndrome. Reassurance and support are critical.

Leading Causes of Spinal Cord Injuries

About 10,000 spinal cord injuries are reported each year. According to researchers, another 4,860 people with spinal injuries die before reaching a hospital.

CAUSES	% OF INJURIES
Vehicle collisions	44
Violence (primarily gunshot wounds)	24
Falls	22
Sports	8
Other	2

Spinal Cord Injuries

The spinal cord is protected by rings of bone (vertebrae) but can be injured when the bones are broken or displaced. If many neurons (nerve cells) are damaged, this often leads to loss of sensation or muscle movement. Doctors have not yet learned how to reattach severed nerve endings to make the circuits work again. Without treatment, and sometimes in spite of treatment, damage to the spinal cord can worsen with time; it often takes as long as 6 months to determine how much function a person is likely to recover.

The symptoms of a spinal cord injury depend on the location of the damage. Below the level of the spinal cord injury, the body is paralyzed and left without sensation. Therefore, the higher (or closer to the head) the injury, the more devastating the effect.

Damage to the cervical (neck) area of the spinal cord, for example, can produce quadriplegia (loss of sensation and movement in all four limbs). Damage to the lower back region can cause paraplegia (paralysis of the lower portion of the body and both legs), along with impaired or complete loss of bladder, bowel, and sexual function.

SYMPTOMS

Pain may not be a prominent feature of spinal cord injury, especially if injury has caused loss of sensation. However, intense pain may occur in adjacent areas. The degree of disability depends mainly on the location and severity of the injury.

Weakness, numbness, or

The Two Types of Spinal Cord Injuries

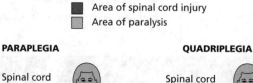
■ Area of spinal cord injury
■ Area of paralysis

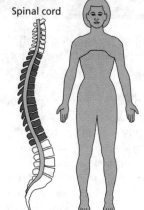
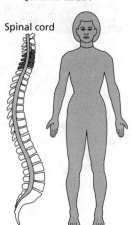

Paraplegia (left) is paralysis of both legs and sometimes part of the torso. Injury is in the middle or lower region of the spinal cord. Quadriplegia (right) is paralysis of the torso, both arms, and both legs. Damage is to the lower neck region of the spinal cord.

How Spinal Cord Damage Occurs

Your spinal cord can be severely injured in many different ways, including compression (such as diving into shallow water), stretching, or tearing (caused by a foreign object or a piece of bone from a vertebra). What often determines if an injury will have permanent effects is the amount of secondary damage, the result of the body's inflammatory response to the injury in the first 8 hours.

Cells in the region of the injury try to fight potential infection and prepare for wound healing by releasing certain chemicals. In the spinal cord, this response paradoxically can be harmful to nerves. The injured area may also swell because of internal bleeding and plasma leaking from injured blood vessels.

Just like the inside of the brain, there is not much room for swelling within the bony cage that surrounds the spinal cord, and pressure can build up quickly. Within a few hours the nerves can start to die. Because nerves that control the breathing muscles can be affected, immediate medical intervention is critical to restore blood flow to the spinal cord.

Restoring Movement to Paralyzed Arms Through Implants

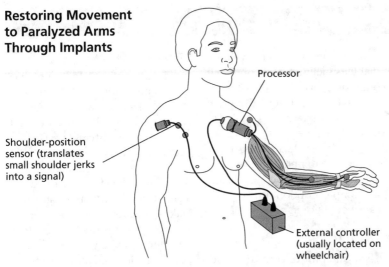

Processor

Shoulder-position sensor (translates small shoulder jerks into a signal)

External controller (usually located on wheelchair)

Most people who have quadriplegia lose the ability to use their hands. An electrical-stimulation hand-grasp system may help, although it has not been tested extensively. The system substitutes for the brain's nerve impulses. Shoulder movements send signals to the sensor and to the processor, which send electricity down wires, giving instructions to the muscles of the hands. Different shoulder movements can cause the thumb and fingers to grasp.

---

paralysis of the muscles may occur immediately below the point of injury or may occur progressively as fluid accumulates near the damaged area.

TREATMENT OPTIONS

The care of a person with a spinal cord injury begins at the site of the accident. Unless the person is in danger, he or she should never be moved; movement can cause further damage to the spinal cord. Life-sustaining measures may be required, such as connection to a respirator to assist in breathing.

Corticosteroid drugs (see p.895) may be injected to reduce swelling and restore blood flow to the injured nerves. An example is a drug called methylprednisolone, which can restore some function when injected within 6 hours of the injury.

Images of the spine, vertebrae, and brain are obtained as soon as

possible, using x-rays, computed tomography (see p.149), and magnetic resonance imaging (see p.151). If pressure on the spinal cord can be relieved within 2 hours of injury, there can be some recovery of spinal nerve function.

Surgery may be necessary to reconstruct fractured vertebrae, to drain the spinal cord of excess fluid, or to remove any fragments of bone or foreign bodies that have been embedded in the spinal cord. Traction is sometimes used to immobilize the body.

The ultimate goals are to treat complications that arise from the injury and plan a rehabilitation program. If the person recovers some sensation or movement within a week, it can be a sign that he or she will recover function fully.

Loss of bladder control is treated with drug therapy, catheterization (insertion of a narrow tube into the urethra to

collect urine), and, sometimes, surgery to create an artificial bladder. Bladder problems leave the individual vulnerable to urinary tract infection, which can be treated with antibiotic drugs.

Physical therapy begins while you are still in the hospital and may continue once you are moved to a rehabilitation center. Physical therapists manually move muscles to maintain muscle tone, avoid atrophy (weakening), and improve circulation. Occupational therapists will teach you how to perform practical tasks and use a wheelchair and will help reorganize your home.

Electrical stimulation (see illustration above), in which electrodes generate electrical impulses, is being used to excite muscles to move in people who have lost function. In addition, scientists are investigating several experimental drugs designed to restore spinal nerve function.

THINKING DISORDERS

One of the most disturbing symptoms a person can experience, or witness in someone else, is a disturbance in the ability to think. Our ability to think is what sets us apart from other living things. One class of thinking disorder is the psychoses (see p.409), in which reality is distorted in bizarre ways. Other kinds of thinking disorders—confusion and delirium, dementia, and Alzheimer disease—are discussed here.

While they can sometime include distortion of reality, these disorders are mainly characterized by an inability to think with normal clarity or speed.

Confusion and Delirium

Confusion is the inability to maintain a coherent stream of thought or action. All of us have periods of temporary confusion. They become abnormal when they last for several hours or longer.

Delirium is a state of confusion that is often accompanied by agitation—increased heart rate, sweating, dilated pupils, trembling, and sometimes hallucinations (see p.409). These changes in mental function superficially resemble those of dementia (see next article), but there are two significant differences: the speed of onset and level of consciousness (see Confusion/Delirium Versus Dementia, right).

Delirium is a medical emergency. It often signals an acute, life-threatening illness (especially in frail elderly people) such as infection, heart attack, heart failure, kidney disease, liver failure,

dehydration, poorly controlled diabetes mellitus, or alcohol or other drug overdose or withdrawal (such as from barbiturates or the antianxiety drugs called benzodiazepines).

Elderly people are especially susceptible to delirium after surgery. Many medicines (including nonprescription drugs) can cause delirium in older people.

SYMPTOMS

The symptoms of confusion and delirium often come on rapidly, over a few days or hours. Consciousness may be clouded, and the person may be drowsy or hyperalert. Symptoms can include restlessness, agitation, trembling, urinary incontinence (see p.826), fear and suspiciousness, hallucinations, and slurred, rambling, or incoherent speech.

The essential abnormality is the inability to focus on one subject or task while keeping other ideas and thoughts from becoming distractions. Alternatively, the person may simply be drowsy or difficult to arouse.

TREATMENT OPTIONS

The doctor will perform a physical examination and ask questions, which may need to be answered by a close friend or relative. Any underlying medical conditions must be treated. If the agitation is severe, antianxiety medicines may be prescribed to calm the person until treatment takes effect. Alternatively, the presence of a supportive relative or friend can be very helpful in dealing with the confusion and agitation.

Dementia

Dementia is a progressive loss of memory and mental capacity that interferes with the ability to function. Although it is more common among people of advanced age, dementia is not an inevitable or normal consequence of aging.

There are several major types of irreversible dementia. Alzheimer disease (see p.363) is by far the most common cause, accounting for up to 70% of cases.

Confusion/Delirium Versus Dementia

Confusion and delirium may be symptoms of dementia but may also be distinct conditions. The differences are outlined below.

CONFUSION/DELIRIUM	DEMENTIA
Often develop abruptly	Develops slowly
Can usually be reversed	Cannot always be reversed
Are of short duration	Persists for many months or years
Consciousness may come and go	Does not affect consciousness
Have a precise time of onset	Has a vague date of onset

The next most common form is vascular dementia, in which abnormalities of blood flow to the brain cause permanent damage. One common kind of vascular dementia (multi-infarct dementia) comes from a series of tiny strokes. Each stroke affects such a small area of the brain that it produces no permanent loss of function (such as loss of strength on one side of the body or problems speaking). However, the accumulation of small infarcts eventually affects enough brain tissue to impair thinking.

The third major cause of irreversible dementia comes from a degenerative disease of the brain such as Parkinson disease (see p.371) or Huntington disease (see p.369).

The fourth, extremely rare, irreversible dementia is caused by an infectious agent called a prion that attacks the central nervous system. The result is Creutzfeldt-Jakob disease, which causes dementia, movement problems, seizures, coma, and death within a year.

Reversible dementias are caused by a variety of conditions that also produce other symptoms besides dementia. Reversible dementias are less common than irreversible dementias; proper diagnosis and treatment may return the person to normal mental function.

Conditions that can cause reversible dementia include depression (see p.395), reactions to some medicines, thyroid disease, vitamin B_{12} deficiency (see p.717), head injury, alcoholism, enlarged brain ventricles (hydrocephalus), and infections (such as Lyme disease, syphilis, or human immunodeficiency virus).

Forgetfulness or Dementia?

Everyone has occasional moments of forgetfulness, regardless of age. Misplacing the car keys, forgetting a name, and other memory lapses seem to occur with greater frequency with age, and many people fear that these lapses are signs of Alzheimer disease or another type of dementia. There are significant differences, however, between normal forgetfulness and dementia.

Normal forgetfulness is neither progressive nor disabling. These memory problems may surface when you are under stress, tired, ill, distracted, or trying to remember too many details at once. The forgotten information is often recalled later. Written reminders and other memory-jogging techniques can be helpful. In dementia, the memory loss is severe enough to interfere with your ability to function in everyday life.

A certain increase in forgetfulness seems to be a normal by-product of aging, perhaps as a result of the gradual loss of myelin and brain cells over a lifetime and the 15% to 20% reduction in blood flow to the remaining cells that occurs between ages 30 and 70. In general, elderly people require more time and effort to learn new information. However, once they learn it, they retain it as well as a younger person.

Brain tumors (see p.357) also can cause dementia, but treating the tumor does not always reverse the dementia.

SYMPTOMS

People with dementia usually experience a decline in intellectual function as well as memory loss. As a result, they may become impaired in judgment, language, performance of complex physical tasks, or recognizing objects or people. These changes occur gradually.

Dramatic and sudden changes in mental abilities are not typical of dementia; they should be brought to your doctor's attention immediately because they can indicate another condition such as delirium, a subdural hemorrhage (see p.352), a stroke (see p.342), or a bleeding brain tumor.

TREATMENT OPTIONS

Since the treatment of dementia depends on the cause, a thorough evaluation is crucial. The doctor will first look for conditions that could cause reversible dementia, performing blood tests and brain scans such as computed tomography (see p.149) or magnetic resonance imaging (see p.151).

See Alzheimer Disease (below) for treatments for irreversible dementia. See also Helping a Person With Severe Dementia (p.367).

Alzheimer Disease

Alzheimer disease is a type of dementia (a progressive, degenerative disease of the brain) that results in memory loss, impaired thinking, and personality change. After the symptoms first appear,

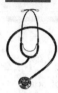

Dementia: *When You Visit Your Doctor*

Your doctor may ask the questions listed here to help diagnose dementia. There are several simple questions that help your physician assess different aspects of thinking and independence. The answers to some of these questions are scored, and the final score is used not only for diagnosis but also to evaluate the disease's effect on quality of life. This can be very helpful in focusing treatment on areas where a person needs help the most.

Questions commonly asked to assess a person's level of function and ability to live independently include those that gauge the person's ability to use the telephone, get to places farther than walking distance, prepare meals, do housework, do laundry, take medicines reliably, and manage money.

For people with more advanced dementia, an assessment is made of the ability to perform the basic activities of daily living such as eating, bathing, dressing, moving about, and controlling urination and bowel movements.

A SIMPLE TEST FOR DEMENTIA

The questions at right help your doctor evaluate mental status. A correct answer to each question or part of a question counts as 1 point. A score of 24 or lower is considered abnormal. The results of this test are not perfect. Some people with low scores are not demented and some with scores above 24, after more extensive testing, are found to have dementia. While the test has proved useful for doctors, its usefulness has not been established when the test is performed by a friend or family member.

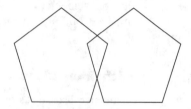

QUESTIONS	TOP SCORE
The person is asked what season, day of the week, year, month, and date it is.	5
The person is asked what state, county, town or city, and hospital he or she is in and what hospital floor he or she is on.	5
The interviewer slowly names three objects (for example, "cat," "boat," and "television") and the person is asked to repeat the names of the objects.	3
The person is asked to subtract 7 from 100, and then subtract 7 from the answer five more times. Or the person is asked to spell "world" backwards.	5
The person is asked to recall the three objects he or she named a few questions back.	3
The interviewer shows the person a pencil and asks him or her what it is.	1
The interviewer shows the person a watch and asks him or her how it is used.	1
The interviewer says: "No if's, and's, or but's" and asks the person to repeat the phrase correctly.	1
The interviewer asks the person to take a paper in his or her right hand, fold it in half, and put it on the floor, giving all three instructions at once. The person gets 1 point apiece for performing each act accurately.	3
The interviewer writes down an instruction (such as "Close your eyes") and the person is asked to read and perform the action.	1
The person is asked to write a sentence.	1
The person is asked to copy the drawing at left.	1

Degenerative Changes in Alzheimer Disease

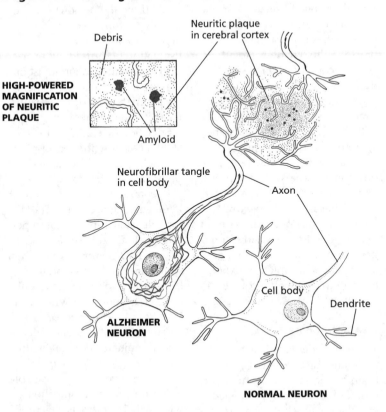

HIGH-POWERED
MAGNIFICATION
OF NEURITIC
PLAQUE

Debris

Neuritic plaque
in cerebral cortex

Amyloid

Neurofibrillar tangle
in cell body

Axon

Cell body

Dendrite

ALZHEIMER
NEURON

NORMAL NEURON

Two abnormalities, which can be seen when the brain is examined under a microscope, are characteristic of the brain damage caused by Alzheimer disease. The first is neuritic plaque, a clump of pieces of dead neurons containing an insoluble substance called amyloid, which is thought to cause much of the nerve cell destruction. The second abnormality is a neurofibrillar tangle, a tightly twisted strand of insoluble proteins inside the nerve cell.

When this protein is not made correctly by brain cells, the cells are damaged, particularly in areas of the brain that are critical for memory and thinking. Several other proteins that are made in brain cells (called presenilins) or are carried to the brain from elsewhere in the body (including a protein called apolipoprotein E4) also can increase the risk of Alzheimer disease, probably through their effects on beta amyloid.

people may live from 2 to 20 years in an increasingly dependent state.

About 4 million Americans have Alzheimer disease, the most common form of dementia. It predominantly affects people over 65 and the risk rises with age. About 10% of people with Alzheimer disease have the early-onset form, which affects people in their 40s and 50s and is inherited.

Great progress has been made in understanding the causes of Alzheimer disease, although this progress has not yet led to breakthrough treatments. A combination of brain cell death and depletion of the neurotransmitter acetylcholine is responsible for the symptoms of Alzheimer disease.

An important cause of cell death is the protein beta-amyloid.

Can Alzheimer Disease Be Prevented?

Some recent studies indicate that the chance of getting Alzheimer disease may be reduced by taking daily doses of nonsteroidal anti-inflammatory drugs. Hormone therapy with Prempro or Premarin does not prevent Alzheimer disease (see p.363). Some studies suggest the herbal therapy, the use of ginkgo, may reduce the chance of getting Alzheimer disease, but the evidence is not strong. In animals with a brain disease like Alzheimer disease, immunization against the beta-amyloid protein caused dramatic reduction in neuritic plaques. One small study of this immunization in humans also reduced the number of plaques and may have improved mental functioning, but side effects stopped the study. Efforts are under way to alter the technique slightly in hopes of achieving the same benefits, without the side effects.

SYMPTOMS

Progressive memory loss is the hallmark of Alzheimer disease. Initially, only short-term memory is impaired, and the person seems merely forgetful. This can interfere with the ability to interact socially and perform work. Long-term memory may be retained, often in great detail, but eventually becomes fragmented as the disease progresses.

Cognitive abilities—the higher "thinking" activities such as reasoning, making decisions, or exercising judgment—become progressively worse. The change may be subtle. A person with Alzheimer disease may do poorly at activities that were once performed well. Poor judgment can lead to accidental injuries.

Early in the disease, people with Alzheimer disease may lose track of time. Later, their disorientation becomes more pronounced and extends to places and people. They may ultimately not recognize members of their own family, or even themselves when they look in the mirror. As time goes on, the person with Alzheimer disease forgets how to perform basic skills such as dressing or eating.

Changes in mood and personality are often the most convincing evidence to families that something is wrong. Depression (see p.395) is common, partly as a result of chemical changes in the brain caused by the disease and partly as a psychological reaction to the loss of mental abilities.

Previously pleasant people can become increasingly withdrawn, irritable, or stubborn. As time goes on, they may become inexplicably hostile, resist care, refuse to give up unsafe activities, shout obscenities, exhibit inappropriate sexual behavior, urinate in unsuitable places, and so on. In some people, these symptoms become worse as the day draws to a close, a condition called sundowning.

It is not possible to predict exactly how Alzheimer disease will affect each person since the symptoms and rate of progression vary widely. Some people develop severe psychiatric problems, while others do not. A symptom can show up early in the disease or not at all. For most people, the decline is slow and gradual over a decade or longer; in rare cases, people can experience a rapid downhill course ending in death within 3 years.

TREATMENT OPTIONS

There is no diagnostic test for Alzheimer disease, short of a brain biopsy (which is only done if other brain surgery is needed) or an autopsy. The diagnosis of Alzheimer disease, in part, involves looking for and ruling out other conditions that can cause dementia, some of which can be treated and cured (see Dementia, p.362).

The diagnostic evaluation includes an interview of the person to determine how well he or she performs daily functions. It also includes a complete physical examination, including a detailed examination of the nervous system and often blood tests. Various techniques for taking pictures of the brain, such as computed tomography (see p.149), magnetic resonance imaging (see p.151), and electroencephalograms (see p.136), may also be used.

Testing often takes more than a day (tests are spread out to avoid tiring the person) and are usually performed on an outpatient basis. It is important that the evaluation be carried out by a doctor (usually a neurologist or geriatrician) experienced in diagnosing Alzheimer disease. Your local chapter of the Alzheimer Association (see p.1229) or a local medical school or hospital can help you find a qualified physician.

Mental status testing is crucial in diagnosing dementia. The doctor will ask the individual to perform mental exercises to assess orientation, memory, comprehension, language skills, and the ability to perform simple calculations (see Dementia: When You Visit Your Doctor, p.364).

Treatment of Alzheimer disease is multifaceted, ranging from lifestyle measures to medicines. There are several drugs available to improve memory in patients with Alzheimer disease: tacrine, donepezil, and galantamine. These drugs increase the amount of the neurotransmitter acetylcholine in the brain. Recently, a different drug, memantine, has also shown modest efficacy. None of these medications slows progression of the disease, nor do they cause dramatic improvement in mental functioning. They yield the best results when used early in the course of the disease. Intensive research is under way to develop drugs that reduce the production of the destructive beta amyloid protein, in hopes that they will both treat and possibly prevent Alzheimer disease.

Studies have found that high doses of vitamin E, and the herbal remedy ginkgo biloba may slow the progress of Alzheimer disease. Medicines can also treat behavioral problems that trouble the person and his or her family.

People with Alzheimer disease should be motivated to remain active, which helps prevent mental decline. This includes participating in regular mental and physical exercise, interacting socially, and ensuring proper nutrition to prevent weight loss. Establishing a daily routine in familiar surroundings may help delay cognitive deterioration.

For people with more advanced cases of Alzheimer disease, more supervision is necessary. People with Alzheimer disease, and the people who care for them, need support. Start by reading Helping a Person With Severe Dementia (below). Also, contact the Alzheimer Association, which helps families cope with the demands of the disease.

Helping a Person With Severe Dementia

If you are giving care to a person with severe Alzheimer disease or another form of dementia, these guidelines may help. See also Caregiving for a Person With Alzheimer Disease or Other Dementia (p.1136).

BATHING

- Follow the person's established routines as much as possible.

- Prepare everything in advance (lay out towels and soap and have the water ready).

- Avoid discussing whether or not a bath is needed. If the person refuses to get into the tub or shower, suggest an alternative

such as a sponge bath. If all else fails, do not force the issue; try again later.

- Be calm, gentle, and unhurried. Many demented people are frightened by bathing. It may help to cover genitals with a towel.

- Encourage the person to do as much as possible without your help. Talk the person through each step.

- Check the skin for rashes and sores and report anything unusual to the doctor.

DENTAL CARE

- Prepare the toothbrush and demonstrate how to get started.

- Try offering a foam applicator (available at drugstores) or a cloth moistened with mouthwash if the person will not brush and refuses assistance.

- Offer apples and other fresh fruit to help clean the mouth if the person refuses to cooperate with toothbrushing.

DRESSING AND GROOMING

- Avoid offering the person choices. Remove clothes that are out of season or seldom worn from closets and drawers. Lay out clothes in the order they are to be put on.

- Select simple clothing the person can manage without assistance; avoid buttons, hooks, snaps, and ties, and be wary of tight-fitting necklines and waists. Choose clothing with large zippers or self-closing fasteners or replace difficult closures with easier-to-use ones.

- Keep in mind the person's past fashion choices and grooming

habits (for instance, a certain hairstyle or if a man has worn a beard in the past). However, modify them to keep grooming simple. Have the person's hair cut in an attractive, easy-to-maintain style.

- Compliment the person on his or her looks—self-esteem remains important.

- Avoid high heels or shoes with slippery soles, pants or dresses that are too long or billowy, and sleeves that are too long or puffy.

MEALTIMES

- Do not give the person too many food choices; playing with food may be a signal the person is faced with too many choices.

- Reduce the person's sensory confusion by making sure the meal area is well lit. Use a plate color that contrasts with the food; remove salt, pepper, and other condiments; and eliminate distractions such as the television.

- Cut food into small, manageable pieces. If the person chokes easily, offer soft foods. Curved spoons, divided plates, and flexible straws can enable the person to feed himself or herself.

- Do not serve foods that are too hot; the person may not be able to sense temperatures.

TOILET NEEDS

- Put a colorful sign or reflective tape on the bathroom door to make it easy to find.

- Dealing with buttons, zippers, or panty hose can be a barrier to using the toilet. Slacks with elastic waists are easier to manage.

- Keep a diary of when the person urinates and moves his or her bowels, and remind him or her at these intervals to use the bathroom.

- Help the person get into a comfortable position on the toilet.

- Restrict fluids 2 hours before bedtime to reduce the chance of wetting the bed at night.

- Use incontinence aids such as disposable briefs and (for men) condom catheters if the doctor has done an evaluation of the incontinence and recommended them.

SLEEPING

- Discourage long naps during the day. An afternoon walk or other exercise may promote a better night's sleep.

- The sleeping area should be kept dim but not dark. Keep a night-light on in the bedroom and bathroom.

OTHER DEGENERATIVE DISEASES

Amyotrophic Lateral Sclerosis

Amyotrophic lateral sclerosis (ALS), also known as Lou Gehrig disease (in honor of the baseball player who died of it in 1941), is a progressive, degenerative disease caused by the destruction of the nerve cells (neurons) in the spinal cord and brain that control the ability to use muscles. ALS is characterized by a gradual weakening and wasting of the muscles and, eventually, complete paralysis.

More men than women are affected by the disease, which affects about 5,000 people in the United States each year and usually starts after age 40. A small fraction of affected people have inherited a defective gene that causes the disease. For others, the cause is not known.

SYMPTOMS

ALS affects the muscles of the legs, arms, face, and tongue (which affects speech), the swallowing mechanism, and, eventually, the person's ability to breathe. It does not affect logical thought; intelligence; touch, taste, smell, hearing, or sight; eye movements; involuntary muscles of the heart, bowel, or bladder; or sexual function.

TREATMENT OPTIONS

Doctors diagnose ALS based on symptoms, physical examination, and laboratory tests. These usually include a nerve conduction study and electromyography (see p.162), which tests the nerves and muscles of the limbs.

There is no cure or good treatment for ALS. The drug riluzole has extended the time before a person requires a machine to assist breathing and the time before a person dies of the disease. Other treatments are being tested.

Multiple Sclerosis

Multiple sclerosis (MS) is an autoimmune disease (see p.870) in which the body mistakenly attacks the substance called myelin, which covers the nerve fibers.

The attack on the myelin can be partially compensated for, causing some symptoms to come and go. However, the attack of the immune system also kills some nerve fibers (axons), leading to permanent loss of function. The word "multiple" represents the multiple areas of scarring (called plaques) that occur from the immune system attack.

No one knows exactly what causes MS or triggers the immune system's response. The disease sometimes runs in families, and researchers have found more than 19 gene regions that contribute to MS susceptibility. They theorize that people who have genes associated with MS may develop the disease years after exposure to a virus or that some other environmental factor triggers the disease.

MS is much more common in women than in men, in temperate than nontemperate climates, and among people of northern European background.

SYMPTOMS

Because MS attacks constantly change and affect different areas of the central nervous system, symptoms vary greatly from one person to the next and in an individual over time. Many people recover completely or nearly completely between attacks, but some suffer progressive loss of function. The first symptoms often affect vision, producing double vision and loss of vision due to optic neuritis (see p.442).

Other common symptoms include tingling or numbness in the limbs. Some people with MS do not have any permanent loss of neurological function but are debilitated by fatigue. Others lose strength in an arm or a leg. In some people the symptoms are mild and in others they are severe. In some, the symptoms come and go, while in others the symptoms are progressive, leading to increasing disability and, sometimes, death.

The most extreme symptoms include complete paralysis of an arm or leg, impaired speech and/or memory, difficulty walking or maintaining balance, tremor, impaired coordination, stiffness, and problems with bowel or bladder control.

TREATMENT OPTIONS

MS can be diagnosed in some people by the symptoms and the results of a physical examination; this is the main basis for a diagnosis of MS. However, other diagnostic tests, such as magnetic resonance imaging (see p.151), evoked potentials (see p.162), and chemical tests of the spinal fluid, can be very helpful.

In others, the diagnosis can be uncertain and remain that way for years. Some doctors do not mention MS is a possibility when the diagnosis is not certain for fear of causing undue concern.

Treatment involves treating the symptoms of an acute flare-up, and using treatments to reduce the frequency of flare-ups. Acute flare-ups of MS are often treated with intravenous

What Happens in Multiple Sclerosis?

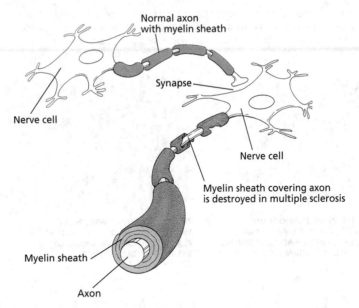

Healthy nerve cells (neurons) transmit electrical impulses to other nerve cells via their tail-like axons (top). The axons are covered with a protective sheath of myelin. The synapse is the place where the impulse passes from one nerve cell to another. In multiple sclerosis (bottom), the body's immune system mistakenly destroys its own myelin, making it harder for the nerve cell to transmit electrical impulses.

and/or oral corticosteroid drugs (see p.895); these medicines can shorten the duration of an attack, but do not change the long-term outcome. Medicines such as baclofen and tizanidine help reduce stiffening of the muscles, which can be severe enough to cause painful, uncontrollable spasms.

Other drugs have been found to reduce the frequency of relapses. Interferon beta-1a is given as injections into muscles and interferon beta-1b and copolymer 1 are given as injections beneath the skin. None of these drugs, however, halts or reverses disability, and they are

effective only in people with mild to moderate conditions. It is not known if these treatments need to be continued for the rest of the person's life.

Support groups are available to help those with the disease and provide the person and his or her family with news about research.

Huntington Disease

Also called Huntington chorea, Huntington disease is a rare, inherited disorder in which a progressive degeneration of nerve cells in the brain results in involuntary, writhing movements

Benefits and Risks of Interferon Beta for Multiple Sclerosis

Treatment with interferon beta can improve the condition of people with the remitting-relapsing form of multiple sclerosis, although it is not a cure and does not work for all people. In about 3 of 10 people, antibodies against interferon beta develop after about 1 year, causing the medicine to lose its effectiveness.

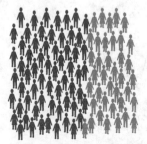

62 OF 100 PEOPLE WHO HAVE MULTIPLE SCLEROSIS AND TOOK INTERFERON BETA HAD WORSENING OF SYMPTOMS DURING A 2-YEAR STUDY

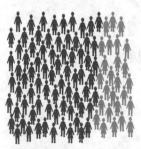

74 OF 100 PEOPLE WHO HAVE MULTIPLE SCLEROSIS AND TOOK PLACEBO HAD WORSENING OF SYMPTOMS DURING A 2-YEAR STUDY

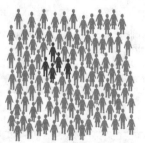

5 OF 100 PEOPLE WHO HAVE MULTIPLE SCLEROSIS AND TOOK INTERFERON BETA PROGRESSED TO SEVERE DISABILITY

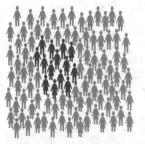

14 OF 100 PEOPLE WHO HAVE MULTIPLE SCLEROSIS AND TOOK PLACEBO PROGRESSED TO SEVERE DISABILITY

(chorea) and mental deterioration.

When one parent has the disease, even if the other does not, a child has a 50% chance of acquiring the disease. Genetic testing (see p.132) can be performed on a fetus to determine if the gene has been inherited.

SYMPTOMS

Symptoms usually begin between ages 20 and 40; they start almost imperceptibly and advance slowly. Vague emotional symptoms may be the first to appear, including irritability, depression, and personality changes. Over time, these cognitive problems progress to dementia (see p.362), with memory loss and failure of other mental abilities.

Physical symptoms soon follow; these include involuntary and random twitches in the face, arms, and trunk. A person with Huntington disease often has unusual facial expressions and walks with a wide, uneven stride.

TREATMENT OPTIONS

There is no cure for Huntington disease. Treatment with medicine such as chlorpromazine or haloperidol can help with the movement and mood disorders but does not stop progression of disease. People with Huntington disease ultimately suffer from complications resulting from the decline in their mental and physical abilities.

Like any person with dementia, they become more prone to infection and illness and become physically weaker and more debilitated because they have problems protecting their respiratory tract from infection and obtaining adequate nutrition through eating.

Neurofibromatosis

Neurofibromatosis is a group of rare genetic disorders that affect the skin and the nervous system and can cause mental retardation. Genetic testing can determine if a person or a fetus carries the gene for neurofibromatosis.

One form is characterized by benign (noncancerous) fibrous growths called neurofibromas that develop on the skin and spinal cord. In other forms, the tumors occur in the eye and other organs and can sometimes be malignant. There are coffee-colored areas called café au lait spots on the skin.

There may also be hydrocephalus (see p.981), scoliosis (see p.622), high blood pressure (see p.644), deafness, cataracts (see p.430), epilepsy (see p.375), and mental retardation, depending on the form of the disease.

Parkinson Disease

Parkinson disease is one of several illnesses that cause parkinsonism, a condition characterized by rigid or slow movements, and tremors. Parkinsonism can be caused by things other than Parkinson disease, such as drug side effects, viral infection, or metal poisoning.

Parkinson disease rarely occurs in people under 30 and becomes more common after age 55. It affects men and women equally.

Parkinson disease results from the death of nerve cells and the depletion of the neurotransmitter dopamine (see p.341) in a small area of the brain called the substantia nigra, which is essential for smooth, normal movement. By the time the symptoms of Parkinson disease develop, at least half of these dopamine-producing cells have died. Symptoms worsen as more cells die.

SYMPTOMS

The first symptoms of Parkinson disease can include listlessness, tremor, or frequent unexplained falls. As the disease progresses, it almost always produces three signs: tremor, rigidity, and bradykinesia (slowness or lack of movement).

The first symptoms may be a subtle tremor when writing—letters appear shaky and become smaller toward the end of a sentence, paragraph, or page. Later, the tremor becomes more apparent, occurring in an arm or leg that is at rest.

Muscle rigidity will be more apparent to a doctor than it is to the person with Parkinson disease. When the doctor bends the person's arm, it will seem to "catch" at regular points throughout its range of motion. This rigidity is caused by the inability of muscles to relax as opposing muscle groups contract. The tension can produce pain in the back, neck, shoulders, temples, or chest.

Bradykinesia slows the pace of walking and eating and makes the face much less expressive.

People with Parkinson disease may sometimes be seen as unfriendly or to have sour personalities because they do not smile or show much emotion; this is because their facial muscles do not allow it. They are no different than most people in appreciating humor and feeling emotion—they simply cannot show it.

Often when people are diagnosed with Parkinson disease, which typically is later in life, they and their friends and family realize that they have had subtle indications of Parkinson disease for many years.

In addition, people with Parkinson disease may develop one or more symptoms that can affect many parts of the body.

Dopamine Production and Parkinson Disease

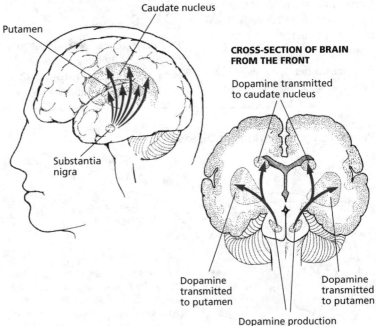

Dopamine is made by cells in the substantia nigra and is transmitted to the caudate nucleus and the putamen, which are the parts of the brain that are critical for creating smooth movement. Parkinson disease destroys dopamine-producing cells, causing less dopamine to be transmitted to the caudate and the putamen, impairing normal, smooth movement.

The following symptoms usually develop gradually (any sudden worsening of symptoms can signal a different underlying problem that may need immediate medical attention):

Gait disturbances Many people develop a walk in which they hunch forward and take small, shuffling steps. They are more likely to lose their balance since they cannot make their muscles move quickly to adjust or correct their position.

Speech The person's speech can lose its tonality and inflection and is gradually replaced by a soft monotone. This is caused by rigidity of the chest muscles, which can no longer force the breath.

Dementia (see p.362) A loss of mental function occurs in 15% to 20% of people with Parkinson disease.

Eye problems Eye movements decrease since the loss of dopamine affects all muscles, including the eye muscles. Less blinking results in dry eye (see p.428) or conjunctivitis (see p.427).

Swallowing Swallowing may be deliberate and slow, creating a buildup of saliva, which causes drooling, and increasing the danger of choking when eating.

Elimination People with the disease are vulnerable to hemorrhoids and constipation due to slower movement of the intestinal muscles.

Sensory illusions Some people experience sensations of unpleasant cold or heat in certain body regions.

Sleep disturbances Sleep problems affect about 70% of people with the disease.

TREATMENT OPTIONS

Parkinson disease is difficult to diagnose early because its onset is so gradual. If you suspect that you have it, ask your doctor to refer you to a neurologist who has extensive experience with the disease. He or she will review your medications (to rule out drug side effects as a cause of the symptoms) and perform a neurologic examination.

Laboratory tests and imaging techniques such as computed tomography (see p.149) or magnetic resonance imaging (see p.151) may be performed to look for the different possible causes of parkinsonism. Positron emission tomography scans show the disease clearly (p.140).

There is no cure for Parkinson disease, but medicines and surgery can be beneficial. A combination of levodopa and carbidopa is the most widely used medicine. This combination supplies the building blocks for dopamine to the brain cells in the substantia nigra. The brain cells use the building blocks to make dopamine.

However, after a while the drug combination becomes less effective. Following a "honeymoon period" lasting an average of 5 years, the response becomes erratic. People often suddenly become as if frozen. They either have great difficulty moving or suddenly have a worsening of excessive and uncontrollable movements. Using lower doses of the levodopa and carbidopa combination may extend the duration of time the medicine works.

Several other drugs (including bromocriptine, pergolide, and the newer medicines tolcapone and ropinirole) enhance the effects of the levodopa and carbidopa combination. However, each has side effects that limit its use. Low doses of the drug clozapine can improve the symptoms of psy-

Pallidotomy for Parkinson Disease

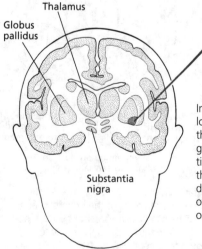

Thalamus

Globus pallidus

Electrode destroys hyperactive cells

Substantia nigra

In Parkinson disease, the progressive loss of dopamine-producing cells in the substantia nigra causes cells in the globus pallidus to become hyperactive. In a pallidotomy, surgeons locate the cells in the globus pallidus and destroy them with an electrode. This often reduces abnormal movements on the opposite side of the body.

chosis (see p.409) that sometimes are caused by levodopa treatment.

For these reasons, physicians disagree over when an affected person should begin taking levodopa. Some prescribe it early and keep the dose low in the hope of extending the duration of the honeymoon period. To keep the dose low, several other drugs are used. Most doctors delay giving levodopa for as long as possible, usually prescribing other drugs for people who have been newly diagnosed and for those with mild symptoms.

Surgery can help people whose symptoms are worsening despite trying all available medicines. One form of surgery (called pallidotomy or thalamotomy) involves destroying a tiny part of the brain, which brings at least partial relief of rigidity, bradykinesia, and tremor in over 90% of people.

Another surgical technique involves placing wires in a particular area of the brain and stimulating that area with a small electrical current. Research is underway to transplant cells from the substantia nigra of miscarried fetuses (or from the person's own adrenal gland) into the brain. These transplanted cells make enough dopamine, at least for a while, to improve symptoms in some people.

There are many practical problems that people with Parkinson disease face every day. People who have the disease and their families can learn valuable information from support groups (see p.1235).

OTHER NERVOUS SYSTEM DISORDERS

Bell Palsy

Bell palsy, also called facial palsy, is a disorder in which damage to the nerve that supplies the muscles of the face causes partial or total paralysis of one side of the face. Inflammation damages the facial nerve, inhibiting its ability to conduct nerve impulses. This nerve also controls some taste sensations and the muscle in the eardrum that dampens loud noises.

The cause of Bell palsy is uncertain, but it may be due to the virus that causes herpes infections of the mouth and genital organs. It affects about 1 of 70 people over the course of a lifetime and usually does not recur.

SYMPTOMS

Symptoms come on suddenly, sometimes preceded by a day or two of pain behind the ear.

About 50% of all people who get Bell palsy have partial or full paralysis of the face within 48 hours, nearly all within 5 days. Symptoms include drooping of the corner of the mouth, flattening of the creases and folds in the skin, and an inability to close the eyelid. The lower lid may also sag, which allows tears to spill onto the cheek.

The paralysis can cause food to collect between the teeth and lips, and saliva may dribble from the corner of the mouth. A heaviness or numbness develops on the affected side, sometimes causing it to ache, but sensation is not lost. Some people are painfully sensitive to loud sounds.

TREATMENT OPTIONS

If you suspect that you have Bell palsy, it is important to see your doctor as soon as possible. Your doctor or a neurologist must examine you to make sure you are not having a stroke (see p.342).

In addition, prednisone, a corticosteroid drug (see p.895), can be given during the first week of symptoms to reduce nerve swelling and relieve pain. Prednisone cannot immediately reverse the symptoms but can decrease the severity of the pain and paralysis and the time to recovery.

About 80% of people with Bell palsy begin to improve within a few weeks and have full function within a few months. If you cannot completely close your eye, your doctor may recommend an eye ointment and a temporary patch to prevent eye dryness and infection.

In some people, injury to the nerve is severe and nerve fibers are irreversibly damaged. Plastic surgery is sometimes performed to correct uneven facial muscles.

Coma

Coma is a state of unconsciousness. It is distinguished from sleep by the inability of the comatose person to awaken (or respond in any way) to noise, touch, or other stimulation. Coma occurs when the areas of the brain that control consciousness (including parts of the brainstem and the cerebrum) are damaged. Coma can result from many different diseases or drugs or from a head injury.

SYMPTOMS

In a light coma, people do not move but can breathe on their own. Some minor responses, such as grunting or blinking, may occur with vigorous stimulation. A person in a deep coma generally does not respond to any stimuli but breathes without assistance. Some automatic reflexes, such as eye movements, can occur in a deeply comatose person if the brainstem is still functioning.

TREATMENT OPTIONS

Treatment involves maintaining vital functions, such as breathing, as well as relieving or reversing the underlying cause of the coma. For example, a person with a head injury may require injections of corticosteroids (see p.895) or other drugs to minimize swelling.

A person can remain in a comatose state for years as long as the brainstem is functioning. If the brainstem is damaged, the person requires help breathing and swallowing.

If a person has been in a coma for 24 hours and the pupils of his or her eyes do not get smaller when a light is shined on them, the outlook is poor. One of 10 people in this condition will survive. It is extremely rare for people who have been in a deep coma for many months or years

to ever come out of the coma. If they do, they almost always have dementia (see p.362) and some kind of paralysis.

Encephalitis

Encephalitis is inflammation of the brain tissue that is usually caused by a virus infection, particularly the herpes simplex virus that causes cold sores. Encephalitis can also be caused by the human immunodeficiency virus (see p.872), a virus transmitted by an insect (as with West Nile virus or equine encephalitis), or an immune reaction after a common viral infection such as mumps or measles.

Sometimes the membranes covering the brain (the meninges) are also inflamed, a condition called meningitis (see p.377). In meningoencephalitis, the meninges and the brain are usually inflamed at the same time.

SYMPTOMS

Symptoms can be very mild—causing only fever and headache (two of the first symptoms) and lethargy. However, severe symptoms such as delirium, abnormal behavior, loss of memory, diminished speech function, clumsy movements, and seizures may also occur.

The affected person may lose consciousness and fall into a coma. When the meninges are affected, the neck may become rigid and the person may shun bright lights. Vomiting, drooping eyelids, crossed eyes, and double vision can also occur.

TREATMENT OPTIONS

If you experience symptoms of encephalitis, see a doctor immediately. A diagnosis of encephalitis is confirmed by magnetic resonance imaging (see p.151), recordings of brain activity through an electroencephalogram (see p.136), and testing a sample of spinal fluid to determine what is causing the encephalitis. The herpes virus can be treated with antiviral medicines such as acyclovir, but other viruses cannot be treated with drugs.

If you have a mild case, your doctor will recommend that you rest and may prescribe corticosteroids (see p.895) to limit brain swelling. The prognosis depends greatly on the type of infection that is causing the encephalitis.

The great majority of people who get encephalitis from the Epstein-Barr virus, the California virus, and the Venezuelan equine encephalomyelitis virus experience a full recovery. On the other hand, encephalitis from the herpes virus often causes permanent injury, even with treatment. Approximately 8 of 10 people who get encephalitis from the eastern equine encephalomyelitis virus have severe and permanent brain damage.

Epilepsy and Seizure Disorders

Epilepsy, a seizure disorder, is a state of recurring seizures. A seizure is a temporary malfunction in the brain that occurs when the usually organized flow of electrical signals is disturbed by a sudden, electrical discharge that disrupts normal brain function.

The result is an immediate

onset of nervous system symptoms including (depending on the type of seizure) disturbed sensations, uncontrollable jerking movements, and loss of consciousness.

Most people with epilepsy can live completely normal lives through the use of medicines.

An estimated 1 million people in the United States have some form of seizure disorder, the vast majority of which began in childhood. Other seizure disorders tend to start after age 60.

Some people with epilepsy have only a few seizures in their lifetime. The average child who experiences one seizure never experiences another. However, an adult who has experienced two seizures has more than a 50% chance of having more seizures.

The causes of epilepsy vary. In two thirds of people, there is no identifiable problem in the brain. One third can be traced to an underlying problem such as brain damage at birth, a tumor, head injury, stroke, or alcohol abuse. Seizures may be provoked by a number of situations, including fever, withdrawal from drugs, sleep deprivation, infection, starvation, dehydration (inadequate fluid intake), injury, flashing lights or intermittent noise, and menstruation.

There are many different types of seizures, but doctors categorize them into two groups: primary generalized seizures and partial seizures. Primary generalized seizures cause loss of consciousness and include grand mal seizures and petit mal seizures (also called absence seizures).

Grand mal seizures cause convulsions; petit mal seizures do

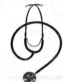

Epilepsy:
When You Visit Your Doctor

ISSUES TO DISCUSS WITH YOUR DOCTOR

■ What are the goals of my treatment? When can I expect to be free from seizures? Could I someday stop taking medicines if my seizures do not recur?

■ Are there activities I should not do because of my epilepsy?

■ When is it safe for me to drive a car? Is it legal for me to drive in my state?

■ How can I decrease my risk of injury from a seizure?

■ Could any of the anticonvulsant medicines I take cause birth defects?

■ If you have had a seizure since last seeing your doctor, describe what you were doing, how long you were unconscious, if you injured yourself, and where you were when you awakened.

TESTS THAT MAY BE PERFORMED PERIODICALLY

■ Blood tests to measure the levels of anticonvulsant medicine you are taking

■ Bone density tests for osteoporosis (if you are a woman and approaching or past menopause)

not. Grand mal seizures usually begin between ages 6 and 12.

In partial seizures (also called focal seizures), the person remains conscious, but there may be disturbances in thinking or mood or uncontrollable jerking movements.

Partial seizures involve only part of the brain but can sometimes spread to other areas of the brain and become secondary generalized seizures. Partial seizures are more likely to indicate a serious underlying brain disorder than generalized seizures.

SYMPTOMS

Secondary generalized seizures are sometimes preceded by an aura, which can include hearing sounds or smelling smells that are not there, abdominal discomfort, or a feeling of pressure in the head.

Generalized grand mal seizures begin with a sudden loss of consciousness. The body is rigid; it can become straight as a rod or even arch backward. A series of jerking movements of the arms, legs, and torso follows, along with clenching of the teeth. Some people have uncontrollable urination or bowel movements. The entire seizure usually lasts no longer than 2 minutes.

After a seizure, the person may feel confused and exhausted for several hours and may have a headache and want to sleep. People do not recall having a seizure, but may remember the aura preceding it.

If several grand mal seizures occur in succession without the person waking up in between, get immediate medical help. This is called status epilepticus and can be life-threatening.

In absence seizures (which occur more often in children), there is a momentary (from several seconds up to 30 seconds) loss of consciousness with no

abnormal movement of the body. Children may be accused of daydreaming during this type of seizure because they stare blankly for a few seconds, unaware of what is happening around them. This type of seizure can be inconspicuous and occur many times a day. The child does not remember the episodes.

Partial seizures usually begin in one part of the brain; symptoms depend on the part of the brain affected. If the seizure remains in only one part of the brain, consciousness may not be lost. If the seizures do not affect the quality of consciousness (for example, if the only symptom is uncontrolled twitching of a body part), they are called simple partial seizures.

If consciousness is affected, they are complex partial seizures. Complex partial seizures may produce abnormal behaviors such as anger, laughter, or picking at cloth for no apparent reason. Complex partial seizures were once (inaccurately) called temporal lobe seizures or psychomotor seizures.

TREATMENT OPTIONS

The diagnosis of a seizure is often obvious. With partial seizures, particularly those that involve the temporal lobe and odd behavior, the diagnosis may be more difficult. Your doctor will order an electroencephalogram (see p.136), which can show an underlying instability in the electrical activity of the brain.

Even when the diagnosis is clear, the cause of the seizures may not be, and the doctor will use computed tomography (see p.149) or magnetic resonance imaging (see p.151) to look for a tumor or other abnormality.

Treatment of seizures may include anticonvulsants (medicines that reduce the tendency of the brain to have seizures). The older anticonvulsant medicines, used for many years, include phenytoin, phenobarbital, carbamazepine, and valproic acid.

Many newer drugs have become available, including gabapentin, lamotrigine, felbamate, and topiramate. These newer medicines are used mainly to treat partial seizures that are not well controlled by one of the older drugs. Treatment with one medicine at a time is preferred to minimize side effects.

For people who still have frequent seizures despite taking

How to Help Someone Who Is Having a Seizure

Seizures look frightening but are not usually harmful. The person may cry out just before the seizure occurs. Stay calm and follow these steps:

■ If the person is in immediate danger (such as in the street), get him or her to a safe location. Otherwise, do not move the person.

■ Move furniture and other objects out of the way so the person does not harm himself or herself.

■ Do not restrain the person or put anything into his or her mouth.

■ Ensure that the person can breathe during the seizure (see Breathing Difficulties, p.1198). Turn the person on his or her side, so that vomit will not collect in the windpipe and cause choking.

■ Stay with the person until the seizure is over (most seizures last less than 2 minutes).

■ Afterward, the person may appear disoriented or sleepy. If he or she does not awaken, have someone get help or call 911 or your local emergency number.

■ If the seizure lasts longer than 2 minutes or another seizure begins, it is a medical emergency; call 911 or your local emergency number.

medicines, a new treatment called vagus nerve stimulation is gaining popularity. A small box, similar to a cardiac pacemaker (see p.679), is placed under the skin. Every few minutes it sends an electrical current to the vagus nerve, which reduces the frequency of seizures in some people.

In a few people, neither medicines nor the box can control the seizures. Surgery may be necessary to cut away small areas of the brain where the epileptic discharge starts, or to cut the nerves connecting one half of the brain to the other in order to prevent the spread of a seizure. Such surgery is performed mainly in a few specialized centers around the country.

Guillain-Barré Syndrome

Guillain-Barré syndrome develops from inflammation of the myelin sheath that covers nerve fibers. It causes weakness that usually starts in the legs, and then moves rapidly, over a period of days, up the body to cause weakness in the arms and, sometimes, in the muscles of the chest, preventing breathing. It can also cause pain and tingling sensations. The symptoms can be mild or severe; muscular paralysis can be life-threatening.

The cause of Guillain-Barré syndrome is not known, although doctors think it is related to the immune system's reaction to a viral or bacterial infection. It can also occur after a tick bite and in people infected with the human immunodeficiency virus.

The syndrome usually develops several weeks after an apparent infection, such as after a cold, cough, or a bout of diarrhea. It is believed that the same antibodies fighting the infection mistakenly attack the nerve sheath as well (see Autoimmune Diseases, p.870), which leads to the damaging inflammation. Guillain-Barré syndrome is uncommon, affecting fewer than 4,000 people each year.

Gamma globulin, which consists of antibodies that block the disease-causing antibodies, may be used to treat the disease. Plasmapheresis, which can filter harmful antibodies from your blood similar to the way a kidney dialysis machine filters blood (see p.815), may be performed to decrease the severity and duration of symptoms.

In severe cases, a breathing machine may be required, and a feeding tube may be used to provide nutrition. Most people completely recover movement and sensation within weeks to months.

Meningitis

Meningitis is inflammation of the meninges, the three membranes that encase and protect the brain and spinal cord. Meningitis is most commonly caused by infection with a virus or bacteria.

Infection usually originates in another part of the body and travels via the bloodstream to the meninges. Infection can also spread directly from the sinus cavities or ear to the brain.

Viral meningitis is the more common and milder form, affecting primarily children. Bacterial meningitis is a medical emergency; it is fatal if not diagnosed and treated.

SYMPTOMS

The symptoms of viral and bacterial meningitis are similar but differ in their severity and the rate at which they progress. Symptoms include fever, nausea, vomiting, severe headache, aversion to light, and a stiff neck.

Viral meningitis causes mild symptoms and clears up on its own within a week. Bacterial meningitis is more severe and can develop within a few hours. Severe neck pain and stiffness, particularly when touching the chin to the chest, can be followed quickly by confusion, loss of consciousness, and death.

TREATMENT OPTIONS

If you suspect that you or your child has meningitis, see a doctor immediately. He or she may perform a lumbar puncture (in which a sample of spinal fluid is extracted through a needle inserted into the lower back) to identify the cause.

Viral meningitis does not require treatment. Bacterial meningitis requires immediate treatment with antibiotics given by intravenous injection. Vaccinations against one bacterium, *Haemophilus influenzae,* has dramatically reduced attacks of meningitis by that bacterium.

In people whose immune systems are impaired (such as people with acquired immunodeficiency syndrome or cancer, or recipients of transplanted organs), meningitis may be caused by fungus infections or parasites.

Myasthenia Gravis

Myasthenia gravis is a rare autoimmune disorder (see p.870)

The Meninges: Protection for Brain and Spinal Cord

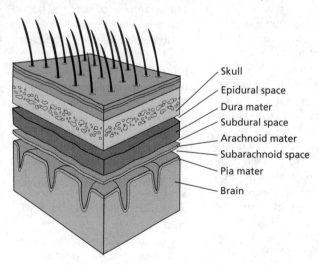

Skull
Epidural space
Dura mater
Subdural space
Arachnoid mater
Subarachnoid space
Pia mater
Brain

The meninges are three membranes that encase the brain and spinal cord. The dura mater lines the skull and encircles the spinal cord. The arachnoid mater forms the middle layer, lying atop the subarachnoid space, which is filled with the cerebrospinal fluid. The innermost membrane is the pia mater, a thin layer covering the brain itself. When the meninges become inflamed (often due to infection), the condition is called meningitis.

affecting muscles. A muscle normally contracts when it receives a message from a nerve. The chemical that delivers the message is called acetylcholine, and the muscle receives the message by a receptor for acetylcholine on the surface of the muscle cell. In myasthenia gravis, the immune system mistakenly makes antibodies that attack these receptors. As a result, the muscles do not receive the message to contract, and they become weak.

The weakness is particularly great in muscles of the face, arms, and legs. Myasthenia gravis affects women more frequently than men. In women, it usually occurs between 20 and 30; in men, it tends to start after age 50.

SYMPTOMS

Myasthenia gravis does not follow a predictable course. It can unfold gradually or progress quickly. It is a disease of acute periods (flare-ups) followed by periods of complete recovery (remissions).

Muscles tire abnormally quickly. For example, repeated attempts to hold a heavy object result in the grip becoming progressively weaker. Most people also notice weak, droopy eyelids and double vision because the muscles that move the eyes are also weak.

Weakness can also occur in the face, throat, voice, and neck muscles, which creates difficulty speaking (such as slurred speech) and eating or swallowing (caus-

ing choking or coughing). Some people have weak arms and legs. Severe myasthenia gravis can cause weakness in the muscles that control breathing. Certain conditions—such as menstruation, stress, or infections—can cause flare-ups.

TREATMENT OPTIONS

See your physician if you have symptoms of myasthenia gravis. He or she will examine you and may perform blood tests to look for the autoimmune antibodies that cause the disease. A further test for diagnosis involves injection of edrophonium, which increases the level of the neurotransmitter acetylcholine at the nerve/muscle junction, and temporarily improves muscle strength. Electromyography (see p.162) is also usually used to help make the diagnosis.

Treatment depends on the severity of the disease. In mild cases, symptoms can often be controlled (and most function can be restored) with long-acting medicines such as pyridostigmine.

People with more severe illness may be helped by removal of the thymus gland, which directs the damaging autoimmune attack. Removing the gland can bring about permanent remission.

High doses of corticosteroid drugs (see p.895) help reduce inflammation and slow the immune system's attack. Other drugs that dampen the immune system are also used; in severe cases, plasmapheresis (in which harmful antibodies are filtered out of your blood) may be required.

Neuralgia

An irritated or damaged nerve can produce periods of pain that vary in intensity; this nerve pain is neuralgia. Often described as a stabbing, burning, or shooting pain, neuralgia has many possible causes, ranging from injury to infection.

Neuralgia caused by herpes zoster, the virus that causes chickenpox and shingles, is called postherpetic neuralgia (see Shingles, p.537). Glossopharyngeal neuralgia is located in the throat, ear, and back of the tongue. Speaking, swallowing, or eating may trigger pain.

Other forms of neuralgia are trigeminal neuralgia (pain in the face) (see p.1119), occipital neuralgia (pain in the back of the head), intercostal neuralgia (pain between the ribs), and the neuralgia associated with migraine headaches.

In many cases, the source of pain is not known. Treatment, usually with over-the-counter painkillers such as aspirin or acetaminophen, may control the pain, but other medicines, such as certain anticonvulsants and antidepressants, may be very helpful. In rare cases, surgical destruction of the affected nerve may be needed to relieve severe and unremitting pain.

Peripheral Neuropathy

Peripheral neuropathy involves damage to the peripheral nerves, the extensive network of nerves that links your brain and spinal cord to the rest of your body. The causes of peripheral neuropathy are numerous (see Common Causes of Peripheral Neuropathy, right), ranging from alcoholism to diseases such as diabetes mellitus to exposure to certain toxic chemicals. Some inherited conditions also produce progressive neuropathy.

SYMPTOMS

Symptoms of peripheral neuropathy vary depending on the site and extent of nerve damage. Almost all forms begin with mild tingling and progress slowly over months or years to numbness. Numbness of the feet, which is a very common and serious problem in people with diabetes, puts you at risk for serious infection or injury because you are unable to feel bumps, bruises, or early symptoms of infection. Most often, the symptoms affect the feet and lower legs; however, other parts of the body can also be affected.

Damage to the peripheral nerves can also cause blurred vision, low blood pressure, difficulty urinating, an enlarged stomach, intestinal cramps, and impotence (see p.1092).

TREATMENT OPTIONS

If you have any symptoms of peripheral neuropathy, see your doctor, who may refer you to a neurologist. Tests may be done to determine the cause of your peripheral neuropathy, if it is not already known. If your doctor is uncertain about whether you have peripheral neuropathy, an electromyogram (see p.162) can help.

Medicines can treat the pain or decrease other symptoms; the most commonly used are heterocyclic drugs (see p.400). Controlling or reversing the underlying condition can slow the progression of symptoms or may result in permanent cure.

Polio and Postpolio Syndrome

Polio (more correctly called poliomyelitis) is a viral infection that can attack the brain and spinal cord, causing permanent paralysis and death due to paralysis of the muscles that control breathing.

Once easily transmitted and widespread among young children, polio is now extremely rare in developed nations due to the development of the polio vaccine in the 1950s. However, polio still occurs in developing countries where standards of hygiene are lower and vaccina-

---

Common Causes of Peripheral Neuropathy

Damage to the peripheral nerves can result from many conditions. The following are some of the more common causes:

- Alcoholism
- Diabetes mellitus
- Malignant tumors
- Uremia (see End-Stage Kidney Failure, p.814)
- Vitamin B_1, B_6, or B_{12} deficiency
- Lead poisoning
- Periarteritis nodosa (see p.902)
- Hypothyroidism (see p.848)
- Guillain-Barré syndrome (see p.377)

tion is not as common. If you are traveling to a developing country, ensure that you have been vaccinated.

Postpolio syndrome is the rare recurrence of symptoms in people who had fully recovered use of their weakened or paralyzed muscles.

SYMPTOMS

The first symptoms of polio—headache, fever, vomiting, and sore throat—can easily be mistaken for a bad case of flu. After a few days, muscle weakness begins, often affecting the legs and lower trunk. The most serious consequence of polio is infection of the brainstem, which controls the muscles that regulate breathing. If breathing stops and the person is not connected to a machine that supports breathing, the person will die.

TREATMENT OPTIONS

Polio vaccination is given during infancy to produce immunity throughout life. There is no drug that can kill the polio virus. Treatment of paralysis depends on the muscles that are affected. Damage to paralyzed muscles can be prevented with physical therapy.

More than 50% of people who are paralyzed recover completely, and less than 25% suffer lifelong disability. Doctors treat postpolio syndrome with gentle physical therapy.

Rabies

Rabies is a serious virus infection of the nervous system, including the brain and spinal cord. Rabies usually affects animals, but it can be spread to humans by an animal bite, or a scratch if the animal's saliva (which contains the virus) enters a break in your skin.

Rabies infects the nerve endings in the skin, and then spreads up the nerves to the brain. It is almost always fatal if it is not treated immediately. It is vital to receive medical attention as soon as possible after coming into contact with the saliva of any wild animal.

In the United States, skunks, raccoons, and bats are the primary carriers. Most dogs are vaccinated against rabies, but unvaccinated dogs can be infected by a wild animal, such as a skunk, and then bite and infect humans.

SYMPTOMS

The symptoms of rabies may not appear for up to 7 weeks after an animal has bitten you. Symptoms include stiff neck and seizures, and you may become anxious and disoriented. Any attempt to drink fluids causes the characteristic symptom of rabies—hydrophobia ("fear of water"). If you attempt to drink, your throat muscles go into spasm and cause gagging and choking. Once symptoms occur, death usually follows within 3 days to 3 weeks.

TREATMENT OPTIONS

Any animal bite should be considered a medical emergency; wash the area with soap and water and see your doctor immediately. Your doctor will start treatment to prevent the development of rabies, if necessary.

First, you will be given antirabies antibodies through shots injected around the animal bite and in the buttocks. Next, you will receive the first of five shots of a rabies vaccine in your buttocks. The rest of the five shots will be given in your arm over the course of 4 weeks. These shots can be quite painful but may save your life.

If possible, the animal should be caught and brought to your doctor. The animal may be killed to examine its brain for evidence of rabies. Sometimes the animal is observed at the same time you are getting the vaccine shots. If the animal shows no symptoms of rabies, the injections are stopped.

Pets should be vaccinated regularly to reduce their chance of acquiring rabies and transmitting it to their owners.

Tics

A tic is a repetitive, involuntary movement that usually affects the muscles of the face or shoulder. Typical tics include eye twitches, shoulder shrugging, and mouth spasms.

Tics often develop during childhood, usually before age 10, and result from minor psychological disturbances. Boys are more commonly affected than girls. Stress can also trigger tics in children and adults. Tics usually resolve on their own by adulthood, but may continue throughout life.

Tourette syndrome is a disorder of the brain characterized by multiple tics, uncontrollable noises, and sometimes cursing. A person with Tourette syndrome may suddenly bark, noisily clear his or her throat, or loudly utter a swear word.

A neurologist will look for and treat potential causes of any tic disorders. Sometimes tic disorders run in families with obsessive-compulsive disorder (see p.404). Medicines such as benzodiazepines, clonidine, heterocyclics (see p.400), and selective serotonin reuptake inhibitors (see p.400) are sometimes used to control severe tics.

Trigeminal Neuralgia

Trigeminal neuralgia, also called tic douloureux, is a disorder of the fifth cranial nerve (trigeminal nerve). It causes severe piercing pain in the lips, gums, cheeks, or chin on one side of the face. The periods of intense pain can be disabling and can last from several seconds to several minutes. The condition usually affects people over 45.

The pain of trigeminal neuralgia may be triggered by touching a certain area of the face or for no apparent reason. Although the underlying cause of the condition cannot always be determined, there is good evidence that viruses (particularly the herpes simplex virus) can infect the nerve and a blood vessel can push on the nerve, both of which can irritate the nerve and cause pain.

Treatment includes painkillers and sometimes anticonvulsant drugs. For people with severe and recurring pain, surgery to move the blood vessel off the nerve, or to actually destroy the nerve, may be performed.

Chronic Fatigue Syndrome

Chronic fatigue syndrome is a condition that involves the sudden onset of severe fatigue and other symptoms. The symptoms of chronic fatigue syndrome must last for at least 6 months and seriously interfere with a person's ability to function for a diagnosis to be made.

Other symptoms (which must also persist for at least 6 months to make the diagnosis) include memory impairment, sore throat, swollen lymph glands, headache, aching muscles and joints, and disrupted sleep. There must also be extreme worsening of symptoms after exertion. Finally, there must be no evidence of a large number of illnesses that can cause fatigue.

The cause of chronic fatigue syndrome is not known. There is evidence that mild, nonpermanent abnormalities occur in the brain, and that there is a low level of activation of the immune system. About half of all people with this illness also experience a psychiatric illness, typically starting after the symptoms of the illness have begun.

There is no diagnostic test for chronic fatigue syndrome, although a large number of tests have been found to be abnormal more often in people with the illness than in people who are healthy. Because this illness has been identified only in recent years, few treatments have been studied, and no medicine has proved to be beneficial.

Cognitive behavior therapy (see p.393) can improve the ability of people to cope with the illness, and various medicines provide symptomatic relief. Light, regular exercise may be beneficial.

What Causes Dizziness?

Dizziness is a term with multiple meanings. It may refer to vertigo (an illusion of motion, such as spinning), a feeling that you are about to pass out (lose consciousness), an instability in walking, or a vague sense of light-headedness. Read the symptom chart Dizziness (see p.177) to learn what disorders can cause dizziness.

Chronic Pain

Chronic pain is pain that lasts at least 6 months and does not respond well to medical treatment. Pain starts with some unpleasant stimulus, such as a joint deformed by arthritis.

The grinding of bone against bone stimulates pain fibers, which send signals to the spinal cord, up the spinal cord to the thalamus in the brain, and then on to the cerebral cortex (see p.338).

At all points along the way, the pain signal is enhanced by certain natural substances (such as substance P) and inhibited by other substances (such as endorphins).

It is in the cortex and limbic system of the brain that the mind reacts to pain. When the sensation of pain generates anxiety, the anxiety amplifies the pain.

Attempts to control chronic pain involve treatments designed to block pain in the nerves in the spinal cord itself and in the nerves in the thalamus and cortex leading to the spinal cord. Unrelieved pain can create a cycle of anxiety, helplessness, and sleep deprivation that can make you demoralized and depressed.

Here are some traditional and some experimental options for pain relief:

Acupuncture is an ancient Chinese technique in which fine needles are inserted into the skin at specific places. Acupuncture has been used to treat a variety of painful conditions, including migraine (see p.355) and back pain (see p.621). It is thought to work by stimulating natural substances in the spinal cord that reduce the intensity of pain. It is important that you find a practitioner who has been trained and who uses packaged, sterile needles.

Anesthetic drugs given in very small amounts in a slow and steady fashion can help people with severe chronic pain. These

---

A Narcotic Lollipop for Severe Pain

People who have severe pain can experience pain that "breaks through" the effects of their painkilling medicine. When this occurs, they need more painkilling medication that acts quickly. If intravenous drugs are not readily available, they can lick a lollipop that contains a narcotic drug to get fast relief. These lollipops must be kept away from children.

---

medicines include lidocaine and mexiletine given as ointments or patches.

Analgesic drugs, or painkillers, play an important role in relieving chronic pain. Aspirin and other nonsteroidal anti-inflammatory drugs are highly effective. Opiate-related compounds such as codeine and morphine also relieve pain but can lead to dependence and even addiction. These drugs work by reducing the pain signal both in the spinal cord and in the brain.

Devices that permit people with severe pain to inject small intravenous amounts of opiate pain medicines when they need it (patient-controlled analgesia) are more effective than taking opiate medicines on a regular schedule; the person also uses less medication.

Antidepressant drugs are sometimes prescribed for pain relief. They may be effective because they increase the supply of the neurotransmitter serotonin, which helps activate the body's natural pain-relief system.

Anticonvulsant drugs such as carbamazepine are prescribed to relieve the pain of conditions caused by damaged nerves.

Behavior modification (see p.394) aims to change the habits, behaviors, and attitudes that can develop in people who have chronic pain.

Biofeedback (see p.395) has been used with success to treat many types of pain.

Corticosteroid drugs (see p.895) help reduce pain in people with bone cancer.

Nerve blocks involve injecting a substance that temporarily or permanently blocks a nerve as it enters the spinal cord.

When pain is coming from one place in the body and is carried by one or a few specific nerves, blocking those few nerves can eliminate pain for a while. However, within a year, pain returns in about half the people who undergo the treatment.

Placebo effect is thought to be a neurosubstance (brain substance) response that results from the belief that pain relief is actually taking place. An estimated 35% of people receiving a placebo experience positive effects.

Psychotherapy (see p.393), particularly cognitive behavioral therapy (see p.393), can help people understand the symbolic meaning of their pain, and achieve new realizations about ways of coping with it.

Relaxation and meditation therapies (see p.90) teach individuals how to relax muscles, relieve anxiety, and disrupt the cycle of pain, anxiety, and tension.

Surgery relieves pain by cutting the nerves that send pain messages to the brain. It may also result in a loss of sensation or movement. In some instances, pain returns. Some procedures use heat or cold treatments to destroy tissue.

Surgically implanted electrodes are placed in the brain to release natural opiates (painkillers). Good results have been reported with this experimental method.

Transcutaneous electrical nerve stimulation is a method of applying pulses of electricity to the skin over pain sites. The electrical stimulation triggers a natural reaction in the spinal cord that lessens the pain. (If you have ever rubbed an injured area anywhere on your body to relieve pain, you have stimulated the same natural pain-relieving reaction in the spinal cord.)

Responses vary, depending on the condition, but some people obtain complete pain relief. A similar technique, called dorsal column stimulation, involves

placing a small electrical transmitter under the skin, with a wire leading to the spinal cord.

SLEEP AND SLEEP PROBLEMS

Dreams

Dreams are images created by mental activity during sleep. Dreaming occurs during rapid eye movement (REM) sleep, which has been described as a "hyperactive brain in a paralyzed body." The brain races, thinking and dreaming as the eyes dart back and forth rapidly behind closed eyelids, but the muscles that control movement of the head, arms, and legs are still. Body temperature rises. The penis or clitoris becomes erect. Blood pressure increases, and heart rate and breathing speed up to daytime levels.

Just as deep sleep restores the physical body, scientists believe that periods of dream sleep restore the mind, perhaps by clearing out irrelevant information. In fact, REM sleep is necessary to feel rested.

Nightmares and Sleep Terrors

Nocturnal attacks of fear or panic interrupt sleep in some people. Nightmares, which usually occur early in the morning, are bad dreams that become so threatening that you awake in a state of fear or agitation. Like all dreams, nightmares occur mainly during rapid eye movement (REM) sleep. When people are able to

recall nightmares, the terrifying plots often incorporate elements of their lives.

Bad dreams can be induced by medicines, including antihypertensives, antiarrhythmics, corticosteroids (see p.895), and drugs that affect neurotransmitters.

Sleep deprivation or withdrawal from alcohol, stimulants, sedatives, or anticonvulsants may also bring on frightening dreams.

In a sleep terror, the sleeper may scream, sit bolt upright, and attempt to fight or run. During an episode, which may last as long as 15 minutes, the person may seem confused and agitated. After the spell is over, the person is likely to fall back to sleep and forget what happened.

Sleep terrors usually occur in the first hour after going to sleep. They appear to run in families, and affect children more than adults. Adults with sleep terrors tend to be more agitated, anxious, and aggressive than children who have sleep terrors. Episodes can involve violent or injurious behavior.

Treatment is not always necessary, but psychiatric evaluation can be helpful. Some doctors prescribe medicines, such as benzodiazepines, which suppress deep sleep. Hypnosis (see p.394) helps some people.

Insomnia

Insomnia is difficulty falling asleep, unwelcome awakenings during the night, fitful sleep, and the resulting daytime drowsiness. Although it is the most common sleep disturbance, insomnia is not a disorder, but a symptom like fever or pain. Over the course of a year, up to 40% of adults have periods of insomnia.

Doctors label it transient insomnia if it lasts only a few days, short-term insomnia if it continues for a few weeks, and chronic insomnia if the problem persists. The causes of transient and short-term insomnia are usually apparent to the sufferer—the death of a loved one, anxiety about an upcoming event, jet lag (see p.385), or discomfort from illness or injury.

The most common form of sleeplessness is called learned insomnia. After experiencing a few sleepless nights, some people become very apprehensive about whether they will be able to sleep. They also feel sleepy in the daytime, which sets up several vicious cycles. First, they try to wake up by drinking coffee. Since the effects of coffee can last up to 16 hours, drinking coffee after 10:00 AM can interfere with sleep later that night.

Some people try to induce sleep by having an alcoholic

How Much Sleep Do You Need?

Most adults sleep 7 to 8 hours a night. After age 60, people tend to spend a little less time sleeping. Studies have shown that people who regularly sleep fewer than 4 hours or more than 9 hours a night do not live as long as people who sleep an average of 4 to 9 hours a night. However, it is not known if these people would improve their life expectancy if they forced themselves to sleep more or less.

drink before bedtime. But while drinking alcohol can make you sleepy initially, within a few hours it will disrupt sleep. Also, a nightcap can cause a poor quality of sleep.

Finally, after a few sleepless nights, some people feel so tired that they skip exercise. Since exercise improves the quality of sleep, this only compounds the problem.

TREATMENT OPTIONS

For people with chronic insomnia, lifestyle modification is usually recommended. An evaluation by a sleep expert (ask your doctor for a referral) can help identify habits that keep you awake at night. Once your problem has been identified, your doctor may suggest one or more of the following solutions:

Sleep restriction People with insomnia often find that spending less time in bed promotes more restful sleep. Some sleep experts recommend beginning with 3 or 4 hours of sleep. If the alarm is set for 7:00 AM, a 4-hour sleep restriction means that, no matter how sleepy you are, you must stay awake until 3:00 AM. Once you are sleeping well during the allotted hours, add another 15 or 30 minutes until a healthy amount of sleep is achieved. Once you have accomplished this, try to go to bed and wake up at about the same time every day, 7 days a week.

Reconditioning With this approach, you train your body to associate bed with sleep instead of sleeplessness and frustration. You should use your bed only for sleeping or sex, and go to bed when you are sleepy. If you are unable to sleep, get up and go to another room. When you are sleepy again, return to bed. You should also get up at the same time every day and not nap.

Relaxation techniques (see p.90) These help some people unwind. In biofeedback, immediate feedback from equipment makes you aware of involuntary body states, giving you insight into how various thoughts or relaxation maneuvers affect tension, and enabling you to gain voluntary control over the process.

Medicines can help with sleep problems, but sometimes only for a short time. Benzodiazepines can be helpful if taken only occasionally or for a few weeks at a time. If used for longer periods, they may become ineffective. The same is true of barbiturates. However, because they produce more dangerous side effects, barbiturates are prescribed much less often.

In 2004 the FDA approved a new sleeping agent, eszopiclone. Not a benzodiazepine, this agent appears safe for chronic use and for use by the elderly. Another similar agent, indiplon, is awaiting approval by the FDA.

Heterocyclic antidepressants (see p.400) can help you spend more hours in deep sleep each night, and their effect does not wear off after a few weeks. Other antidepressant drugs, such as

Is Melatonin Safe?

Humans make melatonin each night. Synthetic forms of this hormone have been studied and, in some cases, found to improve sleep. This and a long list of other benefits have been touted by melatonin manufacturers.

Because melatonin is classified as a dietary supplement rather than a drug, its manufacture is unregulated. As a result, there are no standards for quality, purity, or dosage, and its safety cannot be guaranteed.

Some melatonin manufacturers employ rigorous standards. However, it can be difficult to identify the manufacturer of a product, since the name on the label is usually that of the distributor. If you are considering trying melatonin, ask your physician for his or her opinion.

selective serotonin reuptake inhibitors (see p.400), can worsen the quality of sleep.

Drugs called imidazopyridines help enhance the sleep-inducing activity of the neurotransmitter gamma-aminobutyric acid. Occasionally, people have paradoxical sleep reactions to "sleep" medicines, though it is not understood why some people have more trouble sleeping when taking medicines that help most people sleep.

Melatonin is a hormone produced by the pineal gland each night. The gradual fading of daylight triggers the production of melatonin, which regulates the sleep-wake cycle. Among the many claims for the synthetic form of this product is improved sleep. Some studies have found that melatonin may help sleep problems in the elderly, and may help adjustment to jet lag. However, the Food and Drug Administration has not approved melatonin as a treatment for insomnia.

Jet Lag

Many people who cross several time zones find that light and other environmental cues disrupt their sleep-wake cycle, a condition known as jet lag. In addition to having headaches, upset stomach, and difficulty concentrating, you may experience shallow and fitful sleep. Younger people usually adapt more quickly to jet lag.

Most people have more difficulty traveling eastward (against the direction of the sun) than westward (following the direction of the sun). Sometimes older people have more symptoms traveling westward.

To Nap or Not to Nap?

Napping can be a restorative tonic or a troublemaker. Naps can help reduce sleepiness after a night of sleep deprivation but can rob you of much-needed sleep the next night. The only way to know if napping is right for you is to try it if you do not nap, or stop napping if you do. Do the opposite of what you normally do for a week and see how you feel. Keep a sleep diary each day and record the number of hours you slept, when you slept, and how you felt afterward. Overnapping can be just as detrimental as lack of sleep. Too much light sleep can cause you to wake up feeling unrefreshed.

The best way to handle jet lag is to try to sleep only at night and to get up early in the morning. It takes about a day to adjust for every time zone crossed. Other approaches include:

- On a brief trip (just one or two time zones away), it may be possible to wake up, eat, and sleep on home time. Schedule appointments for times when you would be alert at home.

- Before you leave, move mealtimes and bedtime closer to the schedule of your destination, an hour at a time. Even a small change may make the trip easier. For example, several days before your trip if traveling eastward (into later time zones), get up and go to bed earlier and earlier until you are getting up and going to bed at the same time as you will be in the eastern time zone.

- On a long trip, do not go to bed until it is bedtime in the new time zone. For the first day or two, spend as much time outdoors as possible to let daylight reset your internal body clock.

- On your trip, drink plenty of fluids, but avoid caffeine and alcohol. They cause dehydration, worsen physical symptoms of jet lag, and can disturb sleep.

Narcolepsy

Narcolepsy is a disorder of sleep-wake regulation whose hallmark is profound daytime sleepiness. Abnormalities in rapid eye movement (REM) sleep are present. Instead of occurring normally after a steady progression through the other stages of sleep, REM sleep intrudes at unusual times—for example, as soon as you lie down, immediately after sleep begins, or during daytime activities.

About 1 of 2,000 people have narcolepsy, which affects men and women equally. A genetic factor is involved; virtually all people with narcolepsy have specific genetic markers. An environmental factor may bring out the genetically determined tendency.

SYMPTOMS

Symptoms of narcolepsy usually begin in childhood or young

Sleep Clinics

For every 20 Americans with a sleep disorder, only one seeks and gets professional help. If your daytime function is compromised by sleep deprivation for more than a month, get medical advice. Most people with common sleep problems do not require a visit to a specialized sleep center. However, when a doctor suspects a more serious condition (such as narcolepsy or sleep apnea), a formal sleep evaluation is often recommended. (See p.1236 for a list of organizations that can refer you to a qualified sleep center.)

The sleep center will request medical records and may send you a sleep questionnaire and sleep diary to use for 1 to 2 weeks before your visit. You may be instructed to change your sleep habits before scheduling a visit. If this corrects the problem, there is no need for a consultation.

When spending the night in a sleep laboratory, you will wear your own nightclothes and may use a pillow from home. The lab usually provides a bed in a private room with a bathroom. In some settings, you are monitored day and night, but you can move around freely. Some of the procedures you can expect include:

Polysomnography (see illustration below), in which wafer-thin electrodes are positioned on specific sites on the body to record your sleep patterns.

Audiotape and videotape recordings, in which snoring, sleeptalking, and movement are recorded.

Multiple latency sleep test, in which you are instructed to try to fall asleep during the day while monitors measure how long it takes you to fall asleep.

Maintenance wakefulness test, in which you are instructed to try to stay awake while monitors measure how long it takes you to fall asleep.

The results of these evaluations are analyzed by sleep experts. A report outlining specific steps you can take to promote sleep is given to you and your doctor.

Polysomnography: Sleep Evaluation in a Laboratory

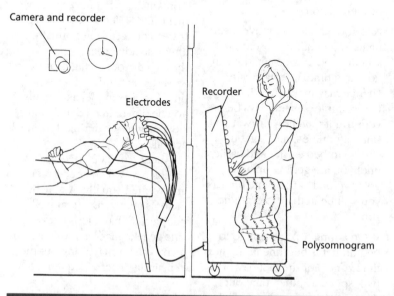

Camera and recorder

Electrodes

Recorder

Polysomnogram

Polysomnography is the recording of brain waves and other functions to evaluate sleep problems. During the procedure, small electrodes are secured to the scalp and other parts of the body to monitor physical symptoms during the night. Laboratory staff assess the data recorded on a printout (the polysomnogram) in a nearby control room.

adulthood, and last throughout life. The symptoms of narcolepsy vary widely and may include any of the following several groups of symptoms:

Sleep attacks A person may suddenly fall asleep for 5 or 10 minutes during waking hours, no matter what else is going on—for example, while eating dinner.

Cataplexy is a condition in which the normal paralysis of muscles that occurs during REM sleep occurs during the day. It usually follows laughter, anger, or other strong emotions. Muscles suddenly become paralyzed, causing the affected person to fall. Sometimes serious injury can result.

Sleep paralysis is a temporary paralysis that normally occurs during the transition between wakefulness and sleep. It can be terrifying but is not serious.

Hypnagogic hallucinations are vivid and often frightening images, smells, or sounds that are difficult to distinguish from reality and occur just as a person is falling asleep.

Disturbed nighttime sleep is unwelcome awakening at night, making people feel as if they barely slept.

Automatic behavior is acting on "automatic pilot" during the day while partially asleep, without recollection.

TREATMENT OPTIONS

There is no cure for narcolepsy. Treatment is geared toward improving wakefulness during the day and preventing the REM-related symptoms. Most people require stimulant medicines like methylphenidate hydrochloride to counter sleep attacks and drowsiness.

Heterocyclic antidepressants (see p.400) or selective serotonin reuptake inhibitors (see p.400) that suppress REM sleep can prevent cataplexy and other REM-related symptoms in some people. Even with medicine, however, people are never as alert as they would be without the condition.

Shift-Worker Sleep Disorder

Almost 20% of Americans work an evening or night shift and about 70% of them experience sleep disturbances related to their working hours. Shift-worker sleep disorder can be eased by incorporating scheduled breaks into your shift, and by rotating shifts gradually from day to evening and then to night (rather than working the day shift, night shift, and evening shift on successive days).

Shift workers should reserve the bedroom for sleep and sex only, keep the bedroom cool and comfortable, relax before falling asleep, and maintain a regular routine of preparing for bed. Dark curtains or shades should be used to keep daylight out; eyeshades also are helpful. A running fan or other "white noise" can help block external noise.

Light therapy (see Seasonal Affective Disorder, p.406) or the short-term use of sleep medicines is sometimes recommended to help people get used to a new schedule.

Sleep Apnea Syndrome

Sleep apnea is a potentially life-threatening condition in which breathing stops hundreds of times each night. It is most common among overweight men. You wake up briefly each time breathing stops and then fall asleep again, never knowing you have awakened. This significantly disturbs sleep.

Over time, you will experience the fatigue, lethargy, and headaches that are common with many sleep disorders. A sleep partner may be the first to notice this stop-and-start pattern of breathing or very loud snoring.

There are two different types of sleep apnea: obstructive sleep apnea and central sleep apnea. Obstructive sleep apnea is more common and occurs when the upper airway is blocked by excess tissue such as a large uvula (the appendage that hangs at the back of the throat), tongue, or tonsils. When sleep causes muscles to relax, the excess tissue tends to fall into the airway and obstructs breathing. People at risk for obstructive sleep apnea include those who snore or have high blood pressure (see p.644) or thick necks. Half of all people with collar sizes of over 17½ inches suffer from sleep apnea.

Central sleep apnea occurs when an important part of the brain fails to send the necessary messages to control the muscles that automatically breathe for you at night (when awake, you breathe without these particular brain messages).

In addition to the symptoms that can accompany any sleep disorder, people with sleep apnea can have overworked

Obstructive Sleep Apnea

SLEEP APNEA

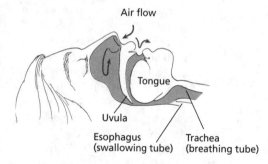

RECEIVING CONTINUOUS POSITIVE NASAL AIRWAY PRESSURE FOR SLEEP APNEA

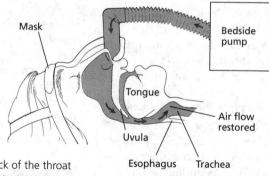

Obstructive sleep apnea (left) occurs when the tissues at the back of the throat temporarily block the flow of air. Continuous positive nasal airway pressure (right) pumps air through a mask or through prongs in the nose. The pressure opens the airway, allowing air to enter the trachea and lungs.

hearts because the heart tries to pump blood harder when it senses low oxygen levels at night.

People with sleep apnea syndrome also risk death from failure to breathe at night and have a higher risk of stroke (see p.342), heart attack (see p.663), and congestive heart failure (see p.683). Sleeping pills should not be used because they can interfere with the natural impulse to wake up. See Treating Sleep Apnea Syndrome (right).

Snoring

When you inhale, air rushes past the upper part of your throat and down your windpipe. Snoring occurs when dangling tissues vibrate during breathing. One of 4 adults snores regularly, and almost half of all adults snore at least occasionally. The source of snoring depends on which tissues are flapping or impeding airflow.

When a person's nasal pas-

Treating Sleep Apnea Syndrome

Doctors may recommend one or more of these treatments to help people with sleep apnea syndrome:

TREATMENT	DESCRIPTION
General treatment measures	Maintain a healthy weight, avoid alcohol and sedatives, and try different sleeping positions.
Continuous positive airway pressure (see illustration above)	The most effective device used to keep the airway open. It uses a compressor to deliver pressurized air through a mask that fits snugly over the nose.
Bilevel positive airway pressure	Used to treat people who have difficulty exhaling against the pressure of continuous positive airway pressure. It delivers air under high pressure as the sleeper inhales and switches to lower pressure during exhalation.
Uvulopalato-pharyngoplasty	Removal of excess tissue from the uvula, tonsils, and a rim of loose tissue at the edge of the soft palate. Helps about 50% of people; others may need more upper airway surgery.
Corrective jaw surgery	Moves the upper or lower jaw forward to enlarge the upper airway. Considered only if other methods fail.
Tracheostomy	Creates a small passageway for insertion of a tube in the lower neck. Considered only if other methods fail.

sages are swollen due to a cold or allergies, temporary snoring may occur. A large uvula (the bell-like appendage of skin hanging at the back of the throat), tonsils, adenoids, or tongue (or a very small jaw) can cause snoring, as can poor muscle tone in the tissues around the upper airway, frequently caused by excessive alcohol use. Excess fat in the neck area may press on the airway and promote snoring.

Many women snore late in their pregnancies due to hormone-related swelling of airway tissues. Before menopause, women snore less than men; snoring increases after menopause.

Although snoring is rarely life-threatening, sleep specialists take snoring seriously. Someone who snores heavily should have a thorough examination of the

throat, mouth, palate, tongue, and neck.

There are hundreds of devices on the market that claim to help the snorer; they should be avoided. Always get a doctor's evaluation and his or her recommendations.

The remedy for your snoring might be as simple as changing your sleeping position from your back to your side since many people snore only when lying on their backs. This can be encouraged by sewing a marble, golf ball, or tennis ball into the backs of pajamas, making it uncomfortable to sleep in that position.

Other remedies include raising your head slightly by using another pillow or raising the head of the bed. An overweight snorer may benefit by losing

weight and improving muscle tone.

Other helpful measures include quitting smoking and avoiding alcohol, sleeping pills, and tranquilizers, which slow breathing.

Sleepwalking

Sleepwalking occurs during partial awakening from deep sleep. Some sleepwalkers carry out complex tasks; others simply pace or sit on the edge of the bed, moving their legs repeatedly. Episodes are not harmful and are usually brief. Scientists once believed that sleepwalkers were acting out their dreams, but experts now know that sleepwalking does not occur during a dreaming stage of sleep.

Sleepwalking is common in children and probably occurs because the brain has not yet mastered regulation of sleep and waking. A sleepwalking child should be gently guided back to bed. Although people are more likely to sleepwalk when they are anxious or fatigued, there is little correlation between sleepwalking and psychological problems.

If the condition continues past puberty, the sleepwalker should be evaluated by a doctor to determine if sleepwalking is the result of nighttime epilepsy (see p.375) or is a reaction to medicine or extreme stress.

Restless Legs Syndrome

Restless legs syndrome is a very common problem that interferes with sleep. As you relax (often in the evening before bedtime), you

What Causes Snoring?

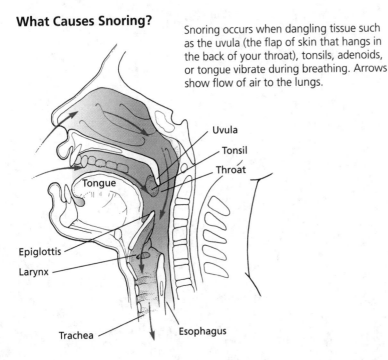

Snoring occurs when dangling tissue such as the uvula (the flap of skin that hangs in the back of your throat), tonsils, adenoids, or tongue vibrate during breathing. Arrows show flow of air to the lungs.

feel unpleasant tingling sensations in your legs (and sometimes your arms). These sensations persist as you try to fall asleep, interfering with falling asleep and staying asleep.

The cause of this condition is unknown, but it runs in families. It may be more common during pregnancy. Several medicines can be effective, including levodopa, bromocriptine, pergolide, the benzodiazepines, and opioids.

Teeth Grinding

Teeth grinding, or bruxism, is the habitual clenching or grinding of teeth during sleep. It can be so loud that it awakens a bed partner, and your jaw may be clenched so hard that the grinding wears away at the tooth's enamel and loosens teeth.

Teeth grinding usually is caused by stress or tension and is treated by addressing the underlying stress through psychotherapy (see p.393), stress reduction, or correcting your bite. Your dentist can create a dental guard that you wear at night to help prevent damage to the teeth.

Restless Legs Syndrome: Dr Winkelman's Advice

Up to 5% to 10% of adults may have restless legs syndrome (RLS), and yet most people have never heard of it, and many doctors know little about it. Most people I see with this condition have had the symptoms for a long time, but figured it was just the "normal aches and pains" of growing older. RLS causes "achy" legs, which feel as if they need to be stretched, most often at night when the legs are at rest, rather than when the legs are being used. In childhood, "growing pains" may be the equivalent of RLS, and so it may be common in kids as well.

Regular use of medications can be remarkably effective for adults. In children, an occasional acetaminophen and avoiding sleep deprivation are all that is needed. An excellent source of support and information is the Restless Legs Syndrome Foundation, Inc. You don't need to tolerate this common, bothersome condition; it can be successfully treated.

JOHN W. WINKELMAN, MD, PHD
BRIGHAM AND WOMEN'S HOSPITAL
HARVARD MEDICAL SCHOOL

Behavioral and Emotional Disorders

The mysteries of the mind are considered by many to be the final frontier of medicine. Recent scientific advances, such as techniques for taking pictures of the working brain (see Functional MRI, p.139), have begun to explain how we think, store memories, and experience emotion.

Scientific advances are also changing how we view illnesses that affect behavior or emotions. For several hundred years in Western civilization, the concept of the mind has been separated from the concept of the body. In particular, illnesses of the mind often have not been regarded as legitimately as have illnesses of the body. Illnesses of the mind historically have not been viewed as diseases, but more as character flaws—things that people could overcome if they had enough willpower.

That view has changed. Most disorders of emotion or behavior are caused by physical factors in the brain interacting with a person's life experiences, along with current stressful situations.

The most important physical factors involve the activity of critical chemicals in the brain. The brain contains billions of nerve cells called neurons that "talk to each other" using chemicals as signals (see Neurotransmitters: Neurons Talking to Neurons, p.341).

The chemical messengers travel between nerve cells, stimulating or diminishing electrical impulses. Important examples of these chemicals, which are called neurotransmitters, are norepinephrine, dopamine, gamma-aminobutyric acid, and serotonin.

In many emotional or behavioral disorders, it is believed that there is either too much or too little of specific neurotransmitters in critical areas of the brain. Neurochemical activity underlies everything your brain does, including thought processes, the experience of emotions, memory, and all the sensations.

Sometimes predispositions to mental disorders are inherited. With some mental illnesses, an inherited component is significant. For example, studies show that, if one identical twin suffers from bipolar disorder, there is an 80% chance that the other twin will as well. Even with identical twins who have been raised separately since birth by different parents and exposed to different life experiences, if one twin develops bipolar disorder, the other is more likely than the average person to develop it also. Strong hereditary tendencies have also been found to be associated with depression, anxiety, and substance addiction and abuse disorders.

At the same time, it is clear that inherited physical factors involving brain chemistry do not explain all behavioral and emotional disease. A person's relationships with family and friends, the financial and employment situation, and stressful events play a major role in bringing on a behavioral or emotional disorder, even if the disorder also has a physical basis. Simply, the chemical makeup of your brain can make you vulnerable to certain emotional disorders, but events in your life bring out the vulnerability.

There can be a fine line between an emotional disorder and a normal life experience. Many people have periods of significant anxiety or depression in response to stress or loss. Sometimes behavioral and emotional reactions are strongly influenced by an individual's family or cultural upbringing.

Psychiatric professionals regularly assess their field and publish an extensive set of criteria—called the Diagnostic and Statistic Manual (DSM)—for diagnosing behavioral and emotional disorders. Much of this section draws on the fourth edition of DSM (DSM IV) diagnostic criteria. In this section, you will find descriptions of the more common behavioral and emotional problems, as well as the most widely accepted treatments.

TREATMENT

The changes in brain chemistry that are found in many mental disorders serve as targets for treatment. Medicines that normalize disordered brain chemistry have led to major improvements in the treatment of mental illnesses.

However, medicines are not the sole answer to behavioral and emotional disorders and, for some illnesses, they are not very effective. For many people, behavioral therapy, cognitive therapy, psychotherapy, and psychoanalysis (see Types of Therapy, p.393) are valuable adjuncts to drug therapy and are sometimes helpful without medicines.

The word "psychotherapy" means "healing of the soul" in Greek. Psychotherapy takes many forms. Psychoanalysis, counseling, family therapy, and group therapy are all forms of psychotherapy.

Schools of psychotherapy vary widely, so it is wise to first investigate the theoretical orientation of your therapist (see Questions to Discuss With a Prospective Therapist, p.393).

Therapists can be many different kinds of health professionals. Your doctor can recommend an appropriate specialist to help you evaluate your problem and prescribe the right treatment.

Where to Turn for Help

If you have recurring, stressful thoughts and feelings that affect your everyday functioning or if you have difficulty sleeping, concentrating, or relating to friends and relatives, talk to your doctor. Sometimes mental distress is a sign of a physical illness, and your doctor may conduct tests to rule out another disease or disorder. You may also need an evaluation by a psychiatrist. The success of psychotherapy hinges on a good relationship with your therapist. For this reason, ask your doctor for the names of two or three therapists who might work well with you and interview each of them before making a decision (see Questions to Discuss With a Prospective Therapist, p.393). This is a partial list of the physicians and nonphysicians who treat behavioral and emotional disorders:

THERAPIST	QUALIFICATIONS AND APPROACH
Psychiatrist	Medical doctor (MD) or osteopathic doctor (DO) with a degree in medicine plus 4 years of post-graduate study (residency) in psychiatry. Often has subspecialty in a specific area such as addiction, adolescence, childhood, or geriatrics. Is usually certified by the American Board of Psychiatry and Neurology, which requires that members meet professional requirements. Can prescribe medication and admit individuals to the hospital.
Psychoanalyst	Psychiatrist or psychologist who has training in psychoanalysis, a form of psychotherapy based on the idea that emotional problems are caused by life experiences. Psychoanalysts who are MDs can prescribe drugs and admit individuals to the hospital.
Psychologist	Person who has a degree and advanced training in emotional issues but is not an MD. Licensing requirements vary from state to state; however, most psychologists have a doctorate (PhD) and some postdoctoral training. May use psychotherapy and other techniques, such as hypnosis, but may not prescribe drugs or perform physical exams.
Psychiatric social worker	Person who may have special training in specific areas of therapy, such as substance abuse or family therapy, but is not an MD. Licensing requirements vary from state to state. May not prescribe drugs or perform physical exams.
Psychiatric nurse	Registered nurse (RN) with advanced degree who may be trained and licensed to practice in a range of psychotherapies and may practice independently or under the supervision of a physician.

TYPES OF THERAPY

Psychotherapy

Psychotherapy can take several forms. Psychoanalysis is based on the idea that traumas (usually involving rejection or loss) that occur in early childhood become repressed but resurface throughout life as emotional problems.

Psychoanalysis is designed to help you recall unconscious conflicts and, in so doing, help release their hold on you. The process of psychoanalysis usually involves meeting with a therapist more than once a week for several years. Often the psychoanalyst will be seated out of sight behind you while you are lying on a couch. Psychoanalysis is seldom covered by health insurance.

In psychodynamic psychotherapy, you usually meet with the therapist once or twice a week. It is particularly helpful in dealing with low self-esteem, difficulties with intimacy or authority, or continuing depression or anxiety. Usually with this form of psychotherapy, the psychotherapist and you will sit facing each other. For more complex, persisting problems, treatment may continue for several years. As in psychoanalysis, the psychotherapist often concentrates on the influence your past experiences have had on your current life.

Interpersonal therapy borrows some techniques from psychoanalysis but concentrates on your current social environment and personal relationships rather than the past. It usually lasts for 3 or 4 months of weekly sessions and is often used to deal with problems of low self-esteem.

Cognitive Therapy

Cognitive therapy is based on the idea that erroneous thoughts cause unhappy feelings. In cognitive therapy, a person is taught to reinterpret situations in ways that are more positive. It usually requires less than 6 months of weekly sessions, sometimes followed by another 6 to 12 months of monthly meetings.

You may be asked to rehearse certain situations and describe your thoughts and feelings. In this way, habitual thoughts that dominate your behavior are made explicit so you can see they are exaggerated. For example, a shy person may avoid greeting an acquaintance on the street, feeling anxious and wanting to avoid being hurt. Cognitively, the person may be anticipating a snub, so he or she avoids contact. By

---

Questions to Discuss with a Prospective Therapist

Whatever form of therapy you choose, ask your primary care doctor for recommendations. You should feel comfortable with the person to whom you will reveal intimate information, so it is common to interview several therapists before making a commitment. You will likely be charged for each interview. Here are some questions to consider asking the therapist:

■ **What form of therapy do you practice?** If you want to learn more about the particular form of therapy, ask the therapist to recommend a book on the subject.

■ **What will a typical session be like?** The answer should give you an idea of whether you will feel comfortable with how the sessions are structured. For example, some therapists are generally passive listeners, while others are more active and confrontational. Similarly, therapy can take place with you and the therapist alone or in a group setting.

■ **Approximately how long will the course of my treatment be?** How often will we need to meet?

■ **Do you recommend and can you prescribe medications for my problem?**

■ **What education do you have to perform this type of therapy?** Certain therapists (see Where to Turn for Help, p.392) must meet educational requirements to be licensed to practice their form of therapy.

■ **Do you accept my health insurance plan?** Because insurance plans vary widely in how much and what type of psychiatric care they provide, it is wise to consult with your insurance carrier.

Hypnosis

Hypnosis is a technique that can help you focus your attention, rethink problems, relax, and respond to helpful suggestions. There is no magic in hypnosis. It relies mainly on your ability to concentrate and on the trust you have in the therapist. Hypnosis can alter your perception of pain and other sensations and help you gain some control over your emotional and physical responses. There is little evidence that hypnosis can be relied upon to retrieve childhood memories accurately.

Hypnosis can help people control chronic cancer pain, menstrual pain, and headaches; make labor and childbirth more comfortable; decrease the amount of medication needed during surgery; and shorten surgical recovery time. It has been shown to alleviate the symptoms of irritable bowel syndrome and, in some cases, those of asthma.

Using hypnosis, some people can gain control of unwanted behaviors such as tobacco smoking, bed-wetting, nail biting, teeth grinding, phobias, overeating, and difficulty sleeping. Skin conditions such as psoriasis, urticaria, and warts can also be helped by hypnosis.

If you are interested in hypnosis, discuss with your doctor or psychologist whether hypnotherapy might be helpful for you. Two of the professional societies in the United States whose members are trained health professionals skilled in the use of hypnosis are the Society for Clinical and Experimental Hypnosis and the American Society of Clinical Hypnosis.

understanding the thoughts underlying the feelings, the person can reinterpret the situation and behave differently.

Behavior Therapy

Behavioral psychotherapy shares similarities with cognitive psychotherapy but focuses on the rewards and unpleasant consequences that underlie all behaviors.

The main theory of behavior therapy is that you learn to behave in certain ways because you have been rewarded in the past for doing so. All actions are learned or conditioned through positive reinforcement, and they can be unlearned and replaced by different behaviors through positive reinforcement. In this type of therapy, people may be helped to repeatedly practice a behavior that they fear and, in doing so, positively reinforce their ability to master it.

For example, if a child refuses to go to bed on time and stays up to get attention, a behavioral psychotherapist might design a several-part plan. A reward, such as a bedtime story, will be offered if the child cooperates in the bedtime routine. A negative reinforcement might also be used.

Group and Family Therapy

In group therapy, the therapist helps a group of people who share a common problem. For some people, group therapy causes less anxiety and is more effective than individual therapy since groups can provide a support system.

Group therapy can also help alleviate isolation and self-preoccupation by showing that other people share the same challenges and problems. Others in your group may express feelings and experiences that give you insight into your past and present experiences and relationships.

The presence of the therapist ensures that the group is safe and supportive. Psychoanalytical, interpersonal, behavioral, or cognitive methods can be used in group therapy.

In the most common form of group therapy—family therapy—the group includes members of the same family. Family therapists help family members learn how the way they interact may adversely affect them all, including the person in the family who initially brought the family together for therapy. That person is often not the only family member in need of help. Sometimes the roles of all family members need to be adjusted before the person can change.

For example, family therapy might reveal that a young adult who is having trouble becoming independent has parents who are having conflicts in their relationship. The parents might have feelings of not wanting their daughter or son to mature into an adult and leave home because they would have to face their own conflicts more directly.

In other circumstances, family members need help coping with the effects of a family member's mental illness on their own lives.

Drug Therapy

Mood-regulating drugs are effective in treating a wide range of symptoms, from mild depression and anxiety disorders (see p.402) to severe depression (see below), obsessive-compulsive disorder (see p.404), panic disorder (see p.404), bipolar disorder (see p.401), personality disorders (see p.407), and psychoses (see p.409).

Biofeedback

Biofeedback is a term used to describe methods that measure specific body responses (such as heartbeat or breathing) and feed them back to you in the forms of

sounds or lights so that you can become aware of your body's responses and learn to control them. You then use relaxation and cognitive techniques to regulate your own responses.

Relaxation Therapy

This form of stress management is described on p.90.

Electroconvulsive Therapy

Electroconvulsive therapy (ECT)—also known as electroshock therapy or, popularly, as "shock treatments"—has a role in the treatment of severe depression (see below), the manic phase of bipolar disorder (see p.401), and, occasionally, schizophrenia (see p.409). It also has been used in emergencies to prevent suicide (see p.397).

Before therapy, you are given

a muscle relaxant and are made unconscious by injection of a general anesthetic. Other drugs are used to control heart rate, and oxygen is administered to prevent damage from interrupted breathing.

Two electrodes are placed on the scalp and a small current, lasting 1 to 2 seconds, is passed between the electrodes; this causes a seizure. When you awaken 20 minutes later, you may have sore muscles and a slight headache.

The treatment is repeated two or three times a week for a few weeks until your condition improves. Mild memory loss is the most common side effect.

Because you are unconscious during ECT, you have no memory of going through the therapy. Although researchers cannot explain exactly how it works, studies show that ECT cuts down on episodes of depression or mania in many people.

MOOD AND ANXIETY DISORDERS

Depression

Many people experience a passing depressed mood, or a period of normal sadness, after a loss. Most of us recover within days or weeks without severe disruption of our daily lives. For other people, however, depression is an acutely distressing, debilitating, and at times life-threatening illness. Suffering from depression also may increase the risk of death in people who also have other illnesses, such as heart disease or cancer.

If you are depressed, you are not alone. More than 1 of 5 adults

experience severe depression at some point in their lives and, in any year, 2% to 4% of men and 4% to 8% of women suffer from depression (see The Gender Gap in Depression, p.397).

Depression often occurs during major transitions in life, such as divorce or the passage from adolescence to adulthood. In some people, depression occurs after the death of a loved one as the normal sadness and loss (see Bereavement, p.1145) becomes prolonged and debilitating. In some people, there is no precipitating event. In others, depres-

sion is a recurring disease.

After one episode of depression, half the people who do not receive treatment suffer a relapse. Chances of a relapse become progressively greater after each episode. Today, there are potent treatments available for depression.

There are several forms of depression: major depression, bipolar disorder, seasonal affective disorder, and dysthymia. Dysthymia, which is Greek for "bad state of mind," is a less severe form of depression that does not disrupt daily life as much as

Depression Questionnaire

If you are unsure about whether you have depression, answer the following questions yes or no:

1 I feel downhearted, blue, and sad almost all of the time.

2 I do not enjoy the things that I used to.

3 I have felt so low that I've thought about suicide.

4 I feel that I am not useful or needed.

5 I am losing weight.

6 I have trouble sleeping through the night.

7 I am restless and cannot keep still.

8 My mind is not as clear as it used to be.

9 I get tired for no reason.

10 I feel hopeless about the future.

You may be suffering from major depression if you answered yes to the first two questions and if your symptoms have persisted for at least 2 weeks. If you have been feeling depressed and answered yes to at least two of questions 4 through 10, you may have a mild form of depression. Talk to your doctor.

Regardless of how you answered the other questions, if you answered yes to question 3, call your doctor or a suicide hotline (look in the Yellow Pages of the phone book under "Crisis Intervention") immediately for help (see Warning Signs of Suicide, p.397).

major depression but often lasts longer (2 years or more). People with dysthymia have many of the same symptoms as sufferers of major depression, but with less intensity. However, those with dysthymia are at risk for more severe depression.

WHO SUFFERS FROM DEPRESSION?

People most susceptible to depression include:

■ People under severe stress, such as those who have experienced the death of a loved one or a dramatic and negative change in lifestyle such as loss of a job.

■ People with depressed family

members, suggesting a genetic (inherited) link. Family upbringing and social relationships may also play a role.

■ People with other psychological disorders such as anxiety (see p.402), obsessive-compulsive disorder (see p.404), drug and alcohol abuse (see p.411), nicotine

Risks of Recurring Depression Without Treatment

These charts show your chances of having another episode of depression if you have had depressive episodes in the past and are not taking antidepressants.

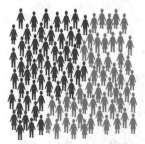

50 OF 100 PEOPLE WHO HAVE HAD ONE EPISODE OF DEPRESSION AND ARE NOT TAKING ANTIDEPRESSANTS WILL HAVE ANOTHER EPISODE OF DEPRESSION

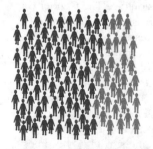

70 OF 100 PEOPLE WHO HAVE HAD TWO EPISODES OF DEPRESSION AND ARE NOT TAKING ANTIDEPRESSANTS WILL HAVE ANOTHER EPISODE OF DEPRESSION

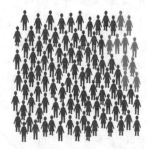

90 OF 100 PEOPLE WHO HAVE HAD THREE EPISODES OF DEPRESSION AND ARE NOT TAKING ANTIDEPRESSANTS WILL HAVE ANOTHER EPISODE OF DEPRESSION

Warning Signs of Suicide

Suicide is one of the 10 most common causes of death in all age groups. If someone you know talks about killing himself or herself, take it as a serious call for help. Many people who threaten or attempt suicide are extremely lonely, and the presence of a concerned friend may be enough to dissuade them. You may fear that you are infringing on individual privacy, but you may be saving a life.

Stay in close contact with the person and urge him or her to see a doctor. If he or she does not, take the lead yourself and contact your doctor, a psychiatrist, or a local suicide hotline.

Most suicide victims are adults, but teen suicide is increasing at an alarming rate. Adult suicides more frequently occur in people who suffer from depression (see p.395), panic disorder (see p.404), schizophrenia (see p.409), or substance abuse. However, thousands of suicide victims are not known to have suffered from any of these conditions.

If you feel that suicide is an option:

■ Call your doctor, a suicide hotline, or go to a hospital emergency department and ask for help.

■ Ask your doctor to refer you to a psychiatrist for therapy. Psychiatrists are trained to help you sort through problems that may seem insurmountable but in reality can be resolved.

Some people never outwardly say that they are contemplating suicide, but they may exhibit warning signs. If you know a person who exhibits any of these signs, take the initiative to get them help. The warning signs are:

■ **Depression** Signs of depression such as fatigue, sadness, and loss of interest in normal activities may precede a suicide attempt.

■ **Moodiness** An extreme change in mood, especially from depression to calm resolve, may be a sign that the individual is ready to take some form of action.

■ **Crisis** In a person who is depressed, a distressing event may initiate suicidal thoughts.

■ **Withdrawal** Seek help if you, or someone you know, has withdrawn from normal activities and seems to avoid all social contact.

Risk of Suicide With Major Depression

The lifetime risk of committing suicide for people in the United States is much higher for those who suffer from major depression.

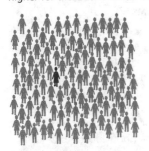

1 OF 100 PEOPLE IN THE GENERAL POPULATION WILL COMMIT SUICIDE

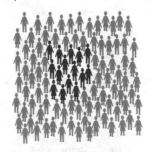

15 OF 100 PEOPLE WHO HAVE MAJOR DEPRESSION WILL COMMIT SUICIDE

addiction (see p.56), posttraumatic stress disorder (see p.406), or eating disorders (see p.1024).

■ People with severe physical illness.

■ People taking medicines that can trigger depressive symptoms, such as sedatives and drugs used to regulate blood pressure and heart rate.

THE GENDER GAP IN DEPRESSION

Women are twice as likely as men to suffer from both mild and major depression. The gender difference is seen in all parts of the world and at all levels of income and education. Scientists have been unable to determine a reason for this pattern. There is

Relieving Depression

BEFORE MEDICATION

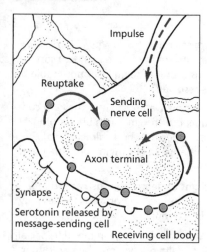

AFTER MEDICATION

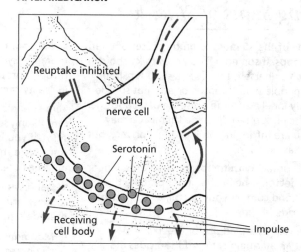

People who are depressed may have diminished amounts of the neurotransmitter serotonin available to activate brain cells. At left, the end of one nerve cell releases serotonin. Some serotonin travels across the synapse and activates the second cell. The message-sending cell also reabsorbs some serotonin, making it unavailable to the receiving cell, so the receiving cell does not get enough serotonin. At right, a selective serotonin reuptake inhibitor (such as fluoxetine) slows reabsorption of serotonin by the sending cell, which increases the amount of serotonin available to the receiving cell, restoring the imbalance.

---

no convincing evidence that genes or hormones explain the discrepancy.

Many women experience a brief depressed mood after giving birth (see Postpartum Depression, p.944), though actual postpartum depression is rare. Women may also experience brief depression around the time of their menstrual periods (see Premenstrual Syndrome, p.1046). Men may be less likely than women to seek help when they feel depressed, making depression appear to be more common in women.

THEORIES ABOUT DEPRESSION

Psychoanalysts believe that depressed adults are grieving from the loss of a parent, either through death, separation, or withdrawal of affection. Later in life, any rejection or loss may trigger a kind of delayed grief reaction.

Behavioral therapists regard depression as the result of learned behavior; they contend that depressed people have learned through upbringing and experience that they cannot change anything, so they stop trying.

Cognitive theory contends that most depression stems from people having false beliefs that they are worthless, the world is hostile, the future is hopeless, and every misfortune is a judgment on themselves.

For more information about these theories, and their respective treatment approaches, see Types of Therapy, p.393.

SYMPTOMS

An episode of major depression may last several weeks to several years. Severely depressed people experience inconsolable misery, despair, guilt, and feelings of worthlessness. They have no hope for the future and may ruminate about death and suicide. They sometimes develop psychotic delusions (see Psychoses, p.409) of being punished for grave sins or dying of an incurable disease.

Sometimes depressed people simply withdraw from human contact, lose all interest in life,

Depression: Dr Brotman's Advice

All of us feel depressed from time to time. The difference between normal mood variation and a clinical depression has to do with the duration and consistency of the symptoms. Changes in sleep, appetite, energy level, concentration, or motivation; an inability to take pleasure in things; and thoughts of death are indications for treatment if they persist consistently for 2 weeks or more. Knowing why you feel depressed (such as losing your job or the breakup of a relationship) is no longer considered relevant as to whether treatment is useful. A depression is responsive to treatment with antidepressant medications irrespective of whether it is "understandable" or "out of the blue." Recovery rates generally approach 80%. However, depression can be ongoing or recur, especially if other members of your family also suffer from depression. Recurring depression often requires long-term treatment.

ANDREW W. BROTMAN, MD
BETH ISRAEL DEACONESS MEDICAL CENTER
HARVARD MEDICAL SCHOOL

and become incapable of feeling pleasure. People with depression may become fretful, irritable, and unable to concentrate or make even minor decisions, turning the same few ideas over and over in their minds. They may become demoralized or guilty about the depression-caused inability to act, thus feeding into a vicious cycle of increasing depression.

Half of all people with major depression and 90% of the most severely depressed have physical symptoms. The most common are loss of appetite (although some sufferers have a ravenous appetite), insomnia (although some tend to oversleep), backache, headache, upset stomach, constipation, and fatigue.

About 15% of people with major depression have psychotic symptoms—usually delusions (irrational thoughts such as being chased by the police) but also sometimes hallucinations or incoherent thinking. The delusions often involve imaginary poverty, physical illness, or moral transgressions.

Agitation, physical immobility, constipation, anxiety, and insomnia are more common in psychotic than nonpsychotic depression. The risk of suicide (see p.397) is also greater.

TREATMENT OPTIONS

If you are depressed, your primary care doctor can often help you through a combination of conversation and medicine. Some people need to see a mental health professional. Treatment works. Medication and psychotherapy can shorten episodes of the illness and reduce the chance of relapse. For a more detailed discussion of therapy, see Types of Therapy, p.393.

ANTIDEPRESSANT DRUGS

There are a wide variety of antidepressant drugs that are very effective. The conditions of about two thirds of the people who use them improve within 3 weeks, but these medicines vary in cost and side effects. Many other types of medications are also prescribed to treat mood disorders, and medicines may be prescribed in combination.

Your doctor will help you

Living with Depression

"I had now reached that phase of the disorder where all sense of hope had vanished. The mornings themselves were becoming bad now as I wandered about lethargic, following my synthetic sleep, but afternoons were still the worst, beginning at about 3 o'clock, when I'd feel the horror, like some poisonous fog bank, roll in upon my mind, forcing me into bed. There I would lie for as long as 6 hours, stuporous and virtually paralyzed, gazing at the ceiling and waiting for that moment of evening when, mysteriously, the crucifixion would ease up just enough to allow me to force down some food and then, like an automaton, seek an hour or two of sleep again."

William Styron. *Darkness Visible: A Memoir of Madness*. New York: Random House, 1990. Page 58.

Withdrawal Symptoms for HCAs and SSRIs

People who have taken heterocyclic antidepressants (HCAs) or selective serotonin reuptake inhibitors (SSRIs) for long periods and who stop the medicines suddenly can experience withdrawal symptoms. For HCAs, these symptoms include dizziness, nausea, headache, fatigue, vivid dreams, irritability, and vertigo. For SSRIs, the symptoms include any of these, in addition to sweating, difficulty sleeping, shooting pains, and memory loss. For these reasons, gradual tapering of these medications will usually be recommended by your physician. If you experience these symptoms after you stop taking these medicines, call your doctor.

decide on the best treatment, which usually lasts for 6 to 12 months. If depression recurs, your doctor may recommend that you stay on a maintenance dose of the drug indefinitely.

The three main classes of antidepressant drugs—selective serotonin reuptake inhibitors, monoamine oxidase inhibitors, and heterocyclic antidepressants— are described here.

Selective serotonin reuptake inhibitors (SSRIs) enhance the activity of the neurotransmitter serotonin by delaying its reuptake at nerve endings. Widely used SSRIs include fluoxetine, paroxetine, and sertraline. SSRIs are as effective as (but no more effective than) heterocyclic antidepressants (see below right).

Like other antidepressants, SSRIs usually take several weeks to reach full effectiveness. Side effects may include agitation, delayed ejaculation and orgasm, and reduced sexual interest and response. It is best to take these medicines in the morning because they can disrupt sleep if taken at bedtime.

Monoamine oxidase inhibitors (MAOIs) are rarely the first choice in treating depression because of their potentially serious side effects. MAOIs can cause dizziness, insomnia, and impotence. They can also produce dangerously high blood pressure in people who eat tyramine-containing foods such as red wine, pickles, and certain cheeses. The MAOIs that require avoiding certain foods include phenelzine, tranylcypromine, and isocarboxazid.

MAOIs are helpful in treating those whose depression is not improved by other drugs, especially people with panic disorder (see p.404). A newer group of MAOIs—including selegiline and moclobemide—does not require that you restrict the tyramine-containing foods in your diet.

Heterocyclic antidepressants (HCAs), previously known as tricyclic antidepressants, were introduced in the 1960s and have been widely used. Commonly prescribed HCAs include amitriptyline, imipramine, desipramine, nortriptyline, doxepin, protriptyline, and trazodone. HCAs enhance the effects in the brain of two neurotransmitters, norepinephrine and serotonin. From 65% to 85% of depressed people improve substantially when taking HCAs. Several of the HCAs are sedating, so they should be taken at night.

HCAs usually begin to work within a few weeks, although sleep patterns and appetite may improve sooner. The dose is sometimes adjusted according to the concentration of the drug in the blood. Compared to SSRIs, HCAs are as effective, generally

Alternative Medicine: St. John's Wort

St. John's wort is an herbal medicine that is commonly recommended as a "natural" treatment of depression. Although it has no serious side effects, there are also no scientific studies clearly confirming its benefit. In some European countries, this herbal medicine is more widely used to treat depression than conventional antidepressants. If you decide you want to try St. John's wort, talk to your doctor. If you then decide to stop it, let your doctor know.

less expensive, more likely to cause side effects, and more dangerous if taken as an overdose. The most common side effects are dry mouth and blurred vision.

Other side effects include weight gain, constipation, difficulty urinating, and postural hypotension (dizziness caused by a reduced blood flow to the brain when you stand or sit up suddenly). HCAs usually are not prescribed for people with heart disease since they can disturb heart rhythm. Different HCAs have different side effects, so your doctor may switch your drug if you have disturbing side effects.

Bipolar Disorder

Bipolar disorder, previously known as manic-depressive disorder or manic depression, is a form of depression in which periods of deep depression alternate with periods of hyperactivity and uncontrolled elation (mania).

People with bipolar disorder differ from those with other depressive disorders in that their moods swing from depression to mania, often with periods of relatively normal mood between the two extremes.

The disorder usually begins with a depressive episode in adolescence or early adulthood. The first manic phase may not follow until several years later. The length of the cycle, from the heights of mania to deep depression, varies from person to person. The risk of suicide is high among people with bipolar disorder; an estimated 1 of 4 people attempt suicide, and 1 of 10 succeed.

Heredity is an important factor in bipolar disorder. Close rela-

tives of people suffering from bipolar disorder are much more likely to develop it or some other form of depression than the general population. Other studies point to environmental factors, such as troubled family relationships, as a factor that aggravates this disorder.

SYMPTOMS

Bipolar disorder is a recurring disease that goes in cycles. One part of the cycle is marked by symptoms of depression (see p.395). In the other, manic phase, people are cheerful, outgoing, talkative, and energetic. Until the mania gets out of control, affected

people can be extremely productive and wonderful company.

As the mania becomes greater, people become unproductive and talk loudly, rapidly, and continuously, jumping from thought to thought. They need little sleep and may call friends at all hours. They may develop exaggerated self-confidence and grandiose delusions of power and wealth.

People in the manic phase may invest money foolishly or spend it wildly, suddenly initiating vast projects and just as quickly abandoning them. This reckless, expansive cheerfulness can quickly turn to irritability, rage, and paranoia. Mania often

Living with Mania

"I decided I wanted to go someplace else. Michael wanted to visit his family in New Jersey and I thought, 'Why not?' I did not want to travel on a regular airliner, so we rented a Lear jet. We went to Chicago, then to New Jersey, then to New York, where I wound up on *The Dick Cavett Show*. Meanwhile the Lear jet I had rented sat in an airport in New Jersey with the meter running. I forgot it was there because I was off doing 12 other crazy things.

"On the show, I told Dick Cavett and I do not know how many millions of other people that I was pregnant and that I was going to build an ark in the desert between Barstow and Bakersfield. I humiliated myself in front of a national audience.

"Cleaning up the debris of that episode did not stop the mania. I decided to rent a house in Palm Springs for a couple of months and calm down, but I wound up flying to Las Vegas again, for what reason I do not know, on another rented plane with the meter running. And I met a woman who was a stewardess on this little plane and she told me a sad story about how she did not have anyplace to live with her little baby. So she and the baby moved in with me. Before long, another girl, an artist whom we met in a restaurant, came to live with us. Now I was running a commune. There was no money, but that did not stop me from writing checks."

Patty Duke and Gloria Hochman. *A Brilliant Madness: Living with Manic Depressive Illness*. New York: Bantam Books, 1992. Pages 26-27.

leads to alcohol and other drug abuse, loss of jobs, bankruptcy, indiscretions, infidelity, and divorce.

Untreated, the manic phase can last as long as 3 months. As it abates, the sufferer may have a period of normal mood and behavior that lasts for weeks to years. Eventually, the depressive phase of the illness sets in.

About 10% to 20% of sufferers develop "rapid cycling," with more than four episodes of mania and depression a year. The chance that there will be future attacks rises with each new episode.

Even with treatment, relapse is common. In one study, people who were treated with lithium and continued to take it averaged 1½ weeks a year when they were severely ill, whereas people who discontinued the medicine averaged 13 weeks a year of severe illness.

The symptoms of bipolar disorder are not always easy to distinguish from other serious conditions. At its height, mania can be difficult to distinguish from schizophrenia (see p.409). People who take amphetamines or corticosteroid drugs (see p.895) or people with overactive thyroid glands (see p.844) have symptoms similar to those of people with the manic phase of bipolar disorder.

TREATMENT OPTIONS

If you or someone you are close to is experiencing the symptoms of bipolar disorder, medical attention is urgently needed. The person in a period of mania often does not know that he or she is behaving strangely and in need of medical attention. A complete evaluation by a psychiatrist is critical to arriving at an accurate diagnosis, which is the first step toward an appropriate treatment plan. Sometimes, manic people are so out of control that they pose a threat to themselves and others and need to be involuntarily hospitalized.

Bipolar disorder is highly treatable with medication and psychotherapy. Lithium is the most frequently prescribed medicine. It prevents the mania and, to a lesser extent, the depression, although its mechanism of action is unknown.

Seventy percent of those who take lithium experience fewer and less intense manic episodes. In about 20% of people with bipolar disorder, lithium completely relieves symptoms.

However, lithium is not a cure. The mood cycle often emerges again if treatment is stopped, even after many years of treatment. Lithium use must also be monitored carefully. Its side effects include weight gain, hand tremors, drowsiness, excessive thirst, and frequent urination.

Because lithium can injure the heart, kidneys, or thyroid gland, your doctor will perform a physical examination and blood tests before prescribing it. Usually the dose is increased gradually until the drug begins to work and is then periodically adjusted. Blood levels of lithium are checked regularly; it is ineffective if the level is too low and risky if the level is too high.

In the early stages of mania, antipsychotic drugs (see p.1160) may be recommended, since lithium takes several weeks to become fully effective. Some people also need an antidepressant drug (see p.399) for depression, along with lithium for mania.

Anticonvulsant drugs such as divalproex may be used instead of lithium, especially when the mood cycle is very rapid. In severe cases, electroconvulsive therapy (see p.395) may be recommended. Psychotherapy can provide valuable emotional support to the affected person and family.

Generalized Anxiety Disorder

Every human being experiences normal anxiety at some point—usually in response to physical stress (such as being nearly run over by a car) or psychological stress (such as having your boss threaten to demote you). For some people, however, feelings of apprehension occur for no specific reason. If a troubling sense of uneasiness persists for at least 1 month, without other psychological symptoms, the problem may be generalized anxiety disorder (GAD).

Normal anxiety has its roots in fear—an emotion that serves an important function. When you face a dangerous or stressful situation, fear helps motivate the body to take action by activating the flight or fight response: the heart beats faster, sending more blood to the muscles, breathing becomes heavier, and muscles tense in readiness for movement.

This defensive mechanism provides the body with the necessary energy and strength to cope with threatening situations. When our prehistoric ancestors saw a tiger lying in wait for them, they needed to run. With generalized anxiety, the same physical and emotional mechanisms are set in motion, even though there is no physical threat to contend with.

Abnormalities (which are often inherited) in the brain's neurotransmitter gamma-aminobutyric acid may make a person susceptible to GAD. Life events, both early life traumas and current life experiences, are probably necessary to trigger the episodes of anxiety.

SYMPTOMS

In addition to a troubling and free-floating worry, you may feel restless and irritable. Your heart may beat faster, your breathing may become shallow and rapid, and your hands may tremble. Rapid breathing sometimes sets the stage for hyperventilation (heavy breathing accompanied by a sense of gasping for air, faintness, and numbness). You may perspire more (even without exertion), have trouble swallowing due to dry mouth, and have insomnia.

Physical symptoms such as upset stomach (cramps, nausea, and/or diarrhea), headache, and general aches and pains may be

Anxiety: Dr Rogers' Advice

There's a difference between "normal" anxiety, which everyone experiences from time to time, and a true anxiety disorder, which affects roughly 15% of the population. When we are being tested or challenged in some way, normal anxiety warns of potential danger and prepares us to deal with it. In contrast, abnormal anxiety disorders go off like a false alarm, out of the blue, creating a false sense of danger and causing us to unnecessarily avoid certain situations. The good news is that a combination of medication and psychotherapy, particularly if focused on specific behaviors and thoughts, is quite effective. Sometimes, doctors fail to recognize the symptoms of an anxiety disorder, and sometimes people with the disorder refuse to take treatment because they are embarrassed to have an "emotional" problem. These are the biggest barriers to treatment. If you think you may have an anxiety disorder, talk to your doctor. Successful treatment could change your life.

MALCOLM P. ROGERS, MD
BRIGHAM AND WOMEN'S HOSPITAL
HARVARD MEDICAL SCHOOL

so prominent that sufferers and their doctors focus on the physical symptoms and overlook the underlying anxiety.

Identifying the right treatment hinges on ruling out physical disorders such as an ulcer (see p.752), asthma (see p.505), an

overactive thyroid gland (see p.844), or the effects of overuse of caffeine, diet pills, or decongestants and exploring the possibility that the symptoms have an emotional source.

Many people with GAD also have another psychiatric disorder, most often depression (see p.395) or dysthymia, a less severe form of depression. People with GAD are more likely to suffer from alcohol or other drug abuse (see p.63). Also, the effects of these drugs or the symptoms of withdrawal from them can raise the level of anxiety.

TREATMENT OPTIONS

If you have symptoms of GAD, talk to your doctor. A combination of treatments (medications and psychotherapy) may be recommended. The most effective drugs for short-term treatment

Chances of Recovering From Generalized Anxiety Disorder

Your chances of recovering from generalized anxiety disorder, if treated properly with medicines and psychotherapy, are very good.

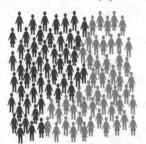

50 OF 100 PEOPLE WHO HAVE GENERALIZED ANXIETY DISORDER AND RECEIVE PROPER TREATMENT WILL SHOW AN IMPROVEMENT WITHIN 3 WEEKS

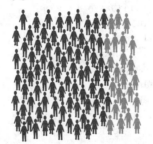

77 OF 100 PEOPLE WHO HAVE GENERALIZED ANXIETY DISORDER AND RECEIVE PROPER TREATMENT WILL SHOW AN IMPROVEMENT WITHIN 9 MONTHS

are benzodiazepine drugs, which calm symptoms of anxiety in about half of people with GAD.

For long-term treatment, antidepressants (see p.399) and the antianxiety drug buspirone may be prescribed to prevent relapse.

Like many drugs for mood disorders, buspirone and antidepressants are not effective immediately; it often takes 2 to 3 weeks before the anxiety-reducing effects are apparent. Short-term psychotherapy is more effective than no therapy and at least as effective as antianxiety medicine without psychotherapy.

Performance Anxiety

Some people experience the physical symptoms of anxiety when they perform, take examinations, or have to make public appearances or presentations. The symptoms of rapid heartbeat, excessive perspiration, trembling hands or voice, breathlessness, and even difficulty concentrating may make it difficult to perform well. Cognitive-behavioral therapy may be useful in learning relaxation and coping skills. In addition, beta-blocker medicines may be effective in controlling the physical symptoms.

Obsessive-Compulsive Disorder

People with obsessive-compulsive disorder (OCD) are plagued by obsessions and compulsions. Obsessions are persistent, unwanted, and distasteful thoughts— often about aggression, sex, religion, or loss—that are the source of much anxiety.

Compulsions—persistent, ritual

behaviors—may accompany obsessions as a means of reducing anxiety. While people with an obsessive disorder do not always suffer from compulsive behaviors, those with compulsions almost always have obsessions.

OCD often begins during adolescence or early adulthood and may be accompanied by anxiety or depression. Without treatment, it can persist throughout life.

The cause of OCD is not known; it is known that the disorder is beyond the control of most people who suffer from it unless they get help.

Many experts believe that OCD involves a disorder of brain chemistry. Others believe that obsessions and compulsions stem from unresolved conflicts during infancy or childhood that need to be identified and resolved during psychotherapy. Behavioral and cognitive therapists assert that compulsions and obsessions are learned behaviors that can be unlearned with proper treatment.

SYMPTOMS

Most often, obsessions focus on a fear, such as the fear of being infected or contaminated by normal contact with the world. This constant fear is terrible for someone to live with. It also can lead to behaviors that other people find strange, such as an unwillingness to shake hands or to go into old buildings.

Because people with OCD may have strange actions or mannerisms, they can be rejected by others, making their lives lonely.

Compulsive rituals are actions that are repeated over and over, sometimes hundreds of times a day. Examples include counting

every step while walking or constantly cleaning one's hands or one's living space. Compulsions usually are performed with the belief that the actions will avert or create a specific consequence. Other times, there appears to be no link between a person's compulsive behaviors and his or her obsessive thoughts.

TREATMENT OPTIONS

If you think that you or someone close to you has OCD, get medical attention. Often, people with OCD do not recognize that their thoughts and compulsive behaviors are strange, and it can be difficult to convince them to seek help. But you need to try.

Treatment can be effective. Without it, affected people may be unable to function adequately at home or at work because of their constant preoccupation with obsessive fears and their compulsive acts.

Besides psychotherapy, desensitization therapy (see Phobias, p.405) may also be helpful. Many people experience relief from symptoms within 3 months of beginning treatment with medications. The heterocyclic antidepressant clomipramine and selective serotonin reuptake inhibitors (see p.400) can help reduce anxiety enough for people to benefit from psychotherapy and begin to function more normally.

Panic Disorder

In panic disorder, the sufferer has sudden attacks of intense fear or anxiety for no apparent reason. The attacks can occur several times a day. Panic disorder is fairly common and tends to run

Risk of Attempting Suicide with Behavioral/Emotional Disorders

The risk of a person with a behavioral/emotional disorder attempting suicide, compared to a person with no psychiatric disorder, can be quite high.

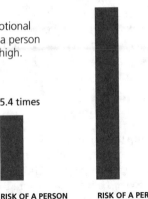

14.3 times

5.1 times

5.4 times

RISK OF AN AVERAGE PERSON WHO DOES NOT HAVE A PSYCHIATRIC DISORDER ATTEMPTING SUICIDE

RISK OF A PERSON WHO HAS ONLY MAJOR DEPRESSION ATTEMPTING SUICIDE

RISK OF A PERSON WHO HAS ONLY PANIC DISORDER ATTEMPTING SUICIDE

RISK OF A PERSON WHO HAS PANIC DISORDER PLUS MAJOR DEPRESSION ATTEMPTING SUICIDE

in families, though the cause is not known. The first attack usually occurs when a person is 20 to 30 years old, although it can come at any time of life.

Personal loss, major change, or illness often set the stage for panic disorder. In some people, panic attacks are more likely to occur in crowds or confined spaces.

Women are two to three times more likely to be affected than men. When a panic attack occurs, a particular area in the limbic system of the brain suddenly becomes very active, requiring increased amounts of nutrients (such as sugar and oxygen).

SYMPTOMS

Psychiatrists have developed the following criteria to identify panic disorder:

■ Intermittent, unexpected periods of sudden intense fear or anxiety during which at least four of the following symptoms occur abruptly, reach a peak in about 10 minutes, and subside

within 30 to 60 minutes: pounding heartbeat, sweating, trembling, difficulty breathing, choking sensations, chest pain, nausea, dizziness, fear of dying, fear of going crazy, feelings of unreality, numbness or tingling in the extremities, and chills or hot flashes.

■ Constant anxiety about having another panic attack.

■ Significant behavior change, such as avoiding certain situations or becoming reliant on alcohol or other substances.

Because the symptoms of panic are similar to those of some other illnesses, such as hyperthyroidism (see p.844) or pheochromocytoma (see p.858), your doctor should rule out other possible causes. People with symptoms of panic disorder may fear that they have a physical illness, such as heart trouble, and may see numerous doctors without receiving a diagnosis. Along the way, they may be considered hypochondriacs and fail to receive proper treatment. The rate of sui-

cide is high among people with panic disorder, making it especially important to recognize and treat this disease.

TREATMENT OPTIONS

Medications and psychotherapy can be effective when used together, relieving symptoms completely in 80% to 90% of those treated. Your doctor may recommend an antianxiety drug initially to help you overcome fear of the panic attacks themselves. Other helpful medicines include heterocyclic antidepressants (see p.400) and selective serotonin reuptake inhibitors (see p.400). Relaxation techniques (see p.90), biofeedback, supportive therapy, and cognitive therapy (see Types of Therapy, p.393) are frequently used to treat panic disorder.

Phobias

A phobia is an irrational sense of fear when a person is confronted by a common object, activity, or situation, leading the person to avoid the thing that is feared.

Phobias are the most common form of anxiety, affecting between 5% and 13% of Americans of all ages and all levels of income. Women of all ages are most subject to phobias, followed by men older than 25.

SYMPTOMS

A phobia can disrupt all aspects of your life, including your ability to work and socialize. Symptoms include sudden, persistent, and irrational panic, dread, horror, or terror when confronted with the object or situation. You usually recognize that the fear is not normal or rational, but you cannot control it.

A common phobia is agoraphobia, which is fear of being in a public place from which you feel you cannot escape. Acrophobia is an irrational fear of heights and claustrophobia is an irrational fear of enclosed spaces. Some people have extreme fear of certain animals, often snakes and spiders.

Many people have a mild degree of fear or discomfort in any of these situations, which is normal. However, when the fear and anxiety become uncontrollable and affect your daily life—for example, if you refuse to ever be in public places or to ever ride in an elevator—it is considered a phobia and requires medical attention.

TREATMENT OPTIONS

If you suspect you have a phobia, ask your doctor to recommend a therapist. The vast majority of phobias can be completely eliminated with treatment. Unlike many other mental disorders, phobias, once overcome, are usually resolved for life.

The most effective form of therapy is called desensitization therapy, or exposure therapy, in which you are exposed to the object of fear either in small increments (systematic desensitization) or all at once (flooding). The affected person is taught relaxation techniques and then visualizes the anxiety-provoking situation while practicing the relaxation techniques in the therapist's office. These exercises are repeated, and may involve using pictures or videos to imagine the feared act.

Finally, the person encounters the feared situation, often with the therapist nearby, and practices relaxation techniques if needed. Most phobias are treated without medications.

Posttraumatic Stress Disorder

Posttraumatic stress disorder (PTSD) is a group of symptoms that can occur in people who have survived a traumatic event involving intense fear, loss of control, and the threat of death. Such events include natural disaster, war, physical or sexual assault, or even sudden, severe illness.

Different types of trauma have different rates of causing PTSD. Natural disasters can cause PTSD in 3% to 16% of people who experience them, whereas rates of PTSD in prisoners of war and concentration camp survivors can be much higher (47% to 50%).

Many experts believe there are factors that make certain individuals more vulnerable to PTSD, such as personality type, history of other traumas, and the availability of social support. PTSD can cause chronic pain, substance abuse, anxiety, depression, and suicide.

SYMPTOMS

PTSD is a syndrome—that is, a collection of symptoms. People with PTSD may relive the distressing event repeatedly in thoughts, dreams, or flashbacks. They are sometimes overly sensitive to loud noises. Emotional numbness, in which little interest is shown in old friends or formerly important activities, may

occur, along with a feeling of being cut off from other people. The emotional trauma also may leave people with PTSD tense and irritable. Difficulty sleeping and concentrating may grow to the point that they interfere with daily life.

TREATMENT OPTIONS

If you have recently experienced major trauma, supportive therapy can prevent PTSD. Ask your doctor to recommend a therapist who has experience in this area. For people in whom PTSD has already developed, psychotherapy combined with medications, including antidepressants (see p.399) and occasionally tranquilizers, can help relieve fear and anxiety and restore normal sleep patterns. Psychoanalysts, psychotherapists, and cognitive and behavioral therapists all treat PTSD.

A highly controversial approach is to use hypnosis to recover memories, with the intent of confronting them directly. Whether such memories are factually correct or represent subconscious fears or even posthypnotic suggestion is difficult to ascertain.

Seasonal Affective Disorder

In seasonal affective disorder (SAD), people experience sadness, depression, and fatigue that comes on in the late fall and subsides in the spring. It is brought on by a lack of sunlight, especially in the most northern and southern regions of the world, where nights are longest in winter. An estimated 10 million Americans suffer from SAD, with women outnumbering men 4 to 1. People most often develop symptoms in their 20s, although SAD sometimes affects children.

Scientists are not sure what causes the condition. One popular theory is that sufferers have too much melatonin, a hormone that communicates signals from the body's internal clock. Other investigators believe that people with SAD suffer from an imbalance in the neurotransmitters serotonin and dopamine (see p.341).

SYMPTOMS

In addition to feeling depressed and lethargic during winter months, you may have headaches and an increased appetite. You may lose interest in activities you once found pleasurable, sleep excessively, become withdrawn, and feel irritable or unable to concentrate. Symptoms must occur for at least 2 successive years to be SAD.

TREATMENT OPTIONS

SAD can be effectively treated with antidepressant drugs, especially selective serotonin reuptake inhibitors (see p.400). Light therapy (phototherapy) may be just as effective, with fewer side effects. Treatment is by supplementing winter's meager supply of sunshine by sitting about 3 feet away from a special bright light source. You are exposed to the light source and occasionally look directly at it. The intensity of prescribed light ranges from 5 to 50 times brighter than ordinary indoor light. There is evidence that greater intensity of light leads to more rapid improvement of SAD.

Most people with SAD report feeling better within 2 to 14 days after starting light therapy. People usually relapse quickly if light treatment is stopped.

Although light therapy appears to be safe for most people, it sometimes leads to eyestrain, headaches (see p.354), insomnia (see p.383), or irritability. Cutting back on the time of exposure or sitting farther away from the light often solves the problem. Treatment can be supplemented by daily walks during the hours with the most sunlight.

PERSONALITY DISORDERS

People with personality disorders see the world differently, and therefore behave differently from what is expected in their culture. No one knows what causes personality disorders—whether a person is born with a tendency to have the disorder or whether it is the result of life experiences. In general, medications are not very useful.

People with personality disorders cope with the world in ways that are often counterproductive and inflexible. However, they do not realize it and do not seek help unless a person they respect tells them they need to change.

Antisocial Personality Disorder

People who have antisocial personality disorder are egocentric and manipulative and consistently display behavior that flies in the face of the norms and rules of society; they lack empathy and remorse. In the past, the terms sociopath and psychopath were used to describe people with this disorder. Perhaps 1% of the population has an antisocial personality disorder. As many as 15% or 20% of prison inmates are thought to have it.

Antisocial personality disorder is used to describe people over 18. Antisocial behavior frequently begins in childhood, however, often involving truancy, rule-breaking, stealing, substance abuse, running away, and vandalism.

As adults, people with antisocial personality disorder may break the law, be physically abusive, fail to fulfill personal responsibilities, lack empathy, and show little remorse for their actions.

They are often unable to maintain close relationships for any length of time. Despite these antisocial behaviors, people with the disorder can be temporarily charming and seductive in order to manipulate others. Once they get their way, the charm disappears.

The goal of treatment is to rehabilitate the individual, either through behavioral therapy or psychotherapy (see Types of Therapy, p.393). Medications are not effective.

Obsessive-Compulsive Personality Disorder

Obsessive-compulsive personality disorder is marked by extreme perfectionism. As in obsessive-compulsive disorder (see p.404), there may be persistent or recurring thoughts or impulses. However, the thoughts are not as intrusive, and the compulsive behaviors are not as uncontrollable.

Obsessive-compulsive personality disorder often emerges in early childhood. Affected people can be such perfectionists about their work and their possessions that they fail to attend to personal relationships. They are preoccupied with performing tasks perfectly yet are often plagued by indecisiveness.

Obsessive-compulsive personalities tend to be moralistic and critical, with an unyielding sense of the correct way of doing things. They tend to be emotionally reserved, stingy, and have difficulty parting with possessions, regardless of value. Cognitive-behavioral therapy (see p.393) sometimes helps the sufferer understand and keep his or her perfectionism from being destructive.

Passive-Aggressive Personality Disorder

People with passive-aggressive personality disorder resent people with authority over them. They express this resentment by subtly resisting demands, rather than actively confronting them. Their passive resistance is an expression of hidden aggressive feelings.

Passive-aggressive personality disorder usually begins in early adulthood. Affected people often procrastinate and conveniently forget to fulfill obligations, whether social or work-related. At the same time, they balk at the weight of their responsibilities and believe they are underappreciated for their efforts. When they fail at a task, they are quick to blame others.

A passive-aggressive personality can thwart personal and social relationships, undermine professional advancement, and make it difficult for individuals to achieve personal goals. Depression (see p.395) often accompanies and aggravates the symptoms. Treatment focuses on counseling that aims to make the person aware of the destructive behaviors in an effort to change them. Psychotherapy (see p.393) may also focus on uncovering and understanding the repressed aggression that drives the destructive behavior.

Paranoid Personality Disorder

People who have paranoid personality disorder are preoccupied with the sense that others are trying to undermine them or do them harm. Unlike people with paranoid schizophrenia, people with paranoid personality disorder do not have delusions. They do not, for example, believe the police are after them. They are suspicious of almost anyone and scrutinize situations and people for hidden motives, which leads to a tendency to be secretive, easily offended, humorless, and guarded.

Quick to blame others and to defend their own importance, people with paranoid disorder have difficulty with personal relationships; their fear of persecution limits the depths of their emotional ties with others.

Symptoms of paranoia may also occur in people with brain damage, substance abuse, and mental illness such as bipolar disorder (see p.401) and schizophrenia (see p.409).

Paranoid personality disorder is difficult to treat because affected people are often unaware of a problem; it frequently takes the urging of family or friends before they seek treatment. Approaches include behavioral therapy or psychotherapy (see Types of Therapy, p.393).

Borderline Personality Disorder

People with borderline personality disorder are almost always in a state of crisis or instability. They have a severe lack of self-confidence and have turbulent relationships. They are often angry at others for abandoning them. Affected people have chronic feelings of emptiness and often act out in manipulative, self-destructive ways; they may even attempt suicide. At times, their thoughts may become highly disordered and may even seem psychotic. At other times they may have feelings of being separated from everyday reality.

Treatment can be difficult. People with borderline personality disorder can have great difficulty entering into any kind of relationship with a therapist because of intense fears that, subsequently, they will be abandoned by the therapist.

PSYCHOSES

Psychoses, also known as thought disorders, are characterized by gross distortions of reality. A psychotic person will often have:

- **Delusions**—fixed beliefs that are false, or even impossible, such as that he or she is a historical figure (like Joan of Arc).

- **Hallucinations**—hearing or seeing things that are not real.

Brief Reactive Psychosis

Brief reactive psychosis is a disorder in which the affected person has delusions or hallucinations (see above) or behaves in a very illogical way, but only for a short time (no longer than a month) before returning to his or her normal behavior.

Brief reactive psychosis is usually a reaction to a very stressful or traumatic event, such as physical or sexual abuse, death of a loved one, war, or disaster. It most often affects young people between the teenage years and early adulthood. Sufferers may be forgetful, even about events that occurred minutes before, and sometimes dress bizarrely. After the psychotic period stops, affected people may feel depressed and anxious.

Antipsychotic drugs, including chlorpromazine and haloperidol, may be prescribed to help eliminate psychotic symptoms. Psychotherapy (see p.393) can provide vital emotional support in dealing with the event that triggered the psychosis.

Schizophrenia

Schizophrenia is a severe mental illness characterized by delusions and hallucinations (see left), a loss of emotional expressiveness, and confused thought and speech. It is the most common type of psychosis.

A person with untreated schizophrenia generally withdraws from everyday relationships into a world of fantasy and bizarre behavior. Schizophrenia usually starts during the teen years or in young adulthood; it affects about 1% of the population worldwide, men and women equally.

Doctors classify schizophrenia into three categories: (1) paranoid schizophrenia, which is characterized by delusions of being persecuted or delusions that are grandiose ("I am the king of the world") and auditory hallucinations; (2) catatonic schizophrenia, in which the sufferer may stop moving or talking and suddenly becomes very excitable; and (3) disorganized (or undifferentiated) schizophrenia, in which the sufferer is incoherent and either shows inappropriate emotions or is expressionless.

The cause of schizophrenia is not known. There is an important hereditary component: a child of two schizophrenic parents has a 40% chance of becoming schizophrenic (the average risk is 1%). For reasons that are not clearly understood, being born in February or March may also increase the risk.

Brain structure and chemistry are abnormal in affected people. The brain either produces too much of the neurotransmitter dopamine (see p.341) or is overly sensitive to its effects. The most successful medicines for schizophrenia reduce dopamine production. Many psychiatrists once believed that schizophrenia resulted from an abnormality in the interaction between child and parents; few currently hold this theory.

Schizophrenia: Dr Dorwart's Advice

I have found that many parents confuse the early symptoms of schizophrenia, which often become apparent between the ages of 15 and 25, with normal teenage rebellion, or perhaps the use of drugs. Since research has shown that this disease responds much better to treatment if identified early, I suggest that if parents see a sudden, marked change of behavior in their son or daughter, they should consider a professional consultation with their family doctor, who may then recommend a consultation with a psychiatrist. It is better to be too careful than overlook a potential problem.

ROBERT DORWART, MD
CAMBRIDGE HOSPITAL
HARVARD MEDICAL SCHOOL

SYMPTOMS

The symptoms of schizophrenia usually develop gradually (although they can occur suddenly), often first manifesting as an unkempt appearance, social withdrawal, or deterioration of performance at work or school.

Schizophrenia gets worse and better in cycles. During a relapse, thoughts become psychotic. People with schizophrenia may have delusions of grandeur in which they believe they are capable of superhuman feats or are famous, heroic figures. They may have auditory hallucinations in which voices insult them or command them to do things.

Affected people may develop delusions that others are listening to and "stealing" their thoughts. They may make rapid and illogical shifts from one topic to another, talk in nonsensical rhymes, or make up words. Those affected may remain withdrawn, exhibit socially inappropriate behavior, and show little emotional spontaneity.

When schizophrenia is most severe, affected people may hurt themselves, attempt suicide, or become violent toward others.

There is a common misconception that people with schizophrenia have a "split personality" in which they alternate between being two or more different people. There are rare instances of people who have such split personalities, but this is not what schizophrenia is.

TREATMENT OPTIONS

If the person seems very disturbed, do not leave him or her alone. In some cases, the only way for a person with schizophrenia to become stabilized may be to be hospitalized against his or her will.

Antipsychotic medicines, such as haloperidol and chlorpromazine, have greatly improved the outlook for schizophrenia, although it still remains a serious illness that cannot always be treated successfully. Antipsychotic drugs are effective in reducing the hallucinations and delusions and in helping to maintain logical thoughts, but it can take time and persistent adherence to medication for these drugs to do their best job. Medications help to prevent relapse.

During the first few weeks, side effects of antipsychotic medicines can include dry mouth, blurred vision, and, in some people, difficulty urinating. After long-term use, the most serious side effect is a disorder of movement called tardive (meaning late onset) dyskinesia (meaning movement disorder).

What Does It Mean to Have a "Nervous Breakdown"?

The old-fashioned phrase "nervous breakdown" was once applied to people who became psychotic, and sometimes to people who were severely depressed or anxious and unable to function. The phrase has no value and is not used today by mental health professionals.

Psychosis and Violence: Dr Borus's Advice

When someone has a psychosis—when they lose touch with reality, imagine things that aren't true, see or hear things that aren't there— their disordered thinking on rare occasion can lead them to commit a violent act against another person. And when this happens, it often makes headlines. But what doesn't make the headlines is the fact that of the millions of people in the United States who suffer from mental disorders, including psychosis, only a tiny few ever commit a violent act. We fear psychotic people, and shun them, but without reason. Our fear further isolates them, and makes it harder for them to get the help they need. Of course, if you see someone preparing to act violently—whether they are psychotic or not—get help. But there's no need to be fearful of people just because they have a psychosis.

JONATHAN F. BORUS, MD
BRIGHAM AND WOMEN'S HOSPITAL,
HARVARD MEDICAL SCHOOL

Tardive dyskinesia is characterized by continual chewing movements of the mouth and tongue, with the tongue suddenly darting out of the mouth. It develops in about 15% to 20% of people taking antipsychotic drugs for long periods. There is no reliable treatment for this condition, which eventually subsides for many people once the drug is stopped.

Lower doses of the traditional antipsychotic medicines than were once used are as effective as higher doses in minimizing the psychotic thinking of schizophrenia and are less likely to cause tardive dyskinesia.

A new generation of drugs—including clozapine, risperidone, olanzapine, and quetiapine—do not appear to cause tardive dyskinesia but cause other side effects. These drugs typically have been used to treat people who have not responded to the more traditional antipsychotic medicines, but they now are being used by some physicians as first-line treatment.

People with schizophrenia may also benefit from stabilizing influences such as group homes and sheltered workshops. Fewer than 20% are able to work full-time. Family support therapy has also been found to be helpful in preventing relapse.

The best prognosis (outlook) seems to occur with a combination of family involvement, psychotherapy, and strict adherence to medication. While psychoanalysis (see p.393) is not useful, periodic contact with a trusted therapist may be very helpful. Many people with schizophrenia have difficulty establishing and maintaining supportive relationships with family and friends; a therapist may be the affected person's only connection to the world.

OTHER BEHAVIORAL AND EMOTIONAL DISORDERS

Substance Addiction and Abuse

People engaging in substance abuse have begun a practice that is entirely in their control. They then repeat the practice and become addicted. Thereafter, they are unable to control their use of addicting substances, including those that are legal (such as alcohol) and illegal (such as heroin).

Abuse of the substance can cause medical complications or negative social consequences—including serious problems with family, friends, coworkers, job, money, and the law—but still use of the substance continues.

Addiction is a physical dependence on a chemical substance. The dependence leads to unpleasant symptoms, called withdrawal, when a person stops using the substance. People often begin using an addicting substance because it initially gives them pleasure. However, by the time addiction has developed, the pleasure is gone. The driving force behind continued use of the substance is a need to avoid the unpleasant symptoms of withdrawal.

There is a strong hereditary component to addiction. For example, children raised apart from alcoholic biological parents have four times the risk of becoming alcoholics than the general population.

The hereditary nature of addiction means that different people have different susceptibilities to becoming addicted. Why one person can have a drink or two each day and not become addicted to alcohol, whereas another becomes addicted, remains a mystery. It appears that people with a tendency to become addicted to one substance also have a tendency to become addicted to other substances.

Environmental factors such as physical and sexual abuse or disadvantaged social status and other factors also play an important role, although people from all walks of life are vulnerable to addiction.

While addiction fosters personality changes over time, there are no specific personality characteristics that predict a person will develop addictive behavior. However, some substance abusers suffer from personality disorders and other psychiatric conditions and may use substances to relieve symptoms.

The most common addictions involve the use of alcohol, tobacco, other legal and illegal drugs, and other mood-altering substances. The use of substances may not only be physically and psychologically harmful to the user but may lead to antisocial behavior. Antisocial behavior can lead to crime, which can occur both when a person is high on a substance or when a person is fighting withdrawal and needs money to obtain the substance to which he or she is addicted.

Depression is unusually common in people who engage in substance abuse.

ALCOHOLISM

Generally, people follow one of three patterns of alcohol abuse. They drink and become intoxicated daily; they drink at specific but predictable times; or they stop drinking for extended periods that end in binges of constant drinking that can last for several days, weeks, or months.

Chronic alcoholism is a progressive disease that develops in stages, usually beginning between the ages of 20 and 40.

The first stage involves using alcohol to relieve tension. It is during this time that a physical dependence on the drug begins to emerge. During the second stage, the alcoholic becomes more and more preoccupied with obtaining alcohol; he or she loses control, suffers blackouts, and forgets alcohol-related events.

In the third stage, behavior and personality changes start to take place, including aggressive behavior and a complete lack of insight into the problem. Finally, in the late stages, the persistent use of alcohol begins to affect the person's physical and emotional health, causing serious deterioration in ability to function.

Physical complications can include inflammation of the stomach (see Gastritis, p.752), inflammation of the liver (see Hepatitis, p.758), permanent nerve and brain damage (forget-fulness, blackouts, or problems with short-term memory), and inflammation of the pancreas (see Pancreatitis, p.768).

Long-term use also can increase the risk and severity of pneumonia (see p.496) and tuberculosis (see p.504); can damage the heart, leading to heart failure (see p.683); and can cause cirrhosis of the liver, leading to liver failure (see p.765).

Alcohol intoxication is a major cause of motor vehicle collisions and other injuries, often with fatal consequences. Alcohol consumption by pregnant women can cause fetal alcohol syndrome (see p.975), which can cause mental retardation.

Withdrawal from alcohol carries its own risks, including restlessness, agitation, hallucinations, delirium, and seizures. In its most severe form, alcohol withdrawal can be life-threatening and the alcoholic should be hospitalized. See p.63 for further discussion of alcoholism and its treatment.

TOBACCO ADDICTION

Chewing tobacco or smoking cigarettes, pipes, or cigars are all forms of nicotine addiction. About 45 million people in the United States use nicotine in some form. More than half of smokers light their first cigarette within a half hour of waking up, and 30% have never stopped smoking for as long as a week.

Most of them wish they had never started; only 5% succeed in quitting on the first attempt, and only 3% to 5% are able to remain abstinent for a year. Nicotine is one of the most addictive of all drugs; the addiction develops quickly and is persistent. Habitual drug addicts say it is easier to give up cocaine and heroin than to stop smoking.

In our society, it is easier for human beings to become and remain dependent on tobacco than virtually any other drug. In comparison with other addicting substances, tobacco is relatively inexpensive and easily available.

It does not make you high and so it does not interfere with your ability to function. Smokers quickly become tolerant of any unpleasant effects (such as bad taste or odor). The cigarette is a highly effective drug-delivery device. Nicotine goes straight to the lungs, where it is absorbed by the blood, sent to the heart, and pumped into the arteries and the brain. The habit is performed regularly and often—75,000 puffs a year at a pack a day—thereby reinforcing the behavior.

Everyone knows the health reasons for quitting. Tobacco accounts for about 1 of 7 deaths in the United States, 1 of 3 between the ages of 35 and 70. Smoking causes chronic bronchitis (see p.517) and emphysema (see p.517). Women who smoke during pregnancy have a higher rate of miscarriage (see p.928).

More on Addiction and Abuse

Addiction, abuse, and ways to quit harmful substances are discussed further on these pages:

- Alcohol (p.63)
- Tobacco (p.56)
- Prescription drugs (p.1157)
- Illegal drugs (p.67)

Tobacco use greatly increases the risk of cancers of the lung (see p.524), lip (see p.489), tongue, throat, cheek, esophagus (see p.749), cervix (see p.1067), and bladder (see p.822).

The role of smoking in causing heart disease leads to even more deaths than from cancers caused by smoking. Cigarette smoking raises blood pressure (see High Blood Pressure, p.644), makes blood clot too easily (see Platelets, p.709), reduces the heart's oxygen supply (see p.652), and damages the walls of arteries (see Atherosclerosis, p.653). Each of these adverse effects increases the chance of heart attacks. For more about nicotine addiction and its treatment, see p.56.

COMPULSIVE GAMBLING

Some people become addicted to certain behaviors, rather than to chemical substances. The behaviors stimulate the release of natural substances in the brain that are like opiate painkillers. The person becomes mildly addicted to these natural painkillers in the same way people become addicted to painkilling pills.

One usually healthy example of such addiction (which can occasionally be carried to unhealthy extremes) is compulsive high-level physical-fitness training. One unhealthy example is compulsive gambling.

Compulsive gamblers, like most people with an addiction, are preoccupied with gambling to the exclusion of other activities in their lives. In the United States, the number of compulsive gamblers has risen threefold over the past 20 years.

Gambling compulsions are more common among men. In a characteristic pattern, gambling moves from being an occasional activity to a habitual one, and the size of the wagers steadily increases. Compulsive gamblers may shirk daily responsibilities and loved ones, sell personal property to finance their bets, lie to hide their losses, and engage in illegal activity to support their habit.

Compulsive gamblers often have other psychiatric disorders as well, including panic disorder (see p.404), depression (see p.395), bipolar disorder (see p.401), and substance abuse, particularly alcoholism.

If you know someone who shows signs of being addicted to gambling, attempt to convince him or her to see a doctor for psychotherapy (see p.393) or to attend Gamblers Anonymous (see p.1232), which is modeled after Alcoholics Anonymous.

TREATMENT OPTIONS

Support groups (12-step programs) are considered a mainstay of the treatment of many forms of substance use. Participants attend a program based on frequent, regular meetings with others who share the problem and are urged to be honest in describing their problems. Members of the group look to each other for support and for ideas about how to deal with their problems.

Most support groups are not run by health professionals. For this reason, there are few research studies evaluating their effectiveness. However, 12-step programs have existed for many years, clearly have helped many people, and are encouraged by most professionals as part of the treatment of addictions, along with a combination of supportive and behavioral psychotherapy.

There are also growing numbers of medicines that are helpful in overcoming addiction to alcohol (see p.66), tobacco (see p.61), and some illegal drugs.

Anorexia Nervosa and Bulimia

Anorexia nervosa (its Greek and Latin roots mean "lack of appetite of nervous origin") involves dieting or not eating to the point where weight is 15% below ideal body weight. It is characterized by an obsessive fear of becoming overweight, an inaccurate perception that one is overweight, and the use of compulsive rituals to lose weight.

Bulimia, also called bulimia nervosa or binge-purge disorder, is binge eating (rapid consumption of large quantities of food) followed by self-induced vomiting and/or overuse of laxatives. Both disorders usually begin in early or middle adolescence.

About 90% of those with anorexia nervosa are women; about 0.7% of all women in the United States are affected.

Bulimia is much more common. Studies of female high school and college students have found 4.5% to 18% have had bulimia.

Like many psychiatric disorders, anorexia and bulimia seem to run in families. The rate of anorexia among mothers and sisters of anorectic women may be as great as 10%. Theories about the origins of eating disorders vary widely, including peer and societal pressure to be thin, fear of sexuality, and family conflicts.

Some doctors think that there is also an important hereditary, biological component.

Anorexia and bulimia may cause many serious complications, including hormonal abnormalities, with loss of menstrual cycles, osteoporosis (see p.596), and imbalances of several minerals; the latter can trigger serious heart rhythm disturbance and even death.

SYMPTOMS

Affected people begin to eliminate foods from their diet and to skip meals; sometimes they also exercise obsessively. They may feel they look fat, although they may be gaunt. Periods of not eating may alternate with periods of binge eating. Menstrual periods may stop.

As their weight drops and their health deteriorates, skin begins to look pale or yellow. Other symptoms include brittle nails and hair, constipation, anemia, swollen joints, feeling cold all the time, sores that do not heal, and difficulty concentrating and thinking.

Over a 10-year period, up to 5% of anorexic women die of complications, including infection, heart rhythm disturbance, and suicide.

People with bulimia also fear weight gain, but unlike people with anorexia, they often realize that their behavior is not normal. They may have depression after a binge-purge episode.

The physical effects can be serious, including fatigue, weakness, constipation, bloating, swollen salivary glands, erosion of tooth enamel or sore throat from exposure to stomach acids by repeated vomiting, dehydration, loss of potassium, and tearing of the esophagus from vomiting. Overuse of laxatives can cause dangerous loss of fluid and minerals.

TREATMENT OPTIONS

Treatment for both disorders is more successful the earlier it is started. If you suspect that you or someone you know is anorexic or bulimic, seek medical help as soon as possible. A doctor may recommend hospitalization if body weight is more than 30% below the ideal.

Cognitive therapy seeks to convince people that their view of themselves as overweight is wrong, and their attempts to lose weight are not rational. Behavioral therapy involves developing a contract with the person to gain weight in exchange for certain rewards (such as more autonomy at home or special privileges).

Family therapy is important to help families understand the illness. Medication may be prescribed so that those with depression or compulsive habits can cope. Many young women with anorexia nervosa or bulimia continue to see a psychiatrist even after their weight has stabilized to resolve emotional issues.

Conversion Reaction

Conversion reaction is a psychological illness in which troubling emotions are converted into physical symptoms without any detectable physical cause. Common conversions include paralysis, inability to speak, vomiting, blindness, and false pregnancy.

The symptoms are usually related to deep-seated psychological conflicts. For example, sudden paralysis may be a person's way of avoiding a particular action.

If you suspect conversion reaction in someone close to you, urge that person to seek medical care. A doctor will perform a thorough medical evaluation to exclude serious physical illness and may recommend the person seek the help of a psychiatrist.

Antidepressant drugs (see p.399) are sometimes prescribed, often along with psychotherapy (see p.393). Stress reduction techniques (such as regular exercise and relaxation) may also help reduce symptoms.

Somatization Disorder

In somatization disorder, the affected person experiences a group of specific physical symptoms for which there is no physical explanation. Frequently, a person with somatization disorder also is suffering from depression (see p.395), anxiety (see p.402), or a past experience of physical or sexual abuse.

More common in females, the disorder usually starts during the teenage years. If you or someone you know appears to have somatization disorder, see a doctor. Psychotherapy (see p.393) can help the affected person understand hidden conflicts that may be contributing to the symptoms. The doctor may also prescribe medication.

Eyes

Of all our senses, it may be sight that most informs the mind. The eye and brain translate light waves into the sensation we call vision. Here is how it happens. Light first passes through the outward-curving cornea, the transparent layer that coats the front of the eye. The shape of the eye is maintained by the pressure of aqueous humor, a fluid that fills the front (anterior) chamber of the eye. The pressure inside the eye is determined by how much aqueous humor is produced, and by how much is reabsorbed into the body through a tiny drainage canal called the canal of Schlemm. Abnormally high fluid pressure occurs in glaucoma.

The cornea starts the process of focusing light waves so that a crisp image is presented to the back of the eye; this process is called refraction. The most common eye problems involve errors of refraction. Light then passes through the pupil, the circular hole in the colored iris. The pupil can change its diameter, closing to about 0.06 inch when light is brightest, and widening six times to about 0.33 inch when light is dimmest.

Emotions also can change the diameter of the pupil; anger generally causes it to narrow, while positive feelings (and some drugs) cause it to open up. Melanin in the iris gives eyes their color. If you have dark eyes, your irises have a high concentration of melanin; a scant quantity results in green or blue eyes.

Light then passes through the lens, which, when healthy, is a clear disc. A process called accommodation (see Focusing Problems, p.420) can change the shape of the lens, which helps the eye focus, just like the lens of a camera. The focused light travels through a thick, gelatinous fluid called the vitreous humor to land on the retina, the multitiered screen of light-sensitive cells in the back of the eye.

The retina ("net" in Latin) is aptly named. Its layer contains millions of light-sensitive cells called rods and cones. Rods detect light; cones detect color. When the rods and cones encounter light, a chemical reaction takes place that generates an electrical impulse. The electrical impulse travels from the retina through the optic nerve to the brain; you experience this sensation as sight. One of the chemicals involved in the chemical reaction is a derivative of vitamin A called retinol. This is why a deficiency of vitamin A can cause night blindness (see p.441). Dysfunction or absence of cones causes color blindness (see p.445).

The eye has other structures that can become diseased. The white of the eye (the sclera) is covered by a transparent film called the conjunctiva, which can become infected and inflamed in the common disorder conjunctivitis (see p.427).

Movement of the eyes is controlled by a group of muscles that

Cross-Section of Eye

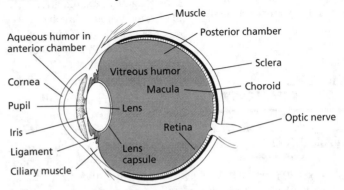

Rays of light are bent as they pass through the cornea, lens, and vitreous humor, ultimately coming to focus on or near the retina. The retina has light-sensitive cells that capture light energy and send it as electric impulses via the optic nerve to the brain. You experience this as sight.

Eye Anatomy

The eyeball is surrounded by fat and muscles and rests in the bony orbit. Six extraocular muscles control the eye's movement. The outermost surface of the eyeball includes the cornea (a clear dome that helps focus light) and the white sclera (which protects the eye).

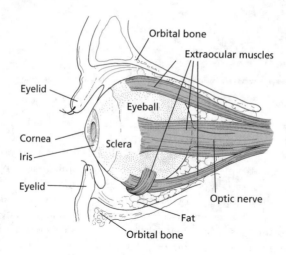

Orbital bone
Extraocular muscles
Eyelid
Eyeball
Cornea
Sclera
Iris
Eyelid
Optic nerve
Fat
Orbital bone

normally move in a coordinated fashion. Some people are born with poorly coordinated eye movements, which can cause visual problems.

Tears are made by the lacrimal glands, located underneath the bone of the outer part of the eyebrow. In some eye conditions, not enough tears are made; in others, the tears do not drain properly.

The most common disorders of the eye are focusing problems (see p.420)—nearsightedness, astigmatism, farsightedness, and presbyopia. Infections, structural problems, and tumors can also occur.

SEEING THE OPHTHALMOLOGIST

Periodic eye examinations by an ophthalmologist are the best defense against eye disease. Your primary care physician can recommend an examination schedule that best suits your needs. Generally, children and

people over age 65 should have regular eye examinations (see below).

If you have been diagnosed with an eye condition, such as diabetic retinopathy (see p.434), macular degeneration (see p.440), or glaucoma (see p.435), you should be examined more frequently. See also Warning Signs of Eye Problems, p.419.

What Happens During an Eye Examination?

A thorough eye examination by an ophthalmologist involves a series of evaluations, some of which are done in a darkened room. Some or all of the following may be conducted:

Medical history Before the examination, the ophthalmologist will ask you about your current and past health, including general well-being, diseases in childhood, allergies, and personal and family medical problems. All of these factors can affect your eyes.

Snellen test for visual acuity

The doctor will test your visual acuity—the sharpness of your vision—with a Snellen chart, which has rows of letters and numbers that diminish in size. If you wear corrective lenses, your vision will be tested with your current prescription.

You will be scored according to how well you see. Excellent eyesight is expressed as 20/20, which means you can see at a distance of 20 feet what an individual with excellent vision sees at 20 feet. If you have 20/30 vision, you see at a distance of 20 feet what a person with excellent vision would see at 30 feet. The higher the second number, the worse your vision.

If the test indicates the need for corrective lenses or a prescription adjustment, the doctor will use an instrument to measure the amount of correction needed. To confirm that reading, he or she will test you with a variety of lenses to ascertain which ones give you the best sight.

Peripheral vision evaluation

How well you see peripherally—that is, at the sides of each eye—is evaluated by covering one eye and fixing the other eye on a point straight ahead. Your doctor will move an object (such as a pen) back and forth at the outer edges of your visual field and ask you to note when you see it moving.

External eye exam The doctor examines your outer eye—the lids, lashes, and the bony socket called the orbit. The appearance of your eyeballs will be studied and the doctor will note whether your pupils dilate (open) and

Who Should Care for My Eyes?

Your primary care doctor can treat many common diseases of the eye, but other eye problems require a specialist. The health professionals listed here have widely varying medical training, but each may be involved in helping you care for your eyes.

Ophthalmologists are medical doctors trained to diagnose and treat all eye disorders. Ophthalmologists go through 4 years of college, 4 years of medical school, and a minimum of 4 more years of specialized education and training in diseases of the eyes. They perform surgery on the eyes and are licensed to prescribe drugs, glasses, and contact lenses. Some ophthalmologists specialize further in a specific disease (such as glaucoma), in a part of the eye (such as the retina), or in a type of person (such as children).

Optometrists receive 4 years of training after completing college and are licensed to diagnose and treat vision problems and prescribe glasses and contact lenses. They are not medical doctors and therefore cannot perform surgery. In some states, they are licensed to prescribe drugs and treat eye diseases.

Opticians are technicians trained to prepare and fit glasses after an ophthalmologist or an optometrist has examined your eyes and prescribed the vision correction you need. Opticians do not examine eyes for vision problems or disease.

---

contract (close) normally in response to light.

Eye muscle check Checking the coordination of the six muscles in each eye to ensure that your eyes move together is an important part of the exam. To test the alignment of your eyes, you will be asked to focus on a target and, at the same time, to cover and uncover each eye. This test can detect a tendency for either eye to drift.

In a separate test, the doctor will ask you to follow a penlight with your gaze to determine whether your range of motion is normal and if your eyes move together.

Anterior eye exam Ophthalmologists and optometrists use a slit-lamp to examine the structures of the front of your eyes. A slitlamp is an instrument that combines a powerful microscope with a narrow beam (or slit) of light.

As you keep your head steady on a chin rest, light is projected onto and into the eye. The doctor can clearly see your cornea, anterior (front) chamber, lens, and vitreous humor. With extra lenses, the doctor can also see the retina.

Your doctor may also use eyedrops to dilate (open) your pupils to get a better view of the interior of your eyes. The effects of the drops take time to wear off, so you may experience sensitivity to light and difficulty in focusing for several hours (unless you are given eyedrops that reverse the dilation). It is wise to avoid driving while your pupils are dilated.

Retina and optic nerve evaluation Your doctor will use a hand-held instrument with a focusing lens called an ophthalmoscope to examine each part of the eye: cornea, aqueous humor, lens, vitreous humor, optic nerve, and retina.

Tonometry Tonometry is a painless test that measures the pressure of the fluid in your eye to detect signs of glaucoma (see p.435). After the eye is numbed with anesthetic drops, the doctor touches the cornea with an instrument called a tonometer to measure the eye's resistance.

Normal pressure is 10 to 22 millimeters of mercury (mm Hg). However, if eye pressure falls within this range, glaucoma can still develop. Likewise, people who have elevated pressure may not get glaucoma. Some optometrists use another kind of tonometer that measures pressure after delivering a puff of air to the cornea. This technique is less accurate.

EYELIDS

Blepharitis

Blepharitis is inflammation of the eyelids. In many people it is a recurring condition that causes irritation, itching, flakiness, crusting, and redness. Blepharitis is sometimes accompanied by a bacterial infection. People with rosacea (see p.535), seborrheic dermatitis (see p.551), oily skin, dandruff, or dry eyes are most susceptible to blepharitis. While unsightly, blepharitis does not cause permanent damage to eyesight.

SYMPTOMS

It is common for people with blepharitis to awaken to find mucus in the corners of their eyes. Both the upper and lower lids may appear greasy and may be crusted with scales that cling to the lashes. This debris sometimes gets into the eyes, causing a grainy feeling when you blink; in some people this leads to conjunctivitis (see p.427).

Your eyes may also become red and swollen. In severe cases of blepharitis, tiny ulcers develop along the edges of the eyelids, eyelashes fall out, or an ulcer develops on the cornea (see Corneal Ulcer, p.429) in response to the inflammation.

TREATMENT OPTIONS

Use this home remedy, in the morning and at night:

- Place a clean washcloth dampened with warm water over closed lids for 5 minutes to loosen crusts and oily debris.

- Fill a small dish with 2 to 3 ounces of warm water and three drops of baby shampoo.

- Moisten a washcloth or cotton-tipped applicator with the baby shampoo solution and rub the base of the eyelashes to remove loosened scales.

- Rinse the lids with warm water and pat gently with a clean, dry towel.

If your condition does not improve, talk to your doctor. He or she may prescribe an ointment containing antibiotics to clear up the infection. Eyedrops containing a corticosteroid drug (see p.895) are also sometimes prescribed.

Ectropion

Ectropion is a condition in which the lower eyelid turns outward and does not touch the eye. Without the protection of the lid, the inside of the eyelid and the eye itself become dry, irritated, and inflamed. Additionally, the out-turned lid can prevent the tears that lubricate your eye from draining properly, resulting in a watery eye.

The main cause of ectropion is relaxation of the muscles and tendons in the lower lid, which normally hold the lid close to the eye; this is most common in the aging eye. Ectropion can also be caused by any condition that pulls down the lower lid, such as tightening of scar tissue or a facial nerve disorder.

Untreated ectropion can lead to mucous discharge and crusting, infection, impaired vision, and damage to the cornea due to inadequate lubrication.

To restore moisture, your doctor may recommend artificial tears or lubricating ointments. He or she may also recommend a simple surgical procedure to reposition the lower lid; it is performed on an outpatient basis using a local anesthetic (see p.168).

Entropion

Entropion is a condition in which the eyelid and eyelashes (usually of the lower lid) turn inward toward the eye, causing the lid and lashes to rub against the cornea and conjunctiva. This is not only painful but can cause excessive tearing, mucous discharge, and crusting. More serious consequences include impaired vision, conjunctivitis (see p.427), and corneal ulcers (see p.429) caused by the rubbing.

Entropion most often affects older people whose lower eyelid tissues have become lax. The weakness of the tissues can lead to abnormal contraction of the muscle at the edge of the eyelid, resulting in a pulling of the lid toward the eye. When entropion is present at birth, the eyelids sometimes return to normal on their own.

Your doctor may suggest that you use adhesive tape to tape your lower eyelid down to your cheek in an effort to pull the lid back to its normal position. Soothing eyedrops and ointments may also be helpful. If these approaches are not successful, your doctor may recommend a surgical procedure in which the eyelid is repositioned so that it does not touch the eye

Warning Signs of Eye Problems

If you have any of the symptoms listed below, schedule an eye examination. The last five symptoms may indicate a more serious problem and require immediate attention. Remember that some eye diseases have no early warning signs, so you should have regular eye checkups even if you have no symptoms. Early treatment can help prevent vision loss or blindness. Call your doctor if you:

- Have particular trouble adjusting to darkness.

- Are highly sensitive to light or glare.

- Have difficulty focusing on near or distant objects.

- Have double vision.

- Have red eyes or crusty, swollen eyelids.

- Have recurring pain in or around your eyes.

- See a change in the color of your iris (the colored part of the eye).

- See a dark spot in the center of your viewing area.

- Have excessive tearing or watering or have very dry, itchy, or burning eyes.

- See spots or ghostlike images.

- Have sudden loss of vision in one or both eyes.

- Have vision that suddenly becomes blurred or hazy.

- See flashes of light or showers of black spots, halos, or rainbows around light.

- Have a loss of vision that looks like a curtain descending.

- Experience any loss of peripheral vision.

---

surface; it is usually performed using a local anesthetic (see p.168) and does not involve a hospital stay.

Bumps on the Eyelid

(See also Color Guide to Visual Diagnosis, p.567)
Lumps and bumps of several types can occur on the eyelids. Skin cancers such as basal cell carcinoma (see p.546) can also occur on the eyelids.

Styes are pus-filled abscesses of the eyelid oil glands that form near eyelashes. They are caused by bacteria that infect the oil-producing follicle (root) of an eyelash. A stye appears as a painful red pustule or a tender red lump on the edge of the eyelid. Several days after forming, it usually bursts and drains, which relieves the pain; the swelling subsides within about a week. People with chronic ble-

pharitis (see p.418) develop styes more frequently.

Begin the following treatment as soon as you feel a stye coming on. Using a clean washcloth, apply warm water compresses to the stye several times a day until the stye opens on its own; do not squeeze it. Once it has opened, wash your eyelid thoroughly to prevent the bacteria from spreading. If you are prone to recurring styes, your doctor may prescribe antibiotics in tablet or ointment form to treat an infection or normalize the secretions of your oil glands.

Chalazions are swellings (usually painless) in the eyelid caused by blockage of one of the oil glands that lubricate the eye. A chalazion may be small, or large enough to blur vision. Small ones often go away on their own without treatment. However, you can accelerate the process by applying a warm water compress using a

clean cloth twice a day for 5 minutes. If the chalazion does not go away, or if it is large and blurs your vision, talk to your doctor. If the chalazion becomes infected by bacteria living on the eyelid, it becomes painful and red.

Your doctor may prescribe antibiotics and/or corticosteroid eyedrops or surgery to remove it. Surgery to drain the chalazion is performed using a local anesthetic (see p.168) and does not require a stay in the hospital.

Xanthelasmas are raised yellow patches on the eyelids (see p.541).

Papillomas are slow-growing, noncancerous bumps that can vary from pink to skin colored. They can occur anywhere on the eyelid. Unsightly or large growths can be surgically removed using a local anesthetic (see p.168).

Cysts of many variations can occur on the eyelids. They are almost always noncancerous.

They should be removed if they grow, disturb vision, or are located where they are subject to recurring injury, bleeding, or irritation.

Ptosis

Ptosis is a drooping of the upper eyelid. It can affect one or both eyes and may partially block vision. Ptosis is caused by a weakness of the thin levator muscle, which is responsible for keeping the upper eyelid open.

The condition seems to run in families. Ptosis that is present from birth may affect only one eye. Babies born with severe ptosis may require surgery to avoid impaired vision development.

Ptosis in adults usually occurs as a normal part of aging as the muscle of the eyelid loses its strength and tone. However, it can also be caused by an underlying disease or by an injury that affects the nerve that stimulates the levator muscle, or that affects the muscle itself.

Diseases that can cause ptosis include myasthenia gravis (see p.377), diabetes mellitus (see p.832), stroke (see p.342), or any condition that causes muscle weakness. When injury or aging muscle tone have caused the condition, outpatient surgery to strengthen the levator muscle

Ptosis

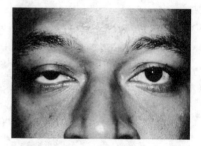

Ptosis (drooping eyelid) can affect one or both eyes and may partially block vision.

and elevate the eyelid is the most common treatment. For ptosis caused by disease, treating the underlying cause can sometimes improve the ptosis.

FOCUSING PROBLEMS

The most common causes of blurred vision come from problems with focusing. This kind of blurred vision comes on slowly, affecting both eyes and the total field of vision.

The process of focusing is called refraction. The eye is like a camera. If the camera lens focuses light directly on the film, the picture is sharp. However, if it focuses light in front of or behind the film, the picture is blurred. It is the same with the eye.

When light rays enter a normal eye, the cornea and lens bend (refract) the rays so that they are focused precisely on the retina. The focal point is the point at which light rays come to perfect focus. Light rays from close objects have a focal point that is farther back in the eye than light rays from distant objects.

The amount of refraction by the cornea is constant, based on the shape of the cornea. The amount of refraction by the lens, however, can be controlled to some degree. Tiny ligaments attach the lens to tiny muscles in the eye called ciliary muscles. By

Myths and Facts: Reading in Dim Light

Myth: Reading in dim light is harmful to your eyes.

Fact: Using your eyes in dim light does not damage your eyes but does cause a temporary strain. Good lighting can make reading and other close work easier.

changing the tension on the ligaments, the ciliary muscles can cause the lens to become more round (which bends light rays more sharply, making the focal point fall closer to the lens) or more flat (which bends light rays less sharply, making the focal point fall deeper in the eye). This process is called accommodation.

There are four common problems with refraction: nearsightedness, astigmatism, farsightedness, and presbyopia.

Nearsightedness

In nearsightedness (also called myopia), objects in the distance are blurred but objects close up can be seen clearly. This is usually because the eyeball is too long from front to back. Thus, while the focal point for close

How the Eye Focuses

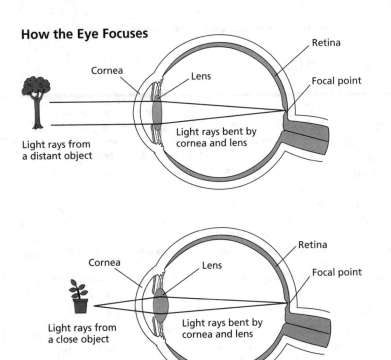

Cornea

Lens

Retina

Focal point

Light rays bent by cornea and lens

Light rays from a distant object

Cornea

Lens

Retina

Focal point

Light rays bent by cornea and lens

Light rays from a close object

When light rays hit the cornea and lens, they bend at a particular angle, which is determined by the fixed curvature of the cornea and the changeable curvature of the lens. Normally, light rays coming from a distant object (top) are parallel and are focused on the retina. Light rays from close objects (bottom) do not come in parallel, but at an angle, and must be focused by increasing the curvature of the lens inside the eye (making it fatter). This happens automatically until age prevents the lens from increasing its curvature as much, a condition called presbyopia.

Common Focusing Problems

NORMAL VISION

Retina

Ciliary muscle

Ligaments

Optic nerve

Focal point on retina

FARSIGHTEDNESS

Retina

Focal point behind retina

NEARSIGHTEDNESS

Retina

Focal point in front of retina

PRESBYOPIA

Retina

Stiff lens

Focal point behind retina

In normal vision, light focuses directly on the retina, producing a sharp image. In nearsightedness, light rays are focused in front of the retina due to either an elongated eyeball or a lens or cornea that excessively bends light rays. In farsightedness, light rays are focused behind the retina, due to a shortened eyeball. In presbyopia, light rays reach the retina before they can be focused (as in farsightedness) because the lens has become stiff and cannot be adjusted by the muscles to bend the rays more sharply.

Computers and Eyestrain: *Dr Bajart's Advice*

Q I spend most of my workday staring at a computer. Does this cause eyestrain or have any other effect on my eyes?

A Working at a computer will not damage your eyes. But many people who look at a computer screen for extended periods blink less often than usual. In one study, people working at computers blinked a third less often than normal. Since blinking helps restore moisture, working at a computer may make your eyes feel dry and irritated, which could contribute to a feeling of eyestrain or tiredness. Refresh your eyes by taking momentary breaks and blinking your eyes several times. Look up from your computer at objects in the distance to relieve eyestrain. Consider using artificial tears before and during prolonged computer use.

ANN M. BAJART, MD
MASSACHUSETTS EYE AND EAR INFIRMARY
HARVARD MEDICAL SCHOOL

Glasses and Contact Lenses

If you need to have your vision corrected, ask your ophthalmologist or optometrist for advice on purchasing glasses, contact lenses, or both.

Glasses are lenses made of glass or plastic that are ground to a shape and thickness that corrects errors of refraction (focusing). Today's lenses can be ground to correct a single overall focusing error, such as nearsightedness, or a combination of focusing problems. Bifocals correct two focusing errors; the top portion is for distance vision and the bottom for close vision. Trifocals contain three different areas of correction: the top part of the lens is for distance vision, the middle for objects 3 to 6 feet away, and the bottom for reading and close work.

Progressive lenses offer the benefits of trifocals without the noticeable dividing line on the lens. Tints, ultraviolet (UV) light protection, scratch protection, anti-reflective coatings, and lenses that darken in bright light (photochromic and transition lenses) are other lens options. Polycarbonate lenses break less easily and have better UV protection. High index lenses are flatter, thinner, and lighter than conventional lenses, offering those who require higher powers a trimmer lens profile and lighter weight.

Contact lenses are thin, transparent, plastic disks designed to fit your eye. They rest on the cornea, floating on the tears that cover the surface of your eye. Eye disorders caused by wearing contact lenses, such as damage to the cornea, are relatively rare, but serious corneal infection can result from improper lens care and hygiene. Wearing contact lenses for too long a period can cause tearing, pain, redness, and blurred vision due to lack of oxygen to the cornea. If you have these symptoms, remove your lenses. If symptoms persist, see your doctor. You may have an infection or you may need refitting or reduction in the number of hours you wear your lenses. Make sure you keep on hand an extra pair of glasses with your most recent prescription to wear in case of emergency. Contact lenses fall into two categories: gas-permeable hard lenses and soft lenses.

Gas-permeable hard lenses offer the clearest vision for some people (particularly those with astigmatism), are the most durable, and require the least maintenance. However, because they are made of hard plastic, they can be less comfortable than soft lenses.

Soft contact lenses cover more eye surface than hard lenses. They are more comfortable but less durable than hard lenses because the thin plastic can be torn. They also require daily cleaning and a once-weekly regimen to remove protein buildup. Extended-wear soft lenses can be worn for a longer period of time because oxygen can pass through them into the cornea, even during sleep. Longer wearing times and improper cleansing places extended-wear lens users at a greater risk for eye infection. Another type of soft contact lens is disposable; you wear a new pair every day. While this reduces the risk of infection, the long-term cost is greater.

objects falls on or near the retina and is in focus, the focal point for distant objects falls in front of the retina and is out of focus. The process of accommodation (in which muscles change the shape of the eye) cannot flatten the lens enough to correct nearsightedness.

Nearsightedness is common and often runs in families; it usually starts during a child's elementary school years and progressively worsens until the late 20s. Eyeglasses or contact lenses can be prescribed to focus the distant light rays properly on the retina by making the focal point for distant objects fall farther back in the eye. However, corrective lenses do not cure, reverse, or slow the progression of nearsightedness.

Astigmatism

In astigmatism, irregularities in the curvature of the cornea or lens cause distorted vision. Some people with astigmatism see diagonal lines out of focus, others see vertical or horizontal lines out of focus. Astigmatism, which may occur with either farsightedness or nearsightedness, tends to remain stable throughout life.

Usually astigmatism can be easily corrected with glasses or toric contact lenses, customized contact lenses that can be made to precisely fit the curves of your cornea. A greater degree of astigmatism may require hard contact lenses.

If you have a more severe case of astigmatism, your doctor may recommend a surgical procedure called astigmatic keratotomy, which is similar to radial keratotomy (see p.425) but requires fewer incisions. In astigmatic keratotomy, bow-shaped incisions are made in the cornea. In the most severe cases, such as when astigmatism is caused by injury to the cornea, a cornea transplant (see p.429) is required.

Purchasing the Right Sunglasses: An Investment in Sight

A link has been established between exposure to ultraviolet (UV) radiation and eye damage, particularly cataracts (see p.430) and age-related macular degeneration (see p.440). The easiest way to protect your eyes from the hazards of the sun's radiation is to wear effective sunglasses.

Neither the darkness of the lenses nor their price is an accurate indication of UV protection. Look for a label from the American National Standards Institute (ANSI), which establishes guidelines for UV protection. There is some evidence that blue light from the sun contributes to age-related macular degeneration; lenses with a red, amber, or orange tint may provide better protection against this light. You will probably have less distortion, however, with gray and green lenses.

Familiarize yourself with the following information before you shop for sunglasses:

UV light has three wavelengths:

- **UV-A** is long, looks almost blue in the visible spectrum, and is responsible for skin tanning and aging; 97% of UV light hitting the earth is UV-A.

- **UV-B** is shorter, more active, and linked to sunburn and skin cancer. A large portion is absorbed by the atmosphere's ozone layer; 3% of UV light hitting the earth is UV-B.

- **UV-C** is short and completely absorbed by the ozone layer.

Sunglasses are labeled according to guidelines for UV protection established by ANSI. There are three categories:

- **Cosmetic** Lightly tinted; good for daily wear. Blocks 70% of UV-B, 20% of UV-A, and 60% of visible light.

- **General purpose** Medium to dark glasses; fine for most outdoor recreation (most sunglasses fall into this category). Blocks 95% of UV-B, 60% of UV-A, and 60% to 90% of visible light.

- **Special purpose** Extremely dark, with UV blockers; recommended for very bright conditions such as beaches and ski slopes. Blocks 99% of UV-B, 60% of UV-A, and 97% of visible light. You can have your regular, nontinted glasses coated with UV block. Glasses made with polycarbonate plastic have UV block automatically.

Surgery to Permanently Correct Focusing Problems

Surgery, using either tiny knives or laser beams to flatten the cornea, is a permanent way to correct problems of refraction—the process of focusing. The flattened cornea makes the focal point for distant objects fall deeper in the eye, on the retina.

Surgery can be performed in the doctor's office or outpatient surgery suite; you do not need to stay in the hospital overnight. Local anesthesia (see p.168) is used, and you may be mildly sedated. You will have to wear a patch over the eye after surgery and may have blurred vision for several days.

No type of surgery can ensure perfect vision; you may still require glasses or contact lenses to treat eye problems that are not fixed by the surgery. In unusual cases, infections complicate the surgery, or vision may worsen. Before undergoing any of the following surgical procedures, you should fully understand the potential risks and side effects:

Radial keratotomy (RK) is a surgical procedure in which a tiny knife is used to make multiple cuts into the cornea. The cuts radiate outward like the spokes of a wheel. The more severe your vision problem, the more incisions are needed. Complications include fluctuating vision, especially the first few months after surgery; a weakened cornea that is more vulnerable to rupture if hit directly; difficulty fitting and wearing contact lenses if they are needed; glare or haze around lights; and, very rarely, permanent vision loss. If you have presbyopia (see p.425), you will still need glasses for reading after RK.

Photorefractive keratectomy (PRK) uses a laser beam to reshape the curve of the cornea. Most often, it is used to correct nearsightedness by removing a layer of corneal tissue to flatten the cornea. The amount of tissue removed varies according to the severity of the nearsightedness. Some surgeons use PRK to treat farsightedness and astigmatism as well. Complications include infection, delayed healing, undercorrection or overcorrection of the vision problem, and the development of astigmatism (see p.423). Many people experience glare around lights at night for some time after the procedure.

Laser in situ keratomileusis (LASIK) is a more recent version of PRK. In this procedure, the doctor slices the cornea from the side, allowing a laser beam to reshape the tissue of the inner layer of the cornea. Complications can include infection of the cornea and loss of sharpness of vision.

Even more so than other forms of permanent vision correction, LASIK is highly dependent on the surgeon's operating skills. In experienced hands, it has the advantage of more predictable wound healing, more rapid improvement of distant vision, and the ability to treat higher degrees of nearsightedness. It can also treat astigmatism and farsightedness.

Farsightedness.

Farsightedness, also called hyperopia, is a condition in which objects at a distance are seen more clearly than objects up close. In farsightedness, the eyeball is shorter than normal from front to back, causing light rays to have a focal point that falls behind the retina, especially light rays from close objects.

Farsighted children and young adults often do not experience blurred vision with farsightedness because they can compensate for it through accommodation, in which the muscles of the eye make the lens more round, which brings the focal point for close objects forward to the retina, creating a clear image. As a person gets older, the lens becomes less flexible and accommodation becomes harder (see Presbyopia, p.425).

Some people who have uncorrected farsightedness have no symptoms or very few. However, others who can still see close objects clearly may get headaches or eyestrain when reading, presumably because the ciliary muscles are overworking to try to correct the problem through accommodation. Most farsighted people require corrective eyeglasses or contact lenses by middle age. In a few people who are farsighted, the angle between the iris and the inside surface of the cornea is narrowed, placing them at greater risk of closed-angle glaucoma (see p.438) in middle age.

Farsightedness is easily cor-

Correcting Nearsightedness

RADIAL KERATOTOMY

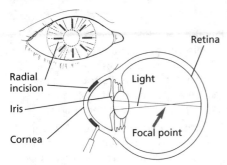

PHOTOREFRACTIVE KERATECTOMY

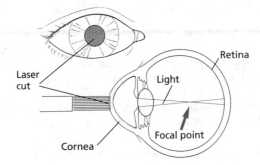

AFTER EITHER TREATMENT

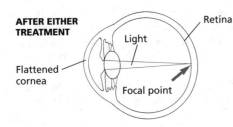

In nearsightedness, light converges just in front of the retina rather than directly on it. In radial keratotomy (top left), four to eight incisions are made in the cornea to reshape it. In photorefractive keratectomy (top right), laser beams remove a thin layer from the center of the cornea. Both procedures flatten the central curvature of the cornea so that light focuses on the retina (left).

---

rected with glasses or contact lenses that have thicker centers and thin edges. These convex lenses bend light from close objects before it hits the lens and retina so that the focal point moves forward to fall on the retina.

Presbyopia

Presbyopia—the Greek word for "old sight"—is the loss of the lens's ability to change the focus of the eye through the process of accommodation, in which the muscles of the eye change the shape of the lens. Presbyopia starts when people are in their early 40s and it eventually affects everyone.

The main difficulty is the same as in farsightedness: light rays from nearby objects have a focal point that lands behind the retina

and is out of focus. In farsightedness, this is because the eyeball is shorter than normal. In presbyopia, it is because the aging lens becomes more rigid and less flexible, making it hard or impossible for accommodation to bend the light rays more sharply to move the focal point forward to fall on the retina.

One of the earliest signs of presbyopia is the need to hold printed material at arm's length to read it. The exhaustion of the ciliary muscles in trying to cause the eyes to focus on close objects also causes some other problems. After reading it may be temporarily hard to see things in the distance clearly, because accommodation is also needed to focus on distant objects.

Reading may also be more difficult in the evening when you

are tired or reading in poor light. Presbyopia occurs regardless of whether you are nearsighted, farsighted, or have astigmatism.

The only remedy for presbyopia is optical correction—reading glasses or contact lenses. People who already wear corrective lenses for nearsightedness may need bifocals (in which the upper portion of the lens is used for distance vision and the lower portion for close vision) or two pairs of glasses, one for distance vision and one for close work.

Many drugstores carry magnifying reading glasses that may help you focus on close work. Talk to your doctor about an appropriate strength before purchasing a pair of magnifying glasses.

Because presbyopia becomes progressively worse, frequent

The Aging Eye

Just as hair turns gray and skin starts to wrinkle, your eyes age. However, except for focusing problems, most people never develop eye disease. A diet rich in vitamin A and antioxidants such as vitamins C and E may slow aging of the eyes. It is important for people of all ages to wear hats and sunglasses that block ultraviolet rays in the sun. Problems of the aging eye include the following:

Lid muscles weaken and the skin becomes thinner and more flaccid, losing its tone. This can cause the skin or muscles of the upper eyelid to droop and/or the lower lid to sag (see Ptosis, p.420; Ectropion, p.418; Entropion, p.418). In some people, when the skin above the eyelid droops, it can interfere with sight; a surgical procedure called blepharoplasty (see p.578) removes some of the excess tissue.

Tear production decreases (see Dry Eyes and Artificial Tears, p.428) and may be compounded by a decrease in the oil component of tears, which causes tears to evaporate more quickly. These changes may make the cornea dry, causing irritation or an uncomfortable, gritty sensation.

The conjunctiva thins and becomes more fragile and may take on a yellow tinge from an increase in elastic fibers. The white sclera also assumes a yellow hue, due to collections of fat deposits. Your cornea may develop an opaque white ring of fats around its edge. These color changes do not affect vision.

The gelatinlike vitreous humor liquefies, allowing tiny harmless clumps of collagen called floaters (see p.425) to move freely back and forth with eye movement.

The lens hardens and loses its elasticity, making it more difficult to focus on near objects (see Presbyopia, p.425). Night vision may also be poorer because the pupil no longer dilates (opens) as easily, the iris takes longer to react to variations in light, and changes in the lens may block some of the light rays. These changes usually occur simultaneously in both eyes.

Certain eye diseases are increasingly likely as a person gets older, including presbyopia, cataracts (see p.430), glaucoma (see p.435), and macular degeneration (see p.440).

changes in prescription may be required until about the age of 65, at which time presbyopia usually stabilizes. By age 65, the eye's focusing ability has virtually ceased because the lens is inflexible; at this point, near vision is totally dependent on glasses. However, nearsighted individuals often find they can remove their distance glasses and see well for close work.

Double Vision

If you have double vision (also known as diplopia), you see two images of an object instead of one when looking at the object with both eyes. Double vision is

most often a symptom of crossed eyes (see p.445), in which the eyes do not focus in tandem and the brain receives and registers two different images. Double vision may also be a symptom of a serious underlying disorder that affects the nerves to the eye muscles or the eye muscles themselves such as myasthenia gravis (see p.377), diabetes mellitus (see p.832), multiple sclerosis (see p.368), bulging eyes (see p.427), an aneurysm (see p.698), or a tumor.

If you have double vision, see your doctor. He or she will examine you for any underlying disorder and treat it, which may clear up the double vision. You

can temporarily stop seeing double by covering one eye with a patch. Glasses with prisms may be required to achieve single vision.

Sudden Impairment of Vision

A partial or complete inability to see that starts suddenly, even if it is temporary, requires immediate medical attention. Sudden loss of vision can be caused by a neurologic or eye disorder.

There are many causes of sudden impairment of vision. Emergency eye conditions include bleeding into the fluid that circulates through the eye (known as hyphema), bleeding into the vitreous gel of the eye as occurs in diabetic retinopathy (see p.434), retinal detachment (see p.442), uveitis (see p.444), optic neuritis (see p.442), and temporal arteritis (see p.900).

Emergency brain conditions that can cause loss of vision include transient ischemic attacks (see p.342), small strokes (see p.342), and brain tumors (see p.357). Treatment depends on the cause.

A migraine headache is another possible cause of sudden impair-

ment of vision. In this condition, vision loss usually lasts less than 15 minutes and is often accompanied by flickering lights or dark spots, followed by the headache. If you know that your temporary loss of vision is caused by migraines, you probably do not need to see a doctor immediately.

OUTER SURFACE OF THE EYE

Bulging Eyes

In this condition, also known as exophthalmos or proptosis, one or (more commonly) both eyes bulge forward in their sockets; you may also feel pressure around the eyes. If you have bulging eyes, they may feel dry and gritty due to exposure of an abnormally large surface of the eye to the air. Bulging eyes can also keep you from closing your eyes completely because the lid cannot cover the eyeball.

The most common cause is Graves disease (see p.844). Other causes include inflammation of the tissue behind the eyeball due to infection, orbital cellulitis (see p.446), or tissue growth in the

eye socket, which can inhibit the movement of your eyes and cause double vision. If swelling is severe, the pressure of the protruding eyes can block the blood supply and interfere with the function of the optic nerve, resulting in blurred vision or blindness. A tumor behind the eyeball or an aneurysm (see p.698) can also lead to bulging eyes.

If you have bulging eyes, see your doctor. He or she will examine your eyes and their sockets and may also use x-rays, computed tomography (see p.149), or blood tests to determine the cause, which directs the treatment. Treating Graves disease sometimes resolves the bulging eyes, but taking corticosteroids (see p.895) may also be required. Surgery on the eyelid may be performed to prevent ulcers from developing on the cornea (see Corneal Ulcer, p.429) due to its increased exposure to air.

Conjunctivitis

(See also Color Guide to Visual Diagnosis, p.567)
Conjunctivitis means inflammation of the conjunctiva—the transparent membrane that cov-

ers the white of the eye and lines the inside of the eyelids. Also called pinkeye, it causes redness, irritation, a gritty feeling in the eye, and a discharge. Conjunctivitis can be caused by infection with a virus or bacteria, or by an allergy. It is an uncomfortable disorder but, in adults, does not threaten sight.

Newborns can acquire a form of conjunctivitis called neonatal ophthalmia from the mother's cervix during childbirth. Neonatal ophthalmia can occur when the mother's genital organs are infected with the herpes virus (see p.890), chlamydia (see p.892), or gonorrhea (see p.891).

SYMPTOMS

In all types of conjunctivitis, the white part of the eye turns pink or red and feels gritty when you blink; there is also a discharge from the eye.

Bacterial conjunctivitis, the most common form, is highly contagious and is usually transmitted by hand-to-eye contact or by coming into contact with a washcloth or towel that an infected person has used. It is very common in schools and other places where children congregate. Bacterial conjunctivitis usually

Bulging Eyes

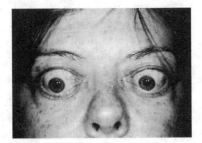

Bulging eyes may be caused by Graves disease, a disorder of the thyroid gland.

Dry Eyes and Artificial Tears

Tears are produced by the lacrimal gland. With every blink, they protect, lubricate, and cleanse the surface of the eye. Sometimes the lacrimal glands do not produce enough tears, or the three layers that make up the normal tear film (see right) are out of balance, causing faster evaporation of tears.

Dry eyes occur when the tear film that coats the eye breaks down and patches of the cornea dry out. Symptoms include stinging or burning, scratchiness, stringy mucus in or around the eyes, eye fatigue after short periods of reading, and difficulty wearing contact lenses.

Aging is the most significant cause of dry eyes but other factors include exposure to sun, wind, smoke, indoor heating, and air conditioners, as well as a disruption in the blink reflex, eyelid dysfunction (see Ectropion, p.418; Ptosis, p.420; Entropion, p.418), and bulging eyes (see p.427).

There are two treatments for dry eyes: replacing the tears or conserving them. Mild cases can usually be treated successfully with over-the counter artificial tears, which are eyedrops that mimic the natural tear film. If drops do not relieve symptoms, inserting tiny plugs into the tear drainage ducts may be recommended.

People with dry eyes can also take simple steps to slow the evaporation of tears. If you smoke, quitting provides considerable relief. It also helps to avoid direct wind, air conditioning, and hair dryers. A

Tear Film

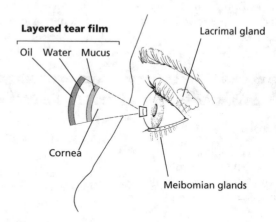

A healthy tear film has three components: the superficial oily layer produced by meibomian glands, the watery middle layer produced by lacrimal glands, and the innermost mucous layer, which helps the watery layer spread evenly over the cornea.

humidifier can add moisture to dry indoor air during the winter. Consciously blinking repeatedly helps spread your own tears more evenly. If you awaken with scratchy, dry eyes, ask your doctor if he or she would recommend a lubricating ointment at bedtime.

causes a thick yellow discharge. Sufferers often awaken to find their eyelids stuck together by the crusted discharge.

Viral conjunctivitis is caused by a virus that affects the upper respiratory tract; it is also very contagious. Along with the redness and a gritty feeling, viral conjunctivitis usually produces a watery discharge. It may be accompanied by a sore throat and swelling of the small lymph glands in front of your ears.

Allergic conjunctivitis produces redness, swelling, and itchiness, along with a clear discharge. You may also have a runny nose. This form of conjunctivitis occurs when you are exposed to a substance, such as cosmetics or pollen spores, to which you have an allergic reaction. Your body perceives the substance as a foreign invader and produces the inflammation and discharge in an attempt to fight back.

TREATMENT OPTIONS

If you have symptoms of conjunctivitis, call your doctor and follow the prevention guidelines below to keep from infecting others. Your doctor will examine you to determine what type of conjunctivitis you have.

With bacterial conjunctivitis, your doctor should advise you to wash the eye with warm water and rub gently to remove the dried discharge. Applying a clean washcloth soaked in warm water as a compress may help relieve discomfort. Your doctor may prescribe antibiotic eyedrops or an ointment for you to use for a week or two.

Viral conjunctivitis usually goes away on its own within a week or two. If you have allergic conjunctivitis, your doctor may recommend over-the-counter antihistamine eyedrops. Avoiding the offending substance, if you can identify it, is the best treatment.

To prevent the spread of conjunctivitis, wash hands frequently, make sure the infected person uses his or her own towels and washcloths (change them daily), launder sheets and pillowcases in hot water, and use a clean pillowcase each night. Keep hands away from eyes and do not share cosmetics of any kind.

Neonatal ophthalmia is very serious and can cause blindness if not treated. The law mandates that all babies receive a preventive treatment for neonatal ophthalmia caused by a gonorrhea infection, but not for neonatal ophthalmia caused by the herpes virus or chlamydia.

Subconjunctival Hemorrhage

A subconjunctival hemorrhage is leakage of blood from the tiny blood vessels of the eye into the space between the conjunctiva and the sclera (the white of the eye). It is common and can cause an alarming bright red patch but is rarely serious.

Subconjunctival hemorrhage may be caused by injury or by coughing, sneezing, or another activity that raises the pressure of the veins in your head. Other causes include inflammation of the iris, scleritis, or episcleritis (see p.430) or use of anticoagulant drugs (see p.1160).

If you have pain with the hemorrhage, call your doctor immediately. Otherwise, be patient and wait for it to gradually go away over several days; the condition usually does not require treatment.

Corneal Ulcer

A corneal ulcer is a sore or break in the surface layer of the cornea. Usually it starts with a scratch or other injury to the cornea, which becomes vulnerable to infection with bacteria, a virus, or a fungus. However, these infections can occur without an injury to the cornea. For example, the eye can be infected with the herpes simplex virus (see p.487), which can originate in the mouth as a cold sore and be spread by touching your eyes.

People who have other eye problems such as dry eyes (see p.428), ectropion (see p.418), entropion (see p.418), or bulging eyes (see p.427) may be more susceptible to ulcers on the cornea because the tear film that bathes the eye is compromised in these conditions. The risk of infectious corneal ulcers is

---

Cornea Transplants

Permanent damage to the cornea usually interferes with vision. A cornea transplant may correct the problem. For this transplant, the central, diseased part of the cornea is cut out and replaced with a cornea from a donor. People who have just died, and who have agreed to give their corneas for transplantation, are the donors. Before their organs are used, the health of the donors is determined through tests, including tests for the human immunodeficiency virus (HIV) and hepatitis.

You will be advised not to eat or drink anything for at least 6 hours before the transplant. Immediately before surgery, you will be given an anesthetic medicine that will make you sleep for a few minutes while numbing medicine is injected around your eye. The surgery takes about 1 to 2 hours and usually does not require an overnight hospital stay.

After surgery, you will wear a patch over your eye for about a day. When the doctor removes the patch, you will see lights and shapes and colors, but you will not see clearly for many months (it takes about a year for the new cornea to heal). Your doctor will examine you regularly and you will use eyedrops for at least 6 months, and possibly for the rest of your life. After complete healing has taken place, you will still need glasses or contact lenses. Avoid rubbing or putting pressure on the eye for several months; wearing a protective shield over your eye will protect it during sleep.

If at any time you have increased redness, sensitivity to light, pain, or worsening vision, call your doctor immediately. Your body's immune system could be trying to reject the transplanted cornea; rejection can be successfully treated if treatment is started immediately.

higher in those who use extended-wear contact lenses.

SYMPTOMS

Symptoms of corneal ulcers typically include pain, redness, sensitivity to light, and blurred vision. Often you cannot see the ulcer; even your doctor may need to use a special dye and viewing instruments to see it clearly.

TREATMENT OPTIONS

If you suspect you have a corneal ulcer, call your doctor immediately. Untreated corneal ulcers can result in scarring and a permanent decrease in vision. If your doctor thinks the ulcer may be caused by the herpes simplex virus, he or she will apply fluorescent drops to reveal the characteristic dendritic ulcer (which looks like a tree branch).

Treatment is with eyedrops or ointments containing antiviral drugs. Corneal ulcers caused by the herpes virus tend to recur. For bacterial infection, antibiotic eyedrops or ointment may be prescribed. In severe cases, antibiotic

drugs may be administered several times an hour around the clock. Fungal infections are treated with antifungal eyedrops. If the ulcer has severely scarred the cornea, you may need a cornea transplant (see p.429).

Scleritis and Episcleritis

Scleritis is inflammation of the sclera, the white of the eye. Episcleritis is inflammation of the episclera, the transparent tissue that covers the sclera and lies underneath the eye's outermost layer, the conjunctiva.

Scleritis is an uncommon disorder that primarily affects people between ages 30 and 60. It sometimes occurs with an autoimmune disease, such as rheumatoid arthritis (see p.606), or with inflammatory bowel disease (see p.787). Episcleritis is a milder inflammation that usually affects young adults. These disorders can affect one or both eyes.

SYMPTOMS

Both conditions cause a violet-red patch or small bump on the white of the eye; the blood ves-

sels in your eye may be inflamed and red. If you have scleritis, you may also have an aching pain in your eye. If scleritis occurs at the back of your eye, you may have some loss of vision or blurred vision. Talk to your doctor immediately if you suspect either of these conditions. Episcleritis is rarely harmful and goes away on its own after about a week but may recur periodically. Untreated scleritis can lead to further inflammation of the sclera, which can lead to a perforation in the eye's tissue.

TREATMENT OPTIONS

To treat episcleritis, your doctor may prescribe anti-inflammatory drugs in eyedrop or pill form to reduce the inflammation. To treat scleritis, you may need to take corticosteroids (see p.895) as eyedrops or tablets to reduce inflammation. Severe cases of scleritis sometimes require treatment with immunosuppressive drugs, which quiet the immune system. If a perforation has occurred, you may need surgery to repair it.

INSIDE THE EYE

Cataracts

A cataract is a clouding of the normally transparent lens of the eye. The lens looks like a dirty pane of glass when a cataract develops. It usually takes years for the clouding of the lens to keep light from reaching the retina or to distort the light rays, both of which cause loss of vision.

Contrary to what many people

believe, a cataract is not caused by cancer or a film that covers the eye, is not related to overuse of the eyes, and does not spread from one eye to the other (although both eyes may be affected). With aging, the lens becomes less resilient, less transparent, and thicker. Fibers in the lens become compressed, and the lens becomes more rigid. In addition, protein particles in the

lens begin to clump together. The change in the lens is similar to what occurs when egg white is boiled, turning from clear to opaque.

The causes of cataracts, in addition to age-related changes, include heredity, eye injuries, some medications (particularly corticosteroids, see p.895), and health problems such as diabetes mellitus (see p.832). Drinking

Cataracts: *Dr Bajart's Advice*

Cataracts are a "normal" part of the aging process. If you live long enough, you will eventually develop cataracts. However, you will not necessarily require surgery. You should consider surgery only when the cataract interferes with your visual functioning, such as driving at night, reading, following a golf ball, or seeing into oncoming light. At the same time, once the cataract starts to interfere with vision, I tell my patients that the best time to remove it is sooner rather than later. This is because a cataract is safer and easier to remove when it is immature. Later on, the cataract becomes dense and hard, making it more difficult to remove.

ANN M. BAJART, MD
MASSACHUSETTS EYE AND EAR INFIRMARY
HARVARD MEDICAL SCHOOL

Ages at Which Many People Will Need Cataract Surgery

This chart shows the number of people in different age groups who will need cataract surgery.

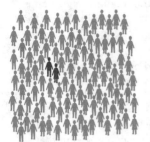

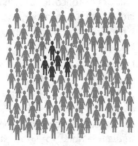

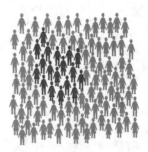

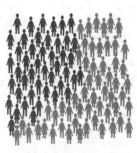

2 OF 100 PEOPLE 45 TO 54 YEARS OLD WILL NEED CATARACT SURGERY

5 OF 100 PEOPLE 55 TO 64 YEARS OLD WILL NEED CATARACT SURGERY

18 OF 100 PEOPLE 65 TO 74 YEARS OLD WILL NEED CATARACT SURGERY

45 OF 100 PEOPLE 75 TO 85 YEARS OLD WILL NEED CATARACT SURGERY

Risk of Developing Cataracts

Your risk of developing a cataract that affects your vision during your lifetime increases if you are in one of these higher-risk categories.

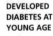

	1.5 times	2 times	2 times	3 times	3 times	3 times	5.8 times
AVERAGE RISK	ARE FEMALE	USE ALCOHOL EXCESSIVELY	CURRENTLY SMOKE CIGARETTES	HAVE BEEN EXPOSED TO HIGH LEVELS OF ULTRAVIOLET RADIATION	HAVE SISTER OR BROTHER WITH CATARACT	DEVELOPED DIABETES AT YOUNG AGE	HAVE USED CORTICO-STEROIDS FOR A LONG TIME

alcohol, smoking, and long-term sun exposure may also contribute to higher risk. In rare cases, if a pregnant woman develops German measles in the first trimester, the infant can be born with a cataract.

SYMPTOMS

Cataracts are painless and progress slowly. Vision usually becomes blurred or dim, and glare from lights and the sun is disturbing. You may experience a distorted image. In the early stages, you may become more nearsighted (see p.420), because the denser lens creates greater refracting power, causing light to focus even more in front of the retina. Night vision worsens, and colors are less vivid.

Because most cataracts develop very slowly, many people do not sense that something is wrong until the decline in visual sharpness forces them to seek changes in their eyeglass or contact lens prescription.

TREATMENT OPTIONS

Surgical extraction of cataract, in which the clouded lens is removed and replaced with a plastic lens implant, is the only effective cure. However, diagno-

---

Cataract Removal and Lens Replacement

Cataract surgery is considered one of the safest surgeries and is very common. Over 1 million operations are performed in the United States each year; 98% are successful in restoring good vision, assuming that there are no other problems with the eye. The operation is usually performed using a local anesthetic (see p.168) without an overnight stay in the hospital.

More than 98% of people who have cataract surgery also have a plastic lens called an intraocular (inside the eye) lens implanted to replace the eye's natural lens. Before surgery, the ophthalmologist measures the curvature of your cornea and the length of your eye to calculate the power of the lens implant needed.

The surgery usually lasts less than an hour. While you may be aware of the presence of the surgical team, you will not feel pain and may not even be able to tell if your eye is open or closed.

REMOVING THE CATARACT

The surgeon makes an incision in the eye with the aid of a magnifying microscope. There are several approaches to surgery. In extracapsular cataract surgery, a semicircular incision (1/3 to 1/2 inch long) is made around the edge of the cornea in the white sclera, under the upper lid. The cataract is removed, leaving the rear capsule of the lens intact; this provides support for the lens implant and reduces the risk of complications with the retina. The incision is closed with several fine stitches that dissolve on their own. This operation can create or increase astigmatism of the cornea.

In a newer technique called phacoemulsification (see illustration), high-frequency ultrasound waves are used to break up the cataract so it can be vacuumed out through a needle-thin tube. This reduces the size of the incision considerably (to 1/8 inch) and eliminates the need for stitches, leaving a wound that heals faster with less astigmatism.

INSERTING THE LENS

Once the lens is removed, the eye becomes extremely farsighted and loses its ability to focus. A plastic lens is permanently inserted in the eye. It requires no care and usually produces good vision. Most often, the lens is placed behind the iris; this is called a posterior (rear) chamber lens. When inserted in front of the iris, it is called an anterior (front) chamber lens. Tiny plastic loops hold the implants in place.

In phacoemulsification, a folding lens made of silicone or acrylic is introduced into the tiny incision after the clouded lens has been sucked out; the new lens unfolds fully on its own. If a conventional lens is to be used after phacoemulsification, the surgeon must enlarge the incision to insert the implant.

sis of cataract does not always mean you need immediate surgery. If your vision is only slightly blurred, an adjustment in your vision correction prescription and stronger lighting may suffice. Medicine that dilates the pupil also helps some people. Many people successfully delay cataract surgery for years, and others never need it. With newer surgical techniques, it is no longer necessary to wait for a cataract to "ripen" (become totally opaque) before removal.

If you are faced with a decision on whether to have surgery, ask your ophthalmologist to discuss the risks and benefits of surgery. Base your decision on your degree of vision loss and your ability to function. If visual impairment interferes with your daily activities, such as driving or maneuvering stairs, consider surgery. For people who have cataracts in both eyes, the denser cataract is usually removed first. The second eye is not operated on until vision is stable in the first eye.

Your doctor may recommend cataract removal if you have other eye conditions—such as diabetic retinopathy, retinal holes, or a retinal detachment—

AFTER SURGERY

The surgeon may place a bandage and shield over your eye and you will rest for a while before you go home. With the newest surgery, using very small incisions and no stitches, vision improves in a few days; with larger incisions and stitches, it may take several weeks. Most people can resume normal activities within a few days, but ask your doctor for guidelines.

It is important not to rub your eye and not to jar your head. Itching, sticky eyelids, mild tearing, and a sensitivity to light are normal for a few hours after surgery, but severe pain and a sudden change in vision are not. Call your doctor immediately if they occur. Minor discomfort can be relieved by taking a nonaspirin substitute (aspirin can cause bleeding) every 4 to 6 hours.

For several weeks, you may need to apply antibiotic and anti-inflammatory eyedrops or ointments (to prevent infection and limit inflammation). Clean your eyelids with sterile water to remove any crusted discharge, avoid sunlight, and wear a protective metal shield at night over the eye that was operated on.

Cataract Surgery

A

Clouded lens

B

Clouded lens

Iris

Lens capsule

Cornea

C

Posterior capsule

Lens removed through tube

D

Plastic lens implant

When a lens develops a cataract, it loses transparency and becomes clouded (A and B). In phacoemulsification (C), ultrasound is used to break up the cataract so it can be sucked out through a tiny tube. The posterior (rear) capsule remains and provides support for an artificial lens. The lens implant (D) is supported by the back wall of the lens capsule and by two springlike plastic arms that stick out from its sides.

even if your vision is not severely impaired. A cataract can impede proper examination and treatment of these conditions. Almost all people with lens implants find their vision restored to what it was prior to the cataract. Some people still require glasses to see most clearly (for instance, for reading or for seeing distant objects).

Diabetic Retinopathy

Diabetic retinopathy is deterioration of the blood vessels of the retina in people with diabetes mellitus (see p.832). It usually occurs in both eyes. The longer a person has had diabetes, or the younger a person is when the diabetes starts, the greater is the risk of diabetic retinopathy.

SYMPTOMS

Diabetic retinopathy can progress to an advanced stage without your noticing any symptoms. However, changes that indicate the presence of the disease can be seen by your ophthalmologist; for this reason, regular eye examinations are critical for people with diabetes. Your ophthalmologist detects retinopathy by a dilated fundus examination, in which eyedrops are inserted to dilate (widen) your pupils and your retina is examined through an ophthalmoscope.

Your physician may also use a test called fluorescein angiogra-phy, in which dye is injected into a vein in your arm. The dye travels to the blood vessels of the retina and photos are taken to determine whether the vessels are leaking fluid.

In nonproliferative retinopathy (also called background or simple retinopathy), existing blood vessels become narrowed, blocked, and deteriorate, reducing the supply of vital oxygen to the retina. As a result, tiny yellow spots called exudates may form on the retina. The remaining blood vessels may hemorrhage (leak blood) into the retina, causing a reduction in the sharpness of vision. If blood leaks into the macular region of the eye—the part responsible for central

Treatments for Diabetic Retinopathy

PROBLEM	TREATMENT	HOW IT WORKS AND WHERE IT IS PERFORMED
Leaking blood vessels and swelling of the macula	Laser surgery (photocoagulation)	Powerful laser beam light is focused on damaged retina to seal ruptured vessels. Performed in office or clinic using local anesthesia (see p.168).
Development of new and fragile blood vessels (neovascularization)	Laser surgery	Laser beam is scattered on the retina to create scars that inhibit growth of blood vessels and secure retina to back of eye. Performed in office or clinic using local anesthesia (see p.168).
Clouded vision from bleeding (with either proliferative or nonproliferative retinopathy)	Freezing therapy (cryotherapy)	Helps shrink new blood vessels until blood settles and laser surgery can be used. Performed in office or operating room using local anesthesia (see p.168).
Advanced proliferative retinopathy	Removal of vitreous gel (vitrectomy)	Removes blood-filled vitreous gel and replaces it with clear solution. Performed under powerful microscope in operating room, often using local anesthesia (see p.168).
Retinal detachment (see p.442)	Retinal repair surgery	Reattaches retina to back of eye. Performed in operating room.

Blurred Vision in Diabetics

The most serious cause of blurred vision in people with diabetes is diabetic retinopathy. However, the most common causes of blurred vision in diabetics are the common problems of focusing (see p.421) and the effects of blood sugar on the lenses of the eyes. Sugar from the blood gets into the fluid of the eyes and can cause temporary changes in the shape of the lenses. Diabetics whose blood sugar is not in control can have periods of blurred vision. People with diabetes should generally avoid getting fitted for new glasses until blood sugar has been in control for 3 to 4 weeks; otherwise, their glasses may give them good vision only when their sugar level is not in control.

vision—macular edema (swelling) may occur, making it difficult to read or do detailed work.

Additionally, new fragile blood vessels may form and grow over the retina; this is called proliferative retinopathy. The new vessels often leak blood into the vitreous humor, the gel-like substance of the eyeball, causing cloudy vision. In an attempt to repair the ruptured vessels, the body may generate scar tissue; this can pull on the retina, resulting in retinal detachment (see p.442) and loss of vision.

TREATMENT OPTIONS

Keeping your blood sugar levels (see p.838) under tight control decreases the long-term chance and progression of retinopathy and the need for surgery by 50%. Controlling any high blood pressure is also essential. If you have nonproliferative retinopathy, your ophthalmologist may recommend that you have a dilated fundus examination every 2 to 6 months, depending on how severe the condition is. If you have proliferative diabetic retinopathy, your doctor may recommend that you have the exam every month. With careful monitoring, treatment (see Treatments for Diabetic Retinopathy, p.434) can begin before your sight is affected.

Glaucoma

Glaucoma is like a thief in the night; it can take a person's vision very gradually, without being noticed. In glaucoma, there usually is increased pressure in the aqueous humor, the fluid that fills the chambers of the eyes. This pressure causes damage to the optic nerves. Glaucoma is a major cause of blindness. However, if it is diagnosed and treated early, vision can almost always be spared.

The aqueous humor circulates between the front and back chambers of the eye through the pupil, nourishing the lens and the cells that line the cornea. It then drains through a sievelike system of tissue (called the trabecular reticulum or meshwork) and empties into a drainage channel, located where the iris and the cornea meet; this area of the eye is known as the drainage angle. From the drainage channel, the fluid is directed into the canal of Schlemm and then into nearby veins, where it flows into the

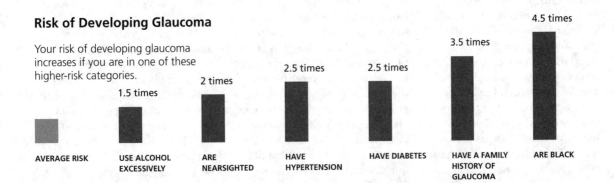

Risk of Developing Glaucoma

Your risk of developing glaucoma increases if you are in one of these higher-risk categories.

AVERAGE RISK	USE ALCOHOL EXCESSIVELY	ARE NEARSIGHTED	HAVE HYPERTENSION	HAVE DIABETES	HAVE A FAMILY HISTORY OF GLAUCOMA	ARE BLACK
	1.5 times	2 times	2.5 times	2.5 times	3.5 times	4.5 times

Glaucoma

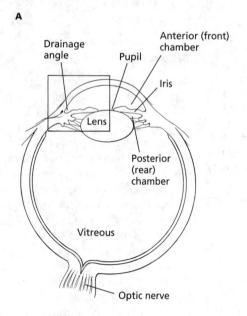

A

Drainage angle
Pupil
Anterior (front) chamber
Iris
Lens
Posterior (rear) chamber
Vitreous
Optic nerve

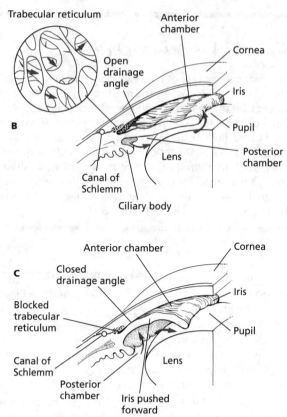

B

Trabecular reticulum
Anterior chamber
Cornea
Open drainage angle
Iris
Pupil
Posterior chamber
Lens
Canal of Schlemm
Ciliary body

C

Anterior chamber
Cornea
Closed drainage angle
Iris
Blocked trabecular reticulum
Pupil
Canal of Schlemm
Lens
Posterior chamber
Iris pushed forward

A, Structures at the front of the eye that are involved in glaucoma. **B**, Structures at the front of the eye in a person with open-angle glaucoma. Normally, the ciliary body continuously produces aqueous humor, a liquid that circulates from the posterior (rear) chamber around the iris through the pupil to the anterior (front) chamber (arrows). Fluid helps maintain the shape of the outer eye, nourishes the lens and cornea, and drains through the trabecular reticulum into the canal of Schlemm and into small veins to join the bloodstream. In chronic open-angle glaucoma, the sievelike trabecular reticulum becomes blocked, fluid accumulates, and pressure increases. **C**, Structures at the front of the eye in a person with closed-angle glaucoma. The drainage angle in the anterior chamber has been narrowed to the point of closure by the forward-bending iris. The fluid cannot exit the eye, which causes a severe rise in pressure, pain, blurred vision, and injury to the optic nerve.

blood. This process works continuously. Aqueous humor is always being produced and excess fluid is always being eliminated through the canal of Schlemm to keep a healthy balance of pressure in the eye.

In glaucoma, the drainage system becomes blocked and pressure rises, which places pressure on the blood supply of the optic nerve. If the pressure continues, the nerve fibers that carry the optical messages die and vision begins to fade. Loss of vision may also be caused by the obstruction of tiny blood vessels that feed the retina and optic nerve. Nerve fibers on the outer edge are affected first, so vision loss begins with peripheral vision and gradually closes in until the cells supplying central vision are killed. The damage that occurs in glaucoma is not reversible, which is why identifying it early is so important.

Why glaucoma appears to affect older people is not clear, but the eye's drainage system seems to become less efficient with age (the risk of glaucoma nearly doubles every 10 years after the age of 50). Glaucoma runs in families; defects in a particular gene cause some cases of open-angle glaucoma.

Glaucoma Medicines and Their Effects

Most ophthalmologists start with the lowest possible effective dose of glaucoma medication to minimize potential side effects. People who take medicine for glaucoma must see their ophthalmologists regularly, sometimes every 3 months, to ensure that a consistent reduction in the eye's pressure is being maintained.

MEDICATIONS	EFFECTS	POSSIBLE SIDE EFFECTS
Timolol and betaxolol hydrochloride	Lower pressure by reducing amount of aqueous humor produced by the eye.	**Eyes:** Stinging, burning, tearing, itching **General:** Slowing of the heart rate, asthma or shortness of breath, depression, fatigue, headache, dizziness, decrease in libido (men)
Pilocarpine and echothiophate iodide	Constrict the pupil to widen the drainage angle and facilitate outflow of fluid.	**Eyes:** Blurred vision, aching brow, eye discomfort, red eyes, tearing, change in peripheral vision, reduced vision in dim light **General:** Abdominal cramps, diarrhea, weakness, sweating, increased salivation, asthma attacks
Epinephrine, dipivefrin, and epinephryl borate	Lower pressure and may dilate pupil briefly.	**Eyes:** Irritated eye surface **General:** Irregular or increased heartbeat, high blood pressure, sweating
Dorzolamide hydrochloride	Lower pressure by slowing aqueous fluid production in the eye.	**Eyes:** Eye discomfort, burning, stinging, tearing, foreign body sensation **General:** Bitter taste
Latanoprost	Lower pressure and increase drainage of fluid.	**Eyes:** Eye discomfort, burning, stinging, tearing, foreign body sensation; can change eye color (from blue or green to brown) **General:** Aching muscles, chest pain, rash, bitter taste
Apraclonidine hydrochloride	Lower pressure by decreasing fluid production.	**Eyes:** Redness, irritation **General:** Dry mouth, sleepiness
Brimonidine tartrate	Lower pressure by decreasing fluid production and increasing fluid outflow.	**Eyes:** Burning, stinging, redness, blurred vision, bumps on conjunctiva **General:** Dry mouth, fatigue

SYMPTOMS

There are several types of glaucoma, each with its own set of symptoms.

Open-angle glaucoma (also known as chronic glaucoma or simple glaucoma) is the most common form, accounting for 90% of all cases. In this form, the angle in the anterior (front) chamber of the eye remains open, yet the aqueous humor drains out too slowly, leading to fluid backup and a gradual but persistent elevation in pressure.

This type of glaucoma may get worse with few or no symptoms until it reaches an advanced stage. Blind spots and diminishing peripheral vision may occur but may be too insignificant to notice initially. Occasionally, people are alerted to the disease by repeatedly needing new eyeglass prescriptions or having trouble with night vision. However, these symptoms generally occur later in the disease.

Low-tension glaucoma, a less common type of open-angle glaucoma, is characterized by damage to the optic nerve in a pattern typical of glaucoma; however, it occurs under normal eye pressure. Low-tension glaucoma probably develops when the blood supply to the optic nerve is reduced by some other condition, such as atherosclerosis (see p.653). Under that circumstance, even normal pressure on the optic nerve is enough to further reduce blood supply and cause damage to the nerve.

Closed-angle glaucoma (also known as acute glaucoma, angle-closure glaucoma, or narrow-angle glaucoma) is characterized by a rapid rise in eye pressure over hours as the drainage angle suddenly becomes blocked, preventing the outflow of fluid.

Sometimes this occurs when the angle narrows and the iris is pushed forward, effectively closing off the drainage path. The eyeball quickly hardens and the pressure causes pain, blurred vision, rainbow haloes around lights, headaches, nausea, and vomiting. This is a serious condition that can rapidly lead to blindness. The onset of symptoms requires immediate treatment by an ophthalmologist.

TREATMENT OPTIONS

If glaucoma is suspected, your doctor will conduct a number of tests. He or she will look at your optic nerve using an ophthalmoscope. If the optic disc—the heart of the optic nerve—is affected by glaucoma, a condition known as cupping may be observed. In cupping, the disc appears deeply indented, with the center of the disc being much deeper than the rim. The disc color—normally pinkish—may be pale and more yellow because advancing disease has hindered blood flow to the area.

If your doctor refers you to an

Laser Trabeculoplasty for Open-Angle Glaucoma

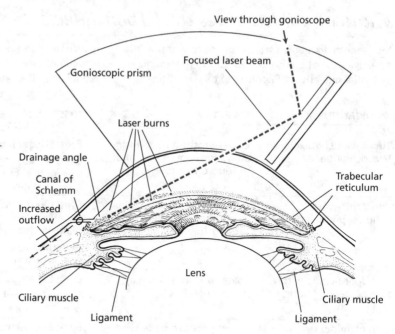

In laser trabeculoplasty, a high-energy beam of light makes small holes in the trabecular reticulum, improving fluid outflow from the eye. A slitlamp microscope and a gonioscopic prism allow a detailed view of the drainage angle.

Laser Iridotomy for Closed-Angle Glaucoma

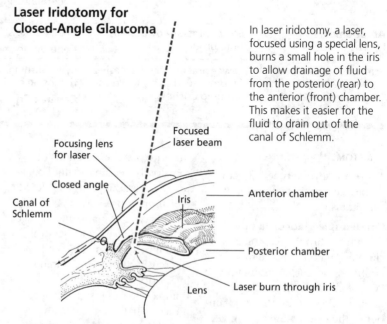

In laser iridotomy, a laser, focused using a special lens, burns a small hole in the iris to allow drainage of fluid from the posterior (rear) to the anterior (front) chamber. This makes it easier for the fluid to drain out of the canal of Schlemm.

Glaucoma and Blindness:
Dr Hutchinson's Advice

"Will I go blind?" is the most common and principal worry of patients with newly detected glaucoma. Glaucoma is an eye disease in which pressure inside the eye is too high and damages the optic nerve, which carries the eye's pictures to the brain. Although glaucoma causes blindness if not detected early and properly treated, all of the many types of glaucoma can be controlled without further visual loss with eyedrops, laser treatment, or surgery. Early visual loss due to glaucoma is not noticed by most people. Anyone with a family history of glaucoma and everyone by 40 years of age should have the periodic painless eye examination that will detect glaucoma. The keys to preserving your vision are: early glaucoma detection; regular, faithful treatment; and periodic examinations to insure control.

B. THOMAS HUTCHINSON, MD
MASSACHUSETTS EYE AND EAR INFIRMARY
HARVARD MEDICAL SCHOOL

Side Effects of Glaucoma Eye-drops: Dr Hutchinson's Advice

Eyedrops for glaucoma can cause side effects in the eye, such as blurring of vision, eye pain, floaters, itching, redness, tearing, and swelling. What you might not know is that medicines in the eyedrops also are commonly absorbed into your system—from the surface of the eye and also through your tear ducts into the nose and throat. If you develop unusual weakness or tiredness, shortness of breath, rashes, dry mouth, diarrhea, nervousness, tingling of fingers and feet, or even a decrease in your sex drive after starting glaucoma eyedrops, it could be a side effect of the drops. If so, your doctor can almost always find another kind of eyedrop for you to use. Read the information that comes with your medications and discuss any new symptoms with your ophthalmologist and your general medical doctor.

B. THOMAS HUTCHINSON, MD
MASSACHUSETTS EYE AND EAR INFIRMARY
HARVARD MEDICAL SCHOOL

ophthalmologist, he or she will do the same examination, but will also use a slitlamp and perform tonometry (see p.417). The ophthalmologist may also perform an examination called gonioscopy, in which a special lens is used to see whether the drainage angle is open, narrowed, or closed.

The goal of treatment is to control eye pressure and stop progression of the disease. For open-angle glaucoma, treatment usually begins with topical medications (eyedrops or ointments), which are administered once to several times a day; pills are also sometimes prescribed. Usually drug therapy keeps glaucoma in check. However, when it does not, your doctor may recommend surgery called laser trabeculoplasty, which improves fluid drainage. It is usually performed in a clinic or the ophthalmologist's office using anesthesia in the form of eyedrops.

In this procedure, a high-energy laser beam is used to burn tiny holes on the surface of half the trabecular reticulum. This lets fluid flow more easily out of the anterior chamber. You may see flashes of green or red as the laser is focused and fired up to 50 times to make the openings. There is no pain, and treatment takes less than 5 minutes to perform.

While laser surgery is helpful, it may need to be repeated on the other half of the trabecular reticulum if the pressure in your eye is not low enough. Pressure increases after about 2 years in more than half of all people who have undergone laser treatment.

Sometimes, the iris moves forward and further narrows the

drainage angle. Laser iridotomy may be used to treat closed-angle glaucoma or narrow angles that may potentially close. Using a laser, the surgeon creates a small opening in the outer edge of the iris to facilitate drainage of the aqueous humor from the posterior (rear) chamber to the anterior (front) chamber. This reduces pressure in the posterior chamber that would have pushed the iris forward into the drainage angle. In cases where a laser cannot be used, a piece of the iris is surgically removed with scissors in a procedure called iridectomy. Iridectomy accomplishes the same goal as iridotomy but requires surgically opening the eye to reach the iris. This carries greater risk of hemorrhage, infection, and other complications than iridotomy.

Trabeculectomy may be recommended if lasers or medication fails. In this procedure, a flap of tissue from the sclera (the white of the eye) is opened to create a new passageway for fluid to drain from the anterior (front) chamber into a space created underneath the conjunctiva. Alternatively, a plastic valve may be implanted to provide drainage for outflowing fluid.

For open-angle glaucoma, diagnosis is nearly always made after some damage to vision has occurred. Your doctor will eliminate other possible causes of optic nerve damage and vision loss. If none is found, lowering the pressure of the fluid in your eye even further with medicine and/or through surgery usually stabilizes the condition.

Ischemic Optic Neuropathy

Ischemic optic neuropathy results when there is ischemia (insufficient blood flow) to the optic nerve. It can cause sudden, painless vision loss. There are two forms of ischemic optic neuropathy: arteritic and nonarteritic. In the arteritic form, which occurs with temporal arteritis (see p.900), the arteries leading to the optic nerve are inflamed. It occurs most often in people over 65. In addition to vision loss, symptoms are those of temporal arteritis. Treatment includes corticosteroid drugs (see p.895) to reduce inflammation of the optic nerve and the surrounding blood vessels.

In the nonarteritic form, the most common symptom is vision impairment. It may be associated with diabetes mellitus (see p.832) or high blood pressure (see p.644). There is no known treatment but treating the diabetes mellitus or high blood pressure may prevent it.

Age-Related Macular Degeneration

Age-related macular degeneration (ARMD) is a disorder in which the macula—the area on the retina responsible for sharp, central vision—deteriorates, gradually causing blurred vision, difficulty reading, and finally a blind spot in the central area of vision.

ARMD is the leading cause of blindness in people over 60. In addition to advanced age, risk factors include cigarette smoking, exposure to bright sunlight and UV radiation, light-colored eyes, farsightedness (see p.424), hypertension (see p.644), high cholesterol (see p.669), and coronary artery disease (see p.652).

SYMPTOMS

ARMD occurs in two forms: dry and wet. The majority of people have the dry, or atrophic, form, which causes a thinning of the tissues of the retina and decay of the light-sensitive cells in the macula. The symptoms of dry ARMD may affect only one eye at first, producing a gradual distortion of vision, particularly blurring of central sight. In the dry form, blurred vision and difficulty reading or distinguishing faces are among the first symptoms. It is common for the second eye to eventually be affected as well.

As the disease advances, a blind spot may develop in the center of the visual field. With time, this area may enlarge and hinder sight. However, some people who have ARMD in only one eye do not realize they have any vision loss because the healthy eye compensates so well.

Wet ARMD, which is more severe, results when abnormal blood vessels develop in the choroid layer (the backmost layer of tissue) under the retina and extend like tentacles toward the macula. These new vessels are prone to leak fluid and blood, which injures tissue and photoreceptor cells. The result is internal scarring and vision loss.

Distorted vision is one of the early signs of wet ARMD. Straight lines may appear wavy and shapes may look deformed. Colors may seem faded and a blind spot may develop in the center of the focusing area. Wet ARMD progresses faster than the dry

Age-Related Macular Degeneration

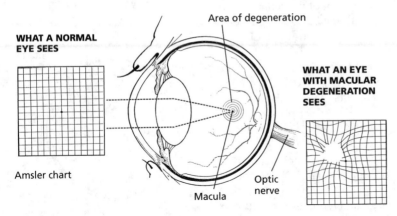

WHAT A NORMAL
EYE SEES

Amsler chart

Area of degeneration

WHAT AN EYE
WITH MACULAR
DEGENERATION
SEES

Macula

Optic
nerve

Age-related macular degeneration (ARMD) results from deterioration of the light-sensitive cells of the central retina (macula). To demonstrate ARMD effects, you will be asked to look at a dot on an Amsler chart (far left). If lines near the dot appear wavy (far right), ARMD may be the cause. In people with ARMD, the center of the visual field may become blurred or develop a blind spot. Straight lines may appear wavy or broken, colors may fade, objects may look larger or smaller than they should, and letters within a word or sentence may seem distorted or may seem to disappear.

form. People with ARMD do not go totally blind; they retain peripheral vision.

TREATMENT OPTIONS

If you have any of the symptoms of ARMD, see your doctor immediately. ARMD is diagnosed by an eye exam, including a Snellen test (see p.416) to determine how well you can see at different distances and light levels. Color tests may also be performed to see how well the cone cells in the retina are functioning.

Your doctor may suspect dry ARMD if there are clusters of drusen (small yellow deposits that build up under the macula) or clumps of pigment visible through a hand-held ophthalmoscope.

The use of an Amsler chart is a crucial part of the exam because it can identify the dis-

torted vision caused by ARMD. You will be instructed to look at a central spot on a grid whose pattern resembles graph paper. If the lines near the dot appear wavy, you may have ARMD. Wet ARMD is diagnosed with the aid of fluorescein angiography, which reveals whether leaking blood vessels in the retina can benefit from laser treatment (see below).

There is currently no proven treatment for dry ARMD. However, this form of the disease progresses very slowly and people are often able to manage well in their daily routine even with some loss of central vision.

Laser surgery called laser photocoagulation is effective for some people with wet ARMD. A laser beam is aimed at the leaky blood vessels to seal them and prevent further seepage. The pro-

cedure is most effective when it is performed on newly formed vessels that have not yet grown over the fovea, the central part of the macula. However, it is not a cure and cannot restore lost vision; it merely halts the progression of the disease.

The procedure takes about half an hour and can be done in the doctor's office using local anesthesia (see p.168). Recurrences happen in about half of those treated, requiring more laser treatments.

Your doctor may recommend that you monitor your condition at home using an Amsler chart. By regularly testing each eye, you can check to see if the condition is getting worse. People who have had laser surgery may be alerted to renewed leakage in their blood vessels. There is evidence to suggest that a diet high in carotenoids (spinach, collard greens, and leafy vegetables) and antioxidant vitamins (such as vitamins C and E) may halt the progression of ARMD.

Night Blindness

Night blindness is an inability to see well in low-intensity light. Many people with this condition have no other eye problems or disease. Although rare in the United States, a vitamin A deficiency can cause poor night vision; treatment includes increasing your intake of foods that contain vitamin A (see p.42) and taking supplements.

Other people inherit a defect of the retina that causes difficulty seeing at night. Night blindness may be a warning sign of retinitis pigmentosa, an uncommon disorder that can be inherited.

In retinitis pigmentosa, there is a degeneration of the rods and cones of the retina, usually in both eyes, that results in progressive loss of visual sharpness and peripheral vision, leading to tunnel vision and ultimately blindness. Symptoms usually do not appear until adolescence. If you have retinitis pigmentosa, your doctor will be able to see a dark pigmentation on your retina.

There is no known treatment for this uncommon, inherited condition, but it can be detected in children by about age 10. If you have poor night vision, talk to your doctor so that he or she can identify the cause.

Optic Neuritis

Optic neuritis is inflammation of the optic nerve. When the optic nerve swells, it can block the signals to the brain, which interferes with sight. Optic neuritis can produce blurred vision and vision loss over a period of several days. Some people also have pain when they move their eyes or eyes that are tender to the touch.

Optic neuritis is sometimes caused by infection of the tissues around the optic nerve. In other people, it accompanies multiple sclerosis (see p.368).

Most cases of optic neuritis clear up on their own, although optic neuritis can recur, especially when it occurs with multiple sclerosis. Though corticosteroid drugs are sometimes prescribed, they are of unproven value in improving recovery. Most people regain their sight without any treatment, usually after 6 weeks.

Detached Retina

Detachment of the retina occurs when the retina—the light-sensitive surface at the back of the eye—lifts away from the inner layer of blood vessels called the choroid. Retinal detachment may occur after injury to the eye. However, in most people it occurs spontaneously. If not treated early, the lifting away continues until the retina barely hangs onto the ciliary body and optic nerve. It can affect one or both eyes. A detached retina is a serious condition that can lead to permanent loss of vision.

Middle-aged and older people are the most likely to experience retinal detachment. Nearsightedness increases the chances for detachment because the eyeball's shape is already elongated lengthwise, which places stress on the retina. Cataract removal also places individuals at greater risk of retinal detachment.

SYMPTOMS

Flashes of light and floaters (see p.443), specks that drift across your field of vision, are early symptoms. However, these can also occur without retinal detachment. Other symptoms include a reduction in vision from one side, much like a curtain hanging across your field of vision. If the macula (the area responsible for sharp central vision) detaches, central vision quickly diminishes.

TREATMENT OPTIONS

Retinal repairs done at an early stage of deterioration lead to greatest vision improvement. A thorough exam (see p.416) with dilated pupils and an ophthalmoscope can determine the extent

Detached Retina

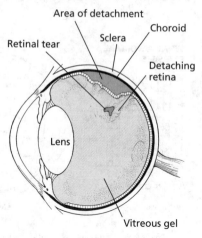

A hole or tear in the retina allows fluid to seep between the choroid and the retina, detaching the retina. This causes loss of vision, like a shade drawn over peripheral vision. As the detachment progresses, central vision is also lost. Floaters (little black spots) occur if the tear causes bleeding.

of detachment, the location of any holes, and the best way to treat the problem.

Several types of surgery can be performed, depending on the severity of the detachment. The goal is to repair any rips in the retina and prevent them from recurring. Holes that have not yet caused detachment may be repaired through cryotherapy by applying freezing probes that form scar tissue and permanently seal the breaks. Laser photocoagulation (see p.434) can be used for the same purpose. Both procedures may be performed in a doctor's office using a local anesthetic (see p.168).

If the retina has already started to pull away from the choroid layer and the gap has filled with fluid, the situation may call for a

Floaters and Flashes: *Dr Bienfang's Advice*

Q Recently I've been seeing a lot of spots drifting across my line of vision. What are they?

A The spots are called vitreous floaters. Floaters are tiny clumps of material in the vitreous gel that fills the inside of the eye. Most often, they are part of the natural aging of this gel over time. What you are actually seeing are shadows of these particles cast on the retina. If the shadows have been present for several months, there is usually no cause for concern. However, any solid material in the vitreous gel can also cast such a shadow. Prominent floaters of recent onset could be caused by a small hemorrhage in the eye or a small tear of the retina. If your floaters are of recent onset, or a noticeable change from what you had been seeing previously, you should be evaluated by an ophthalmologist.

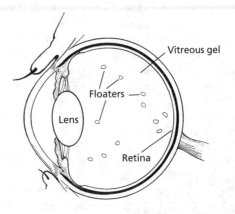

Q Occasionally I see flashes of light that look like stars. Are they dangerous?

A If the flashes of light are reliably located in one spot of the field of vision, they should be evaluated by an ophthalmologist. They may represent a small hole in the retina or a retinal hemorrhage. If the flashes of light cover a large area of your field of vision, there are two possibilities: (1) migraine attack, in which the lights typically are bright and shimmer or (2) temporary poor circulation to the eye similar to

what you may experience when standing up after having been bent over, but which may be a sign of poor circulation to the eye.

Another type of light flash occurs in an arc or semicircular shape at the far extreme of the side vision in one eye and usually appears when the eye moves. This is usually due to the vitreous gel pulling off the peripheral retina. Because this can indicate a retinal hole or a small detachment of the retina, it should be evaluated by an ophthalmologist.

DON C. BIENFANG, MD
BRIGHAM AND WOMEN'S HOSPITAL
HARVARD MEDICAL SCHOOL

---

procedure called scleral buckling. This involves making a hole to drain the fluid so that the retina falls back against the choroid. The hole is sealed and the sclera (the white of the eye) is tucked or indented slightly to make better contact with the retina and then secured with a silicone buckle that is stitched around the circumference of the eyeball. In a newer technique called pneumopexy, gas is injected into the vitreous cavity to press the retina to the choroid.

Some complicated cases require vitrectomy, which is removal of the vitreous humor. In this delicate surgery, fragments of the gel are cut and aspirated (vacuumed out) from the front or back section of the eye. Because the body does not replace its own vitreous fluid, a saline solution or other substance is inserted as a permanent substitute.

Vision often returns to normal if surgery is performed before the detachment is complete. However, in advanced cases that

affect central vision, you may continue to have blurred vision. Regular visits to your ophthalmologist are essential to prevent recurrences.

Tumors of the Eye

Tumors inside the eye are rare and usually do not cause symptoms until they grow large enough to see, cause pain, or disturb vision. Like tumors elsewhere in the body, eye tumors may be benign (noncancerous) or malignant (cancerous and likely to spread).

Malignant melanoma (see p.543) is a cancer that can occur in the eye as well as the skin. People of middle age or older are most susceptible. Malignant melanoma is the most common eye tumor. It affects the pigment-containing cells (called melanocytes) in the iris or choroid layer—the thin membrane that lies between the sclera and the retina. The choroid is rich in blood vessels and supplies nutrients to the retina. There are usually no symptoms early in the tumor's development, but the malignant melanoma eventually causes the retina to detach (see p.442) and compromises vision.

Your doctor may simply monitor an eye tumor by watching its growth. Alternatively, he or she may treat the tumor using surgery, standard radiation therapy, or proton beam radiation, which delivers tumor-killing doses of radiation precisely to a small area, minimizing damage to nearby healthy tissue. If the tumor has metastasized (spread) to other parts of the body, treatment is a subject of scientific controversy because there is little clinical evidence that surgery, radiation, or removing the eye produces a better outcome than doing nothing.

Retinoblastoma is a rare, usually inherited, malignant tumor of the retina that can affect one or both eyes. It occurs in young children, usually between ages 2 and 3. Often there are no symptoms, but a child with retinoblastoma may have crossed eyes (see p.445). The affected pupil looks white instead of black because it reflects light off the tumor. Report any suspected abnormality in your child's vision to your doctor immediately.

If retinoblastoma runs in your family, your child should be examined by an ophthalmologist soon after birth. If the tumor is diagnosed in its early stages, treatment may include radiation therapy (see p.741), laser therapy, or freezing, all of which can be very effective. If discovered in a more advanced stage, your doctor may recommend removing the eye to prevent the tumor from spreading. Couples who have a family history of retinoblastoma may choose to have genetic counseling before considering a pregnancy, to understand the risk of having an affected child.

Secondary eye tumors can develop when cancer affecting another part of the body spreads to the eye. These tumors usually occur in the later stages of the primary (original) cancer. If a tumor begins to grow behind the eye, it can cause bulging of the eye and sometimes affect vision. Secondary eye tumors may be treated with radiation therapy.

Uveitis, Iritis, Cyclitis, and Choroiditis

Uveitis is inflammation of the uvea, which is made up of three parts: the colored iris, the ciliary body, and the choroid, a sponge-like membrane between the sclera and the retina. Uveitis affecting the iris is called iritis; inflammation of the muscles that focus the lens is called cyclitis; and inflammation of the choroid is called choroiditis.

For most people with uveitis, the cause is unknown. However, it can result from an autoimmune disorder (see p.870). It can also occur with infection by the herpes simplex virus (see p.487) or the herpes zoster virus, such as with shingles (see p.537). People with acquired immunodeficiency syndrome (AIDS) develop uveitis due to infection with cytomegalovirus (see p.871).

SYMPTOMS

Symptoms of uveitis include sensitivity to light, blurred vision, pain, and redness of the eye. In iritis and cyclitis, these symptoms can begin abruptly and last up to several months. With choroiditis, the onset of symptoms is more gradual and may last longer.

Inflammation of the uvea can have serious consequences—including glaucoma (see p.435), cataract (see p.430), neovascularization (formation of new, abnormal blood vessels; see Diabetic Retinopathy, p.434), and blindness—if it is not treated. Prompt evaluation of your symptoms is critical.

TREATMENT OPTIONS

Treatment of uveitis and iritis may include eyedrops or an ointment containing a corticosteroid drug to reduce inflammation and pain. Eyedrops that dilate the pupil may also be used; this prevents the inflamed iris from moving, which helps relieve pain. Your doctor will treat separately any complications caused by glaucoma, cataract, or neovascularization.

OTHER EYE CONDITIONS

Black Eye

Usually the result of an injury, a black eye is a bruising of the tissues that surround the eye. Like any bruise, a black eye is the result of blood seeping out of the surface blood vessels and collecting under the skin. Because the skin is so thin around the eyes, bruising in this area can be darker than on other parts of the body.

To ease the pain and reduce inflammation, apply cold compresses to the area as soon as possible after the injury. If your black eye is accompanied by other symptoms, such as double vision, flashing lights, or "floaters," call your doctor immediately.

Color Blindness

Color blindness is an abnormality of the eye's ability to distinguish colors; it is common and not a threat to vision. True color blindness, in which everything appears in shades of black, gray, and white, is very rare. More common are inherited conditions in which the retina lacks one type of cone (the color-sensitive cell in the retina) or in which the cone cells themselves are defective. In the most common type of color blindness, people cannot distinguish green from red.

Most color blindness is caused by an inherited defect on the X chromosome (see p.128); ten times as many men as women are color blind, although women can carry the defect and pass it on to their children. Acquired color blindness may develop as a result of injury or disease of the retina or optic nerve. Most sufferers are not aware that they have color blindness until another person questions their color discrimination (such as pointing out that their socks do not match) or until the color blindness is revealed during color vision testing.

There is no treatment for hereditary forms of color blindness; color blindness caused by disease is treated by addressing the underlying problem.

Crossed Eyes

Crossed eyes, also called strabismus, is a defect in the coordination of the muscles that move the eyes, causing the eyes to be misaligned and point in different directions. Normal eyes move in unison so that they focus on an object together, which is necessary for clear vision.

Strabismus most often occurs in infants and young children. Infants in the first several months of life are still learning to focus their eyes, and a wandering eye is common at this time. Most babies outgrow the condition by the age of 6 months. If they do not, medical treatments are essential to protect against loss of vision.

In adults, strabismus usually develops as a result of a disorder that affects the brain, such as a stroke (see p.342); the nerves that control the eye muscles; or the eye muscles themselves. Strabismus can accompany diabetes mellitus (see p.832), multiple sclerosis (see p.368), or disorders of the thyroid gland (see p.844).

SYMPTOMS

The main symptom of strabismus in adults is double vision and an eye that does not move in a coordinated fashion with the other eye. The misalignment may take different forms: one eye may look straight ahead while the other turns inward (esotropia), outward (exotropia), downward, or upward (vertical strabismus).

Sometimes the lack of coordination is intermittent, sometimes it is continuous. Squinting in bright sunlight, or tilting the head to align the eyes, is also common. Faulty depth perception frequently occurs.

TREATMENT OPTIONS

Children should be monitored closely during infancy and the preschool years to detect potential eye problems, particularly if a relative has strabismus. If there is any question about a child's ability to see or about the muscle alignment of his or her eyes, the child should see an ophthalmologist. The earlier treatment is pro-

Crossed Eyes

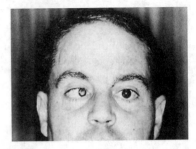

Crossed eyes are a visual defect in which eyes are misaligned and point in different directions.

vided, the better the chances for normal vision.

If strabismus persists beyond the age of 6 months, the brain reacts to the double vision and begins to ignore signals from the weak eye. If this goes on for long, the brain will lose the ability to recognize signals from the weak eye even if the strabismus is later corrected with surgery.

A child under age 10 should be made to use the weak eye through a variety of approaches: an eye patch may be worn over the normal eye, eyedrops may be used to temporarily blur the vision of the normal eye, exercises may be prescribed to strengthen specific eye muscles, and/or glasses may be used to correct vision in the weak eye. Forcing the child to use the weak eye can reinforce the connection between the eye and the brain and improve sight.

Usually, surgery to tighten or loosen specific muscles is required to realign the eyes. Occasionally, surgery can be avoided by injecting a drug into one or more of the eye muscles to temporarily paralyze them, allowing the opposite muscle to tighten and correct the misalignment.

Orbital Cellulitis

Orbital cellulitis is infection of the tissues of the eye socket, the bony cavity of the skull that contains and protects the eyeball. It usually occurs when bacteria spread from infected sinuses (see Sinusitis, p.464) or from a boil on the eyelid to the tissues of the eye. Because orbital cellulitis can quickly deteriorate into a very serious condition or spread to the brain (see Menin-

gitis, p.377), immediate treatment is critical.

SYMPTOMS

The first signs of orbital cellulitis include pain in the area of the eye, redness and swelling of the eyelid and the skin around the eye, difficulty moving the eyes, decreased sharpness of vision, and fever. The swelling of the tissues can push the eyeball forward (see Bulging Eyes, p.427).

TREATMENT OPTIONS

Your doctor will examine the eye and may perform blood tests to confirm the presence of infection. You may require strong doses of antibiotics (see p.868) to combat the infection. In addition, your doctor may recommend computed tomography (see p.149) to determine if the original source of the infection is located in your sinuses. Infected sinuses, and any abscesses in the eye socket, may need to be drained.

Watery Eyes

Constant tearing can be caused by a foreign body in the eye or chronic irritation of the eye. It also can be caused by injury to the bone of the nose, leading to scarring of the nasolacrimal tear ducts—the ducts responsible for draining tears out of the eye into the nose.

Blockage of the tear ducts is rare but can lead to an infection of a duct from bacteria, causing painful red swelling of the nose near the infected duct. It is usually treated with antibiotics in eyedrop or tablet form.

Some people have a watery eye as a symptom of sinusitis (see p.464) or from the irritation

Location of Tear-Producing Glands

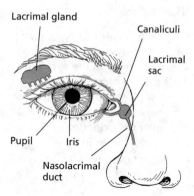

Lacrimal gland

Canaliculi

Lacrimal sac

Pupil   Iris

Nasolacrimal duct

Lacrimal (tear-producing) glands are located under the brow bone behind the upper lids at the edge of the eye socket and, to a lesser degree, in the lids. Tears course over the eye surface and keep it lubricated, well nourished, and clear of foreign matter. Tears drain through the canaliculi at the innermost corners of the lids, collect in the lacrimal sac, and empty into the nose through the nasolacrimal duct. When you blink, the lacrimal sac compresses, actively pumping excess tears away from the eye and down the nasolacrimal duct.

of a dry eye. In many people, the cause of watery eyes is unknown. If you have an eye that waters persistently, talk to your doctor. If you have a blocked tear duct you may require surgery to create a new duct.

Some infants have a blocked tear duct when they are born, which can cause the eye to water. The blockage often disappears on its own by 9 months of age. If it does not, the infant may require minor surgery to open the duct. In advanced cases, an artificial duct to drain fluid is surgically created.

Ears, Nose, and Throat

Although they serve very different purposes, the ears, nose, and throat are physically closely linked. Primary care doctors care for most of the problems of the ears, nose, and throat, but sometimes a specialist's help is required. Otolaryngologists, sometimes called (not surprisingly) ear, nose, and throat (ENT) doctors, are the specialists who treat disorders of and perform surgery on the ear, nose, and throat.

EARS

If a great inventor, like Thomas Edison, had been asked to design a machine for hearing, his invention would not have been nearly as clever as our ear. The outer, middle, and inner ear work together to transform sound waves into electrical impulses that transmit sound messages to the brain. Sound waves travel through the ear canal of the outer ear and strike the eardrum, which causes three tiny middle ear bones—the hammer (malleus), anvil (incus), and stirrup (stapes)—to vibrate. These vibrations bend tiny hairs that lie inside a snail-shaped organ in the inner ear called the cochlea.

When the hairs bend, they transform sound-wave vibrations into electrical signals that travel along the cochlear nerve to the brain, where they are perceived as sensations of pitch and loudness.

Your ears also help maintain your sense of balance. Besides the cochlea, the inner ear contains a mazelike compartment composed of the utricle, saccule, and three semicircular canals. The utricle and saccule provide the brain with information about the body's position at rest; the semicircular canals track the body in motion. All three organs

Cross-Section of Ear

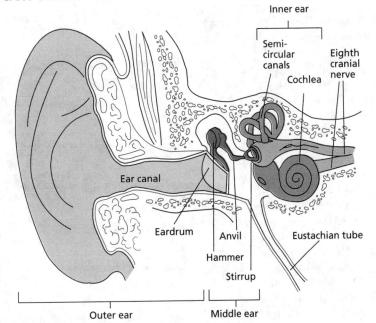

Ears allow you to hear by processing sound waves that travel through the air. The three parts of the ear—the outer ear, middle ear, and inner ear—work together to transform these sound waves into electrical impulses that transmit sound messages to the brain. Ears also play a key role in your sense of balance.

contain fluid and minute hairs; as the body's position changes, the fluid shifts, moving the hairs in a particular way. Your brain knows your position by the electrical signals that are sent by the vestibular nerve, generated by movement of the hairs. Together, the cochlear nerve and vestibular nerve form the eighth cranial nerve.

NOSE AND SINUSES

The nose performs three functions: it smells, it helps keep foreign matter out of your lungs, and it warms and humidifies the air you breathe in. Smell is a reaction your body has to substances in the air. Buried in the inner lining of the nose are millions of nerve endings that are triggered to make electrical impulses when they encounter a substance. These impulses travel up the olfactory (smelling) nerve to the brain, where they are recognized as the sensation of smell.

The two nostrils are lined with cells that have hairlike projections and cells that produce mucus. Particles in the air passing through the nostrils get stuck in the mucus. The hairs then move the mucus to the back of the nose and throat where it is either swallowed or spit out.

The nasal passages open into the throat and also into the sinuses, which are air-filled cavities in the skull bones. Given all the trouble they cause us (see Sinusitis, p.464), we assume we were provided with sinuses for a reason. Scientists guess that human beings developed sinuses to help give the voice power and lighten the skull. Who knows?

THROAT, MOUTH, AND LARYNX

The mouth takes in food, drink, and the air you breathe. The mouth also begins the process of digesting food. The throat is lined with many immune system cells (especially in the tonsils and adenoids) that serve as sentries, guarding against incoming germs.

The mouth also allows you to taste. Like smell, taste is the sensation created when substances in the food you eat trigger the millions of taste nerve endings located in your tongue. Electrical impulses travel from the tongue to the brain, generating the sensation of taste.

A tiny tube, the eustachian tube, runs between the back of the nose and the ears. This tube provides ventilation for the middle ear and is normally closed. It opens when you yawn or blow your nose, sometimes causing a pop or crackle in your ear as the air reaches the ear. Various microorganisms can travel through this tube to cause infection. When the lining of the nose and throat becomes swollen, such as from allergies or colds, the eustachian tube can become blocked. This may increase the

Cross-Section of Nose and Throat

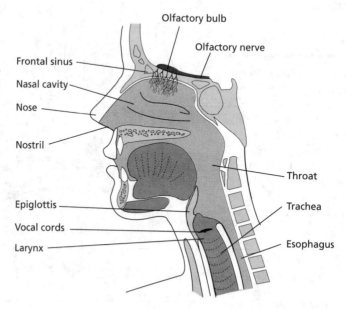

The nose is composed of two nostrils that are separated by the septum, a plate made of cartilage and bone. Each nasal passage opens into the four sinuses on that side of the head. The nose gives us a sense of smell and filters out foreign matter from the air we breathe. The epiglottis directs food and liquids away from the passage to the lungs and down the esophagus. Vocal cords allow us a wide range of vocalization, including talking, shouting, whispering, and singing.

chance of ear infections and can produce a popping sensation or a feeling that your ears are blocked.

The larynx performs two important functions: it aids in speech and provides a passage for air between the throat and the trachea, the tube leading toward the lungs. Speech is created when the lungs exhale air across the vocal cords, the membranes that vibrate to create sound waves. Those waves are further altered by the position of your tongue, palate, and lips to create spoken words. The larynx also helps prevent food from falling into the lungs.

EARS

Acoustic Neuroma

An acoustic neuroma is a slow-growing, benign (noncancerous) tumor of the eighth cranial nerve, which connects the inner ear to the brain. Early symptoms include feeling unsteady or dizzy, hearing noises in your ear, and having a gradual loss of hearing. In advanced cases, the tumor compresses the facial nerve, resulting in weakness of the muscles of facial expression. Evaluation to look for the tumor may include an audiometry (see Hearing Tests, p.452), magnetic resonance imaging (see p.151), or a computed tomography (see p.149) scan of your head. Your doctor may refer you to a specialist for evaluation. Treatments include surgery to remove the tumor and a single session of radiation therapy.

Barotrauma

Barotrauma means injury to the ear from changes in barometric air pressure. It occurs when the eustachian tube (see Cross-Section of Ear, p.447) becomes partially or completely blocked. The tube functions to keep the pressure in the middle ear similar to the pressure outside of the ear.

Some people have eustachian tubes that do not function well or have tubes that become temporarily blocked by a cold, allergy, or infection. In such cases, when there is a sudden change in air pressure (such as when an airplane lands or during scuba diving), problems can develop. There is an imbalance in the pressure between the middle ear and air outside the ear. The eardrum is sucked inward as a result of the relatively increased outside pressure.

SYMPTOMS

Symptoms, which are mild most of the time, consist of blockage and a feeling of pressure in the ear or a feeling that you need to "pop" your ear. More severe symptoms include hearing loss, dizziness, accumulation of fluid or bleeding in the middle ear, severe pain, and possibly even rupture of the eardrum, with blood and fluid running out of the ear.

TREATMENT OPTIONS

If you have recurring barotrauma, or have pain or pressure when you fly in an airplane, take a decongestant pill and use a

Flying or Scuba Diving with Nasal Congestion: Dr Ota's Advice

If you have an ear infection, you should not fly in an airplane or scuba dive because you could develop barotrauma (see left). If you have a cold, allergy, or nasal congestion and want to know if you will be able to fly or scuba dive without causing barotrauma or discomfort, try this test: Take an elevator to the top of a tall building. On the way down, try to equalize the pressure in your ears with the pressure outside your ears by performing the techniques discussed under Barotrauma (left). If you cannot make your ears pop, you should not fly or scuba dive. If descending from the top to the bottom of the building in the elevator has caused any pressure or pain that you cannot alleviate, go back up the elevator and come down several floors at a time to give the pressure in your ears a chance to equalize.

H. GREGORY OTA, MD
MASSACHUSETTS EYE AND EAR INFIRMARY
HARVARD MEDICAL SCHOOL

Preventing Hearing Loss

Many types of hearing loss are preventable. However, once they occur, they are often irreversible. Hearing loss is most often caused by exposure to loud noises, which permanently damage the hair cells in the cochlea of the inner ear that receive sound vibrations and transform them into electrical nerve signals. Damage to the hair cells accounts for most nerve deafness later in life.

Avoid sounds that cause you pain, produce ringing in your ears, cause you to temporarily lose hearing, or are stressful. The most common recreational cause of serious hearing loss is gunshot noise such as rifle fire. The affected ear is most often on the side opposite the shoulder the rifle rests on since the ear on the same side is somewhat shielded by the butt of the gun.

Extremely intense sound can rip the delicate hair cells of the inner ear completely off the membrane on which they sit, kill the cells, or simply injure them permanently. While one very loud noise can damage the inner ear, continuous noise over 85 decibels (see Decibel Levels of Common Sounds, p.452) tends to be more damaging. Many work environments demand long-term exposure to loud noise such as that caused by power looms, welding equipment, power saws, and jackhammers. Large machines or vehicles used on construction sites or in military operations also generate loud noise, as do aircraft. Machines used around the house or yard, including power tools, vacuum cleaners, power mowers, wood chippers, chain saws, snowblowers, and some kitchen appliances, can also be noisy, as can loud music, power boats, and snowmobiles.

If you are exposed to loud noise on a regular basis, wear earplugs or earmuffs, which bring high decibel levels down to lower levels, and see your doctor regularly to have your hearing checked. Early detection and treatment can prevent further hearing loss. If your hearing loss is due to job-related noise, your employer may be required to provide noise-protection devices.

decongestant nasal spray an hour before your flight. Continue the medicines in the recommended dosage until you have landed. Drink lots of liquids, but avoid alcohol, caffeine, and tobacco.

Stay awake during descent so you can equalize the pressure in your ears. Yawning, chewing gum, sucking on hard candy, and swallowing will help open the eustachian tube when you feel pressure. If these measures do not help, try to pop your ears by performing the Valsalva maneuver. Take a breath, pinch your nose, close your mouth, and gently blow your nose without letting air escape. Stop when your ear pops. Do not use excessive force; this could rupture your eardrum.

If you have severe pain for several hours, or drainage or bleeding from your ears, see your doctor immediately. Also, if you have other, milder symptoms, or the barotrauma persists for more than a few days, see your physician.

Cholesteatoma

A cholesteatoma is a cyst or overgrowth of skin of the eardrum into the middle ear. The growth can become infected or can grow and damage the delicate bones of your middle ear. You may be born with a tendency to form a cholesteatoma, or it may be caused by repeated infection of the middle ear or repeated blockage of the eustachian tube.

Symptoms include hearing loss, dizziness, pressure in your ear, earache, and drainage of pus from the affected ear. If not treated, a cholesteatoma can cause your face muscles to become weak or paralyzed. Your doctor may refer you to an otolaryngologist, who will examine your ear and use medicines to control any infection. You will need either minor or major surgery, typically performed while you are under a general anesthetic (see p.168), to remove the growth completely and reconstruct any damaged bones or a damaged eardrum.

Cholesteatomas can recur; for this reason, your doctor should examine the ear every year for signs of recurrence.

Home Remedies for Unblocking Earwax

The ear canal has glands that produce a wax called cerumen, which helps trap dust and other substances, keeping them from reaching the eardrum. Accumulated wax usually dries up and moves out of the ear on its own, bringing the debris with it. Sometimes earwax accumulates faster than the body removes it, which can result in hearing loss, a plugged sensation, or an earache.

Never put any solid object like a cotton-tip swab (or, even worse, a paperclip) into your ear canal. The skin of the canal and the eardrum itself are very fragile and can be easily injured, and you may pack the wax down into the canal, making it harder to remove.

Ask your doctor for help in removing earwax if you have a hole in your eardrum or if you have had surgery on your ear. Otherwise, it is usually easy to unblock the wax yourself by following these instructions:

■ Get a medicine dropper and any of the following substances (available at any drugstore): liquid docusate sodium, baby oil, mineral oil, any nonprescription earwax remover liquid, or hydrogen peroxide.

■ Tilt your head so the affected ear points upward.

■ Drip any of the liquids into the affected ear canal with the medicine dropper until your ear is full.

■ Keep your head tilted, with the affected ear canal up, so that the liquid stays in the ear canal for 5 minutes. Then, holding a washcloth or small towel to your ear, tilt the affected ear canal down so that the liquid and its contents drip out.

■ If necessary, repeat one to two times a day for several days to fully remove wax from the ear.

If you are not successful at removing the wax, see your doctor, who may attempt to flush out the wax, extract it with an instrument, or vacuum it out.

Hearing Loss

Partial or complete loss of hearing can be caused by a wide variety of conditions, including blockage of the ear canal by earwax, aging, loud noise, injury, drugs, infection, and birth defects. Age-related hearing loss (called presbycusis) occurs in one third of all people over 65. It can start as early as age 40 and become progressively worse, particularly affecting your ability to hear high-frequency sounds.

Sensorineural hearing loss is caused by damage to the cochlea and the eighth cranial nerve. It occurs when the tiny hair cells (which cannot repair themselves or grow back) of the cochlea in the inner ear die from aging or become damaged. Damage is usually due to prolonged exposure to loud noise, but can also be a result of injury, disease or

Earwax Removal

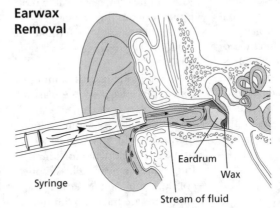

Syringe

Eardrum

Wax

Stream of fluid

Your doctor can safely remove earwax by directing a stream of warm fluid into your ear canal. Earwax is loosened and comes out of the ear with the fluid. Doctors also use suction or instruments to pull wax out of the ear.

infection, toxic drugs, or an inherited condition. As a result, sound reaching the cochlea is not properly processed and inadequate nerve signals are sent to the brain.

Sensorineural hearing loss is permanent and usually affects both ears. Occasionally, sensori-

neural hearing loss develops suddenly. It is important to see your doctor; immediate treatment, sometimes with corticosteroid drugs (see p.895), may be helpful.

When sound waves are blocked or obstructed in the outer or middle ear, the condition is called conductive hearing loss.

Decibel Levels of Common Sounds

The chart below shows the approximate decibel levels of some common sounds. Wear hearing protection anytime you are exposed to 80 decibels for more than a few hours.

DECIBELS	SOUND	DECIBELS	SOUND
20	Watch ticking	90	Lawn mower; convertible ride on free-way
30	Whispering		
40	Leaves rustling; refrigerator humming	100	Blow-dryer; diesel truck; subway train; chain saw
50	Neighborhood street; average home		
60	Dishwasher; normal conversation	110	Car horn; snowblower
70	Car; alarm clock; city traffic	120	Rock concert; propeller plane
80	Garbage disposal; noisy restaurant; vacuum cleaner; outboard motor	130	Jet engine plane (100 feet away); air-raid siren
85	Factory; electric shaver; screaming child	140	Shotgun blast

Conductive hearing loss is caused by damage to the ear canal, eardrum, or tiny bones of the middle ear. Blockage can result from wax buildup or from inflammation of the outer ear or middle ear caused by ear infections, cholesteatoma (see p.450), otosclerosis (see p.458), or a foreign object in the ear. An eardrum damaged by injury or infection can also cause this type of hearing loss.

SYMPTOMS

Read the Hearing Loss Quiz (see p.453) to learn about the most common symptoms of hearing loss. Less commonly, you may also have ringing or rustling noises in your ear, earache, discharge, dizziness, or nausea.

HEARING TESTS

Hearing tests help your physician determine what type of hearing loss you have and to what extent it is affecting your hearing. The simplest hearing tests, called the Rinne test and the Weber test, use a tuning fork to determine what kind of hearing loss you have.

In the Rinne test, the tuning fork is placed against the mastoid bone behind your ear (to test bone conduction of sound) and then near your outer ear canal (to test air conduction of sound). In conductive hearing loss, bone conduction is better because the vibrations are traveling through the bone to the cochlea, bypassing the problems in the outer or middle ear.

In a healthy ear or one with sensorineural hearing loss, air conduction is better than bone conduction because sound is transmitted more efficiently through the healthy apparatus of the middle ear than through bone.

In the Weber test, which is used to diagnose one-sided hearing loss, a vibrating tuning fork is held against the middle of your forehead. If you have conductive hearing loss, you hear the sounds better in the ear with poor hearing because the ear is not distracted by environmental sounds (which do not get through as well because of the abnormalities in the outer and middle ear).

Audiometry is a more sophisticated test that must be performed by a specialist. For audiometry, you wear padded headphones in a soundproof room and listen to sounds transmitted to one ear at a time. The frequency of the sounds is increased gradually (from low to high), as is the volume, until you can hear them. You are also tested to see if you can distinguish words that sound alike, such as distinguishing the word "pin" from "fin."

Impedance testing measures

Hearing Loss Quiz

Take this quiz to determine whether or not you have hearing loss. Review the possible responses in the key and record your points for each answer. Then total your points and follow the recommendations in the results section.

KEY

Almost always	3 points
Half the time	2 points
Occasionally	1 point
Never	0 points

1. I have trouble understanding people over the telephone.
2. I have to strain to understand conversations, or have trouble hearing when two or more people are talking.
3. People complain that I turn the TV volume too high.
4. I have difficulty hearing conversations when there is a lot of noise in the background.
5. I get confused about where sounds are coming from.
6. I often misunderstand some words in a sentence, especially when a woman or child is speaking.
7. I have worked in a noisy environment (such as on an assembly line or near jackhammers or jet engines).
8. Many people seem to mumble.
9. People seem annoyed that I misunderstand what they say.
10. I have a blood relative with hearing loss (3 points).

RESULTS

0–3 points	Your hearing is probably fine.
4–6 points	You may want to discuss hearing loss with your doctor.
≥ 7 points	Make an appointment with your doctor and tell him or her you are having trouble hearing.

your eardrum's ability to reflect sound waves and can indicate whether a middle ear problem is causing your hearing loss. If the pressure on the inner side of the eardrum is too high or too low, the eardrum cannot reflect and conduct sound well. Impedance testing measures the eardrum's mobility with a probe placed in your ear that sends sound waves to the eardrum. Simultaneously, the pressure of the ear canal is changed. A microphone in the probe registers the sounds returned from your eardrum as the pressure changes.

TREATMENT OPTIONS

Once your doctor has determined the cause of your hearing loss, he or she may refer you to a hearing specialist. Age-related hearing loss is permanent; a hearing aid (see below) may be recommended. Infection can be treated with antibiotics, though sometimes the infection must be drained and the pressure relieved by myringotomy, in which a tiny opening is made in the eardrum. Reconstructive surgery is used to correct or replace damaged middle ear structures.

HEARING AIDS

A hearing aid is an electronic device that amplifies sound and transmits it to the ear canal to improve hearing by intensifying sound so the inner ear can detect it. Most age-related hearing loss can be corrected only with a hearing aid.

Hearing aids consist of a tiny microphone that coverts sounds to electrical impulses, an amplifier that boosts this signal, a speaker that changes the signal into sound, a battery, and a volume control. Hearing aids must be made to fit your ear properly. Different types of hearing aids have different features; they differ by how large and visible they are, by the quality of the sound you hear, and by the ease with which you can control the sound.

If you have hearing loss in both ears, a hearing aid is usually tried first in the ear with the worst hearing loss. Even if you have only a modest loss of hearing in the other ear, a second hearing aid in that ear can help you hear better because you will be able to locate where sounds

Hearing Aids and Sound Transmission

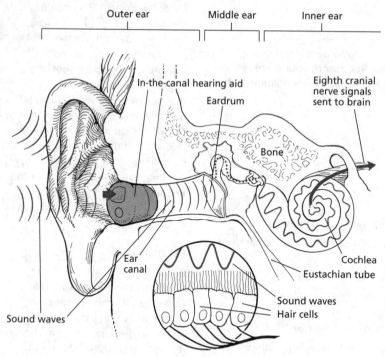

A hearing aid contains a tiny microphone that picks up sound waves and amplifies them, sending the sound waves down the ear canal. Tiny hair cells in the cochlea send the signals along the eighth cranial nerve to the brain, where they are perceived as sound.

are coming from more easily.

Medicare and many private insurers will not cover the cost of hearing aids, but some state Medicaid programs will. The basic types are grouped according to how you wear them, as follows:

On-the-body hearing aid This hearing aid is carried in a pocket or clipped onto clothing. It resembles a transistor radio and contains a battery, an amplifier, and a microphone. A cord connects the case to a speaker that snaps onto a custom plastic ear mold. This model has the greatest power because of its large speaker and battery; it is excel-

lent for people with severe hearing loss. Its main advantages are that the chance of feedback (an echoing of sound waves from microphone to speaker that causes a buzzing noise) is low because the microphone and speaker are far apart, its volume controls are easiest to handle (important for people who have arthritis of the hands or problems with dexterity), and it is less expensive than many other types of hearing aid. Nevertheless, the pocket-style hearing aid is less popular because some people regard it as cumbersome, old fashioned, and cosmetically unat-

tractive. Costs range from $200 to $800.

Behind-the-ear hearing aid All of the electronic components in this model are contained in a plastic case that fits behind the ear. This type of hearing aid is slightly less visible than the on-the-body hearing aid. A thin tube carries sound from the case to a custom ear mold. Next to the on-the-body hearing aid, this model is the most reliable, easiest for you to adjust volume, and easiest to repair.

In-the-ear hearing aid This device is made from a hollow acrylic shell that is created from an impression of your ear. Advantages of this type include better reproduction of high-pitched sounds and less wind noise than external models. It is also less visible than the on-the-body or behind-the-ear models. It has controls that allow you to adjust the volume, although they are not quite as easy to use as those of the behind-the-ear models. The primary disadvantage is that the proximity of the microphone to the receiver makes feedback more likely. Prices range from $600 to $900.

In-the-canal hearing aid This model is custom-made to fit mostly inside the ear canal, making it less visible than the in-the-ear models. Its volume controls are somewhat harder to use than the in-the-ear models. Costs range from $700 to $1,000.

Completely-in-canal hearing aid This model is custom-made to fit entirely inside the ear canal, where it is essentially invisible. You must have an adequately large ear canal to use it, and you cannot adjust its volume. It may

Cochlear Implant for Hearing Loss

A cochlear implant (below) is a hearing device for those with severe sensorineural hearing loss, which affects about 200,000 people in the United States. It occurs when the cells with the hairlike structures that receive sound waves and translate them into electrical messages to send up the eighth cranial nerve to the brain have been destroyed. A standard hearing aid that merely amplifies sound is of little value for people with this type of severe hearing loss because even amplified sound waves cannot be recognized.

Cochlear implant surgery is performed under general anesthesia (see p.168). Although the implant does not restore normal hearing, it restores enough to enable most people to better discriminate speech, which, along with lipreading, helps them communicate. The ultimate effectiveness of a cochlear implant depends on how long your hearing has been affected prior to implanting the device and on the current health of your remaining inner ear nerve fibers. Your motivation is also very important since you will have to work hard (with the aid of a therapist) to learn to interpret the sounds you will hear.

Cochlear Implant

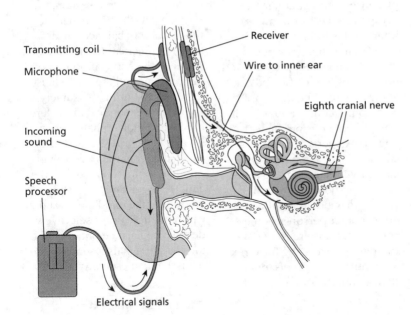

Transmitting coil

Microphone

Incoming sound

Speech processor

Electrical signals

Receiver

Wire to inner ear

Eighth cranial nerve

A cochlear implant consists of several pieces of electronic equipment. A small microphone is worn behind the ear to capture incoming sound, which is sent down a wire to a small box called a speech processor. The speech processor, which is usually worn on a belt or in a pocket, translates sound waves into electrical signals that are sent back up the wire to a transmitting coil located behind the ear. The transmitting device sends radio waves that travel through the skull to a receiver implanted in the skull. The receiver has wires that run to the inner ear, stimulating the eighth cranial nerve to send information (which is interpreted as sound) to the brain.

take several fittings to get the fit just right. Costs range from $1,200 to $1,500.

Digital hearing aid This newest type of hearing aid has a tiny digital computer that can be programmed for different acoustic environments (such as a noisy restaurant versus a quiet room) by using a remote control. It can also be programmed to compensate for the specific type of hearing loss you have (such as high-frequency or low-frequency hearing loss). Prices for these models range from $1,500 to $3,000.

It can take several weeks or months to adapt to using a hearing aid and to adjust to the sound, which will differ from what you are accustomed to. Start out using your hearing aid in a quiet environment until you become used to it; then try it in different environments and on new sounds. Wear your hearing aid daily to establish a routine.

Labyrinthitis

Labyrinthitis is an infection and inflammation of the labyrinth, the fluid-filled passages in the inner ear that control balance. It is almost always caused by a viral infection. In rare cases, it is caused by bacteria that have spread to the inner ear from a middle ear infection (see p.457).

Symptoms include vertigo (a spinning sensation) and loss of balance, nausea, vomiting, involuntary movements of the eyes, and loss of hearing in one ear. Although the most severe symptoms can be frightening, they usually do not last for more than a few days, and there are treatments that help.

Your doctor will inspect your ear and ask if you recently had an ear infection. If the labyrinthitis is due to a bacterial infection, you will need to take antibiotics. Antibiotics cannot help a viral infection. For both types of labyrinthitis, your doctor may recommend antinausea drugs to alleviate the vertigo. Dizziness usually dissipates within several days to several weeks. Lack of balance, especially when you move quickly, can last several weeks or even months. It is rare for labyrinthitis to recur.

Ménière Disease

Ménière disease is a recurring and sometimes disabling disorder of the inner ear that causes periods of vertigo (a spinning sensation), dizziness, nausea and vomiting, fluctuating hearing loss,

and noise in the ear (see Tinnitus, p.459). In most cases, only one ear is affected.

Ménière disease is caused by a fluid accumulation in the inner ear. Doctors do not know why the fluid accumulates. Because of the excess fluid and the rupture of delicate membranes of the inner ear, the balance center sends chaotic signals to the brain, which causes vertigo and imbalance.

SYMPTOMS

The symptoms of Ménière disease can be dramatic and disabling. The worst symptom is vertigo, sometimes accompanied by nausea and vomiting. The vertigo may last for minutes to hours and is followed by a sense of imbalance that may persist for days. You may feel pressure and hear noises in the affected ear. Some degree of hearing loss is common. It comes and goes; in some people it is permanent. You may experience one or several attacks of symptoms that may vary in duration and severity; your experience with the disease may be quite different from another person's. Sometimes symptoms are frequent and highly distressing for weeks or months and then disappear almost entirely for months or years.

TREATMENT OPTIONS

There is no cure for Ménière disease, although your doctor may prescribe medicines to prevent vertigo or to relieve nausea and vomiting. Diuretics may also be prescribed to reduce fluid retention (and thus fluid buildup in the inner ear). Reducing your intake of salt, nicotine, alcohol,

and caffeine is occasionally recommended, although there is no research to prove the effectiveness of this course of action.

Several types of ear surgery can reduce or halt attacks of vertigo with varying degrees of risk and success. The most successful operations are destructive, meaning that they purposely destroy structures in the ear (which results in total deafness) in order to halt the vertigo. These surgeries are usually performed only on people who experience severe dizziness and have little or no hearing in the affected ear.

In an operation called selective vestibular nerve section, the surgeon cuts the nerve that carries the body's balance signal from the inner ear to the brain. To reach the nerve, a portion of the bone around the nerve must be removed during the surgery.

In a newer surgical procedure called an endolymphatic shunt, a small hole is made in the inner ear to drain out the excess fluid. Another approach is to instill the antibiotics gentamicin or streptomycin into the middle ear via the eardrum; these drugs selectively destroy the balance organ (and the chaotic signals it sends to the brain) while preserving hearing.

Outer Ear Infection

Also called otitis externa and swimmer's ear, this is infection and inflammation of the outer ear canal. The infection, which can be caused by bacteria or fungi, also sometimes affects the external part of the ear. Outer ear infection due to bacteria can cause a boil or abscess. Skin disorders such as dermatitis can also

Preventing Swimmer's Ear: Dr Randolph's Advice

Drying your ears thoroughly can help prevent swimmer's ear. If you get water in your ears while swimming, showering, bathing, or washing your hair, first dry them thoroughly. Next, if you do not have a perforated eardrum and have not had recent ear surgery, mix equal amounts of rubbing (isopropyl) alcohol and white vinegar in a small bowl. (The alcohol dries out the ear and the vinegar changes the acidity of the ear canal, making it less likely that bacteria will grow.) Lie down with one ear up. Instill three to four drops of the mixture with a medicine dropper. Keep the ear with the liquid in it upright for several minutes. You can help the drops get farther down into your ear canal by pulling on your earlobe and by opening and closing your mouth. After several minutes, tip your head over to allow the drops to come out. Repeat the procedure in the other ear.

GREGORY W. RANDOLPH, MD
MASSACHUSETTS EYE AND EAR INFIRMARY
HARVARD MEDICAL SCHOOL

cause inflammation of the outer ear structure and can make the ear more prone to infection.

Outer ear infection is often caused by water getting into the ear canal. Symptoms include itching, swelling, pain, and a yellow discharge from the ear; you may also have hearing loss from the inflammation or discharge, which can block the ear canal. In time, the ear may become painful to the touch and infection may spread to other ear structures. See your doctor if you have these symptoms. Diabetics can develop serious infections from outer ear infection and should see a doctor as soon as symptoms develop.

Your doctor will inspect your ear with a viewing tool called an otoscope and prescribe medicine, usually in the form of eardrops. Antibiotics help clear up bacterial infections, antifungal drugs kill

fungus, and anti-inflammatory drugs reduce swelling. It is important not to get moisture in your ear while the infection is clearing, which usually occurs within a week. The best way to keep water out of the canal (such as when you are showering) is to use a ball of cotton covered with a layer of petroleum jelly. Remove the cotton after showering and air out your ear canal.

Middle Ear Infection

Infection of the middle ear, also called otitis media, is common in children. It can cause severe pain in the affected ear. There are three types of middle ear infection: acute otitis media, otitis media with effusion, and chronic suppurative otitis media.

Acute otitis media is caused by a bacterial infection of the

middle ear. Viruses may also play a role. Symptoms include the sudden development of earache, pain, fever, and the feeling of being generally sick and irritable. Sometimes it is brought on by an upper respiratory, sinus, or throat infection. Complications of acute otitis media include rupture of the eardrum (with drainage of blood and pus from the ear), mastoiditis (an infection in the bone behind the ear, causing redness and painful swelling), or meningitis.

Mastoiditis and meningitis are rare complications. However, both require immediate hospitalization, and mastoiditis may require surgery. A ruptured eardrum permits the pressure in the middle ear to be released, relieving the pain; healing usually takes place in a few days.

Various antibiotics, along with eardrops, are used to treat acute otitis media. Although decongestants or antihistamines have not been proven to affect the course of infection, they can make the person more comfortable if there are allergic symptoms and nasal congestion. When antibiotic treatment does not help acute otitis media, a hole is made in the eardrum using a needle or scalpel to allow infected fluid in the middle ear to drain out of the ear canal.

Acute otitis media tends to recur in some children. If your child has three or more episodes in 6 months or less, it may be beneficial to search for other underlying causes. Environmental allergens, food allergies (such as to milk), immune deficiencies, enlarged adenoids, chronic sinusitis, exposure to tobacco smoke, and other causes can make a child more susceptible to recurrent infections. Immunization to two bacteria that cause otitis media, *Streptococcus pneumoniae* and *Haemophilus influenzae,* may help.

If no underlying cause of the recurring infections can be identified, your child's doctor may recommend low daily doses of antibiotics for several weeks or months. If antibiotic treatment fails, the doctor may suggest that tubes be inserted through the eardrum to drain fluid that collects in the middle ear.

Otitis media with effusion is the presence of fluid in the middle ear without the infectious symptoms of acute otitis media. Most often, this occurs after an acute infection has cleared, but the fluid persists. Other causes are poor eustachian tube function that is usually caused by a cleft palate (see p.970), colds, or barotrauma (see p.449).

One month after treatment, up to 40% of children with acute otitis media still have fluid in the middle ear; 10% have it up to 3 months after treatment. Antibiotics may be recommended if the fluid persists for 2 to 3 months or if antibiotics have not yet been used. Corticosteroid medicines (see p.895) may also be prescribed.

The most serious problem with persistent effusion is hearing loss. In a young child, hearing loss may lead to delays in speech and language development. Ventilation tubes should be inserted if your child has had fluid in both ears for 3 months, despite taking antibiotics, or if fluid persists in one ear for 6 months.

Chronic suppurative otitis media causes drainage from the ear for 6 or more weeks. There may also be a cholesteatoma (see p.450). Your doctor may prescribe antibiotics and eardrops to treat the drainage. If treatment fails, intravenous antibiotics and diagnostic tests, including an audiogram and a computed tomography (see p.149) scan, may be necessary. Surgery may be recommended if the problem persists.

Otosclerosis

Otosclerosis is abnormal bone growth of the middle ear bones or the bone surrounding the inner ear. When this abnormal bone affects the delicate middle ear bones, it eventually immobilizes them so that they do not vibrate and therefore do not transmit sound. The most common location of the abnormal bone growth is the stapes. Hearing loss occurs because the stiffened stapes can no longer vibrate and pass sound waves through the ear canal to the inner ear. Otosclerosis tends to run in families and affects more women than men.

The main symptom is hearing loss that occurs gradually in one or both ears. You may also have noises in your ear (see Tinnitus, p.459) and dizziness. Consult your doctor if you develop these symptoms; he or she may refer you to an otolaryngologist, who will perform hearing tests (see p.452). Tell the otolaryngologist if anyone in your family has had otosclerosis. If you are diagnosed with otosclerosis, a hearing aid may help.

Stapedectomy is the most common surgery for otosclerosis

and is usually successful. In this operation, most of the rigid stapes bone is replaced with an artificial piston made of wire or stainless steel; this piston conducts the vibrations that the stapes bone used to conduct. You may have some dizziness after surgery, but it usually disappears within a few days.

Although less than 1% of stapedectomies result in total loss of hearing, your doctor may recommend operating on one ear first to determine how much hearing is restored before operating on the other ear.

Ruptured Eardrum

A ruptured or perforated eardrum is a hole or tear in the membrane that separates the outer ear canal from the middle ear. Most ruptured eardrums are caused by infection of the middle ear (see p.457). An explosion or open-handed slap to the head (which produces a sudden change in pressure) or inserting a foreign object, such as a cotton-tipped swab or paper clip, in the ear are other ways of rupturing the eardrum.

Rupture can produce partial hearing loss, minor bleeding or discharge from your ear, and earache. Take a painkiller to help ease the pain and see your doctor, who will use an otoscope (a viewing instrument) to look for a torn portion of eardrum. If a rupture has occurred, your physician may prescribe antibiotics to ensure that infection will not develop. Some small tears heal on their own.

It is important to keep water out of your ear until the perforation heals completely; you should also avoid blowing your nose. Blowing your nose creates pressure in the ear that can damage the thin tissue that is growing to replace the hole in the eardrum. If the eardrum does not heal within 2 months, your doctor may recommend a minor operation called a tympanoplasty, in which tissue is used to patch the tear.

Injury to the Outer Ear

Injury to the external part of the ear can occur anytime, but especially during some sports such as wrestling or boxing. This can lead to bleeding (hematoma) or a collection of clear fluid (seroma) beneath the skin of the outer ear. If untreated, this can cause a permanent deformity that is sometimes called cauliflower ear. If an injury to the external ear has caused swelling, see your doctor. He or she may refer you to an otolaryngologist, who may perform a minor procedure to drain the fluid. This can prevent permanent deformity.

Tinnitus

Tinnitus is the sensation of hearing noises in your ears when there are no sounds present in the environment. The sounds you hear may be loud or soft and can be steady or intermittent. The noise is often described as a ringing, tinkling, roaring, whistling, hissing, or buzzing. If you have tinnitus, see your doctor, who may refer you to an otolaryngologist. Your doctor or the otolaryngologist may perform hearing tests, as well as a computed tomography (see p.149) scan or

Alternative Medicine: Tinnitus

Although it is unproven, many European doctors and a growing number of doctors in the United States use the herb ginkgo biloba, available at most drugstores or health food stores, to treat tinnitus. Any ginkgo preparations specifying 24% ginkgo or bearing the designation "standardized extract" or "German Kommission E" should be adequate. They are usually sold as 40-milligram tablets or capsules and are taken three times a day with meals.

magnetic resonance imaging (see p.150).

Causes of tinnitus include diseases of the eustachian tube or ear or underlying diseases such as allergy, high blood pressure (see p.644), heart disease (see p.652), and anemia (see p.713). Hearing loss due to an infection can also cause tinnitus, as can blockage of the ear canal with earwax (see p.451) or with a foreign object. Injury to the head or neck and some medicines such as aspirin and other nonsteroidal anti-inflammatory drugs, antibiotics, and sedatives may also cause tinnitus.

If a blockage is causing the tinnitus, removing it usually resolves the condition; treating an ear infection also usually brings a cure. If the cause is unknown, self-help measures can help you cope with the noise. Self-help measures include avoiding exposure to loud noises, ensuring your blood pressure is in normal range, decreasing salt intake, and exercising to improve your circulation.

Some people mask the noises with other sounds, such as

"white noise" tapes or steady sounds such as a ticking clock. Using a hearing aid to amplify environmental sounds can also help mask the tinnitus.

Positional Vertigo

Vertigo, the sensation of spinning or having objects spin around you, is a result of a disturbance in the part of your ear that controls balance. In positional vertigo (medically known as benign paroxysmal postural vertigo), you feel an extreme spinning sensation when you bend your head back to look up or when you are lying on your side. During such an episode, your eyes may move from side to side without your control. Positional vertigo usually lasts only about a minute, even when you maintain the position that originally caused it.

Positional vertigo may be due to atherosclerosis (see p.653), ear canal damage that occurs with advancing age, middle ear infection (see p.457), infection of the inner ear canal (see Labyrinthitis, p.456), head injury, or ear surgery. It may also be a symptom of multiple sclerosis (see p.368) or viral infection.

See your doctor if you have positional vertigo. Often, simply avoiding the body positions that bring on an attack is the only treatment required. Your doctor may recommend a physical maneuver of the head and neck, called the canalith repositioning maneuver, which can realign inner ear structures and improve dizziness. Alternatively, physical therapy to improve your balance may be recommended.

NOSE

Common Cold

Officially known as nasopharyngitis or an upper respiratory infection, the common cold affects people an average of twice a year, mostly in the winter. Colds are not acquired from exposure to drafts or cold weather. A cold is caused by one of hundreds of viruses, which are transmitted by direct contact, such as shaking hands with someone who has one or more of the viruses on his or her hands and then touching a mucous membrane (such as your eyes, mouth, or nose) with your infected hand.

You also can catch the viruses by breathing in the infected droplets of someone who has coughed or sneezed in your direction. A cold virus can survive outside the body for up to 3 hours.

People who have weakened immune systems due to chemotherapy (see p.741) or human immunodeficiency virus (HIV) (see p.872) may be more susceptible to colds. Children have one cold after another because they have not built up immunity to the viruses that cause colds. Antibiotics cannot cure a cold because they are not effective against viruses. Even antiviral medicines do not kill the viruses that cause the common cold.

SYMPTOMS

Everyone knows what the symptoms of a cold are, but you may not know why you have those symptoms. By and large, the symptoms are the body's way of countering the viral attack. Mucus is produced to trap the virus, and coughing and sneezing expel it. Symptoms usually begin 2 to 3 days after infection and include runny or stuffy nose, sneezing, dry cough, burning eyes, scratchy throat, husky voice, headache, ear and sinus discomfort, fatigue, and low-grade fever. Most people

The Nose's Role in Smell and Taste

Both odors and taste are detected by hairlike receptors in the roof of the nasal cavities. Stimulation of these receptors sends electrical signals to nerve fibers connected to the receptors. The nerve fibers pass through tiny holes in the roof of the nasal cavity to enter the olfactory bulbs. Electrical signals that convey the sense of smell travel via the olfactory nerve to the smell center in the brain.

Home Remedies for the Common Cold

There is no cure for a common cold, but some of the following remedies may help you feel better. The only way to prevent catching a cold is to stay away from people and surfaces that are infected with a cold virus. You can minimize your chance of infection by keeping your distance from a person who has a cold (because a cough or sneeze can propel infected droplets up to 10 feet) and by not kissing, touching, or sharing utensils. Wash your hands frequently.

REMEDY	EFFECTIVENESS	WHEN TO USE
Zinc tablets	Some scientific studies show that zinc tablets may shorten the duration of a cold.	Use at the earliest sign of a cold.
Hot vapor or chicken soup	Breathing in the vapors from a bowl of hot water or during a steamy shower or sipping a bowl of hot soup helps stimulate the flow of mucus, offering temporary relief from congestion.	Use to relieve a stuffy nose.
Liquids	Drinking lots of liquids (at least eight glasses a day) helps your body get rid of infected secretions.	Use throughout your cold, especially to relieve congestion.
Vitamin C	There is no scientific evidence that vitamin C helps prevent or treat the common cold.	Not recommended to relieve cold symptoms, but may have more general health value (see p.42).
Gargling	Gargling with salt water provides temporary relief of a scratchy or sore throat.	Use to relieve a sore throat.

recover completely within 5 days. For every hundred sufferers, only one or two go on to develop complications such as sinusitis (see p.464) or ear infection.

TREATMENT OPTIONS

There is no cure for a cold, but acetaminophen or aspirin (people under 20 years old should not take aspirin because of the risk of Reye syndrome; see p.1017) can help relieve headache and a general achy feeling. Take it easy and get enough rest when you have a cold. The decongestant medicine pseudoephedrine, an ingredient in several cold remedies, helps shrink blood vessels and open clogged passages in the upper respiratory tract, making it easier to breathe.

Decongestant medicines may also help reduce the small risk of developing ear or sinus infection, although they can produce side effects such as a racing heart and insomnia.

Nonprescription nasal sprays of various decongestant medicines may also be helpful, although you should not use them for more than 5 days since prolonged use can make the symptoms worse. A prescription medicine called ipratropium, available in a nasal spray, can also improve symptoms.

Check with your doctor before taking any of these drugs, especially if you are taking any other medicines or have high blood pressure, glaucoma, urinary problems, diabetes, cardiovascular disease, or hyperthyroidism.

Practical measures to prevent transmitting your cold to family members and coworkers include washing your hands frequently, covering your mouth with a tissue when coughing or sneezing (and then disposing of the tissue immediately after use), avoiding touching your eyes, and being vigilant about keeping surfaces in the kitchen and bathroom clean.

Deviated Septum

The nasal septum is a wall of tissue between the two sides of your nose. Frequently, it deviates significantly to one side or the other, narrowing or blocking the nostril on one side. The cause is usually unknown, although sometimes it follows injury to the nose. Chronic cocaine use can also damage the nasal septum, sometimes opening a hole through it.

In most cases, a deviated septum poses no serious medical problem. However, some people experience difficulty breathing, a blocked or stuffy nostril, frequent nosebleeds (see p.1198), headaches, or sinus infections. Your doctor may refer you to an otolaryngologist, who will examine your nasal cavities. If the deviation is causing problems, surgery to realign your septum may be recommended.

Allergic Rhinitis (Hay Fever)

Allergic rhinitis is nasal allergy to many substances, the most common being pollens, molds, dust, or animal dander. More than 35 million Americans have allergic rhinitis. Like any allergy, it is triggered by exposure to a substance called an allergen. Some people are born with a tendency to react very strongly to allergens.

The tissues of the nose, throat, and eyes of all people contain white blood cells that make immunoglobulin E (IgE) antibodies. In allergic people, IgE antibodies cause another group of white blood cells (the mast cells) to produce substances, including histamine, that produce inflammation and excessive mucus.

When allergic rhinitis is triggered by particular pollens in a particular season, it is called hay fever. People who are sensitive only to pollens find that their reactions are seasonal. Tree pollens are most common in spring, grass pollens in summer, and weed pollens in summer and early fall.

Many people have allergic rhinitis all year. These people may be affected by indoor allergens, such as dust (which contains microscopic insects called mites that produce irritating substances, especially in warm, humid air), molds, or hair and skin cells. The hair and skin cells (or the saliva on the hair and skin cells), better known as dander, is shed by animals.

However, in most people who have allergic rhinitis throughout the year, no clear allergen can be found. The allergens that cause allergic rhinitis almost always come from the air. Only rarely do food allergies cause allergic rhinitis. Allergic rhinitis tends to become less intense as people reach age 50.

SYMPTOMS

Symptoms include a stuffy and runny nose; eyes that become red, itchy, watery, and may produce mucus; frequent sneezing; and irritated throat and skin.

TREATMENT OPTIONS

See your doctor if you find your symptoms difficult to live with. He or she will discuss your symptoms, and ask about any prescription medicine you take (beta blockers, oral contraceptives, and thyroid hormones can cause nasal symptoms) as well as hobbies or work that may expose you to allergens. Your doctor will examine your nose for polyps (see p.464) or inflammation of the sinuses (see Sinusitis, p.464).

If allergy is suspected, skin testing (either the scratch test or an injection of the possible allergen just under the surface of the skin) may confirm it. Blood tests for IgE antibodies to particular allergens also may be helpful in diagnosing your allergy.

There are many nonprescription medicines for allergic rhinitis. Decongestant pills with the medicine pseudoephedrine can also be useful, but you should check with your doctor before taking pseudoephedrine if you have high blood pressure, diabetes, coronary artery disease, narrow angle glaucoma, or difficulty urinating.

Nonprescription antihistamines such as chlorpheniramine or diphenhydramine are inexpensive and very effective, although, in some people, they can cause drowsiness, blurred vision, difficulty urinating, or other side effects. For most people below the age of 50, however, they are worth trying.

If they produce unacceptable side effects, your doctor may prescribe much more expensive (but no more powerful) nonsedating antihistamines, including cetirizine, loratadine, and fexofenadine. These medicines are less likely to produce drowsiness. Your doctor may prescribe a sedating antihistamine such as chlorpheniramine or diphenhydramine at bedtime and a nonsedating type in the morning.

Two older nonsedating antihistamines, terfenadine and astemizole, can cause potentially fatal heart-rhythm abnormalities

Preventing Nasal Allergies

You can prevent nasal allergies if you can avoid allergens—the substances to which you are allergic. This is easier said than done, but here are some tips that can help:

A common indoor allergy is to dust mites—microscopic insects that live in most homes. To reduce your exposure to dust-mite allergens:

- Minimize the amount of carpeting and rugs in your home, and have someone other than the allergy sufferer vacuum frequently. A vacuum with a special allergen filter is best.

- Do not use rugs on cement floors; they are particularly likely to become infested with mites.

- Have someone (not the allergy sufferer) change bed sheets and blankets weekly and wash them in water that is hotter than 100°F.

- Replace feather pillows with synthetic polyester pillows.

- Cover mattresses with plastic casings.

- Use air conditioners and dehumidifiers frequently; dust mites thrive in warm humid air.

Another common cause of allergies is animal dander, saliva, and urine. Take these steps:

- Get a pet that sheds less dander.

- Keep your pet outdoors as much as possible.

- Wash your hands every time you touch your pet.

- Have someone (not the allergy sufferer) wash your dog every week. But be sure to ask your veterinarian if weekly washing is bad for your dog's skin, and always carefully dry the dog.

- Have someone (not the allergy sufferer) wash your cat every week with a special preparation that neutralizes the cat's saliva on its fur. This can be difficult, since most cats hate being washed. Starting to bathe the cat while it is still a kitten sometimes makes it easier.

Molds are common indoor allergens. Like dust mites, they thrive in warm, moist air. To reduce your exposure to indoor molds:

- Use dehumidifiers and air conditioners when the air is warm and humid.

- Minimize your exposure to those parts of a house that attract molds; old paper products such as old books, newspapers, or magazines; humidifiers; houseplants; and fish tanks.

- Have someone (not the allergy sufferer) dust and clean (especially the above items) frequently.

Molds and pollens are also common outdoor allergens, particularly between early spring and the middle of autumn. To reduce your exposure to outdoor molds and pollens:

- Minimize activities such as lawn mowing or leaf raking.

- Avoid being outdoors on a day when the mold or pollen count is high.

- Close the windows on days when the mold or pollen count is high (and run an air conditioner on hot days).

---

in people who have severe liver disease or who take certain antibiotics or antifungal drugs. Other potentially dangerous side effects include asthmalike symptoms such as tightness in the chest and wheezing.

Your doctor may also recommend various nonprescription nasal sprays. Decongestant nasal sprays can offer relief for several days, but continuing to use them beyond 4 to 5 days can lead to a rebound—an increase in symptoms. Other nasal sprays include cromolyn sodium, which blocks the release of an irritating substance called histamine from mast cells, and ipratropium, which blocks a natural substance called acetylcholine that is important in the production of mucus. Finally, your doctor may prescribe a nasal spray that contains low doses of corticosteroid drugs (see p.895). This spray can avert an allergy attack but takes a week or more to reach maximum effectiveness.

If prescription-strength antihistamines, nasal sprays, and environmental controls (see Preventing Nasal Allergies, p.463) do not work, or the medicines cause troublesome side effects, you may want to consider immunotherapy (allergy injections). For immunotherapy to work, your doctor must be able to identify the allergen causing your symptoms. At first, small amounts of the allergen are injected under your skin. Then increasingly higher doses are injected at roughly weekly intervals; treatment may need to be continued for several years.

The allergens for which immunotherapy has been shown to work best are ragweed, grass, dust mites, and cat dander. Symptoms usually subside within 6 months to a year; doctors recommend the treatments be continued for 4 or 5 years. However, immunotherapy does not always help.

Nasal Polyps

Nasal polyps are benign (noncancerous) tumors that grow, often on a stalk, from the lining of the nose or sinuses. Most polyps are not a threat to health, but they can obstruct the flow of air in one or both nostrils. They also can block the sinus openings and interfere with the drainage of sinus secretions, leading to infection.

Polyps may occur more often in people who have allergies (see Allergic Rhinitis, p.462) or recurring nasal infections, although they can occur for no apparent reason.

Nasal polyps are almost always present in both right and left nasal cavities. If the blockage is only on one side, you should see an otolaryngologist to be sure you do not have another type of growth

that can cause blockage. Some of the other growths are of little concern, but cancer is always a possibility. For example, a growth that looks like a polyp called an inverted papilloma can grow and destroy bone; it can also turn into cancer of the sinuses.

SYMPTOMS

Polyps may grow large enough to block the nostril, causing a stuffed feeling and loss of smell. Polyps bleed easily. A polyp that is blocking a sinus that has become infected can cause pressure or pain in your face.

TREATMENT OPTIONS

See your doctor, who may refer you to an otolaryngologist. He or she will examine the inside of your nose to check for polyps. A computed tomography (see p.149) scan may be used to assess the size and location of the polyps. Some doctors try to shrink polyps with sprays containing corticosteroid drugs (see p.895) and, if necessary, corticosteroid pills.

If this does not work, polyps that are inhibiting your ability to breathe properly may need to be surgically removed. Often, this requires simply snipping them off with scissors; sometimes a stitch is needed to stop bleeding. An endoscope (see p.142) may be used to remove polyps farther back in the nose. However, polyps have a tendency to recur, so you may need repeated treatments.

Postnasal Drip

Postnasal drip is an accumulation of mucus that moves down the back of the nose into the throat. Your body makes mucus every

day as part of its effort to trap dust and other foreign particles. In postnasal drip, your body produces thick mucus, often as a result of allergic rhinitis (see p.462).

Increased mucous production can also be caused by cold temperatures and very dry environments, some foods and spices, pregnancy, nasal inflammation not caused by allergy, and a variety of drugs (including birth-control pills and high blood pressure medicines).

Symptoms can include stuffy nose, coughing up phlegm, and a persistent sore throat. Postnasal drip can cause hoarseness and the feeling that you have something in your throat.

Treatment depends on the cause. When no cause can be found, your doctor may suggest measures aimed at thinning the secretions so that they pass more easily, such as increasing your intake of fluids (especially for older people). Avoid caffeine and diuretics (fluid-eliminating drugs), which thicken the secretions, if they are not necessary for medical reasons.

Nasal sprays containing corticosteroids (see p.895) or ipratropium may also be helpful. Nasal saline spray and mucus-thinning agents may also be recommended.

Sinusitis

Sinusitis means inflammation of the sinuses, the air-filled spaces above, behind, and below the eyes. These normally sterile cavities are lined with a thin membrane that produces mucus. Hair cells sweep the mucus along to flush out foreign particles and

Location of Sinuses

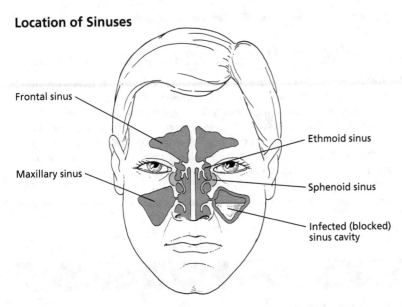

Frontal sinus

Maxillary sinus

Ethmoid sinus

Sphenoid sinus

Infected (blocked) sinus cavity

There are four pairs of sinuses (the air-filled spaces above, behind, and below the eyes). Maxillary sinuses are located beneath your cheeks, to the sides of your nose. Frontal sinuses are located in the bone just above your eyes. Ethmoid and sphenoid sinuses lie deeper in the skull than the other sinuses.

Home Remedies for Sinusitis

To prevent an allergy or cold from progressing to chronic sinusitis and to keep your nasal passageways clear, follow these home-remedy guidelines:

- Blow your nose gently to keep passages clear.

- Drink lots of fluids (at least eight 8-ounce glasses a day) to keep mucus thin and flowing.

- Avoid flying when congested. Changes in air pressure can force mucus into the sinuses. If you must fly, use a decongestant beforehand and use a decongestant nasal spray about 30 minutes before the plane begins its descent.

- Avoid scuba diving until your sinusitis is completely cleared.

- Apply warm facial packs or inhale steam (take a hot shower; have a hot bowl of soup; or inhale the steam from a pan of hot water, using a towel to form a tent over the steam source).

Sinusitis can be a complication of a seasonal allergy. Lower your risk of sinus infection by determining what causes your allergy and doing what you can to avoid it.

organisms, such as bacteria, viruses, and dust. The mucus normally drains through small openings from the sinuses into the nose. Sinusitis starts when this normal system of drainage is blocked.

An infection or allergies cause the normally thin sinus membranes to swell. They can block the openings from the sinuses into the nose, causing pressure, discomfort, and a feeling of congestion in the head. The sinuses can also develop a bacterial infection; mucus builds up in the sinus and becomes a breeding ground for bacteria.

SYMPTOMS

Chronic allergic sinusitis or temporary sinus blockage from a virus infection can cause stuffiness, postnasal drip (see p.464), headaches, and a dazed feeling. Bacterial sinusitis usually causes fever, green discharge from the nose, pain and a red flush over the infected sinus, and aching in the teeth just below the sinus. In extreme cases, bacterial sinusitis can also cause high fevers, shaking chills, and weakness so intense the person is bedridden.

TREATMENT OPTIONS

Your doctor will examine your mouth, throat, and nasal passages. For sinusitis that does not involve a bacterial infection, he or she may prescribe decongestant pills or nasal sprays to shrink swollen mucous membranes and allow drainage, or antihistamine pills or nasal corticosteroid (see p.895) sprays to reduce inflammation. If there appears to be a bacterial infection, an antibiotic will be prescribed.

When sinus infections recur

despite treatment, surgery to enlarge the narrowed sinus openings may bring relief. A computed tomography (see p.149) scan of your sinuses can show whether, after treatment, you still have sinus obstruction. The surgery is done with tiny endoscopes (see p.142) that are placed through the nostrils and into the sinus passages. There are no incisions on the skin of the face. The surgery widens the sinus openings to improve sinus drainage.

Nosebleeds and Dry Nasal Passages

Nosebleeds often occur during winter, when indoor air is overly dry due to heating. The dry air causes the membranes of the nose to become dry and cracked and bleed more easily. To prevent nosebleeds caused by dry air, use a humidifier. If your nose seems particularly dry, before bedtime place a small drop (the size of a pea) of petroleum jelly in the front of each nostril and let it melt back up into your nose. You can also use a nonprescription nasal saline spray throughout the day to keep your nasal passages moist and free from bleeding. To stop a nosebleed, see p.1198.

THROAT

Tumors of the Vocal Cords

A tumor of the vocal cords—small, muscular structures in the larynx—may be benign (unlikely to spread) or malignant (cancerous). Cancerous tumors occur much more often in people who smoke or drink. Benign tumors are generally either polyps, which are usually caused by overusing the voice, or papillomas, which are growths caused by a virus. Men 60 and older are ten times more likely to develop tumors of the vocal cords than are women.

SYMPTOMS

All vocal cord tumors can cause hoarseness. If they are large enough, vocal cord tumors can cause breathing difficulties as well. A growing cancerous tumor of the vocal cords can cause progressive hoarseness, swallowing difficulties, and a lump in the neck. If you have hoarseness that lasts for more than 4 weeks, see your doctor.

TREATMENT OPTIONS

Your doctor will examine you and may refer you to an otolaryngologist. He or she will examine the outside of your neck and your throat and larynx. If a growth is discovered, a biopsy of the growth (tissue removed for examination under a microscope) will be performed to discover whether the tumor is benign or malignant. Polyps and papillomas can be removed by surgery performed under general anesthesia (see p.168).

A cancerous growth has a better chance of being cured if detected early. Depending on the stage of the cancer, chemotherapy (see p.741), radiation therapy (see p.741), and surgery—separately or in combination—may be recommended. If only a part of the larynx is removed, you will retain part of your ability to speak.

In more advanced cases, the entire larynx may be removed to prevent cancerous cells from spreading to other parts of your body. If the entire larynx is removed, your vocal cords will

also be removed and a hole will be created in your neck for you to breathe through (your windpipe will stop at the hole in your neck).

In order for you to speak, your doctor may recommend surgery to place a small valve into another hole that is made between your trachea (windpipe) and esophagus (the tube through which food passes down on its way to the stomach). When you want to speak, you plug the hole in your neck, which opens the valve and sends air into and up your esophagus. The vibrations from air moving up your esophagus create sound, and that sound can be shaped by your mouth to create speech. Your voice will not be the same as it was before the operation, but the speech is comprehensible.

Laryngitis

Laryngitis is inflammation of the larynx (voice box), often due to irritation or infection. It causes either a hoarse voice or makes you lose your voice. Normal speech occurs when you force air up from the lungs through the vocal cords, the small muscular structures in the larynx. The force of air causes the vocal cords to vibrate, making a sound. You can control and shape this sound by both the tension you put on the vocal cords and by shaping the sound with your tongue, mouth, and lips.

In laryngitis, the membrane covering the vocal cords in the larynx is inflamed and swollen; it vibrates less easily and therefore produces less sound.

Irritation of the larynx can be caused by the common cold (see p.460), regurgitated stomach acid (see gastroesophageal reflux, p.747), bronchitis (see p.494), influenza (see p.875), or pneumonia (see p.496). Other causes include shouting, talking too much, breathing polluted air or chemicals, or excessive drinking or smoking. Viral laryngitis usually clears up on its own within 1 to 3 weeks.

Regardless of the cause, you should rest your voice, inhale steam, and drink warm liquids to soothe any irritation. If your laryngitis is due to drinking, smoking, excess stomach acid, or improper use of your voice, eliminate the offending substance or activity. A voice coach can help you prevent laryngitis that stems from speaking incorrectly.

Common Sore Throat and Strep Throat

Irritation and soreness of the throat (also called pharyngitis) occurs when your throat is infected. Viruses probably cause most sore throats, although bac-

teria also infect the throat. The best known bacterial infection— strep throat—is caused by streptococcus bacteria. However, in recent years it has been learned that other bacteria are actually more common causes of sore throat. Canker sores, postnasal drip, inhaling irritants (such as tobacco smoke), and breathing extremely dry air can also cause sore throat.

Most sore throats are caused by mild, temporary infections, but occasionally infection is severe or threatening.

SYMPTOMS

Sore throat often starts as a slight tickling sensation in the throat and rapidly progresses to painful irritation, often with other symptoms. Most sore throats get better without treatment. Call your doctor if you have a severe sore throat that lasts longer than a week; if you have difficulty breathing, swallowing, or opening your mouth; if you have joint pains, earache, rash, and fever over 101°F; or if you have a sore throat and have recently been exposed to someone with strep throat.

TREATMENT OPTIONS

After examining your throat, your doctor may take a throat culture (see p.159), which can detect most but not all kinds of bacteria. If you have a persistent sore throat, your doctor may want to take special cultures.

Alternately, your doctor may perform a "rapid strep" test. This is useful if it is positive, because the doctor can tell right away if you have a strep infection and you can start treatment promptly (results of a rapid strep test are

available in about 5 to 15 minutes).

However, if the test is negative, it could mean that you have some other bacterial infection besides strep. Your doctor may prescribe antibiotics even if the throat culture comes back negative for bacteria, based on an assessment of your overall condition and symptoms.

It is important to treat strep throat not only to relieve pain but because untreated strep throat can lead to nephritis (see p.1015) or rheumatic fever (see p.697). Although these complications are far less common than they were 50 years ago, they still occur. If your doctor prescribes antibiotics, it is essential that you take the full course, even if you feel better. Stopping the medicine early gives the bacteria an opportunity to regroup and can allow serious complications to develop.

There is no cure for sore throats due to viral infection. However, unless you have mononucleosis (in which case your sore throat may last much longer), sore throats usually clear up without treatment within 1 to 2 weeks.

Home treatments to ease discomfort include inhaling steam, using throat lozenges, gargling with salt water, and taking aspirin (do not take aspirin if you are under 20 because of the risk of Reye syndrome) or acetaminophen for pain.

Tonsillitis, Peritonsillar Abscess, and Epiglottitis

Tonsillitis is inflammation of the tonsils, the two mounds of immune system (lymph) tissue located where the back of the mouth meets the throat. Tonsilli-

Breathing and Swallowing

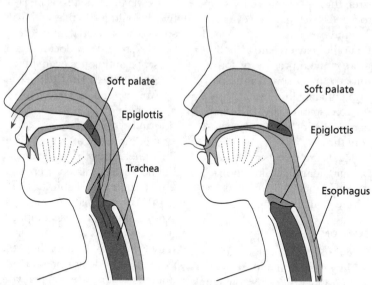

When you breathe (left), your soft palate and epiglottis move so that your trachea is open. When you swallow food or liquids (right), the soft palate moves to prevent backflow up your nose and the epiglottis folds down to close the opening to the larynx and trachea—to keep you from breathing in food and liquids, which are directed down the esophagus to the stomach.

tis is a common cause of sore throat and can cause flulike symptoms such as sudden fever and chills, headache, an achy feeling, and swollen glands. Your tonsils will be red and enlarged and, often, covered with a yel-lowish creamy substance or with white patches of debris. A throat culture should be taken any time there is a substance on your tonsils; infection with streptococcus or another bacterium is likely.

A more severe form of tonsilli-tis is peritonsillar abscess. In this condition, the infection spreads deep underneath your tonsils into the surrounding tissue, and a pocket of pus (an abscess) forms. Your throat will be very sore, and it may hurt to swallow saliva. With peritonsillar abscess, you have difficulty opening your mouth and your speech changes (you sound like you are speaking with a mouth full of hot pota-toes). See your doctor if you have these symptoms; in addition to antibiotic treatment, you may need a minor surgical procedure to have the pus drained.

An even more severe form of sore throat is epiglottitis. In this rare condition, the epiglottis, the flap that covers the windpipe, becomes infected. It enlarges and can block the windpipe, leading to sudden asphyxiation and death.

Epiglottitis can reach a serious stage in a matter of hours. If you suddenly have a severe sore throat, fever, difficulty breathing when lying down, or noisy breathing, see your doctor imme-diately. You need immediate treatment with antibiotics and may need to remain in the hospi-tal until the condition is cured.

Teeth, Mouth, and Gums

TEETH

Your teeth are living tissues infused with a pulp containing blood and nerves. There are normally 32 permanent teeth in the adult mouth. Children have 20 primary, or "baby," teeth (see p.965) that precede the permanent teeth.

The crown is the part of the tooth that shows above the gums; it is covered with enamel, the hardest material in the body. The shades of enamel vary widely from person to person, determined partly by genetics, diet, and other activities such as smoking. Even given its strength, enamel is vulnerable to the acids produced by dental plaque (see Preventing Tooth Decay and Plaque, p.470), which contributes to tooth decay and periodontitis (see Gingivitis and Periodontitis, p.474).

Dentin makes up most of the tooth. Though harder than bone, dentin is a sensitive tissue that is subject to piercing pain if its protective covering of enamel is broken. The tooth's root is embedded in bone and covered with cementum, a softer material that protects it. Teeth have one to three roots. At the core of a tooth is the pulp, the living root tissue that consists of blood and lymph vessels (which provide nourishment and disease protection), nerves, and connective tissue.

MOUTH

The mouth is the point of entry for food, where it is first tasted and digested. It is also where we voice our thoughts and sentiments. The mouth includes the tongue, lips, and palate at the roof of the mouth—along with the teeth and gums. It is lined with delicate tissue that is kept moist by saliva.

The lips consist of skin on the outside, muscles in the middle, and mucous membrane on the inside. The muscles of the lips help shape the mouth for purposes as disparate as swallowing food, giving a speech, and kissing a baby. Lips can become dry and chapped and are subject to blisters (see p.487) from herpesvirus and other infections.

The tongue is made up of a special group of muscles that give it the flexibility to change size, position, and shape. The tongue's muscles manipulate food of dif-

Your Mouth

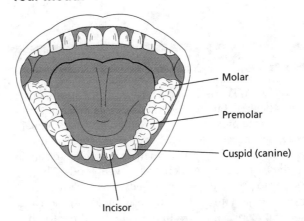

- Molar
- Premolar
- Cuspid (canine)
- Incisor

The mouth consists of the teeth, gums, soft tissues, and tongue. Molars and premolars grind food, incisors have a sharp edge for cutting, and the cuspids (canines) tear food. The health of your teeth is closely linked to the health of your gums, which should be pink, firm, and wrapped closely around the bottom of the teeth (the root). A healthy tongue is pink and smooth.

Cross Section of Tooth

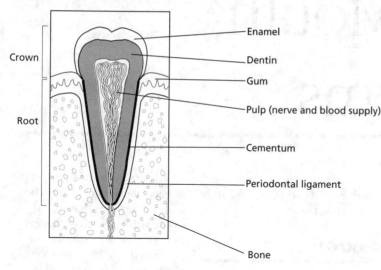

Teeth are composed mainly of two parts: the crown and the root. The pulp is the living core of the tooth, and is encased in the hard substance dentin. The root is covered by cementum, which attaches to the periodontal ligament. Above the gum line, pulp (the living core of the tooth) is protected by dentin and by the outermost tooth surface, enamel.

ferent sizes and textures, and shape an extensive variety of sounds. The top of the tongue can identify an estimated 10,000 different flavors through taste buds that surround tiny protuberances called papillae. A healthy tongue is pink and textured.

The inside of the mouth is kept moist by saliva, which is pro-duced by three sets of salivary glands: the parotid, sublingual, and submandibular glands. Saliva also lubricates food for digestion and contains a digestive enzyme called amylase, which helps break down food and digest carbohydrates. It is also helpful in preventing tooth decay, since undigested carbohydrates on the teeth lead to the formation of plaque (see Preventing Tooth Decay and Plaque, below).

GUMS

Teeth are surrounded by the gums (gingivae), the visible pink tissue that covers the bone. The gums are attached directly to the teeth, and above this attachment at the gum line is a small sulcus, or moat. This area is vulnerable to infection, usually by bacteria that collect on plaque that is not brushed and flossed out of the gum line. Gum disease (see Gingivitis and Periodontitis, p.474) is the leading cause of tooth loss in adults.

PREVENTING TOOTH DECAY AND PLAQUE

Your dentist can do a lot to keep your teeth and gums healthy, but the person who can do the most is you. Tooth decay, also called dental caries or cavities, occurs when bacteria on the tooth surface metabolize sugar to produce acid. The primary cause of tooth decay is plaque, a coating of saliva on teeth that harbors bacteria. The bacteria produce acid that eats away at the minerals in enamel, creating tiny pitted areas on the surface of the tooth. Over time, the bacteria create an acid that causes decay of the enamel. As the cavity nears the tooth's pulp, there is increased sensitivity to cold and sweet foods. The cavity can expose the pulp to bacteria, leading to infection and death of the tissue. If the tooth dies, root canal surgery (see p.484) may be needed. A buildup of plaque is also responsible for gingivitis and periodontitis (see p.474), also called gum disease. The good news is that you can remove plaque through regular brushing and flossing.

Brushing, Flossing, and Rinsing

To prevent the formation of dental plaque, brush your teeth with a soft-bristle brush at least twice a day, in the morning and before bed. If possible, also brush after

Abnormal Tooth Development

Teeth can develop abnormally due to a number of factors, including heredity and general health. This chart provides a brief description of various problems and recommended courses of action.

ABNORMALITY	DESCRIPTION	RECOMMENDED ACTION
Delayed eruption	Teeth that do not appear after expected date of eruption (see p.965).	Ask dentist's advice. You may need to have dental x-rays to evaluate status of the teeth.
Abnormal enamel	Developmental defects in enamel. Caused by poor nutrition, nondental diseases, or an inherited disease called amelogenesis imperfecta, which causes thin tooth enamel, pitted and discolored teeth, and a higher susceptibility to cavities.	Cosmetic options (see p.486) and restorations can help improve the appearance of the teeth, especially the permanent teeth.
Abnormally spaced teeth	Cosmetically troubling gaps between teeth. Caused by premature loss of baby teeth before permanent teeth have erupted, or by small teeth or loss of teeth at any age.	Consult your dentist who, depending on the severity of the problem, may suggest one of the following options: orthodontics (see p.479), crowns (see p.482), bridges (see p.482), or dental implants (see p.483).
Nursing bottle caries	Tooth decay (cavities) in infants and young children. Caused by sleeping with a bottle of milk or juice, or by prolonged nursing.	Filling cavities and removing teeth may be necessary. Prevent by not allowing prolonged nursing or children to sleep with bottles.
Fluorosis	Discoloration of tooth enamel. Caused by taking in too much fluoride during tooth formation (usually from drinking overly fluoridated water).	Prevent by having the fluoride level of your water checked. Cosmetic options, such as bleaching (see p.486), can help mask the discoloration.
Abnormally shaped teeth	Caused by heredity or injury.	Treatment depends on the severity of the problem. Options include crowns (see p.482) and smoothing edges.

every meal or snack. Replace your toothbrush every 3 to 4 months. Your toothpaste should contain fluoride, a mineral that helps prevent cavities. Toothpastes that contain ingredients that control calculus (the hard material—also known as tartar—that forms when plaque is not removed by brushing and flossing) may be helpful for people who tend to form heavy calculus deposits. However, these toothpastes can also irritate your gums, so it is best to ask your dentist what he or she recommends.

The mechanical act of brushing your teeth does most of the cleaning work. When done properly, brushing also stimulates your gums, which helps prevent gingivitis and periodontitis (see p.474). Water jets (which are helpful for removing debris, but not plaque) and rubber-tipped probes may help you more thoroughly clean your teeth and mouth and stimulate your gums. However, they are not necessary.

To clean the outer surfaces of your teeth, gently press a soft-bristle brush at a 45-degree angle where your gums meet your teeth until the bristles flare. Gently move the brush up and down using short strokes. Keep the bristles angled against the gum line. Brush the surface of every tooth, including hard-to-reach back teeth in your upper and lower jaw.

To clean the inner surfaces of your front teeth, hold the brush vertically and use gentle up-and-down strokes. Excessive scrubbing, especially with a hard brush or in a horizontal position, can damage delicate gums. Brush for at least 3 minutes. Finish by brushing your tongue and rinsing with water.

Flossing is as essential as brushing; you should floss at least once a day, but ideally after every meal. Devices that aid in the use of dental floss can help people who have difficulty managing dental floss. The action of flossing removes particles of debris from between teeth and the edge of the gums, reducing the amount of plaque in your mouth. Flossing is especially important in preventing gum disease (see Gingivitis and Periodontitis, p.474), the major cause of tooth loss and cavities between teeth.

Flossing technique is more important than the type of floss you use. Guide the floss between your teeth, using a gentle motion to run the floss up and down both sides of the tooth edges; never snap floss into your gums. When the floss reaches your gum line, curve it into a C shape against one tooth and gently rub with an up-and-down motion. Flossing is a learned skill. If you are just starting to floss, have patience; it will get easier.

Mouthwashes serve several purposes. Fluoride mouth rinses may help prevent decay; antiseptic mouthwashes may temporarily kill some odor-causing bacteria.

Sealants and Fluoride

Sealants are one of the best ways to prevent tooth decay in children. Tooth decay usually starts in the pits and fissures of the tops and sides of the back chewing teeth called molars. Your dentist can apply a plastic coating called a sealant to these surfaces; it forms a physical barrier that prevents food and bacteria from lodging in tiny imperfections in the tooth enamel.

Fluoride is another useful means of preventing decay. It occurs naturally in the water supply in some communities and is added to the water supply in others. Children benefit greatly from fluoride-containing water because the fluoride is taken up by developing teeth and incorporated into the teeth themselves.

If your child is not drinking fluoride-enriched water, he or she should take fluoride drops or tablets after 6 months of age; ask your dentist to recommend a fluoride product.

Your dentist or hygienist also can paint fluoride directly on the teeth at 6-month intervals. These topical fluoride treatments may also be recommended for adults who have dry mouths due to disease, medicine, or radiation treatment.

Diet and Lifestyle

Your diet has a significant influence on your overall health and the health of your teeth and gums. The digestive process, which starts in your mouth, forms an acid that can dissolve tooth enamel, especially after eating carbohydrates (which include sweets and starchy foods). The best course of action is to remove the acid by brushing after every snack or meal.

In addition to the significant overall health risks, smoking or chewing tobacco also can cause stained teeth, periodontitis, and oral cancers. Teeth stained by tobacco can promote bacterial growth and, thus, tooth decay. Quitting is the best medicine.

Some dental injuries (see p.485) can be prevented by lifestyle changes. Playing some sports can increase the risk of mouth injury. Make sure mouth guards are worn as a part of standard athletic equipment.

Dental Checkups

A dental examination permits your dentist to evaluate all parts of your mouth, including the lips, gums, tongue, teeth, and the bones that support your teeth. Schedule a dental examination twice a year so that your dentist can check your teeth for decay and the buildup of plaque, and your gums for overall health. He or she will also look for other diseases of the mouth. Children should have their first complete dental checkup no later than age 3 (see p.966).

If you are seeing the dentist for the first time, you will be asked to complete a form about

What X-Rays Can Reveal

X-rays can show decay, bone destruction, and other problems in their early, more treatable, stages. Most dentists take a complete set of mouth x-rays during the first appointment. The frequency of subsequent x-rays depends on the health of your teeth. If you have good oral health, you need a complete set of x-rays only every 5 to 10 years; bitewing x-rays are recommended every 2 to 4 years. People with gum disease and those who have had root-canal treatment may need x-rays more frequently to monitor treatment or the progress of disease. Mouth injuries and major dental procedures such as crowns, bridges, or dental implants may require additional x-rays to provide clear views of the surgical site.

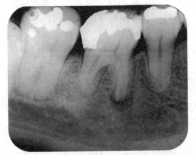 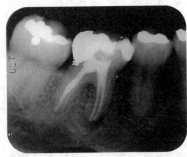 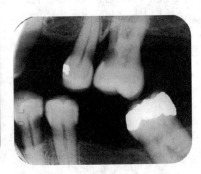

The two periapical x-rays above reveal detailed images of teeth, gums, and bones.

Bitewing x-rays show the crowns of teeth.

Panoramic x-rays depict the entire mouthful of teeth and supporting structures.

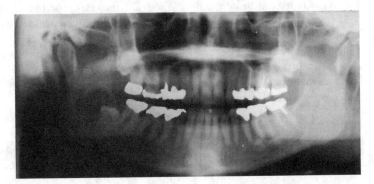

Safety of Dental X-Rays: Dr Sonis's Advice

My patients often express concerns about the safety of having dental x-rays. When I was a kid, dental x-ray machines did expose the body to more radiation than was necessary. Modern dental x-ray machines and film minimize your exposure in two ways. First, they focus the radiation just on the teeth, and virtually eliminate any scatter of x-rays to other parts of your body. Second, dentists now use "fast film" that requires much less radiation to get a good picture. When dental x-rays are taken of children, the dentist should use a lead collar to protect the thyroid gland in the neck and a lead apron to protect the rest of the body. With modern equipment, there should be no risk to a pregnant woman or her fetus from dental x-rays. Nevertheless, I like to avoid x-raying pregnant women, unless a dental emergency requires it. Although many dentists still put lead aprons on adults during dental x-rays, this may not be needed.

STEPHEN T. SONIS, DMSc
BRIGHAM AND WOMEN'S HOSPITAL
HARVARD MEDICAL SCHOOL

your medical history. Some medical conditions require a change in dental procedures. It is especially important to tell your dentist if you have any allergies, especially to antibiotics. If you have heart disease or heart valve problems (see p.689), you may need to take antibiotics before several types of dental procedure (see p.481). Your dentist may also ask if you have any other chronic diseases because they can affect the bacterial content of the saliva as well as the general health of the gums and other soft tissues in your mouth.

The dentist will examine your face and lymph nodes for any swelling, which is a sign of infection and can indicate a dental abscess (see p.477). He or she may also examine your temporomandibular joint, which connects your jaws and contributes to the way your teeth come together when you bite, for any sign of temporo-

mandibular joint dysfunction (see p.476).

Using a mirror, the dentist will examine your tongue and the other soft tissues that line your mouth, looking for sores or other abnormalities. A sharp, pointed instrument called an explorer helps your dentist probe each tooth for minute cavities and examine the condition and location of fillings and crowns. If you wear a denture, your dentist will ensure that it fits correctly.

An instrument called a periodontal probe is used to measure the depth of any gaps between your gums and teeth, which can signal gum disease (see Gingivitis and Periodontitis, below). Gums that are red, swollen, and/or bleed easily may indicate gingivitis or more advanced periodontitis. Your oral hygiene is reflected in the amount of plaque and calculus that accumulates on your teeth. Periodic x-rays (see p.473) of your teeth and support-

ing ligaments can reveal hidden areas of decay, periodontitis, impacted teeth, cysts, abscesses, tumors, and bone diseases. Based on the examination, your dentist may recommend further dental work or changes in your oral hygiene routine.

Regular professional cleaning is vital to maintaining healthy teeth and gums. Your dentist or a dental hygienist will recommend a cleaning schedule for you (usually once or twice a year). A primary objective of cleaning is to remove plaque, the soft material that collects along the edge of your teeth near the gums, and calculus (also called tartar), the hard material that forms when plaque is not removed by brushing and flossing. Calculus is scraped away with an instrument called a scaler, and your teeth are then polished using a mild abrasive tooth cleanser and a rotating polishing device. Finally, the dentist or hygienist will floss your teeth.

COMMON DENTAL PROBLEMS

Gingivitis and Periodontitis

Gingivitis means inflammation of the gums; it is a precursor to periodontitis, which is commonly called gum disease. Periodontitis is inflammation of the gums and destruction of the bone and ligaments that support your teeth.

Gum disease is the most common reason for loss of teeth in adulthood. The term "periodontal" is derived from Greek words that mean "around the tooth." It refers to the structures that support the teeth, including the bony

socket and the collagen-filled substance called periodontal ligament that connects the roots of the teeth to the bone.

The primary cause of gingivitis and periodontitis is dental plaque, which is composed of bacteria and other organisms. The organisms secrete toxins that progressively damage the ligament. As a result, the gums become inflamed and pull away from the teeth, creating a pocket that traps more plaque. Over time, the toxins can damage the gums, the outer layer of the roots of the teeth, and, finally, the bone.

The progression of periodontitis depends not only on which organisms are present, but also on the response of your immune system to them. Prevention, which involves regular brushing, flossing, and professional cleaning to minimize bacterial buildup on the surfaces of the teeth, is the best approach to these diseases.

SYMPTOMS

The early stages of gingivitis may cause no symptoms or only subtle changes in the appearance of your gums. However, the symptoms of advanced gingivitis are

Gingivitis and Periodontitis

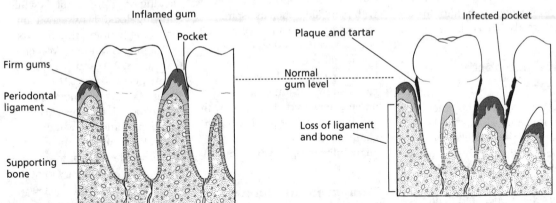

Healthy gums (far left) are firm, pink, and tight against the teeth. When gingivitis (above) develops, the gums become inflamed and red and a pocket starts to form. In periodon-titis (right), supporting bone and ligaments break down and pull away from teeth, creating pockets where debris accumulates and infection begins.

obvious—swollen, shiny, painful, bleeding gums, and unpleasant breath. Gingivitis can be triggered by changing hormone levels (due to pregnancy, puberty, menstrual cycles, menopause, or taking oral contraceptives); by antidepressants and antihistamines, which reduce levels of saliva and disrupt the protective bacterial ecosystem in the mouth; and by anticancer drugs.

In periodontitis, the symptoms of gingivitis are present and the protective covering (called cementum) of the roots of the teeth may become exposed, leading to toothache on contact with hot or cold foods or beverages. Signs of more advanced periodontitis include loose teeth, a bad taste in your mouth, and bleeding gums. Sometimes, an abscess (see p.477) forms in the pocket between the gums and a tooth.

Less common forms of periodontal disease include juvenile periodontitis (a disease that appears in adolescence that affects the first molars and incisors), acute necrotizing periodontitis (also called trench mouth, a bacterial infection of the gums), and gum conditions that accompany disorders involving the white blood cells. People with diabetes are at greater risk for gum disease because their immune systems are less able to fight the mouth bacteria that lead to periodontitis.

TREATMENT OPTIONS

Your dentist treats gingivitis by physically removing the buildup of plaque and tartar with a dental instrument in a process called scaling; the surfaces of the teeth are then polished. Scrupulous dental hygiene and regular examinations can help prevent gingivitis.

Periodontitis is not as easily cured. The aim of treatment is to prevent progression of the disease. Scaling and planing are usually the first approaches to periodontitis. In scaling, calcified deposits are removed from the roots of the teeth; in planing, the surface of the root is smoothed.

However, once deep pockets have formed, your dentist may be unable to clean deeply enough to remove the buildup of plaque; periodontal surgery may be required.

The most common operation involves cutting the gum on either side of the tooth and pulling down the resulting flap to expose the roots of the teeth and the supporting bone. The root is cleaned and any decayed material removed. The bone may also need to be reshaped. When the root surface is clean and smooth, the flap is stitched back into place to form a tight enclosure around the teeth. After surgery, your dentist will pack a protective substance around the teeth and gums for 7 to 10 days so they can heal. You must be vigilant about brushing and flossing your teeth to avoid recurrence. Regular visits to your dentist to monitor the disease are also advised.

Sensitive Teeth and Gums

Teeth are protected by their hard outer enamel surface; under the enamel is a softer substance called dentin, which surrounds the nerve and extends to the roots of the teeth. When the enamel is eroded and dentin is exposed, stimuli such as hot and cold or sweet and sour foods or drinks or even the touch of a toothbrush can trigger pain.

Sensitive teeth can also be caused by poor brushing techniques. If you use a hard toothbrush, or if you brush your teeth too vigorously, you can wear away the surrounding gums and expose the sensitive dentin or the root surface. Gum disease (see Gingivitis and Periodontitis, p.474) can also cause gums to pull away from teeth, exposing the sensitive roots. Tooth decay and broken fillings can also cause pain.

Talk to your dentist if you have a sensitive tooth or sensitive gums. Special toothpastes are available to relieve sensitive teeth, but it is most important to see your dentist so that any underlying disease can be treated.

Toothache

Toothaches are common and can be caused by many of the same conditions that cause sensitive teeth (see above). The quality of pain can range from searing and sharp to dull and throbbing, de-

pending on the cause. A dental abscess (see p.477) can also cause pain with swelling. A toothache can often be temporarily treated with painkillers such as aspirin, ibuprofen, or acetaminophen until you can arrange a dental appointment. Call your dentist if you have persistent and severe pain. He or she will want to see you immediately if you have pain with swelling, with fever, with swollen glands, or that is accompanied by an inability to open your mouth.

Temporomandibular Joint Dysfunction

Temporomandibular joint dysfunction (formerly known as temporomandibular joint syndrome) is a collection of painful symptoms affecting the jaw joints. The joints are formed by the temporal bone of the skull and the jawbone (mandible) and the jaw muscles.

SYMPTOMS

Symptoms include difficulty chewing or opening your jaw, clicking or popping noises while chewing, locked jaws, jaw pain, throbbing temples, ringing ears, and aching shoulders. Women in their teens, 20s, and 30s are most often affected.

This condition is not fully understood. It may be caused by problems with the jaw muscles, particularly stress on jaw muscles from gum chewing or tooth grinding (see p.390); by joint disorders such as arthritis (see p.605); by dislocation of the jaw joint; by tumors of the bone or soft tissue; by neurologic conditions in which pain messages continue to be transmitted to the brain after the source of pain is removed; or by psychological factors that exacerbate chronic pain.

To obtain a diagnosis, your doctor or dentist will perform a

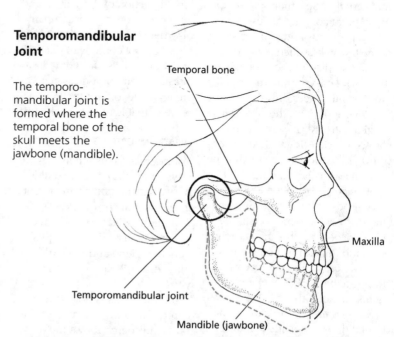

Temporomandibular Joint

The temporomandibular joint is formed where the temporal bone of the skull meets the jawbone (mandible).

Temporal bone

Maxilla

Temporomandibular joint

Mandible (jawbone)

thorough examination of your face and jaw, paying particular attention to your jaw's range of motion and looking for other potential causes of your pain.

TREATMENT OPTIONS

Pain of the temporomandibular joint rarely signals a serious disease and usually goes away on its own. Treatment aims to address the underlying cause.

Take steps to manage stress (see p.90), which may contribute to tooth grinding and, thus, the condition. Try to avoid foods that are difficult to chew or necessitate opening your mouth extremely wide. Switch to a diet of soft foods for several weeks and see if you feel an improvement.

Painkillers such as aspirin can help relieve pain; warm, moist compresses applied to the painful area may help reduce muscle spasms. Muscle relaxants and low doses of antidepressant drugs are effective treatments for some people. Biofeedback (see p.395) is helpful in some instances; other people benefit from psychotherapy (see p.393). Dental appliances such as bite guards to prevent tooth grinding may also be helpful.

If your disorder is caused by degenerative joint disease, your doctor may recommend surgery to alter the structure of your jaw. Treatments for temporomandibular joint dysfunction that have not been carefully studied and have not been proven helpful include wearing braces or retainers to realign the teeth; grinding down teeth and fitting them with crowns; or extracting teeth.

Dental Abscesses

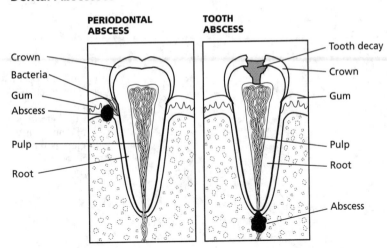

There are two types of dental abscess, or pouch of infected tissue. In a periodontal (gum) abscess (left), the abscess may form when bacteria grow between the gum and tooth. A tooth abscess (right) may be caused by a fracture in the crown of the tooth that permits microorganisms to enter the pulp and travel down to produce an abscess at the bottom of the tooth.

Dental Abscess

A dental abscess is a pouch of infected tissue that can occur in one of two locations. A periodontal (gum) abscess forms when gum disease produces pockets between the teeth and gums, and bacteria grow into the pocket. A tooth abscess forms when advanced tooth decay or a fractured tooth (see Dental Injuries, p.485) permit bacteria to invade the pulp of a tooth, causing it to die and the bacteria to spread to nearby gum tissue and bone.

Dental abscesses can ache or throb and are very painful when you bite. The lymph glands under your jaw or in the front of your neck may become swollen and you may have a fever due to the infection. Take aspirin, acetaminophen, or ibuprofen for the pain and call your dentist or doctor immediately if you think you have a dental abscess.

Periodontal abscesses are treated by inserting a probe into the infected area to relieve the pressure, and then cleaning out the infected pocket. A tooth abscess is treated by drilling a hole in the tooth to release the pressure and cleaning and disinfecting the infected pulp. A root canal (see p.484) is then performed. If the infection persists, the tooth may need to be pulled (see p.479). Because of the infection, you may need to take antibiotics before either procedure.

Impacted Wisdom Teeth

Any tooth can be impacted—that is, fail to fully emerge from beneath the gum. Wisdom teeth, the last teeth in the back of your

Impacted Wisdom Tooth

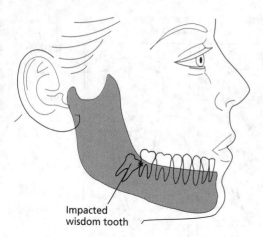

An impacted tooth fails to fully emerge from under the gum due to obstruction or overcrowded teeth. If the tooth cannot emerge, it can put pressure on nearby teeth, causing pain.

Impacted wisdom tooth

Removing Impacted Wisdom Teeth: Dr Donoff's Advice

Most of us develop four wisdom teeth. Usually, they grow straight, break through the gums, and serve as the main teeth we use to grind food before swallowing it. Sometimes, though, wisdom teeth grow crooked, don't break through the gums, and therefore can't be used for chewing. All they can do is cause trouble. They can push against other teeth, and cause pain. They can also lead to a common infection termed "pericoronitis"—the flap of gum over a partially impacted lower wisdom tooth traps food or other debris and the bacteria living in the mouth feed on the food, multiply, and cause infection. If the pain of an impacted tooth persists, or if the infection keeps recurring, your doctor may recommend removing the wisdom tooth.

BRUCE DONOFF, MD, DMD
HARVARD SCHOOL OF DENTAL MEDICINE
HARVARD MEDICAL SCHOOL

mouth, usually erupt in the late teenage years (although some people have no wisdom teeth) and often become impacted, or stuck, beneath the gum, sometimes with little adverse effect.

Complications can arise, however, when a wisdom tooth only partly breaks through the gum;

the broken gum can act as a trap for bacteria, which cause infection with swelling and pain when you bite down. Your ability to open your mouth may be limited and, if the infection spreads, you could have trouble swallowing or breathing.

If a wisdom tooth is infected,

call your dentist; you may need to take an antibiotic drug for the infection and possibly have the tooth pulled (see p.479). X-rays will help your dentist determine the position of the wisdom tooth. He or she may perform the extraction or refer you to an oral surgeon. You can treat a mildly impacted wisdom tooth by taking aspirin, ibuprofen, or acetaminophen. Gargle with warm salt water to help soothe the gums.

Discolored Teeth

Teeth can become discolored for many reasons. Stains on the enamel's surface from outside sources are relatively easy to prevent and remove; stains that emerge from the tooth's internal structure are permanent.

External stains include a black-brown coloring caused by tobacco use or caffeine consumption, and a yellow coloring produced when plaque on the tooth's surface is stained by foods. Other external stains include those caused by ingesting metals found in some medicines or by inhaling metallic dust; the metals can stain the teeth brown (iron), greenish (copper), or black (mercury).

A professional cleaning and scaling can remove many external stains. Tooth whiteners and bleaching products (see p.486) can also help fade stains.

Stains from the internal structure include the natural darkening of teeth as you age. Teeth may blacken after injury or after the pulp is removed during root canal surgery. Blackening can also occur if the pulp (the tooth's life-giving source) dies and the decomposing red blood cells

What Causes Bad Breath?

- Failure to regularly brush and floss your teeth
- Raw onions, garlic, and alcoholic beverages
- Bacteria-causing plaque and gum disease

- Medicines (such as some antidepressant drugs) that encourage the growth of bacteria in your mouth by reducing the amount of saliva your body makes
- Infections of the mouth, sinuses, or lungs

---

from the dead pulp move into the outer layers of the tooth. Taking the antibiotic drug tetracycline can cause yellow, blue, or gray coloration of primary (baby) and permanent teeth when teeth are still developing in childhood.

Another internal stain occurs when too much fluoride is ingested during childhood. Stains that emerge from the tooth's internal structure may require treatment by your dentist. In a procedure called bonding (see p.486), a plastic, acrylic, or porcelain covering is secured to the enamel to cover the discoloration.

COMMON DENTAL PROCEDURES

Dental Extraction

Your dentist may recommend pulling a tooth for a variety of reasons, including a badly broken or decayed tooth or because of a dental abscess (see p.477) or overcrowding. Most tooth extractions are performed in the office of a dentist or oral surgeon after the administration of a local anesthetic (see Killing the Pain of Dental Procedures, p.480).

If more than one tooth must be pulled or the extraction procedure itself is difficult (such as for some impacted teeth), your dentist may recommend sedation or even general anesthesia to make you more comfortable during the procedure.

Teeth are usually extracted using dental forceps, which grasp the crown of the tooth and cut the ligaments that support the tooth in the socket. The socket is gradually opened and the tooth is pulled out. After the extraction, bleeding is controlled by biting on gauze pads placed over the surgical site; the pressure causes the bleeding to stop within about 30 minutes. For pain after surgery, your dentist will recommend a painkiller such as acetaminophen, which does not affect the ability of the blood to clot. Aspirin and ibuprofen can interfere with clotting and prolong the bleeding.

Your dentist may advise you to refrain from any vigorous rinsing of your mouth or from drinking through a straw for 24 hours after the procedure to avoid dislodging the clot. Thereafter, gently rinsing your mouth with warm salt water can promote healing at the extraction site. Call your dentist if you have any prolonged bleeding or severe pain after the extraction. The site is usually completely healed within 7 to 10 days.

Orthodontics

Orthodontics is the dental specialty concerned with the correction of all forms of misaligned (crooked or out-of-place) teeth, spacing problems, and discrepancies in the alignment of the jaws. Orthodontic treatment may be needed to correct problems with biting, chewing, swallowing, pronouncing words, and tooth crowding, or for improving appearance.

Orthodontic correction can be started during childhood but definitive treatment often cannot be completed until after the permanent teeth have emerged (after about age 12).

Malocclusion, an abnormal relationship between the upper and lower teeth when biting, is easiest to correct in childhood or the early teenage years, when the teeth and jaw are still developing. Misaligned teeth and spacing

Killing the Pain of Dental Procedures

There are three methods dentists use to eliminate or reduce pain during dental procedures: local anesthesia, sedation, and general anesthesia.

Local anesthesia deadens only the area being treated and is injected or applied directly to the gums. It is often used for procedures for which the dentist must drill into a tooth, such as for a filling, and for procedures that involve the living pulp of the tooth, such as root canals or other oral surgery. A local anesthetic may also be used for teeth cleaning if you are especially sensitive.

Sometimes, injecting a local anesthetic into the area being treated is not possible (or may be too painful due to inflammation, infection, or pain). In these cases, your dentist may use a peripheral nerve block, in which the anesthetic is injected into a nerve near the site being treated. This results in the temporary numbing of a larger area.

Sedation and premedication Many people have some anxiety when they go to the dentist. If you find that your anxiety is preventing you from getting regular dental treatment, ask your dentist about sedation and premedication. Sedation may include the use of nitrous oxide, a safe gas that is breathed through the nose, or intravenous drugs. Premedication consists of drugs taken before your dental appointment.

General anesthesia causes loss of consciousness and is not often used in general dental practices. Some oral surgeons use general anesthesia (induced by drugs given intravenously) for short office procedures, such as wisdom tooth removal. However, because general anesthesia carries risks, it is usually used only for people who are in good health and only along with sophisticated monitoring of the patient. More complicated dental surgery may be performed in an operating room with the person under general anesthesia.

---

problems can be caused by heredity, thumb-sucking, or pacifier use (see p.986), or premature loss of a child's baby teeth, causing the permanent teeth to move into spaces they would not normally occupy.

There are three main categories of orthodontic treatment: preventive, interceptive, and comprehensive. Preventive treatment, usually reserved for children, minimizes the degree of future problems by correcting habits such as thumb-sucking. Preventive treatment also includes putting devices called space maintainers into the spaces created when a baby tooth is lost early, to keep the space open for the permanent tooth when it comes in.

Interceptive orthodontic treatment includes procedures on primary (baby) and permanent teeth to avoid future problems; they are usually performed between the ages of 6 and 12. For example, some people are born with a tendency to have unusually big teeth that create overcrowding of teeth. Interceptive treatment may extract teeth and redirect other teeth to relieve overcrowding in the future.

Comprehensive orthodontic treatment usually employs orthodontic appliances, such as braces and retainers.

BRACES

Braces are devices applied to the teeth to slowly move the teeth into new positions. If you need braces, your dentist will take a full-mouth x-ray, which will show your permanent teeth (including any that have not erupted) as well as your bones,

to determine the relationship between your upper and lower jaws. Your dentist will also make a plaster reproduction of your teeth. This is accomplished by having you bite into a soft clay-like substance to leave an impression; after it is removed, plaster is poured into the impression, creating a permanent cast of your teeth and bite.

In some cases of overcrowding, your dentist may recommend pulling one or several teeth to make room for others. Braces may then be used to move the crowded teeth into the open spaces created by the extracted teeth.

Braces may be worn for as long as 3 years. When there is a less severe problem, they may be worn for a shorter time. Several types of braces are available.

How Braces Work

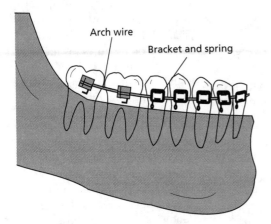

Arch wire

Bracket and spring

Braces are metal or plastic brackets cemented onto the outside or inside of the teeth; they contain slots to hold wires called arch wires. The brackets also feature tiny springs so that your dentist can tighten the arch wires regularly to guide teeth into their new position.

One type features stainless steel rings that encircle each tooth and are cemented into place. Another type features a small bracket that is cemented onto the front or back of the tooth. Wires, rubber bands, and springs are attached and manipulated to apply pressure in the direction the orthodontist wants the teeth to move. Your orthodontist adjusts the tension of the braces every month.

Having braces applied or adjusted can cause some short-term discomfort; painkillers such as ibuprofen, acetaminophen, or aspirin (those under age 21 should not take aspirin) can help ease the pain.

In addition to braces, your orthodontist may recommend that you wear an external device known as headgear that attaches to the back molars to apply pressure at night to accelerate the alignment process.

Once your braces have been removed, you will need to wear a retainer for several months or years to help keep your newly positioned teeth from moving back to their original position. A retainer is a removable device whose wires encircle your teeth; it is anchored by a plate that fits in your mouth.

Orthodontic appliances such as braces and retainers are ideal traps for food, and can cause plaque, tooth decay, and gum disease. Brush, floss, and rinse your mouth thoroughly twice a day, after every meal, and between meals if you snack. Ask your dentist or orthodontist to show you the best way to keep your braces scrupulously clean.

Fillings

The placement of a dental filling is a process by which a chipped tooth, or an area of tooth damaged by tooth decay (cavities), is

Antibiotics Before Dental Work

Some dental procedures—such as having gum surgery, dental implants, root canal therapy, or a tooth pulled—can cause tiny cuts in the gums. These cuts can permit bacteria living in your mouth to enter your bloodstream. In people who have certain heart conditions, the bacteria can cause a serious infection of the lining of the heart called bacterial endocarditis (see p.695).

The most common heart conditions requiring antibiotic treatment are previous artificial heart valve surgery (see p.694), previous bacterial endocarditis, damaged or malfunctioning heart valves (such as from rheumatic fever, see p.697), hypertrophic cardio-myopathy (see p.682), and mitral valve prolapse when it has caused thickening or regurgitation of the heart valves.

If you have any of these conditions, your doctor or dentist may require you to take antibiotics 1 hour before undergoing any of these dental procedures. Some doctors and dentists also recommend antibiotic treatment for people who have had artificial joint replacements, but the value of this is uncertain. Tell your dentist if you have any of these heart conditions, and ask your physician about having antibiotic therapy before dental work.

restored with a hard substance. When the enamel of the tooth—the hard outer surface—is damaged by decay or injury, bacteria can enter and cause further erosion and damage, sometimes to the tooth's central pulp, where blood vessels and nerves lie.

To fill a tooth, your dentist first administers a local anesthetic (see p.480) to numb the area in and around the affected tooth; he or she then cleans the tooth thoroughly and removes any decaying material with a drill. If the sensitive pulp is uncovered during drilling, your dentist may apply a sedative paste to prevent the pulp from causing pain once the tooth is filled. If the decay has destroyed a great deal of the tooth, a metal band may be positioned around the tooth to hold the filling in place.

The filling material is mixed and applied firmly into the hole or the space created by the metal band, and the surface is then smoothed. It hardens in several minutes. For front teeth, a tooth-colored plastic material is used. For teeth that do not show, an amalgam (a metallic mix of silver, mercury, or other minerals) or gold is used as a filling.

Amalgam fillings may break down after about 10 years; gold fillings last longest, but are more expensive. Newer composite materials and porcelain materials are also used for fillings, although amalgam remains the most common filling material. Some people have asserted that mercury in dental fillings may leak out and poison the rest of the body. Research to date has not found any evidence to support this theory.

Dentures

Dentures are prostheses that are usually made to replace multiple teeth. There are two types of dentures: partial and full. Partial dentures position false teeth between your own teeth, to fill the gap where a real tooth used to be. Full dentures replace all of the upper teeth, all of the lower teeth, or both.

Partial dentures typically have a metal base, and metal clasps that hold the denture to the teeth. Full dentures are usually made of a plastic (acrylic) that is colored to match your teeth and gums. The base plate is colored like the gums and sits on the gums; the upper plate stays in place, in part, by suction.

Sometimes temporary dentures (also called immediate dentures) are made before any teeth are extracted; they are placed in the mouth immediately after tooth removal to fill the empty spaces. Temporary dentures usually must be replaced later by permanent dentures.

Making dentures requires several visits. First, impressions are made of your mouth. This gives the dentist a copy of how your mouth is built, so that he or she can make the denture to fit precisely. A wax version is often made before the final plastic denture, to ensure that the false teeth have a shape and size that look right and work correctly. Since the bone that supports dentures changes over time, you will need to make periodic visits to your dentist to be sure the dentures still fit correctly and that the tissues underneath them remain healthy.

DENTURE CARE

Your dentures are as vulnerable as your natural teeth and must be cleaned daily. Plaque and tartar build up on dentures (as they do on original teeth) and can spread to living teeth and gums, causing cavities and gum disease.

After you remove your dentures, rinse your mouth thoroughly with water to remove any debris. Soak your dentures overnight in a half-and-half solution of lukewarm water and white vinegar or soak them in a denture cleaner. If your dentures have metal clasps, use water only. Soaking loosens plaque so you can brush it off more easily.

After soaking, brush your dentures with a denture-cleaning toothpaste using a denture brush. Always clean your dentures over a sink filled with water so that, if they drop, they will not break.

Crowns and Bridges

A crown is a replacement for the top (visible) portion of a tooth; dentists use crowns to replace decayed, cracked, or broken areas of the tooth. Bridges are one or more false teeth usually made of metal alloy (often platinum or gold) covered with porcelain; they are used to fill gaps in the mouth caused by missing teeth.

Crowns are made of porcelain for front teeth, or a combination of porcelain and metal to withstand the pressure of chewing for back teeth. A local anesthetic (see p.480) is usually required when you are being fitted for a crown.

Making a Crown

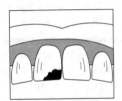

Tooth needing a crown

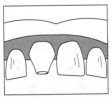

Tooth filed down to a
stub (crown preparation)

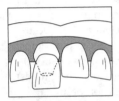

Crown fitted over and
cemented to crown
preparation

For a crown, your dentist makes an
impression of the natural shape of
your tooth. The tooth is then filed
down to a stub (the crown preparation). The crown has a hollow core
that fits precisely over the crown
preparation, onto which it is
cemented.

CROWN

Your dentist makes the crown by
first creating an impression of the
crown of the tooth that is to be
replaced. You are asked to bite
into a soft substance that looks
like clay; this leaves an imprint of
the shape of the original tooth.
Then, a drill is used to shape the
tooth into a stub (still naturally

attached to the underlying bone)
that will receive the crown. This
stub is called a crown preparation, and another impression is
made of its shape.

From the impressions of both
the crown that is to be replaced
and of the crown preparation, an
artificial tooth is created that has
a crown that matches the original
tooth, and which fits tightly on
top of the crown preparation.

While the crown is being
made, a temporary crown is positioned over the stub so there is
no empty space in your mouth.
During a second visit to your
dentist, the manufactured crown
is cemented onto the crown
preparation.

BRIDGE

A bridge consists of one or more
false teeth. Unlike dentures (see
p.482), bridges are not attached
to a plate that fits in the roof of
your mouth. Instead, a bridge
has a metal frame that attaches it
to the teeth adjoining the space
being filled.

These adjoining teeth (even
if they are healthy) must first be
prepared to receive crowns (see
above) because the adjoining
teeth anchor the bridge into place.
The bridge, like a crown, may
have a cover of porcelain so that
it resembles natural teeth. Creating a bridge can take several visits to your dentist.

If you have a crown or bridge,
you have a greater risk of gum
disease (see Gingivitis and Periodontitis, p.474) because the artificial teeth can attract plaque. In
addition to brushing and flossing,
use a rubber-tipped gum stimulator to clean the gum line near
crowns and bridges. Your dentist
may also recommend that you

use an interdental brush, which
is a brush with a small tip, to
thoroughly clean the area. A
device called a floss threader can
be used to clean under the bridge-
work.

Dental Implants

Dental implants are a way to
replace missing teeth by anchor-
ing false teeth to bone in the jaw,
instead of to adjacent teeth using
a metal frame, as is done with a
bridge (see left). Bone is a living
tissue that grows around an
implant, joining with it to create
a secure anchor.

As is done for a crown or a
bridge, an impression is made of
the tooth or teeth to be replaced.
These teeth are then removed,
and the implant is ready to be
inserted into the bone. After
administering a local anesthetic,
the dentist makes an incision in
the gum, and the gum is gently
lifted to expose the bone.

Using a series of drills, the
dentist then creates a hole in the
jawbone into which he or she
inserts a metal screw called an
implant fixture. The gum is then
replaced over the implant fixture,
which is left to integrate with the
bone for about 4 to 6 months.
During this period, a temporary
tooth or denture is placed over
the area so that you do not have
a space in your mouth.

After the implant fixture has
integrated with the bone, the gum
above the fixture is cut open
(after the dentist has administered
a local anesthetic) and a small
metal cylinder called an abutment
is attached to the top of the fixture. The abutment is what will
support your new crown.

After the gum has healed

Dental Implants

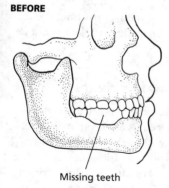

BEFORE

Missing teeth

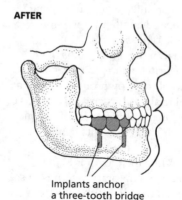

AFTER

Implants anchor
a three-tooth bridge

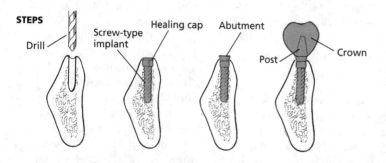

STEPS

Drill

Screw-type
implant

Healing cap

Abutment

Post

Crown

For dental implants, the dentist drills a hole in the jawbone (one for each implant) and inserts a screw, topped with a temporary healing cap, into the hole. The gum is stitched over the healing cap and bone grows around the screw, making a solid connection between bone and metal. After several months, the dentist makes an incision, removes the healing cap, and screws in a small metal cylinder (an abutment), onto which the custom-made crown or denture will be attached.

around the abutment (about 1 month), the dentist makes an impression of the abutment. The laboratory uses the impression of the crown of the tooth that is to be replaced, and the impression of the abutment, to create an artificial crown. That crown is then cemented onto the abutment. For people who have no teeth, implants may be used to support and secure dentures.

The 10-year success rate for implants is about 95% for the lower jaw in the chin area, 85% for the back of the lower jaw, 90% for the upper jaw under the nose, and 70% to 75% for the upper back jaw. Because healing is impaired in heavy smokers, heavy drinkers, and people with poorly controlled diabetes or a weakened immune system, failure is more common in these groups. Some people do not have enough bone to secure the screw.

Dental implants are inserted by a periodontist or oral surgeon, and crowns or dentures are made by a general dentist or prosthodontist. Complications from dental implants are rare but, just like your own teeth, they require diligent care from you and your dentist. Not all dental insurance plans pay for implants; check with your insurer before deciding on implants.

Root Canal Surgery

Root canal surgery replaces the pulp—the living tissue at the center of a tooth—with a filling material. A root canal is performed when the pulp has become infected or has died, often due to tooth decay or injury.

Before the procedure, your dentist will take x-rays to determine how many roots need to be treated. Incisors (front teeth) have a single root, premolars have two canals, and molars have three or four canals. A local anesthetic (see p.480) is given and a sheet of rubber called a rubber dam is fitted around the tooth to be treated to protect the underlying tissue.

In root canal treatment, the first objective is to remove the pulp from the tooth. To gain access, a hole is drilled into the tooth and the pulp is removed using an instrument called a broach. Then a series of tiny files is used to clean the sides of the canal. Once a clean root canal has been created, your dentist flushes the area with an antibacterial solution and then dries it.

Some dentists fill the tooth immediately; others fill the root

Root Canal Surgery

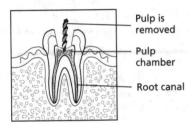

In root canal surgery, the area around the tooth is made numb by an anesthetic and a hole is drilled into the tooth. The infected pulp is removed and the pulp chamber and root canals are cleaned by filing their sides.

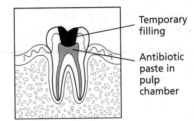

The pulp chamber is filled with a temporary filling (and occasionally with an antibiotic paste to kill any bacteria left in the pulp chamber and root canals). Later, the filling is removed and the dentist ensures the pulp chamber is sterile.

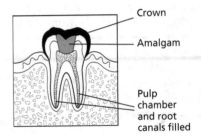

The pulp chamber and root canals are filled with solid material. An amalgam filling is inserted and a crown is applied.

canal during a second appointment to ensure that the tooth is no longer painful. The prepared canal is filled with a material called gutta-percha. Generally, the tooth then requires a crown (see p.482) to strengthen it and keep it from breaking. Root canal treatment may be performed by your dentist or by a specialist called an endodontist.

DENTAL INJURIES

Loose Teeth

In children, a loose tooth from the first set of teeth (called the primary teeth or baby teeth) usually is an indication that the tooth is ready to fall out. Do not pull out a loose baby tooth; it will usually come out on its own. In some cases, a baby tooth must be pulled by a dentist to make way for a secondary tooth. In adults, a very small amount of tooth looseness is normal. Otherwise, loose teeth are usually caused by external injury; injury to the teeth from an abnormal bite (malocclusion) or from grinding the teeth at night (see p.390); infection; or gum disease (see Gingivitis and Periodontitis, p.474). See your dentist if you have a very loose tooth. Treatment depends on the underlying cause, and the extent of the tooth's mobility.

Treating a Split Lip or Bleeding Gums

A split lip or cut to the gums can cause profuse bleeding. Flush the area with water to clean it. If the cut was caused by a fall or other injury, check to see if any teeth are broken; bits of broken teeth could be imbedded in the lip. Use a clean piece of gauze or paper towel to absorb the blood. Then apply ice wrapped in gauze or a washcloth (using some pressure) to the affected area for about 15 minutes. This should stop the bleeding and prevent swelling. Call your dentist or doctor if the cut is deep or will not stop bleeding. The cut might need stitches.

Repairing a Fractured or Chipped Tooth

Fractured (broken) and chipped teeth are classified according to their degree of severity. In a class I fracture, only the enamel (the hard, outer layer of the tooth) is broken or chipped; the dentin (the next, deeper layer) is not affected. Your dentist can smooth any sharp edges using a polishing instrument.

A class II fracture involves the dentin, but not the pulp (the living root of the tooth that contains blood vessels). To treat this type of fracture, your dentist may bond the tooth (see below right) by first roughening it with a weak acid and then covering it with a smooth plastic resin.

If the fracture exposes the sensitive pulp (a class III fracture), or if the root is involved (a class IV fracture), root canal surgery (see p.484) may be required. After initial treatment, all classes of fractures can be definitively repaired with bonding techniques using plastic materials. Your dentist can treat a broken filling by completely removing the filling and refilling the tooth.

COSMETIC IMPROVEMENT OF TEETH

Bleaching

Bleaching is a dental treatment that lightens teeth that have darkened due to tobacco or food stains or as a consequence of age. This painless procedure is the least expensive of the professional whitening treatments. In bleaching, your dentist paints your teeth with a bleaching solution, and then exposes your teeth to heat or light, which activates the whitening process. The light is applied with a small gun. Alternatively, your dentist may apply the bleaching solution by inserting a mouthpiece containing the solution, or by mixing the solution with toothpaste and brushing it on. The treatment lasts 6 to 12 months, but you can prolong the effects with home supplements.

TOOTH-WHITENING KITS AND HOME BLEACHING

Tooth whiteners available for home use remove stains by abrasion or by bleaching. Their safety and effectiveness vary according to the type used. Kits that contain abrasive agents can make teeth look whiter initially by removing surface stains, but they can be harmful over the long run because they accelerate the natural aging process, in which the enamel of teeth is slowly worn away to reveal the yellowing dentin behind it.

Bleaching is a more effective and safer way to remove stains at home, as long as it is done under your dentist's supervision. There are a variety of systems available, most of which feature hydrogen peroxide or another bleaching agent as active ingredients. Side effects include irritation of gums; making teeth more sensitive to heat and cold; and diarrhea, nausea, and sore throat from swallowing the whitening solution.

Your dentist will take an impression of your mouth that will serve as a mold for a soft plastic appliance called a nightguard. You will be instructed to add a bleaching solution to the nightguard and wear it for 6 to 8 hours a day, usually while you sleep. The device serves two purposes: it delivers the bleach to your teeth and protects the gums and soft tissues of the mouth. It can take 6 weeks to complete a bleaching. During that time you will need to visit your dentist periodically to allow him or her to monitor the effects.

Bonding

Bonding involves applying a coating to teeth to help cover stains, disguise cracks, or fill gaps. For bonding, a composite resin (a plasticlike material) is painted onto the tooth and hardened by exposing it to a special curing light. Repairs last for 3 to 5 years.

Veneers

Veneers are thin shells that are attached to the surface of the tooth to correct uneven, stained, or chipped enamel. Your dentist first removes the enamel of the tooth with a drill and then applies the shell-like veneer with a soft plastic powder; the tooth is then shaped and polished. The procedure is painless. Veneers last from 3 to 12 years.

SORES OF THE MOUTH, LIP, AND TONGUE

Canker Sores, Cold Sores, and Other Mouth Sores

(See also Color Guide to Visual Diagnosis, p.567)

Canker sores, also called aphthous ulcers, are small (about 1 to 2 millimeters) and usually develop on the inside of the lips and cheeks and, in rare cases, on the gums or hard palate (the roof of your mouth). They are not contagious and often occur in women around the time of their menstrual period and in adolescents.

Canker sores start out as a single, small, yellow spot ringed in red, and often first cause pain when you eat something spicy. They may appear in clusters and usually go away within a week to 10 days.

Rinsing with salt water may make canker sores less sore. Avoid hot foods and drinks, as well as spicy and acidic foods. True canker sores should go away within 14 days. If a mouth sore has not gone away in 14 days, contact your doctor or dentist. If canker sores continue to recur, your doctor may want to perform blood tests to look for vitamin deficiencies (particularly of folic acid or vitamin B_{12}) or a low level of white blood cells.

Cold sores are caused by the herpes simplex virus (HSV) types 1 and 2. HSV type 1 is the most common cause of cold sores. Type 2 more often causes herpes infection of the genital organs (what most people mean when they say they have "herpes," see

p.890), but it can also cause cold sores.

At least half of all adults are infected with HSV. Once you are infected with either type of HSV, you have the infection permanently. The virus lies dormant inside the nerves, causing no symptoms most of the time. In some people, the virus periodically "wakes up" and causes cold sores.

Doctors do not understand exactly what activates the virus. The following conditions or circumstances seem to bring on a recurrence: emotional anxiety, exposure to sunlight, hormonal changes (before a menstrual period, during pregnancy or menopause, or while taking oral contraceptives), physical exhaustion, and infections in other parts of the body.

Cold sores most often occur on the edge of the mouth, and they usually appear in the same place every time (because the virus lives in the nerves that lead to that spot on the skin). A cold sore usually begins with a slight tenderness or tingling, which develops into a painful, swollen, red lump. During this time, the virus in the sore is highly contagious (when the virus is dormant in the nerves, it is not contagious).

After a day or two, the area blisters, bursts, and crusts over. Then the yellow crust peels away and secretes a clear liquid. It can take as long as 2 weeks for the sore to heal.

Most experts do not think that antiviral medicines such as acyclovir make the cold sore go

away faster than it would without treatment in healthy people. Therefore, the use of antiviral medicines is not recommended. Some people have experienced success in shortening or averting full-blown cold sores by applying ice or taking the amino acid L-lysine, which is available in pill form at many health-food stores. Talk to your doctor about the various treatments for cold sores.

Mouth ulcers, caused by injury to the mucous membrane lining of your mouth, are called traumatic ulcers. They can be inflicted by vigorous tooth brushing, by biting your cheek, or by a rough tooth or denture. Talk to your dentist if you think a sharp tooth or dental appliance is causing the traumatic ulcer. These ulcers usually heal within a week once the cause is resolved.

Mouth Blisters

The mouth is subject to several diseases that can cause blisters. The diseases are not contagious.

Oral lichen planus is a very common condition, of unknown cause, that can take three forms. The most common form is characterized by thick white streaks on the inner lining of the cheeks or on the sides of the tongue. The second form causes painful, eroded areas and blisters of the gums. The final form is the most severe and produces painful blistering sores throughout the mouth. The condition affects women more than men and usually affects people between ages

40 and 60. Some people also develop a skin rash.

Lichen planus tends to be a chronic (long-term) condition that may come and go. If you have the most common form of oral lichen planus, it may not require treatment. If you have either of the other types, your dentist or doctor may prescribe corticosteroid drugs (see p.895). Your dentist or doctor may also recommend a biopsy to confirm the diagnosis.

There is a controversy as to whether having oral lichen planus predisposes you to cancers of the mouth (see p.489). If you have lichen planus, it is prudent for your dentist to check your mouth regularly for signs of oral cancer.

Pemphigoid and pemphigus are autoimmune diseases (see p.870). Large mouth blisters can occur alone or along with similar blisters elsewhere on the skin in pemphigoid. Pemphigus, another uncommon but serious disease that involves both the skin and mouth, causes blisters that usually start in the mouth (and sometimes remain only in the mouth) and then usually appear on the skin. The fragile blisters break easily, forming painful areas that crust over and can become infected. If not treated, the blisters can spread, causing extensive skin loss, and even death.

If your doctor or dentist suspects that you have pemphigoid or pemphigus, he or she will take a small sample of a blister for examination under a microscope. Treatment of both diseases includes prescription corticosteroid drugs (see p.895) and, in some cases, immunosuppressive drugs, which quiet the immune system. Antibiotics may be needed for any infection that accompanies the blisters.

Erythema multiforme is a relatively uncommon autoimmune disease (see p.870). Young adults, particularly men, are most susceptible to it. Unlike other blistering conditions in the mouth, erythema multiforme has a severe and explosive onset in which dramatic blisters and ulcers develop in the mouth and may extend onto the lips. A rash on the skin develops in about half the people with the condition; it is characterized by sores that look like an archery target.

A more severe variant of erythema multiforme produces sores in the mouth, on the genitals, and in the eyes. Flulike symptoms such as fever, headache, cough, and sore throat may occur about a week before the outbreak. The sores tend to last between 2 and 6 weeks. Treatment of milder forms is usually unnecessary; more severe forms require treatment with corticosteroid drugs (see p.895).

Oral Thrush

The fungus *Candida albicans* is a natural inhabitant of your mouth, where helpful bacteria normally keep it in correct balance with other microorganisms. However, when your resistance to infection is low, or you take antibiotic drugs or corticosteroid drugs, the natural balance of organisms is upset and the fungus may proliferate, causing oral thrush.

Sore, yellow-white, raised patches in the delicate lining of the mouth and throat are the main symptom. If the patches are rubbed off during toothbrushing or eating, areas of painful skin are exposed. Sometimes *C albicans* can cause your tongue to burn even without the white patches or sores in your mouth.

Oral thrush is not serious but it tends to recur. Chronically ill people—including those with an infection caused by the human immunodeficiency virus (HIV) or acquired immunodeficiency syndrome (AIDS) or people who are undergoing chemotherapy—are more prone to oral thrush, but children and elderly people also are affected.

If you think you have oral thrush, see your doctor or dentist. He or she will examine you and may take a small sample of the affected area to confirm the diagnosis. Antifungal drugs applied directly to the patches usually cure the condition, although oral medicine may be needed in stubborn cases to eradicate the fungus from your system.

CANCEROUS AND PRECANCEROUS CONDITIONS OF THE MOUTH

Leukoplakia

Leukoplakia means white plaque; it is a condition that produces a white patch in the mouth or on the tongue or gums. Leukoplakia is the most common type of precancerous growth (p.564) in the mouth and can have several causes, including repeated irritation from a sharp tooth or a broken denture.

Other causes include irritation from chewing tobacco, lupus (see p.898), kidney failure (see p.811), lichen planus, and tertiary syphilis (see p.893).

In its early stages, leukoplakia is rarely painful and appears as a gray or white patch of any size. The patch becomes progressively stiff and rough.

If you have any thickening or hardening in your mouth that does not heal within 2 weeks, see your dentist or doctor. The first line of treatment is to repair any physical cause of the leukoplakia such as an abrasion from a rough denture. If you smoke, your doctor will advise you to stop. A biopsy (p.161) may be required to rule out the possibility of cancer. If cancer is found, prompt surgical removal (after the administration of a local anesthetic) is essential.

Mouth and Lip Tumors

(See also Color Guide to Visual Diagnosis, p.567)

The mouth is a common site for benign (noncancerous) tumors. Benign tumors are growths that are not likely to spread but are often irritating. The most common is a tumor called a fibroma. It is caused by chronic irritation, often from the teeth rubbing up and down against the delicate tissues of the mouth, and is usually white. Another type of benign tumor that looks something like cauliflower are papillomas; they are thought to be caused by viruses.

Many people have a series of bony, round bumps on the roof of their mouth. The bumps most often are due to a somewhat unusual bone formation called torus palatinus and are nothing to worry about. There is a wide range of other benign growths; your dentist may remove them for diagnosis and to avoid irritation.

Mouth cancers (also called oral cancers) are not rare and are almost always associated with tobacco use, which increases your risk of oral cancer in any form. The combination of tobacco and alcohol increases the risk of oral cancer dramatically. Mouth cancer may begin as a nonhealing ulcer or sore, a white patch (often with areas of red), or a lump.

The key to curing oral cancer is early diagnosis. Tell your dentist or doctor if you have a white area or lump or a sore that lasts more than 2 weeks. He or she may remove a sample for exami-

Preventing Cancers of the Mouth and Tongue

About 8% of all cancers occur in the mouth and on the tongue. Most can be prevented and most can be completely cured if treated early. Take the following steps to help prevent cancer and improve your overall health:

- Quit smoking.
- Stop chewing tobacco.

- Limit your intake of alcohol to no more than two drinks a day.

- Wear lip balm with a sun protection factor (SPF) of 15.

- See your doctor or dentist immediately if you detect a white or discolored area, a sore that does not heal after 2 weeks, or an unusual lump in your mouth or on your lips or tongue.

The Sense of Taste

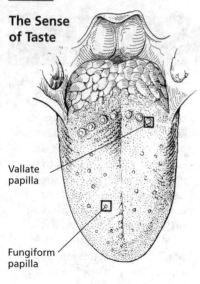

Vallate papilla

Fungiform papilla

Humans can identify four basic tastes—sweet, sour, bitter, and salty—and at least 10,000 different flavors, each of which is a combination of the four basic tastes. Throughout the mouth, and especially on the front two thirds of the tongue, are tiny taste buds, located in the walls of bumps on the tongue called the vallate and fungiform papillae. Taste buds for bitter substances are located mainly toward the back of the tongue, sour taste buds along the edges, sweet taste buds at the tip, and salt taste buds on the top. Many nerve endings run into each taste bud and then travel to the brain, where your consciousness recognizes the messages as a particular taste.

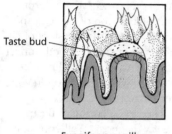

Taste bud

Fungiform papillae

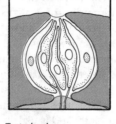

Taste bud

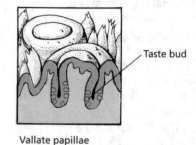

Taste bud

Vallate papillae

---

nation under a microscope. Surgical removal is the most common treatment. Radiation therapy (see p.741) may be used to kill remaining cancer cells. Chemotherapy (see p.741) is helpful if your doctor believes that the tumor has metastasized (spread) to other parts of your body.

TONGUE VARIATIONS

The tongue is covered with tiny projections called papillae that house taste buds and give the tongue a bumpy texture. Your tongue is a reflection of your general health. A white or yellow coating may appear when you have a viral or bacterial infection, clearing up when the infection is cured.

Inflammation of the tongue, called glossitis, may make the tongue feel sore, swollen, and painful and look red. Glossitis can be caused by infection, smoking, irritation of the mouth by a rough tooth or denture, spicy foods, and vitamin or mineral deficiencies (such as vitamin B or iron). Geographic tongue is a form of glossitis in which the redness and swelling occur only on small areas on the tongue; its cause is not known. It occurs in 1% to 3% of the population, more often in women.

Correcting any known causes usually clears up the condition

within several weeks. Gargling with salt water can also help. If you are concerned, talk to your doctor, who can help you resolve any underlying problem. The tongue can easily become discolored by foods it helps to chew and digest. Coffee, tea, and smoking can stain the tongue a darker color, as can some medicines. Sometimes the papillae become elongated, resulting in another temporary condition called hairy tongue. In some people, creases form in the tongue. No treatment is necessary for these conditions, but brushing your tongue with a toothbrush and rinsing with an antiseptic mouthwash will help keep your tongue clean and free of debris.

PROBLEMS OF THE SALIVARY GLANDS

Salivary Gland Infections

The salivary glands can become infected with viruses and bacteria. The mumps virus (see p.950) is the most common cause of salivary gland infection; it causes the glands to become swollen and painful.

Blocked salivary ducts may lead to bacterial infections, which are more serious and can even be fatal, especially in dehydrated, elderly people. Salivary duct stones (see below) are the most frequent cause of blockage, although tumors may obstruct the ducts as well. Symptoms include painful swelling of the gland, especially before eating. Pus from the duct may cause a bad taste in your mouth.

Treatment with antibiotics usually helps. If the duct is blocked, your doctor may insert a thin metal probe to try to remove the obstruction. A gland that has been chronically infected and is irreversibly damaged may need to be removed.

Salivary Duct Stones

Salivary duct stones, also called calculi, block the salivary duct from secreting saliva. The stones are produced when calcium deposits form around debris in the duct, blocking passage of saliva into your mouth and causing painful swelling. Stones are most common in young and middle-aged adults. Salivary duct stones are an uncommon source of infection in the submandibular gland, which is the salivary gland located at the juncture of your jaw and neck.

See your doctor if you have pain or swelling under your jaw; he or she may take an x-ray to

Location of Salivary Glands

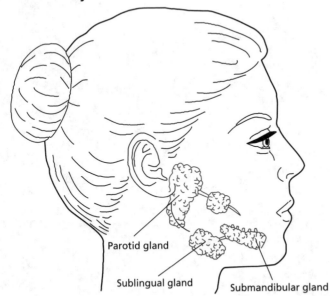

Parotid gland

Sublingual gland

Submandibular gland

Three pairs of salivary glands help produce moisture (saliva) and enzymes for digesting food and lubricating the mouth. The parotid glands, located just in front of and below the ear, drain into the mouth through ducts that empty into the inner cheeks. The submandibular glands are located under the back of the jaw and drain into the mouth through ducts located just behind the lower front teeth. The sublingual glands also lie in the floor of the mouth and drain through a series of small ducts there.

view the duct. If this does not yield a clear explanation, computed tomography (see p.149) or ultrasound (see p.148) may be performed. Small salivary stones may pass on their own by stimulating saliva production. Larger stones may need to be removed surgically.

Salivary Gland Tumors

Of all the salivary glands, the parotid glands are most susceptible to tumors. These tumors are slow growing, unlikely to spread, but often recur. Swollen salivary glands are the main (and often the only) symptom. If you have any pain or swelling in your sali-vary glands, talk to your doctor, who may perform a biopsy (see p.161), magnetic resonance imaging (see p.151), or computed tomography (see p.149). If a tumor is diagnosed, your doctor may recommend surgical removal. If the tumor is malignant (cancerous), you may also require radiation therapy (see p.741).

Lungs

The survival of the human body hinges on receiving an uninterrupted supply of oxygen and on disposing of the body's waste products, including carbon dioxide. The amount of air you require depends on your level of activity. At rest, the lungs move about a half liter of air in and out with each breath, or 8 liters per minute. During maximal exercise, the lungs can move 80 to 120 liters of air each minute—10 to 15 times as much.

Delivering oxygen to each cell requires the cooperative efforts of the lungs, heart, trachea (windpipe), and bronchi, the airways that connect the trachea to the lungs.

How you breathe Before reaching the lungs, air is inhaled through the nose or mouth, where larger impurities are filtered out. Oxygen then moves through the bronchial tree: the trachea, which is about as wide across as your thumb, somewhat smaller pipes called bronchi, and then a branching system of ever-smaller tubes that lead finally to the alveoli (a network of hundreds of millions of microscopic air sacs).

Surrounding these air sacs are millions of tiny blood vessels called capillaries. Oxygen passes through the wall of the alveoli and enters the bloodstream. In exchange, carbon dioxide leaves the blood, enters the alveoli, and is exhaled through the lungs. The oxygen-rich blood then travels to the heart for distribution throughout the body.

The act of breathing—inhaling and exhaling—is directed by the brain, which sends signals to the respiratory muscles. One of these muscles is the diaphragm, a flat muscle that separates the chest from the abdomen. When it moves down, air is pulled into the lungs; when it moves up, air is pushed out of the lungs. In addition, there are muscles between the ribs that help expand the rib cage, also pulling air into the lungs.

Dealing with impurities in the air The air you breathe is not pure. It is filled with dust, dirt, smoke, and other substances and microorganisms that we cannot see. Your lungs have an elaborate system for filtering out these impurities before they reach and damage the delicate air sacs, the alveoli. The lining of the bronchial tree contains glands that make mucus, a thick liquid that traps particles. In addition, the tubes of the bronchial tree are lined with tiny hairs called cilia that beat upward toward the mouth. The bronchial tubes are thus well-equipped to carry mucus (and any particles that have been caught) up to the mouth and nose to be coughed or sneezed out. The last line of defense is the white blood cells of the immune system (see p.865), stationed in the lining of the bronchial tree and the alveoli where they can engulf particles or kill germs.

Your Lungs

Air is inhaled through the nose or mouth and moves through the trachea, through small bronchial tubes and even smaller bronchioles into millions of tiny air sacs (alveoli). Next to the alveoli are capillaries (blood vessels). The close proximity of the alveoli and capillaries allows carbon dioxide from the blood to be exchanged for oxygen in the lungs. Oxygen enters the lungs and then the blood, and carbon dioxide is released by the blood and exhaled through the lungs.

Trachea (windpipe)

Bronchial tube

Right lung

Left lung

Bronchioles

Bronchiole

Alveoli

Capillary (blood vessel)

Common Lung Tests

Here are some tests your doctor may use to diagnose lung diseases and disorders:

Chest x-ray An x-ray (see p.145) of your chest provides a picture of your lungs. It is one of the first tests your doctor may recommend if he or she suspects a problem. To make a chest x-ray, you stand in front of the x-ray machine, take a deep breath to expand your lungs, and hold your breath while pictures are made from the front and the sides. The x-ray picture can confirm that you have an infection such as pneumonia and can show a tumor larger than half a centimeter.

Percutaneous needle aspiration (biopsy) When cells from a lung need to be examined under the microscope, they may be collected by a method called percutaneous ("through the skin") needle aspiration. This procedure avoids the need to perform an operation to open the chest for a simple biopsy.

Instead, the biopsy needle is inserted after numbing the skin with a local anesthetic (see p.168) and then guided to the proper spot by using the imaging technique computed tomography (see p.149). A sample of tissue is taken and the needle is withdrawn.

Examination of pleural fluid Pleural fluid can collect in the space (the pleura) between the outside of the lungs and the inside of the chest wall. Samples of pleural fluid may be taken to look for infection or cancer cells. During thoracentesis, local anesthesia is used to insert a needle into the chest wall, and a small amount of pleural fluid is withdrawn for evaluation.

Sputum evaluation A phlegm (sputum) evaluation can reveal the source of infection or the presence of cancerous cells. Your doctor will ask you to cough vigorously to bring up a sample of phlegm. If this is not possible, a solution of salted water can be sprayed into your throat to make you cough, a procedure called sputum induction.

Pulmonary angiography Pulmonary angiography is most often performed to look for clots, or pulmonary embolisms (see p.512), in the blood vessels of the lungs. In this procedure, you receive a sedative and your skin is numbed at the point of injection, usually your arm or groin. A hollow tube called a catheter is inserted into a vein and guided by x-ray toward the main pulmonary artery. Then a contrast medium (which can be seen inside the blood vessels on x-rays) is injected, and x-rays are taken of the artery and its smaller branches in your lungs to look for blockages. The contrast medium may produce a warm sensation.

Radionuclide scan A radionuclide scan (see p.137) of the lungs is also called a lung scan or ventilation-perfusion (VQ) scan. It is usually used to identify the presence of a pulmonary embolism (see p.512) in the lungs. After you inhale an aerosol containing a tiny amount of radiation, a gamma camera takes pictures

---

Despite the presence of an elaborate defense system, the lungs do not cope well with tobacco smoke. In smokers, the mucous glands make too much mucus, which clogs airways and makes it difficult to breathe. Smoking weakens the immune system, making the lungs vulnerable to infections such as pneumonia.

Smoking also damages the delicate alveoli, making it hard to breathe and often leading to emphysema. In addition, smoke particles cause lung cancer and many other diseases. Secondhand smoke (smoke from other people's cigarettes) can affect the lungs of nonsmokers, especially children.

Acute Bronchitis

Acute bronchitis is an infection and inflammation of the lining of the bronchial passages, the large airways that connect the windpipe to the lungs. Although bronchitis makes you cough, it is not an infection of the lungs like pneumonia (see p.496). However, when acute bronchitis does not get better, it can develop into pneumonia.

Acute bronchitis often begins with an upper respiratory infection (involving the nose, sinuses, ears, or throat) that is usually caused by a virus. Infection with bacteria can sometimes follow a viral infection.

Infants, young children, elderly people, smokers, and people with lung or heart disease are

of where the flow of air goes in your lungs. Next, another small amount of radiation is injected into a vein in your arm, and the flow of blood through your lungs is recorded by the gamma camera.

The images are compared to see if the air and blood travel to the same places, which they do in healthy lungs. If a lung area fills with air but not with blood, a pulmonary embolism may be blocking the flow of blood.

Bronchoscopy A bronchoscope, one type of endoscope (see p.142), is a thin, hollow, flexible or rigid tube that contains a tiny magnifying camera and light. A channel allows instruments to be inserted through the bronchoscope to remove foreign objects or collect samples of tissue (biopsies) or secretions. Images of the structures viewed by the camera in the bronchoscope are transmitted to a monitor.

You will be asked not to eat or drink before the procedure, which requires either local anesthesia (to numb your throat to keep you from coughing or swallowing) or general anesthesia (to put you to sleep). The bronchoscope is inserted through the nostrils or mouth.

Mediastinoscopy Mediastinoscopy is the evaluation of the mediastinum—the central portion of the chest that contains the heart, trachea, and esophagus—with a viewing instrument called an endoscope (see p.142), usually to obtain a sample of tissue for biopsy.

Using general anesthesia (see p.168), the doctor makes an incision at the base of the neck and inserts the endoscope. The tissue sample is removed, the endoscope is withdrawn, and the incision is stitched closed.

Pulmonary function tests These tests involve blowing into a machine called a spirometer, which measures how much air you can hold in your lungs, and how easily you can move air through your lungs. Pulmonary function tests are valuable in determining the severity of some lung diseases, particularly chronic bronchitis, emphysema, and interstitial diseases of the lungs (see p.522).

Video-assisted thoracic (chest) surgery (VATS) VATS is an endoscope (see p.142) technique used to diagnose and treat lung disease. Using general anesthesia (see p.168), three small incisions are made in the side of the chest, and a rigid tube with a camera and light is inserted into the space between the lungs and the chest wall. A video image is transmitted to a monitor, guiding the physician's use of various instruments as he or she takes samples of tissue for examination or removes segments of diseased lung tissue.

VATS has largely replaced open surgery for lung biopsy because it can be performed with much smaller incisions, which permits quicker recovery.

more vulnerable to developing acute bronchitis from upper respiratory infections. They are also more likely to develop pneumonia from bronchitis. When symptoms persist or recur at frequent intervals (which usually occurs in smokers), the condition is called chronic bronchitis (see p.517).

SYMPTOMS

A cough is the main symptom of bronchitis. It may be a dry cough or produce phlegm (sputum), a collection of mucus and puslike

material containing white blood cells, which fight the infection. When the phlegm is yellow-green, a bacterial infection is more likely.

Fatigue, wheezing, sore throat, low-grade fever, and chest discomfort are other common symptoms. You may also feel short of breath. Even after the infection clears, sometimes a dry, hacking cough persists for several weeks because the airway lining is still irritated.

TREATMENT OPTIONS

Acute bronchitis usually clears up after 4 or 5 days without antibiotics. If you have a fever, take aspirin or an aspirin substitute. Rest and drink plenty of fluids—eight to 12 glasses a day—to thin the phlegm and make it easier to cough up.

Breathing in warm, moist air also helps loosen the discharge. If you do not have a vaporizer or humidifier, stand in the bathroom and run a hot shower or bath, or run hot water in the sink and drape a towel over your head while breathing in the steam.

If you smoke, avoid smoking for at least the duration of your illness. The most important step you can take is to quit smoking altogether (see p.59).

Call your doctor if you have a fever for more than 3 days or a high fever that does not come down with aspirin or if you have chills that shake your body uncontrollably. You should also call your doctor if you become short of breath or if your cough gets worse and produces thick mucus that is bloody or smells foul.

Symptoms of acute bronchitis that occur in infants, elderly adults, and people who are chronically ill (especially those with lung or heart disease) should be reported to a doctor immediately.

Your doctor will perform a physical exam that includes listening to your chest through a stethoscope and taking samples of sputum so they can be examined under a microscope for bacteria. If a bacterial infection is suspected and does not seem to be going away, an antibiotic (usually in tablet form) may be prescribed to help treat the infection.

In some cases of acute bronchitis, a bronchodilator drug may be prescribed, usually in inhaler form, to open your airways. Ask your doctor which nonprescription medicines he or she recommends to loosen phlegm or suppress coughing to help you sleep at night.

Pneumonia

Pneumonia is an infection of the lungs. Because pneumonia affects the lung's air sacs, it can seriously interfere with the exchange of oxygen and carbon dioxide in the alveoli, the lung's smallest air sacs.

Many infections can cause pneumonia, including infection with different kinds of bacteria, viruses, mycoplasma, chlamydia, fungi, and parasites. Some are very common, while others, such as pneumonia caused by fungi or parasites, are rare.

Pneumonia is an illness that can range from mild to very severe. It may be so mild in some people that neither they nor their doctor even know they have it, and it passes quickly. Some people feel very ill for a week or two, but they fully recover. In others, pneumonia is fatal.

What makes some cases of pneumonia mild and others severe? The type of microorganism causing the pneumonia and the person's underlying health are the most important factors. Generally, bacteria produce more severe pneumonia than most viruses, mycoplasma, or chlamydia. Some bacteria tend to produce worse infections than others (for example, infections with staphylococcal or pseudomonas bacteria usually are more severe than other bacterial lung infections).

In general, however, the severity of illness depends more on your health at the time of infection than the kind of microorganism causing the infection. People who are bedridden have a harder time clearing lung infections because the cough reflex becomes weaker and infected sputum tends to accumulate in the lungs. Infants are at risk because their immune systems are not fully developed.

Elderly adults are five times as likely to die of pneumonia as younger adults because their immune systems are not as vigorous, they are more likely to be malnourished, and the defense mechanisms of their lungs are weaker (even if they have never smoked and do not have chronic lung disease).

Young people with chronic lung diseases—most often smokers who have developed chronic bronchitis and emphysema (see p.517)—more easily develop infections of the lungs because the defense mechanisms used to clear the lungs of infections are impaired.

People with diabetes (see p.832) tend to get more severe pneumonia because diabetes weakens the ability of some types of white blood cells to fight infections. Those with heart disease, especially congestive heart failure (see p.683), also often have more severe pneumonia.

Pneumonia is also more common in people exposed to environmental toxins, which increase mucous secretions and impair the lung's ability to remove them. Finally, people with serious immune system problems—for example, those recovering from cancer treatment, those who have AIDS, or those taking medicines after receiving organ transplants—develop unusual and serious kinds of pneumonia (see Pneumonia in People With Impaired Immune Systems, p.500).

Pneumonia that develops from exposure in the home or workplace is often caused by different microorganisms than pneumonia that develops in a hospital or other institution that houses the sick.

How Common Types of Pneumonia Are Transmitted

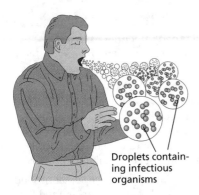

Droplets containing infectious organisms

Common kinds of pneumonia are often transmitted in close quarters when an infected person sneezes or coughs, releasing droplets containing the infectious organism.

Certain kinds of pneumonia are sufficiently different from the more common types that they are discussed separately: see Tuberculosis (p.504), Fungal Infections (p.503), Hantavirus Pulmonary Syndrome (p.501), aspiration pneumonia (see p.498), and SARS (see p.501).

SYMPTOMS

The main symptoms of pneumonia are coughing; shortness of breath; feeling ill, tired, or achy; and fever. The cough may produce phlegm (sputum) or may be dry. The phlegm may be white or clear or may be yellow, brown, or green.

Sometimes pneumonia develops after an initial infection of the nose, throat, ears, or sinuses, and then travels down into the lungs. In this case, sneezing, runny nose, congestion, pain in the nose and sinuses, earache, and sore throat may all precede pneumonia symptoms.

Pneumonia sometimes leads to a sharp pain in your chest when you breathe deeply (see Pleurisy, p.502) or causes you to cough up blood. Especially with pneumonia caused by bacteria, you can develop a high fever and uncontrollable chills or shaking. Some people get so sick that they become confused or even lose consciousness.

Elderly people in particular can become lethargic, confused, or unresponsive as a result of pneumonia. Because they may not be coughing or having shortness of breath, the doctor may not initially suspect pneumonia.

DIAGNOSIS

Your doctor will determine if you have pneumonia by first asking you about your symptoms. If pneumonia seems likely, he or she will establish the type of pneumonia you have, based on your symptoms and other factors.

For example, has someone you are in contact with been sick? Have you traveled out of the country recently, where you may have acquired an unusual type of pneumonia? Do you have other conditions—such as chronic bronchitis, cancer, or other illnesses—that make you vulnerable to specific types of pneumonia?

Your doctor will then examine your lungs by listening to your chest with a stethoscope placed on your back while you breathe. A person with pneumonia often produces delicate crackling noises or wheezing in the area of the lung affected by pneumonia.

Percussion, in which the doctor taps on your back and listens to the sound produced, may also

reveal areas of infected lung. In a healthy lung, the air-filled lung creates a highly resonant sound. In a lung with pneumonia, the sound can be dull or muffled because the air sacs are filled with fluid instead of air.

Your doctor may take a chest x-ray to confirm a diagnosis of pneumonia. He or she may look at your phlegm under the microscope to see if there is evidence that bacteria are causing the pneumonia, and what type of bacteria are most likely. A sample of your phlegm may also be sent to the laboratory for a culture (see p.159), to see if the cause of the infection can be identified. This can take a day or two. However, in at least 40% of people, tests cannot identify the microorganism that is causing the pneumonia.

Blood tests can show if you have a lot of white blood cells fighting the infection. Sometimes the blood is cultured to see if bacteria from your lungs have moved into the blood.

TREATMENT OPTIONS

Antibiotics are the primary treatment for pneumonia caused by bacteria, mycoplasma, and chlamydia. You can be treated at home with antibiotics taken by mouth if you are under 50 years old, do not have a major chronic disease, have relatively mild symptoms, and if you or someone else can fix meals and perform other necessary chores. Sicker people may need to be hospitalized for closer observation and to receive intravenous antibiotics, assistance with breathing, and oxygen.

All people with pneumonia should get plenty of rest and

drink lots of liquids. Fluids make it easier for you to cough up infected phlegm, an important way for the lungs to clear themselves of infection.

However, cough-suppressing medicine is sometimes prescribed, particularly if the cough is not bringing up infected phlegm and is making it difficult to sleep. Discuss with your doctor what types of nonprescription medicines might be helpful, especially at night.

If your condition takes longer than 3 weeks to resolve, your doctor may want to further evaluate your lungs with additional x-rays or other tests, such as computed tomography (see p.149) or a bronchoscope (see p.525), to check for other conditions such as lung cancer or tuberculosis.

BACTERIAL PNEUMONIA

Pneumonia caused by bacteria occurs more commonly during the winter months. Many different kinds of bacteria can cause pneumonia, but by far the most common is *Streptococcus pneumoniae* (also called pneumococcus). The next most common bacterium that infects the lungs is *Haemophilus influenzae*, followed by *Moraxella catarrhalis* (which mainly causes pneumonia in people with chronic bronchitis), group A streptococci, *Staphylococcus aureus* (also called "staph"), and a group of bacteria called gram-negative bacteria.

All of these tend to cause high fevers, shaking chills, severe fatigue, lethargy, and a cough that produces green phlegm. A bacterium called *Pseudomonas aeruginosa* is more common in hospitals and other institutions that house the sick. It causes a

Types of Pneumonia

Doctors classify pneumonia into three broad categories: community-acquired pneumonia, hospital-acquired pneumonia, and aspiration pneumonia.

Community-acquired pneumonia Most pneumonia is community-acquired pneumonia, meaning that the microorganism was picked up in a setting such as the home or workplace. Community-acquired pneumonia affects about 3 million Americans each year and causes the death of 50,000 of those people. Most of these deaths occur in people with other chronic illnesses, such as heart disease, kidney failure, diabetes, or cancer.

Community-acquired pneumonia tends to be spread when someone who has bronchitis or pneumonia coughs and you breathe in the air (and the droplets containing infectious organisms) they have coughed out. The most common causes are *Streptococcus pneumoniae, Haemophilus influenzae, Mycoplasma pneumoniae,* and *Chlamydia pneumoniae.*

Hospital-acquired pneumonia People who are in the hospital can develop hospital-acquired pneumonia, which is caused by bacteria that tend to be present in the hospital environment. The most common causative bacteria are *Pseudomonas aeruginosa, Staphylococcus aureus,* and gram-negative bacteria.

Pneumonia acquired in the hospital tends to be more serious than pneumonia acquired in the community, partly because the bacteria in the hospital are more likely to be resistant to various antibiotics. This pneumonia can produce life-threatening illness in people who are already weakened by whatever condition originally brought them to the hospital.

Aspiration pneumonia Aspiration pneumonia occurs from aspirating (breathing in) material from the crevices of the teeth (especially when dental health is poor) or regurgitated matter or vomit. The matter drops down into the trachea (windpipe) and into the lung.

Aspiration tends to occur in people who have periods of impaired consciousness due to alcohol or other drug use, a seizure disorder, or dementia, or in those under general anesthesia. It also can affect people who have a problem with the muscles that facilitate swallowing, which can occur with a nervous system disorder or after a stroke.

The damaged lung has more difficulty fighting off infection caused by the breathed-in bacteria, leading to a secondary bacterial pneumonia. Inhaling acid material from the stomach can also cause chemical damage.

Aspiration pneumonia is easily treated with antibiotics; if it is not treated, it can progress to a serious life-threatening illness. If you have aspiration pneumonia, your doctor may perform tests to check your swallowing reflex in order to diagnose and treat any problem and thus prevent further episodes of aspiration pneumonia.

Preventing Pneumonia:
Vaccines for Pneumonia and Influenza

Because pneumonia has many potential causes, such as viruses, bacteria, or fungi, it is impossible to immunize against all of them with a single vaccine. However, there is a vaccine against the most common form, pneumococcal pneumonia, which is caused by *Streptococcus pneumoniae*.

The vaccine is primarily given to people who are more likely to develop life-threatening pneumonia. Most likely to benefit from the pneumococcal pneumonia vaccine include those who:

■ Are over age 60

■ Have serious lung disease

■ Are over 50 and abuse alcohol

■ Have one of the following conditions or live in the same household as someone with these conditions (you get immunized to prevent giving an infection to the person with the condition):

  □ Cancer

  □ Human immunodeficiency virus (HIV) infection

  □ Treatment to suppress the immune system because of organ transplantation

  □ Kidney disease

  □ Liver disease

  □ Blood disease

  □ Diabetes

  □ Persistent lung problems (such as chronic bronchitis, pneumonia, or tuberculosis)

  □ Spleen removed

Because the influenza virus also can cause pneumonia, getting a flu vaccine is another important part of preventing pneumonia. The influenza vaccine is changed each year (and a new shot is required each year) to fight the anticipated strains of influenza virus. It is recommended that a flu shot be given each year to adults who:

■ Are age 50 or older

■ Live in a long-term care institution, regardless of their age

■ Have diabetes mellitus; chronic disease of the heart, lungs, liver, or kidneys; or certain blood disorders

■ Have a weakened immune system due to HIV/AIDS or treatments that weaken the immune system

■ Are women who will be pregnant during influenza season

■ Health workers or others who are in close contact with people at risk for serious influenza

■ Anyone else who wants to reduce their chance of catching influenza

Flu shots prevent or lessen the symptoms of influenza but do not prevent colds or other mild viral illnesses that are sometimes called "the flu." By preventing influenza, you also prevent a predisposition to get bacterial pneumonia along with the influenza.

---

very serious form of pneumonia that can be resistant to many antibiotics.

VIRAL PNEUMONIA

Many cases of pneumonia, particularly in younger and healthier people, are caused by viruses. One of the most common and best known viruses is the influenza virus, the virus that causes "the flu."

Some viruses cause pneumo-

nia only infrequently, but the pneumonia they cause is very severe. An example is the varicella-zoster virus, which causes chickenpox; it causes pneumonia mainly in adults. There are antiviral drugs that can help treat this form of pneumonia.

Another severe form of viral pneumonia is caused by the hantavirus (see Hantavirus Pulmonary Syndrome, p.501), for which antiviral drugs have not

clearly been shown to be effective.

Viral pneumonia causes the typical symptoms of pneumonia (see p.496). The cough usually does not produce phlegm. Most cases of viral pneumonia last only a week or so, although it may be several weeks before you feel completely healthy.

On occasion, a lung weakened by viral pneumonia becomes more easily infected by bacteria (a condition called "bacterial superinfection"). This happens most often with pneumonia caused by the influenza virus. Such bacterial superinfections can produce severe illness.

MYCOPLASMAL PNEUMONIA

Mycoplasma pneumoniae, the microorganism that causes mycoplasmal pneumonia, is different from bacteria or viruses but can be treated with antibiotics. It is a very common cause of pneumonia, particularly in teenagers and young adults, although it can affect people of all ages.

Mycoplasmal pneumonia is most common in the late summer and early fall but can occur any time of year. The infection usually starts as a sore throat for 1 or 2 days and is followed by a cough and fever. You may also have a bad headache. Mycoplasmal pneumonia is highly contagious.

Current diagnostic tests for *M pneumoniae* are not very accurate and do not give results promptly. For this reason, doctors usually make the diagnosis and begin treatment based only on a physical examination. Usually, mycoplasmal infections respond to antibiotic treatment, both with erythromycin and related macrolide antibiotics and with tetracycline and quinolone antibiotics. However, even after starting antibiotics, your cough may persist for several days or even weeks.

CHLAMYDIAL PNEUMONIA

Chlamydia pneumoniae is a microorganism that is different from bacteria, viruses, or mycoplasma but can be treated with antibiotics. It is related to, but

Should Healthy Young Adults Get Flu Shots?: Dr Sax's Advice

I agree with the official recommendations for who should get flu shots, but I think there is increasing evidence that flu shots should be recommended for most healthy young adults as well.

Flu shots are very safe; you may feel a little aching in the area of the shot for a few days. However, studies have shown that you are no more likely to feel weak, tired, or sick than people who get a placebo shot. One study found that healthy young adults who get flu shots have more than 40% fewer sick days and doctor visits for respiratory infections in the months following the shot than people who do not get a flu shot.

By preventing influenza, you also prevent a predisposition to getting bacterial pneumonia on top of the influenza. So, although it's not yet the official recommendation, I and a growing number of doctors recommend an annual flu shot for most healthy young adults.

PAUL SAX, MD
BRIGHAM AND WOMEN'S HOSPITAL
HARVARD MEDICAL SCHOOL

different from, the kind of chlamydia that causes genital infections (see p.892).

People of all ages can acquire it but young and middle-aged adults are most commonly affected. The infected person may remain ill for 1 to 2 weeks. There are no widely available diagnostic tests for chlamydia. Treatment with erythromycin, other macrolide antibiotics, tetracycline, or quinolone antibiotics usually cures the infection.

PNEUMONIA IN PEOPLE WITH IMPAIRED IMMUNE SYSTEMS

A number of conditions can seriously injure the immune system: infection with the human immunodeficiency virus (HIV) with or without full-blown acquired immunodeficiency syndrome (AIDS), undergoing cancer chemotherapy or radiation, taking corticosteroids, and taking immunosuppressive drugs (usually after organ transplantation).

People with HIV infection often get bacterial pneumonia, but they also get an unusual fungal infection called *Pneumocystis carinii* pneumonia (PCP), along with infection with other fungi. PCP usually produces pneumonia of a gradual onset, with significant shortness of breath and a dry cough.

People with cancer, especially those being treated with corticosteroid drugs (see p.895), are also more prone to PCP and fungus infection.

Diagnosing pneumonia in people with impaired immune systems can be challenging because the symptoms may or may not include fever, and the cough is usually dry.

Hantavirus Pulmonary Syndrome

Hantavirus pulmonary syndrome is an uncommon but very serious type of pneumonia (lung infection) caused by the hantavirus, a virus transmitted by the droppings and urine of infected rodents, most often deer mice.

Infection is most common among people who live in the southwestern United States, but it has occurred in more than 20 states, mostly in the western and northeastern parts of the United States.

The infection begins with fever, headache, muscle aches, cough, dizziness, and shortness of breath. Sometimes gastrointestinal symptoms (such as nausea and vomiting) occur. Infected people then experience a rapid heart rate, low blood pressure, and lung symptoms such as cough, fluid in the lungs, and pain, which leads rapidly to shock (see p.645) and respiratory failure (inability to breathe). About half the people who acquire hantavirus die of it.

If you live in an area where the hantavirus has been found, it is particularly important to take preventive measures against getting the syndrome, including disinfecting all areas in your home that mice or mouse droppings could have touched and preventing mice from entering your home by patching holes and other entryways.

Call your local public health office or the Centers for Disease Control and Prevention (CDC) (see p.1238) for more prevention information.

Legionnaires Disease

Legionnaires disease is a type of pneumonia (infection of the lungs) caused by a genus of bacterium called legionella—because the first recorded outbreak of the disease killed 29 people at an American Legion convention in 1976.

However, it is now known that the bacterium has been affecting people for many years; it has been identified in autopsy specimens of people who died of pneumonia many years ago.

People acquire this bacterium from contaminated water, not from a person who has the infection. The bacterium is found in most water supplies but is usually kept under control by chlorination. It can multiply in plumbing systems where water pools (such as in showerheads) and in large, water-cooled air-conditioners.

Symptoms appear about 1 week after infection. Sudden weakness, headache, and sore muscles are typically followed by abdominal pain, diarrhea, sore throat, and dry cough. Over the next few days, fever, chills, drowsiness, breathing difficulties, and delirium may develop, and some people cough up thick phlegm (sputum). Like other types of pneumonia, the illness gets worse unless it is treated.

Pneumonia caused by legionella is often severe, and affected people often require hospitalization. It cannot be definitely diagnosed by symptoms and a physical examination alone; a diagnosis is made from tests on a sample of sputum, blood, or urine. Because test results may take several days to come back, your doctor may treat you for Legionnaires disease before the diagnosis is known for certain.

Treatment is with antibiotics, most often erythromycin, azithromycin, or a fluoroquinolone antibiotic initially given intravenously in high doses; later you can take the antibiotics by mouth.

SARS

Severe acute respiratory syndrome (SARS) is a newly defined infectious disease that emerged from China. It became evident in 2003 and rapidly spread around much of the world. A remarkable, international cooperative research effort involving the latest scientific technology, and using the Internet to instantly communicate information, led to the discovery of the cause of SARS in just a few weeks—a modern medical triumph.

SARS is caused by a coronavirus. It seems to be spread to humans from an animal reservoir. In China, one reservoir is an animal called the civet. Human-to-human transmission is common and it is likely that contaminated water may cause transmission also.

People who develop SARS have high fever, pneumonia, kidney damage, and other abnormalities. About 10% have died. No antibiotic or antiviral agent has been proven effective so far. Therefore, when a case is suspected, the patient is quarantined. In 2003, the city of Toronto quarantined itself from outsiders for several weeks. This most extraordinary event shows how serious SARS is. Much work is currently being done to develop a vaccine, and to find effective antiviral therapies.

Pneumonia from Bioterrorism

Bioterrorism has become a concern in many parts of the world. The deliberate release of highly infectious biological agents, such as anthrax and plague, has caused pneumonia and death. There currently is a vaccine for anthrax. The U.S. government has recommended that it be given to emergency health care workers and other citizens who would be involved in the first lines of defense against such an attack. There are antibiotics that treat anthrax, but they must be started at the first sign of symptoms in order to be optimally effective. (Other potential bioterrorism agents include Ebola virus and the Marburg virus, which cause hemorrhagic fevers. These latter agents affect multiple organ systems and have a high mortality rate.)

Pleurisy

Pleurisy is inflammation of the two membranes (pleura) that cover the lungs and line the chest wall. Healthy lung membranes are lubricated and slide easily over each other as you breathe in and out. In pleurisy, inflammation makes the membranes rub against each other, causing a sharp pain when you breathe in deeply.

The pain is usually focused on one spot in the chest but sometimes is felt in the shoulder.

Pleurisy often is a complication of pneumonia (see p.496) when the lung inflammation

Percussion

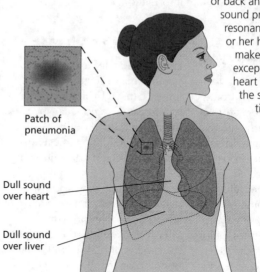

Patch of pneumonia

Dull sound over heart

Dull sound over liver

In percussion, your doctor taps your chest or back and listens to the quality of sound produced and feels the resonance of the sound with his or her hand. A healthy lung makes a resonant sound except in the areas over the heart and upper liver, where the sound is dulled by normal tissue. A dull sound in any other part of the lung indicates that fluid has collected in the area, such as from pneumonia or a pleural effusion.

caused by the pneumonia extends out to affect the pleura. It also can be caused by a viral infection of the pleura or by other inflammatory conditions such as systemic lupus erythematosus (see p.898) or a blood clot in a lung (see p.512).

Antibiotics are prescribed if the inflammation is caused by an underlying bacterial infection; anti-inflammatory pain medicines are prescribed if the cause is not a bacterial infection.

Lung Abscess

A lung abscess occurs when infection destroys lung tissue, creating a cavity that contains fluid with bacteria, pus, and lung tissue. An abscess is often caused by inhaling material contaminated with bacteria that live around the teeth. This occurs most often in people who are bedridden; are under general anesthesia; have had a stroke, seizure, or other loss of con-

sciousness; have problems swallowing; or are abusers of alcohol or other drugs.

A lung abscess can also form when infection develops behind a blocked air passage. In adults, the blockage is most often caused by a tumor. Children sometimes inhale objects that block the air passages; this can be detected by computed tomography (see p.149) or bronchoscopy (see p.495).

Symptoms include fever, a cough that produces blood- or pus-containing phlegm (sputum), or, more rarely, chills. If a foreign object has been inhaled, bronchoscopy can be performed to remove it, after which antibiotics are required to clear up the infection; 4 to 6 weeks of treatment may be required.

Bronchiectasis

Bronchiectasis is a lung condition in which the airways (bronchi) that connect the windpipe to the lungs are weakened by years of recurring bacterial infections; the infections usually occur during childhood.

The weakened walls of the bronchi cause them to form little balloonlike sacs that look like clusters of grapes attached to the bronchi. These little sacs are a breeding ground for bacteria.

Though rarely fatal, bronchiectasis is a common cause of recurring respiratory infections in adults, often in the same part of the lung. The first symptoms often occur after a person has apparently recovered from bronchitis, pneumonia, or another lung infection. A persistent cough may develop that produces copious quantities of foul-smelling phlegm. A chest x-ray (see p.145) and computed tomography (see p.149) can confirm the diagnosis.

Samples of phlegm help identify which microorganisms are causing the infection. Treatment includes antibiotics and physical therapy to drain pus out of the sacs in the bronchi. In severe cases, surgery may be necessary to remove damaged areas of the lung.

Fungal Infections

Fungal infections of the lungs are caused by inhaling the spores of a variety of fungi that live in the world around you (you cannot catch a fungal infection of the lungs from another person). Healthy people inhale fungus spores all the time, and the spores are usually destroyed by the immune system.

In people whose immune systems are compromised, however, the spores can survive and reproduce, causing pneumonia and also sometimes spreading to the bloodstream and causing severe fungal infections elsewhere in the body.

If your doctor suspects a fungal infection in the lungs, he or she will examine a sample of your phlegm (sputum) and may have a lung specialist perform a lung biopsy or bronchoscopy (see p.495) to identify the causative fungus and determine the proper treatment.

The fungal infections that most commonly cause pneumonia are aspergillosis, coccidioidomycosis, cryptococcosis, and histoplasmosis. Each of them causes somewhat different symptoms.

Aspergillosis is caused by inhaling spores of aspergillus fungi, which are widely present in the environment, mostly in decaying material such as dead leaves and old building materials. Aspergillosis, which occurs most often in people who have impaired immune systems, often starts out with symptoms of fever, cough (sometimes with blood in the phlegm), and breathlessness.

The aspergillus fungus can also infect a lung cavity in a person with a healthy immune system. If this happens, the fungus grows into a ball that fills the cavity.

Treatment is with intravenous antifungal drugs. Lung surgery often is required to remove the fungus ball.

Other people develop an allergic reaction to the fungus, with coughing and wheezing that requires treatment with corticosteroid drugs (see p.895) such as prednisone.

Coccidioidomycosis is caused by inhaling spores of the fungus *Coccidioides immitis*, which lives mainly in desert environments of Arizona, New Mexico, and the central valley of California. Symptoms include fever, a dry cough, aching, chest pain, weight loss, and skin rash. Most people recover with no permanent damage to their lungs, but in some the infection spreads to the brain, causing chronic meningitis (see p.377). Treatment is with antifungal drugs.

Cryptococcosis is a relatively rare infection caused by inhaling the fungus *Cryptococcus neoformans*. This fungus is found in pigeon droppings and in soil worldwide. Most infections with cryptococcosis occur in people with impaired immune systems, especially people with acquired immunodeficiency syndrome (see p.872).

You may have flulike symptoms, chest pain, shortness of breath, weight loss, or a phlegm-producing cough. The infection commonly spreads to the fluid surrounding the brain, causing meningitis (see p.377). Treatment is with antifungal drugs.

Histoplasmosis is caused by inhaling the fungus *Histoplasma capsulatum* from soil or other areas that have been contaminated by the droppings of birds or bats. Symptoms include a mild cough, chest pain, and (sometimes) aching joints. If you have a healthy immune system, your body will fight off the infection within about 2 weeks, but tiny scars on the lungs, which can be seen on a chest x-ray, are common.

Some people are susceptible to a long-term form of histoplasmosis in which serious lung dis-

Cough Medicines:
Dr Fanta's Advice

Q When should I take a cough syrup?

A It's fine to take a nonprescription cough syrup when you have a minor cough, particularly one that interferes with sleep. But when you have had a cough for at least 2 weeks, or if the cough is producing yellow-green material, you should contact your doctor, and not simply use a cough syrup. You may have a more serious condition that the cough syrup will hide but not cure.

Q What kind of cough syrup should I use?

A Use an over-the-counter cough syrup that contains guaifenesin (to loosen thick airway secretions) and/or dextromethorphan (5 to 30 milligrams per dose) to suppress your cough. If you have nasal congestion, use one that also has an antihistamine or a decongestant. If you have pain (such as from a sore throat or sinus congestion), use one that also has acetaminophen.

CHRISTOPHER H. FANTA, MD
BRIGHAM AND WOMEN'S HOSPITAL
HARVARD MEDICAL SCHOOL

ease develops. For the severe form, antifungal drugs are prescribed. Most people with the mild form do not require treatment.

Tuberculosis

Tuberculosis (TB) is an infectious and potentially life-threatening bacterial infection caused by *Mycobacterium tuberculosis*. TB once was incurable but, in the 1950s, effective antibiotics were developed and the number of cases of TB dropped by 75%. Public health officials projected that TB could be eradicated from the United States by the year 2010.

However, in an unexpected reversal of this trend, the incidence of TB took an upturn in 1985. This was largely due to the spread of TB in people with the human immunodeficiency virus (HIV) or acquired immunodeficiency syndrome (AIDS). People with HIV or AIDS are especially vulnerable to TB, and can readily transmit it to others, including people with healthy immune systems.

Increased public health efforts have caused the number of TB cases once again to fall. However, in developing countries, TB is still a huge problem that is made worse by the global AIDS epidemic. TB is one of the most common causes of death in the world.

TB is very contagious. It is spread primarily when people with active lung disease expel bacteria from their lungs into the air through coughing. Other people breathe the infectious droplets into their lungs, where the bacteria land and begin to multiply.

Although it is relatively easy to catch the bacteria that cause TB, in most people the lung infection is short-lived because the immune system contains it. In a few people, however, a serious pneumonia called progressive primary TB develops shortly after the initial infection. This infection can spread to the lymph glands, into the bloodstream, and throughout the body.

In all people who become infected with TB, some bacteria lie dormant in the lungs for many years; the immune system has contained them, but not eliminated them. In about 5% to 10% of these people, the bacteria become active again, causing pneumonia and sometimes spreading elsewhere in the body.

This is called secondary TB (or reactivation TB). Secondary TB is more common than primary TB and tends to occur as people's immune systems become weakened (such as from developing a chronic illness, or from aging).

In addition to people infected with HIV, other people susceptible to TB include those living in crowded conditions—such as dormitories, shelters, prisons, or nursing homes—and health care workers who are in prolonged or close contact with people who have TB.

Also at risk are those who are chronically malnourished, including homeless people, alcoholics, people whose immune systems are suppressed for other reasons (such as those taking corticosteroid drugs), and some elderly people. The elderly represent 25% of those who have TB today.

SYMPTOMS

A nagging cough is a prominent symptom of TB, along with fatigue and weakness, unexplained weight loss, loss of appetite, persistent low-grade fever, sweating at night, chest pain, and blood-stained phlegm.

DIAGNOSIS

Diagnostic tests are used to determine if you have ever been infected with the TB bacterium; other tests are used to see if you have an active infection with TB. TB skin tests, chest x-rays, and examination of samples of phlegm (to see if they contain TB bacteria) are commonly performed.

TB skin tests can determine if you have ever been infected with the TB bacterium but they cannot tell you if you have an active infection. In a skin test, a small amount of protein extracted from killed TB bacteria is injected under the skin of your forearm. The test result is positive if a small bump forms at this site over the next 2 to 3 days.

People with positive skin test results who do not have an active infection are not contagious to others. If you have a positive skin test result, your doctor may suggest you take the antibiotic isoniazid to decrease the chance that you will develop active disease.

This is particularly true if you are under 35 years old, if you have diabetes or another condition that impairs the immune system, or if you previously had a negative skin test result but

recently have had a positive test result.

Chest x-rays can reveal scars in the lungs and lymph nodes of the chest that suggest you may have been infected with TB in the past. Occasionally, the scars are difficult to distinguish from cancer, and further tests are required. A chest x-ray can also show signs of an active TB infection.

Samples of phlegm can be examined for the TB bacterium itself. If the bacterium is in your phlegm, you have an active infection and can transmit that infection to others when you cough. The sputum is usually cultured (see p.159) to see if TB bacteria grow.

If these common tests do not give an answer, your doctor may perform a bronchoscopy (see p.495) to remove a tiny sample of lung tissue for analysis.

TREATMENT OPTIONS

Most people can be cured by taking a combination of at least three different antibiotics every day for 6 months or longer. The

mainstays of therapy, usually given at the same time, include isoniazid, rifampin, pyrazinamide, and rifapentine. When these drugs fail, others such as ethambutol and streptomycin are sometimes added to the mix. Sometimes as many as four drugs are given at once.

Stopping your medicines early—or taking them only occasionally—causes serious problems. First, it increases the chances of a relapse. Second, it sets the stage for drug-resistant bacteria to develop in your body. The problem of drug resistance (a state in which microorganisms are no longer killed by once-effective antimicrobial drugs) is on the rise. Some TB bacteria currently in circulation are resistant to virtually all the antibiotics that once killed TB; this is called multi–drug-resistant TB.

Asthma

Asthma is an inflammatory disorder of the airways that is marked by recurring bouts of breathless-

---

What Happens in Allergic Asthma?

About 90% of children and 50% to 70% of adults who have asthma have allergic asthma. In allergic asthma, the allergen (allergy-causing substance) is breathed into the lungs, where it attaches to an antibody called immunoglobulin E (IgE) that is on the surface of mast cells in the lung.

This attachment causes mast cells to explode, releasing irritating substances (including histamine and leukotrienes) that make blood vessels dilate, stimulate glands to produce mucus, and cause bronchial tubes to tighten. The result is the coughing, breathlessness, and wheezing that are characteristic of asthma.

These reactions are controlled by immune system chemicals called cytokines. Blocking the cytokines, particularly one called IL-13, is a promising but unproven approach to treatment.

How Airways Narrow in Asthma

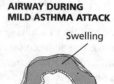

HEALTHY AIRWAY

Smooth muscle

Airway

Normal mucous lining

AIRWAY DURING MILD ASTHMA ATTACK

Swelling

Mucus

Muscle contraction

AIRWAY DURING SEVERE ASTHMA ATTACK

Mucus

Inflammation

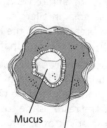

In a healthy airway (left), the passageway is unrestricted and airflow is normal. During a mild asthma attack (center), the airway walls thicken with inflammation and muscles in the walls contract, narrowing the airways. The airways also begin to fill with mucus, further interfering with the flow of air. Wheezing and coughing develop as airflow deteriorates. During a severe asthma attack (right), the combination of wall thickening and increased mucus in the airway can block airflow severely.

ness and wheezing. The symptoms are caused when the breathing tubes of the lungs clamp down and fill up with sticky mucus, making it harder to move air in and out of the lungs.

Asthma affects an estimated 15 million Americans, almost a third of whom are children. Despite the availability of more effective and safer treatments, asthma and asthma-related deaths have increased dramatically over the past 20 years.

Doctors and researchers do not fully understand what causes asthma. Factors in the environment (see Common Triggers of Asthma, p.507), especially allergies, play an important role. In addition, people with asthma are probably born with a genetic tendency to develop an allergic reaction when allergens enter the airways (bronchi) of the lungs.

In children, asthma tends to improve as years go by, either clearing up completely or at least becoming less burdensome. In some people, the damage caused by severe asthma in childhood can leave permanent effects in the lungs. Lung capacity is reduced by about 10% in adults who had severe asthma as children.

Sometimes asthma begins only later in life, in your 40s or 50s. Some doctors think that this kind of later-life asthma may have different causes and a worse prognosis than childhood asthma, but there is no strong evidence of this.

SYMPTOMS

The main symptoms of asthma are cough, breathlessness, and wheezing. An asthma attack can come on at any time, day or night. Asthma is mild in some people and life-threatening in others, marked by periods of wheezing and coughing that can

Preventing Asthma Attacks

Prevention is extremely important in avoiding the triggers that can cause an asthma attack. Follow these suggestions:

Take precautions before exercise Exercise-induced asthma can often be prevented by breathing warm, humidified air while you exercise. Medications are also effective. See Treating Exercise-Induced Asthma (p.507).

Inhale steam Open your airways by inhaling the warm mist from a hot shower or bath or by placing a towel over your head while inhaling the steam from a pot of hot water. Inhaling steam can also help prevent an asthma attack.

Avoid pollutants Do not smoke and avoid secondhand smoke. Prohibit smoking in your home and patronize restaurants that ban it. Other environmental pollutants can be more difficult to escape. Listen to the news for air-quality reports, and minimize the time you spend outdoors when pollution and ozone levels are high.

Eliminate allergens Eliminating allergens (see p.463) from your home or workplace is very important.

Common Triggers of Asthma

Some common triggers of asthma include:

ALLERGENS

■ Cockroaches and tiny insects called dust mites (see p.463)

■ Feathers, molds, animal dander and saliva, or pollen

■ Foods, particularly those containing sulfites (widely used in wine, beer, salad bars, and dried fruits), or coloring dyes such as tartrazine

STRENUOUS EXERCISE

■ Especially in cold, dry air

POLLUTED OR COLD AIR

■ Outdoor air pollution

■ Wood or tobacco smoke

■ Indoor pollutants such as fumes from dry cleaning, new carpeting, cleaning products (particularly mixing bleach and ammonia), and wood-refinishing products

MEDICINES

■ Aspirin and other nonsteroidal anti-inflammatory drugs such as ibuprofen or indomethacin

■ Beta blockers

■ Cholinergic drugs used to promote bladder contraction and in eyedrops for glaucoma (see p.435)

VIRAL RESPIRATORY TRACT INFECTIONS

■ The flu

■ The common cold

OCCUPATIONAL SUBSTANCES

■ Metal salts

■ Wood or vegetable dusts

■ Some solvents or plastics

STRESS OR EMOTIONAL UPSET

■ Can also worsen an impending asthma attack (see Alternative Medicine: Asthma, p.511)

Treating Exercise-Induced Asthma

Most people with asthma occasionally have an asthma attack while exercising, particularly in cold, dry air. Even many people who do not have asthma cough and wheeze a bit when exercising in cold, dry air. The wheezing often develops not while a person is exercising but several minutes after stopping.

Exercise-induced asthma can often be prevented by breathing warm, humidified air while you exercise. Use a heated indoor pool or gym during cold weather and allergy season, walk in an indoor mall, or exercise at home. In addition, the following medicines are effective:

Inhaled corticosteroids In people with asthma, the regular use of inhaled corticosteroids often reduces or eliminates exercise-induced wheezing. However,

inhaling corticosteroids before you exercise (without using them on a regular basis) does not help.

Inhaled beta$_2$-agonists Inhale albuterol 15 minutes before exercising.

Cromolyn sodium and nedocromil Inhale either of these medicines 15 minutes before exercising.

Montelukast Taking the leukotriene antagonist montelukast once daily provides relief for many people, but does not work for everyone.

For people who spend many hours outside exercising each day (a reality for many children with asthma), repeated treatments with albuterol, cromolyn, or nedocromil may be necessary. If this proves to be difficult, then using montelukast or the longer-acting beta$_2$-agonist salmeterol is preferred.

Treating Asthma

Asthma treatment has four components: assessment, medication, environmental control measures, and education:

ASSESSMENT

Assessment is the use of objective measures of lung function (including lung capacity and lung volume) to gauge the severity of asthma and to monitor the course of treatment. Periodic examinations, performed in the doctor's office and at home, can help track general trends and predict a downward decline over several months. Many doctors recommend that people take an active part in monitoring their own lung function with a simple device called a peak flow meter (see p.509).

MEDICATION

Medication can prevent and reverse inflammation and treat narrowed airways. Medicines for long-term control help achieve and maintain a better level of lung function and decrease recurring attacks of asthma. Medications for quick relief treat attacks of breathlessness or wheezing and include anti-inflammatories (such as corticosteroids, leukotriene antagonists, and cromolyn sodium and nedocromil), bronchodilators (such as beta$_2$-agonists and methylxanthines), and immunotherapy.

Anti-inflammatories include the following:

■ *Corticosteroids* (see p.895), in tablet or liquid form, are used to treat flare-ups of asthma until lung function is normalized. Inhaled corticosteroids are reserved for day-to-day treatment. Potential adverse effects (which primarily occur with oral corticosteroids) include suppression of the immune system, weight gain, high blood pressure, cataracts, weakening of bones (see Osteoporosis, p.596), muscle weakness, and swelling. Inhaled corticosteroids can cause candidiasis of the mouth (see p.488), but do not usually cause the complications of corticosteroids taken by mouth.

■ *Cromolyn sodium and nedocromil* are used to prevent (rather than treat) attacks of asthma caused by allergies. You use these agents if you know you were exposed to something that will predictably trigger an attack.

■ *Leukotriene antagonists* are a newer class of anti-inflammatory drug. They work by reducing inflammation in the airways and by producing relaxation of

the muscle that lines the airways. Since they are newer medicines, their optimal use is still being determined. They have been useful in treating people with mild asthma, asthma triggered by exercise, and those with severe asthma that responds only to corticosteroid drugs because they reduce the need for daily corticosteroid pills.

Bronchodilators are designed to open the airways by relaxing the smooth muscle of the bronchi. The two types of bronchodilators are:

■ *Beta$_2$-agonists* are adrenalinelike drugs that relax the smooth muscle of the airways. They can be taken in tablet or liquid form; by injection (for emergencies); or by inhalation (for acute flare-ups and to prevent exercise-induced asthma) via metered-dose inhalers, dry-powder capsules, or compressor-driven nebulizers (see p.510).

■ *Methylxanthines* are a class of drugs that include theophylline, which is used primarily to treat difficult-to-control asthma or to treat people who cannot tolerate other medicines. Long-acting theophylline provides 24-hour control and is sometimes used along with beta$_2$-agonists for extra control. Side effects may include stomach pain, nausea, vomiting, insomnia, and nervousness. There are also many drugs that adversely interact with theophylline-type medicines.

Immunotherapy involves injecting small amounts of allergens to create a tolerance or resistance to allergens that trigger asthma flare-ups. The amount of the allergen is increased over time to reduce or eliminate allergy symptoms. A new class of agents inhibits the release of leukotrienes and thus interrupts the inflammatory process that causes asthma.

ENVIRONMENTAL CONTROL MEASURES

Environmental control measures help you prevent or abolish factors that bring on asthma flare-ups (see Preventing Asthma Attacks, p.506).

EDUCATION

Education about your disease can improve your quality of life or even save your life. Become aware of the factors that trigger your asthma attacks, the medicines available, and the educational resources (such as the American Lung Association, see p.1236) that can keep you informed of the most recent innovations.

Benefits of Inhaled Corticosteroids for Asthma

Flare-ups of asthma can often be prevented with treatment. Inhaled corticosteroids are preferred over corticosteroids taken as pills for preventing asthma because they produce fewer serious side effects.

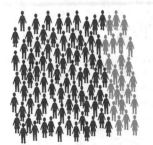

78 OF 100 PEOPLE WHO HAVE MODERATE TO SEVERE ASTHMA AND DO NOT INHALE CORTICOSTEROIDS HAVE FLARE-UPS OF ASTHMA WITHIN 2 MONTHS

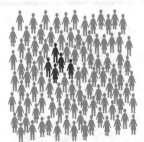

5 OF 100 PEOPLE WHO HAVE MODERATE TO SEVERE ASTHMA AND INHALE CORTICOSTEROIDS HAVE FLARE-UPS OF ASTHMA WITHIN 2 MONTHS

lead to sudden, severe difficulty breathing. In some people, one attack of asthma may be mild, while the next attack may be severe. You can often hear your own wheezing, and a doctor can almost always hear it with a stethoscope.

A moderate or severe asthma attack is frightening. You cannot breathe. Partly because of the fear and partly because you are working so much harder to breathe, other symptoms develop, including rapid heartbeat, sweating, and light-headedness.

In between asthma attacks you may feel perfectly normal or have some degree of limitation. You may suffer from extended colds and flu, be particularly vulnerable to bronchitis (see p.494), or become easily winded after normal physical activity or exercise.

TREATMENT OPTIONS

If you experience attacks of wheezing and breathlessness, see your doctor. Even if the attacks you have had are mild, it is important to see your doctor to prevent more severe attacks. A primary care doctor can take care of most people with asthma, though some people are referred to a lung specialist or an allergist.

A diagnosis of asthma is usually not difficult to make, particularly if you are having a moderately severe attack. Your physician will examine your chest, airways, and skin; listen for wheezing; and watch your muscles contract as you breathe. Most likely, several tests will be performed.

The forced expiratory volume in 1 second (FEV_1) test measures how much air you can exhale in 1 second. The peak flow test (see Using a Peak Flow Meter, p.510) measures how forcefully you can exhale; during this procedure, you will exhale forcibly through a mouthpiece connected to a machine.

Normal FEV_1 and peak flow values can be determined based on your age and height. In people with asthma, the values are lower because expiration is slowed by narrowed airways.

The amount of oxygen in your blood may be measured, either with a device called an oximeter that attaches to your finger or by taking a sample of blood from an artery (which also can test the amount of carbon dioxide and acid in your blood).

Benefits of Self-Monitoring for Asthma Using a Peak Flow Meter

People with asthma who monitor themselves daily with a peak flow meter have better control of their asthma.

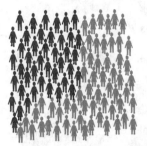

42 OF 100 PEOPLE WHO HAVE ASTHMA AND DO NOT MONITOR THEIR PEAK FLOWS AT HOME REQUIRE DAYS OFF FROM WORK WITHIN 4 MONTHS

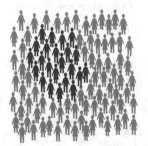

23 OF 100 PEOPLE WHO HAVE ASTHMA AND MONITOR THEIR PEAK FLOWS AT HOME REQUIRE DAYS OFF FROM WORK WITHIN 4 MONTHS

You may also be asked to cough up a sample of phlegm for examination. In addition, blood tests may be performed to determine whether you have signs of allergies (as reflected by an increase in the quantity of specific white blood cells called eosinophils) or of infection (as reflected by an increase in the number of white blood cells called neutrophils).

If you are seeing your doctor for the first time about the possibility that you have asthma (but you are not currently having an asthma attack), he or she will ask you about your symptoms, their severity, the factors that trigger them, and how often they occur.

You may be asked to keep a diary of your asthma symptoms and to record where and when your asthma attacks occur, such as during work (suggesting substances at work), in the spring (suggesting pollen), or at home at night (implicating feathers or dust mites in your bed). You may be asked to regularly measure your own breathing at home with a handheld peak flow meter.

ALLERGY TESTING

If your allergies are severe and difficult to control, your doctor may recommend testing for specific allergies. To identify allergies that may be causing your asthma, a blood test called the radioallergosorbent test (RAST) (see p.157) may be performed to identify antibodies to specific allergens.

Allergy skin testing, also called patch testing, may be used to identify specific allergens that you should avoid. In this test, a variety of allergens is administered either by pricking the skin with the allergen or by applying the allergen to a patch that is taped to the skin for several days. A raised, red patch of skin (wheal) indicates sensitivity to a particular allergen.

USING A PEAK FLOW METER

One measure of asthma severity is the peak expiratory flow rate. It is determined using a peak flow meter—a simple, portable, and inexpensive device that you can use at home to take daily

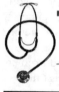

Asthma: *When You Visit Your Doctor*

QUESTIONS TO DISCUSS WITH YOUR DOCTOR:

- How is your breathing? Do you currently feel short of breath?

- How often have your asthma symptoms interfered with your functioning?

- How often have you used each of your inhalers since your last visit?

- Do you feel your medicines are helping you?

- Have symptoms improved or worsened since your last visit?

- Have you had to go to an emergency department or urgent care center since your last visit?

- What have your peak flow readings been since your last visit?

- Do you feel you know how to use your inhaler and peak flow meter?

- Has your asthma had a financial or personal impact on you? If yes, how so?

YOUR DOCTOR MIGHT EXAMINE THE FOLLOWING FUNCTIONS AND BODY SYSTEMS:

- Vital signs (by taking your temperature, blood pressure, pulse, or respiratory rate)

- Nose, ears, and throat

- Lymph nodes in the neck

- Chest and lungs

- Heart

YOUR DOCTOR MIGHT ORDER THE FOLLOWING LAB TESTS OR STUDIES:

- Peak flow (see p.495) or spirometry

- Immunoglobulin E (IgE)

- Radioallergosorbent test (RAST) (see p.157)

- Eosinophil count (a blood test)

Alternative Medicine: *Asthma*

Medicines are just one way to improve breathing during an asthma attack. Breathing exercises, biofeedback, the relaxation response, and hypnosis can help you learn to relax and control your breathing. The techniques described here should not be used as a substitute for your inhaler if you take medicine. Discuss the best combination of drugs and alternative therapies with your doctor.

Breathing exercises help you relax and breathe more effectively. When you relax your breathing, many body systems relax (including your mental state), which can be valuable if you respond to an asthma attack with fear and anxiety. Becoming anxious can set in motion physical effects that can further constrict your airways. Practice these exercises daily and use them when you feel an asthma attack coming on:

1 Inhale gently but deeply so that your abdomen expands, and allow the expansion to continue up to your chest. As soon as you reach full capacity, inhale gently a bit more and exhale slowly to a count of five. The longer you exhale, the more relaxed you will become. Repeat five times.

2 Breathing normally, place one hand comfortably on your chest near your collarbone, and the other on your lower abdomen. Without changing your breathing pattern, simply note how you breathe for a minute or two. Then begin to breathe from your abdomen—that is, so that the hand over your abdomen moves more than the one on your chest. Continue with this relaxed breathing for as long as you like. Focus your concentration on the exhalation and on releasing tension.

Biofeedback (see p.395) uses a machine to measure the activity of certain body systems (such as the lungs) and to feed that information back to you so that you:

■ Become more aware of how your breath changes during different circumstances.

■ Learn ways to control your breathing.

■ Use these techniques during times of stress. It may be possible through biofeedback to relax your airways before an asthma attack, minimizing its effects.

The relaxation response is described on p.90.

Hypnosis (see p.394) is a technique that can help you focus your attention, rethink problems, and relax. For example, if your normal response to an impending asthma attack is fear and anxiety, hypnotherapy can help you substitute calming thoughts that may lessen the episode's severity.

---

measurements of your peak expiratory flow rate.

When you are in the middle of an asthma attack, it takes more time and medicine to return your lungs to normal function. By using a peak flow meter regularly, you may be able to avoid an attack by taking early action.

Peak flow is measured by inhaling deeply and then exhaling as forcibly as possible through the mouthpiece of the meter. Falling peak flow readings can provide early warning of the need to take your medicine or see your doctor. When you compare your readings with your ideal or normal peak flow level, you can determine how well-controlled your asthma is.

Your doctor may recommend that you first take measurements when you are feeling good and breathing well. This value will reflect your baseline or ideal level—the goal against which you can gauge the severity of your condition in the future. Measure your peak flow level daily.

Various levels are described here in terms of zones:

■ **Green zone** (80% to 100% of your ideal level) Your asthma is under good control and you probably are not experiencing symptoms. Take your medicines as usual.

■ **Yellow zone** (50% to less than 80% of your ideal level) Your asthma may not be under good day-to-day control. You may or may not have symptoms. Take your asthma medicine right away. Your doctor may recommend changes in your medicine.

■ **Red zone** (less than 50% of your ideal level) You are having an asthma attack. Take your medicine immediately. Contact your doctor or go to the nearest hospital emergency department.

USING INHALED ASTHMA MEDICINES

Inhalers and nebulizers are devices that deposit medicine directly into the lungs. Inhalers are used by almost anyone with asthma. Nebulizers are primarily used by people who have more severe asthma.

Learn to use your inhaler or nebulizer correctly. The goal of inhaler treatment is for all of the medicine you inhale to penetrate as deeply as possible into the lungs. If you use your inhaler incorrectly, much of the medicine can be lost in the air or deposited in your mouth, where it does no good.

Inhalers There are two types of inhalers: metered-dose inhalers (MDIs) and dry-powder inhalers (DPIs). When you press the top of an MDI canister, an aerosol spray containing the drug is released. With a DPI inhaler, a capsule containing a powdered form of the drug is placed between two prongs and is pierced when you press the top of the canister.

Spacers Spacers are tubes several inches long. You seal your lips around one end of the tube and the other end is connected to the inhaler. Using a spacer with your inhaler makes using an inhaler somewhat easier, and directs more of the medicine into your lungs. Spacers are particularly rec-

ommended for children and older adults, but anyone can use them. Talk to your doctor about whether you need a spacer.

Here are some tips on how to inhale properly:

- Exhale completely before pressing your inhaler.

- When you inhale, make sure you are inhaling through your mouth, not your nose.

- If you are not using a spacer, hold the inhaler 4 inches away from your mouth, and have your mouth wide open.

- If you are using a spacer, seal your lips around the spacer.

- Begin inhaling at exactly the same moment that you press the inhaler, and keep pressing the

---

How to Use a Metered Dose Inhaler

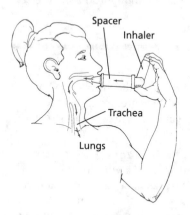

Before putting the inhaler in your mouth, exhale deeply once or twice to completely empty your lungs of air. With the inhaler in your mouth, start taking a deep breath while pressing down on the button at the top of the inhaler. This draws the medicine deep into your lungs. Hold your breath for 5 to 10 seconds to allow the medicine to settle in your lungs and then exhale.

Pulmonary Embolism

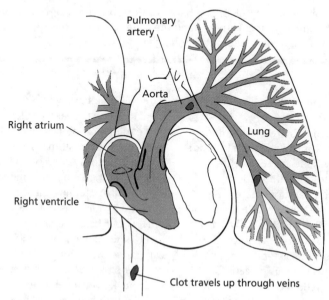

Clot travels up through veins

A pulmonary embolism is caused by a blood clot that lodges in the pulmonary arteries that supply the lung. Usually, the blood clot has formed in veins in the legs or pelvis, becomes dislodged, and travels in the veins up to the right side of the heart and then out into the arteries of the lung.

Benefits of Blood-Thinning Drugs for Blood Clots in the Legs

Blood clots in the deep veins of the legs (deep venous thromboses) are treated with blood thinners such as warfarin. Warfarin helps prevent blood clots from forming again and reduces the chance that a piece of clot will break free and travel to blood vessels in the lungs, causing a potentially fatal condition called pulmonary embolism. Six months of warfarin treatment is more beneficial than 3 months in people who have developed a blood clot. If you develop a second or third clot, treatment with warfarin is usually continued for the rest of your life. The main side effect of warfarin is bleeding. The risk of bleeding is higher with lifelong warfarin therapy than with short-term treatment.

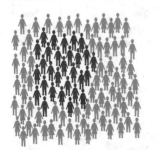

29 OF 100 PEOPLE WHO HAVE BLOOD CLOTS IN THEIR LEGS AND ARE NOT TREATED WITH WARFARIN DEVELOP A SECOND BLOOD CLOT

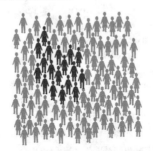

18 OF 100 PEOPLE WHO HAVE BLOOD CLOTS IN THEIR LEGS AND ARE TREATED WITH WARFARIN FOR 6 WEEKS DEVELOP A SECOND BLOOD CLOT

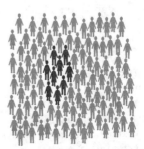

9 OF 100 PEOPLE WHO HAVE BLOOD CLOTS IN THEIR LEGS AND ARE TREATED WITH WARFARIN FOR 6 MONTHS DEVELOP A SECOND BLOOD CLOT

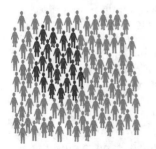

21 OF 100 PEOPLE WHO HAVE BEEN DIAGNOSED WITH A SECOND BLOOD CLOT AND TAKE WARFARIN FOR ONLY 6 ADDITIONAL MONTHS DEVELOP ANOTHER BLOOD CLOT

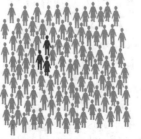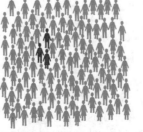

3 OF 100 PEOPLE WHO HAVE BEEN DIAGNOSED WITH A SECOND BLOOD CLOT AND TAKE WARFARIN ALL THEIR LIVES DEVELOP ANOTHER BLOOD CLOT

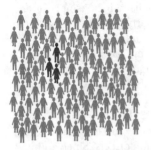

3 OF 100 PEOPLE WHO TAKE WARFARIN FOR ONLY 6 MONTHS HAVE A MAJOR BLEEDING EPISODE

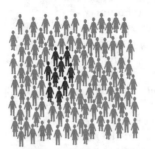

9 OF 100 PEOPLE WHO TAKE WARFARIN ALL THEIR LIVES HAVE A MAJOR BLEEDING EPISODE

inhaler until you have finished inhaling.

■ Inhale as slowly (take about 5 seconds) and as deeply as you can. Inhaling too rapidly or too shallowly will not deposit as much of the medicine into your lungs.

■ Press your inhaler only once while you are inhaling.

■ Continue to hold in your breath for 5 to 10 seconds, so that the medicine can deposit inside your lungs before you start exhaling.

■ If you are to take several puffs of the inhaler at a time, wait 1 minute between each puff to improve the penetration of the medicine.

Nebulizers Nebulizers are machines that deliver medicine as a spray (aerosol) through a face mask. The device consists of a mask, a chamber containing the drug, and a compressor pump. It is operated either by electricity or by hand. Activating the nebulizer sends air across the chamber that contains the medicine. The stream of air scatters the drug into a fine mist, which is sent to the face mask and then inhaled.

Pulmonary Embolism

Pulmonary embolism is the blockage of one or more portions of the pulmonary arteries in the lungs by a blood clot (embolus) that has traveled via the bloodstream. Most often the clot forms in a vein in the pelvis or legs and has dislodged. The clots are often a complication of deep vein thrombosis (see p.703), in which blood tends to clot in the deep veins of the legs because of sluggish blood flow or an increased tendency of the blood to clot.

When such clots form, there is a risk that they may break off and travel to the lungs.

A large embolus can create a life-threatening chain of events. It can cut off the circulation of blood to the lungs, causing the heart's right ventricle to pump harder—potentially leading to heart failure (see p.683), shock (see p.645), and sudden death. A small pulmonary embolus produces milder symptoms.

Pulmonary embolism affects between 500,000 and 750,000 Americans each year and causes the deaths of up to 30% of these people. The condition affects women more frequently than men. At greatest risk are people who are inactive or immobile due to surgery, illness, obesity, or a leg or hip fracture. Those who are vulnerable to stroke (see

p.342), heart disease (see p.652), or deep vein thrombosis are also at greater risk of pulmonary embolism. For women over 35, smoking while taking oral contraceptives raises the risk.

Several inherited disorders that make blood clot more easily (hypercoagulable disorders) have been discovered in recent years. If you have one of these disorders, you are vulnerable to forming blood clots in the veins of your legs and pelvis, which can make you more susceptible to a pulmonary embolism.

The most common of these disorders is factor V Leiden disorder. This condition makes your blood resist the effects of a natural blood-thinning substance called protein C. Less often, you can be born with a tendency to make lower-than-normal amounts of protein C and two other natural blood-thinning substances— protein S and antithrombin III.

SYMPTOMS

The size and location of the pulmonary embolus determine the symptoms. Blockage of blood to the lungs results in sudden shortness of breath and chest pain when you inhale. You may cough up blood-streaked phlegm (sputum).

You may also feel faint or dizzy, have heart palpitations, and perspire heavily, which may be signs of low blood pressure and impending shock. A small embolus may not produce any symptoms. However, if you have recurring small emboli, over time they can lead to a lung disease called pulmonary hypertension (see p.515).

TREATMENT OPTIONS

See your doctor if you have any of these symptoms, especially if you have been immobile or inactive. Your doctor will conduct a number of tests. Blood tests may include a d-dimer level and a measure of the amount of oxygen in your blood. Imaging tests of your chest may include a chest x-ray, a radionuclide scan of your lungs (see p.137), or a special CT angiogram of your lungs or a pulmonary angiogram (see p.147). Imaging studies of your legs, to look for the source of blood clots, may include an ultrasound Doppler study of the veins of your legs (see p.148) or a venogram.

An electrocardiogram (see p.135), which records the heart's electrical impulses, may also be needed to differentiate your symptoms from other causes of chest pain, such as a heart attack.

If your doctor diagnoses, or even strongly suspects, pulmonary embolism, you need immediate intravenous treatment with the strong anticoagulant medicine heparin to prevent more clots from forming in your legs and pelvis.

A newer type of heparin called low molecular weight heparin is being used increasingly often, particularly for blood clots in the legs that have not yet caused pulmonary embolism. It has several advantages over the older heparin; it can be given as an injection into the muscle once a day (whereas the older heparin is given intravenously) and it has fewer side effects. Since an intravenous medicine is not required, you can often be treated at home, without going to the hospital.

For large clots that are causing

a major blockage in the arteries of the lung, rapid clot-dissolving drugs such as tissue-plasminogen activator (TPA) and streptokinase may be used, although they carry a small risk of causing excessive bleeding. In very rare situations, surgical removal of the clots may be necessary.

The effects of heparin or low molecular weight heparin last about a week. After that point, a second blood-thinning medicine (warfarin) that you take as a pill can replace heparin. Warfarin treatment is continued for up to 2 years, or longer, to help prevent the formation of new blood clots. You can help keep emboli from developing by staying active, by walking regularly, moving around after surgery, and moving around every hour when traveling by car, train, or air.

If you are bedridden, prevent blood from pooling in your legs by keeping them elevated. If you have had a blood clot in the veins of your legs or pelvis, with or without a pulmonary embolus, you should be tested for the genetic disorders that make your blood clot more easily.

If you have one of these disorders, your risk for having another pulmonary embolus after stopping warfarin is higher than if you do not have one of these disorders. For this reason, some doctors advise that warfarin be used for much longer periods, possibly for the rest of your life.

Pulmonary Hypertension

Pulmonary hypertension is a condition in which the increased resistance to blood flow through the lungs raises the blood pressure in the pulmonary arteries, which lead to the lungs. Pulmonary hypertension affects both men and women but affects more men over 40.

When the underlying cause is not known, the condition is called primary pulmonary hypertension. Primary pulmonary hypertension may be an inherited condition. It is twice as common in women as in men.

Most often, an underlying condition in the lungs causes pulmonary hypertension. When this occurs it is called secondary pulmonary hypertension. By far the most common lung conditions that lead to secondary pulmonary hypertension are chronic bronchitis and emphysema (see p.517). However, chronic left heart failure (see p.683), rheumatic heart disease that has damaged the mitral valve (see Mitral Stenosis, p.692), interstitial diseases of the lungs (see p.522), and recurring small pulmonary emboli (see Pulmonary Embolism, p.512) also can cause secondary pulmonary hypertension.

SYMPTOMS

In its early stages, there are usually no symptoms. Symptoms develop when the right side of the heart (which pumps blood from the veins of the body to the lungs) has to produce a high pressure to push blood through the narrowed, thickened pulmonary arteries. The high pressure causes the heart to struggle and fail. When it fails, blood backs up in the veins, and fluid starts to leak out of the blood and into the tissues, causing swelling.

The swelling is most prominent in those parts of the body that are nearest the ground, such as the legs and feet, because gravity pulls the fluid downward. The veins of the neck also bulge. In advanced cases, the liver and abdomen become enlarged.

TREATMENT OPTIONS

Symptoms of pulmonary hypertension should be reported to your doctor, who will conduct a medical history and physical exam. In addition, he or she will take samples of your blood for laboratory examination and perform chest x-rays, which in the later stages of disease can show an enlarged pulmonary artery. An electrocardiogram (see p.135) can show if the right side of the heart is enlarged or failing.

The main treatment for secondary pulmonary hypertension is treatment of the condition that is causing it. Several newer treatments that are at least temporarily effective in treating primary pulmonary hypertension include calcium-blocking pills, prostacyclin (given intravenously), adenosine, and an inhaled gas called nitrous oxide. These medicines relax the constriction of the pulmonary arteries, reduce the pressure, and, in some cases, reduce the thickening of the walls of the pulmonary arteries.

Your doctor may recommend that you have oxygen therapy. He or she may prescribe diuretics to reduce the accumulation of fluid (and hence the pressure), digitalis to increase the strength of heart muscle contractions, or vasodilators to open blood vessels and improve blood flow. If these treatments fail, a heart-lung transplant (see p.516) may be needed.

Lung Transplantation

Lung transplantation is the removal of a diseased lung and the insertion of a healthy lung from another person. In some cases, when there is severe disease of both the heart and lungs, both the heart and the lungs are transplanted together. Transplantation of a single lung or two lungs has been tried in the last stages of some lung diseases with modest success. A lung transplantation is an extremely complicated surgical procedure that lasts for many hours.

As with all organ transplantation, healthy donor tissues are scarce and precious. For these reasons, lung transplantation is considered only for people who could not otherwise survive and who are healthy enough to withstand the physical and mental stress of surgery and the healing required afterward. Transplant candidates include young adults with cystic fibrosis, emphysema, primary pulmonary hypertension, or interstitial diseases of the lungs.

One of the greatest challenges involved in lung transplantation is finding a healthy donor lung. The lung must not only be disease-free (which is rare) but it must match the recipient's size, blood type, and tissue.

Surgery carries its own risks. A large surgical incision is required in the chest. The specific type of incision varies, depending on whether a single lung, double lung, or heart-lung transplant is being performed. Some people are connected to a heart-lung machine, which takes over the function of the heart and lungs during surgery. This massive surgical procedure often requires several months of healing, close surveillance, and supportive therapy because the lungs are so vital to the function of the entire body.

Complications include airway obstruction and infection, as well as organ rejection (an attack by the recipient's immune system on the foreign transplanted lung). In recent years, the immediate success rate from surgery has improved, but organ rejection remains a major problem. Immunosuppressant drugs are administered for life to prevent rejection of the transplanted organs by the recipient.

Pleural Effusion

Pleural effusion is an accumulation of fluid between the two-layered membrane (pleura) that covers the lungs and lines the chest. There is normally a small amount of lubricating fluid between the membranes.

Many lung conditions can cause pleural effusion, including pneumonia, pulmonary embolism (see p.512), heart failure (see p.683), or a cancer that has spread to the pleura. Your doctor can diagnose the condition with a chest x-ray and may take a sample of the fluid or pleural tissue for examination.

Treatment of pleural effusion involves addressing the underlying cause. If there is so much fluid that it pushes on the lung and your breathing is impaired, your doctor will drain the accumulated fluid. If you continue to have a recurring and significant buildup of fluid, your doctor may inject irritating substances into the pleural space to scar the pleura and prevent fluid from reaccumulating.

Pneumothorax

In pneumothorax, air leaks from the breathing tubes of the lungs into the space between the pleura (the double membrane that covers the lungs and lines the chest cavity). Normally these two membranes touch each other, with no air between them. As air builds up in the space, it pushes on the lung. This can lead to a collapsed lung and respiratory failure.

A pneumothorax can occur when an object—such as a knife or a broken rib—tears the outer surface of the lung or punctures the lung. More often, it occurs spontaneously (spontaneous pneumothorax). Some people, particularly those with emphysema or asthma, have sacs of air (called bullae or blebs) about the size of large grapes on the outer part of their lungs. If these sacs rupture, air escapes into the pleural space and causes pneumothorax.

Thin adults are most prone to spontaneous pneumothorax, and men are more vulnerable than women. Spontaneous pneumothorax can also be a complication of emphysema (see p.517), asthma (see p.505), cystic fibrosis (see p.1003), or tuberculosis (see p.504). If you have had one episode of spontaneous pneumothorax, you are at high risk for another one.

SYMPTOMS

Symptoms of spontaneous pneumothorax include pain in the chest (usually on the side of the collapse) that comes on abruptly or breathlessness that gets worse over time.

TREATMENT OPTIONS

A diagnosis of pneumothorax is made with a chest x-ray. A minor case of pneumothorax does not require treatment. It usually resolves on its own. However, your doctor needs to monitor your condition carefully to ensure that the size of the space filled with air outside your lung is not enlarging, and may need to give you supplemental oxygen to breathe.

If you have another lung disease or disorder, even a small amount of air outside of the lung may require the same treatment as a more serious lung collapse. Your doctor will remove the air from between the membranes by placing a suction tube in your chest and drawing out the air. If you have a recurrence, your physician may inject the pleura with a substance that irritates the membranes and causes them to stick together as they heal. In severe cases, surgery may be required to remove the ruptured area or to fuse the pleural membranes together.

Acute Respiratory Distress Syndrome

Acute respiratory distress syndrome is a life-threatening condition that usually develops in people whose lungs have been damaged by injury or disease. It often leads to respiratory failure, in which the life-sustaining exchange of oxygen and carbon dioxide in the lungs is disrupted.

In acute respiratory distress syndrome, the air sacs of the lung tissue become filled with fluid and cannot exchange oxygen and carbon dioxide. It can be caused by pneumonia (see p.496); severe bacterial infections in other parts of the body; inhaling vomit, water, or irritants; drug overdose; or severe injury.

In most people, death occurs if the condition is not treated. Even with treatment, the survival rate is only 50%.

SYMPTOMS

For most affected people, the first symptoms are those of the underlying problem that is causing the damage to the lungs. Once acute respiratory distress syndrome begins, rapid, shallow, and labored breathing are the main symptoms. As the disease advances, skin may have a blue tinge (called cyanosis) because the tissues are not getting enough oxygen.

TREATMENT OPTIONS

See your doctor immediately if you develop symptoms. He or she will perform blood tests to measure the amount of oxygen and carbon dioxide in your blood. A chest x-ray will also be performed. If the condition is

diagnosed, you will be admitted to the intensive care unit of a hospital for treatment. If your condition deteriorates, you may need to be attached to a mechanical ventilator (see p.520) to help you breathe. You may also receive antibiotics and corticosteroids intravenously.

Chronic Bronchitis and Emphysema

Chronic bronchitis and emphysema are together also known as chronic obstructive lung disease. They produce a progressive and ongoing blockage of the flow of air into and out of the lungs.

Chronic bronchitis and emphysema affect 15.4 million Americans. Both are diseases of longtime smokers: 82% of those who die of these diseases are smokers, and smokers are ten times more likely than nonsmokers to die of them.

The prevalence of and death rates from chronic bronchitis and emphysema are soaring. Since 1982, the number of cases has increased 41%. These are the only lung diseases that disproportionately affect whites, and the only ones for which the death rate for whites exceeds that for blacks.

The main symptoms of chronic bronchitis and emphysema—coughing up phlegm and breathlessness—are often ignored until the diseases have reached an advanced state. People often alter their lifestyles, either consciously or unconsciously, over months or years in an effort to reduce their symptoms. However, by the time most people see their doctors, their lungs have been

Benefits of Oxygen Therapy and Positive Pressure Masks for Chronic Bronchitis and Emphysema

Inhaled oxygen therapy has been shown to reduce the risk of death in people who have chronic bronchitis and emphysema along with low blood oxygen levels.

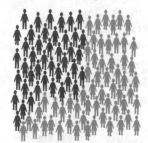

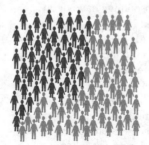

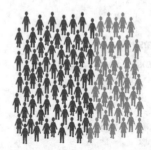

42 OF 100 PEOPLE WHO HAVE CHRONIC BRONCHITIS AND EMPHYSEMA ALONG WITH LOW BLOOD OXYGEN LEVELS REMAIN ALIVE AFTER 3 YEARS IF THEY USE OXYGEN INFREQUENTLY

44 OF 100 PEOPLE WHO HAVE CHRONIC BRONCHITIS AND EMPHYSEMA ALONG WITH LOW BLOOD OXYGEN LEVELS REMAIN ALIVE AFTER 3 YEARS IF THEY USE OXYGEN 12 HOURS A DAY

62 OF 100 PEOPLE WHO HAVE CHRONIC BRONCHITIS AND EMPHYSEMA ALONG WITH LOW BLOOD OXYGEN LEVELS REMAIN ALIVE AFTER 3 YEARS IF THEY USE OXYGEN 24 HOURS A DAY

seriously damaged. At this point, affected people are already more vulnerable to developing other serious conditions, such as pneumonia (see p.496), pulmonary hypertension (see p.514), or heart failure (see p.683).

CHRONIC BRONCHITIS

Chronic bronchitis is persistent inflammation of the lining of the bronchial tubes (airways) of the lungs. In comparison to acute bronchitis (see p.494), which lasts several days and is caused by infection, chronic bronchitis is the presence of a phlegm-producing cough most days of the month, for 3 months out of the year for at least 2 successive years. Chronic bronchitis is not caused by infection.

Smoking is the most common cause of chronic bronchitis. It develops when the bronchial tubes are subject to steady and unrelenting irritation, such as

from tobacco smoke. In an effort to expel the irritants, the body mounts a defense that includes inflammation (when white blood cells are drawn to the area), swelling of the lining of the airways with subsequent narrowing, and a constant production of mucus

in an effort to rid the body of the irritating smoke particles.

Unless exposure to smoke stops, the lining of the airways will thicken and scar. In addition, smoke damages the tiny hairs called cilia that move mucus along the airways to be coughed

Destruction of Air Sacs in Emphysema

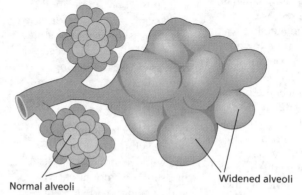

Normal alveoli

Widened alveoli

Emphysema involves destruction of the walls of the alveoli, the air sacs in your lungs. The damaged alveoli merge to form fewer, larger sacs. These larger sacs are less efficient in exchanging oxygen and carbon dioxide in the lungs.

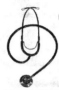

Chronic Bronchitis or Emphysema:
When You Visit Your Doctor

QUESTIONS TO DISCUSS WITH YOUR DOCTOR:

- Are you still smoking cigarettes?
- Have your symptoms improved or worsened since your last visit?
- How is your breathing?
- Have you had a fever? Have you been sweating at night?
- Have you lost your appetite or lost weight since your last visit?
- How have you been sleeping?
- Have you had any chest discomfort since your last visit?
- Have you noticed swelling of your ankles or feet since your last visit?
- Do you feel your medicines are helping you?
- If you use inhalers, do you know how to use them?

YOUR DOCTOR MIGHT EXAMINE THE FOLLOWING FUNCTIONS AND BODY SYSTEMS:

- Vital signs (by taking your temperature, blood pressure, pulse, or respiratory rate)
- Nose, ears, and throat
- Lymph nodes in the neck
- Skin
- Hands and feet
- Chest and lungs
- Heart
- Abdomen

YOUR DOCTOR MIGHT ORDER THE FOLLOWING LAB TESTS OR STUDIES:

- Oxygen saturation by oximetry (particularly after exercise)
- Chest x-ray (if symptoms are worsening)
- Phlegm culture (if cough has developed or worsened)

---

out. Because the damaged cilia are less able to clear mucus out of the body, mucus remains in the airways. The large amounts of mucus and the damaged airways lead to an irritating cough, difficulty breathing, and an ideal environment for infection. Damage to lung tissue can be permanent.

People with chronic bronchitis regularly cough up phlegm, may wheeze, and become increasingly limited in their capacity to exercise. Ultimately, breathlessness increases, and many people with chronic bronchitis cannot exert themselves at all without breathing supplemental oxygen. In others, fluid retention causes the ankles and abdomen to swell. They gain weight, appear bloated, and have a blue tinge to their lips due to low levels of oxygen in their blood.

EMPHYSEMA

Emphysema can occur along with or independently of chronic bronchitis. In emphysema, the walls between the air sacs (alveoli) are destroyed, creating fewer and larger air sacs. These merged air sacs do not have as much surface area for the exchange of oxygen and carbon dioxide.

The lung tissue also loses its resilience and is unable to stretch and recoil, leaving air trapped in the air sacs. The damaged lungs cannot absorb as much oxygen and cannot release as much of the body's waste product, carbon dioxide.

Symptoms of emphysema include breathlessness when you exert yourself. In advanced disease, you will feel breathless after taking several steps and you will eventually require oxygen to breathe even when you are at rest. You may lose weight as the work of breathing consumes a greater portion of the calories you take in and as breathlessness makes it more difficult to eat.

Smoking is the most common

Acute Respiratory Failure

Acute respiratory failure is the failure to breathe enough air into and out of the lungs to supply the body with vital oxygen or to get rid of high levels of carbon dioxide.

People with chronic bronchitis or emphysema (see p.517), pneumonia (see p.496), or asthma (see p.505) are especially vulnerable to acute respiratory failure, although any lung condition that interferes with the healthy exchange of carbon dioxide and oxygen in the lung tissue can cause it.

Respiratory failure can also occur because of problems with the parts of the brain that control breathing or with the muscles of the chest that move air in and out. Hospitalization, usually in an intensive care unit, is required, and a lung specialist (pulmonologist) may be involved in your care.

Symptoms of acute respiratory failure include an increased or decreased rate of breathing, blue-tinged skin and nails, and anxiety or confusion. Blood from an artery is tested to see how high the level of carbon dioxide and how low the level of oxygen are. If this test shows that you have acute respiratory failure, it means you cannot breathe adequately by yourself and need the help of a ventilator (see below).

One of the greatest threats of respiratory failure is respiratory arrest, a life-threatening situation in which breathing suddenly stops. Once the lungs stop breathing, all of the body's tissues quickly become deprived of oxygen, a condition called anoxia. This leads to death within minutes. Immediate cardiopulmonary resuscitation (see p.1201) and emergency artificial respiration are required.

Ventilator

A ventilator, sometimes referred to as a respirator, is a machine that takes over breathing function, inflating and deflating the lungs, moving oxygen in and carbon dioxide out. Using a ventilator requires the placement of a tube through the mouth or nose into the throat and down into the trachea (windpipe). If the tube needs to remain in place for a long time, a surgical opening is made in the throat (tracheostomy) and the tube is placed through the opening, down into the windpipe.

After inserting the tube, your doctor can adjust the amount of oxygen delivered, the pressure of inflation of the lungs, and the volume of air delivered—all of which are required for the delicate balance of breathing.

Using a ventilator can be lifesaving; it allows the body time to heal and recover the ability to breathe without mechanical support. However, in people with severe chronic illnesses, the ventilator may prolong life for only days or weeks in an intensive care unit, with little chance of survival or of a meaningful life

after survival. Family members are often placed in the difficult and painful position of deciding about the use of a ventilator.

If you or a relative has a severe or chronic illness, it would be useful to discuss your feelings about artificial breathing now—before the need arises. Consider asking your doctor the following questions:

- Under what conditions would you recommend a ventilator for me?

- In such a situation, would the ventilator successfully treat the complication and allow a return to independent functioning for a reasonable length of time?

- What are the risks involved in using a ventilator (as they relate to the illness)?

If you believe that you (or your relative) would not want to have a ventilator used, make these wishes known to the doctor and your family by preparing an advance directive (see p.1142). This document can save family members from having to make difficult decisions about ventilator use or withdrawal.

cause of emphysema. About 2 million Americans have emphysema: 61% male and 39% female. As the number of women who smoke increases, the number of women with emphysema also increases.

Causes Cigarette smoking is by far the most common cause of both chronic bronchitis and emphysema. Smoking also greatly increases the risk of death due to both conditions. Passive smoking, outdoor air pollution, and indoor air pollution (due to wood-burning fireplaces and other sources) also contribute to chronic bronchitis and emphysema.

Coal miners, grain handlers, factory workers who work with cotton to manufacture textiles, and metal molders develop chronic bronchitis more readily if they also smoke. In addition, they are susceptible to lung diseases called pneumoconioses (see Interstitial Diseases of the Lungs, p.522).

Treatment options If you have slowly worsening shortness of breath or a chronic cough that produces phlegm (sputum), see your doctor. He or she will take a medical history and perform a physical exam. Depending on the findings, your doctor may also order chest x-rays and tests of your breathing (see Common Lung Tests, p.494). A machine called an oximeter may be connected to your finger to estimate the amount of oxygen in your blood.

Sometimes a sample of blood in an artery (usually an artery in your wrist) is taken to get a more precise measure of the oxygen

and carbon dioxide in your arterial blood—a measure of how effectively your lungs are working. You may be asked to produce a sample of your phlegm; the phlegm will be examined under a microscope to look for evidence of inflammation or infection, and may be sent for a culture to identify bacteria that are possibly causing a chronic infection.

Quitting smoking is the most important step you can take to treat chronic bronchitis and emphysema. You can reverse these diseases in their early stages by stopping now. Ask your doctor for help in finding a technique (see p.60 for smoking cessation options) to help you quit.

You also need to eliminate your exposure to irritants other

than tobacco smoke. If your job puts you in contact with lung irritants, your doctor may suggest that you change your work environment.

Since people with chronic bronchitis and emphysema have damaged lungs that are vulnerable to infection, your doctor will recommend that you be immunized annually against influenza virus ("the flu") and against the most common cause of bacterial pneumonia, *Streptococcus pneumoniae* (pneumococcus) (see Preventing Pneumonia: Vaccines for Pneumonia and Influenza, p.499).

In addition to recommending that you quit smoking, your doctor may prescribe medicines to open up the airways and help

Value of Pulmonary Rehabilitation: Dr Weinberger's Advice

I am quite enthusiastic about having my patients enter an outpatient pulmonary rehabilitation program. Almost all my patients find it to be an extremely valuable part of their overall care. Such programs include regular aerobic exercise and patient education, and may also include breathing exercises and instruction as well as involvement in a patient support group.

The programs really work—they decrease your symptoms, improve your ability to exercise and your overall sense of well-being, and decrease the need for hospitalization.

If you are considering such a program, understand that the program cannot directly improve lung function; what it can do is improve your overall physical conditioning and quality of life. In other words, the program does not improve your lungs, but it improves your ability to live with your lungs.

STEVEN E. WEINBERGER, MD
BETH ISRAEL DEACONESS MEDICAL CENTER
HARVARD MEDICAL SCHOOL

you cough up phlegm. Broncho-dilators, usually taken through an inhaler, relax the muscles around the bronchial tubes to increase the flow of air, but do not reverse the course of the disease. Bronchodilators include beta$_2$-agonists and anticholinergic medicines.

Anticholinergic drugs are not as fast acting as beta$_2$-agonists, but they produce fewer side effects. Another bronchodilator that is most often swallowed as a pill or liquid is theophylline.

Corticosteroids calm inflammation of the bronchial tubes and improve the disease in about 30% of people. Corticosteroids are best administered as metered-dose inhalers (see p.512), which deliver the medicine directly to the inflamed lung tissue and cause fewer side effects than when taken regularly in pill form. Sometimes, however, it is necessary to take pills or even injected forms of corticosteroids during flare-ups. Antibiotics may be prescribed to prevent or treat infection.

Some people need constant supplemental oxygen, which is delivered through small plastic tubes (nasal prongs) in the nose or a plastic face mask. These people need to keep portable tanks of oxygen at home. Constant use of oxygen by people who have severe disease and low levels of oxygen in their blood reduces the chance of developing pulmonary hypertension (see p.514) and failure of the right side of the heart (see p.683). It also prolongs life.

Exercise is another aspect of treatment. The increased breathing you do during exercise helps clear the mucus from your airways. In addition, aerobic activity strengthens your heart and other

muscles and increases the ability of your body to utilize oxygen. Work with your doctor to establish a daily exercise program. However, avoid exercising near high-traffic areas or when air-pollution levels are high.

Your doctor may also recommend a formal pulmonary rehabilitation program, run by a team of health professionals, to help you cope with the physical, psychological, and social challenges of living with these diseases. For people with severe disease, lung transplantation (see p.516) may be necessary.

Lung volume reduction surgery is a relatively new procedure in which a surgeon removes some of the areas of the lung that are most damaged by emphysema. This enables the remaining, less damaged areas of lung to work more effectively.

Recent studies indicate that only certain patients with chronic bronchitis and emphysema benefit from lung volume reduction surgery: those with upper-lobe emphysema and low base-line exercise capacity. It may be harmful to other patients. The procedure is done best by surgeons and institutions with considerable experience.

Interstitial Diseases of the Lungs

There are more than 200 conditions that can affect the delicate air sacs of the lungs (alveoli), the smallest breathing tubes (bronchioles), the smallest arteries (arterioles), and particularly the tissue in between (interstitium).

These interstitial diseases are characterized by an excessive and abnormal pattern of inflam-

Home Remedies for Hiccups

Fetuses hiccup in the uterus and adults hiccup throughout life—no one really knows why. Most hiccups disappear on their own after a short time, but this has not stopped people from seeking cures. If one of the following home remedies does not work, try another. By the time you have made your way halfway down the list, your hiccups will either have been cured or they will have vanished as mysteriously as they arrived.

■ Hold your breath.

■ Pull hard on your tongue.

■ Chew and swallow dry bread.

■ Suck on a lemon wedge soaked with bitters.

■ Gargle with water.

■ Take a teaspoon of dry sugar and hold it on the back of your tongue, pressed against the roof of your mouth.

■ While bending over, drink a glass of water from the opposite side of the cup.

■ Use the relaxation response (see p.90) to refocus your attention.

mation and scar tissue formation (fibrosis) that interferes with the exchange of oxygen and carbon dioxide in the lungs. While not rare, interstitial diseases are less common than obstructive diseases such as asthma and chronic bronchitis and emphysema.

Asbestosis is abnormal scarring of the lungs caused by inhaling asbestos fibers, a building material that was widely used to insulate buildings until the mid-1970s.

Asbestos has put more than 9 million workers (ranging from miners to electricians to do-it-yourself renovators who work on old buildings) at risk. Asbestosis usually does not develop until 10 years after exposure and may lead to cancer (see Cancers That Originate in the Lining of the Lungs, p.526).

Silicosis, caused by inhaling silica dust, also takes many years to produce symptoms. It is the most prevalent occupational disease worldwide. Black lung disease, or coal miner's pneumoconiosis, also occurs after about 10 years of breathing in coal products.

Other conditions that lead to interstitial pulmonary fibrosis are thought to be due to an autoimmune reaction, in which the body's immune system mistakenly attacks its own tissues, leading to inflammation and scarring.

Sarcoidosis is one of the most common of these conditions and typically affects people between the ages of 20 and 50. The cause is unknown. Although the disease often improves on its own, some people have persistent or even progressive and debilitating disease of the lungs and of other parts of the body.

Pulmonary fibrosis of un-

known cause (idiopathic pulmonary fibrosis) is a disease affecting middle-aged to older people in which inflammation and scarring of the lungs develop. Many experts believe that this is another example of autoimmune lung disease.

SYMPTOMS

Interstitial lung diseases usually develop slowly and insidiously. You may first experience mild shortness of breath only when you exert yourself. Over time you feel tired and out of breath with less exertion. Other symptoms include dry cough and chest pain. As scarring of the lung tissue increases, you may lose weight.

TREATMENT OPTIONS

Your doctor may perform a chest x-ray, computed tomography (see p.149), spirometry (see p.495), or possibly lung biopsy (see p.494) to help make a diagnosis.

Treatment depends on the underlying condition and the extent to which the lungs have stiffened. In severe cases, as in chronic bronchitis and emphysema, you need to have a constant supply of oxygen delivered through nasal prongs or a face mask.

For conditions caused by occupational exposure, you will probably be advised to eliminate your exposure to the agents. For idiopathic pulmonary fibrosis, corticosteroids (see p.895) or other drugs to suppress inflammation may help. For sarcoidosis, treatment is based upon the severity of disease and its course over time. Corticosteroids may be prescribed. If, despite treatment, your condition deteriorates, lung

transplantation (see p.516) may be an option.

Atelectasis

Atelectasis is a collapsed lung caused by blockage of the airways or one of the arteries of the lungs (pulmonary arteries). The amount of lung collapsed depends on the extent and location of the obstruction. There are no symptoms in mild cases.

One of the most common causes of blockage is mucous buildup in the lungs due to asthma (see p.505), but it can also be caused by chronic bronchitis (see p.517), inhaling a foreign object, a tumor in the lung, or immobility (commonly after surgery).

Adults can often compensate for a partially collapsed lung and can continue breathing. In infants, however, the blockage may be life-threatening. Atelectasis can usually be seen on a chest x-ray. It is important that even small areas of collapsed lung be opened up as soon as possible to improve breathing and to prevent infection.

Most collapsed lungs can be opened up by deep breathing, coughing, chest clapping (pounding on the chest to loosen mucus), and postural drainage (extending the body at a downward angle to help drain mucus).

Bronchoscopy (see p.495) can remove an inhaled object or a mucous plug. The lung usually expands on its own once the blockage has been removed, but some people are left with areas of permanent scarring.

Spots on the Lungs

A spot on the lung is any small area that looks different from surrounding parts on a chest x-ray. Hearing that you have a spot on your lung can be alarming, but keep in mind that this finding does not necessarily mean that you have lung cancer.

Many causes are not serious. For example, spots commonly occur on lungs after infection with tuberculosis (see p.504). This kind of spot may have been there for a long time and is rarely cause for concern.

Depending on the size, shape, and location of a spot, your doctor will decide whether to take another chest x-ray in a few months or obtain further studies to determine the cause.

LUNG CANCER

Cancers That Originate in the Lungs

A cancer that originates in the lung (primary lung cancer) may remain limited to an airway of the lung, where it can block the passage of air into the lungs, or may spread to other parts of the body. Primary lung cancer is the leading cause of death due to cancer in both men and women in the United States; 85% of lung cancer is caused by cigarette smoke.

The risk of cancer increases with the number of cigarettes smoked over a lifetime. Anyone who has smoked more than one pack of cigarettes per day for 40 years is at high risk for developing lung cancer. The risk for cigar and pipe smokers is not as high as for cigarette smokers, but it is

significantly higher than for non-smokers.

Other factors besides tobacco smoke that cause lung cancer are exposure to asbestos, radon, and uranium. Scarring of the lungs caused by interstitial diseases of the lungs (see p.522) and chronic infections such as tuberculosis (see p.504) may also increase the risk of primary lung cancer.

The outlook for people with lung cancer is not good. Approximately 85% of people in whom lung cancer is detected die within 5 years of diagnosis. For those in whom the tumor is very localized (without evidence of spread to the lymph nodes in the chest), surgery can offer up to a 60% chance of long-term survival. However, most cancers are not discovered before they spread.

Lung cancer is highly preventable by never smoking or by stopping as soon as possible. When you quit smoking, your risk of lung cancer gradually drops. After you have stopped smoking for 10 to 15 years, your risk of lung cancer approaches that of people who never smoked.

TYPES OF PRIMARY LUNG CANCER

There are many different types of primary lung cancer, but four predominate:

Squamous cell carcinoma represents 30% to 35% of all lung cancers. These cancers originate on the surface of the lining of the larger airways (bronchioles) and thus are usually found in the central part of the lung. They are slow growing, but they spread (metastasize) early to lymph glands near the lungs and to other organs.

Adenocarcinoma, represent-

Lung Cancer's Spread

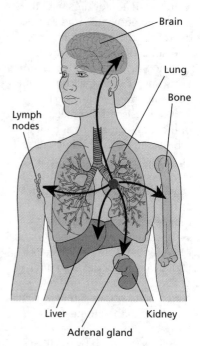

Lung cancers that start in the lung can spread (metastasize) to other parts of the body. Cancer cells travel from the lung through the blood vessels and lymph vessels to different organs. The most common places for lung cancer to spread are the brain, bones, liver, and adrenal glands.

ing 35% to 40% of lung cancer cases, frequently originates in the smaller airways and is therefore found in the periphery of the lungs. It often spreads to the lymph glands near the lung area where it has originated and to other organs.

Large cell carcinoma is responsible for 10% to 20% of lung cancers. These tumors often spread inside the lung before spreading to other parts of the body.

Small cell carcinoma (also known as oat cell carcinoma

Bronchoscope

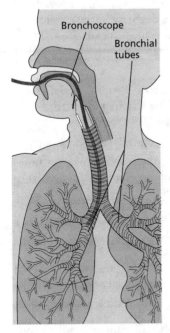

Bronchoscope

Bronchial tubes

A bronchoscope permits your doctor to view the inside of your bronchial tubes. It is threaded into your lungs via the nose or mouth and has a light on one end. It can accommodate a variety of instruments, such as those used for grasping an inhaled object or taking a tissue sample from a growth.

because the cancerous cells are shaped like oats) represents 20% to 30% of lung cancers. It occurs primarily in the large airways and almost always spreads (metastasizes) to other organs from the original tumor in the lung.

Although it is more likely to metastasize widely throughout the body than the other kinds of primary lung cancer, small cell carcinoma is more likely to respond to chemotherapy (see p.741). However, the response is usually temporary and not curative.

Preventing Lung Cancer

If you smoke, stop. If you do not smoke, never start. This is the most effective way to prevent lung cancer. Ten to 15 years after you quit smoking, your risk of lung cancer approaches that of a person who never smoked at all. See p.60 for recommendations on how to quit. Here are some other ways to prevent lung cancer:

■ Strive for a smoke-free environment at home and at work.

■ Test your home for radon (see p.86).

■ If you are exposed to industrial dusts and fumes in your work environment, follow all safety rules and wear protective gear.

SYMPTOMS

Symptoms almost always include coughing, sometimes with blood-tinged phlegm or shortness of breath. You may also have chest pain. Your speech may become raspy or you may lose your appetite. Sometimes, cancer causes repeated periods of pneumonia (see p.496) or produces a pleural effusion (see p.516).

In more advanced disease, you may experience symptoms of the cancer's spread to other organs, such as pain in your bones or neurological disturbances due to its effect on the brain. Occasionally, the first signs of primary lung cancer are tumors that have spread to other parts of the body.

TREATMENT OPTIONS

If you experience symptoms of lung cancer, see your doctor immediately. He or she will conduct a physical examination and take a thorough medical history. Your doctor will ask whether and how much you have smoked tobacco, and also will ask about your possible exposure to other causes of lung cancer.

You will have a chest x-ray, which usually reveals the presence of any cancer. Computed tomography (see p.149) is generally also done (particularly when a cancer is in the large breathing tubes in the center of the lung); it is particularly helpful in showing

White Mass on Lung X-Ray

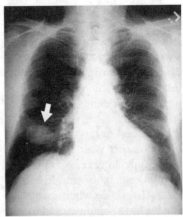

In this chest x-ray of the lungs, a white mass (arrow) is clearly visible. While this looks like a cancerous tumor on the x-ray, it could also be an infection. A biopsy is required to confirm the diagnosis.

if the tumor has spread to lymph glands in the chest.

A definitive diagnosis is based on a laboratory examination of phlegm or a sample (biopsy) of tissue from your lungs obtained during bronchoscopy (see p.495), percutaneous needle biopsy (see p.494), video-assisted thoracic surgery (VATS) (see p.495), or open lung biopsy. The type of biopsy depends on the location of the tumor. Mediastinoscopy (see p.495) is sometimes used to obtain a biopsy because samples of lymph node tissue can be taken at the same time.

VATS, mediastinoscopy, and open biopsies are performed with the person under general anesthesia (see p.168) in either an outpatient or inpatient setting. Bronchoscopy and percutaneous needle biopsies are done using local anesthesia. There is a small risk of collapsed lung (see Pneumothorax, p.516) with any of these procedures.

Upon diagnosis, your physician may refer you to an oncologist (a doctor who specializes in cancer treatment), who will determine the stage of the cancer and the best type of treatment. The stage is based on the size of the tumor, whether it has spread to the lymph nodes in the region, and whether there is evidence that the cancer has spread to other areas of your body. Most commonly, lung cancer spreads to the bone, brain, and liver.

To determine whether the cancer has spread beyond the lung (a process called staging), your doctor may order blood tests, a bone scan (see p.622), computed tomography, or magnetic resonance imaging (see p.150) of the brain, lungs, or abdomen.

For cancers other than small cell carcinoma, surgical removal of part or all of the affected lung is the best method of achieving long-term survival or cure. However, it is an option only for cancers that are confined to one area of the lung or, at most, that have extended to the lymph nodes on the same side of the chest as the tumor. About 50% of cancers are discovered at this stage.

Surgery may involve removal of a single lobe (lobectomy) or the entire lung (pneumonectomy), depending on the location and extent of disease. Both procedures require up to 10 days of hospitalization and several months' recovery.

Surgery cannot be performed in people whose lungs have been severely damaged by other conditions. In rare cases, radiation therapy (see p.741) may be used to treat very small cancers in people who cannot tolerate surgery. Radiation may also be used to control some of the complications that result from lung cancer.

In general, treatment extends life for an estimated two thirds of people. However, only about 15% of people survive 5 years. Chemotherapy (see p.741) may be recommended either alone or in combination with other forms of therapy, but the responses are temporary and not curative.

Small cell carcinoma almost always has spread by the time it is detected. For this reason, surgery is rarely recommended, unless the tumor is discovered when it is very small and thus has not spread. Treatment combines radiation and chemotherapy, which helps most people to some degree, but only a small percentage achieve long-term survival.

Cancers That Originate in the Lining of the Lungs

Mesothelioma is an uncommon cancerous tumor that arises from the pleura (the membranes that cover the outside of the lungs and the inside of the chest wall).

It is almost always caused by exposure to asbestos fibers, a heat-resistant and insulating material that was commonly used until the mid 1970s. People who worked in occupations that exposed them to asbestos (such as asbestos mining, building construction, and home renovation) are at greatest risk, and smoking increases the risk. The tumor may not develop until many years after exposure.

A noncancerous form of mesothelioma can also occur; it remains isolated to one part of the pleura. The cancerous form spreads throughout the pleural lining. If you work or have worked in contact with asbestos dust, you should have regular chest x-rays to look for changes in your lungs.

SYMPTOMS

Asbestosis (see Interstitial Diseases of the Lung, p.522), a disease caused by inhalation of asbestos dust, often precedes mesothelioma. Symptoms of asbestosis include shortness of breath, dry cough, and difficulty breathing.

Mesothelioma may develop

without symptoms or cause the same symptoms as asbestosis. In addition, mesotheliomas may cause chest pain.

TREATMENT OPTIONS

If you have worked near asbestos in the past, contact your doctor any time you have a new cough, persistent chest pain, or difficulty breathing. In addition to a chest x-ray, he or she may perform computed tomography or take a sample of your phlegm to examine under a microscope to look for cancerous cells. It may be necessary to remove a sample of pleural tissue to look for mesothelioma.

If the tumor is confined to one spot on your pleura, your doctor will remove it surgically; the out-look is very good. Extensive and radical surgery is occasionally performed, and sometimes radiation is used to reduce pain.

Cancers That Spread to the Lungs

The lungs are a target for many cancers that start elsewhere in the body and spread to the lungs via the bloodstream. These are called secondary lung cancers.

The cancers most likely to spread to the lungs include those of the breasts, thyroid gland, bone, and kidneys.

The symptoms of secondary lung cancer are the same as the symptoms of primary lung cancer. You may have a cough, shortness of breath, and wheezing. You may also cough up blood. Most cancers that have spread to the lungs cause symptoms in other locations before the secondary lung cancer is found.

If you have cancer in other parts of your body, your doctor will probably determine what stage your disease is in by performing a number of tests to identify potential sites of spread (metastasis), including the lungs.

Treatment generally includes chemotherapy (see p.741) directed toward the primary cancer. In some cases, these cancer-fighting drugs are combined with radiation therapy (see p.741) directed at the tumors in the lungs.

Skin, Hair, and Nails

SKIN

Your skin consists of several different types of tissue that perform a variety of essential functions for your body. Skin helps regulate your body temperature by sweating in response to heat and decreasing blood flow to the skin in response to cold (thereby keeping the heat deeper inside the body).

The skin's pigment shields your body from dangerous ultraviolet rays. Nerve endings in the skin pick up and relay information about the surrounding environment to your brain, where it is translated into the sensations of touch, pressure, heat, or cold. Cells known as Langerhans cells are part of the immune system and help the skin fight infection. The skin also makes vitamin D from sunlight, which is essential in making bones strong.

Perhaps most important, your skin forms a physical barrier to injury and infection. The most significant part of this barrier is the top layer of skin, called the epidermis. At the very top of the epidermis, dead cells called keratinocytes (which contain a chemical called keratin) form a soft, protective sheet. The dead cells come from younger, living cells in the lower part of the epidermis, where they are constantly produced.

Young cells rise to the surface as they age, die, and are sloughed off by friction. That friction stimu-lates the growth of new cells and causes the epidermis to thicken, which is why skin is generally thicker on the bottoms of your feet and the palms of your hands. It is also why a callus—rough, thickened skin on any part of the body—forms on areas that are rubbed excessively. The skin you see on your body today may look familiar, but it has been completely renewed over the course of a month.

The pigment in the skin that helps protect the body against ultraviolet rays is called melanin. This protein is made primarily by cells called melanocytes but is also present in the keratinocytes. In general, skin color is a hereditary characteristic determined not by the number of melanocytes but by their degree of activity.

People with darker skin have more active melanocytes, resulting in more melanin. The ultraviolet rays in sunlight stimulate the activity of melanocytes to produce more melanin, causing skin to darken, thereby defending the

Cross Section of Skin and Hair

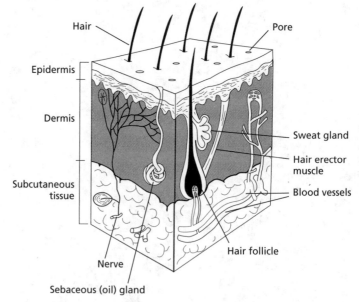

The skin consists of the epidermis (the thin, outer layer made up mostly of dead cells) and the dermis (the thicker layer containing blood vessels, nerves, oil glands, and hair follicles). A subcutaneous (literally "under the skin") layer forms the base.

body against the damaging effects of the sun.

If the top layer of skin is totally replaced every month, why does skin age? Skin aging occurs, in part, because the layer of skin beneath the epidermis, called the dermis, gradually loses its supply of two substances—elastin and collagen. Long fibers of elastin give the skin its elasticity, while collagen fibers provide strength. Over time and with repeated exposure to ultraviolet light (mainly sunlight), these fibers deteriorate.

The dermis also contains four sets of glands:

Sebaceous (oil) glands, primarily located in the ducts containing shafts of hair, secrete an oil called sebum. The sebaceous glands are highly active during adolescence because of the hormone changes that occur at this time, which contribute to the higher likelihood of acne.

Ceruminous glands are the ear's version of sebaceous glands and are the source of earwax (cerumen).

Sweat glands called eccrine or exocrine glands are found all over the body's surface. They are most numerous on the soles, palms, upper lip, and forehead. Sweat is important in maintaining a comfortable and healthy body temperature. When the body gets heated or is under stress, it produces sweat, which evaporates and cools the body.

Apocrine glands are located mainly in the underarm and genital areas; they may release a smelly liquid in response to physical or emotional stress.

Below the dermis is the subcutaneous tissue, consisting of connective tissue and fatty (adipose) tissue. This layer lies between the dermis and underlying muscles or bones. The subcutaneous tissue is richly supplied with blood vessels, which expand or contract to help keep a constant amount of heat inside the body. This tissue also contains white blood cells, which are always on patrol to fight off infectious organisms that manage to break through the top layers of skin. The adipose tissue not only cushions and insulates the internal tissues, but also helps store nutrients.

While marvelously effective and efficient, the skin is far from invincible. Disorders of the skin are common and varied. If the recommendations in the following section do not work, or if your condition is severe, consult your doctor, who can care for most skin conditions. If necessary, he or she will refer you to a dermatologist, a doctor who specializes in treating skin disorders.

HAIR

Though the hair follicles are located in the dermis (the second layer of skin), the composition and function of hair is similar to that of the top layer—the epidermis. Hair is made of keratin, the same substance that forms nails and the barrier at the top of the skin. Cells that make keratin and melanin live at the root of the hair, where they die—leaving their keratin and melanin to give substance and color to the hair.

Like other parts of the skin, hair helps protect the body. Eyelashes and eyebrows shield the eyes from sun, dust, and perspiration. Nasal hair helps reduce your intake of dust and other foreign bodies. Hair on the scalp provides some insulation. However, as the human species has evolved and become more sophisticated in protecting itself from extremes of temperature, it has less need for body hair. When we get goose bumps, we are seeing an evolutionary remnant of a once-critical ability to thicken our "fur" in response to cold.

NAILS

Nails are thickened and hardened forms of epidermis. Nail cells are created in the base of the nail bed and then die. Nails are composed of dead cells that are, in turn, composed of a strong form of keratin. The nail bed is alive and continuously produces new nail. Thus, a nail is simply a much harder and thicker mat of keratin than the topmost layer of skin.

Cross Section of Nail

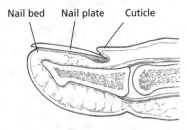

Nail bed   Nail plate   Cuticle

Nails are thickened, hardened plates made up of dead cells from the epidermis, the outer layer of skin. The nail bed is alive and continuously produces new cells, which die, stick together into a hard substance, and form the nail. The cuticle protects the base of the nail from infection-causing bacteria and fungi.

SKIN

FUNGAL INFECTIONS

Tinea

(See also Color Guide to Visual Diagnosis, p.561)

Tinea is a fungal infection of the skin, hair, body, or nails. All fungal infections thrive in moist areas but can affect any part of the body. They can also spread from one part of the body to another. You can catch a fungus from an infected person or animal or from contaminated floors, showers, or bathtubs. See also Fungal Infections of the Nails, p.560.

Athlete's foot is the most common form of tinea. It is spread by direct contact, which commonly occurs when bare feet come in contact with moist areas, such as locker rooms, bathrooms, and pool areas. Symptoms include redness, swelling, scaling, cracking, burning, and intense itching between the toes. The skin may look white and puckered. Many people with athlete's foot also have toenail fungus (see Fungal Infections of the Nails, p.560).

Jock itch is a fungal infection of the groin, which is the second-most common site for a fungal infection. Men are more prone than women to this infection, which appears as itchy, burning, scaling, reddened patches that extend over the genital area and in the creases and folds of the upper thigh (although usually not on the penis or scrotum). The fungus that causes jock itch can also infect other moist areas, such as the armpits and under the breasts.

Ringworm is another fungal infection of the skin that is most often acquired by direct contact with an infected person or household pets. Ringworm begins as small, circular, red patches that enlarge. The inner circle heals first, leaving an outer ring of redness. The itchy scales can affect different parts of the body. Usually, multiple patches develop, but seldom more than five at a time.

Tinea infection of the scalp is more common in children and is widespread in some urban areas, where overcrowding leads to the spread of infection. Signs and symptoms include itching, inflammation, and round, scaling patches of hair loss on the scalp.

Tinea versicolor is a skin condition that usually causes oval, flaking patches, spots, and pimplelike bumps on the chest, shoulders, and back. The infection can appear darker on light skin, and lighter on dark skin. Tinea versicolor can be made worse by sunlight. The fungus that causes this infection lives on the skin of many people without causing symptoms. It is frequently spread by sexual contact or in locker rooms on contaminated towels.

TREATMENT OPTIONS

There are many effective over-the-counter antifungal creams and ointments for athlete's foot, jock itch, and ringworm. If your fungal infection recurs or becomes severe, see your doctor. A prescription antifungal medicine in tablet form may be required.

Preventing Fungal Infections

Fungi travel easily from one part of the body to another, and they tend to recur once they find a hospitable environment. The state of your general health helps determine how friendly a host you are to fungi. An underlying illness can make you more susceptible to fungal infection.

Taking antibiotic drugs (see p.868) can upset your body's natural balance of bacteria and fungi, causing normally harmless fungi to proliferate and cause infection. To prevent a fungal infection from spreading—and returning—take these preventive measures:

- Keep your body clean and dry. Infectious fungi thrive in warm, dark, moist areas.

- To prevent athlete's foot, keep your feet dry, and dry each toe individually.

- Wear protective footwear in moist areas, such as locker rooms, gyms, and near pools.

- Never share personal items, such as towels, combs, or brushes, with others.

Tinea infection of the scalp is treated by taking a prescription antifungal drug in tablet form for up to 2 months, along with treating the hair and scalp with antifungal creams.

Heat and humidity encourage the growth of tinea versicolor. Treatment involves applying antifungal creams or ointments that contain pyrithione zinc to the upper torso—thighs, trunk, arms, and neck—to clear the condition and prevent reinfection. Bed linens and pajamas should be laundered daily while the condition is active.

See Preventing Fungal Infections (p.530) for advice on preventing and stopping the spread of fungi.

Candida

(See also Color Guide to Visual Diagnosis, p.561)

Candida is another kind of fungus. Candida infection causes beefy red discoloration of moist areas of the skin under the breasts, under the arms, around the vagina, or in the groin. It also can appear in the mouth and on the tongue, in the vagina (see p.1066), and on the area around the rectum.

Candida infections are treated by keeping the moist area as dry as possible by using drying powders, drying the area with towels frequently, and applying creams containing an antifungal drug.

With groin infections, it is helpful to wear loose-fitting cotton underclothes and to avoid tight-fitting wool or nylon underclothes.

Where Candida Infections Occur

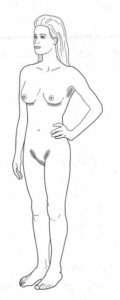

Candida, a type of fungus, thrives in warm, moist areas such as under the armpits and breasts, the groin, and the vagina. It causes a beefy, red discoloration.

BACTERIAL INFECTIONS

Impetigo

(See also Color Guide to Visual Diagnosis, p.562)

Mostly a childhood condition, impetigo is a highly contagious bacterial infection that usually appears around the nose and mouth, although it can appear anywhere on the skin. Bacteria enter the skin through breaks caused by cold sores, cuts, or scrapes and then multiply and spread. Impetigo can also be a complication of scratching itchy skin conditions such as eczema (see p.550).

SYMPTOMS

Impetigo often begins with a reddened area of skin. Within a day or two, a group of small blisters crops up. Often, because the blisters are so small and fragile (and thus, break easily), they are not noticed. Sometimes, impetigo causes small bumps and not blisters. When the bumps or blisters of impetigo burst, moist areas of tender, red skin appear underneath and secrete a clear liquid.

Eventually, a scabby, honey-colored crust, which may itch, forms over the reddened area. In severe cases, impetigo may be accompanied by fever, and the lymph glands in the face or neck may swell. Young children are especially prone to complications of impetigo, such as inflammation of the kidneys (see Glomerulonephritis, p.810) and infection of the blood (see Bacteremia, p.878).

TREATMENT OPTIONS

It is essential to avoid touching the affected area because the infection can easily spread. Talk to your doctor if you or your child has impetigo. The doctor may prescribe an antibiotic pill, injection, or a skin cream such as mupirocin. All are very effective, clearing up the infection in about a week.

The following scrupulous sanitary practices are an important part of treating and preventing the spread of impetigo:

■ Wash sheets and pillowcases daily.

■ Keep personal items, such as soap and towels, away from other family members.

■ Wash the area around the blisters with soap and water (showering is especially effective for doing this). Gently wash away the scabs themselves with water and an antiseptic solution such as chlorhexidine and then dry the area. This gives the topical preparations better access to the infection.

■ Because impetigo is highly contagious, children who have it should be kept away from others until the infection clears.

Folliculitis, Furuncles (Boils), and Carbuncles

(See also Color Guide to Visual Diagnosis, p.562)

Folliculitis is an inflammation of hair follicles that can occur anywhere hair grows. The inflammation is your immune system's response to the invasion of bacteria, usually *Staphylococcus aureus*. In the process of fighting the bacteria, the immune system deploys helpful white blood cells to the infected site, causing inflammation.

When combined with bacteria and dead cells at the follicle, the white blood cells form pus. The result is a boil, or furuncle. When the boil is severe and large, or when several boils merge, it is called a carbuncle.

There is little risk associated with boils or carbuncles except in rare cases when pus spreads below the skin's surface. The boils and carbuncles caused by folliculitis occur most often on the buttocks, thighs, groin, scalp, armpits, and face.

SYMPTOMS

A red, warm, tender bump in the skin emerges first. Within a day, bacteria proliferate, the bump

enlarges, and, because the contents are encased in skin, the swelling creates painful pressure. Nearby lymph glands may become swollen. Usually, the boil forms a head and bursts, allowing the pus to drain and the skin to heal. Less commonly, the boil dissipates under the skin on its own, relieving the pain.

Diseases such as diabetes mellitus (see p.832)—or other conditions that can make your immune system weaker than normal—increase your risk of having recurring boils. Talk to your physician if you have a chronic problem.

TREATMENT OPTIONS

Never squeeze or open the boil yourself; this can cause a more severe infection and encourage the infection to spread. To help the boil or carbuncle come to a head faster, wash the infected area and apply warm, moist compresses every 2 or 3 hours. For every application, use a clean washcloth soaked in hot water.

The boil should go away on its own within 3 weeks. If it does not, or if it is severe, consult your doctor, who may lance the boil and drain it. He or she may also prescribe antibiotics, especially if you have a recurring problem.

While shaving, men can get small skin cuts that become infected. To help this type of folliculitis heal, avoid shaving for several days, since the razor can spread the bacteria from one part of the skin to another.

Some people have a chronic staphylococcus bacterial infection of the nose, which can cause more frequent boils or folliculitis on the face and neck. One preventive treatment is to regularly

apply an antibiotic ointment called mupirocin to the inside of the nose (this can sometimes cause a burning sensation).

Cellulitis and Erysipelas

(See also Color Guide to Visual Diagnosis, p.562)

Cellulitis and erysipelas are two bacterial infections of the skin; they are often caused by the same types of bacteria. Both cellulitis and erysipelas are potentially dangerous infections—each can spread to the blood and the infection can then affect other organs. They are particularly dangerous in infants, the elderly, people who have a weak immune system, and those with abnormal or artificial heart valves (because the infection from the skin can settle on the valves and produce serious heart disease).

SYMPTOMS

With both infections, the skin becomes red, tender, and warm over the course of a few hours or a few days. You may also feel generally ill and develop a fever, shaking chills, swollen lymph glands near the area of the infection, and red streaks leading from the red area of skin to the nearby swollen lymph glands.

Cellulitis usually occurs in the legs, often following a break in the skin that permits bacteria living on the skin's surface to enter the inner layers of skin, where they can more easily cause infection. Breaks in the skin of the feet are sometimes responsible for cellulitis of the leg.

With cellulitis, there is usually one large area of redness that feels unusually firm and thick.

You can often see in the reddened area the break in the skin that led to the cellulitis.

Erysipelas is usually located in one of three places. It often occurs on the bridge of the nose, spreading across the upper cheek and causing swelling of the eye on one side of the face. It also can develop in a part of the body where lymph vessels have been cut, such as in the arm after radical mastectomy surgery for breast cancer. Finally, it can occur where veins have been cut, such as in people who have had veins in their legs removed as part of heart surgery. This latter kind of erysipelas is often confused with cellulitis.

In erysipelas (in contrast to cellulitis), there are often several different red patches of skin that are not connected to each other, and the red skin is not as raised as it is in cellulitis.

TREATMENT OPTIONS

If you suspect you have cellulitis or erysipelas, call your doctor immediately. Treatment with antibiotics to kill the bacteria (usually streptococcus or staphylococcus) that cause these conditions cures the infection, but a cure takes longer if treatment is delayed. Hospitalization is usually not required. During treatment for cellulitis of the leg, keep the affected leg elevated. Doctors sometimes recommend keeping an infected arm elevated by a sling attached to a pole that is on wheels so that you can walk with it.

OTHER SKIN CONDITIONS

Acne

(See also Color Guide to Visual Diagnosis, p.562)

Acne is a common skin condition that occurs most often during the hormonal changes that accompany adolescence, but it can occur at any age. It is so common among teenagers (about 80% have it) that it is considered a natural part of growing up.

Acne occurs in adolescence because various hormones—mainly androgen (which increases the amount of skin oil produced)—circulate in higher levels in the blood. It also can occur or become worse with other conditions that involve hormonal changes, including menstruation, pregnancy, or use of birth-control pills, and sometimes during early menopause.

The severity of acne varies. Some people have only mild, sporadic outbreaks of a few annoying whiteheads or blackheads. Others have severe eruptions of pimples and cysts that can leave permanent scars. Acne usually clears up on its own by the late teens or early 20s in men, and somewhat later in women.

Acne occurs in the sebaceous glands and the hair follicles to which they are attached. The sebaceous glands make an oil called sebum. Normally, this oil, along with dead skin cells, moves up from the bottom of the gland through the pore (opening) on the surface of the skin, spreading across the skin, where it is washed away.

Acne: Dr Stern's Advice

Q I'm 16 years old and my acne seems to be getting worse, especially around my period. My mom says I'll outgrow it. Will I?

A Most teenage girls with acne notice that flare-ups tend to occur about a week before their periods. Your body's hormonal changes trigger an increase in the production of sebum (oil made by tiny glands in your skin), which contributes to acne. Your mother is right about your acne diminishing as you get older. For most people, it largely disappears or greatly diminishes by the late teens or early 20s, although for some people acne persists longer or even first develops in their 20s or 30s.

Q Some of my friends say that french fries and chocolate cause acne. Is it true?

A No. There is no relationship between what you eat and acne flare-ups. However, too many french fries and too much chocolate are bad for your health in other ways.

ROBERT S. STERN, MD
BETH ISRAEL DEACONESS MEDICAL CENTER
HARVARD MEDICAL SCHOOL

In acne, the sebum and dead cells plug up the opening of the sebaceous gland and its hair follicle. This plug is called a comedo. Sometimes the opening of the comedo is not visible; there is just a bump underneath the skin. This is called a closed comedo. Other times the opening at the top of the plug is visible (open comedo).

When the plug of sebum and cells is white, it is called a whitehead. Sometimes the pigment melanin in the dead cells makes the plug dark (which is sometimes mistaken for dirt); this is called a blackhead. Generally the plug in closed comedos is not dark, while open comedos usually have a dark plug.

The bacteria *Propionibacterium acnes* live inside the hair follicles. They use sebum for their nutrition. When the bacteria digest the sebum, they produce waste material (fatty acids) that can be very irritating to the skin. Most of the time these fatty acids are pushed up to the surface of the skin and washed away. However, when the glands get plugged and filled with sebum, these fatty acids accumulate inside the sebaceous gland, causing inflammation.

SYMPTOMS

Acne falls into two categories: inflammatory and noninflammatory. Both types usually occur on the face, but may also appear on the upper chest, back, neck, and buttocks. Most people have noninflammatory acne, which consists of comedos that have no surrounding redness or tenderness. Inflammatory acne occurs when fatty acids cause plugged

Acne

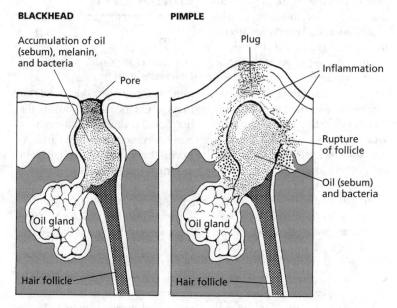

BLACKHEAD

Accumulation of oil (sebum), melanin, and bacteria

Pore

Oil gland

Hair follicle

PIMPLE

Plug

Inflammation

Rupture of follicle

Oil (sebum) and bacteria

Oil gland

Hair follicle

Blackheads result from the accumulation in a hair follicle of oil, bacteria, and the pigment called melanin (which gives skin its color). The pore is exposed, revealing a pigment-darkened area. Pimples emerge under an enclosed pore; they result from inflammation and rupture of a follicle filled with oil and bacteria, causing a red bump in the skin.

follicles to become inflamed, forming pimples and pus-filled nodules. Severe inflammatory acne may create nodules that leave deep, pitted scars that can be disfiguring.

PREVENTING COMPLICATIONS

It is difficult to prevent acne, but you can take steps to prevent its complications. Wash your face twice a day with ordinary soap and water; this is the only cleanliness measure that is necessary.

Using cosmetic creams or oils on your face can plug pores and make you susceptible to acne; choose products labeled "oil-free." Taking oral contraceptives or illegal "muscle-building"

steroids (see p.1024) can also bring on acne.

Do not scratch or squeeze pimples or cysts; this can lead to scarring that is often permanent. There is no evidence that any foods or sexual activity have any effect on acne.

TREATMENT OPTIONS

Talk to your doctor if you have acne. There are three general approaches to treatment: preventing the pores from getting plugged with sebum; causing the whiteheads and blackheads to dry up more rapidly; and using antibiotics that kill the *P acnes* bacteria. It usually takes time for acne to improve. In some people the condition worsens before it gets better.

Mild noninflammatory acne, with relatively few open comedos, is often treated by a cream or lotion that contains benzoyl peroxide, which helps keep pores open. If you have many whiteheads and blackheads, the medicine tretinoin (which comes as a cream, lotion, or gel) can open them up and let the material drain onto the surface of the skin, where it can be washed away. Ask your physician which medication is best for your acne.

If your acne includes inflammation (redness and tenderness around the whiteheads or blackheads), your physician may recommend antibiotics. For milder degrees of inflammation, the antibiotics can be taken as creams, lotions, or gels to rub on the face.

For more severe inflammation, antibiotics in pill form such as tetracycline, doxycycline,

minocycline, or erythromycin are used. Antibiotics mainly prevent the formation of new acne, and do not help very much with existing acne; thus, improvement typically takes several months. Antibiotics are often given for at least 6 months, although the dosage may be reduced with time.

For the most severe forms of acne in which there are cysts and great inflammation and when the treatments above have not been effective, two additional treatments are possible. Your doctor may inject anti-inflammatory corticosteroid medicines (see p.895) directly into the inflamed cysts.

Alternatively, the drug isotretinoin, taken as a tablet, is very effective against acne. However, isotretinoin should never be taken by a woman who is pregnant or could become pregnant, because it can cause severe birth defects and miscarriage.

Rosacea

(See also Color Guide to Visual Diagnosis, p.562)

Rosacea causes spidery blood vessels and flushing of the face. Although it shares some features with acne (see p.533), it is a different condition and occurs primarily in middle-aged adults.

SYMPTOMS

The predominant symptoms are flushing and visible spidery blood vessels called telangiectasias on the face. However, rosacea may also appear as pimples (but not whiteheads or blackheads) on the forehead, cheeks, nose, and chin.

Early symptoms, beginning with brief periods of facial flushing, may go unnoticed. Eventually, the redness persists and telangiectasias appear just below the surface of the nose and cheeks. Small, raised bumps with a yellow top and a red rim called

Dry Skin

Dry skin can occur at any age, but it is more common as you age. Sun exposure, cold weather, indoor dry heat, and irritating soaps or chemicals can strip the skin of its natural oils. As a result, skin becomes dry, flaky, and can appear more wrinkled. The goal of treatment is to minimize moisture loss:

- Try substituting warm (not hot) showers for baths.
- Use soaps with a heavy fat content, glycerin bars, or soap substitutes.
- Avoid highly alkaline soaps.

Moisturizers work best when applied while your skin is still damp. All moisturizers are either water-in-oil lubricants or lighter, oil-in-water preparations. Some

products include substances like glycerin, urea, pyroglutamic acid, and sorbitol that draw moisture to the skin. Others containing lactic acid, lactate salts, or alpha-hydroxy acids are particularly good for extremely dry, scaly skin. Moisturizers that contain fats not only preserve but may even increase the water content of the outer layer of skin (the epidermis).

When you buy over-the-counter products, read the labels for additives. Avoid preparations with alcohol, which dry the skin. Lanolin can cause an allergic reaction in some people. Sometimes dry skin is so severe that a prescription-strength lotion or cream is required; if you have extremely dry skin, ask your physician for advice.

pustules (because they are filled with pus) may also form.

In rare cases, the soft tissues of the nose, especially the sebaceous glands, become heaped up, yielding a bulbous nose (the comedian W.C. Fields had a nose that was made bulbous by rosacea).

TREATMENT OPTIONS

To minimize flushing, avoid the things that cause blood vessels to open up, including rapid temperature extremes and sunlight. Daily use of sunscreen may also help. Since rosacea involves a widening of the small blood vessels, try to avoid drinking hot beverages or alcohol or eating spicy foods, all of which can make you flush, aggravating the condition.

The strongest medicines for rosacea pustules are antibiotic pills such as tetracycline, minocycline, or doxycycline. An antibiotic called metronidazole, in the form of a gel rubbed into the face, is also effective in treating less severe rosacea. Avoid acne medicines containing resorcinol, salicylic acid, or benzoyl peroxide; they can irritate your flushed skin.

Once you start treatment for rosacea, have patience; it usually takes weeks or months for the condition to improve.

The spidery blood vessels called telangiectasias can be covered with makeup. They also can be eradicated using a technique similar to that used on spider veins of the legs (see p.583) in which a tiny needle is inserted into the veins and an electrical charge passed through the needle to cauterize (seal) the veins. Laser treatment (see p.582) is also effective. Since the vessels

interconnect, it may take several treatments to eliminate all of the visible telangiectasias.

If you have excess nose tissue caused by rosacea, ask your doctor about surgery, which is usually performed with a laser.

Birthmarks

(See also Color Guide to Visual Diagnosis, p.562)

Birthmarks are areas of discolored skin that are present at birth. They range in hue from light pink to blue-black on people with light skin. On people with dark skin, birthmarks may exist but not show, since the pigment in the top layer of skin effectively hides the color of birthmarks below the skin. The two most common varieties of birthmarks are hemangiomas (malformations of blood vessels) and moles.

Birthmarks may appear alone or in a group on any part of the body. Hemangiomas include strawberry marks, port-wine stains, and salmon patches. Strawberry marks are raised purple-red blemishes that can be very small or up to several inches in diameter; most disappear by age 10.

Port-wine stains are purple, raised, and persist throughout adulthood; they can grow to be quite large over time. Salmon patches, also called stork bites, are small, flat patches of pink-red marks located primarily near the eyes and nape of the neck. Moles that you are born with (see p.544) are usually brown or blue.

Birthmarks need to be removed only if they are bothersome or unsightly to you. A variety of methods is available, depending on the size and loca-

tion (see Removing Skin Growths, p.542). Plastic surgery may be used to remove birthmarks. Laser treatments are effective in fading port-wine stains. Special cosmetics are available to conceal flat birthmarks. Talk to your doctor to determine the best option for you.

Your doctor should examine moles regularly and may recommend removal if they are in a location where they are likely to be constantly rubbed or if the moles look as if they might be cancerous or precancerous (p.543).

Hives

(See also Color Guide to Visual Diagnosis, p.562)

Hives, also called urticaria, is a common skin condition that causes itchy, raised areas and inflammation of the skin. An allergic reaction is one cause of hives but, often, the cause of hives is unknown.

Substances that can bring on hives include foods, drugs, insect bites, plants, or metals. Some people break out in hives after perspiring or after being in extreme cold or out in the sun. Emotional stress can trigger hives or make the condition worse in people who are susceptible.

SYMPTOMS

Hives causes itchy, inflamed, raised areas of skin. After exposure to the causative substance, the skin responds by producing the chemical histamine, which sets in motion a chain of immune system reactions that result in skin inflammation.

Foot Odor

Foot odor starts when the sweat glands in your soles create perspiration. Bacteria that like moist environments feed on dead skin, thrive, and produce the odor. Anything that makes the feet moist—such as exercise and wearing shoes that are not properly ventilated—can make the odor worse. To remedy foot odor, practice good foot hygiene:

- Change your socks regularly and wash your feet at least once a day.
- Apply moisture-absorbing foot powders (but not cornstarch, which feeds some of the bacteria that cause the smell) to your feet and toes.
- Use an antiperspirant directly on your feet.
- Allow your shoes to dry by airing them out thoroughly after you take them off.
- Try using odor-absorbing shoe inserts that contain charcoal.

The appearance of hives varies widely in shape and size, but usually the rash is round. The spots may merge to form a large white and red patch with irregular borders. Other forms of hives include dermatographism (see right) and angioneurotic edema (see p.562).

TREATMENT OPTIONS

Hives cannot be cured, but you can prevent it by avoiding allergens (allergy-producing substances) that cause it. Soothing preparations that you apply to your skin to relieve itching are available at drugstores. Antihistamine drugs can also relieve itching; some (such as diphenhydramine or chlorpheniramine) are available in drugstores without a prescription.

Antihistamines make some people sleepy. Your doctor can prescribe an antihistamine drug that is less likely to make you sleepy. To treat more severe cases of hives, your physician may prescribe corticosteroid drugs (see p.895).

Dermatographism

Dermatographism (also known as dermagraphy) means "skin writing." It is a type of hives (see p.536) in which scratching or rubbing the skin causes a raised, pale area with a red halo in the exact path of the scratching or rubbing. The raised area may itch and last for hours. If itching becomes bothersome, calamine lotion can help soothe it.

Rashes

(See also Color Guide to Visual Diagnosis, p.563)

Rash is a general term used to describe redness or spots on the skin. Rashes take a variety of different forms, depending on the cause. Most rashes are short-lived and nonthreatening, such as the rashes that occur with common childhood infections (see p.568).

However, in some instances, a rash indicates a serious underlying problem, such as lupus erythematosus (see p.898), Lyme disease (see p.884), or meningitis (see p.377), and requires prompt treatment by your doctor. Other rashes can be caused by an allergic reaction to a drug (see below). Rashes may also be recurring, uncomfortable, and cosmetically annoying.

Treatment depends on the origin of the rash and on the cosmetic problems it causes. See also Rash in Infants and Children (p.304), Hives (p.536), Dermatitis (p.550), Psoriasis (p.551), Shingles (below), Lichen Planus (p.538), and Fungal Infections (p.530).

Drug Rash

(See also Color Guide to Visual Diagnosis, p.563)

An allergy to a medicine can cause a rash that may occur within hours or even days of taking the drug. Your skin may get slightly red, either all over your body or only in limited areas. Sometimes the rash is very severe and sometimes it goes away on its own, even if you continue to take the medicine that caused it. Call your doctor if you have a rash that began shortly after you started taking a new drug, including any nonprescription drugs. Your doctor may be able to substitute a medicine that does not give you a rash.

Shingles

(See also Color Guide to Visual Diagnosis, p.563)

Shingles, also known as herpes zoster, is a virus infection of the nerves that causes a painful, blistering rash. The virus responsible for shingles, the varicella-zoster virus, is the same virus that causes chickenpox.

Where Shingles Blisters Occur

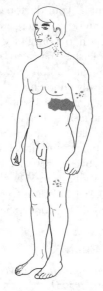

Shingles blisters, which are often accompanied by a burning pain, erupt on the skin along nerve pathways. They are especially common on the trunk and limbs, but can affect the neck, face, and eye. Sometimes pain occurs in an area but the blisters never develop.

By age 30, most Americans have been exposed to chickenpox. After the initial exposure, the virus lies dormant in the spinal nerve and, for most people, remains inactive throughout life. But for some people—particularly those over age 50 or those with a weaker immune system—the varicella-zoster virus "reawakens" and causes shingles.

The virus can be spread to nonimmunized people through direct contact with the weeping skin blisters. Immunization against the varicella-zoster virus is now recommended for chil-dren (see p.947) and adults who have never had chickenpox. It will protect many children against chickenpox and shingles, but cannot help people who already have been infected with the virus.

SYMPTOMS

Shingles starts as sharp, burning pain near the surface of the skin. The pain precedes a rash of red sores by several days. The sores turn to itchy blisters loaded with the virus, and the blisters form distinct patterns along nerve pathways, often appearing in a band over the ribs on one side of the body, or on the face.

The blisters usually disappear after 7 days, crusting over and sometimes leaving scars. Pain may persist for weeks or, less commonly, for several months. The affected area can become so sensitive that even light bed sheets or clothing cause intense pain, a condition called postherpetic neuralgia.

Postherpetic neuralgia is a result of damage to nerves and is more common in people over 60 and in those with weaker immune systems. It often disap-pears on its own.

TREATMENT OPTIONS

If shingles affects your eyes it can cause blindness. If your immune system is seriously weakened, the complications of shingles can be life-threatening. If you suspect that you have shingles, see your doctor immediately. He or she may recommend analgesic drugs or corticosteroid drugs (see p.895) to minimize the pain and an antiviral drug to reduce nerve damage.

Lichen Planus

(See also Color Guide to Visual Diagnosis, p.563)

Lichen planus is a rash that affects people in different ways. In many people the rash first appears as pinhead-sized, blue-red blemishes that, over time, may coalesce into rough, scaly patches. The rash commonly occurs on the arms, wrists, and legs, as well as in the vulva. It can also occur in the mouth. Lichen planus may also cause ridges on the nails.

Although the cause is un-known, there is some evidence that emotional stress can trigger lichen planus. Your physician may prescribe corticosteroid drugs (see p.895) to relieve the itching and inflammation of the rash; only high-potency forms of the drug help.

Lichen planus can resemble skin cancer; your doctor may perform a biopsy (removing a small piece of tissue for examina-tion in the laboratory) to diag-nose it. Lichen planus that affects the vulva is sometimes treated with corticosteroid drugs taken by mouth.

Pigment Changes

(See also Color Guide to Visual Diagnosis, p.563)

Changes in skin color are com-mon and usually harmless. Skin color is determined by melanin, a protein made by cells called mel-anocytes. Darker skin has a higher concentration of melanin; light skin has less. Your melanin level is genetically determined, but exposure to the sun also plays a major role. In an effort to protect skin from the sun's harm-

Help for Aging Skin

Aging takes its toll on the dermis (the deepest layer of skin) as the number of fibroblasts, its principle constituent cell, declines. In addition, molecules of collagen, the connective protein that forms the skin's supportive structure, become stiffer.

Sun exposure also speeds up the aging of skin—compare the skin on the back of your hand to the skin on your buttocks or breasts to see the effects of sun damage. As a result of exposure to the sun, the skin loses the resilience of youth, eventually taking on the appearance of tissue paper.

The most important thing you can do for your skin is to keep it out of direct sunlight, especially in late spring and summer, when sunlight is most intense. When you are in the sun, cover your skin by wearing a hat, tightly woven clothing, and a sunscreen that has a sun protection factor (SPF) of at least 15. Smoking also accelerates the skin's aging process.

The treatments listed here are helpful for some people; ask your doctor to give you more information about them. In addition, dermabrasion, chemical peels, laser surgery, and face-lifts (see Cosmetic and Reconstuctive Surgery, p.570) can mitigate the passage of time, but not without some risk from surgery.

TREATMENT	PROS	CONS
Water-in-oil lubricants and oil-in-water lubricants	Temporarily replace moisture.	Can be very expensive; have no long-term effect on skin structure.
Tretinoin and other derivatives of vitamin A	Help reduce age spots (liver spots), birthmarks, and other dark pigmented areas; reduce delicate wrinkles and skin roughness; produce thickening of the outermost layer of skin; decrease melanin (skin pigment) content.	May bleach normal skin as well as pigmented areas; can cause skin peeling, irritation, and redness; make skin more susceptible to sun damage; prescription needed.
Alpha-hydroxy acids	Are available in different forms and concentrations; reverse delicate wrinkles; improve skin tone; smooth rough skin; no prescription needed for lower concentrations.	Redness and stinging (at first); high concentrations (above 14%) carry greater risks, including skin burns; need to be applied by a doctor; generally, higher risk of side effects in higher concentrations; concentrations not always given on package; make skin vulnerable to sunburn.

ful ultraviolet rays, melanin levels increase, darkening the skin.

INCREASE IN PIGMENT

Several conditions can cause darker areas of skin:

Melasma is a condition in which dark areas appear on the cheeks, forehead, and above the lips. It can be caused by the hormonal changes of pregnancy or menopause and by taking oral contraceptives or hormone replacement therapy. Melasma usually fades when hormones stabilize.

Liver spots, also called age spots, are darkened spots that often occur on the hands and other sun-exposed areas. They arise when aging skin becomes more fragile and more vulnerable to the sun's ultraviolet light. Areas of the skin exposed to perfumes or scented cosmetics along with sunlight can also temporarily become darker.

These conditions may be bothersome but are not harmful. Other increases in pigment may warrant your doctor's attention. Skin that seems to tan without being exposed to the sun may be

Why Aging Skin Tears Easily

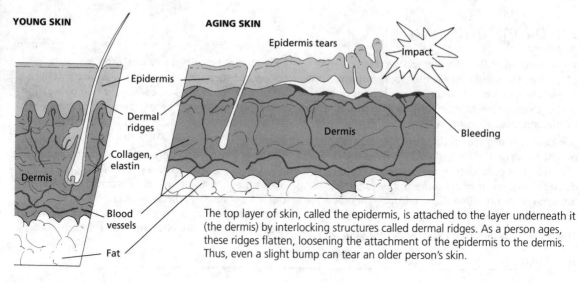

YOUNG SKIN

Epidermis

Dermal ridges

Collagen, elastin

Dermis

Blood vessels

Fat

AGING SKIN

Epidermis tears

Impact

Dermis

Bleeding

The top layer of skin, called the epidermis, is attached to the layer underneath it (the dermis) by interlocking structures called dermal ridges. As a person ages, these ridges flatten, loosening the attachment of the epidermis to the dermis. Thus, even a slight bump can tear an older person's skin.

a sign of an underlying disease, such as Addison disease (see p.856) or Cushing disease (see p.857). Moles also can occur or change due to exposure to sunlight (see Cancerous Skin Growths, p.543); tell your doctor about any change in a mole so that he or she can rule out cancer.

DECREASE IN PIGMENT

Vitiligo causes patches of skin to become lighter. In vitiligo, parts of the skin stop producing melanin. The result is symmetrical white patches that often occur on the face, hands, armpits, and groin. In some people, the patches begin producing pigment again without treatment. The cause of vitiligo is not known, but it may be an autoimmune disorder (see p.870) that affects melanocytes, the cells responsible for making pigment.

Albinism is a rare, inherited dis-

ease in which melanin, which colors the skin, hair, and eyes, is absent from birth. People with albinism have extremely pale skin and hair and often have eye problems, including extreme sensitivity to sunlight.

Phenylketonuria, a genetic condition, causes lower melanin levels and fairer, but not white, skin and hair.

Psoriasis and other scaly skin conditions may leave the skin melanin-deficient after treatment to remove the scales.

Tinea versicolor (see p.530) may bring on a similar lack of pigment.

TREATMENT OPTIONS

Normal pigmentation gradually reappears when psoriasis or tinea versicolor are effectively treated. Depigmenting creams can help lighten dark areas in other condi-

tions, although they should be applied carefully since they lighten normal skin as well.

For vitiligo and age spots, you can also cover areas of increased or decreased pigmentation with a cosmetic. Your doctor may recommend psoralen, a drug that makes skin more sensitive to light, and ultraviolet light (in combination, called PUVA) for vitiligo. The drug tretinoin in cream form may help lighten the skin discoloration of melasma. Laser treatments (see p.582) are also available to lighten dark patches of skin. See also Help for Aging Skin, p.539.

Stretch Marks

Stretch marks, also called striae, are thin red lines that appear on the skin of the thighs, abdomen, or breasts. They are caused by a thinning of the skin, usually brought on by changes in skin elasticity. Over time, the red lines fade from purple to silver-white.

Hormonal changes and stretching of the skin during pregnancy and adolescence are thought to cause the skin to become thinner and more vulnerable to stretch marks. About 90% of women develop stretch marks during pregnancy. Pregnancy-related stretch marks tend to be more prominent with greater weight gain, are red-purple when new, and become lighter than normal skin several months after delivery; they often fade with time.

Stretch marks that are purple also develop in people who have Cushing syndrome (see p.857). There is no proven way to prevent or treat stretch marks, although one study found that a tretinoin cream may be helpful.

Xanthelasma and Xanthoma

(See also Color Guide to Visual Diagnosis, p.563)

Xanthelasma is a harmless skin condition, common among elderly adults, in which yellow fatty deposits appear around the eyelids. Xanthomas are yellow fatty deposits that appear on the elbow or buttocks and are much less common than xanthelasma.

Xanthomas are harmless, but may be a warning sign of elevated cholesterol (see p.669) and another kind of fat (triglyceride). If you have xanthomas, your doctor should check the levels of cholesterol and other fats in your blood. Lowering your levels of cholesterol can make the xanthomas smaller. If the deposits are cosmetically bothersome, they can be removed.

NONCANCEROUS SKIN GROWTHS

Warts

(See also Color Guide to Visual Diagnosis, p.564)

Warts are noncancerous skin tumors caused by the human papilloma virus (HPV). Warts are very common, most often occurring in children, teens, and young adults, and can spread through physical contact. There are more than 40 types of HPV, resulting in a variety of warts. Flat warts—the kind that crop up on the face, neck, chest, forearms, and legs—are common in children.

SYMPTOMS

The appearance of a wart depends on its location:

Common warts may be light-colored to brown and are found mostly on the hands.

Plantar warts tend to press into the sole from the pressure of standing and can be very painful.

Genital warts (see p.891) appear around the genitalia, as well as in the vagina and cervix in women.

Cervical warts may be precursors of cervical cancer (see p.1068).

Warts can itch or bleed and become infected with bacteria or fungi. Any wart that looks suspicious should be evaluated by your doctor to rule out skin cancer (see Cancerous Skin Growths, p.543). People who have weakened immune systems should be especially vigilant in having a physician examine any odd-looking growth.

Monitor Your Moles: Shape, Surface, Color

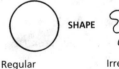
NORMAL MOLES

MOLES YOUR DOCTOR SHOULD EXAMINE

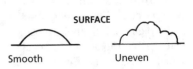

SHAPE

Regular   Irregular

SURFACE

Smooth   Uneven

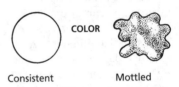

COLOR

Consistent   Mottled

Use this visual guide to look for suspicious moles.

TREATMENT OPTIONS

If a common wart or plantar wart is painful, or if you are bothered by its appearance, try one of the wart-removal preparations available at most drugstores. Since these medicines destroy normal as well as abnormal skin cells, do not use them for warts on your face or in genital areas; see your doctor about removal in these areas.

Also see your doctor if your wart does not respond to treatment. He or she can use a variety of methods—electricity, laser surgery, cryosurgery, or surgery with a scalpel—to remove the wart (see Removing Skin Growths, below right). Several treatments may be needed. In some people, warts return despite treatment.

Seborrheic Keratoses

(See also Color Guide to Visual Diagnosis, p.564)

Seborrheic keratoses are one of a group of harmless skin conditions caused by skin cells called keratinocytes. These cells contain some pigment but, unlike melanocytes (other pigmented skin cells, which cause malignant melanoma, see p.543), keratinocytes do not cause cancer.

Seborrheic keratoses can appear on any part of the body as crusty patches of light-colored to dark skin that range in size from tiny to larger than 3 inches. They look frightening but are harmless. Talk to your doctor if you are concerned or if you note a change in the appearance of a patch of affected skin (especially if it becomes inflamed).

Treatment, which attempts to improve cosmetic appearance, includes alpha-hydroxy acid creams and cover-up cosmetics available at most drugstores.

Molluscum Contagiosum

(See also Color Guide to Visual Diagnosis, p.564)

Molluscum contagiosum is a harmless skin infection caused by a virus. It appears as groups of tiny, pale, pearl-like lumps on the skin. If squeezed, a cheesy material often can be expressed from the central pore. In children, in whom it is common, the bumps usually occur on the face, trunk, and limbs; they are spread by direct contact.

In adults, the most common mode of transmission is sexual contact, and the infection occurs in the genital area, lower abdomen, and inner thighs. Molluscum contagiosum usually disappears within 2 to 12 months. If desired, your doctor can remove the lumps by scraping or freezing.

Skin Tags

(See also Color Guide to Visual Diagnosis, p.564)

Skin tags are harmless, small, skin-colored (or sometimes brown on white skin) growths that emerge without reason. They usually occur on the neck, in the armpits, or in the groin. They occur more frequently in people who are overweight and during pregnancy. Skin tags can also appear on the anus in conjunction with hemorrhoids (see p.795).

Skin tags usually do not go away on their own, but your doctor can remove them by curettage (scraping) or by cutting them off. Sometimes, accompanied by a local anesthetic (see p.168), they are clipped, frozen, or burned off with a small electrical instrument.

Removing Skin Growths

If you have a suspicious growth on your skin, your doctor may want to remove part of it for examination in a laboratory by performing a biopsy (see p.161) or remove the growth altogether. Several methods of removal are commonly used, depending on the site, type, and extent of the skin growth:

- **Cryosurgery** is a painless way to remove a skin growth. The growth is sprayed with very cold liquid nitrogen, or an instrument with a frozen tip is pressed against it.

- **Curettage** means scraping. It involves using a curet—a sharp, concave instrument—to scrape off all or part of the growth for biopsy.

- **Electrosurgery** (or electrodesiccation) involves using a probe to direct an electric current into the growth to destroy it. Electrodesiccation may cause redness around the treated area. It also is somewhat painful in comparison to cryosurgery.

- **Surgery** involves the use of a small, sharp knife called a scalpel to cut out the growth (using local anesthesia).

- **Lasers,** which are powerful beams of light that vaporize skin, may be used to remove skin growths.

- **Radiation therapy** (see p.741) may be used alone, or after surgery, to destroy malignant (cancerous) cells or reduce the size of an incurable tumor. Side effects can include redness and ulceration of the skin and hair loss.

Cysts

(See also Color Guide to Visual Diagnosis, p.564)

Cysts are areas of swelling that are filled with fluid, semifluid, or solid matter. Cysts usually arise from an obstruction of a duct (such as a sebaceous gland in the skin). Although usually harmless, cysts can be extremely painful if they become infected, and they may be cosmetically bothersome.

Complications may also arise. For example, sebaceous cysts may become infected with bacteria, causing redness, swelling, and intense pain. Treatment depends on the type of cyst and its complications; your doctor can drain, scrape, or remove a skin cyst. Skin cysts are not cancerous.

Cysts can also occur deep inside the body. Although all cysts are balloonlike circular structures, cysts inside the body can be much larger, and sometimes are part of a cancerous tumor or other serious condition. See also Ovarian Cyst (p.1080); Fibrocystic Breast Disease (p.1062).

Ganglion

A ganglion is a potentially painful, noncancerous lump that develops on a tendon or on connective tissue, most frequently on the wrist. The cyst contains synovial fluid (which lubricates joints and tendons) and can vary widely in size, from pea-sized to much larger. A ganglion may go away on its own. Treatment for a persistent and bothersome ganglion consists of either drawing out the fluid from the cyst with a needle (recurrence is likely with this approach) or surgically removing the cyst (recurrence is less frequent).

Lipomas

(See also Color Guide to Visual Diagnosis, p.564)

Lipomas are harmless, painless, movable, rubbery, fatty masses under the skin. They often appear in a group. Lipomas can occur in many different parts of the body but are mostly found on the neck, trunk, forearms, and back of the neck. They do not usually require removal, although your doctor can remove them by cutting them out (using local anesthesia) if they are annoying or unsightly.

PRECANCEROUS SKIN CONDITIONS

Two common skin conditions, actinic keratoses and leukoplakia (see p.489), can sometimes turn into cancer and therefore are called "precancerous" skin conditions. Certain kinds of moles can also turn into the skin cancer called melanoma (see below right) or can signal you to be alert for melanoma elsewhere on your body.

If you suspect that you have any of the following skin conditions, see your doctor. By rigorously following the suggestions under Preventing Skin Cancer (p.548), you can help prevent precancerous growths altogether.

Actinic Keratoses

(See also Color Guide to Visual Diagnosis, p.564)

Thousands of people each year are diagnosed with actinic keratoses, also called solar keratoses because they are caused by accumulated long-term exposure to the sun. They are usually pink or red-brown, scaly growths. While actinic keratoses themselves are harmless, they sometimes itch or become slightly painful. Moreover, actinic keratoses fit into the category of "precancerous" growths because they can develop into squamous cell carcinoma (see p.547), a type of malignant (cancerous) skin growth.

In fact, having actinic keratoses signals that you are at higher risk of skin cancer, including the deadliest form, malignant melanoma (see below). Ask your doctor to check any scaly, eroded area of skin that persists for more than a month. The best insurance is prevention (see Preventing Skin Cancer, p.548).

Because actinic keratoses are slow to develop into cancerous growths, your doctor may recommend only that you carefully monitor any existing patches. When necessary, individual keratoses can be eradicated in several weeks using daily applications of a prescription cream containing a drug called fluorouracil, either alone or in combination with liquid nitrogen treatments to freeze the growth.

Your doctor may also use laser resurfacing (see p.582) or a chemical peel (see p.585) to remove actinic keratoses.

CANCEROUS SKIN GROWTHS

Melanoma

(See also Color Guide to Visual Diagnosis, p.565)

Melanoma, the deadliest form of skin cancer, occurs when the pigment-making skin cells called melanocytes begin reproducing

Preventing and Identifying Melanoma

Doctors call freckles, age spots, and common moles "pigmented spots." Most pigmented spots are neither precancerous nor cancerous; most are harmless. Melanomas are the least common type of pigmented spot, but they are the most lethal and must be distinguished from the many harmless pigmented spots.

Familiarize yourself with the warning signs of malignant melanoma below. Nearly all skin cancers are related to sun exposure. Prevention is the best course of action. See Preventing Skin Cancer, p.548, for information on limiting your sun exposure and examining your skin.

THE ABCD'S OF MOLES

Most moles are "common moles," meaning the pigmentation in the mole is evenly distributed, the mole is symmetrical, and its borders are crisply defined. Moles have certain features that indicate they are more likely to be, or to become, dangerous melanomas. Use these guidelines to check your moles and see your doctor if you have a suspicious mole:

A Asymmetric One half of the mole does not match the other half.

B Border irregularity The edges are ragged, notched, or indistinct.

C Color Pigmentation is uneven and includes black, blue, or gray.

D Diameter Mole is larger than a pencil eraser (especially if there are more than two of this size) or has increased in size.

DYSPLASTIC MOLES

Dysplastic (or atypical) moles are not melanomas, but they can sometimes turn into melanomas. If you have one or more dysplastic moles you have an increased risk of a melanoma developing somewhere on your body; ask your doctor to examine any dysplastic moles. Dysplastic moles have the following features:

■ They are large (usually greater than 6 millimeters, or greater than the size of a pencil eraser).

■ Their borders are fuzzy, not crisp, although their shape is usually symmetrical.

■ They vary in color; usually they appear in various shades of brown and pink (but usually not black, blue, or gray).

EVALUATING YOUR RISK OF MELANOMA

Use the guidelines on p.548 to examine your skin for suspicious moles. In addition, there are three factors that are important in evaluating your risk of melanoma: your skin color, your hair color, and whether close relatives have had melanomas (see Risk of Melanoma, p.545). If you are at moderately increased risk, have your doctor examine your skin within the next several months and, after that, every year or two.

If you have one of the three general warning signs listed on p.546, or are at significantly or highly increased risk according to the Risk of Melanoma chart, have your moles examined promptly and every 6 months thereafter. Your doctor may take photographs to record the appearance of your moles so that even the subtlest change can be detected and new moles monitored.

---

uncontrollably to form a life-threatening tumor. Melanomas are painless and can form from an existing mole or develop on apparently unblemished skin. They can occur anywhere, including under nails and inside the eye.

Melanoma rarely occurs before age 18. However, the risk of melanoma rises rapidly in young adulthood, making it one of the most common life-threatening forms of cancer in people between the ages of 20 and 50. After age 50, the risk of melanoma rises more slowly with advancing age.

The incidence of malignant melanoma is now many times higher than in 1935 in the United States. It is estimated that, by the year 2000, 1 of 75 people will develop melanoma. This is presumed to be due to increased sun exposure in childhood.

SYMPTOMS

Melanomas are usually larger than 1/4 inch in diameter (about the size of a pencil eraser), but

Risk of Melanoma

Review the risk categories below to determine your risk of malignant melanoma. **Moderately increased risk** equals 25 to 50 common moles greater than 2 millimeters (mm) wide; two to nine common moles greater than 5 mm wide; recent growth of moles; light skin; blond hair; blue eyes; and/or a father, mother, sister, or brother with melanoma. **Significantly increased risk** equals 50 to 100 common moles greater than 2 mm wide; one to five dysplastic moles; previous skin cancer; and/or red hair. **Highly increased risk** equals more than 100 common moles greater than 2 mm wide; more than five dysplastic moles; and/or a family history of melanoma.

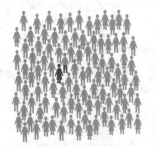

1.3 OF 100 PEOPLE ARE AT NORMAL RISK OF MELANOMA

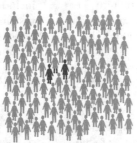

2.2 OF 100 PEOPLE ARE AT MODERATELY INCREASED RISK (LESS THAN TWO TIMES THE RISK) OF MELANOMA

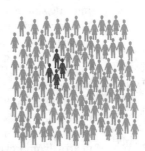

4 OF 100 PEOPLE ARE AT SIGNIFICANTLY INCREASED RISK (TWO TO FOUR TIMES THE RISK) OF MELANOMA

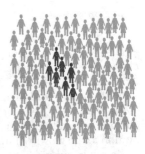

6.7 OF 100 PEOPLE ARE AT HIGHLY INCREASED RISK (GREATER THAN FOUR TIMES THE RISK) OF MELANOMA

Your Chances of Surviving Melanoma

Your chances of surviving the deadliest form of skin cancer—melanoma—depend on how deep the melanoma is. The deeper a melanoma, the less your chance is of being alive 5 years after the diagnosis.

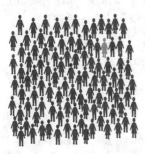

99 OF 100 PEOPLE WHO HAVE A MELANOMA THAT IS LESS THAN .03 INCHES DEEP WILL BE ALIVE IN 5 YEARS

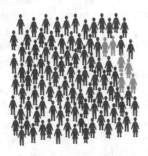

94 OF 100 PEOPLE WHO HAVE A MELANOMA THAT IS .03 TO LESS THAN .07 INCHES DEEP WILL BE ALIVE IN 5 YEARS

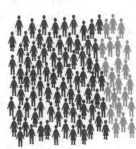

78 OF 100 PEOPLE WHO HAVE A MELANOMA THAT IS .07 TO LESS THAN .15 INCHES DEEP WILL BE ALIVE IN 5 YEARS

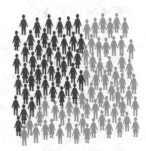

42 OF 100 PEOPLE WHO HAVE A MELANOMA THAT IS .15 INCHES OR MORE DEEP WILL BE ALIVE IN 5 YEARS.

they can be smaller. The most common sites are the face (especially in older people), upper trunk (especially in men), and legs (especially in women). There are three general warning signs of melanoma. If you have any of the following, discuss them with your doctor.

GENERAL WARNING SIGNS
OF MELANOMA

■ A mole that has recently changed its size or shape, even if it does not fit all the ABCD criteria in Preventing and Identifying Melanoma (see p.544). Moles in children normally grow in proportion to the growth of the child, so do not be worried about a mole that slowly doubles in size as your child doubles in size.

■ A mole that fits any of the ABCD criteria in Preventing and Identifying Melanoma (see p.544).

■ A mole that has been present since birth. Such moles have a greater chance of turning into melanoma. Depending on their size, color, and location, they may need to be removed.

TREATMENT OPTIONS

The first thing a melanoma does is invade the tissue immediately below the skin. How deeply it invades the adjacent tissue affects the prognosis (outlook). When the melanoma has invaded only adjacent tissue, it can be cured. But if the cells break away and travel through the lymph vessels to nearby lymph nodes and then spread (metastasize) to other organs, the disease can be fatal.

Diagnosing melanoma requires a biopsy that removes the entire suspicious area of skin. Under the microscope, the doctor can

tell the difference between a harmless mole and a melanoma and can also tell how deeply the melanoma has invaded the adjacent tissue. If the biopsy shows that it is a melanoma, your doctor may perform another biopsy that removes more tissue from around the melanoma. Melanomas that have grown deeply into the skin may require skin grafting to minimize scarring.

Determining whether the melanoma has spread to the nearby lymph glands is very important. If it has not, the chance of a cure is much greater. Your physician may be able to feel that the cancer has spread to a nearby lymph gland by feeling the enlarged gland with his or her fingers.

However, even if no enlarged lymph gland can be felt, the cancer may still have spread. In such cases, special tests are needed. Dyes or radionuclide materials (see p.137) may be injected at the site of the melanoma. These materials travel to, and thereby identify, the closest nearby lymph node. That lymph node is removed surgically, using local anesthesia, and examined under the microscope.

If there is no cancer in it, nothing further usually is done. If there are cancerous cells in it, then all of the nearby lymph nodes are removed by surgery, in hopes that the tumor will have spread only to those nearby nodes and not yet spread elsewhere.

More recently, techniques for identifying cancer-related genes in lymph nodes have improved the accuracy of biopsies in determining the prognosis of melanoma.

If the cancer has progressed

beyond the lymph nodes, the tumor is usually incurable. Chemotherapy (see p.741), surgery, and radiation therapy (see p.741) may be performed to increase survival time. More recent treatments, called immunotherapy, are designed to strengthen the immune system's capacity to fight the melanoma. These treatments include the use of the immune system chemical called interferon. Many doctors believe that immunotherapy will become more significant in the treatment of melanoma.

Basal Cell Carcinoma

(See also Color Guide to Visual Diagnosis, p.565)

Each year about 750,000 people in the United States learn that a small growth on their body is basal cell carcinoma (also called epithelioma)—the most common skin cancer. Repeated long-term exposure to sunlight is the primary cause. Light-skinned middle-aged people who spent a lot of time in the sun as children are especially susceptible. X-ray treatments for acne and exposure to arsenic and hydrocarbons (industrial pollutants) also increase your risk of basal cell carcinoma.

SYMPTOMS

A basal cell carcinoma begins as a painless bump or nodule that grows slowly. Later, it becomes an open ulcer with a hard edge. Nearly 90% of basal cell carcinomas occur on the face, but they can appear on any part of the body that is sometimes exposed to the sun—the face, ears, neck, back, chest, arms, and legs.

Although the tumors almost

never spread to other organs and are rarely fatal, they can invade surrounding tissue and be very disfiguring if they are not treated.

TREATMENT OPTIONS

Basal cell carcinoma is curable, but prevention is the best medicine. To prevent this skin cancer, avoid exposure to strong sunlight, wear a hat, and use a sunscreen (see Preventing Skin Cancer, p.548).

Your doctor can diagnose basal cell carcinoma by examining your skin and performing a biopsy. Basal cell carcinomas must be removed. Methods include surgery (cutting), cryosurgery (freezing), radiation therapy (see p.741), electrosurgery (which uses electrical current to kill cells), and curettage (scraping). A painstaking procedure called Mohs fresh tissue chemosurgery technique minimizes the amount of tissue removed and often is performed when the cancer is located in the skin folds around the nose, at the corners of the eyes, and around the ears.

Regular checkups are recommended for 5 years after removal to ensure the cancer has not returned. If you have had one basal cell carcinoma, you are at higher risk of developing others.

Squamous Cell Carcinoma

(See also Color Guide to Visual Diagnosis, p.565)

Squamous cell carcinoma is a life-threatening skin cancer that sometimes develops from a precancerous skin growth called an actinic keratosis (see p.543). The risk is highest among fair-skinned and fair-haired people who have

repeatedly been exposed to strong sunlight.

If you had freckles as a child, have blue eyes, or are over age 40, your risk is also greater. Other risk factors include taking immunosuppressants (drugs that weaken the immune system) and being exposed to arsenic or to hydrocarbons such as tar and industrial oils. Squamous cell carcinoma can also occur on the penis or vulva. Having had genital warts in the past is a major risk factor for genital squamous cell carcinomas.

SYMPTOMS

Squamous cell carcinoma starts out as a small, red, painless lump or patch of skin that slowly grows and may ulcerate. It usually occurs on areas of skin that have been repeatedly exposed to strong sunlight, such as the head, ears, and hands. Your doctor can diagnose squamous cell carcinoma by skin biopsy (removing a piece of tissue for examination in the laboratory).

Tumors are staged (a designation that refers to the progression of the cancer) by the number of abnormal cells, their thickness, and the depth of penetration into the skin. The higher the stage of tumor, the greater the chance of it metastasizing (spreading) to other organs of the body.

Squamous cell carcinoma on sun-exposed areas of skin (such as the face) usually does not spread. However, squamous cell carcinoma of the lip, vulva, and penis are more likely to spread. You should contact your doctor about any sore in these areas that does not go away after several weeks.

TREATMENT OPTIONS

Squamous cell carcinoma can be prevented by avoiding exposure to sunlight (see Preventing Skin Cancer, p.548), arsenic, and hydrocarbons. Treatment involves removing the tumor by cutting it out (after administering a local anesthetic), cryosurgery (freezing), or radiation therapy (see p.741). Advanced cancer may require chemotherapy (see p.741). Most people who are treated early for squamous cell carcinoma make a complete recovery, but your doctor may recommend regular checkups for several years to ensure that the tumor does not recur, and that new tumors do not form.

Kaposi Sarcoma

(See also Color Guide to Visual Diagnosis, p.565)

Kaposi sarcoma starts out as a slow-growing skin tumor that is unlikely to spread, but in its later stages may become an aggressive skin cancer that spreads throughout the body. The most common type of Kaposi sarcoma in the United States occurs in people infected with the human immunodeficiency virus (HIV) (see p.872); this type takes an aggressive course and cannot be cured.

Kaposi sarcoma also occurs in people taking immunosuppressant drugs after an organ transplant. In transplant patients, the tumors often disappear when treatment with the immunosuppressant drugs is discontinued. However, prolonged therapy with high doses of immunosuppressants can cause a more aggressive form of Kaposi sarcoma, similar to that found in people who are HIV-positive.

Preventing Skin Cancer

The source of warmth, light, and life—there are few images more positive than the sun. But when it comes to skin cancer, the sun is anything but wholesome. Nearly all skin cancers are related to sun exposure. Prevention is the best course of action.

RISK-REDUCING STRATEGIES

Here are some steps you should take to keep skin cancer from developing:

■ **Check your medicines.** Some prescription drugs and over-the-counter preparations make skin more vulnerable to sun damage. These include alpha-hydroxy acids; acne medications such as tretinoin; antidepressants; diuretics; and some antibiotics, antihistamines, and sedatives. Ask your doctor if your medication increases your risk in the sun.

■ **Be aware of your history.** Light skin and hair, childhood exposure to sunlight, and a family history of skin cancer increase your risk of skin cancer (see Risk of Melanoma, p.545).

■ **Monitor your moles.** Watch existing moles closely for any changes that could indicate malignant melanoma (see Preventing and Identifying Melanoma, p.544).

■ **Examine your skin regularly.** Use a mirror to help you examine your whole body, including your face (check underneath any facial hair), neck, arms, back, buttocks, legs, feet (including the soles), and under your fingernails and toenails. Use a blow dryer to part your hair so you can examine your scalp. See your doctor immediately if you find any new moles or suspicious-looking areas.

■ **Get regular exams.** If you are at risk (see Risk of Melanoma, p.545), make sure you get regular checkups.

■ **Practice safe sunning.**

  □ Minimize direct sun exposure, particularly between 10 AM and 2 PM.

  □ Use a sunscreen (see below), even in winter and on cloudy days.

  □ Wear a broad-brimmed hat and sunglasses.

  □ Wear sunglasses with ultraviolet (UV) light protection.

  □ Wear long sleeves and long pants.

SCREENING OUT THE SUN

In your effort to prevent skin cancer, make a decision to stop tanning your body. Sunscreens are an essential tool. There are two different types of sunscreens:

Chemical sunscreens contain substances that mimic the skin pigment melanin (the body's own defense against skin cancer) and may even reverse some sun damage. Sunshine contains UV rays that damage the skin. UV-A rays cause tanning and long-term skin damage, but not sunburn. UV-B rays cause tanning, sunburn, and skin damage.

Sun protection factor (SPF) is a standardized measure of a product's effectiveness. Here are some guidelines for selecting the correct chemical sunscreen:

■ SPF 15 is adequate for most people. Protection above SPF 15 is marginally better but seldom justifies the increased cost. An SPF under 15 is rarely enough for people with light skin.

■ Select a broad-spectrum sunscreen that covers both UV-A and UV-B rays.

■ If you are prone to acne, choose a waterproof product with a gel base. Oil-based products may clog pores and make acne worse.

■ Choose fragrance-free products to avoid an allergic reaction and to avoid attracting insects.

■ Apply sunscreens before you go outside and reapply every hour if you are in the water.

Physical sunscreens, also known as sunblocks, create an opaque, and therefore visible, barrier against UV rays. Zinc oxide is an example of a widely available sunblock.

An uncommon and relatively harmless type of Kaposi sarcoma, called European Kaposi sarcoma, occurs most often in elderly Jewish or Italian men.

SYMPTOMS

In people with HIV, Kaposi sarcoma can occur anywhere—in the mouth, on the skin, or inside the body. Other forms of Kaposi sarcoma often begin as a purple, brown, or red nodule on the ankles and feet that spreads up the legs, and then appears on other parts of the body. The nodules start out soft and spongy, become hard and solid, and then enlarge and swell.

TREATMENT OPTIONS

Your doctor diagnoses Kaposi sarcoma by a biopsy (removing a small piece of tissue for examination in the laboratory). Treatment depends on the course of the disease. In people with HIV, individual nodules can be removed, or injected with anticancer drugs. Tumors often respond well to radiation therapy (see p.741), although they frequently recur within months. In people with the less aggressive form of the disease, this treatment often provides a cure.

INFESTATIONS WITH INSECTS

Lice

Human lice are tiny bloodsucking insects that live in the hair of the head (head lice) and in pubic hair (see Crabs, right). Head lice can spread from person to person during daily activi-

Lice

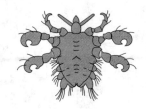

ties. They can also be transmitted by sharing hats and other head coverings (such as helmets), as well as by sharing combs and brushes. Lice spread easily among children at school or in day care.

SYMPTOMS

The first indication of lice infestation is itching. Small red bumps (lice bites) may be evident on the scalp, neck, and shoulders. If not treated, the bumps can become crusty and ooze and the hair may become matted. Infection, accompanied by swollen glands, occurs in rare instances.

TREATMENT OPTIONS

You can confirm the presence of lice and their eggs by looking at the infested person's scalp. The eggs of lice, called nits, look like tiny white flecks clinging to hair shafts (and sometimes to clothing). Lice themselves are minute but visible. If you think you or your child may be infested with head lice, see your doctor. If your child is infested, notify his or her school.

Your doctor will recommend one of several shampoos or hair rinses containing the medicine permethrin, which kills lice and their nits. After treatment, remove the lice and nits with a fine-toothed comb. Disinfect or soak

hats or other head coverings and grooming supplies in insecticide, or wash them in hot water and dry in a hot dryer. Clothing and linens should also be thoroughly washed and dried to rid them of lice.

Crabs

Also called pubic lice, crabs are a variety of lice that live in pubic hair, where they suck blood from skin. They are transmitted primarily by sexual contact. Crabs can also inhabit hair at other sites, such as the anus, eyelashes, and eyebrows.

In addition to intense itching, which occurs mainly at night, the bites of these tiny insects cause blue spots. The eyelids may become inflamed if the eyelashes are infested. Crabs easily elude detection. Less than 3 millimeters long, they cling tightly to hair shafts, where they lay barely detectable white eggs, known as nits, to hatch.

If you have itching, or see evidence of crabs, see your doctor as soon as possible. He or she will recommend a cream rinse that kills both crabs and nits (normal washing with soap and water does not remove them). Clothing and linens should be washed in

Crabs (Pubic Lice)

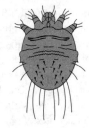

hot water and dried in a hot dryer for 30 minutes. You should also inform all sexual partners that they might have crabs so they also can be treated.

Scabies

(See also Color Guide to Visual Diagnosis, p.566)

Scabies is another kind of insect infestation and is highly contagious. Infestation with scabies causes intense itching. The pregnant females burrow into the top layer of skin (usually on the buttocks, genital area, wrists, hands, and armpits—although usually not on the face, scalp, neck, or palms).

In the burrows, the females deposit two to three eggs each day for a month. After about 2 weeks, the eggs mature. The adults emerge, mate with each other, and then reinvade the skin. The pregnant females spread from one person to another during close physical or sexual contact and through contact with infested bed sheets or clothing.

SYMPTOMS

Infestation with scabies causes intense itching. The burrows the females make appear as dark wavy lines on the skin that end in a small round lump. A symmetric rash of tiny red lumps resembling small insect bites often appears around the burrows.

The main symptom, an intense itching, especially at night, results from a reaction to the insect's excrement. As a result, the first infestation may not be noticed for a month or longer, and itching may persist for weeks after the mites are eradicated. Scratching is

Scabies Mite

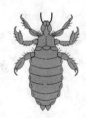

one of the body's best defenses against scabies because they cannot survive out of their burrows. Scratching can cause the lumps to crust over, resembling psoriasis (see p.551).

TREATMENT OPTIONS

See your doctor if you think you have scabies. He or she will recommend a prescription medicine that is applied from the neck down after bathing. Your doctor may also recommend a prescription drug taken by mouth. Antihistamines, mild painkillers, and/or calamine lotion may also be needed to control the itching.

Clothing and bedding should be washed in hot water and dried in a hot dryer to avoid reinfestation. Sexual partners and family or friends with whom you have been in close physical contact should be treated even if they do not have symptoms.

SCALING AND ITCHING CONDITIONS

Dermatitis and Eczema

(See also Color Guide to Visual Diagnosis, p.566)

Dermatitis and eczema are interchangeable terms for several conditions that cause inflammation

of the skin. The most common of these conditions are listed below. Each has a different cause but similar symptoms—red areas of skin, raised red lumps, and/or blisters that sometimes join to form patches. In severe cases, the areas may become infected (see Impetigo, p.531). In long-standing cases of dermatitis, the skin becomes dry, thick, and scaling.

Atopic dermatitis, or atopic eczema, is often called the "itch that rashes." The rash causes an itch, the itch promotes scratching, and scratching leads to further irritation and increased rash, and so on in a continuous cycle. If you have this form of eczema, it is likely that a family member has some type of allergy such as asthma or hay fever or a food allergy.

The rash changes with age. It is common in infancy, when it appears as inflamed, weeping patches or crusty areas on the face, neck, and groin. In childhood and adolescence, the rash is found mainly in the folds of the skin. Atopic dermatitis generally goes away on its own. In adults, it usually becomes limited to one area of the body, such as the hands.

Contact dermatitis arises after contact with a substance that either irritates the skin or, less commonly, causes an allergic reaction. In both cases, depending on how long the skin has been in contact with the substance, the skin is itchy and may swell or become marked by blisters. The pattern of the rash corresponds directly to the area exposed to the irritant.

Causes of contact dermatitis

include laundry detergents, metal from jewelry or clothes fasteners, some rubber products such as gloves and condoms, some cosmetics, plants (such as poison ivy) (see p.1214), and some drugs. The reaction almost always occurs 1 or 2 days after exposure.

Stasis dermatitis occurs on the lower extremities—calves, ankles, and feet—in people who have varicose veins, chronic swelling of the feet, or circulatory problems. Symptoms include mild redness and swelling, as well as itching. As the disorder progresses, the affected area becomes redder. If the swelling is not treated, the rash may become crusted and leak fluid. Infection can occur, and injury to the area can lead to ulceration (see Varicose Ulcers, p.556). Treatment of stasis dermatitis starts with wearing compression stockings.

Seborrheic dermatitis is typified by scales over red patches, which most commonly appear on the scalp in the form of dandruff (see p.558). However, it also affects the eyebrows, eyelids, ears, and the folds near the mouth and nose, causing flaky, red, burning, and itchy patches. Infants often get a form of seborrhea called cradle cap (see p.972), which can persist for several months before going away on its own. The cause of this extremely common condition is not known.

Perioral dermatitis is often confused with rosacea (see p.535) or acne (see p.532). The small red papules and pustules are limited to the skin surrounding the mouth and, less commonly, can appear around the nose and under the eyes. It primarily

affects young women and its cause is unknown. The dermatitis usually clears in 1 to 2 months with the use of antibiotics such as tetracycline, erythromycin, or minocycline. Antibiotic gels rubbed onto the dermatitis may also be effective.

TREATMENT OPTIONS

You can treat most kinds of dermatitis yourself. Hydrocortisone cream and skin moisturizers, available at any drugstore without a prescription, can cure many cases of contact dermatitis and seborrheic dermatitis. Antihistamine tablets or capsules (such as chlorpheniramine or diphenhydramine), also available without a prescription, can relieve the itching but may also make you feel drowsy. Try to identify and avoid any substances that may be causing the irritation.

Dandruff is best treated with a medicated shampoo. Apply the shampoo to your wet hair and

rub it into all areas of the scalp with your fingers. Let it remain on your scalp for at least 2 minutes before rinsing your hair.

Psoriasis

(See also Color Guide to Visual Diagnosis, p.566)

Psoriasis begins when certain areas of skin produce new skin cells much more rapidly than normal, thus causing a thickening and scaling of the skin. Although the exact causes of psoriasis are not known, the immune system is involved and heredity may play a role; at least 1 of 3 people with psoriasis has an immediate relative with the disease.

The characteristic scaly, red patches of skin caused by psoriasis affect men and women of all ages equally and can erupt anywhere on the body, clear up for months at a time, and then reappear. Prevalence increases with age.

 Preventing Dermatitis

Dermatitis is inflammation of the skin. As you get older, your skin becomes more vulnerable to irritation. Here are some recommendations for coping with dermatitis:

- Identify and avoid the irritants. Your doctor may want to perform a patch test (see Skin Tests, p.162) if allergies are suspected.

- Substitute short showers for baths and avoid very hot water.

- Use soaps with a high fat or glycerin content, or use soap substitutes.

- Apply a rich moisturizer to your skin while it is still damp.

- Try moisturizers containing lactic acids and lactate salts.

- Avoid products with perfumes and dyes that may cause a sensitivity reaction.

- If these measures fail, try an over-the-counter corticosteroid cream or an oral antihistamine tablet to control itching, especially at night.

Psoriasis can be triggered by a strep throat infection, heavy alcohol consumption, stress, some medicines (such as beta blockers and lithium), injury to the skin, and infection with the human immunodeficiency virus (HIV).

SYMPTOMS

Psoriasis appears as reddish patches of skin covered with silvery scales; they may or may not cause discomfort. Psoriasis takes several forms. The most common is plaque psoriasis, in which patches appear on the trunk and limbs, especially on the elbows and knees, and on the scalp. Fingernails and toenails may become thick, pitted, and separated from their nail beds.

Pustular psoriasis is characterized by small pustules, spread all over the body. Guttate psoriasis causes many teardrop-sized areas, more prominent on the body than on the face. It often develops after a strep throat infection or an upper respiratory tract infection.

Fifteen percent of people with psoriasis develop psoriatic arthritis, an autoimmune disease (see p.870) that causes inflammation of the joints.

TREATMENT OPTIONS

Psoriasis is a chronic condition for which there is no cure. However, there are many treatments available to help keep it from flaring. Exposure to sun and ultraviolet lamps help clear up psoriasis; on the other hand, a bad sunburn can make symptoms worse. If your symptoms are mild or moderate, try one of the over-the-counter ointments containing corticosteroids (see p.895) or tars.

For severe outbreaks, the goal is to help slow down the production of skin cells and treat the inflammation. Your physician may recommend prescription-strength corticosteroids and/or calcipotriene, a relatively new drug related to vitamin D, both of which can be very helpful.

Psoralens, agents that sensitize the skin to light, along with ultraviolet therapy (a combination called PUVA) is often used to treat psoriasis. Methotrexate, an anticancer drug that slows down cell division, is primarily prescribed for people who have severe psoriatic arthritis. Retinoid drugs can be effective, but they must be used carefully since they can cause severe birth defects.

Each of these treatments requires close supervision by your doctor to monitor side effects. Most people who have psoriasis find that it comes and goes throughout their lives.

Lichen Simplex Chronicus

The rash-itch cycle of dermatitis (see p.550) often results in lichen simplex chronicus. Repeatedly scratching an itchy area leads to a thickened, itchy surface, and more scratching.

Symptoms include well-defined areas of red skin or skin that is made pale by loss of pigment and a hard, scaly, or thickened surface on the feet, ankles, elbows, and the back of the neck. The aim of treatment is to interrupt the rash-itch cycle.

Your doctor may recommend a high-potency corticosteroid (see p.895) preparation that you apply to your skin to relieve the itching. If this does not help, he or she may apply a corticosteroid drug and then bandage the area to help ensure penetration of the corticosteroid and prevent it from rubbing off. In some cases, a

Living with Psoriasis

"Whenever in my timid life I have shown some courage and originality it has been because of my skin. Because of my skin, I counted myself out of any of those jobs—salesman, teacher, financier, movie star—that demand being presentable. What did that leave? Becoming a craftsman of some sort, closeted and unseen—perhaps a cartoonist or a writer, a worker in ink who can hide himself and send out a surrogate presence, a signature that multiplies even while it conceals. Why did I marry so young? Because, having once found a comely female who forgave me my skin, I dared not risk losing her and trying to find another....

With my admission to the PUVA program, I was no longer alone with my skin. The world's dermatological wisdom had come into the cage with me. In the years since, I have watched my skin fight back. The psoriasis irrepressibly strains against the treatment, breaking out in odd areas like the tops of the feet, the backs of the hands. To my body, which has no aesthetic criteria, psoriasis is normal, and its suppression abnormal."

John Updike, *Self-Consciousness*. New York: Alfred A. Knopf Inc., 1989. Pages 48–49; 78.

Psoriasis

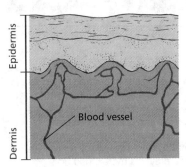

NORMAL SKIN

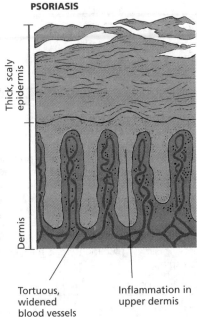

PSORIASIS

Thick, scaly epidermis

Epidermis

Dermis

Blood vessel

Dermis

Tortuous, widened blood vessels

Inflammation in upper dermis

In contrast to normal skin (left), skin affected by psoriasis (right) has scaly, red patches because new skin cells are produced at a more rapid rate than usual and they do not mature normally and die. This causes the epidermis to become a thick, scaly mass of largely dead cells. Inflammation and the growth of new blood vessels in the dermis redden the affected areas.

corticosteroid drug is injected directly into the affected area. Oral antihistamine drugs may also help relieve itching.

Pityriasis Rosea

(See also Color Guide to Visual Diagnosis, p.566)

Pityriasis rosea is a harmless, non-contagious skin condition in which small, round or oval, scaly patches develop, mainly on the trunk and upper arms. For unknown reasons, it primarily occurs during the spring and fall. Pityriasis rosea usually clears up on its

own within a month or two.

Talk to your doctor about treatment, which usually focuses on relieving the mild itching that accompanies the rash. Your doctor may recommend an over-the-counter cream containing a mild corticosteroid (see p.895) or, if itching is bothersome at night, an antihistamine (see p.1160) in tablet form. In severe cases, therapy with ultraviolet light may be prescribed to shorten the duration of the condition and reduce the itching.

INJURIES

Blisters

Blisters are fluid-filled, circular, raised areas on the outer surface of the skin. They form as a protective response to skin injury and can occur with burns, friction (such as from new shoes), and some skin conditions, including eczema (see p.550), impetigo (see p.531), pemphigoid (see p.488), and, in rare cases, porphyria (see p.736). The fluid in the blister is sterile (it is not pus, which indicates an infection); it is released from blood vessels in the skin underneath the blister to help heal the injured area and prevent infection.

The best treatment for blisters is no treatment at all. Do not open the blister or peel away the delicate upper skin; this can cause infection of the tissue underneath.

Blisters caused by viruses, such as the blisters that occur in shingles (see p.537), genital herpes (see p.890), and chickenpox (see p.948), should also be left alone. Avoid touching or scratching them and keep them clean to prevent infection with the viruses they contain. Talk to your doctor if you have large blisters that occur for no known reason.

Bruising

Bruising is dark discoloration of skin that occurs after an injury. The impact of a sharp bump or blow tears small blood vessels in the dermis (the deepest layer of skin) and allows blood to leak out and collect in the epidermis

Bruising

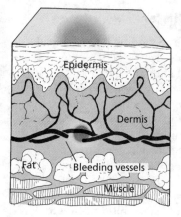

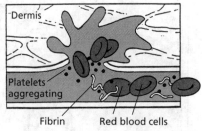

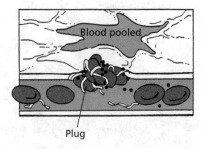

A bruise develops when an injury tears the walls of small blood vessels in the dermis (the second layer of skin) and allows blood to leak out and collect in the epidermis (the top layer of skin) and between cells and fibers in the dermis, fat, and muscle (left). The wall of a blood vessel (center) has been ruptured. Red blood cells spill out into the tissue of the dermis and break apart, coloring the skin purple. Platelets clump together where the wall has ruptured, and clotting factors such as fibrin create a mesh plug that traps red blood cells and platelets. This mesh plug (right) seals the leak and prevents more blood from escaping.

(the thin top layer of skin) and between cells and fibers in the dermis, fat, and muscle.

The body responds quickly to contain the bleeding. Platelets, the blood-clotting cells, begin stemming the flow of blood from blood vessels and a mesh of fibrous threads traps red blood cells and platelets, forming a semisolid plug that prevents more blood from escaping. Within a few days, as the escaped red blood cells are broken down by white blood cells, the bruise takes on a yellowish hue.

If you have bruising that appears for no reason, or a bruise that does not fade within a week, contact your doctor; this can be a sign of an underlying bleeding disorder.

Sunburn

Sunburn is inflammation and reddening of the skin caused by overexposure to the sun. Inflammation is the immune system's response to damaged skin cells and, in some cases, damaged blood vessels.

You can get a sunburn at any time of day in any season, although the intensity of the sun is strongest at noon and in summer. Clouds do little to block ultraviolet (UV) rays. Even the shade does not guarantee protection from UV light. Water, sand, snow, and light-colored pavement reflect it, which is almost as harmful as direct sunlight. Although weaker, the winter sun can burn unprotected skin, especially when reflected by snow and water.

Repeated sunburns increase the likelihood of actinic keratoses (see p.543), which are precursors

to skin cancer (see Cancerous Skin Growths, p.543) and also cause skin to wrinkle prematurely. Ironically, some wrinkle-reducing medicines sensitize the skin to sun damage (see Help for Aging Skin, p.539). Also, certain medicines increase your likelihood of sunburn.

SYMPTOMS

A mild sunburn appears as redness that fades to tan, or peels off. A severe sunburn causes red and tender skin that, like any burn, can blister. The dead skin cells peel off. In severe cases, sunstroke can occur, causing faintness, nausea, and vomiting.

TREATMENT OPTIONS

Apply cool compresses to the burned skin and take aspirin or acetaminophen to relieve discomfort and inflammation. Those under 21 years old should not take aspirin due to Reye syndrome (see p.1017).

If you have a severe sunburn or sunstroke, see a doctor. Do not expose the burned area to the sun. If blisters appear, do not burst them.

To prevent sunburn, avoid the sun during peak burning hours—between 10 AM and 2 PM. Wear tightly woven, light clothing and apply a water-resistant sunblock or sunscreen to all exposed areas; most people need a sunscreen with a sun protection factor (SPF) of at least 15 (see p.548).

Corns and Calluses

Corns are raised areas of thick skin most often found on the toe. They are usually caused by wearing a tight, poorly fitting shoe. Calluses are areas of thickened skin that usually develop on the ball or heel of the foot, but they can occur any place the skin undergoes repeated pressure or friction. Excessive pressure and friction cause both corns and calluses. The skin responds by erecting a tough protective layer made of keratin, a fibrous, strengthening protein.

You can prevent corns by wearing well-fitting shoes, keeping your feet dry, and changing your socks daily. If you have persistent corns and calluses, or if you have diabetes mellitus (see p.832), poor circulation, or an abnormal foot structure, talk to your doctor about foot care.

Corns caused by ill-fitting shoes generally go away on their own once you wear a more comfortable shoe. You can also try a corn pad, available at drugstores, which you place over the corn to reduce pressure. Hard corns and

Corns and Calluses

CORNS

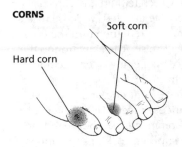

Soft corn

Hard corn

CALLUSES

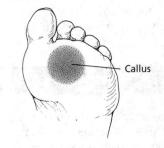

Callus

Excessive pressure and friction on one spot on the foot cause the cells of the outside layer of skin to multiply and then die. This creates a thickened area of skin. Such areas on the side of a toe are called corns. On the underside of the foot they are called calluses.

calluses can be cut away by a podiatrist.

You can also treat corns without a prescription by applying keratinolytic agents containing at least 40% salicylic acid. For soft corns that develop between toes, reduce foot perspiration by inserting lamb's wool padding between your toes.

Bedsores

Bedsores are skin ulcers that occur in people after extended periods of inactivity in bed, often due to prolonged illness. Also called decubitus ulcers and, aptly,

pressure sores, these ulcers develop when the continued weight of the body exerts pressure on specific points.

Bedsores commonly develop where skin makes contact with bedding: heels, ankles, knees, buttocks, spine, hips, elbows, and shoulder blades. The pressure first makes the skin red, painful, and inflamed. Soon, the skin turns purple and breaks down and an ulcer develops. At this point, bedsores are prone to infection.

Untreated bedsores deepen, cause significant pain, and heal very slowly. For information on preventing and treating bedsores, see Caregiving and Eldercare, p.1120.

Keloids

(See also Color Guide to Visual Diagnosis, p.567)

A keloid is an itchy, hard, reddish, raised lump on the skin. Keloids are produced when excess collagen builds up at the site of a healing scar, producing excess tissue.

More likely to occur in people with dark skin, keloids can appear on any part of the body that has been injured or has a blister, vaccination, pimple, or any other type of skin disruption. However, keloids tend to develop on the skin of the shoulder and breastbone. Keloids may continue growing (although they tend to become flatter and less itchy) even after the wound has healed.

Your doctor may inject a corticosteroid drug directly into the affected area, which can help reduce the itching and flatten some scars. Removing a keloid by cutting usually results only in a new keloid.

Varicose Ulcers

(See also Color Guide to Visual Diagnosis, p.567)

Varicose ulcers are shallow ulcers on the legs that occur when circulation in the veins of the legs is made inefficient by varicose veins (see p.706). Varicose ulcers primarily affect older people and, once they form, they tend to recur.

The ulcers usually appear on the inside of the leg over the ankle, although they can occur anywhere on the lower leg; they may secrete fluid and can easily become infected. Varicose ulcers start out red, then turn the color of a bruise. The skin around the ulcer's opening often becomes itchy and flaky.

See your doctor if you have varicose ulcers. He or she may recommend a support bandage or support stockings to improve the circulation in your legs. In more severe or chronic cases, your doctor may advise you to cleanse and bandage the ulcer regularly. For very severe varicose ulcers, your doctor may dress and bandage the ulcer, or recommend a short period of bed rest.

You can help prevent recurrences by keeping your feet elevated when sitting and sleeping; also, avoid standing for extended periods. Walking helps improve circulation. In severe and recurring cases, surgery to remove the varicose veins (see p.708) may be required.

HAIR

The best way to keep your hair healthy is to avoid or minimize use of blow-dryers, bleaching and coloring agents, permanents, straighteners, hair rollers, and sun exposure to your scalp.

Baldness

Baldness is loss of hair. Also called alopecia, the most common form is male-pattern baldness, a gradual process of hair loss that affects many men after puberty. Hair loss also occurs in women, although usually not in the same pattern as men experience.

Most balding men inherit their tendency to baldness. In male-pattern baldness, the growth cycle of hair becomes shorter and the follicles begin to produce thin, downy hair, rather than thicker hair. For most men, hair loss follows a specific pattern, starting at the temples and moving over the crown of the head. In severe cases, hair grows only on the back and the side of the head in a narrow rim.

It is not uncommon for women to experience hair loss. Most women lose some hair all over the top of their head with age. If hair loss occurs when a girl or woman is in her teens or 20s and is accompanied by acne, menstrual abnormalities, and excessive facial hair, it is likely to

Male-Pattern Baldness

For most men, hair loss follows a specific pattern, starting at the temples and progressing to the top and back of the head. In severe cases, hair grows only on the back and the side of the head in a narrow rim. The degree and pattern of balding is often inherited.

Hair Growth

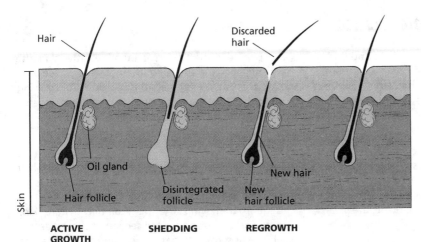

Hair

Oil gland

Hair follicle

Discarded hair

Disintegrated follicle

New hair follicle

New hair

ACTIVE GROWTH

SHEDDING

REGROWTH

Hair in each part of the body has its own cycle of active growth and shedding. Hair in the eyebrows is replaced every 4 months; on the scalp, between 2 and 5 years. After an active period of growth, the follicle disintegrates, the hair is shed, and a new follicle is created.

Skin

be due to elevated levels of the hormone androgen. Rarely, male-pattern balding in a woman can indicate a severe, underlying problem such as a tumor of the ovary or adrenal gland.

Certain conditions set the stage for temporary hair loss. Many women have dramatic hair loss after childbirth and at menopause; hair usually returns to normal thickness 6 months to 2 years later.

Radiation therapy (see p.741) and chemotherapy (see p.741) often produce temporary hair loss. Certain diseases, including anemia (see p.713) and thyroid disease (see p.844), can produce slight hair loss. Skin diseases, such as lupus (see p.898), lichen planus (see p.538), and bacterial infections, may create bald patches.

TREATMENT OPTIONS

Baldness can cause anxiety for men and women. It cannot be prevented, but there are several treatments you can discuss with your doctor. Solutions containing minoxidil, originally developed as a blood pressure–lowering drug, can produce growth of very fine hair in both men and women after 6 months of use, but the new hair falls out as soon as you stop using the drug.

The drug finasteride, taken by many men to ease the symptoms of an enlarged prostate gland (see p.1098), can help men grow hair in bald spots if used constantly (the effects stop when you stop taking the drug). However, it is not very effective in men who are largely bald. Finasteride is taken once a day in pill form.

Side effects include reduced sexual drive and function in about 2% of the men who take it. Finasteride should never be used by women because it can cause abnormalities in the male fetus of a pregnant woman.

Hair transplantation (see p.588), in which sections of scalp and hair are moved into bald spots, is the most effective treatment. If your hair loss is temporary, your best option may be to consult a hair professional about concealing it with a different hairstyle or a wig.

Alopecia Areata

(See also Color Guide to Visual Diagnosis, p.567)

Alopecia areata is a disease in which hair suddenly falls out, leaving bald patches. The hair regrows within a year in roughly half the people affected, although in some people hair never grows back. Recurrences are common.

The cause is still unknown, but scientists suspect it is an autoimmune disease (see p.870). The painless hair loss mainly affects the scalp, but eyebrows and eyelashes may fall out as well.

Several treatments with limited effectiveness exist, including applying creams containing corti-

Removing Unwanted Hair

Excess hair is in the eye of the beholder, and this view often differs dramatically from one culture to another. If you want to remove hair from your body, you have several options. However, only electrolysis is permanent.

SHAVING

Shaving cuts off the hair at the surface of the skin and, therefore, provides the shortest-term hair removal. To avoid skin irritation, use warm water and a lubricating soap, and make sure razors are clean and sharp.

TWEEZING

In tweezing, hairs are removed one by one with tweezers. This method is more suitable for small areas. Like waxing (see below), tweezing removes hair from the root and lasts between a week and a month, depending on how quickly your hair grows.

WAXING

Waxing provides hair removal that lasts between a week and a month, depending on how quickly your hair grows. It can be performed at a salon or at home using a kit available at drugstores. There are two types of waxing—hot and cold, both of which pull the hair root out of its follicle.

With the hot wax method, wax is heated and applied to the hair in strips. While the wax is still moist, a strip of cloth is pressed onto the wax, then quickly pulled away. Waxing may feel awkward at first, but your technique will improve with practice. Small blisters and pimples sometimes crop up on sensitive skin after waxing; applying soothing lotions to the waxed area after treatment minimizes this reaction. Cold waxing is similar to hot waxing, and the strips are less messy, but the results are not as precise.

DEPILATORY CREAMS AND SPRAYS

Depilatory creams and sprays chemically dissolve hairs above skin level and part way to the root. Results are not as long-lasting as waxing and tweezing, but last longer than shaving. The chemicals may irritate skin, so perform a test on a small section of skin to determine your sensitivity before applying to larger areas.

ELECTROLYSIS

This permanent removal process involves inserting a tiny needle attached to an electrical source into the follicle of each hair to destroy the hair root. You may feel slight to sharp pain, depending on where the hair is located (skin is more sensitive under the arms, for example, than on top of the arms). Choose a professional; in many states, practitioners of electrolysis are licensed. If you are uncertain about someone's professional training, have them treat a limited area of skin on the first visit; if irritation and pimples develop in the treated area, choose another practitioner.

Disposable needles should always be used with electrolysis. However, many people who undergo electrolysis treatments keep and bring their own needles so there is no chance of being treated with a needle used by someone else. It may take more than one treatment for permanent hair removal.

costeroid drugs (see p.895) or minoxidil (see Baldness, p.556), injecting corticosteroid drugs directly into bald patches, exposing the bald areas to ultraviolet light, and taking antiviral drugs. Each treatment has been effective for some people, but none is universally successful.

Hirsutism

Hirsutism is a term generally used to describe abnormal hair growth in women. What constitutes a normal pattern of hair growth in women is a subjective judgment. In the United States, hirsutism is broadly considered to be growth of hair in a pattern resembling that of men—thick hair on the face, arms, chest, back, stomach, and/or thighs.

Hirsutism almost always first appears after puberty and often results from diseases that cause increased levels of the hormone androgen. Sometimes no increased level of androgen is found, and it is assumed that the person's hair follicles make increased amounts of hair in response to normal levels of androgen. Hirsutism can also occur after menopause.

Your doctor may recommend that you have blood or urine tests to diagnose the cause of hirsutism. Diseases that cause higher-than-normal androgen levels include polycystic ovary syndrome (see p.1081), Cushing syndrome (see p.857), congenital adrenal hyperplasia, ovarian tumors (see p.1078), or obesity (see p.853).

TREATMENT OPTIONS

Temporary hair removal treatments include bleaching, waxing, tweezing, shaving, and chemical depilatories. Electrolysis is the only permanent method (see Removing Unwanted Hair, p.558). Hirsutism due to tumors disappears when the tumor is removed. Treatment with estrogen is sometimes prescribed for polycystic ovary syndrome in cases of androgen excess. Other prescription medicines include spironolactone.

Dandruff

Dandruff is a very common and harmless condition in which an itchy, dry scalp produces dead skin flakes that appear in the hair or on the shoulders. Dandruff results most often from seborrheic dermatitis (see p.551) and sometimes psoriasis (see p.551). Additionally, very cold or hot, dry air also makes the scalp, like other parts of the skin, more susceptible to flaking and itching.

Dandruff is usually a long-lasting condition that requires ongoing control. Try using an antidandruff shampoo; active ingredients to look for include salicylic acid, selenium, sulfur, and tar. Use the shampoo daily, rinsing with lukewarm (not hot) water. When you take a shower, apply the shampoo to your wet hair and rub it into all parts of your scalp. Let it remain on your scalp for at least 2 minutes before rinsing your hair.

Avoid prolonged use of hot dryers or electric curlers, which cause your scalp to dry out. If your dandruff persists, consult your doctor, who may recommend a preparation containing a corticosteroid drug, which can help loosen scaly flakes.

Ingrown Hair

An ingrown hair is, literally, a hair that grows into the skin. Ingrown hairs can occur anywhere, but two conditions predispose people to them: pilonidal sinus and pseudofolliculitis.

The pilonidal sinus is an indentation located above the cleft of the buttocks; it can become inflamed when one or more hairs cannot grow out of their pores and remain in the skin. A boil-like ulcer develops, and it can secrete pus and cause severe pain. This condition is more common in younger men who have a lot of body hair.

Pseudofolliculitis is a condition most common in black and Hispanic men and other people with curly hair. It is aggravated by shaving and is often called "razor bumps." The condition usually occurs on the face and looks like folliculitis infection (see p.532) or acnelike pimples.

Talk to your doctor if you have either of these conditions. If you have an infection, your doctor will remove the trapped hair and infected fluid. A pilonidal sinus that causes repeated problems often must be cut out. Pseudofolliculitis cannot be treated or prevented; many men with the condition simply stop shaving and grow beards. Your doctor can treat a single ingrown hair by making a small cut to release the trapped hair.

NAILS

Many dietary supplements are recommended to improve the health of your nails but none are of proven value (except vitamins if you have a vitamin deficiency).

The best thing you can do for your nails is minimize their immersion in water, which causes them to expand, dry, shrink, and, over time, become brittle. Take protective measures, such as wearing cotton-lined rubber gloves (the latex in rubber gloves can cause a sensitivity reaction; see Contact Dermatitis, p.550). Avoid exposure to harsh chemicals, including too much nail polish remover. Trim your nails frequently to avoid splitting and accumulation of dirt underneath; avoid cutting the cuticles, which can lead to infection.

Occasionally, brittle nails can be a symptom of an underlying medical condition such as a fungal infection (see p.530), a thyroid problem (see p.844), or a nutritional deficiency—particularly of iron, vitamin A (beta carotene), or protein. If you suspect one of these medical problems, talk to your doctor.

Discolored Nails

Discolored nails may be caused by injury or underlying disease. Yellow or brown-stained nails may result from nicotine in cigarettes or cigars. Green nails suggest bacterial or fungal infections (see right). A black and/or blue spot near the bottom of the nail may be a bruise caused by injury or by pressure. Pale or white nails can indicate anemia (see p.713). Blue-gray nails suggest heart disease (see p.652) or lung disease (see p.493). Pitted brown spots may denote psoriasis (see p.551).

Small, sharp-edged black flecks in the nails most often are caused by a simple injury. On rare occasions, they can be caused by blood-clotting disorders (see p.709) or infection of the heart valves (see p.689).

As with deformed nails, treating the underlying cause of discolored nails usually resolves the problem. It can take several months before the nail returns to normal.

Deformed Nails

Healthy fingernails and toenails are smooth, slightly curved, and rigid. Make sure your shoes allow ample room for your toes; pressure on the toes impedes healthy nail growth and can cause deformities. Talk to your doctor to ensure that any abnormal nail growth is not related to injury or an underlying disease:

Thickened nails may be caused by circulatory problems, which accompany atherosclerosis (see p.653), or injury.

Flat nails may indicate Raynaud disease (see p.706). Flat nails that are thin and spoon-shaped are sometimes caused by a nutritional deficiency, such as a lack of iron.

Raised nails suggest a respiratory problem; they can also result from skin conditions such as psoriasis (see p.551), lichen planus (see p.538), or chronic paronychia (see p.569).

Clubbed nails denote potential lung infection, lung cancer, or congenital heart disease.

Ridges running across nails suggest an infection, such as a cold.

Curved, thick toenails are a common result of aging and pressure to the feet by ill-fitting shoes.

Fungal Infections of the Nails

(See also Color Guide to Visual Diagnosis, p.561)

Fungal infections of the fingernails and toenails are caused by the same fungus that produces athlete's foot (see p.530). Like other infections, fungal infections of the nails are spread by direct contact.

Discoloration and swelling are the primary symptoms, causing the nails to peel and become brittle, thickened, and generally unsightly. In addition, they can be painful due to the pressure of the nail against infected skin.

Fungal infections of the nails are notoriously difficult to treat. One reason for this is that nails grow slowly; it takes 4 to 6 months for a fingernail to grow, and twice as long for a toenail. In addition, ointments cannot penetrate the nail itself, where the fungus lives.

Controlling nail fungus requires help from your doctor (see Treating Fungal Infections of the Nails, p.561). The only cure for nail fungus is prescription drugs. Nails may also be removed surgically, which results in the destruction of the nail bed so that they do not grow back. This procedure is usually reserved for people who have very thick nails that cause a lot of problems.

Ingrown Toenails

Ingrown toenails are nails that grow into surrounding skin, sometimes causing infection and disabling pain. Wearing shoes

Color Guide to Visual Diagnosis

Use this chapter to help identify conditions that make a visible appearance on your body. The photographs on the following pages are intended to help you identify more than 60 skin, hair, nail, mouth, and eye disorders. This section is not intended as a substitute for diagnosis by your physician. If you or a family member has one of the conditions listed here, read the full article about the condition elsewhere in this book to more thoroughly acquaint yourself with the condition and start any recommended home care. If you have concerns, talk to your doctor.

FUNGAL INFECTIONS

Fungi are simple microscopic organisms that thrive in moist areas. Many are harmless to humans, but some cause skin infections. Others can cause serious infections inside the body.

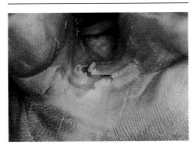

ATHLETE'S FOOT

Athlete's foot appears as reddened, swelling, scaling, puckering, and cracking skin on the foot, especially between the toes and on the soles. It can also cause burning and itching.

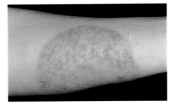

RINGWORM

Ringworm forms round, red, itchy scales on the skin. It starts as small red patches but often grows larger (as shown here).

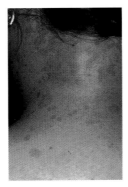

TINEA VERSICOLOR

This fungal infection appears as round flaking patches and pimplelike bumps on the skin of the upper body and arms.

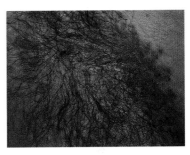

CANDIDA SKIN INFECTION

Also called intertrigo, this infection shows up as dark red discoloration. It often occurs under the breasts or arms (as shown here) and in the groin.

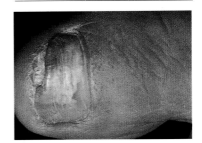

FUNGAL INFECTION OF THE NAIL

This fungus causes discoloration and swelling of the finger and peeling, brittle, and thickened nails.

BACTERIAL INFECTIONS

Bacterial infections are caused by single-celled microorganisms that are found nearly everywhere. Many of the following bacterial skin conditions can be eradicated with antibiotics.

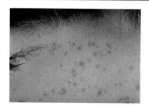

IMPETIGO

Impetigo begins with reddened skin that turns into small blisters that burst, revealing tender red skin that is soon covered by light brown crusts.

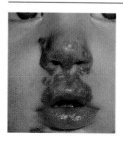

FOLLICULITIS

Folliculitis appears as small red dots. It inflames hair follicles and can occur anywhere hair grows, such as on the chest (as shown here).

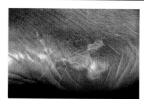

BOIL

A boil appears first as a small red bump and then swells, often creating warmth and painful pressure. This boil has formed on the heel.

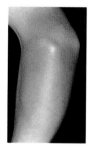

CELLULITIS

Cellulitis causes a large, firm area of reddened skin that may feel warm. It often occurs in a leg (as shown here) and can spread to the blood.

OTHER IMPORTANT SKIN CONDITIONS

Skin problems can arise from a wide range of causes, including food allergies, stress, medicines, infections, or hormonal changes.

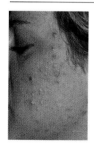

ACNE

Acne occurs when oil and dead skin cells plug the opening of an oil-producing gland and the hair follicle to which it is attached.

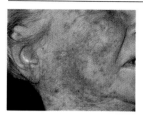

ROSACEA

Rosacea appears as spidery blood vessels and flushing of the face. There may also be small bumps filled with pus, resembling acne.

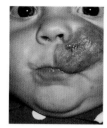

STRAWBERRY HEMANGIOMA

This birthmark, a malformation of blood vessels, appears as a raised, purple-red area that may be very small or several inches wide.

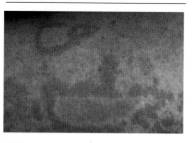

HIVES

Hives appears as itchy, raised areas and inflamed skin. The hives rash is usually round but may take any shape or size.

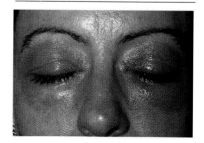

ANGIONEUROTIC EDEMA

A form of hives, this condition causes painless swelling on the face, neck, hands, feet, or genitals. It can be caused by a food or drug allergy, infection, or stress.

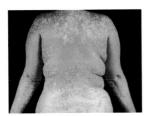

DRUG RASH

A drug rash, caused by an allergic reaction to a medicine, can occur on one small area of the body or all over (as shown here).

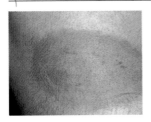

LYME DISEASE RASH

This rash starts as a small red spot where the tick bites, and expands over days or weeks. Sometimes the rash has a clear center and looks like a bull's-eye.

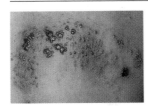

SHINGLES

Shingles causes a burning pain near the surface of the skin. Next, red sores appear and turn into itchy blisters that crust over and may leave scars.

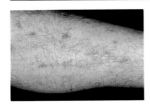

LICHEN PLANUS

This rash appears as tiny, blue-red spots on the skin that may join to form rough, scaly, possibly itchy patches.

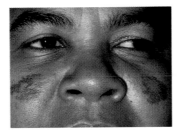

MELASMA

Melasma, which is darkening of the skin, often appears on the face during pregnancy or menopause due to hormonal changes.

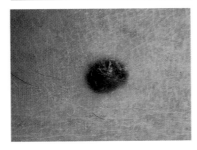

TYPICAL MOLE

Moles are dark spots on the skin that are noncancerous and usually symmetrical, with a clear border and even color throughout.

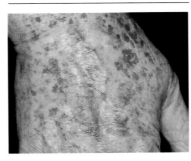

AGE SPOTS

An age spot is a noncancerous brown or black spot on the skin that occurs as a result of sun exposure, usually in middle-aged or older people.

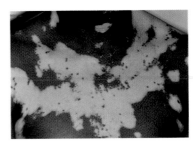

VITILIGO

In vitiligo, sections of skin stop producing the pigment melanin, resulting in white patches of skin on the face, hands, armpits, and groin.

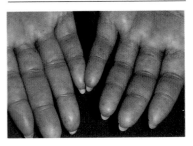

SCLERODERMA

Scleroderma is characterized by hard, stiff skin. In localized scleroderma (as shown here), the skin becomes shiny, uncomfortably tight, dry, and hairless.

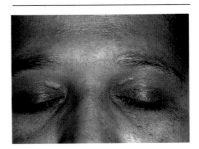

XANTHELASMA

This condition appears as yellow fatty deposits around the eyelids. It may be accompanied by high cholesterol and high triglyceride levels.

NONCANCEROUS (BENIGN) GROWTHS

Noncancerous growths do not have the potential to turn cancerous. Some, however, can cause problems and should be removed by your doctor.

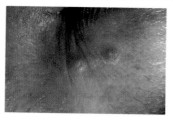

WARTS

Warts can range from light tan to brown. Common warts (as shown here) are usually found on the hands; plantar warts occur on the feet.

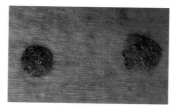

SEBORRHEIC KERATOSES

Seborrheic keratoses can appear on any part of the body as crusty, raised patches of skin. The patches may feel itchy or greasy but are harmless.

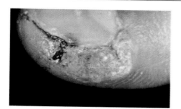

MOLLUSCUM CONTAGIOSUM

This viral infection appears as groups of small, pale lumps on the skin. It can be found everywhere except the palms and soles. When squeezed, the lumps may exude a cheeselike material.

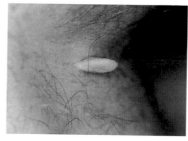

SKIN TAGS

Skin tags are small, harmless growths. They appear on the neck or in the armpits or groin, often in people who are overweight and during pregnancy.

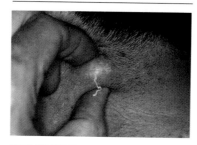

SEBACEOUS CYST

Sebaceous cysts arise when an oil-producing gland in the skin is blocked, leading to a buildup of cheesy material.

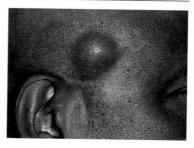

LIPOMA

A lipoma is a painless ball of fat that occurs just under the skin. It is rubbery and movable and often found on the neck, trunk, and forearms.

PRECANCEROUS GROWTHS

Precancerous growths are those that are not now cancerous but could potentially become cancerous. Your physician may recommend that you monitor any precancerous growths for changes and have them removed if they have a worrisome appearance.

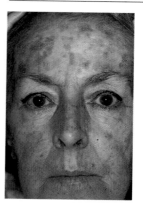

ACTINIC KERATOSES

Actinic keratoses are pink or red-brown, scaly growths that may itch or be slightly painful. They are harmless but can develop into skin cancer.

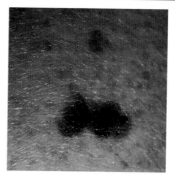

DYSPLASTIC MOLE

Dysplastic moles are usually larger than a pencil eraser and symmetrical, though their borders are fuzzy. They commonly occur in shades of brown and pink. They should be monitored closely by your doctor; often, these moles are removed.

CANCEROUS (MALIGNANT) GROWTHS

Many cancerous skin growths can be cured if they are diagnosed and treated in their early stages. Cancerous moles (melanomas) are the most serious skin cancers; they can be life-threatening. Therefore, it is vital that you regularly examine your skin for changes.

THE ABCDs OF CANCEROUS MOLES

The following characteristics describe a potentially cancerous mole. If you have any questions about a mole, see your doctor immediately.

Asymmetry One half of the mole does not match the other.

Border The borders are ragged, notched, and indistinct.

Color Pigmentation varies and includes black, blue, or gray.

Diameter Mole is larger than a pencil eraser.

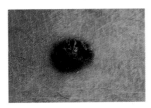

NONCANCEROUS MOLE

A noncancerous mole is symmetrical and has a clear border and even color throughout. Noncancerous moles are usually smaller than a pencil eraser.

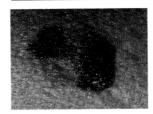

MELANOMA IN SITU

This is a cancerous melanoma in its earliest stage. Note that it fits several of the ABCD criteria: it is asymmetrical, it has an irregular border, and its diameter is larger than a pencil eraser.

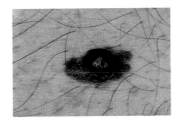

SUPERFICIAL SPREADING MELANOMA

The most common melanoma, this type grows outward and spreads over the skin. Note that it fits several of the ABCD criteria: it is asymmetrical, it has an irregular border, and its diameter is larger than a pencil eraser.

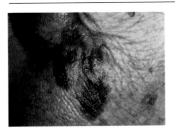

LENTIGO MALIGNA MELANOMA

This melanoma often occurs on the face of elderly people. Note that it fits all the ABCD criteria: it is asymmetrical, it has an irregular border, its color varies, and its diameter is larger than a pencil eraser.

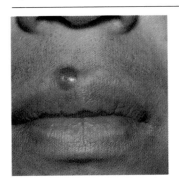

KAPOSI SARCOMA

Kaposi sarcoma begins as soft, spongy nodules that become hard and solid, and may grow larger. The nodules may be purple, brown, or red. They can appear anywhere on the body.

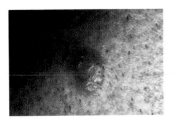

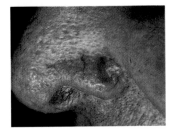

BASAL CELL CARCINOMA

A basal cell carcinoma starts as a painless bump (top) and grows slowly, eventually becoming an open ulcer (bottom). The center may bleed and crust over. Most occur on the face.

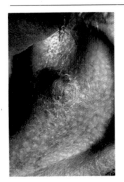

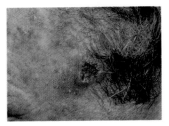

SQUAMOUS CELL CARCINOMA

This skin cancer begins as a small red bump or red patch of skin, usually on sun-exposed areas such as the head, ears (top), and hands. Over time, it grows larger and may form an ulcer (bottom).

INFESTATIONS WITH INSECTS

The first sign of an insect infestation is often itching. Infestations by different insects have different appearances. Your doctor needs to see you to make the diagnosis and prescribe the right treatment.

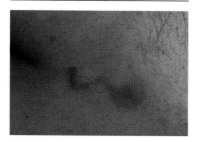

SCABIES

Scabies appears as a wavy line on the skin that ends in a small bump. There may also be a rash of tiny red lumps around the line.

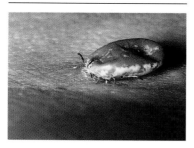

TICK

Ticks bite into the skin to suck blood. Their bodies become engorged with blood. The tick shown has just begun to fill up with blood.

SCALING AND ITCHING CONDITIONS

Scaling and itching are very common symptoms of skin disorders. Scratching can make a skin condition worse so it is best to avoid touching the affected area. If you think you have one of the conditions pictured here, read about it elsewhere in this book to learn whether you can treat it yourself.

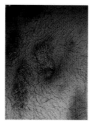

ECZEMA/ATOPIC DERMATITIS

Eczema in adults appears as crusty, dark patches on the skin, often in folds of skin. Here it appears on the abdomen.

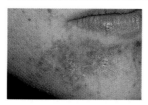

PERIORAL DERMATITIS

This inflammation causes small red bumps and pus-filled blisters around the mouth (which is the definition of "perioral"), although it can occur near the nose and eyes.

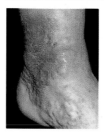

STASIS DERMATITIS

This type of dermatitis causes redness, swelling, and itching. Later the area reddens and the tissue ulcerates.

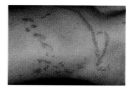

POISON IVY

This rash arises after contact with oils found in the leaves of the poison ivy plant. Poison ivy may be itchy, swell, and have blisters.

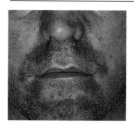

SEBORRHEIC DERMATITIS

Seborrheic dermatitis causes scales on top of itchy, red patches of skin. It is most commonly found on the scalp, where it is known as dandruff.

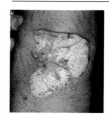

PSORIASIS

Psoriasis causes red patches covered with silvery scales that often appear on the scalp, trunk, and limbs, especially the elbows (shown here) and knees.

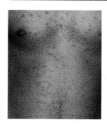

PITYRIASIS ROSEA

This harmless skin condition consists of short-lived, small, round or oval scaly patches on the back or chest and upper arms. It can be slightly itchy.

INJURIES

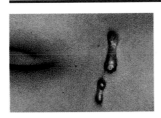

KELOID

A keloid is a hard, raised lump on the skin. It arises when excess collagen builds up at the site of a healing scar.

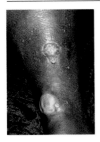

VARICOSE ULCERS

These shallow ulcers, caused by varicose veins, appear on the legs, start out red, then turn darker and may secrete fluid. Nearby skin may be itchy and flaky.

HAIR LOSS FOR UNKNOWN REASONS

Many people experience hair loss as they grow older. However, not all hair loss is normal; it can be a sign of disease.

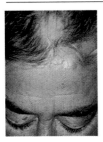

ALOPECIA AREATA

This is a painless condition in which patches of hair fall out. It mainly affects the scalp, but the eyebrows and eyelashes may also fall out.

INFECTIONS OF THE NAILS

The microscopic organisms called fungi that cause problems elsewhere on the body can also affect nails. These nail conditions often need to be treated with prescription medicine.

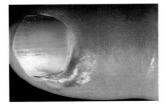

PARONYCHIA

This infection is caused by bacteria (or sometimes a fungus). Symptoms include red, swollen, and painful cuticles and pus-filled sores.

DISORDERS OF THE MOUTH

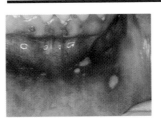

CANKER SORE

A canker sore is a small, sometimes painful sore that develops inside the mouth. It begins as a small yellow spot ringed in red.

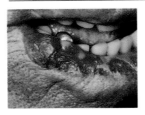

CANCER OF THE LIP AND TONGUE

These cancers are almost always caused by tobacco use. Mouth cancer may begin as a nonhealing sore, a white patch (often with areas of red), or a lump.

DISORDERS OF THE EYES AND EYELIDS

Some eye conditions can be treated with over-the-counter medicines. However, talk to your doctor about any problem that lasts more than a few days.

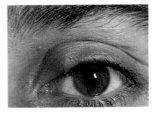

CHALAZION

This small swelling on the eyelid is caused by blockage and inflammation of an oil-producing gland. It may become infected and painful and have a discharge.

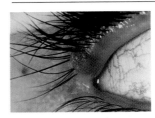

STYE

A stye is a bacterial infection found at the base of an eyelash. The oil-producing gland there becomes hard and tender, with a pus-filled cyst in the center.

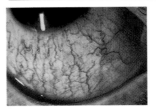

CONJUNCTIVITIS

Also called pinkeye, conjunctivitis causes redness and swelling of the membrane, a thick discharge, and, on awakening, sticky eyelids.

COMMON CHILDHOOD DISEASES

Many common childhood diseases look more alarming than they really are. However, none should be taken lightly; your child should see his or her doctor for a diagnosis.

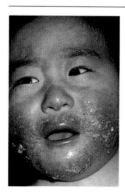

INFANTILE ECZEMA/ ATOPIC DERMATITIS

This condition appears as inflamed, weeping, or crusty patches on the face, neck, and groin. It is often itchy, and scratching leads to further irritation.

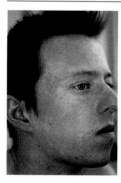

GERMAN MEASLES

Also called rubella, German measles is a viral infection characterized by a pink or red rash that spreads from the face to the rest of the body. Because of immunizations, it is uncommon today.

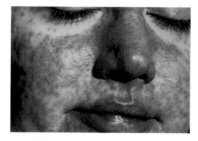

MEASLES

Measles, caused by a virus, causes a blotchy red skin rash that is slightly raised. It first appears around the hairline and ears and then spreads to the torso. Other symptoms are a high fever and cold symptoms. Because of immunizations, it is uncommon today.

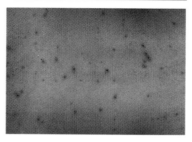

CHICKENPOX

Chickenpox appears as a rash of itchy, dark red pimples that begins on the trunk and spreads to the face, limbs, and other areas.

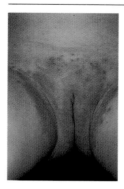

DIAPER RASH

Diaper rash is a painful, reddened area of skin that, if untreated, can become ulcerated. It can be caused by urine, feces, or heat.

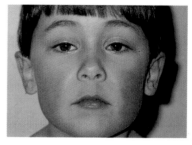

FIFTH DISEASE

Symptoms of fifth disease include fever and a pink flush or rash that begins on the cheeks. It later appears on the arms, thighs, buttocks, and trunk.

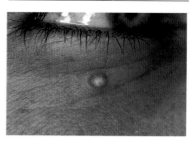

MILIA

Milia are small white cysts that occur when hair follicles or sweat glands are blocked. They are common in infants and disappear within a few weeks.

Caring for Your Nails

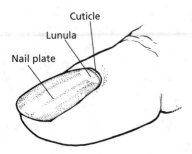

It can take 4 to 6 months to grow a completely new nail; toenails can take a year to replace themselves. Take good care of your nails by following these steps:

■ Trim nails frequently to avoid splitting and accumulation of dirt underneath the nail.

■ Cut nails straight across to avoid damage to skin at corners.

■ Avoid cutting cuticles, which can lead to infection.

■ Keep nails dry to prevent splitting and growth of fungi.

that are too tight or too narrow can lead to this condition. Other causes include injuries, fungal infections (see p.560), abnormalities in foot structure, or repeated pressure and pounding of the feet while exercising.

The most common cause, however, is faulty trimming of the toenails. The best way to trim toenails is to use a toenail clipper (not scissors) and to cut nails straight across so they are slightly longer than the fleshy tips of the toes. Do not cut your nails in a curve or cut them too short.

To ease the pain of an ingrown toenail, apply warm compresses or soak your foot in warm water to ease the swelling and pain; elevating the foot can

also help. Soaking also softens nails enough for you to insert a small piece of cotton between the nail's edge and the skin. This helps decrease discomfort and permits the nail to grow out without pressing on adjacent flesh.

If the skin around the nail becomes infected, see your doctor. He or she may prescribe an antibiotic drug or perform a minor operation in which a small portion of the ingrown nail is cut away.

Paronychia

(See also Color Guide to Visual Diagnosis, p.567)

Paronychia is infection of the skin near a fingernail or toenail. It is caused by staphylococcus and pseudomonas bacteria or by fungi. Most bacteria and fungi have an affinity for sites that are chronically moist and where the skin is broken.

Paronychia occurs most often

in people whose hands are in water frequently; it can develop suddenly or slowly. In acute paronychia, symptoms are more severe and include red, swollen, painful cuticles. The cuticle sometimes rises above the base of the nail, and pus forms underneath. In some people, a very painful pus-filled sore occurs. In chronic infection, the disease often affects more than one nail, and the nail becomes deformed and discolored.

To prevent paronychia, keep your hands and feet dry and clean. Wear rubber gloves when your hands must be in water and do not cut or push back your cuticles; they provide a barrier against infection invading the nail.

See your doctor if you have a pus-filled area. He or she will lance it to relieve pressure and may prescribe an antibiotic or an antifungal drug to eradicate the infection.

Treating Fungal Infections of the Nails

The only way to cure a fungal nail infection is by taking prescription drugs. For decades, the only drug available was griseofulvin, a reasonably safe medicine that prevents new fungus from infecting the nail. However, griseofulvin cannot kill an established fungus, so it must be taken every day until the entire nail is replaced. This can take months for fingernails and more than a year for toenails.

In recent years, two new and more potent drugs have become available: itraconazole and terbinafine. Both are moderately effective, but carry some risks. Itraconazole should not be taken with some drugs, including antihistamines or erythromycin or related antibiotics. Drug interaction is less of a concern with terbinafine, but it has an unpleasant taste and causes intestinal distress, among other side effects. In addition, both can cost hundreds of dollars for a course of treatment. With the help of your doctor, weigh these options against the unpleasant, but harmless and free, alternative—living with the unsightly fungus.

Cosmetic and Reconstructive Surgery

The record of time's passage is visible on our faces and bodies. Some of us accept these changes as a normal part of the aging process. Others find that the face and body in the mirror no longer represent the youthful spirit inside and seek the surgical solutions of plastic surgery. Cosmetic surgery—which includes face-lifts, nose reshaping, fat suction (liposuction), and other procedures done to enhance appearance—is one form of plastic surgery. The other type, reconstructive surgery, is performed to repair birth defects, correct developmental problems such as unusually large breasts, and repair deformities caused by accidents or disease. A sharp distinction between reconstructive and cosmetic surgery is often difficult to make because there is an appearance aspect to virtually all plastic surgery.

If you are considering cosmetic or reconstructive surgery, it is essential that you employ a good surgeon (see Choosing a Plastic Surgeon, p.572). If you are considering elective (not medically necessary) cosmetic surgery, it is also vital that you understand your reasons for having the surgery. Cosmetic surgery cannot make you perfect, restore lost youth, or fix a psychological problem such as low self-esteem. Ours is a culture that places high value on physical beauty and a youthful appearance. Few of us could measure up to the ideal represented by teenage fashion models, even with plastic surgery. Some people resolve conflicts between their appearance and the cultural ideal by deciding that they like themselves just the way they are. Others choose to enhance their appearance with cosmetic surgery. There is no right or wrong answer for everyone—only personal choice.

Sometimes children need plastic surgery, and parents can face considerable confusion in making the choice for them. For most reconstructive procedures, such as cleft lip and palate (see p.970), the benefits are usually clear. Meeting with your child's pediatrician, and with the surgeons and a psychologist, can help you make the best decision for your child. For procedures that have a lesser medical mandate, such as surgery for prominent ears (see Otoplasty, p.580), talk to your child's pediatrician and affiliated medical specialists. Sometimes such surgery helps the child's emotional health as much as his or her physical appearance. It is important to consider your child's feelings and involve him or her in making a decision.

If you decide on plastic surgery, be certain to discuss fees, which vary widely among surgeons and communities. While many reconstructive surgeries are covered by insurance, most cosmetic procedures are not. A representative of your insurance company can tell you what types of procedures are covered.

BREASTS

Breast Enlargement

Breast enlargement, also called breast augmentation, is done by inserting a fluid- or gel-filled implant between the breast tissue and the chest wall. This increases breast size, even though the amount of breast tissue itself does not change. The incision to insert the implant can be made in one of three locations: below the breast, around the nipple, or in the armpit.

Until 1992, most breast implants were filled with silicone gel, a material chosen because it was thought to have no effect on the body. In the early 1990s, several cases were reported of women with silicone gel–filled implants who developed connective-tissue diseases such as scleroderma (see p.897), raising concerns about a possible link

Preparing for and Recovering From Plastic Surgery

Carefully follow your surgeon's directions on how to prepare for surgery. Depending on the type of surgery you will have, there will be restrictions on eating, drinking, smoking, and taking medicines or vitamins. For some types of surgery, you should arrange for someone to drive you home and to assist you with daily activities for at least a day or two afterward; some surgeries require you to have assistance for a longer period. In general, younger people heal faster after plastic surgery than older people because they usually require less extensive surgery, younger tissues are more resilient, and younger individuals are less likely to have chronic medical problems that can impair healing.

between the two. When the product's manufacturers could not provide proof of its safety, the Food and Drug Administration banned the use of silicone gel–filled breast implants in 1992. Subsequent studies have

not proven a relationship between gel-filled implants and connective tissue diseases or any other disease, but silicone gel implants are still used only under very close supervision in clinical trials designed to assess their safety.

Nearly all breast implants used today are filled with saline (salt water), which has never been associated with these illnesses, and researchers are looking for newer, better materials. For information on breast reconstruction after breast removal surgery, see p.1060.

Breast implants do not cause breast cancer, but there is some evidence that cancers are detected at a later stage in women with implants than in those without them. Although breast implants do not usually interfere with breast self-examinations (see p.78), they can change the way a mammogram is performed or reduce the sensitivity of this screening test. If you have

Breast Enlargement Incision Sites

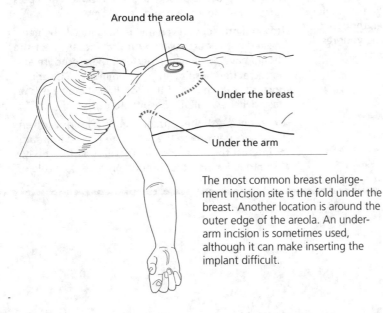

Around the areola

Under the breast

Under the arm

The most common breast enlargement incision site is the fold under the breast. Another location is around the outer edge of the areola. An underarm incision is sometimes used, although it can make inserting the implant difficult.

Choosing a Plastic Surgeon

One of the most important factors in the success of any plastic surgery is the surgeon you choose. Start by developing a list of good candidates, and note doctors who are suggested by more than one person or organization. Consider the following sources as you make your list:

Doctors Your family doctor, internist, general surgeon, or gynecologist may be able to recommend a plastic surgeon. Ask how many people he or she has referred to the surgeon and what feedback was offered. Ask your doctor whether he or she would send a family member to this plastic surgeon.

Hospitals Call a respected hospital in your community and ask for the names of plastic surgeons on staff who are certified by the American Board of Plastic Surgery (ABPS). Ask for doctors who have hospital privileges (official approval) to perform the procedure you are considering.

American Society of Plastic and Reconstructive Surgeons (ASPRS) The ASPRS provides a toll-free Plastic Surgery Information Service. Call 1-800-635-0635 and leave your name, address, and the procedure you are interested in. ASPRS will send you the names of five board-certified plastic surgeons in your area who perform that procedure.

Friends If you know someone who has had the procedure you are considering, and you like the result, ask for the physician's name. Remember, though, that every person and every surgery is unique; your results might be very different from your friend's.

CHECK CREDENTIALS

Once you have compiled your list of candidates, begin checking credentials. While good credentials cannot guarantee a successful outcome, the following can significantly increase the odds:

Training More important than where your surgeon went to school is the type of training he or she received. Has the surgeon completed an accredited residency program specifically in plastic surgery? Such a program includes 2 or 3 years of intensive training in the full spectrum of reconstructive and cosmetic procedures. While your plastic surgeon may choose to concentrate on a limited number of procedures, this comprehensive background gives a solid foundation to his or her skills.

Board certification Everyone has heard the phrase "board-certified," but few people know what it means. Make sure the doctor you choose is certified by the American Board of Plastic Surgery (ABPS). Such a designation indicates that the doctor has graduated from an accredited medical school and completed at least 5 years of additional residency—usually 3 years of general surgery or its equivalent and 2 years of plastic surgery. To be certified by the ABPS, a doctor must also practice plastic surgery for 2 years and pass comprehensive written and oral exams.

Hospital privileges Even if your surgery will be performed in the doctor's own surgical facility, he or she should have privileges to perform the procedure at an accredited hospital in your community. Ask the doctor for the name of the hospital where he or she has privileges. Call the hospital to verify.

Experience Ask the surgeons on your list how often they have performed the particular procedure that is of interest to you, and when they last performed it. Technique is perfected through practice. As a rule of thumb, the surgeon should perform the procedure you are seeking at least several times a month, and have performed the last procedure no longer than 6 months before.

INTERVIEWING PLASTIC SURGEONS

After you narrow your list to two or three surgeons, consider having an initial consultation with each before making your decision. However excellent the doctors' credentials, meeting the candidates in person is worthwhile. You can get a feeling for each one as a person, learn what type of surgical procedure each suggests for you, and see before-and-after pictures of the surgeon's work. Ask for the price of each consultation in advance. At the time of the consultation, discuss surgical, anesthetic, and institutional fees. Take notes. By meeting with several surgeons, you will have a better idea of what is a fair fee for the procedure you are considering. If you feel uncomfortable with a doctor for any reason, choose another one.

QUESTIONS TO DISCUSS WITH A PLASTIC SURGEON

1 What are your professional qualifications and training?

2 How frequently do you perform the procedure?

3 What complications exist, and, in your experience, what is the frequency of each complication?

4 May I see before-and-after pictures—both of your best results and your typical results—of people who have had the same procedure and have given their permission to have their pictures shown?

5 Can you give me the names of a few people who have had the procedure and have agreed to speak to others about their experience?

During the consultation, look for a surgeon who:

■ Explains the procedure thoroughly and answers all of your questions in language you can understand.

■ Asks about your motivations and expectations, discusses them with you, and asks for your reaction to his or her recommendations.

■ Offers alternatives, without pressuring you to consider unnecessary procedures.

■ Welcomes questions about professional qualifications, experience, costs, and payment policies.

■ Makes clear the risks of surgery and the possible variations in outcome. If the surgeon shows you photographs of people or uses computer-imaging to show you possible results, he or she should make it clear that there is no guarantee that your results will match them.

■ Tells you the final decision is yours.

AFTER YOU CHOOSE A PLASTIC SURGEON

During your first visit, the surgeon will want to know your reasons for seeking surgery, analyze the structure of the area to be treated, and help you evaluate whether your goals are realistic. Good surgeons are very frank about what can and cannot be changed by a procedure. The surgeon should also take your medical history, including questions about medical conditions, medicines, past surgeries, allergies, and habits such as smoking or alcohol use.

The surgeon should then provide a step-by-step description of what will take place. You should understand the procedure thoroughly, including the type of anesthesia that will be used, lines of incision, possible pain, time required for surgery, and what to anticipate after the operation. Sign a consent form only after you have read it and understand it.

Location of Implants for Breast Enlargement

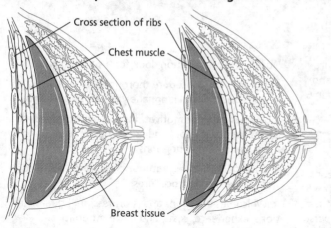

IMPLANT OVER CHEST MUSCLE   IMPLANT UNDER CHEST MUSCLE

Breast implants can be inserted over (left) or under (right) chest muscle.

implants, your mammogram should be performed by technicians skilled in obtaining reliable x-rays in women with breast implants.

THE PROCEDURE

Before surgery, discuss with your surgeon where he or she recommends making the incisions and the risks and benefits of different types of implants. The surgery, which lasts about 2 hours, can be performed on an outpatient basis in a clinic or hospital. Most surgeons recommend general anesthesia (see p.168) but some prefer local anesthetics (see p.168), along with sedatives to make you drowsy.

First, the surgeon makes the incision. The breast tissue is lifted to create a pocket for the implant, either under the chest muscle or on top of it. The incision is stitched closed and taped for support; drainage tubes may also be inserted for several days. A gauze bandage is usually placed over the breast.

RECOVERY AND COMPLICATIONS

After surgery, you may have considerable pain, especially if your implant was placed under the chest muscle. Most people feel tired and sore for a few days after surgery but are active within a day or two. After surgery, you may need to wear a surgical bra, which provides extra support and minimizes swelling. The wound will be evaluated after about a week, at which time your breasts may still be tender, bruised, and swollen. Breast soreness and sensitivity may last for 6 weeks. The scars will fade but never completely disappear.

Care after surgery involves daily stretching of the arm muscles and massaging the breasts. This helps reduce the chance of capsular contracture, which occurs when the scar or capsule around the implant begins to tighten, causing the implant to feel hard. It is the most common reason for dissatisfaction with the procedure. Contracture can be treated by further surgery to cut the scar tissue or remove it, or to replace the implant. Chances that contracture will recur are high.

Other complications include excessive bleeding into the tissue, which may require surgical drainage, or infection around the implant, which may require removal of the implant for several months. These complications occur in 2% to 4% of cases. Oversensitive or numb nipples can also occur, especially if incisions were made around the nipple. Permanent partial or total loss of nipple sensation after breast implant surgery occurs in about 15% of women.

Occasionally, breast implants rupture or leak, which can cause pain, inflammation, and distortion of the breast. If a saline implant breaks, the implant usually deflates over several hours and the salt water is absorbed harmlessly by your body. A slow leak can occur through the valve of the implant; it may take weeks before you notice it. If a gel-filled implant leaks, it can be more difficult to detect and may cause new scarring around the breast. Any break in an implant requires a second operation to remove it.

Breast Lift

Breast lift, also called mastopexy, is a surgical procedure to temporarily reshape and lift sagging breasts. It can also be used to reduce the size of the areola (the darker skin surrounding the nipple). Breast skin can lose its elasticity due to pregnancy, breast-

Breast Lift

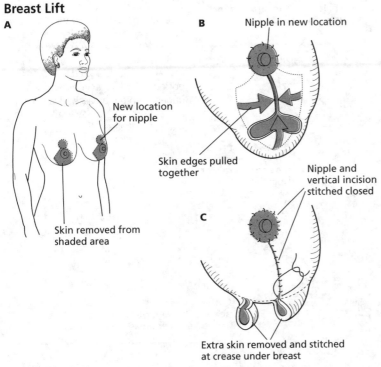

A

New location for nipple

Skin removed from shaded area

B

Nipple in new location

Skin edges pulled together

C

Nipple and vertical incision stitched closed

Extra skin removed and stitched at crease under breast

An incision is made around the nipple and along the natural contours of the breasts and excess skin is removed (A). The nipple and areola are moved to a higher position and skin is brought together under the nipple (B). The incision is stitched around the areola, in a vertical line from the nipple to the crease under the breast, and in the crease under the breast (C).

Recovering From Breast Surgery

Most women need assistance at home during the first 2 days after breast surgery. You can usually return to work 5 to 7 days after surgery. Be vigilant in following your doctor's instructions regarding lifting, exercise, resuming sexual activity, and care of incisions.

feeding, and gravity, causing breasts to lose their shape and firmness. Although a breast lift does not usually interfere with breast-feeding, the surgery is not recommended for women who plan a future pregnancy because increased breast size during pregnancy can reverse the effects of a breast lift.

THE PROCEDURE

The procedure for a breast-lift is described in the illustration above. The surgery takes about 3 hours to complete and can be performed on an outpatient basis in a clinic or hospital. Most sur-

geons recommend general anesthesia (see p.168) but, if smaller incisions are planned, a local anesthetic (see p.168) along with sedatives to make you drowsy may be used.

RECOVERY AND COMPLICATIONS

Plan to spend up to a week recuperating. Your breasts may be bruised, swollen, and uncomfortable for a day or two. You may be given a support bra or elastic bandage to wear over the dressings; this is often replaced by a softer support bra within a few days. You will wear the soft bra day and night for up to a month, although your stitches and bandages may be removed within a week or two. You may notice numbness in your nipples and the skin of your breast. This loss of sensation usually diminishes along with the swelling over about 6 weeks but may last longer or may be permanent. Scars, which are extensive and permanent, may remain lumpy and red for months, gradually fading to thin lines. You should plan to be away from work for about a week after surgery.

Breast Reduction

Breast reduction is the removal of fat, glandular tissue, and skin from the breasts. In most cases, it can also lift the breasts and reduce the size of the areola, the dark skin around the nipple.

THE PROCEDURE

This surgery takes about 3 to 4 hours. It is usually performed in a hospital under general anesthesia (see p.168) and may require an overnight stay in the hospital.

Breast Reduction

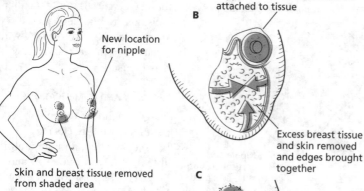

A

New location for nipple

Skin and breast tissue removed from shaded area

Nipple and vertical incision stitched closed

B

Nipple moved to new location attached to tissue

Excess breast tissue and skin removed and edges brought together

C

Extra tissue and skin removed and stitched at crease under breast

An incision that circles the areola, extends downward, and follows the natural curve of the underside of the breast (A) is made. Excess tissue, fat, and skin are removed, and the nipple and areola are relocated to a higher position (B). Skin is brought together underneath the breast and stitched in a line running vertically to the crease under the breast (C).

Excess tissue, fat, and skin are removed, which results in a new and uplifted shape (see illustration). In most women, the nipple and areola are moved to a new position, which may cause a complete and permanent loss of nipple sensation and a loss of the ability to breast-feed. Your surgeon may use liposuction (see p.590) to remove fat from the breasts and under the arms.

RECOVERY AND COMPLICATIONS

After surgery, the incisions are dressed with gauze bandages.

You will be given a surgical bra or elastic bandage to wear over the dressings that is replaced by a softer bra within a few days. The soft bra will need to be worn day and night for up to a month, although your stitches will be removed within 5 to 7 days. A small tube may be placed in your breasts for a day or two to drain fluids and blood. Your breasts may be painful for about a week. Your doctor can prescribe medicine to relieve the pain. Bruising and swelling usually subside after several weeks. Expect your

breasts to swell and be tender during your first menstrual period after surgery. You may feel unusual sensations in your breasts for about a month, as well as numbness in your nipples and the skin of your breasts. The numbness usually subsides but can be permanent. Most women require about 2 weeks of recuperation. The scars from surgery, which are permanent, may be red and quite visible for more than a year, but they usually fade.

FACE

Face-Lift

A face-lift, or rhytidectomy, is one of the most common cosmetic surgery procedures performed. Despite its name, it does not reverse the signs of aging over

the entire face. The procedure creates a more youthful contour primarily of the cheeks and neck by removing excess skin and fat, tightening the underlying muscle and connective tissue, and

pulling tight the remaining skin. It is often combined with liposuction (see p.590) of the face and neck, which permits surgeons to use smaller incisions and do more subtle facial con-

Face-Lift

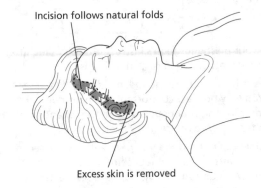

Incision follows natural folds

Excess skin is removed

Incisions are made along or behind the hairline, tracing a path from around the earlobe and back of the ear to the lower scalp. Skin is lifted away and up, excess skin is removed, and the skin is pulled tight against the head and stitched into place.

UNDERMINING

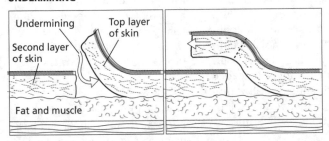

Undermining

Top layer of skin

Second layer of skin

Fat and muscle

In a face-lift, the two top layers of skin are first separated from underlying fat and muscle in a process called undermining.

touring than they could do with the traditional surgical procedure.

Although a face-lift cannot smooth forehead wrinkles or remove creases or bags around the eyes, it can be combined with a browlift (see p.579) and an eyelid lift (see Blepharoplasty, p.578) to combat the effects of aging across the entire face.

It is important to understand that a face-lift can make you look younger, but it cannot restore your face to its original appearance or completely change the way you look. It is also important to realize that a face-lift slows the effects of aging on the face but does not stop the clock. Your face continues to age. The procedure can be repeated, usually after 5 or 10 years.

The ideal candidate for a face-lift is a person whose facial and neck skin has begun to droop but still remains elastic and whose bone structure is well defined. Most people who have a face-lift are in their 40s, 50s, or 60s, although the procedure can be done successfully in older individuals as well.

THE PROCEDURE

A face-lift generally takes several hours. It may be performed in an outpatient surgical unit or in a hospital operating room using local anesthesia (see p.168) to numb the face, with intravenous sedation to make you sleepy and relaxed. Some surgeons prefer to use general anesthesia (see p.168). The placement of incisions and the sequence of surgery depends upon your facial structure and your surgeon's goals and technique (see illustration). Endoscopic techniques are sometimes used to permit smaller incisions (see Browlift, p.579).

RECOVERY AND COMPLICATIONS

Your face will be loosely bandaged and you will stay in bed for several hours or overnight if you are staying in the hospital. Drains and dressings will be removed within 2 days, and stitches will be taken out 3 to 7 days later. Expect your face to look bruised, pale, and puffy for a few weeks. Your doctor will encourage you to stand up and move around after surgery to prevent the formation of blood clots in your legs, but you should not bend over or engage in any strenuous activity for 4 to 6 weeks. Extensive bruising and swelling can last 2 or 3 weeks, and numbness in your cheeks and neck may last up to 6 months.

Serious complications include a hematoma (a blood-filled swelling under the skin) that can cause tissue damage. Other complications include (usually temporary) damage to the nerves that control facial movement, infection, scarring, and poor healing of the skin (which occurs more often in people who smoke).

Blepharoplasty

Eyelid surgery is performed on the lower and/or upper eyelids to reduce creases around the eyes, heaviness over the lids, bags under the eyes, and extra skin. It can also alter the appearance of the epicanthal fold, which is a characteristic of Asian upper eyelids. However, the procedure cannot remove "crow's-feet," totally eliminate dark circles under the eyes, or lift sagging eyebrows (see Browlift, p.579).

In some older people, a drooping upper eyelid can interfere with vision, and some people inherit a heavy upper eyelid that can obstruct vision at any age.

Before having eyelid surgery, you may wish to have a thorough eye exam by an ophthalmologist to ensure that your eyes

are healthy and that surgery will not affect any existing eye problems, such as dry eyes. If you do not have an ophthalmologist, your plastic surgeon will examine your eyelids and refer you to an ophthalmologist if needed. Your plastic surgeon will want to know whether you have any chronic conditions that cause

changes in the eye tissues, such as thyroid disease (see Hyperthyroidism, p.844), diabetes mellitus (see p.832), kidney disease (see p.810), or congestive heart failure (see p.683).

THE PROCEDURE

Most blepharoplasty surgery is performed on an outpatient basis using local anesthesia (see p.168) with a sedative to relax you. Time spent in surgery ranges from 1½ to 2 hours for the upper and lower eyelids. For upper lid surgery, the surgeon makes an incision following the creases of your eyelids. For bags under the eyes and for lower lid surgery, the incision is made just below the lashes of your lower eyelids. Excess skin and fat are removed, and the incision is closed with delicate stitches.

For bags caused by excess fat under the eyes but no excess skin, your surgeon may perform a transconjunctival blepharoplasty, in which an incision is made inside your lower eyelid, fat is removed, and the incision is closed, leaving no visible scar.

Recovering From Surgery on Your Face

Be vigilant in following your plastic surgeon's instructions regarding lifting, exercise, resuming sexual activity, and care of incisions.

Face-lift surgery Most people can get around independently by the second day after surgery. You may not feel comfortable going out in public for about 2 weeks to a month. This is dependent upon the extent of plastic surgery and your tendency to bruise and discolor.

Eyelid surgery Most people can get around independently by the second day after surgery. With sunglasses, you may feel comfortable going out in public after 3 or 4 days. Makeup can usually mask the scars after about a week.

Surgery on Upper Eyelids

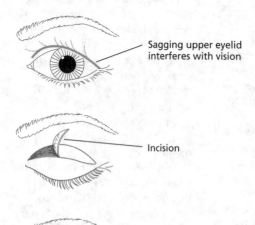

Sagging upper eyelid interferes with vision

Incision

Incision stitched closed

In upper eyelid surgery, two curved incisions are made at the crease above the eyelid, through which excess skin, fat, and muscle are removed. The incision is then stitched closed.

RECOVERY AND COMPLICATIONS

After closing the incisions, your eyes will not be covered with a bandage, but your eyelids will be lubricated with an antibiotic ointment. Your eyelids may feel sore as the anesthesia wears off. After it has completely worn off, you can go home. To help minimize swelling, use cold compresses, applying slight pressure, and keep your head elevated for several days. Your vision may be blurred for a while and your eyes may be gummy due to ointment, tears, and blood. Expect swelling and bruising for about 10 days; they should disappear completely within 6 weeks.

For the first few weeks you may also have excessive tearing, sensitivity to light, numbness at the site of the incision, and temporary changes in your eyesight, such as blurry vision. It may take several months before the incision sites lose their redness and blend into the surrounding skin. Keep this area protected from the sun to minimize scarring. If you wear contact lenses, your doctor may ask that you not wear them for about a month.

The skin incision in blepharoplasty leaves an almost undetectable scar after 3 to 6 months in almost all cases. Most serious complications, which are rare, result from bleeding. If blood pools behind the eye, it can create pressure on the optic nerve, resulting in loss of vision. In the first 48 hours after surgery, be alert to any changes in your vision or to significant asymmetrical swelling around your eyes. Call your plastic surgeon if you are concerned.

Browlift

A browlift, or forehead lift, is a procedure designed to lift drooping brows and reduce horizontal forehead lines by removing or tightening the muscles and tissues that cause the furrowing or drooping. Plastic surgeons use two different approaches: an open surgical method requiring an incision hidden in the hairline or an endoscopic method performed through several small keyhole incisions.

THE PROCEDURE

Most browlifts are performed on an outpatient basis using a local anesthetic (see p.168) and a sedative to relax you. In most people, the incisions are made behind the hairline. In some people, particularly those whose foreheads are very high, the plastic surgeon may make the incision at the hairline. For balding men, the incision is made across the forehead in an existing frown line.

In a conventional browlift, the incision starts above one ear, crosses the top of the forehead, and goes down the other side of the head and ends above the other ear. The surgeon lifts the skin of the forehead to remove the underlying tissues and to release, remove, and alter the forehead muscles. The eyebrows are raised by releasing these tissues from their attachment at the upper edge of the eye socket. Vertical lines are improved by removing the muscles that cause them.

In an endoscopic browlift, the surgeon makes up to five 1-inch-long incisions along the hairline. The endoscope (a pencil-like tube fitted with a tiny camera connected to a monitor) is inserted through one incision. An instrument containing a tiny scalpel is

Botulinum Toxin: How a Deadly Toxin Can Ease Wrinkles

Creases in the forehead and the vertical lines between the eyebrows can be softened, at least for a while, by injecting the underlying muscles with botulinum toxin. This potentially deadly poison is produced by bacteria. If large amounts are inadvertently consumed in spoiled food, death can result. But the same chemical, when applied in very small doses to specific individual muscles, causes temporary paralysis of the immediate area. It does this without altering sensation because it does not travel far from the injection site. Botulinum toxin has been used by dermatologists and cosmetic surgeons to soften wrinkles of the forehead muscles. The effect begins a day after the injection, increases over the first week, and lasts weeks to months; however, it is not permanent. The effects and safety of the toxin are not fully understood. It is very likely that the skill of the doctor doing the injection is a key feature in the result. If you consider this technique, be sure that your doctor is experienced in using it.

inserted through another incision. Watching the monitor, your surgeon views the muscles and tissue and uses the scalpel to lift the forehead skin and remove or tighten the muscles. If your eyebrows are being lifted, they are secured into their higher position by stitches made beneath the skin's surface or by temporary screws placed behind the hairline.

In both procedures, the incisions are closed with clips or stitches and are left either unbandaged or wrapped in gauze padding and an elastic bandage. The stitches and clips will be removed within a few weeks. You may have some swelling, which can also affect your eye and cheek area, for a week or so. People who undergo a conventional forehead lift may have some numbness and itching on their scalp for several years. People who undergo the endoscopic procedure usually have less numbness and itching.

RECOVERY AND COMPLICATIONS

Loss of sensation along, or just above, the incision line is common, especially with the conventional procedure. It is usually temporary, but sensation to the area can be very slow to recover in some people. In rare cases, the nerves that control eyebrow movement may be injured on one or both sides, resulting in a loss of the ability to raise the eyebrows or wrinkle the forehead. Additional surgery may be required to correct the problem. Formation of a broad scar is also a rare complication, in which case additional surgery can usually improve the situation by pro-

ducing a new, thinner scar. Some people lose hair along the edge of the scar. If a complication occurs during an endoscopic browlift, your surgeon may have to abandon the endoscopic approach and switch to the conventional, open procedure. This may result in a more extensive scar.

Otoplasty

Otoplasty is surgery to reposition protruding ears closer to the head or to reduce the size of large ears. It is often performed on children between ages 4 and 14, but many adults also have the procedure. Even if only one ear is very prominent, some surgeons recommend that surgery be performed on both ears to ensure a balanced appearance. Parents are advised to be sensitive about their child's feelings about protruding ears; surgery is usually not done until the child asks for it. Children who feel uncomfortable about their ears and want the surgery are generally more cooperative during the process and happier with the outcome. Because the ear is 80% of its full size by the time a child is 5 years old, most corrective surgery on the ears can safely be done after this age.

THE PROCEDURE

Otoplasty is usually performed on an outpatient basis using intravenous sedation and local anesthesia (see p.168), although young children may tolerate the surgery better with general anesthesia (see p.168). Surgery usually takes from 2 to 3 hours. The most common technique involves

making a small incision behind the ear to reveal the ear cartilage so that the surgeon can cut it and reposition the ear closer to the head. The ear may be held in place with permanent stitches. In another technique, after making an incision behind the ear, skin is removed and stitches are used to fold the cartilage back on itself to reshape the ear without removing cartilage. In severe cases, a combination of techniques may be used.

RECOVERY AND COMPLICATIONS

Most people can leave the hospital soon after surgery, although young children who received general anesthesia may need to stay in the hospital overnight until the effects wear off. The head will be wrapped in a large, close-fitting bandage to ensure proper healing. The stitches dissolve or are removed after about a week, and most people can resume normal work and school schedules at this time. Avoid any activity that could result in a bent ear for about a month. Most people have only a faint scar behind the ear after healing is complete.

Other Ear Surgery

Besides protruding ears, other ear malformations can be helped with surgery, including an ear tip that folds down and forward, a very small ear, and an ear that is missing the curve in its outer rim or its natural folds. Surgery can also correct large, stretched, or creased earlobes. Finally, surgeons can build new ears for infants born without them or for people who lose them through injury.

Rhinoplasty

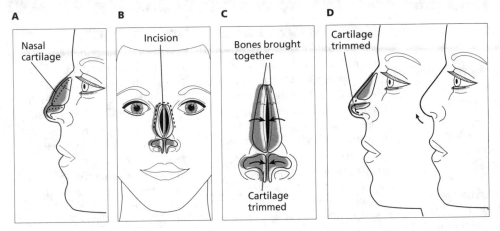

Nose shape is largely determined by nasal bones and nasal cartilage (A). To reshape the nose, an incision (B) is made either inside the nostrils or at the base of the nose. The surgeon chisels or files away bone and cartilage and then brings nasal bones together (C) to make the bridge of the nose more narrow. Cartilage at the tip of the nose may be trimmed to make the tip of the nose turn upward (D).

Rhinoplasty

Nose surgery, which is the most common cosmetic procedure, can make your nose smaller or larger, change its shape, or narrow the nostrils. Occasionally, it is also performed for medical reasons, such as to correct an injury or birth defect, or to relieve breathing problems.

THE PROCEDURE

Rhinoplasty, which takes from 1 to 3 hours, is usually performed on an outpatient basis using local or general anesthesia (see p.168). With local anesthesia, you will be given a sedative to relax you. The anesthetic will numb your nose but you will be somewhat awake throughout the procedure. The surgeon will elevate and separate the skin of the nose from the bone and cartilage, which are then reshaped. The incision is made either inside the nostrils

or, in more complicated cases, across the strip of skin that separates the nostrils. The skin is then pulled over the reshaped bone and cartilage of your nose and stitched closed. To help your nose keep its new shape, the surgeon may place a plastic or metal splint over the nose and place material inside the nostrils to hold the septum (the dividing wall of cartilage between the nostrils) in place. This is particularly useful if the septum has required plastic surgery to improve breathing or appearance.

RECOVERY AND COMPLICATIONS

For the first 24 hours after surgery you may have a dull headache and your nose will be uncomfortable. You may be asked to stay in bed and keep your head upright to minimize swelling. Swelling and bruising around the eyes are normal and

usually disappear within 3 weeks. Applying cold compresses can help ease the pain and diminish the discoloration. Nosebleeds and stuffiness are common for the first week or two after surgery, and your plastic surgeon may ask you to avoid blowing your nose for about a week so the tissues can heal. Nasal packing is usually removed within a few days unless surgery has been done on the septum. The splint is usually removed after a week. If you wear glasses, you may need to tape them to your forehead for a month or two to avoid putting pressure on your nose. After surgery, small burst blood vessels may appear as tiny red spots on the skin's surface. These are usually minor and may fade, but they can be permanent. When rhinoplasty is performed from inside the nose, there is no visible scarring. When an open technique is used, the small scars between the nostrils are usually very minor. It can take up to a year before the full effects of the surgery are apparent.

SKIN

Laser Surgery of the Skin

Lasers are used for skin resurfacing to remove sun-damaged or wrinkled skin in a very controlled fashion. They are also used to remove noncancerous skin growths, blood vessels (including spider veins), birthmarks, and tattoos. Laser treatments, like other surgery, carry a small risk of infection, scarring, or change in the color of the treated skin. Not all physicians who use lasers are trained in every technique. It is especially important to choose a doctor who has experience in the treatment you are considering.

WHAT TO EXPECT

Laser treatment, which is almost always an outpatient procedure, takes place in a special surgical unit designed to prevent fires and other hazards that could accompany the use of a laser. To avoid eye damage from the intense light, you will wear goggles or other protective eyewear. Local anesthesia (see p.168) is most often used unless the area to be treated is very extensive, in which case general anesthesia (see p.168) may be required. You must avoid sun exposure for 3 weeks before surgery because the pigmentation of a tan or sunburn can absorb the light beam and keep it from reaching its target. After surgery, treated skin is very sensitive to the sun. You should wear a sunblock with a sun protection factor (SPF) of 30 and avoid excessive sun exposure.

SKIN RESURFACING

Laser skin resurfacing is used to reduce the appearance of fine lines on the face, particularly around the eyes and mouth. It can also treat sun damage and acne scars. Lasers treat a similar spectrum of skin problems as dermabrasion (see p.584) and chemical peels (see p.585). All three procedures remove the superficial layers of skin but by different means. The laser uses heat, a chemical peel uses strong chemicals, and dermabrasion physically scrapes off the top layer of skin. Lasers can be more precisely controlled than the other techniques, so complications are less common. Laser skin resurfacing is a newer procedure than the others. Ask several physicians if the outcome you want would be best achieved by

Laser Skin Resurfacing

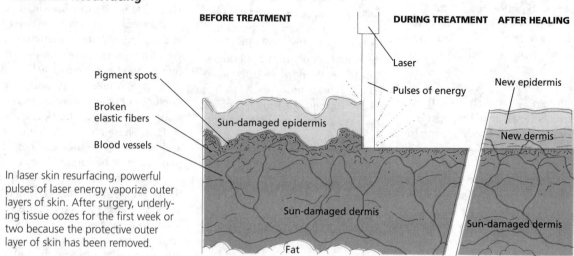

BEFORE TREATMENT

Pigment spots

Broken elastic fibers

Blood vessels

Sun-damaged epidermis

Sun-damaged dermis

Fat

DURING TREATMENT

Laser

Pulses of energy

AFTER HEALING

New epidermis

New dermis

Sun-damaged dermis

In laser skin resurfacing, powerful pulses of laser energy vaporize outer layers of skin. After surgery, underlying tissue oozes for the first week or two because the protective outer layer of skin has been removed.

How Do Lasers Work?

A laser (an acronym for **l**ight **a**mplification by **s**timulated **e**mission of **r**adiation) is an intense light beam of a specific wavelength (for example, color). Different types of laser beams emit light of different wavelengths, each of which is absorbed by a different substance in the skin. The laser can target water; pigments, including melanin (which is heavily concentrated in freckles and moles); or a variety of pigments inserted into the skin by tattooing. When laser energy is absorbed, it is transferred to the target in the form of heat, which causes physical changes in tissues. Heat from the absorbed light can coagulate proteins, break down pigment particles, and boil water in body cells. When carefully controlled, lasers can be used to seal off blood vessels and vaporize tissue in thin layers. Many lasers emit light in pulses as brief as a fraction of a second, which allows the intense heat to dissipate before it is conducted to surrounding tissue, minimizing damage to healthy skin.

laser resurfacing, dermabrasion, or a chemical peel.

Laser resurfacing can be lightly used or used to remove deeper layers of skin. The recovery time is longer for procedures that remove deeper layers of skin. People with darker skin have a slightly higher chance of a skin-color change than do people with fair complexions. Scarring rarely occurs. The procedure usually is performed on an outpatient basis and lasts from several minutes to 2 hours. An anesthetic is first injected to numb the areas being resurfaced. Then, short powerful pulses of laser energy vaporize outer layers of skin. Afterward, the area is rubbed vigorously with gauze pads soaked in salt water. An ointment or cream may then be applied.

After the procedure, the treated area will look and feel as though it had been burned, oozing clear or yellow fluid for 4 to 10 days, depending on the depth of treatment. You are likely to have some redness, swelling, and mild pain. Redness and swelling after resurfacing may last 6 to 8 weeks. Applying ice during the first 48 hours helps relieve swelling. The treated area must be cleaned and dressed several times daily to prevent the formation of scabs, reduce the chance of infection, and permit the skin to regrow.

New pink-red skin will cover the treated area within about 7 days. The red will fade slowly over several months; in people with darker skin, new skin may never match the original color. You must avoid the sun and use a sunscreen with a sun protection factor (SPF) of 15 or higher for up to 10 weeks after surgery. Since the procedure can activate a herpesvirus infection (see p.487), the drug acyclovir is given to anyone with a history of cold sores. It is not known how long the effects of laser resurfacing last, but it is generally believed to be at least 5 to 10 years. However, the process of aging continues and skin remains vulnerable to damage by the sun.

TREATING SPIDER VEINS AND OTHER BLOOD VESSELS

Spider veins, also called telangiectasias, are tiny blue, red, or purple veins that often congregate on the thighs, ankles, and calves. Spider veins can be caused by pregnancy, weight gain, and some medicines; they can also be inherited. They can be treated in one of two ways: sclerotherapy (see Sclerotherapy for Spider Veins, p.584) or laser therapy. Larger, usually purple, blood vessels may respond better to sclerotherapy.

Several types of lasers can be used, but all produce laser light that is absorbed by hemoglobin in blood cells. The resulting heat coagulates the blood, damaging the blood vessel wall and sealing the vessels, which subsequently disintegrate and are absorbed by the body. The laser's pulse feels like the snap of a rubber band; anesthesia is usually not necessary when the treatment area is small. The treated area turns purple after the procedure and will remain so for 10 to 14 days. Then it will change to pink or brown before returning to normal within a few weeks. Discoloration of the skin is common and can persist for up to a year.

TREATING STRAWBERRY MARKS AND PORT-WINE STAINS

Pulsed dye lasers are used to treat port-wine stains (see p.969) and strawberry marks (see p.969) in infants and adults. The pulse of this dye laser feels like a snap from a rubber band. Small areas can be treated without anesthesia; larger areas may require an injection of a local anesthetic (see p.168). As many as eight to ten treatments may be required

Sclerotherapy for Spider Veins

Sclerotherapy for spider veins is performed on an outpatient basis and does not require anesthesia. In the procedure, the skin over the area of spider veins is stretched taut and a saline (salt water) solution is injected into the affected veins, causing them to collapse. The tissues are later absorbed by your body. You will feel a pinprick sensation as a delicate needle is inserted into the vessel, usually followed by 15 to 30 seconds of some mild cramping during the injection. If larger amounts of saline are injected, muscle cramps can develop, lasting up to a minute. Your surgeon will then wrap your leg in compression bandages or hose, which you will wear for several days. The injection site can be tender for 2 or 3 days after treatment and your leg may be bruised and swollen for a week or two. The bruises usually fade within a month, but there may be some darker pigmentation that lasts for up to a year. Complications include formation of blood clots in the superficial veins, local infections, and scarring. Another complication is the development of mats of red or purple blood vessels, which may disappear on their own or require more injections or laser treatment.

to remove a birthmark. The appearance of birthmarks that cannot be entirely removed can be improved.

The treated area will feel like a sunburn and look purple, like a dark bruise, for 10 to 14 days. Care of the treatment site during the first 4 days is important to prevent scabbing and infection and to promote growth of new skin. It may be several weeks before you see a noticeable improvement. Follow-up treatments are usually performed no sooner than 6 to 8 weeks after the first procedure.

TREATING TATTOOS, FRECKLES, AND OTHER PIGMENTED AREAS

There are several specialized lasers used to remove tattoos and sun-induced freckles (typical moles are usually not removed with a laser). Ruby lasers produce red light that is selectively absorbed by melanin (which gives color to skin) and by dye pigments (which are injected in tattooing). This makes the laser well suited for removing tattoos and freckles. Usually no anesthesia is required, although a topical anesthetic (see p.168) may be used. Removing a tattoo may require 6 to 12 separate treatments. Professional and multicolored tattoos require more treatments than amateur and single-color tattoos. Some tattoos can never be completely removed.

Dermabrasion

Dermabrasion is a technique in which the outer layer of skin is essentially sanded away, using a handheld motorized device with a rotating wire brush or a diamond-encrusted wheel. Repeated treatments are usually necessary to produce an optimal result.

Dermabrasion can reduce fine wrinkles, some scars (including acne scars), and other surface irregularities. These conditions can also be treated by laser skin resurfacing (see p.582) or a chemical peel (see p.585). In general, dermabrasion removes deeper layers of the skin than a chemical peel does and is used to treat more obvious wrinkles and acne scars. Dermabrasion can also be used to remove actinic keratoses (see p.543), which are precancerous growths.

THE PROCEDURE

Dermabrasion is an outpatient procedure that is usually performed using a local anesthetic (see p.168) or a refrigerant spray to deaden the tissues of the face. The physician holds the rotating device and scrapes away the surface layer of skin on selected spots or on the entire face while air is directed toward the face to reduce bleeding and to begin formation of a scablike crust. An ointment, wet bandage, dry bandage, or a combination of dressings is then applied to the treated area.

RECOVERY AND COMPLICATIONS

After surgery, your skin will be very red and swollen and you may have burning or aching in your face. The swelling will subside within about a week. A scab, which may itch, develops over the treated area; it falls off to reveal pink new skin, which will fade to a more normal color after several months. You must use a sunscreen with a sun protection factor (SPF) of at least 15 and avoid excessive sunlight, especially in the first year after the

Chemical Peels and Their Uses

	ALPHA-HYDROXY ACID (AHA)—GLYCOLIC ACID, LACTIC ACID, OR FRUIT ACIDS	TRICHLOROACETIC ACID (TCA)	PHENOL
Potency	Mild; produces light peel	Medium; produces medium-depth peel*	Strong; produces deep peel*
What it can treat	Sun damage; uneven pigmentation; acne	Fine surface wrinkles; superficial blemishes; pigment problems of darker-skinned people	Coarse facial wrinkles; blotchy, sun-damaged skin; precancerous growths; areas of dark pigmentation, including freckles
Side effects and potential problems	Red and flaking skin; stinging; increased sun sensitivity	Stinging; mild swelling and discomfort; crust or scab formation; increased sun sensitivity	Severe swelling (eyes may be swollen shut); crust or scab formation; redness and blotchiness for several weeks; inability to eat solid food for several days; complete healing takes several months; skin may never again produce pigment; you must stay out of sun always; not recommended for people with darker skin; absorption may pose risk for those with heart problems
Physician-supervised regimen	10 to 15 minutes per treatment, usually in concentrations higher than 8%; repeated applications needed	15 minutes per treatment; requires two or more applications; may sting on application	1 to 2 hours per treatment
At-home regimen	AHA-based facial cleanser or cream available in concentrations of less than 8%; wear sunblock	Pain medicine if needed; wear sunblock	Pain medicine if needed; wear sunblock

* Depth of penetration depends on the concentration of the chemical used and the application technique.

procedure. The most common complication is a change in skin color, usually a lightening in pigment that is most pronounced in darker skin. Some temporary skin darkening can occur; in rare cases there is infection and scarring.

Chemical Peel

A chemical peel, also called chemabrasion or chemexfoliation, is used to remove delicate wrinkles in the superficial layers of the skin. These are usually the result of sun damage and cannot be removed by surgery. Dermabrasion (see p.584) and laser skin resurfacing (see p.582) are alternative procedures for this purpose.

With a chemical peel, the surgeon applies a chemical solution to the skin to create a controlled burn (much like a severe sunburn) that blisters. Eventually the top layer of skin, the epidermis, and part of the underlying layer, the dermis, peel off, leaving newer skin that is tighter and smoother. Chemical peels can remove fine wrinkles or very superficial acne scars but cannot remove most deep lines or scars that involve deeper layers of the skin. The deeper the peel, the more the appearance of the wrinkles is improved but the greater the tendency for skin discoloration and the greater the risk of scar formation.

A chemical peel can be performed on part of your face, such as the area around the mouth, or on the entire face. In some states, no medical degree is required to perform the most superficial chemical peel. As a result, many inadequately trained practitioners offer the procedure. Never permit any person other than a board-certified plastic surgeon or dermatologist to perform a deep chemical peel.

THE PROCEDURE

Chemical peels are usually performed on an outpatient basis. One of several chemical solutions, which vary widely in strength, is used (see Chemical Peels and Their Uses, p.585). Most doctors do not administer an anesthetic but you will be given a sedative if you are having a deep peel. After your face is cleansed, your physician paints the chemical on the skin, stopping the application at the jawline. Once the chemical has been applied, he or she may

spread an ointment over the treated area to encourage deep penetration.

RECOVERY AND COMPLICATIONS

Treatment with the mildest agent, alpha-hydroxy acid (AHA), is sometimes known as a "lunch-time peel" because it allows you to go back to work immediately. At most, you may have some flaking of skin, redness, and dryness. After a chemical peel using stronger agents such as trichloroacetic acid or phenol, you may have significant swelling and some discomfort. If you have a full-face peel with stronger agents, your eyes may be swollen shut.

In all cases, the outer surface of skin will dry to a crust that will fall off in 5 to 7 days, and the redness of your skin should fade. With a trichloroacetic acid peel, swelling and discomfort usually subside within a week, and within about 10 days the new skin will be apparent under the crusts. After a phenol peel, new skin forms in about 10 days. Your face will be very red at first; the redness will gradually fade in the following months.

You must not expose your face to the sun for 6 months, and you must wear a sunscreen with a sun protection factor (SPF) of at least 15 at all times. The most common adverse effect is skin discoloration such as darkening or lightening. Any color change is usually temporary and is less noticeable on people with fair skin. The most serious complication is scarring due to the chemical penetrating too deeply into the skin.

Soft Tissue Augmentation

A variety of materials called soft tissue fillers can be injected into the skin to fill out wrinkles (especially around the mouth and eyes), enlarge the lips, or diminish acne scars. The injected material adds volume to the tissue lying just below the skin, which may have loosened as a result of gravity, sun exposure, and repeated facial movements such as squinting and frowning. These injections are not effective for treating deep folds and wrinkles.

One commonly used material is collagen, a protein harvested from cows; its effect is temporary after injection, lasting only 3 to 12 months. Another material is body fat, which is removed from one part of your body and transferred to another. If the injected fat picks up a blood supply in its new location, it may last indefinitely. Because this does not always happen, newer materials are constantly being developed. For example, a new gel matrix implant activated by your own blood products may produce effects that last longer than collagen injections.

THE PROCEDURE

Injectable fillers are usually administered in a dermatologist's or surgeon's office. Sometimes a local anesthetic (see p.168) is also used.

With collagen injections, the anesthetic is included in the injection mixture. Purified collagen derived from cows is injected, using a delicate needle, into several different sites along the edge of the part of the body being treated. You may feel some mild burning if you have not received a local anesthetic. Because collagen can cause an allergic reaction, the doctor will perform an allergy skin test several weeks before surgery.

With fat injections, the donor site and injection site are deadened with local anesthetic. Your doctor uses a syringe and suction device to extract fat from the donor site, usually the thighs, buttocks, or abdomen. This is done using local anesthesia. The doctor then uses a delicate needle to inject the fat into the skin at the new site. Injection of fat, also known as autologous fat transplantation or microlipoinjection, does not produce an allergic reaction because the fat is taken from your own body and is therefore not foreign material.

RECOVERY AND COMPLICATIONS

With both procedures, the treated site must be slightly overfilled to allow for some absorption of the material by the body. This can cause temporary puffiness and swelling. You may have pain, redness, swelling, and bruising at the donor site and the injection site, and small scabs may form. These effects usually dissipate within a few days. If a large area of your body has been treated, you may need to rest for several days. In rare cases, complications can occur with both procedures, including infection, open sores, abscesses, scarring, lumpiness, and, in the case of collagen, allergic reactions. Injected fat does not always last and may reabsorb unpredictably.

Surgical Treatments for Scars

Scar revision is the term for surgically improving the appearance of a scar or the function of a scarred area. The goal is to reduce the thickness or width of a scar, enhance skin color, and improve the function of the area if the scar is limiting motion. A number of techniques may be used, depending on the type of scar and its location. No scar can be removed completely. The degree of improvement depends on the size of the scar and the type of skin you have. For all procedures, be vigilant in following your surgeon's instructions on care of the treatment area after surgery.

Z-plasty is a surgical technique used to reposition a scar so that it follows the natural lines of the skin. Z-plasty can also relieve scars that buckle and pucker due to loss of underlying tissue; this often occurs after serious burns. The procedure can make some scars less apparent but it cannot eradicate them. In Z-plasty, the old scar is usually removed and new incisions are made on both sides of the scar, producing triangular skin flaps. These are placed over the wound in a Z-shaped pattern and stitched; stitches are removed several days later. The surgery is performed on an outpatient basis using local anesthesia (see p.168) to deaden the affected area.

Skin grafts and flap surgery are usually performed in a well-equipped office or in an operating room in a hospital. General anesthesia or an overnight hospital stay may be needed. To make a skin graft, a healthy

patch of skin is removed from the donor site and reattached at the injured site. If the graft is successful, it grows new blood vessels in its new location. Scars will form at both the donor site and the injured site. Healing can take several months. A compression bandage that pushes the graft down onto the underlying tissue may need to be worn to prevent uneven healing of the wound.

There are two types of skin grafts: full thickness and split thickness. A full-thickness graft makes a deeper cut, to the bottom of the dermis (see p.528), whereas a split-thickness graft removes only the epidermis and/or a part of the dermis. The advantage of a full-thickness graft is that the graft heals more evenly in the site where it is transplanted, compared to a split-thickness graft. However, the donor site of a full-thickness graft may not heal as well as the donor site of a split-thickness graft. It must be stitched closed edge-to-edge after the graft is removed because no skin remains to close the wound; a split-thickness graft donor site can heal from the bottom up since some skin remains at the donor site. Your plastic surgeon will weigh these and other factors in helping you choose the proper skin graft for you.

Flap surgery is a complex procedure that involves moving skin and underlying fat, blood vessels, and sometimes muscle from a nearby healthy part of the body to the injured site. In a pedicle flap, the blood vessels remain attached to their site of origin. In a free graft, the surgeon completely removes the flap and reattaches the blood vessels at the new site.

Hair Replacement Surgery

Medication can help hair loss in men and women (see p.556). Several surgical procedures are also used to replace lost hair, individually or in combination. Each of these procedures uses your hair and requires that you have a substantial growth of hair at the back and sides of your head; these places serve as donor sites. None of the procedures can completely restore hair loss but they can hide the thin areas.

Hair replacement surgery is usually performed in a physician's office-based facility or in an outpatient surgery center. It rarely requires a hospital stay. Hair replacement surgery, no matter what technique is used, is usually performed using local anesthesia (see p.168) along with sedation to relax you. While the surgery is being performed, your scalp will be insensitive to pain but you may be aware of some tugging or pressure.

GRAFTS

There are various techniques for transplanting a patch of scalp and its hair (a graft) from the hairy part of the scalp to the bald part. Grafts of different sizes and shapes go by different names— punch grafts, minigrafts, micrografts, and slit grafts. Graft surgery usually takes several sessions over several months to allow the sites of previous surgery to heal. Usually grafts are placed about 1/8 inch apart; the spaces between

the first grafts are filled in during later sessions. The grafts must be positioned properly so that the transplanted hair will grow in the correct direction in its new location. Ask your plastic surgeon to explain to you more precisely the technique that will be used.

TISSUE EXPANSION

Tissue expansion has been used for many years to cause new healthy skin to grow into areas that have been burned or severely injured. More recently, this procedure has been used for hair loss. A balloonlike device is placed beneath the scalp at the border between a hairy and a bald area. Over several weeks, the balloon is gradually inflated with salt water, causing the scalp to bulge upward. This causes new, hair-bearing skin to grow over the bulging area. After several months, the new, hairy scalp skin is pulled over to replace the bald scalp skin next to it.

FLAP SURGERY

Flap surgery is used to achieve more substantial hair replacement. In flap surgery, a section of the bald scalp is removed. Then a flap from a similar-sized area of adjacent hair-covered scalp is lifted off the surface of the head and placed where the bald scalp was removed. One end of the flap remains attached to its original skin and blood supply. Over time, the donor site from which the flap came fills in with new skin and hair, and the transplanted flap generally continues to grow hair in its new location.

RISKS OF HAIR REPLACEMENT SURGERY

When the surgeon is qualified and experienced, hair replacement surgery is generally safe. However, as with any surgical procedure, there is a chance of complications such as infection, excessive bleeding, or wide scars (which are most common in flap surgery). Also, sometimes the surgery is unsuccessful because the transplanted tissue does not grow in its new location.

WHAT TO EXPECT AFTER SURGERY

Aching, tightness, or throbbing can occur after surgery but are easily controlled with pain medicine. After the surgery, plan for someone to drive you home, and take it easy for a day or two. After several days, most people feel well enough to go back to work. If you have bandages, they are usually removed the day after surgery. Avoid washing your hair for 2 days and, when you do, wash very gently. If you have stitches, they will be removed in 7 to 10 days. Because strenuous physical activity increases blood flow to the scalp and can cause your incisions to bleed, your surgeon may advise you to avoid vigorous exercise, contact sports, and sexual activity for 1 to 3 weeks.

Do not worry if your transplanted hair falls out during the first 6 weeks after surgery. This is normal, and hair growth should start again within 5 to 6 weeks. After this, hair should grow at about the usual rate—1/2 inch each month.

BODY SHAPING

Abdominoplasty

Abdominoplasty, popularly known as a tummy tuck, is major surgery to remove excess skin and fat from the middle and lower abdomen and to tighten abdominal muscles. A partial abdominoplasty is a less-extensive procedure in which fat is removed only from the area below the navel.

THE PROCEDURE

A complete abdominoplasty may require an overnight stay in a hospital. General anesthesia (see p.168) is required and surgery can last from 2 to 4 hours. Partial abdominoplasty is often performed as an outpatient procedure, using a local anesthetic (see p.168) to numb the surgical area and sedation to make you drowsy. It can take an hour or two to perform.

In a complete abdominoplasty, the plastic surgeon first makes a horizontal incision, from one hipbone to the other, across the lower abdomen. A second incision is made around the navel to separate it from surrounding tissue. Some plastic surgeons use liposuction (see below) at this point to suck out excess fat through the incision around the navel.

The surgeon then separates the skin from the underlying abdominal wall and lifts the large flap of skin to view the two vertical muscle bands of the abdomen. The two sides are overlapped and pulled together with stitches. The skin is then pulled down (somewhat like a window shade), extra skin and fat are cut away, and the lower incision is stitched closed. A new opening for the navel is created and the navel is brought out and stitched into place. Bandages are applied and several tubes are inserted to drain fluid.

A shorter horizontal incision is made for a partial abdomino-

Abdominoplasty

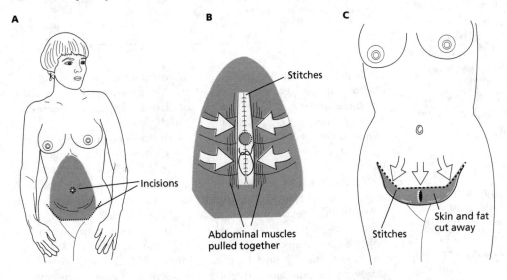

An incision is made across the lower abdomen from hipbone to hipbone (A) and a second incision is made around the navel to separate it from surrounding tissue. Skin is separated from the underlying abdominal wall and the flap of skin is lifted to reveal the two vertical muscle bands of the abdomen. The two sides are overlapped and pulled together with stitches (B). The skin is pulled down, extra skin and fat are cut away, and the incisions are stitched closed (C).

plasty, and the skin is separated only between the incision and the navel. The navel may not have to be separated from the skin as it is in a complete abdominoplasty. The skin is then pulled down, excess skin is cut away, and the flap is stitched into place and drained.

RECOVERY AND COMPLICATIONS

Pain and swelling, which can be helped with painkillers, are common during the first few days after surgery. After a complete abdominoplasty, it may be several days before you can stand upright and a few weeks before you feel ready to return to work. After a partial abdominoplasty, you may need 2 or 3 days before resuming normal activities. The drainage tubes are removed after several days. Stitches are removed after a week. You may need to wear a girdle-type support garment for several weeks to minimize swelling. The scars from abdominoplasty can be prominent for 6 months. They usually fade within a year but never disappear completely. Risks, such as infection at the wound site or a blood clot in the leg or groin, are rare.

Liposuction

Liposuction is a procedure that removes fat ("lipos" is the Greek word for fat) from the body by sucking it out through a tube attached to a vacuum. The ideal candidate is someone who is at or near ideal body weight but has focal areas of fat, such as on the buttocks or thighs, that have resisted diet and exercise and are out of proportion to the rest of

Liposuction

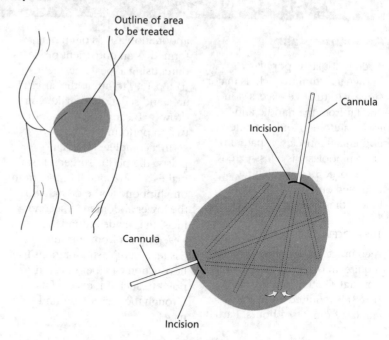

The area to be treated is outlined on the surface of the skin. A small incision is made and a cannula is inserted and manipulated back and forth, dislodging fat cells. Several tunnels are made from the first incision (red lines) and several perpendicular tunnels are made from a second incision.

the body. Liposuction is most effective in younger people (usually those under age 50) whose skin is resilient enough to maintain its shape over the smaller area that results after the fat is sucked out.

If the skin overlying the fat deposit has been stretched out of shape by fat, age, or pregnancy, liposuction alone could lead to floppy skin and an unsatisfactory result. Areas of cellulite (dimpled skin) may become more irregular and look worse after liposuction. In these cases, liposuction may need to be combined with surgery to remove the excess skin. Unlike weight loss achieved

through diet and exercise, liposuction does not reduce the risk of diabetes, hypertension, or elevated cholesterol.

The most common areas for liposuction are the abdomen, thighs, buttocks, knees, and upper arms. Liposuction can be used alone to treat fat deposits in the neck and face, especially in younger people who have very resilient skin, or it can be combined with a face-lift (see p.577) to shape the jawline in people with less-resilient skin. Little is known about the long-term results of liposuction.

The area treated by liposuction can eventually develop more fat than is present immediately after liposuction (but not as much as before treatment).

THE PROCEDURE

Liposuction (see illustration on p.590), which can take from 1 to 3 hours, is usually performed on an outpatient basis using a local anesthetic (see p.168). If the treatment area is large, or if the person or surgeon prefers, general anesthesia (see p.168) may be used. The surgeon first outlines the area to be treated on the skin surface. A small incision is made and a cannula (a narrow, hollow tube that has a blunt tip and is ringed with small holes) is inserted and manipulated back and forth. This action dislodges fat cells, which are sucked through the instrument and deposited into a collecting bottle.

The surgeon repeats the process until enough fat is removed to eliminate the bulge. When the procedure has been completed, the incisions are stitched and bandaged. Because you lose fluid along with the fat during the procedure, you may be given intravenous fluids during the treatment and could even require a blood transfusion.

The tools and techniques of liposuction continue to improve. With the newest and safest method (called the tumescent technique), a large amount of saline (salt water) mixed with a low dose of local anesthetic and epinephrine (a constrictor of blood vessels) is injected into the area to be treated prior to the suctioning. This greatly reduces the amount of blood and fluid

---

Recovering From Body-Shaping Surgery

Be vigilant in following your doctor's instructions regarding lifting, exercise, care of incisions, and resuming sexual activity.

It may take 2 to 4 days before you can get around independently after having abdominoplasty. You may need help for a longer period of time. Recovery is very similar to that of a cesarean section (see p.939). Many people can return to desk jobs after about a week, and to more strenuous jobs after 2 to 4 weeks. Recovery is dependent on the surgeon's technique and the person having the procedure.

After liposuction, depending on the number of areas you have had treated, it may take 2 days before you can get around independently. Many people can return to work after about a week, depending on how many areas were treated and what type of work they do.

---

lost during the procedure and the discoloration after the operation. It also allows more fat to be removed at one time. Even so, because of the loss of fluid and blood, liposuction may not be recommended for people who have severe diseases of the heart, lungs, kidneys, or circulation.

RECOVERY AND COMPLICATIONS

You may feel pain after the anesthesia wears off, which can be relieved with painkillers. The recovery period may last several weeks. If you had liposuction below the waist, you will wear a support garment resembling an extra-firm girdle for 2 to 3 weeks to minimize swelling and bruising and help the treated area heal smoothly. Bruising usually subsides within a week or two, but swelling may last for up to 6 months. Vigorous exercise must be avoided for several weeks after the procedure.

Serious complications are rare,

but deaths have occurred due to extreme loss of blood or fluids or from blood clots that travel to the lungs. Inexperienced surgeons and the removal of excessive amounts of fat appeared to have played a role in these deaths. Overall, liposuction appears to be safe when done by experienced, qualified physicians who carefully limit the amount of fat removed.

According to surveys of people who have had the procedure, minor complications—such as fluid accumulation (which requires draining), sagging skin, uneven skin texture (rippling), or an asymmetrical appearance—occur in up to 20% of cases. Although a symmetrical result cannot be guaranteed, significant asymmetry after surgery often can be improved by a combination of fat resuctioning and reinjection. Even if the outcome is less than perfect, most people are satisfied with the results.

Bones, Joints, and Muscles

BONES

There are 206 bones in your body. Bones perform four critically important functions. First, they provide a strong barrier that protects your inner organs. The brain, for example, is as soft as gelatin. It is shielded by the skull's 26 bones, which, along with the brain, weigh about 15 pounds. The bones of the spine permit some flexibility, but basically they keep you straight and upright, keep your heavy head from dropping down into your chest, and keep your internal organs in proper position.

Second, bones give you strength. The bones of your legs and spine support your weight against the constant pull of gravity.

Third, bone marrow, which lies inside some of your bones, manufactures many types of blood cells (see p.709).

Finally, bones—in conjunction with the joints that connect them and the pulleylike system of muscles attached to them—allow us to move (see How You Move, p.104). The bones in your neck and arms allow you to use your hands—something humans do better than all other animals.

To some degree, the health, integrity, and growth of your bones is inherited. For example, osteoporosis (see p.596), a condition in which bones become thin and brittle, runs in families. Nevertheless, you can do a great deal to keep your bones strong.

JOINTS

Bones meet each other at joints. Flexible joints like knees and elbows have a lining of cartilage on top of the bones. Cartilage is strong but is a softer substance than bone and permits the joint surfaces to move more easily when they rub against each other, with less wear and tear.

Flexible joints also have synovial membrane, an outer sleeve of tissue, which produces the slippery synovial fluid. This fluid fills the joint space, acting as a lubricant to reduce friction. In some kinds of arthritis, such as rheumatoid arthritis (see p.606), the synovial membrane grows and begins to invade the cartilage, damaging and sometimes deforming the joint. Some joints are built to make flexible but strong connections between two bones. For example, your elbow joint allows you to reach out to catch a baseball or lift a forkful of food to your mouth. Different types of joints are described further on p.602.

Bone Strength

The skeleton may look rickety and frail, but bones resist compression with a strength equal to that of cast iron or oak. Although incredibly light—the average adult skeleton weighs only about 20 pounds—bones are capable of bearing tremendous weight. Their strength is necessary to withstand the forces of movement. For example, when you walk at a leisurely pace, each foot strikes the ground with a force about three times your weight. At a brisk walk or run, the pressure generated increases to five or six times your weight. If you weigh 150 pounds, your lower extremities are subjected to 450 to 900 pounds of force during normal activity.

Bones, Joints, and Muscles

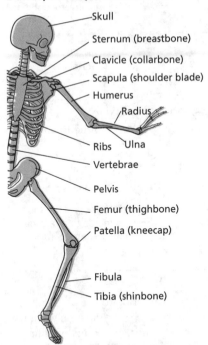

- Skull
- Sternum (breastbone)
- Clavicle (collarbone)
- Scapula (shoulder blade)
- Humerus
- Radius
- Ribs
- Ulna
- Vertebrae
- Pelvis
- Femur (thighbone)
- Patella (kneecap)
- Fibula
- Tibia (shinbone)

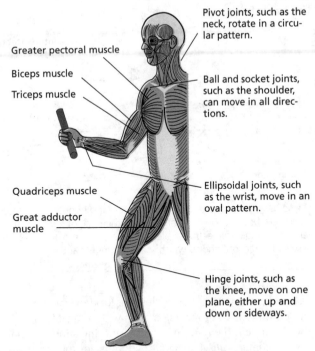

- Greater pectoral muscle
- Biceps muscle
- Triceps muscle
- Quadriceps muscle
- Great adductor muscle

Pivot joints, such as the neck, rotate in a circular pattern.

Ball and socket joints, such as the shoulder, can move in all directions.

Ellipsoidal joints, such as the wrist, move in an oval pattern.

Hinge joints, such as the knee, move on one plane, either up and down or sideways.

The 206 bones in your body protect and support the internal organs. They are living tissue endowed with weight-bearing strength. Like other tissues, they contain blood vessels; many bones also contain bone marrow in their center that forms red blood cells, white blood cells, and platelets.

Of the more than 600 muscles in your body, most are attached to bones by tendons. Voluntary muscles contract on command from the brain; involuntary muscles, such as those in the heart, work automatically. The joints make connections between bones and are stabilized by ligaments.

MUSCLES

Bones attached to each other by flexible joints would flop around if not for the controlled action of muscles. There are more than 600 muscles in your body. Most muscles are attached to bones by tendons, while ligaments connect bones to each other, providing stability. Tendons and ligaments are made of connective tissue. The main structural proteins of connective tissue are collagen (which gives it toughness) and elastin (which gives it elasticity).

Muscles almost always work in groups. It takes the coordinated action of 40 muscles to take one step forward. The muscles that control your eyes are in nearly constant movement, moving about 50 miles a day. Your brain directs the action of muscles by sending a signal down the spinal cord to the nerves, which transmit the signal to the muscles. Inside muscles are special nerve endings that also send signals back to the spinal cord and brain, communicating the extent of muscle stretch and tension. These specialized nerves play a part in your ability to walk in the dark without losing your balance or to climb stairs without calculating each step.

Bone Doctors

Although your primary care physician can take care of most problems that affect your bones, joints, and muscles, sometimes specialists are required. Rheumatologists usually treat such chronic diseases as rheumatoid arthritis (see p.606). Orthopedic surgeons usually evaluate injuries of the bones, muscles, and joints. Both rheumatologists and orthopedic surgeons may take fluid out of joints with a needle (for testing) and may inject medicine into the joints.

Structure of the Vertebrae

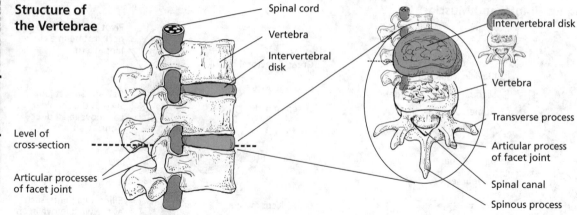

Spinal cord

Vertebra

Intervertebral disk

Level of cross-section

Articular processes of facet joint

Intervertebral disk

Vertebra

Transverse process

Articular process of facet joint

Spinal canal

Spinous process

The spine is composed of cylindrical interlocking bones called vertebrae. A bony ring attached to the back of each vertebra contains projections called processes that project in several directions and to which spinal ligaments and muscles are attached. Between each vertebra is the shock-absorbing intervertebral disk. The vertebrae form a canal through which the spinal cord and its nerve roots run.

Besides the voluntary muscles that permit you to move when your brain tells them to, the body has involuntary muscles that work without any conscious direction. For example, the heart is an involuntary muscle that works automatically, pumping blood every moment of your life without instruction. Your stomach and intestines are lined with muscles that work automatically to help digest food. A muscular action called peristalsis pushes waste out of your body in a wavelike rhythm.

In addition to the physical stresses of everyday life, the muscles, bones, and joints of your body are vulnerable to injury, disease, and, in rare cases, infection. The most common disorders are discussed in this section.

BONES

Fractures

A fracture is a broken bone. Doctors classify fractures into several categories (see Types of Fractures, p.595). In an open fracture, the broken bone protrudes through the skin; in a closed fracture, bone does not break through skin.

(See also Fractured Collarbone or Upper Arm, p.614; Colles Fracture, p.618; Hand Fracture, p.618; Hip Fracture, p.629; Ankle Fracture, p.635; and Broken Bones in the Foot, p.637.)

SYMPTOMS

A broken bone usually causes severe pain that is worsened by moving the broken part or applying any pressure to it. Swelling and bruising may develop over the broken bone and, in serious fractures, the area may look misshapen and function poorly or not at all.

TREATMENT OPTIONS

If you think you have a broken bone, see your physician or go to the emergency department of a hospital immediately to have the bone set. Do not eat or drink anything; you may have to have general anesthesia (see p.168) and it is most safely administered if it has been at least 8 hours since you last ate or drank.

The doctor will examine your injury and, if he or she thinks there could be a fracture, will make images of it by x-ray (see p.145), computed tomography (see p.149), or bone scan (see p.622).

Bone begins to heal immediately after it breaks; for this reason it is essential for a broken bone to be realigned immediately so that the bones do not heal in

Types of Fractures

There are several ways in which a bone can break. Fractures are broadly classified as either open (or compound), in which the broken bone protrudes through the skin, or closed (or simple), in which the broken parts do not break through skin. Other categories describe the way in which the bone breaks, as follows:

- **Greenstick fracture** The bone cracks but does not separate into two distinct parts. This type of fracture often occurs in children, whose bones are more resilient and less likely to break completely.

- **Transverse fracture** The bone breaks cleanly across its width.

- **Oblique fracture** The bone breaks at a slanting angle.

- **Comminuted fracture** The bone shatters into several pieces.

- **Impacted (compression) fracture** One fragment of bone is embedded into another fragment of bone.

- **Pathologic fracture** The bone breaks because it has been weakened by disease, such as cancer or osteoporosis.

- **Stress fracture** A hairline crack occurs in a bone that may be healthy but has been exposed to extensive or repeated stress, such as from jogging.

a distorted fashion. Sometimes this can be done without surgery. After giving you pain medicine, the doctor moves your bones back into alignment and immobilizes the bones (see below).

For other fractures, surgery is necessary; this usually requires a general anesthetic. The surgeon cuts through the skin and puts in metal plates, rods, and screws to hold the bones together.

The next step is to immobilize the fractured bone—that is, hold it in place so it can heal in the correct alignment. Immobilization may involve applying a cast or splint made of plaster, plastic, or resin to hold the bone pieces together. Sometimes traction is used to maintain proper position.

Casts or splints are generally needed when no surgery has been performed and sometimes when surgery has been performed. Sometimes, bones are held together naturally and need no artificial device. For example, a broken rib bone is held to neighboring ribs by the surrounding chest muscles. A broken toe is often taped to a neighboring toe to serve as a splint.

Once the fractured bone has been stabilized, rehabilitation begins. Carefully exercising the injured area helps keep joints mobile and prevents the muscles from losing tone. Your doctor may refer you to a physical therapist who will show you how to perform the exercises.

Many different factors determine the time required for complete healing, including the location and type of fracture and the

age of the injured person. Your doctor may recommend pain-killing medicines, and antibiotic tablets may be prescribed for some open fractures to prevent infection.

Osteomyelitis

Osteomyelitis is a rare condition in which bacteria or fungi infect bone and bone marrow, which . can destroy bone and adjacent tissues. This infection most often arises as a complication of an open wound or open fracture (see p.594), but in some cases it is transmitted to bone via a blood infection.

Osteomyelitis is more common in children, in whom it usually affects the vertebrae and the long bones of the legs and arms. In adults it more often affects the vertebrae and pelvis. Osteomyelitis is rare in the United States because of the general good health of Americans and because of antibiotic treatment for infection.

SYMPTOMS

Symptoms of osteomyelitis include fever, severe pain, tenderness, and swelling of the affected area. A child may not be able to walk if a leg is affected and may feel great pain if the affected part is touched.

TREATMENT OPTIONS

If osteomyelitis is not treated, it can destroy bone and can spread into nearby joints, causing permanent deformity of the joint. See your doctor immediately if you suspect osteomyelitis. He or she may take blood tests and x-rays; a bone biopsy (in which a tiny piece of infected bone is removed for evaluation under a microscope) may also be required.

Treatment includes antibiotics, usually given intravenously but sometimes in tablet form, taken for 3 weeks or more, and immobilization of the affected bone. Surgery is sometimes required when infection has spread to nearby tissues. The extent of surgery depends on the severity of infection.

Osteomalacia

Osteomalacia, more commonly known as rickets, is a rare disease that causes weakening and softening of the bones. It usually results from a lack of vitamin D, which prevents the gastrointestinal tract from absorbing calcium and phosphorus from the diet, interfering with the body's ability to make and strengthen bone (see How Bone Grows, p.600).

Various diseases may contribute to vitamin D deficiency, including chronic kidney failure (see p.812), celiac disease (see p.774), some types of digestive tract surgery, and long-term treatment with antiepileptic drugs. Most people get enough vitamin D from foods such as milk and from exposure of the skin to sunlight.

SYMPTOMS

Symptoms of osteomalacia include pain and tenderness in the bones of the arms, legs, pelvis, and spine. In addition, you may experience fatigue, stiffness, progressive weakness, cramps, and difficulty standing. In severe cases, bones may break.

TREATMENT OPTIONS

Your physician will measure the levels of calcium and phosphorus in your blood and urine, as well as the vitamin D level in your blood. You may also require x-rays and, if the diagnosis is not clear, a bone biopsy, in which a small sample of bone is extracted for laboratory evaluation. In most cases, vitamin D and calcium supplements cure osteomalacia.

Osteoporosis

Literally translated, osteoporosis is "a condition of porous bones." The loss of bone density and mineral content occurs when new bone is not created as quickly as old bone is broken down (see How Bone Grows, p.600).

Osteoporosis is most often caused by an acceleration of the normal changes that occur with age, leading to a loss of bone tissue (and, therefore, density), brittleness, and a higher risk of fracture. Fractures are most likely to occur in the hip, wrist, and vertebrae.

Osteoporosis affects women more often than men (although men are also susceptible), especially during and after menopause, when a woman's production of estrogen, which helps maintain bone mass, decreases.

RISK FACTORS

Although some bone loss is a natural result of aging, the rate at which bone loss progresses varies widely. If you have several of the risk factors listed here, read Preventing Osteoporosis (see p.597) and ask your physician if he or she recommends that you take other steps based on your risk:

Age The risk of osteoporosis increases with age—starting at about age 30, when bone is lost more quickly than the body forms it.

Body type Women who are thin and have smaller frames have less bone to begin with; they are more likely to lose bone density with age.

Heredity Women whose mothers had osteoporosis are at greater risk for osteoporosis. Several genes have been identified that affect a person's risk of osteoporosis.

Race Asians and whites are at higher risk than blacks.

Estrogen loss The female hormone estrogen, which retards bone loss, is produced primarily by the ovaries. Women who are going through or have gone through menopause or those who have had their ovaries surgically removed (see Oophorectomy, p.1081) are at increased risk of osteoporosis because their production of estrogen has decreased.

Low calcium and vitamin D levels Getting an inadequate amount of calcium (see p.44) and vitamin D (which helps your body absorb calcium) can lower blood levels of calcium, forcing your body to draw on reserves in the bone, which leads to bone loss.

Inactivity When bones are at rest, bone formation slows. See Preventing Osteoporosis (p.597) for bone-building exercises.

Smoking Smokers seem to lose bone faster than nonsmokers, possibly because smoking interferes with the body's production of estrogen.

Preventing Osteoporosis

Osteoporosis can be prevented in most people. Women are at particularly high risk of osteoporosis and should take these steps to prevent the disease:

IF YOU HAVE NOT GONE THROUGH MENOPAUSE

The soundest strategy is to concentrate on attaining and maintaining a high bone mass. Some of the same factors that help reduce the risk of osteoporosis also help prevent cancer, heart disease, and type 2 diabetes mellitus. Take the following steps:

■ Get enough calcium and vitamin D.

■ Do weight-bearing exercise. Now is the time to develop exercise habits that will serve you throughout life. Make a point to get at least 30 minutes of weight-bearing exercise five times a week, such as brisk walking, running, or dancing. Lifting weights (see p.54) is another good way to increase bone mass.

■ Avoid cigarettes and too much alcohol. Both decrease bone mass.

■ Find out if either of your parents had osteoporosis. If so, let your doctor know.

■ If you take corticosteroid, antiepilepsy, or thyroid drugs, ask your doctor if you need a bone-density test or treatment to prevent osteoporosis.

IF YOU ARE GOING THROUGH MENOPAUSE

If you are in the early years of menopause, you are beginning the stage of greatest bone loss. All of the suggestions for younger women apply, and you should do the following as well:

■ Assess your risk. If you are at greater-than-average risk for osteoporosis (see p.596 for risk factors), talk to your doctor about treatment options and about having a bone-density test.

■ Consider hormone replacement therapy (HRT) (see p.1049). Although it is not an appropriate treatment for every woman, it prevents bone loss and reduces your risk of fractures.

■ Monitor your intake of calcium (see p.44). Make sure you are getting at least 1,000 milligrams a day (1,500 milligrams if you choose not to have HRT). Your doctor may also recommend that you take vitamin D.

■ Re-evaluate your exercise regimen. Exercise not only builds bone, it increases strength, flexibility, and balance. As you age, it becomes more difficult to maintain muscle mass, and it may be necessary to exercise more frequently. This is a good time to add weights (see p.54) to your routine.

IF YOU ARE 65 OR OVER

At this point, bone loss has tapered off. Estrogen deficiency is not the primary thief of bone mass; that role is usurped by your decreased ability to absorb minerals. All of the previous suggestions for bone maintenance apply, and you should also be vigilant about pursuing the following:

■ Increase your calcium intake. Get 1,500 milligrams every day. Make sure that you accompany it with 400 to 800 international units of vitamin D to enhance absorption.

■ Keep up your exercise routine. This is necessary both for bone preservation and for muscle maintenance. Muscle mass not only exerts extra force on bones (which helps keep them strong), it helps protect your bones if you fall. Consider exercises that improve balance and coordination (to minimize the risk of falling), such as tai chi, an ancient Chinese martial art, or yoga. Lifting weights (see p.1113) is also strongly recommended.

■ Consider preventive medicine. Although taking HRT when you are 65 or older does not increase bone density as much as it does in the first years after menopause, studies have demonstrated that estrogen builds bone mass, even when it is started in your 70s. Medicines such as alendronate and calcitonin are another approach to preventing osteoporosis. Ask your doctor about them. Having a bone density test may help you decide.

Bone Building and Bone Loss

BONE BREAKDOWN

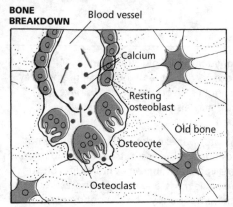

Blood vessel
Calcium
Resting osteoblast
Old bone
Osteocyte
Osteoclast

Bone is in a continual state of flux, alternating between bone breakdown (top left) and bone building (bottom left). The bone-building process relies on calcium, used by the bone-building cells called osteoblasts. Osteoblasts become incorporated into the bone matrix and turn into new bone cells called osteocytes. When blood levels of calcium drop below normal, bone-destroying cells called osteoclasts dismantle bone and release calcium into the bloodstream. If the bone breakdown outpaces bone building, it leaves the skeleton porous and weak, a condition called osteoporosis.

BONE BUILDING

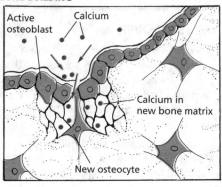

Active osteoblast
Calcium
Calcium in new bone matrix
New osteocyte

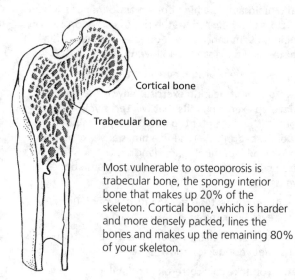

Cortical bone
Trabecular bone

Most vulnerable to osteoporosis is trabecular bone, the spongy interior bone that makes up 20% of the skeleton. Cortical bone, which is harder and more densely packed, lines the bones and makes up the remaining 80% of your skeleton.

Alcohol While a daily cocktail has little effect, more than two drinks a day can hasten bone loss. Heavy drinkers are at greater risk because they often eat poorly, aggravating bone loss. Since heavy drinkers also are accident-prone, they have a greater frequency of fractures.

Certain medicines Long-term use of some medicines, including corticosteroids (see p.895) and antiseizure drugs, can lead to bone loss. Too much thyroid hormone also can cause bone loss;

women taking thyroid pills should have regular blood tests to check the level of thyroid hormones in their bloodstream.

Gastrointestinal surgery Some kinds of surgery on your digestive system can decrease your body's absorption of calcium and other minerals needed for bone growth.

Some medical conditions Conditions that can cause loss of bone mass include anorexia nervosa (see p.413), some cancers, liver disease (see p.758), disor-

ders that affect absorption of minerals such as celiac disease (see p.774), hyperparathyroidism (see p.852), and several rare congenital diseases.

SYMPTOMS

Osteoporosis causes no symptoms (unless a fracture occurs), and progresses slowly but steadily. The first indication of osteoporosis can be a broken bone. In some people, compression fractures occur in spinal vertebrae that have been weakened by osteoporosis simply by lifting a bag of groceries. Small compression fractures of the spine can cause a person to bend forward and become shorter.

TREATMENT OPTIONS

If you have osteoporosis or are at high risk for it, your physician may want to measure the density of your bones to determine the degree of bone loss. The most widely used techniques for measuring bone density are dual-energy x-ray absorptiometry and dual-photon absorptiometry. With each technique, you lie on a table while an imaging device passes over different bones (the spine, hip, and forearm are most commonly measured).

The results express bone density in terms of your bone's deviation from normal, healthy bone for a person of your age. Computed tomography (see p.149) scanning and another x-ray technique called single-photon

Visible Effects of Osteoporosis

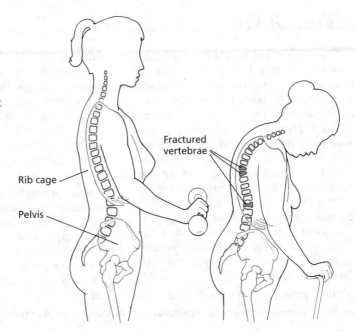

Rib cage

Pelvis

Fractured vertebrae

Osteoporosis sets the stage for fractures of the vertebrae, called compression fractures, that eventually can cause a distortion of the normal spinal curve, a stooped appearance, and loss of height. As support declines and the rib cage sinks toward the pelvis, internal organs can become cramped, creating breathing difficulties and gastrointestinal discomfort.

Compression Fracture of the Vertebrae

Vertebral fractures are more common than hip fractures in women who have osteoporosis. They often occur with little precipitating injury. The simple acts of daily life, such as bending over or lifting a package, are often sufficient to break one or more vertebrae weakened by osteoporosis. The bones of the spine are compressed (see Types of Fractures, p.595) rather than split into pieces.

A compression fracture may be accompanied by pain that is sharp, dull, intense, or radiating around your side. Occasionally, there is no discomfort. The pain may also be felt as spasms in the muscles at the sides of your spine and may come and go for several months, tending to recur after sitting in the same position for a long time.

Most women who have vertebral fractures have one or two, usually in the middle of the back or just above, in the thoracic region. The resulting lack of strength at this location can cause a stooped appearance.

Surgery to repair the fracture is usually not possible because the bones themselves are not strong enough to withstand the insertion of screws or pegs to hold the spine in the proper position. A compression fracture can take several months to heal. Your doctor may recommend that you rest your back by lying flat for several hours every day, and that you avoid lifting. Exercise, calcium supplements, painkilling drugs, and a special corset to support your back can help you maintain your ability to function without pain.

How Bone Grows

Bone is a living tissue that is constantly changing, a process called remodeling. Bone is made up of three layers. At bone's core is the soft bone marrow, where blood cells are made. Encasing the marrow is the honeycomblike tissue called trabecular bone. The cortex, or outer shell, and bone shaft are made up of densely packed hard bone. Both trabecular bone and hard bone are formed from the same fabric—a meshwork of collagen fibers inlaid with calcium and phosphorus that forms a hard substance that gives bone its strength. Ounce for ounce, bone bears as much weight as reinforced concrete. Bone also acts as a storage site for calcium and phosphorus. When the levels of calcium and phosphorus in your bloodstream drop, the bones release a new supply to maintain their balance in the blood.

Your skeleton is a beehive of microscopic activity in which existing bone is continuously broken down and replaced with new bone. The bone demolition process, called resorption, is carried out by cells called osteoclasts that chew into bone, releasing its calcium and other minerals into the blood. Another group of cells called osteoblasts lays down collagen and other proteins into bone spaces to form the bony matrix, a strong fibrous mesh. The osteoblasts eventually become embedded into the matrix they have created.

Calcium, phosphorus, and other minerals from the blood are deposited into the matrix to complete the process of bone formation. In childhood, bone formation outpaces bone breakdown, enabling bones to become longer, denser, and heavier. By your mid-20s, the two processes occur at about the same rate. Starting in your mid-30s, bone loss occurs faster than new bone is made.

absorptiometry may also be used to evaluate bone mass.

Several effective treatments reduce the rate of bone loss and may even help build new bone. Estrogen in the form of hormone replacement therapy (see p.1049) is the oldest and most widely prescribed treatment for osteoporosis in women. Estrogen is thought to be most effective in retarding bone loss when women start taking it during perimenopause or shortly after menopause begins and use it for several years thereafter. A class of medicines called selective estrogen-receptor modulators are slightly less effective than estrogen, but have fewer side effects. Calcium and vitamin D can also reduce the rate of

Benefits of Bone-Density Drugs

When taken by women who have entered menopause, estrogen and progesterone (used in hormone replacement therapy) and alendronate (a bone-building drug) can significantly increase bone density of the hip, compared with a placebo. Large studies have not shown significant side effects over a 2-year period.

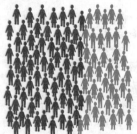

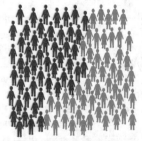

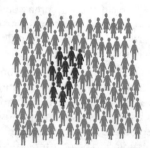

62 OF 100 WOMEN WHO TAKE ESTROGEN-PROGESTERONE HAVE INCREASED BONE DENSITY

50 OF 100 WOMEN WHO TAKE ALENDRONATE HAVE INCREASED BONE DENSITY

10 OF 100 WOMEN WHO TAKE PLACEBO HAVE INCREASED BONE DENSITY

bone loss but are less potent than estrogen.

Another group of medicines called bisphosphonates, including etidronate, alendronate, and pamidronate, are prescribed for women with established osteoporosis. These drugs can increase bone density. Calcitonin (which can be taken as an injection or inhaled in a spray) also reduces the rate of bone loss. Estrogen, raloxifene (a selective estrogen receptor modulator), alendronate, and calcitonin have all been found to reduce fractures.

Paget Disease

Paget disease is a thickening and paradoxical weakening of bone, usually of the pelvis, collarbone, vertebrae, skull, shinbone, thighbone, or humerus (the bone that runs from the shoulder to the elbow). It occurs when the normal balance of bone formation and bone loss, which occurs constantly, is disrupted.

The cause of Paget disease is not known, although it seems to run in families. Mild forms are common among the elderly. Paget disease affects 3% of people over age 40 and the risk increases with age. However, only about 10% of people who have Paget disease experience symptoms, which may include a dull aching pain caused by small fractures or because nerves are compressed by thickened patches of bone. In some people, a visible deformity such as an enlarged skull or curvature of the thighbone or shinbone develops. In rare cases, when the disease affects the skull, thickened areas of the skull can impinge on nerves and cause deafness, numbness of the face, or blindness.

Bone Changes in Paget Disease

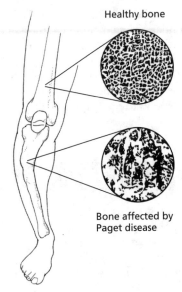

Healthy bone

Bone affected by Paget disease

Healthy bone consists of a meshwork of thin beams called trabeculae that look like a sponge. Bone (the white area in insets) is constantly remodeled by large cells called osteoclasts, which break down bone, and osteoblasts, which form new bone. In Paget disease, it is thought that osteoclasts destroy areas of bone at a faster rate than normal. To make up for this loss, osteoblasts form irregularly patterned new bone that is weaker and contains more blood vessels than normal bone.

If you have pain, nonsteroidal anti-inflammatory drugs (see p.1162) such as aspirin or ibuprofen are usually effective. For more advanced cases that affect the skull or spine, your doctor may prescribe one of several drugs, including calcitonin, bisphosphonates, or plicamycin, which work by inhibiting the activity of osteoclasts, the cells that break down bone.

Bone Tumors

Most bone tumors are malignant (cancerous) and have spread to the bone from cancers elsewhere in the body, such as from the prostate, lung, or breast. Tumors that originate in the bone are rare, and most are benign (noncancerous).

Benign bone tumors include osteochondromas, which most often develop in children and adolescents. They are made up of bone and cartilage, and are usually found near joints such as the knee or shoulder. Osteomas, another benign bone tumor, are hard lumps of bone that usually occur on the skull.

The rare cancerous tumors that originate in bone are called primary malignant bone tumors; the most common are osteosarcomas. A blood cancer called multiple myeloma (see p.731) that begins in bone marrow also affects bone.

SYMPTOMS

Most benign bone tumors are experienced as a hard, usually painless lump on the surface of a bone. The unusual malignant tumors that start in the bone are typically painful. Malignant tumors that spread to the bone often cause pain, although they may sometimes be discovered when a person has a pathologic fracture (see Types of Fractures, p.595).

TREATMENT OPTIONS

See your physician if you have pain that seems to be in a bone, or if you feel any bump on a bone. The doctor will perform a complete examination, including blood tests, x-rays, and possibly other imaging tests such as bone scans (see p.622), magnetic resonance imaging (see p.151), or a computed tomography (see p.149) scan.

Benign tumors often do not require treatment but may be removed if they are causing pain or could cause the bone to break. If cancer is suspected, your doctor may take a biopsy, which involves pushing a sturdy needle into the bone (after the area is made numb) to extract a sample for laboratory evaluation.

Treatment of primary or secondary malignant bone tumors includes radiation therapy (see p.741), chemotherapy (see p.741), or sometimes surgical removal of the tumor. If the tumor does not respond to nonsurgical treatments, the diseased part of the bone may be removed and the site restored by a bone graft (placing a piece of healthy bone taken from another part of the body into the diseased area of bone). Amputating the affected limb to keep the cancer from spreading elsewhere may be necessary when a malignant tumor that has started in the bone is not responding to treatment.

JOINTS

Ankylosing Spondylitis

Ankylosing spondylitis is a disease that causes inflammation of and damage to the sites where ligaments and tendons insert into bone; it most commonly affects the joints of the vertebrae, but also occurs in the pelvis. Inflammation results in new bone growth that extends into the ligaments and tendons. The result is fusion of the joints, which restricts the ability to move. The cause of ankylosing spondylitis is not known. It is much more common in men, typically begins between ages 20 and 40, and seems to run in families.

SYMPTOMS

An early sign of ankylosing spondylitis is a dull ache deep in the buttocks or lower back, sometimes on one side only. Aching pain may come and go but gradually, over a few months, pain becomes constant on both sides.

Some affected people have little or no pain but do have back stiffness, muscle aches, or tenderness over inflamed areas along the breastbone, spine, shoulder blades, pelvis, hips, knees, and heels; the stiffness improves with movement and exercise. For unknown reasons, eye inflammation (see Uveitis, p.444) occurs in about one quarter of people who have this disease. You may also have trouble breathing if it affects your ribs and reduces the mobility of your chest. The diagnosis

How Joints Work

Joints are the connections between two bones. By allowing one bone to move relative to the bone next to it, joints permit a wide range of motion (see How You Move, p.104). The skeletal system has three types of joints:

- **Fixed joints** allow very little movement; thin bands of fibrous tissue connect one bone to the next. A good example is the platelike bones of an infant's skull that allow the skull to expand and accommodate the growing brain. When brain growth is complete, the skull bones fuse and the fibrous joints disappear.

- **Cartilaginous joints** contain tough cartilage plates and allow limited movement. An example is the sacroiliac joint, where the sacrum (the lowest bone of the spinal column) and pelvis meet. The disks between the vertebral bones in the spine are also cartilaginous joints; they are thicker than the sacroiliac joint and allow greater mobility.

- **Synovial joints** are the most mobile joints and include the shoulders, elbows, wrists, fingers, hips, knees, ankles, and toes. They are surrounded by a loose fibrous capsule that is lined with the thin synovial membrane. Synovial membrane produces a thick, lubricating, translucent fluid called synovial fluid (from the Greek word "synovia," meaning "like egg white") that permits frictionless movement. Synovial fluid also helps protect joints by forming a seal that enables adjacent bones to slide freely against each other and keeps them from pulling apart.

Types of Joints

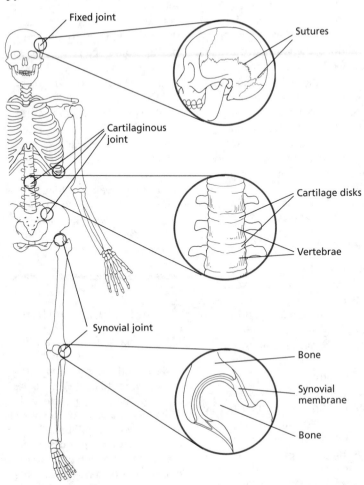

There are three basic types of joints. Fixed joints called sutures connect platelike bones of the skull. Cartilaginous joints, such as the disks between the vertebrae, contain tough cartilagelike plates that bend. The most mobile are synovial joints. They are surrounded by a loose fibrous capsule lined with a thin membrane called the synovial membrane.

of ankylosing spondylitis may be delayed because its symptoms can mimic those of more common back problems.

TREATMENT OPTIONS

Your doctor will examine you and may perform x-rays and blood tests to make a firm diagnosis. He or she may recommend nonsteroidal anti-inflammatory drugs for pain. Severe inflammation and pain may require corticosteroid injections (see p.895), medicines that alter the immune system such as methotrexate, or surgery to replace damaged joints. Rehabilitative approaches include adequate sleep, proper walking positions and posture, and daily stretching exercises after a hot shower to keep your spine limber and strengthen your back muscles. Aerobic exercise and deep breathing are also important to help you maintain normal chest expansion and prevent serious respiratory infections.

Infectious Arthritis

Infectious arthritis is infection of the joints, usually caused by bacteria, that produces significant inflammation. Occasionally, joints are infected by a fungus. Joints may also be infected by viruses, but the symptoms are usually not severe or long lasting. In adults, most bacterial joint infections have spread to the joint from the bloodstream.

Sometimes the joint is the only part of the body that is infected, although some joint infections occur as part of an infection that involves many parts of the body, such as Lyme disease (see p.884).

See your doctor if you experience pain and stiffness in one joint (usually a shoulder, knee, hip, ankle, wrist, or finger) accompanied by a warm sensation, swelling and redness around the joint, as well as chills, fever, fatigue, and/or nausea.

Your doctor may remove some fluid from an inflamed joint for analysis in the laboratory and may also perform tests to look for an infection in the blood. Antibiotics usually clear up bacterial infections. Antiviral drugs are rarely used since most viruses cannot yet be killed by drugs, and since viral infections of joints usually go away on their own.

In most cases, with early diagnosis, infectious arthritis is easily and successfully treated. Your physician may recommend physical therapy to ensure you regain movement and strength in the joint. Untreated infectious arthritis can permanently damage the bone, joint, and surrounding cartilage. In severe cases of joint damage, you may need surgery to rebuild the joint.

Gout and Pseudogout

Gout is a metabolic disorder in which uric acid, one of the body's waste products, accumulates and forms crystals in a joint, causing periods of severe pain and inflammation.

Normally, uric acid is processed by the kidneys and leaves the body in your urine. However, if your body produces more uric acid than the kidneys can process, or if your kidneys are not working well, the balance is upset. Uric acid then builds up in your joints, where it irritates and inflames the synovial membrane and other tissue, causing pain, redness, warmth, and swelling. Gout may run in families and affects men far more often than women, although this gap is less dramatic between elderly men and women.

Pseudogout is a disorder that occurs when a form of calcium crystals, rather than uric acid, is deposited in the joints. It also starts later in life, usually after age 70.

SYMPTOMS

Gout causes sudden severe pain, usually in the base of the big toe, but it can affect any other joint, particularly joints that have been

damaged by another condition, such as osteoarthritis (see p.605). Pseudogout most often affects the knees and wrists. In both conditions, the joint becomes red and swollen and you may have a fever. The pain, which can be unbearable with the slightest pressure, reaches a peak after a day or two. Your first attack may be your only one, but, without preventive treatment, most people suffer recurrences within a few years.

TREATMENT OPTIONS

See your doctor if you experience symptoms of gout or pseudogout, even if your symptoms subside. Aspirin can inhibit your body's ability to excrete uric acid, so do not take it if you think you are having an attack of gout.

Your physician will examine you and may place a needle into the affected joint to obtain a sample of the joint fluid for examination under a microscope; microscopic examination can distinguish gout from pseudogout. In gout, the fluid contains uric acid crystals; pseudogout shows calcium crystals. X-rays may also be taken.

Treatment aims to reduce pain, inflammation, and the risk of damage to the joint. Nonsteroidal anti-inflammatory drugs can relieve severe pain. An alternative approach is colchicine, which should be taken as soon as you have symptoms. Colchicine can greatly lessen the severity of an attack but often causes diarrhea. Finally, your doctor may inject a corticosteroid medicine (see p.895) into the affected joint or into a muscle, or prescribe oral corticosteroids.

Drink plenty of water to dilute the concentration of uric acid in your urine and thereby reduce the risk of kidney stones (see p.818). Your doctor may also suggest that you reduce your consumption of alcohol, which can reduce your body's ability to excrete uric acid, and of proteinrich foods such as liver, kidney, herring, anchovies, and sardines, which can elevate uric acid levels.

If you have multiple attacks of gout or develop kidney stones, your physician may prescribe drugs such as allopurinol to

Living with Gout

Late in the evening, I felt a stiffness in my ankle. I assumed that I had strained a muscle in my lower leg and went to bed. While I was sleeping, the swelling increased dramatically and when I awoke it was the size of a golf ball, and red in color. I phoned my doctor immediately. I have a high pain threshold, but this pain was so extreme it was intolerable. The doctor took some fluid from the swollen joint, gazed at it under the microscope, lifted both arms in the air, and exclaimed, "We have a diagnosis! I see the crystals. You have gout." He prescribed an anti-inflammatory medicine and colchicine. In a week, the pain was gone. Then he had me stop the anti-inflammatory medicine and start taking a medicine called allopurinol. In 6 months, I will discontinue taking the colchicine if I do not have any more episodes. So far, I have had no pain at all.

Don A., 69 years old

lower the levels of uric acid in your blood, along with colchicine in low doses to prevent attacks.

Osteoarthritis

Osteoarthritis, also called degenerative joint disease, is painful and gradual deterioration of the joint cartilage, without much inflammation. It is the most common form of arthritis, affecting more than 16 million Americans.

Symptoms typically emerge before age 45 in men and after age 55 in women. Osteoarthritis affects men and women in equal numbers but men are more likely to have it in their hips, knees, and spine and women in their hands and knees. Women are far more likely to develop hard bony growths called Heberden nodes on the joint nearest the fingertip.

Just as a damaged gasket leads to metal-on-metal contact in a machine, the bones are subject to mechanical friction and irritation. In osteoarthritis, the cartilage that protects the joint surfaces from rubbing together changes and starts to wear away. Without this cushioning, bone surfaces rub directly against each other. The body responds by trying to repair the damage but, instead of generating normal bone, bony protru-

sions called osteophytes or bone spurs form. These can irritate surrounding soft tissues and cause inflammation. People whose joints are severely damaged sometimes have periods of joint swelling.

Osteoarthritis was long considered to be a natural part of aging caused by normal wear and tear on cartilage. Experts now believe that aging is an important factor, but that it does not cause osteoarthritis. Other factors apparently contribute to osteoarthritis, including heredity (it may run in families), obesity, damage to the joints due to injury or other disease, or simply the way people use their joints.

SYMPTOMS

The symptoms of osteoarthritis usually develop slowly over many years. You may first notice pain and stiffness only after engaging in strenuous activity or after overusing the joint. In the

How Osteoarthritis Damages Joints

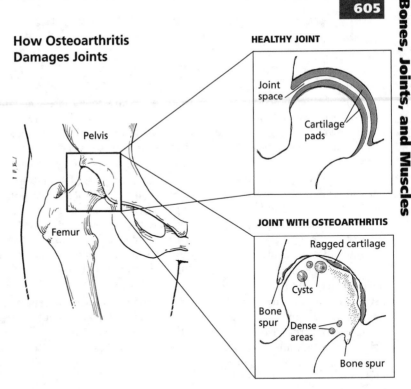

HEALTHY JOINT

Joint space

Cartilage pads

Pelvis

Femur

JOINT WITH OSTEOARTHRITIS

Ragged cartilage

Cysts

Bone spur

Dense areas

Bone spur

In a healthy joint like this hip joint, cartilage (shown in color) covers the ends of bones, reducing friction and absorbing shock. Osteoarthritis damages cartilage and allows bones to rub together. As the disease advances, bone spurs, abnormally decreased density, and cysts may develop.

Alternative Medicine: Chili Peppers for Osteoarthritis

Analgesic creams containing capsaicin, a natural substance found in hot peppers, have helped some people reduce the pain and tenderness of osteoarthritis of the hands. Capsaicin cream is sold at drugstores and many health food stores. Use it according to instructions and do not touch any mucous membranes such as your eyes, nose, or genitals (including the penis) after applying the cream.

morning, the joint may be stiff but loosens up with movement after a few minutes. Cartilage is insensitive to pain, but the synovial membrane in the joints is well supplied with nerves. As cartilage destruction progresses, the synovial membrane is increasingly irritated by even small movement. Some people have continual joint pain that interferes with sleep. Others have mildly tender joints that produce a grating sensation called crepitation.

Osteoarthritis usually affects the joints of the thumbs and those nearest the fingertips; it does not usually involve the large knuckles, which are commonly affected in rheumatoid arthritis (below right). It also may affect the hips, knees, neck, and lower spine. The pain is usually felt directly in the joint, but radiating pain is often the most striking feature of hip osteoarthritis (see Arthritis of the Hip, p.628) and osteoarthritis of the neck and lower back.

TREATMENT OPTIONS

If you experience pain in one or more joints, consult your doctor. He or she will make a diagnosis based on your medical history and symptoms. If your symptoms do not fit the usual pattern of osteoarthritis, further investigation, often by x-ray or other imaging techniques (see p.145), may be necessary.

Physicians focus on three areas when prescribing therapy: pain relief, usually in the form of acetaminophen or nonsteroidal anti-inflammatory drugs; protecting the joint from overuse (which may involve canes, splints, and/or weight loss); and exercise, often with physical therapy to improve muscle tone.

Exercises for Arthritis

Exercise can slow the progressive deterioration of arthritis. However, no single program is right for everyone; your exercise should be tailored to prevent discomfort and aggravation of the arthritis. Ask your physical therapist to provide specific exercises that will benefit you most.

Exercises for people with arthritis fall into three categories. The first consists of daily range-of-motion exercises designed to improve and maintain flexibility (see p.54). The second type is strengthening exercises for muscles (see p.54) to protect and support affected joints. The third category is low-impact aerobic (see p.54) or endurance exercise such as walking, swimming, and stationary bicycling. This kind of activity improves cardiovascular function, tones muscles, helps control weight, and enhances your overall function and well-being. It also maintains the normal function of muscle.

Unless you are experiencing severe joint inflammation, perform your exercises every day, after a hot shower or bath and when your medicine is having the greatest effect.

Sometimes surgery is necessary to relieve extremely painful or misaligned joints. Joint replacement (see Hip and Knee Replacement, p.629) may be an option for people whose mobility is limited, who are in generally good health, and who are not dangerously overweight.

Rheumatoid Arthritis

Rheumatoid arthritis is an inflammatory disease that damages the synovial tissue connecting bones and joints. One of the most crippling forms of arthritis, it affects more than 2.5 million Americans. It is not known what triggers the immune system to produce the substances that cause the inflammation, which can destroy all components of the joint.

In rheumatoid arthritis, the synovial membrane, normally smooth, develops into a rough and grainy tissue called pannus

that invades the joint cavity. The pannus then releases enzymes that eat into the cartilage, bone, and soft tissues. Inflamed tendons can shorten, immobilizing the joint and causing the bones to fuse. If tendons rupture, the result can be loose, floppy joints.

Rheumatoid arthritis can occur at any age but usually begins between 20 and 45. Although the cause is unknown, there may be a genetic link; the disease may run in families.

SYMPTOMS

Rheumatoid arthritis usually begins insidiously with fatigue and flulike aching for several weeks or months before overt arthritis develops. It typically affects multiple joints and is symmetrical, targeting similar joints on both sides of the body, particularly the finger joints, base of the fingers, wrists, elbows, knees, ankles, or feet. Joint pain may be

Joint Changes in Rheumatoid Arthritis

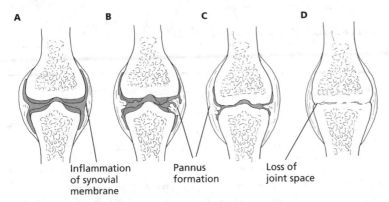

A   B   C   D

Inflammation
of synovial
membrane

Pannus
formation

Loss of
joint space

In rheumatoid arthritis, inflammation begins in the synovial membrane (A). The synovial membrane begins to proliferate and forms extra tissue called pannus (B). Cells in the pannus release enzymes that eat into the cartilage, bone, and soft tissues (C). Finally, the tendons and joint capsule may become inflamed and shorten, causing bone fusion (D).

continuous, even without movement. Morning stiffness that lasts for an hour or longer is common.

The thickening of synovial tissue or the buildup of synovial fluid in the knees, elbows, wrists, or knuckles makes the joints look puffy and red and feel warm and tender when touched. You may experience a flare-up of acute synovitis (inflammation of the synovial membrane) that lasts for several weeks to a few months and then subsides. When there is less inflammation you may feel less fatigued, and better in general.

The most obvious damage occurs in joints, but the disease can affect the entire body—particularly the heart, lungs, blood vessels, eyes, lymph nodes, and spleen. Inflammatory skin nodules may occur at pressure points such as at the elbows, along tendons, or under the toes. These pea- to walnut-sized lumps may go away on their own.

Fatigue, fever, weakness, loss of appetite and weight, and anemia (see p.713) are other common symptoms of rheumatoid arthritis. People with rheumatoid arthritis can develop eye problems, including dryness, redness, burning, and itching (see Uveitis, p.444).

The course of rheumatoid arthritis is unpredictable. Early on, the symptoms may calm down or disappear only to flare up weeks or months later. Occasionally, complete remission occurs, usually within the first year. For some people—usually those who have not been treated—the disease can cause severe disability within a few years.

TREATMENT OPTIONS

If you have symptoms of rheumatoid arthritis, see your doctor for a complete medical evaluation. A blood test sometimes shows a protein called rheumatoid factor circulating in the blood. However, the diagnosis of rheumatoid arthritis cannot be made or excluded based upon the presence or absence of rheumatoid factor or other blood tests.

X-rays can show joint damage characteristic of rheumatoid arthritis, although these changes may not be apparent early in the disease. Extracting the joint's synovial fluid with a needle may help the doctor diagnose rheumatoid arthritis rather than some other condition, such as osteoarthritis or a bacterial infection.

Your greatest chance for relieving symptoms is to take an active part in your treatment. This includes following a therapeutic plan, recognizing flare-ups and drug side effects, and maintaining joint function with regular exercise. Your doctor may refer you to a physical therapist to help with exercises and other treatments, such as heat and cold therapy.

The first medicines used are nonsteroidal anti-inflammatory drugs, particularly aspirin or an aspirin substitute, to reduce pain and inflammation. If these medicines are not effective in the first few weeks of treatment, most doctors add drugs that affect or alter the immune system, such as hydroxychloroquine or methotrexate. In the past, these drugs were used as a last resort; it is now known that low doses of these drugs taken early in the disease can improve treatment.

Other disease-modifying antirheumatic drugs such as gold therapy, penicillamine, and sulfasalazine are also prescribed

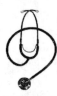

Rheumatoid Arthritis: *When You Visit Your Doctor*

QUESTIONS YOUR DOCTOR MIGHT ASK ON YOUR RETURN VISITS:

- Are your joints stiff or painful in the morning? If so, at what time of day do your joints feel the best?

- How severe is your joint pain?

- Do you have fatigue? If so, how severe is it?

- What limitations do you have in your everyday activities? Have these limitations changed since your last visit?

- How active is your disease?

ASK YOUR DOCTOR THESE QUESTIONS:

- If my disease is active, would I benefit from a different medicine? How much better can I expect to feel?

- How long will it take for this medicine to improve my symptoms? What percentage of people improve on this medicine? What are the common side effects? Which side effects should alert me to call you?

- If joint damage is present, at what point should surgery be considered?

THIS EXAM SHOULD BE PERFORMED REGULARLY:

- Complete examination of joints for presence of active inflammation or decreased range of motion

THESE TESTS MAY BE PERFORMED PERIODICALLY:

- Erythrocyte sedimentation rate or C-reactive protein blood test (elevated levels indicate active inflammation)

- Complete blood cell count (to look for anemia, which is common in many chronic inflammatory diseases) and kidney, liver, or urine tests (especially if medicines are prescribed)

- X-rays of affected joints to evaluate the progression of damage (it takes several months of active inflammation for damage to appear on the x-ray, so your doctor may not order x-rays until you have had arthritis for at least a year)

Living with Rheumatoid Arthritis

When it started, I felt like I was walking on gravel. My wrists were stiff and weak. I could no longer turn the door handle or hold my hairbrush. Within a year of the first symptoms, I was crippled. Medicines would initially relieve the pain, but eventually the arthritis would break through. I had my hip replaced, and my wrist fused with a metal rod. The disease was unpredictable. I could never make plans for tomorrow or next week. One day I would feel well, but the next I would be canceling my dinner party because I could not grip the potato peeler. I wondered if people thought I was lying about the pain to avoid work or unpleasant situations. Most of my friends were encouraging, but they did not know the agony I felt with every movement. Sometimes they would forget, and I would have to say, "I cannot keep up with you—either slow down, or I will have to walk by myself." I am now on an experimental medicine that dissolved the swelling and pain within 2 weeks. I have been born again.

Ellen T., 65 years old

sooner rather than later, and in combination. Corticosteroid drugs (see p.895) are prescribed to treat sudden flare-ups of symptoms and may be recommended in low doses on a daily basis to keep symptoms suppressed. However, regular use of high doses is avoided because of the serious side effects. A new class of drugs has been used with great success in patients unresponsive or partially responsive to the older medications. This group of drugs involves inhibition of TNF-alpha, a protein that causes joint inflammation in rheumatoid arthritis. These drugs have "rescued" patients who were treatment failures, and their use is growing rapidly. They have their downside in that they can cause reactivation of tuberculosis, and patients taking them often have difficulty healing even simple infections.

Another exciting new therapy is leflunomide, a drug you take by mouth. Leflunomide diminishes the activity of immune cells (T cells) that help cause joint damage. It begins to work within 6 to 8 weeks. Side effects include diarrhea, rash, hair thinning, and (in rare cases) liver abnormalities.

When a joint has been severely damaged or deformed, surgery or joint replacement (see Hip and Knee Replacement, p.629) may be necessary.

If you have rheumatoid arthritis, the following issues are important to consider:

Diet Although there is no specific diet for rheumatoid arthritis, some evidence suggests that symptoms may be lessened by consuming more than two servings a week of fish oils rich in omega-3 polyunsaturated fatty acids, which are found in salmon, mackerel, and sardines. It is possible that these fatty acids taken in capsule form may also be beneficial.

Rest and exercise People with rheumatoid arthritis function best when they can adjust their level of rest and activity to match the disease's severity. During episodes of acute inflammation, you may need 8 to 10 hours of sleep at night plus an hour of rest during the day. Rest may have preventive value as well. Some people overdo it when their symptoms recede only to find themselves exhausted. Several short naps during the day may prevent fatigue and allow you to accomplish more.

Regular exercise may help maintain joint function, relieve stiffness, and reduce pain and fatigue. Exercising also increases bone strength. In general, it is better to move joints than not to move them. Thus, balancing rest with exercise is an important goal. (See Exercises for Arthritis, p.606.)

Protecting joints and saving energy Overuse of arthritic joints can lead to pain, swelling, and additional joint damage. An occupational therapist can teach you how to reserve energy and protect your joints while accomplishing daily tasks with greater ease. These recommendations can help you control pain and inflammation:

■ Avoid positions or movements that put extra stress on joints.

■ Avoid being in one position too long.

■ Use your strongest joints and muscles.

■ Plan ahead for activities and simplify your life as much as possible; stress can exacerbate arthritis.

■ Modify your home to make it easier to live in, installing grab bars in the shower and tub and using other assistive devices (see p.1128).

■ Ask for help when you need it.

The emotional side of rheumatoid arthritis People with rheumatoid arthritis often worry about becoming crippled, unable to work, or becoming dependent on others. However, only a very small percentage of people with the disease ever become severely disabled.

Depression is common in people with chronic diseases, including rheumatoid arthritis. A form of treatment called cognitive therapy (see p.393) can enhance your sense of control over disease, reducing depression and stress.

MUSCLES, TENDONS, AND LIGAMENTS

Costochondritis

Costochondritis is inflammation of one or more areas of rib cage cartilage. It causes pain, tenderness, and swelling in the front chest region, where the ribs merge with the sternum (breastbone). In most cases the cause is unknown. Your doctor may prescribe nonsteroidal anti-inflammatory drugs to reduce pain and

Benefits and Risks of Corticosteroids for Rheumatoid Arthritis

Corticosteroid drugs slow the rate of bone damage in the hands of people with rheumatoid arthritis. However, they also can produce serious side effects, such as osteoporosis, bone fractures, intestinal tract bleeding, infections, or cataracts. Your doctor can help you evaluate the risks and benefits of treatment with corticosteroid drugs.

BENEFITS

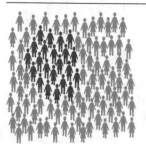 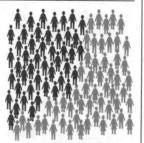

RISKS

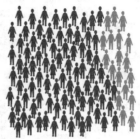 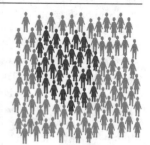

22 OF 100 PEOPLE WHO HAVE RHEUMATOID ARTHRITIS AND TAKE CORTICOSTEROIDS FOR 2 YEARS DEVELOP BONE DAMAGE IN THEIR HANDS

46 OF 100 PEOPLE WHO HAVE RHEUMATOID ARTHRITIS AND DO NOT TAKE CORTICOSTEROIDS DEVELOP BONE DAMAGE IN THEIR HANDS

82 OF 100 PEOPLE WHO HAVE RHEUMATOID ARTHRITIS AND TAKE CORTICOSTEROIDS FOR MORE THAN 2 YEARS DEVELOP SERIOUS SIDE EFFECTS

28 OF 100 PEOPLE WHO HAVE RHEUMATOID ARTHRITIS AND DO NOT TAKE CORTICOSTEROIDS DEVELOP SERIOUS SIDE EFFECTS

Benefits and Risks of Methotrexate for Rheumatoid Arthritis

In people with rheumatoid arthritis, the drug methotrexate offers both considerable relief of symptoms and a slowing of bone damage. Methotrexate produces side effects such as liver damage, nausea and vomiting, headache, rash, and mouth sores.

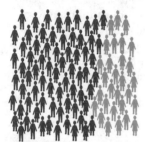 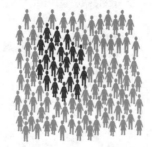 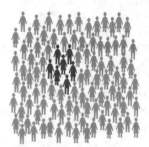

71 OF 100 PEOPLE WHO HAVE RHEUMATOID ARTHRITIS AND TAKE METHOTREXATE HAVE MARKED IMPROVEMENT THAT LASTS FOR AT LEAST 5 YEARS

20 OF 100 PEOPLE WHO HAVE RHEUMATOID ARTHRITIS AND TAKE METHOTREXATE HAVE SIDE EFFECTS BUT CONTINUE TREATMENT BECAUSE IT RELIEVES THEIR SYMPTOMS

7 OF 100 PEOPLE WHO HAVE RHEUMATOID ARTHRITIS AND TAKE METHOTREXATE DISCONTINUE TREATMENT BECAUSE OF SIDE EFFECTS

swelling. If symptoms persist, your doctor may recommend an injection of corticosteroid drugs (see p.895) to reduce the swelling.

Fibromyalgia

The word fibromyalgia literally means "pain of the fibrous tissue (the ligaments and tendons) and muscles." The cause is unknown, although there is some evidence that certain substances in the brain are disordered, leading to a lowered threshold of pain.

SYMPTOMS

The most common symptoms of fibromyalgia are tenderness at certain points in the body, muscle pain, fatigue, and disturbed sleep. You may also have headaches, irritable bowel syndrome (see p.789), temporomandibular joint dysfunction (see p.476), premenstrual syndrome (see p.1046), chest pain, and

depression (see p.395). These symptoms wax and wane and are often exacerbated by stress, illness, and abrupt changes in the weather, and relieved by relaxation. Fibromyalgia shares many symptoms in common with chronic fatigue syndrome (see p.381).

TREATMENT OPTIONS

Treatment can include any or all of the following:

■ **Muscle conditioning** A well-chosen aerobic exercise program may be the most important factor in treating fibromyalgia. Low-impact exercises, such as swimming and bicycling, are recommended for increasing muscle tone and heart strength; stretching exercises can help alleviate stiffness.

■ **Pain relief** Small doses of painkillers such as acetaminophen and nonsteroidal anti-inflammatory drugs such as

aspirin and ibuprofen may relieve pain and stiffness. Other options include biofeedback (see p.395), hypnosis (see p.394), and behavior modification.

■ **Sleep enhancers** Medicines that improve the quality of sleep, particularly heterocyclic antidepressants (see p.400), can be very helpful when taken in very low doses and only at bedtime. Muscle relaxants may also help relieve muscle tension. If your fibromyalgia is accompanied by significant depression, stronger doses of antidepressant medicines may be helpful.

Muscular Dystrophy

Muscular dystrophy is a rare progressive weakening and shrinking of muscles, commonly in the arms, legs, and spine, due to a lack of a key protein necessary for muscle function. Several forms of the debilitating disease occur, but the most common is Duchenne dystrophy, which is passed by a gene on the X chromosome (see p.128) through the mother to males only; it affects about 1 of 10,000 boys. Scientists are trying to use gene therapy to cure this disease.

If you are a woman and Duchenne dystrophy runs in your family, consider genetic counseling (see p.130) before pregnancy. Testing can reveal if you carry the gene. If you do, a male fetus has a 50% chance of being affected. Prenatal tests (see p.917) can determine whether the fetus is affected.

SYMPTOMS

The disease usually is apparent before age 5; muscle weakness in

Tender Points in Fibromyalgia

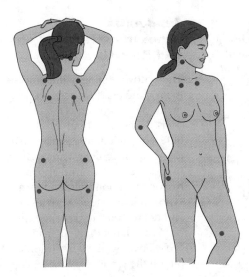

Tissue that becomes painful when pressed, particularly in the locations shown, are called "tender points." They often develop in people with fibromyalgia, occur less frequently in people with other conditions (such as chronic fatigue syndrome), and occur rarely in healthy individuals.

What Do Tendons and Ligaments Do?

Tendons and ligaments are composed of fibers made of collagen, the protein that gives them the strength and flexibility to perform their distinct functions. Ligaments attach bone to bone. For example, the ligaments on either side of your finger joints prevent side-to-side bending, while the ligaments that stretch across your palm keep your fingers from bending too far back. Tendons anchor muscle to bone; when your muscle contracts, it pulls on the tendon (which then pulls on the bone) and you move (see How You Move, p.104). In addition to moving your joints, tendons also stabilize them. The fibrous tissues of tendons and ligaments have little blood supply. As a result, when they are injured, the repair process is slow.

Tendons, Ligaments, and Cartilage

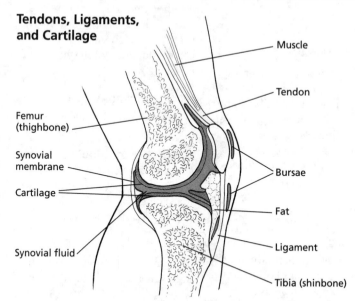

Ligaments bind the bones together and keep them in proper alignment. Muscles and their tendons stabilize joints as well as move them. Cartilage, a tough and somewhat elastic tissue, provides a smooth, slippery surface for movement and cushions the joint. The synovial membrane produces fluid that lubricates the joint (providing frictionless movement) and supplies nutrition to nearby bone and cartilage. Bursae, fluid-filled sacs, cushion the tendon and surrounding tissue.

a toddler manifests itself in several ways, including an apparent lack of coordination, clumsiness, inability to walk or climb stairs, and difficulty raising the arms over the head. Chest infections such as pneumonia (see p.496) commonly occur because the breathing muscles are weakened. In most cases, muscular dystrophy progressively deforms the spine and muscles, confining affected boys to a wheelchair by adolescence.

TREATMENT OPTIONS

If your son shows any signs of the disease, he should see his pediatrician immediately. The doctor will most likely recommend a muscle tissue biopsy, in which a small sample of muscle is removed for laboratory evaluation. There is no cure for muscular dystrophy. Your son's pediatrician may recommend physical therapy to delay muscle deterioration and reduce deformity.

Tendonitis, Tenosynovitis, and Bursitis

The synovial lining, a thin, moist membrane that lubricates movement, often surrounds the tendons. Sometimes tendons lie over little sacs called bursae that cushion their movement. Due to overuse, diabetes, or for no apparent reason, a tendon (tendonitis), its synovial lining (tenosynovitis), and nearby bursae (bursitis) can become inflamed. Inflammation causes pain whenever tension is put on the tendon.

For reasons that are not understood, tendonitis occurs more often with certain tendons than others; see Tendonitis and Capsulitis of the Shoulder (p.615); Rotator Cuff Tear and Bursitis (p.615); Achilles Tendonitis (p.636); Tenosynovitis of the Hand (p.619).

Treatment with nonsteroidal anti-inflammatory drugs often eliminates the symptoms. Sometimes physical therapy, the wearing of shoe inserts, and injections of corticosteroids (see p.895) are recommended. Tendonitis has a tendency to recur in the same tendons, and repeated treatment usually is effective.

NECK, SHOULDERS, ARMS, AND HANDS

Cervical Osteoarthritis

Cervical osteoarthritis is a gradual deterioration of the cervical vertebrae, the bones of the neck. It can cause stiffness and pain. The condition mainly affects people over 50; in fact, most people over 50 have a minor degree of cervical osteoarthritis.

SYMPTOMS

The symptoms usually develop slowly over many years. You may first notice muscular pain and stiffness, and later a grating sensation (called crepitation), in your neck. If a nerve leading from the spinal cord in the neck into the arms is pinched, you may feel pain in the arms and shoulders or tingling or numbness in the hands. A pinched nerve can also occur with a herniated disk (see p.622) in the neck.

TREATMENT OPTIONS

A diagnosis is made with the help of x-rays or magnetic resonance imaging (see p.150), to determine if there is compression of the spinal cord or degenerative changes in your joints. Pain can usually be relieved by anti-inflammatory drugs such as aspirin; in severe cases, injections of corticosteroid drugs (see p.895) may be used. You should protect your neck joints from overuse, which may involve wearing a soft collar around your neck when you have symptoms. Physical therapy, moist heat, or massage may help reduce pain or stiffness. In severe cases, traction may be necessary to immobilize the affected neck area; surgery may be recommended if these treatments fail.

Stiff Neck

Stiff neck is a condition of strained muscles and ligaments in the neck. A stiff neck often occurs from the everyday stress of holding your head in an upright position (your skull and brain weigh 15 pounds) or from holding your head in a stationary position, such as when working at a computer all day. Other common causes include sleeping in an awkward position, twisting your neck suddenly, emotional and psychological stress, and injury.

You may feel a dull or piercing pain, stiffness and soreness, painful muscle spasms, limited neck flexibility, and inflammation (swelling and redness).

Nonprescription medicines to relieve pain and inflammation can help, including aceta-minophen or nonsteroidal anti-inflammatory drugs such as aspirin. Apply cold packs for about 15 minutes four times a day for the first 2 days to reduce inflammation; then apply heat (in the form of a hot water bottle or heating pad) on the same schedule to ease muscle spasms. Rest your head by lying down and by having your neck and upper back muscles massaged.

If your pain persists for more than 3 days, consult your doctor, who may recommend that you wear a soft neck collar to ease the pain and keep your neck from moving, although you should be careful to wear it only a few hours at a time. Some physicians also prescribe muscle-relaxant drugs.

Whiplash Injury

The descriptive term "whiplash" describes the violent whiplike motion that most often occurs when a motor vehicle is struck from behind. If your head is thrown backward beyond its normal range of motion, muscles and ligaments in the neck can be damaged. Although properly positioned headrests can reduce the severity of neck pain after rear-end collisions, the injury can occur even when they are in use.

SYMPTOMS

Usually, whiplash injury is felt as temporary pain and stiffness followed by a period of improvement and the return of pain several days later. The pain may gradually intensify, sometimes moving to the back of the head, chest muscles, and one or both shoulders or upper arms. Your neck may feel tender and swollen and may hurt when you turn it from side to side. Violent whiplash motion can squeeze the disks of the cervical (neck) spine so hard that they bulge out and press on a nerve, causing severe pain. Spinal vertebrae can also be fractured or knocked painfully out of alignment.

How Whiplash Injury Occurs

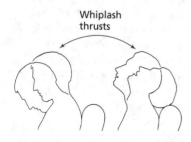

Whiplash
thrusts

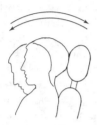

Whiplash injury usually occurs when you stop suddenly in a vehicle, or are hit from behind; the head snaps violently back and forth. A properly positioned headrest limits this motion.

TREATMENT OPTIONS

The mildest forms of whiplash injury get better after a few days of rest; take aspirin or another painkiller for pain. If your neck hurts constantly, if muscle spasms occur when you turn your head, or if pain and spasms spread to your shoulder or upper arm, contact your doctor. Muscle-relaxant drugs and a soft neck collar may be prescribed. The collar takes the weight off your muscles, allowing them to rest.

Avoid sports, carrying heavy groceries, and other physically demanding activities that can interfere with healing, which takes 2 to 3 weeks for muscles and much longer for torn ligaments.

Once healing has begun, your doctor may recommend exercises that move your neck through an ever-increasing range of motions, which may be painful at first. Injured muscles tighten up and, as time passes, they become shorter and more resistant to stretching, so it is vital that you perform the exercises as often as your doctor suggests. For serious abnormalities of alignment or fracture, immediate surgery may be needed.

Dislocated Shoulder

A shoulder dislocation occurs when the ball-shaped head of the upper arm bone moves out of its socket. The shoulder may be dislocated either forward (which is most common), usually due to falling on the shoulder or on an extended arm, or backward, which can occur if the shoulder is hit from the front.

A severe dislocation can cause tearing of the muscles, ligaments, or tendons that support the shoulder. Shoulder dislocations always cause pain; if you have a forward dislocation, your shoulder may look deformed. Your primary care doctor or a bone specialist may take x-rays of your shoulder to make sure it is not also fractured and will reposition the ball of your upper arm back into its socket after giving you painkilling medicine (or, for severe dislocations, a general anesthetic). You will wear a sling for several weeks to permit healing. Rest your shoulder and apply ice packs for about 15 minutes three or four times a day.

After the pain and swelling subside, exercises to strengthen your muscles and restore your shoulder's full range of motion are beneficial. Recurring dislocations can occur if the supporting structures of your shoulder have been damaged; surgery may be required to tighten stretched ligaments or mend torn ones.

Fractured Collarbone or Upper Arm

A break of the collarbone (clavicle) or of the upper arm bone (humerus) most often occurs during a fall on an outstretched arm. If you have great pain in the shoulder soon after a fall or after a hard blow to the shoulder, call your physician immediately. For a collarbone fracture, you will need to wear a sling to keep your collarbone and arm immobilized. For a fracture of the humerus, you will likely need at least a cast, and possibly surgery. See also Fractures, p.594.

Frozen Shoulder

Frozen shoulder, also called adhesive capsulitis, is caused by inflammation and thickening of the joint capsule, the tough, fibrous tissue that surrounds the joint. As a result, movement of the shoulder is stiff, painful, and severely restricted.

Frozen shoulder is often the result of chronic pain in the shoulder, such as from capsulitis (inflammation of the shoulder capsule; see below) or injury, which leads you to limit the motion of your shoulder. Without regular motion, the joint becomes so tight and stiff that the simplest movement, such as raising your arm, is severely restricted. The stiffness and discomfort may be worse at night.

See your doctor if you think you have frozen shoulder. Treatment usually begins with nonsteroidal anti-inflammatory drugs to relieve pain and inflammation, followed by mild stretching exercises and heat applications. Your physician may recommend physical therapy to teach you exercises that can help you keep your shoulder mobile and in use. He or she may also inject a corticosteroid drug (see p.895) directly into your shoulder joint to decrease the painful inflammation.

Rotator Cuff Tear and Bursitis

The rotator cuff is a powerful quartet of muscles and tendons that attach your upper arm bone to the shoulder blade. These structures can be partially or completely torn. This occurs primarily in people over age 50, unless some unusual activity, such as pitching a baseball, puts constant stress on the cuff. Partial tears of the rotator cuff can be confused with subdeltoid bursitis (see Helping Your Doctor Diagnose Shoulder Pain, below). With a complete tear, you cannot lift your arm from your side. Surgery is recommended to repair the tear.

Bursitis (see Tendonitis, Tenosynovitis, and Bursitis, p.612), on the other hand, causes pain when you lie on the affected shoulder or when pressing on a bursa.

Tendonitis and Capsulitis of the Shoulder

Tendonitis (see Tendonitis, Tenosynovitis, and Bursitis, p.612) often occurs in the shoulder. The affected tendon or tendons may become inflamed from excessive use, such as repeated

---

Helping Your Doctor Diagnose Shoulder Pain

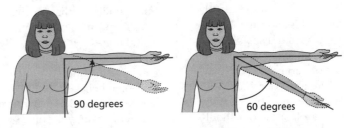

TORN ROTATOR CUFF   90 degrees   **SUPRASPINATUS TENDONITIS OR SUBDELTOID BURSITIS**   60 degrees

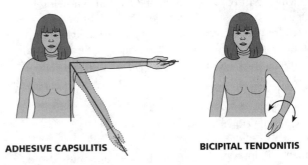

ADHESIVE CAPSULITIS   **BICIPITAL TENDONITIS**

If your **rotator cuff** is torn, you will find it impossible to lift your arm up to the 90-degree position. However, if someone helps you lift your arm up to the 90-degree position, you will be able to hold it there without help. Partial tears may cause pain and milder weakness.

In **supraspinatus tendonitis or subdeltoid bursitis**, you will notice pain when you, or when someone helps you, lift your arm up to the 60-degree position. (Also, it will hurt if the top outer part of your shoulder is pressed.)

In **adhesive capsulitis**, it will hurt when you, or when someone helps you, lift your arm in almost any direction.

In **bicipital tendonitis**, whenever you try to turn your hand it will hurt. (Also, it will hurt when the area in front of the shoulder—where the biceps muscle tendon attaches to the bone—is pressed.)

overhand arm movements or heavy lifting. Tendonitis may also follow an injury such as a fall on an outstretched arm. Often it occurs without a clear reason. Tendonitis can occur at different spots in the shoulder, producing somewhat different symptoms. Capsulitis involves inflammation and shrinkage of the capsule of the shoulder. If capsulitis becomes chronic, it can lead to the development of scar tissue, which transforms capsulitis into adhesive capsulitis (see Frozen Shoulder, p.615).

SYMPTOMS

Both tendonitis and capsulitis produce pain and discomfort in your upper shoulder or the upper third of your arm. The pain may also radiate into your neck. You may be awakened from sleep by pain if you roll onto your shoulder. The factors that aggravate the pain are slightly different depending on which part of the shoulder is affected.

Most often tendonitis involves the tendon on the top of the shoulder (the supraspinatus muscle tendon) that runs under a cushioning sac called the subdeltoid bursa; the tendon can be pinched by the scapula (the triangular bone over the ribs) with certain movements. Pain from inflammation of the supraspinatus muscle tendon and subdeltoid bursa often comes on suddenly and is felt at the top outer part of the shoulder when you lift your arm, in the upper arm, and when someone presses down on the top outer part of your shoulder.

Pain caused by the tendon of the biceps muscle also often

comes on suddenly and is felt in front of the shoulder with certain motions (see Helping Your Doctor Diagnose Shoulder Pain, p.615) and when someone presses where the biceps muscle tendon attaches to the bone.

Capsulitis usually produces pain that comes on gradually. The pain is felt throughout the whole shoulder area and, in contrast to tendonitis, usually is not caused by pressing on a particular spot.

TREATMENT OPTIONS

Your doctor will recommend treatment similar to that for rotator cuff injury—rest, cold applications, and nonsteroidal antiinflammatory drugs to relieve pain and inflammation. Gentle exercises can help restore full range of motion and use. If you have extreme pain, your physician may inject a corticosteroid medicine (see p.895) around the inflamed tendon. Knowing where to inject it involves making the right diagnosis (see Helping Your Doctor Diagnose Shoulder Pain, p.615). X-rays of the shoulder are not usually helpful in making the diagnosis.

Bursitis of the Elbow

Bursitis (see Tendonitis, Tenosynovitis, and Bursitis, p.612) of the elbow causes pain and swelling of the bursa that lies over the bony tip of the elbow, called the olecranon process. The condition is also known as olecranon bursitis. It occurs when the olecranon bursa becomes inflamed, often due to prolonged pressure of the elbow against a hard surface. The bursa may also become inflamed

due to injury of a neighboring joint, infection, or an inflammatory disease such as gout (see p.604).

Symptoms of olecranon bursitis include pain, redness, and swelling in the area of the elbow, along with stiffness of the joint. It often heals on its own within a few weeks if you avoid putting pressure on it; rest helps your body reabsorb the extra fluid inside the bursa. Apply ice for 15 minutes several times a day to help reduce inflammation and take a nonsteroidal anti-inflammatory drug.

If your symptoms continue, see your physician. If inflammation persists, the fluid inside the bursa may need to be removed through a needle. If your condition recurs, your physician may recommend a corticosteroid injection (see p.895) or an operation to remove the affected bursa.

Tennis Elbow

Tennis elbow is a common term for any inflammation and pain near the bone on the outside of the elbow, where tendons connect the muscles of the forearm to the bone. It is caused by overusing the muscles that straighten your fingers and wrist. Fewer than 10% of people develop the condition through playing tennis; more common causes include gardening, job-related lifting, using a screwdriver, or other wrist overuse, but often there is no apparent cause.

If you have tennis elbow, you will have tenderness and sometimes redness where the muscles attach to bone just below the outer part of your elbow. You will often feel pain in that area when you extend your wrist against resistance. You may have pain when handshaking or lifting.

If your pain is severe, see your doctor, who may recommend resting your wrist and elbow and applying ice for 15 minutes at a time several times a day. Nonsteroidal anti-inflammatory drugs can help relieve pain. Ultrasound therapy sends soothing sound waves into the inflamed area, and improves the inflammation (although how this treatment works is not entirely clear).

An elbow strap or air splint (a plastic, inflatable splint) may reduce pain by resting and immobilizing the inflamed tendon. If pain is severe, your doctor may inject a corticosteroid medicine (see p.895) into the inflamed area. Avoid performing the activity that caused your pain for several weeks. Surgery is rarely necessary.

Carpal Tunnel Syndrome

Carpal tunnel syndrome is numbness, tingling, burning, or aching pain in the fingers that occurs when the median nerve is compressed or damaged. The median nerve and a bundle of tendons pass through a narrow channel, which is covered by ligament that lies just below the inner surface of the wrist.

The nerve is vulnerable to compression from a variety of sources, including swelling of surrounding tissue. This can occur with pregnancy, rheumatoid arthritis (see p.606), diabetes (see p.832), an underactive thyroid gland (see Hypothyroidism,

p.848), or pressure caused by bone spurs. Repetitive wrist motions, such as those used in typing on a computer keyboard, seem to be responsible for a growing number of cases; even sleeping with your wrist flexed can cause this condition.

SYMPTOMS

Symptoms include burning, aching, numbness, or tingling of the thumb, index, middle, and ring fingers, and eventually a weakened thumb muscle. The symptoms are worsened by grasping heavy objects. In early or mild cases, the symptoms are intermittent but can become persistent.

TREATMENT OPTIONS

Your doctor may recommend putting your hand in a splint to immobilize the wrist during

the night; nonsteroidal anti-inflammatory drugs help reduce swelling around the nerve. If these treatments are ineffective, or if you develop weakness in your thumb, your doctor may suggest an injection of a corticosteroid medicine (see p.895) into the carpal tunnel to reduce the inflammation that is pinching the nerve.

Once your symptoms have subsided, your doctor may refer you to an occupational therapist who can teach you ways to prevent recurrences. Exercising your hand does not help, and may aggravate, the condition. If these treatments fail, surgery to cut the ligament and relieve pressure on the nerve may be necessary.

When carpal tunnel syndrome is due to thyroid disease, successful treatment of the thyroid condition usually alleviates carpal tunnel syndrome.

Carpal Tunnel Syndrome

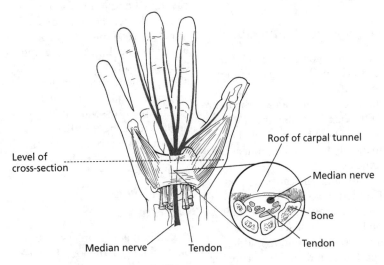

Level of cross-section

Median nerve

Tendon

Roof of carpal tunnel

Median nerve

Bone

Tendon

In carpal tunnel syndrome, the median nerve in the hand is compressed by bones, ligaments, and swollen tendons in the carpal tunnel.

Colles Fracture

Colles fracture is a broken bone in one or both of the arm bones (radius and ulna) just above the wrist. It usually occurs when a person who is falling thrusts out an arm and hand to break the fall. Colles fracture is more common in people whose bones are weakened by osteoporosis (see p.596).

Symptoms include a deformed wrist and hand, swelling, and severe pain that is intensified if you move or put pressure on the hand. If you think your wrist is broken, get medical help immediately. You will receive anesthesia and the broken bone will be realigned and immobilized with a cast or splint. Nonsteroidal anti-inflammatory drugs help relieve pain; your physician may also prescribe antibiotics in tablet form to prevent any infection.

Healing can take more than a month. Once the cast is removed, your doctor will give you exercises to regain the flexibility and strength of your wrist.

Dupuytren Contracture

Dupuytren contracture is a progressive thickening and shortening of the connective tissue situated beneath the skin of the palm of the hand, causing the ring finger and little finger to bend permanently toward the palm at the knuckles.

Although the cause of Dupuytren contracture is unknown, scientists believe it may be hereditary. It seems to be most common among middle-aged men and may be more prevalent among people who have diabetes (see p.832) or who abuse alcohol. Usually it causes no problems, but contact your physician if you are finding it difficult to straighten your fingers. Surgery to cut and release the bands of constricting tissue may be recommended. Physical therapy after the surgery will help you regain the use of your hand.

Hand Fracture

A broken hand or broken fingers usually occur due to a fall on the outstretched hand or a sports activity in which an object strikes the hand with great force. Symptoms include swelling and bruising around the injured area. If you also have deformity of your hand or fingers, difficulty moving your fingers, or pain with any pressure or movement of the affected bone, see your doctor.

Otherwise, see your physician if the injury does not improve within 2 days of using the RICE technique (see p.636). A splint or cast may be required for fractures of hand bones. For fractures of finger bones, taping the broken finger to a healthy adjacent finger (called "buddy-taping") is usually all that is necessary. Sometimes surgery is required. To regain function, it is essential that you begin exercising the affected area as soon as your doctor recommends. (See also Fractures, p.594.)

Ganglion

A ganglion is a harmless cyst or outpouching of the joint lining under the skin, usually on the back or front of the wrist but, in some cases, on the top of the foot. It looks odd, and some people worry that it could be a cancerous tumor. However, a ganglion is simply a cyst filled with a thick fluid that has escaped the tendons or joints that the fluid normally lubricates. It may feel rubbery or hard to the touch and may or may not be painful. A ganglion requires no treatment unless you find it cosmetically annoying or painful. Your doctor may remove the fluid with a syringe or remove the entire ganglion by cutting it off.

Jammed Finger

A jammed finger, also known as baseball finger or mallet finger, is a tear in the tendons that straighten your fingertip. It is caused by a forcible injury to the tip of the finger, such as by an oncoming ball. The top joint of your affected finger will be painful and swollen. You will also find that you are unable to straighten the injured finger.

See your doctor as soon as possible. He or she will take an x-ray of the affected joint to ensure it is not broken and then immobilize the finger with a splint, which you will wear for about 6 weeks. Sometimes a wire is inserted through the bone to keep your finger straight while the tendons heal, which can take several months.

Painkillers and nonsteroidal anti-inflammatory drugs can help reduce inflammation and relieve pain. After the splint is removed, your doctor may recommend that you do exercises to aid flexibility and restore normal use.

Tenosynovitis of the Hand

Tenosynovitis of the hand is known by a number of terms, including repetitive strain disorder or trigger finger. The tendons in your hands and wrists run like cables through your hands to your fingers, permitting the delicate motion of your fingers. The tendons and their synovial sheaths can develop tenosynovitis (see Tendonitis, Tenosynovitis, and Bursitis, p.612), which causes pain, tenderness, and swelling in your hand or wrist. This is often due to repetitive overuse of the fingers, such as in typing or assembly-line work. Sometimes, tenosynovitis is caused by rheumatoid arthritis, diabetes, or infection, but often a person with tenosynovitis has none of these conditions.

SYMPTOMS

You may hear or feel a grating noise when you move the affected area or you may have difficulty straightening a finger or thumb. A soft, clicking sensation (the "trigger finger" effect) can occur when you try to straighten or bend your finger. Once the finger is bent, the straightening mechanism jams for a few moments, and then the finger extends in a jerking motion. Pain and tenderness may result from this triggering effect.

TREATMENT OPTIONS

Your doctor may recommend nonsteroidal anti-inflammatory drugs to reduce the swelling and pain. Rest, a change of work habits, and splinting the hand may also help. Your doctor may inject the painful area with corticosteroid medicine (see p.895) to relieve pain, although frequent injections (more than three injections in a year) can weaken the tendon and make it more vulnerable to tearing. Surgery may be required in persistent cases to release the constricting synovial membrane.

Less commonly, tenosynovitis is caused by an infection that occurs after a puncture wound provides an entry point for bacteria. See your doctor immediately if you have a warm, painful area on your hand after a puncture wound; antibiotic drugs (see p.868) may be needed to eradicate any bacteria that have entered your system. Minor surgery may be required to release pus and limit the spread of the infection. (See also Carpal Tunnel Syndrome, p.617.)

BACK, HIPS, LEGS, AND FEET

Kyphosis

Kyphosis is an abnormal degree of bending of the spine, usually in the upper part of the body, causing a hunched back. Kyphosis may be present at birth if the front portion of several vertebrae have developed abnormally. Kyphosis that develops later in life is usually caused by one or more compression fractures (see p.595), which are common in women who have osteoporosis; they can also be caused by ankylosing spondylitis (see p.602). Your physician may recommend that you wear a corsetlike brace. Surgery is also sometimes recommended, though surgery is not an option for people whose bones have been severely weakened by osteoporosis because there is not enough healthy adjacent bone to which the surgeon can secure supporting rods or screws.

Sciatica

Sciatica is pain along the sciatic nerves, the longest nerves in the body. The pain begins in the lower spine, passes through the buttock, down the back and side of the leg, and into the foot and toes. A herniated disk (see p.622) is one of the most common causes of sciatica, although sciatica can also be brought on by spinal stenosis (see p.625), infection, fractures of the pelvis or thigh, or a tumor. This condition usually affects people in their 40s and 50s, more often those who are overweight.

SYMPTOMS

The main feature of sciatica is one-sided numbness, tingling, or pain in the lower back, buttock, and leg. It can be relatively mild or erupt into violent throbbing pain that grips the back and leg, making any movement excruciating and forcing you to lie down flat. The symptoms are made worse by moving, coughing, or sneezing. Activities that tug on the sciatic nerve, such as bending forward from the waist or flexing

How Muscles Support Your Back

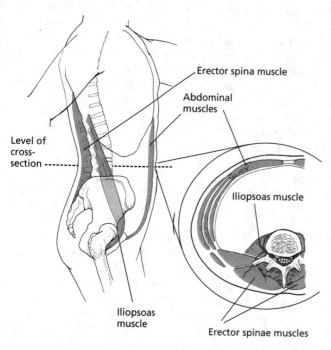

Erector spina muscle

Abdominal muscles

Level of cross-section

Iliopsoas muscle

Iliopsoas muscle

Erector spinae muscles

Your muscles enable you to move, control the motions of your back, and support your spine.

■ Flat abdominal muscles in front are attached to the pelvis below and the ribs above. These muscles form the cavity that contains the stomach and other abdominal organs; they also support the lower back.

■ The two iliopsoas muscles, located on each side of the lower-back vertebrae, are attached to the vertebrae and to the inside of the pelvis. They pass downward in front of the hip joints and attach to the thighbones. These muscles not only support the spine but flex the hips and help balance your trunk while you are standing.

■ The erector spinae (Latin for "upholder of the spine") muscles, located to the left and right of the spine in the rear, are the large muscles visible in the lower part of the back. They are composed of many muscle groups attached to the bony parts of each vertebra, as well as to the pelvis below and the rib cage and the spine above. They are the major supports of the spine during lifting.

Cervical, Thoracic, and Lumbar Regions of the Spine

The spine is made up of 33 bones called vertebrae and is divided into five regions. Vertebrae of the sacrum and coccyx are fused and immobile. The remaining vertebrae provide you with the flexibility to bend, stretch, and lift. The cervical and lumbar spine are the most flexible and are the most common sites of arthritis.

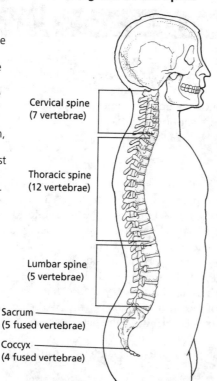

Cervical spine (7 vertebrae)

Thoracic spine (12 vertebrae)

Lumbar spine (5 vertebrae)

Sacrum (5 fused vertebrae)

Coccyx (4 fused vertebrae)

the hips while the knees are straight, aggravate the symptoms.

The pain may be constant, so that you cannot find any comfortable position, or it may be occasional, sharp, and shooting, like an electric shock. In rare cases, when a severely herniated disk and other nerve roots are involved, bladder or bowel function may be affected, and one or both legs may become weak. If unpleasant leg pains seem to bother you only when relaxing, especially in the evening before bedtime or while falling asleep, you may have restless leg syndrome (see p.390) instead of sciatica.

TREATMENT OPTIONS

See your doctor immediately if you are having problems control-

Origins of Sciatic Pain

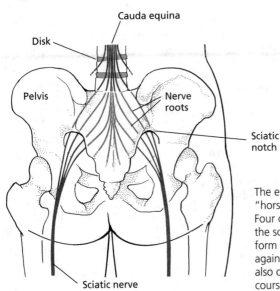

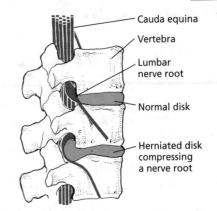

The end of the spinal cord, called the cauda equina (Latin for "horse's tail"), branches into nerve roots along the lower backbone. Four of these roots thread throughout the pelvis and merge to form the sciatic nerves that extend down each leg. In the most common form of sciatica, a herniated disk squeezes a sciatic nerve root against the backbone, causing inflammation and pain. Sciatica may also occur when irritation of the sciatic nerve occurs lower in its course, such as in the buttock where the sciatic notch is found.

ling your bladder or bowels. For most people, the tendency for sciatica to get better on its own makes choosing the best treatment a complicated matter. In half the people with sciatica, the pain goes away without treatment within 4 weeks; fewer than 5% to 10% of people with sciatica require back surgery (see What to Do for Back Pain, p.626).

No matter how painful your sciatica is, your doctor may first recommend up to 3 days of bed rest and nonsteroidal anti-inflammatory drugs to relieve pain and decrease inflammation. Longer periods of bed rest are not recommended; instead, doctors advise that you get up and begin to move slowly to regain motion.

If pain lasts for more than 6 weeks or is so severe that you cannot live with it, your doctor may use magnetic resonance imaging, computed tomography, or a myelogram (see Tests Your Doctor May Perform to Diagnose the Cause of Back Pain, above) to verify that a herniated disk is causing the sciatica.

Weight loss, if necessary, and learning proper posture and preventive exercises (see Preventing Back Pain, p.627), may be recommended. Chemonucleolysis or percutaneous diskectomy (see Two Surgical Techniques for Herniated Disk, p.623) may also be recommended, but generally as a last option.

Alternative Medicine: Acupuncture for Back Pain

In the ancient Chinese physical science and art of acupuncture, extremely thin sterilized needles are inserted for brief periods at precise points along a complex network of body meridians. These "lines of energy" encircle the body like the global lines of longitude and latitude. Acupuncture can help some people with chronic back pain. How it works is not clear; it may block pain signals from reaching the central nervous system or it may stimulate the production of endorphins, natural morphinelike substances produced by the body. A new technique called percutaneous electrical nerve stimulation (PENS) has been shown to be very effective. In PENS, acupuncture needles are placed about an inch into the skin and a tiny electrical current is sent through them.

Tests Your Doctor May Perform to Diagnose the Cause of Back Pain

In the great majority of cases of back pain, no diagnostic tests are necessary. However, if your back pain is not getting better with rest and painkillers, your physician may use one or more of the following tests to exclude the possibility of a more serious disorder:

X-rays Lower back x-rays primarily show the bones and other calcium-containing tissues. While giving some idea of the condition of the vertebrae, they provide little information about the disks, ligaments, muscles, or other soft tissues. But they can help identify fractures, bone tumors, infection, or arthritis. They are not useful in diagnosing most cases of lower back pain.

Magnetic resonance imaging Magnetic resonance imaging (MRI) (see p.150) uses electromagnetic waves to show internal structures. It delineates soft tissues, including disks, the spinal cord and nerves, and tumors. When a test is needed to diagnose back pain, MRI is often the most useful.

Computed tomography In computed tomography (CT) scanning (see p.149), computers instantly analyze and synthesize multiple images of back structures, providing a remarkably detailed composite view in nearly any anatomic plane. CT can identify arthritis (see p.605) or spinal stenosis (see p.625), but may not clearly indicate whether a herniated disk is causing a problem.

Bone scan Bone scans show a tumor, an infection, or a mending fracture as a hot spot on the film. Bone scans help doctors locate abnormalities so that other techniques can be used to make the diagnosis.

Myelography This form of x-ray involves injecting a dye into the fluid-filled sheath that surrounds the spinal cord. Before CT or MRI scans were available, it was the best way to visualize a herniated disk. However, myelography is uncomfortable and sometimes can cause side effects, so it is infrequently used today.

Scoliosis

Scoliosis is an abnormal sideways curvature and tilting of the spine when viewed from the back. The chest and lower back areas are most often affected. Scoliosis is usually painless. In some people, it is caused by congenital (inherited) defects, or polio, but often the cause is not known.

Scoliosis may start as early as infancy, but the first signs of the abnormal curvature usually appear during adolescence, continuing until full growth is achieved. This deformity may remain undetected for many years, due to the absence of pain and its slow progression. In children and adolescents, an S-shaped curvature may develop in the spine as the body compensates for the original curvature.

Your physician diagnoses scoliosis with a physical examination and x-rays of the spine. In mild cases, where there is only a small curve, no treatment is necessary. However, your doctor may want to examine you periodically to ensure that the curvature is not worsening. If it does, immobilization in a brace or plaster jacket may be recommended. In some cases, surgery is required to realign the spinal vertebrae and fuse them together to achieve a straight spine.

Herniated Disk

A herniated disk is also known as a prolapsed, protruded, or ruptured disk. Intervertebral disks serve as small shock-absorbing cushions between each bony vertebra of the spine. They have a jellylike interior and a tougher outer area. Over time, the tough outer part of the disk may start to tear, permitting the jellylike substance to bulge out through the tear. The bulging disk can press on a nerve root as it leaves the spinal cord, causing pain.

SYMPTOMS

The pressure of a herniated disk on a nerve root can cause slight to intense pain, numbness, or weakness. When the herniated disk is in the neck, the symptoms are felt in the neck, shoulder, arm, or hand. When the herniated disk is in the lower back, it may cause sciatica (see p.619). The symptoms are usually made worse by moving.

Herniated Disk

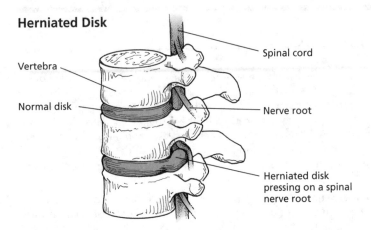

Spinal cord

Vertebra

Normal disk

Nerve root

Herniated disk pressing on a spinal nerve root

The pain of a herniated disk occurs when part of the disk presses on a nerve root in the spine.

Surgery for Herniated Disk

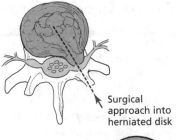

Surgical approach into herniated disk

CHEMONUCLEOLYSIS

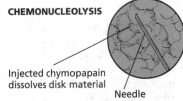

Injected chymopapain dissolves disk material

Needle

PERCUTANEOUS DISKECTOMY

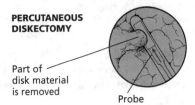

Part of disk material is removed

Probe

LASER DISKECTOMY

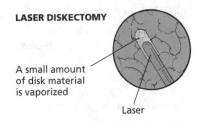

A small amount of disk material is vaporized

Laser

Surgery for Adults with Low Back Pain: Dr Lipson's Advice

As a spine surgeon, I see a lot of patients with low back pain who would like to consider surgery. Most often, I advise against it. Any kind of surgery always involves risks, and you have to be sure that the benefits from the surgery are likely to outweigh the risks. Most cases of acute back pain can be treated successfully with rest, as needed, and simple nonprescription pain medications.

Back pain that is accompanied by loss of control of your bowels and/or bladder represents the one absolute surgical emergency and should be reported to your physician immediately. Not only does it require surgery, it usually requires surgery within the next day or two.

Some patients have recurrent bouts of severe back pain, and don't get adequate relief from back exercises, rest, and medicines. I will sometimes perform surgery in such patients if it is clear from the examination and from tests like an MRI that they have pressure on spinal nerves or instability of the spine. Surgery in these patients often produces relief, but it isn't perfect. Unless I cannot avoid it, I try to let nature provide the healing for back pain and use surgery only if it is likely to be beneficial.

STEPHEN J. LIPSON, MD
HARVARD VANGUARD MEDICAL ASSOCIATES
HARVARD MEDICAL SCHOOL

There are several minimally invasive alternatives to major back surgery for a herniated disk. In chemonucleolysis, an enzyme called chymopapain is injected into the disk to dissolve a portion of it; this procedure can produce serious side effects. In percutaneous (through the skin) diskectomy, a portion of the damaged disk is removed through a small incision in the back. Laser diskectomy, in which a microlaser is used to vaporize part of the disk, is a variation of the percutaneous technique.

Open Surgery for Herniated Disk or Spinal Stenosis

Traditional open surgery, in which a large incision is made in the back to gain direct access to the structures of the spine, may be recommended for back problems (such as herniated disk or spinal stenosis) that do not respond to more conservative treatment. This type of surgery may also be necessary to treat infection, a tumor, or an injury that has caused severe damage to vertebrae and the spinal cord.

After surgery, guidelines for recuperation will depend on the operation, and a specific program for recovery will be planned by your surgeon. You will need pain medicines for the first few days after surgery. It is important for you to be out of bed, sitting up, and walking soon after the surgery. Exercise should be resumed and activities increased gradually. Vigorous activity that puts stress on the lower back should generally be avoided for several months.

A diskectomy involves making an opening in the bones of the spine and removing material protruding from the abnormal disk. Compared to percutaneous diskectomy, open surgery gives the surgeon a better view. Since the problem area is exposed, the risk of damage caused by the surgery to neighboring bone, ligaments, and nerve roots is minimized and the maximum amount of protruding or detached disk material can be cut away by the surgeon. However, recovery may take longer.

Removing portions of intervertebral disks sometimes requires laminectomy, in which parts of each vertebra are cut out to gain access to the herniated disk. The success of disk operations in relieving back pain and sciatica is related to the condition of the disk at the time of surgery.

To treat spinal stenosis, all bony structures contributing to the narrowed spinal channel are cut away. Sometimes the individual vertebrae are fused to permanently hold them in position and prevent future movement of bone that pushes on the nerves.

TREATMENT OPTIONS

A herniated disk usually heals within 2 to 6 weeks with proper rest (sometimes bed rest) and a decrease in activity. Your doctor may recommend nonsteroidal anti-inflammatory drugs to ease the pain. He or she may also suggest physical therapy (including gentle exercises, massage, and alternating heat and ice packs) to reduce pain and inflammation. If the herniated disk is in your neck, you may be advised to wear a soft neck collar to support your head.

If symptoms persist after a month of this conservative treatment, your doctor may take x-rays and, if your pain is severe, may recommend chemonucleolysis or percutaneous diskectomy. Severe, unrelenting sciatica caused by a herniated disk may necessitate a surgical procedure such as diskectomy or laminectomy (see Open Surgery for Herniated Disk or Spinal Stenosis, above).

TWO SURGICAL TECHNIQUES FOR HERNIATED DISK

When other approaches to back pain caused by a herniated disk have not produced a lasting effect, surgery may be the best alternative. The two techniques described here are less invasive than open-back surgery (see above).

Chemonucleolysis In this treatment, the enzyme chymopapain, derived from the juice of the papaya, is injected into the herniated disk. This causes a chemical reaction that dissolves the bulging disk.

Some people have had success with chemonucleolysis, though it is infrequently performed in the United States because it can be followed by several days of severe pain and can cause an allergic reaction to the enzyme itself.

In addition, if chymopapain comes into contact with structures near the disk, serious neurological damage can result. Ask your doctor if he or she recommends the procedure for your disk problem.

Diskectomy In percutaneous ("through the skin") diskectomy, a portion of the damaged disk is removed through a small incision in the back. A hollow tube is inserted through an incision while the surgeon visualizes the site by fluoroscopy, a diagnostic procedure in which x-rays that have passed through the body

Compression of Spinal Nerves

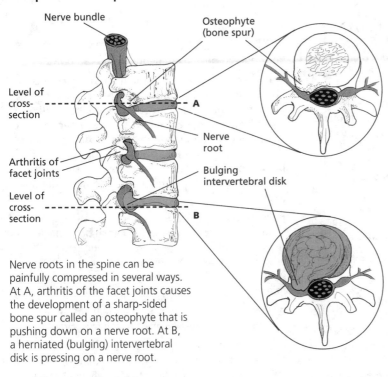

Nerve roots in the spine can be painfully compressed in several ways. At A, arthritis of the facet joints causes the development of a sharp-sided bone spur called an osteophyte that is pushing down on a nerve root. At B, a herniated (bulging) intervertebral disk is pressing on a nerve root.

and, often, sciatica (see p.619) when standing up straight, bending backward, or walking. Pain usually subsides when you sit down or bend forward, such as when pushing a shopping cart.

Sometimes you feel the pain more in your buttocks, thighs, and legs than in your back. It can therefore be confused with poor circulation to the legs, called intermittent claudication (see Atherosclerosis of the Arteries to the Legs, p.701). Spinal stenosis often causes pain when you stand or bend backward, whereas intermittent claudication does not.

TREATMENT OPTIONS

See your doctor if your back pain lasts for more than a few days and your symptoms are severe enough to interfere with your daily activities. The best test for spinal stenosis is magnetic resonance imaging (see p.150). Epidural (around the spinal cord) injections of corticosteroid medicines (see p.895) may provide temporary pain relief.

If your symptoms continue, and tests verify significant narrowing of your spinal canal, surgery may be performed to relieve the constricting pressure on the nerves of your spine. An incision is made in your back and the surgeon cuts out portions of the vertebrae contributing to the narrowing. Sometimes spinal fusion (in which several vertebrae are fused together permanently) is required to prevent the vertebrae from moving in the future.

A majority of the people treated by surgery eventually have good to excellent results; pain is either eliminated completely or can be controlled by

are projected onto a screen, providing a continuous image of the body's internal structures.

The probe is guided precisely through the skin, muscle sheath, and muscle and directed toward the disk's center. An automatic cutting, irrigating, and suctioning tool is inserted through the probe and used to remove some of the disk's contents.

This operation can reduce the pressure and the volume of material inside the disk, relieving the irritation on the nerve root. Percutaneous diskectomy requires only a local anesthetic (see p.168) and you can usually go home the same day.

Laser diskectomy is a variation in which a laser (beam of light) is used to vaporize part of the disk;

there are no good statistics on its effectiveness.

Spinal Stenosis

Spinal stenosis is a reduction in the size of the spinal canal, which puts pressure on the spinal nerves, causing varying degrees of pain and discomfort. Spinal stenosis mostly affects people over 65; however, some people have naturally smaller spinal canals and are more prone to the disorder. Spinal stenosis can also be caused by degenerating and bulging disks (see Herniated Disk, previous article).

SYMPTOMS

Spinal stenosis in the lower back causes lower back pain

What to Do for Back Pain

Back pain that lasts for several days or is severe enough to interfere with your daily routine is reason enough to see your physician. See your doctor immediately if you have had cancer in the past or if the pain is accompanied by fever, weight loss, problems controlling your bladder or bowels, numbness in your groin or anal area, or weakness in your legs. These symptoms can signal nerve damage (which could be irreversible if not promptly treated) or another serious cause.

Your doctor will perform a physical exam and may recommend one of the treatments below. If a physician recommends more invasive treatment—such as puncturing, penetrating, or cutting into your back—to treat your back pain, get a second opinion from another physician.

It is important to remember, even if you are in pain, that 90% of people who have sudden back pain get better within 4 weeks by using the minimal treatments listed here. For the majority of people with back pain, regardless of its intensity, the problem usually is caused by overuse, an unaccustomed activity such as lifting, or an injury.

Your doctor may recommend, or you can try:

■ Lying down on a bed or the floor in any comfortable position: pillows under your head and between your knees when lying on one side, under your knees when lying on your back, or crosswise under your hips when lying on your stomach. These positions reduce the forces that sitting or standing impose on your back, especially on the disks, ligaments, and muscles. Bed rest is generally recommended for a maximum of 3 days.

■ Physical activity helps develop the muscle tone necessary to support the back. Remain in bed only if pain requires it and, even then, try to get up and walk around every few hours even if it hurts a little. As soon as possible, try moderate exercise, such as swimming, riding a stationary bicycle, or walking.

■ Take over-the-counter nonsteroidal anti-inflammatory drugs or acetaminophen to relieve pain.

■ Apply cold and then heat to your back, which reduces discomfort. When your pain begins, use an ice pack to reduce swelling; then apply heat several days later to relax the muscles.

Benefits and Risks of Surgery for Spinal Stenosis

Surgery for spinal stenosis is usually performed only when all nonsurgical treatments have failed to provide enough relief. Surgery brings relief to many people, but it does not help about 25%. Other people require further surgery.

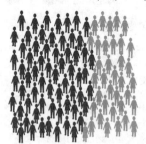

64 OF 100 PEOPLE WHO HAVE SPINAL STENOSIS AND UNDERGO SURGERY HAVE CONTINUED RELIEF OF PAIN 5 YEARS AFTER SURGERY

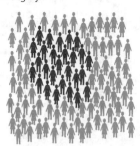

27 OF 100 PEOPLE WHO HAVE SPINAL STENOSIS AND UNDERGO SURGERY RETURN TO THE SAME LEVEL OF PAIN 5 YEARS AFTER SURGERY

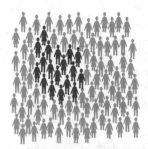

18 OF 100 PEOPLE WHO HAVE SPINAL STENOSIS AND UNDERGO SURGERY REQUIRE A REPEAT OPERATION 4 YEARS LATER

Preventing Back Pain

The best way to reduce the strain on your back is to stay in good physical condition. Concentrate on strengthening your abdominal muscles, which help hold you in an upright position. Lifting weights can strengthen your muscles and the supporting structures in your back.

Integrate exercise and the following preventive measures into your daily routine:

■ Maintain a good posture and avoid sudden or awkward twisting movements.

■ Do not wear high-heeled shoes; they cause your pelvis to tilt forward, increasing the strain on the muscles and ligaments that attach to your spine. Wear well-cushioned, supportive shoes that are flat or have very low heels.

■ At your workplace, check the height of your desk and computer to ensure that you are not overstretching to perform basic tasks. Chairs should provide lower-back support and your feet should rest on the floor.

■ If you sit for long periods, rest your feet on a low stool; if you stand, rest one foot on a low stool. Walk around and stretch periodically.

■ While driving, cushion the small of your back with a pillow. Stop occasionally on long trips to stretch your legs.

■ Learn to lift properly.

■ Learn relaxation techniques (see p.90) to reduce the stress and tension that can contribute to muscle fatigue and poor posture.

Everyday Prevention for Back Pain

Sit up straight; when you lean forward, bend from your hips instead of slouching.

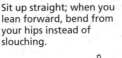

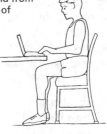

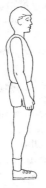

Stand with your head up, your chin in, your back flattened, and your pelvis straight.

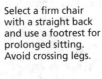

Select a firm chair with a straight back and use a footrest for prolonged sitting. Avoid crossing legs.

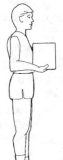

Hold heavy objects close to your body when you lift or carry.

When lifting, bend from your hips and knees, not your back.

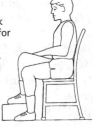

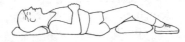

Sleep on a firm mattress. If you lie on your back, place a thin pillow under your knees.

Nonsurgical Approaches to Back Pain

Some people benefit from one or more nonsurgical treatments for back pain. Ask your physician whether he or she can recommend any of the following:

Back exercises Exercises intended to improve body mechanics can play a role in treating back pain. Several different programs with varying objectives exist. The benefits of exercises that are performed conscientiously may be substantial for some people.

"Back schools" These encompass many programs that teach people with back pain how to care for their backs and control symptoms. In good programs, trained instructors lead students through graduated exercise regimens as well as lessons in anatomy, self-care, and prevention. The success of these programs varies greatly.

Spinal manipulation Spinal manipulation is practiced by many health professionals, including chiropractors (practitioners who believe that the normal function of the spine can be restored by manipulating bones and joints), osteopaths (medical doctors who use medicine and surgery in addition to manipulation to treat disease), and physical therapists. For some people, manipulation provides relief from symptoms.

However, it is best performed only if you have had a prior medical evaluation by a physician to rule out infection or tumor of the spine, conditions that can be worsened by manipulation.

Braces A brace may provide relief of symptoms for people who have chronic back pain that does not respond to other treatments and for which there is no surgical solution. Fit and comfort are key criteria.

Traction Produced by weights, ropes, and pulleys, traction pulls on a part of the body and stretches it. It can be applied to the legs, pelvis, and upper body in various ways. The assumption is that stretching out the trunk will reduce pain and enhance recovery. Traction is actually no more effective than bed rest and may require hospitalization.

Transcutaneous electrical nerve stimulation (TENS) In this therapy, small electrodes are placed on the skin at or near sites of pain or dysfunction. They transmit a very low-voltage electric current to underlying tissues to provide pain-suppressing stimulation. Whether TENS has any appreciable benefit for people with lower back pain is controversial, but it is not harmful.

---

over-the-counter painkillers. Physical activity is possible with only minor restrictions. Rehabilitation, which can take 6 months, includes walking, riding a stationary bicycle, and/or swimming for gradually extended periods.

Arthritis of the Hip

Arthritis of the hip is inflammation and gradual deterioration of the hip joint. Osteoarthritis (see p.605) is the most common form of hip arthritis, but rheumatoid arthritis (see p.606) can also affect the hip joint.

SYMPTOMS

The symptoms of osteoarthritis in the hip can take years to develop; the symptoms of rheumatoid arthritis can begin more suddenly. With osteoarthritis, you may first notice muscle pain and stiffness, and later swelling, crackling, and grating (called crepitation), and pain that radiates to your buttocks, legs, knee, or groin.

TREATMENT OPTIONS

The treatment options for arthritis of the hip are generally the same as for osteoarthritis and rheumatoid arthritis. Hip replacement surgery may be required after many years of osteoarthritis, and sometimes in cases of rheumatoid arthritis.

Aseptic Necrosis

Aseptic necrosis develops when the small blood vessels in the ball of the femur, the long bone of the thigh, deliver insufficient blood to the bone, leading to degeneration of the hip joint. It is not known why aseptic necrosis occurs in some people, but it happens more often in people who abuse alcohol, who take corticosteroid drugs (see p.895) for a long time, or after injury. Surgery to repair or replace the damaged hip may be required (see Hip and Knee Replacement, p.629).

⃠ *Preventing Hip Fractures*

Take these three steps to prevent the possibility of hip fracture:

Avoid falling Preventing falls is described on p.1127.

Reduce the severity of a fall At least 90% of hip fractures occur during a fall; the next best thing to remaining upright is to reduce a fall's severity. Scientists have noted the design of football clothing in developing hip pads that reduce the impact of falling. One model involves pads built into a tight-fitting undergarment. A newer model is filled with a gel-like substance that conforms to the body during normal activities but stiffens rapidly on impact, deflecting force away from the hipbone. Ask your doctor about these pads.

Keep bones strong Increasing or maintaining bone density is the basis of preventing fractures. This is described in Preventing Osteoporosis, p.597.

Padded Garments Reduce Hip Fractures

ENERGY-ABSORBING PAD   **ENERGY-SHUNTING PAD**

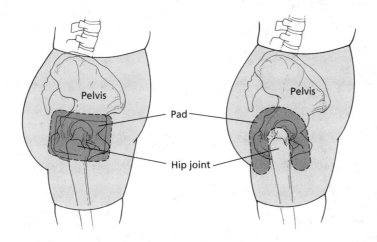

Hip fractures can be greatly reduced when special, tight-fitting undergarments are worn. Those that feature energy-absorbing pads (left) decrease the impact of a fall by absorbing energy in the pad material. Newer types (right) transfer energy away from the bone and into surrounding tissues upon impact. The model on the right has a U-shaped pad that fits over the hip, providing twice the cushioning.

Hip Fracture

A hip fracture is one or more breaks in the thighbone (femur) or pelvis. A broken hip usually results from a fall. However, in people with osteoporosis (see p.596), everyday activities, such as taking a step off the curb, may cause a fracture. Most common are breaks in the bone area between the top of the thigh's shaft and the ball joint of the hip; this causes shortening of the leg and severe pain in the hip that worsens with movement.

A broken hip is always serious; fewer than half of the people who break a hip return to full function or to the state of independence they previously enjoyed. Furthermore, the state of immobility from the hip fracture can lead to complications, such as pneumonia (see p.496) or pulmonary embolism (see p.512), that can be fatal. The outcome usually depends on the state of the bone and the condition of the individual.

A person with a suspected broken hip should go immediately to a hospital emergency department. The area will be x-rayed to confirm the fracture and the bone ends will be realigned and secured with screws or nails during an operation. Some people require hip replacement (see next article) surgery. See also Fractures, p.594.

Hip and Knee Replacement

Joint replacement is a major surgical procedure to replace a damaged joint with a prosthetic substitute. It is recommended when the original joint is so damaged that you cannot use it and it causes severe pain.

Most joints requiring replacement have been ravaged by osteoarthritis (see p.605), but sometimes joints damaged by rheumatoid arthritis or injury are replaced.

On average, the implanted joint components last from 10 to 15 years. Although the hips and knees are the most commonly replaced joints, joint replacement surgery can be performed on other joints, including those of the foot, shoulder, elbow, and finger.

If you are considering a hip or knee replacement:

■ Choose an orthopedic surgeon who is experienced and has a low complication rate. Your primary care physician or the Arthritis Foundation (see p.1229) are good resources to guide referral.

■ Have your surgeon describe the different kinds of prostheses available and explain which one is best for you.

■ Donate blood several weeks before surgery.

■ Attend all meetings with your physical therapist to learn exercises that can help before and after surgery.

■ Ask your doctor if you should look into rehabilitation hospitalization or home health care to help you after surgery.

■ Check your health insurance to see how much coverage you will receive for the joint replacement.

PROCEDURES

General anesthesia is used for both hip and knee replacement surgeries. For a hip replacement,

the surgeon makes a large incision on the outside of the hip and then moves surrounding muscle so that the hip joint is exposed.

The thighbone is removed from its socket to expose the ball of the joint, which is cut off. Next, the socket in the pelvis is enlarged and the pelvic bone is ground down to accommodate the ball that is part of the artificial joint.

For both hip and knee replacements, a metal shaft is driven into the marrow canal (the innermost canal) of the upper leg bone to anchor half of the artificial joint. The other half of the device is attached to the pelvic bone for hip replacement or to the shinbone (tibia) in knee replacement.

At the point of contact between the two halves of the

Artificial Hip and Knee Joints

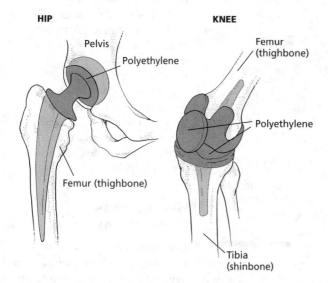

HIP

Pelvis

Polyethylene

Femur (thighbone)

KNEE

Femur (thighbone)

Polyethylene

Tibia (shinbone)

Artificial joints (shown in color) have metal shafts that are inserted into bone and anchored. At weight-bearing points, slick high-density polyethylene is used to reduce friction, as cartilage does in natural joints.

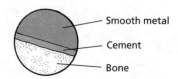

Smooth metal

Cement

Bone

Cement is used to fasten the artificial joint to the bone in many joint-replacement operations.

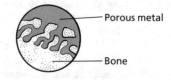

Porous metal

Bone

Cementless implants have a porous surface that bone tissue grows into, holding the prosthesis in place.

Benefits and Risks of Knee Replacement Surgery

Nearly everyone benefits, with minimal risk, from total knee replacement surgery.

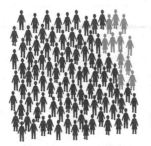

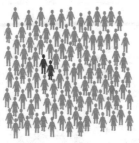

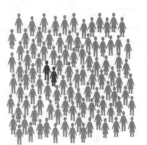

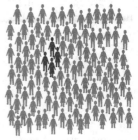

89 OF 100 PEOPLE WHO UNDERGO KNEE REPLACE-MENT SURGERY HAVE IMPROVEMENT IN KNEE PAIN AND FUNCTION

2 OF 100 PEOPLE WHO UNDERGO KNEE REPLACE-MENT SURGERY DEVELOP A SIGNIFICANT INFECTION, WHICH CAN BE TREATED WITH ANTIBIOTICS

2 OF 100 PEOPLE WHO UNDERGO KNEE REPLACE-MENT SURGERY GET BLOOD CLOTS THAT WILL TRAVEL FROM THEIR LEGS TO THEIR LUNGS (SEE P.512)

4 OF 100 PEOPLE WHO UNDERGO KNEE REPLACE-MENT SURGERY WILL HAVE TO REPEAT THE SURGERY BECAUSE OF INFECTION OR MALFUNCTION OF THE ARTI-FICIAL JOINT

metal joint, a coating of high-density plastic is used to reduce friction, much as cartilage does in a natural joint.

Knee replacements are the more complicated of the two procedures. In addition to implanting a new joint between the upper and lower leg bones, the surgeon also must replace or resecure the ligaments, which hold the knee together, so that the joint will be stable while allowing side-to-side movement and rotation.

Artificial joints are fastened to bones in two ways. In one method, the artificial joint is glued to natural bone using a strong adhesive; alternatively, the surgeon inserts an artificial joint made of porous materials, into which new bone cells migrate. Eventually enough new bone is made to hold the shaft firmly in natural bone.

Your age, general health, activity level, and bone quality are taken into account when deciding between the two options.

RECOVERY

Recovery requires time, patience, and work; plan on recovery taking about 6 weeks. Your doctor will encourage you to stand up and walk on your new joint

---

Living with a Joint Replacement

When joint replacement was first suggested to me, I was at one of life's low points. I was not doing the things I wanted to do, and the painful arthritis would keep me awake at night. But I did not like the idea of a foreign object in my knee. It took some convincing. I had my surgery in the middle of August. By September, I was off crutches. Going down stairs is the crucial test. In the second week of October, I made myself do it. I walked down the 27 stairs of the altar in full view of my congregation—without holding the railing.

Next week, I will be skiing in the World Championships, Masters Division. I cannot emphasize enough the importance of doing your flexibility exercises after surgery. Focus on flexibility, not strength. My other suggestion is to have one knee done at a time. There is a great deal of psychological benefit to be gained from having one leg working well. It is hard to focus on your postoperative exercises without one good leg to stand on.

John E., 75 years old

about a day after the operation with the aid of crutches, a cane, or a walker.

If you have a cemented prosthesis, it should be able to bear your full weight on the second day. If it is an uncemented prosthesis, you will need to use crutches or a walker for the first 6 weeks.

Exercise is an essential part of the recovery process. Your doctor and his or her staff will discuss the exercise program that best suits your needs. The risk of dislocating an artificial joint requires that you avoid strenuous activities and certain positions, and that you undergo physical therapy to build muscle.

Arthritis of the Knee

Arthritis of the knee is most often caused by osteoarthritis (see p.605) and less often by rheumatoid arthritis (see p.606). Osteoarthritis usually comes on gradually, whereas rheumatoid arthritis can begin more suddenly.

Symptoms include pain, swelling (which is more prominent in rheumatoid arthritis), stiffness, and a catching or creaking sensation in the knee. Analysis of x-rays and fluid obtained by placing a needle into your knee joint can help your doctor make a diagnosis.

Treatment includes acetaminophen, nonsteroidal anti-inflammatory drugs, and, less frequently, injections of corticosteroids (see p.895) for pain and swelling. Severe arthritis in the knee may require joint replacement (see previous article).

Although osteoarthritis is progressive, symptoms may stabilize

Structure of the Knee

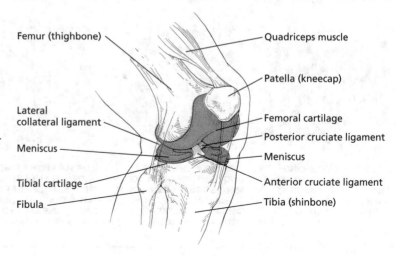

Femur (thighbone)
Quadriceps muscle
Patella (kneecap)
Lateral collateral ligament
Femoral cartilage
Posterior cruciate ligament
Meniscus
Meniscus
Tibial cartilage
Anterior cruciate ligament
Fibula
Tibia (shinbone)

The knee is an engineering marvel but is prone to injury. The meniscus, a type of cartilage sandwiched between the femur and the tibia, may be torn if the knee is twisted too far while it is bearing weight or because the meniscus has become weaker with age. The anterior cruciate ligament in the center of the joint is also prone to twisting injuries.

or even decrease for a time. Exercise, including brisk walking, stair climbing, and weight training, can help improve the stability and function of your knee.

Baker Cyst

A Baker cyst is a fluid-filled swelling behind the knee. It occurs when the fluid inside the synovial membrane (the membrane covering the knee joint) is pushed out to form a cystlike bulge. Baker cysts may accompany an inflammatory condition such as rheumatoid arthritis (see p.606) or occur after a knee injury. The cysts can be painless or they can rupture, causing considerable pain in the back of the

knee and down into the calf. Sometimes they block the veins passing through the knee, causing swelling in the legs and feet.

See your doctor if you feel a cyst. Usually, your doctor will be able to feel any cyst during a physical examination, but ultrasound (see p.148) can help with diagnosis. Your doctor may inject your knee with a corticosteroid medicine (see p.895) or, after numbing the area to be treated, cut out the cyst. Sometimes a Baker cyst goes away without treatment.

Bursitis of the Knee

Bursitis of the knee, also called anserine bursitis, is inflammation and distension of fluid in the

Knee Pain: *Dr Kay's Advice*

Many people who suddenly develop knee pain are told that an x-ray shows osteoarthritis. Particularly if the knee pain bothers a person at rest, that diagnosis is often wrong. A more common cause of knee pain is anserine bursitis, which can cause severe pain on the inner part of the knee that is worse with walking or when arising from a seated position in a chair. It often awakens affected people from sleep and causes them to place a pillow between their knees when going to bed.

Treatment with nonsteroidal anti-inflammatory drugs (NSAIDs) usually cures the problem. If the pills don't work, corticosteroid medicine injected into the bursa itself can fix the problem. Sometimes anserine bursitis is caused by bearing weight on the big-toe side of the foot when walking, causing stress on the inner part of the knee. Patients with this type of knee pain often benefit from the use of an insert in their shoes to correct this abnormality and to prevent recurrence of this painful yet very treatable condition.

JONATHAN KAY, MD
MASSACHUSETTS GENERAL HOSPITAL
HARVARD MEDICAL SCHOOL

bursa, a small, fluid-filled sac that cushions movement. The bursa may become inflamed due to repeated pressure on it, such as by extensive kneeling, infection, or injury. Symptoms include pain and swelling in the area just below the inside of the knee, along with stiffness. The skin over the bursa may feel warm and look red. Unless there is infection, bursitis of the knee usually resolves on its own within a few weeks with rest, which permits the excess fluid to be reabsorbed into the bloodstream. Applying ice and taking a nonsteroidal anti-inflammatory drug can help ease the pain and reduce the swelling. To treat more severe cases, a corticosteroid medicine (see p.895) may be injected into the bursa.

Runner's Knee

Runner's knee is pain at the front of your knee, sometimes with swelling, that is caused by inflammation of the tendons. It is usually caused by overusing or misusing the knee. The most common symptom of runner's knee is a dull pain around or under the kneecap. The pain worsens when walking up or down stairs or hills or while doing other activities that cause the knee to bear weight when straightened. This condition is most common among runners but also occurs in skiers, cyclists, and soccer players and is usually caused by improper technique.

Take nonsteroidal anti-inflammatory drugs for pain, apply an ice pack to your knee several times daily for several days, and

stop exercising the knee for a few days. If pain persists, your doctor may recommend that you switch to exercises that strengthen muscles without high impact, such as swimming, riding a stationary bicycle, and using a cross-country ski machine. In severe cases, an injection of corticosteroids (see p.895) may be used to relieve pain and swelling.

Torn Ligaments in the Knee

Ligaments, which your knee relies on for support, are tough bands of tissue that connect bones. Ligament injuries can range from a minor stretch to a complete tear and usually occur when the knee is twisted or hit hard. Most commonly damaged are the medial collateral ligament, which runs along the inner knee, and the anterior cruciate ligament, which is located in the center of the knee. Injuries to the medial collateral ligament usually heal on their own with a knee brace and rest, but tears of the anterior cruciate ligament do not. This type of injury can cause permanent knee instability, meaning that your knee may give way when it is rotated.

SYMPTOMS

When a ligament is torn, the pain is typically intense and immediate. Do not put weight on the injured knee; see a doctor immediately. Your leg may not be able to bear weight, go through a normal range of motion, or remain stable.

Arthroscopic Surgery

Arthroscopy is the use of a tiny, lighted optic tube called an arthroscope to visualize, diagnose, and treat some disorders inside a joint. In arthroscopic surgery, the doctor makes several tiny incisions (about the size of a buttonhole) and inserts pencil-sized instruments that hold a small lens and lighting system to magnify and illuminate the inside of the joint.

By attaching the arthroscope to a tiny TV camera, the surgeon can see the inside of your body without having to make the large incision that would be required for open surgery. The knee is the joint most often viewed and operated on through an arthroscope, but other joints (including the shoulder, elbow, ankle, hip, and wrist) may also be "scoped."

After administering a local anesthetic to numb the area being examined or, for very painful sites, a general anesthetic to put you to sleep, your doctor makes an incision and maneuvers the arthroscope into position. To increase visibility and enlarge the joint area, a sterile fluid may be injected into the joint. Several other incisions may be made to insert other instruments or to enable better viewing.

Arthroscopic surgery usually takes about an hour. In most cases, you can return home the same day. While you may feel good enough to return to your daily activities immediately, your doctor will advise you to avoid putting pressure on the treated joint for at least a week.

Arthroscopic Knee Surgery

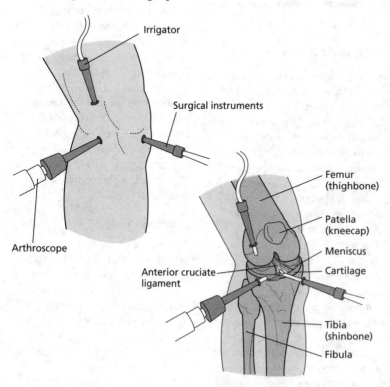

Irrigator

Surgical instruments

Arthroscope

Anterior cruciate ligament

Femur (thighbone)

Patella (kneecap)

Meniscus

Cartilage

Tibia (shinbone)

Fibula

In arthroscopic knee surgery, two small incisions are made to create portals for the arthroscope and irrigator, which infuses sterile fluid into the joint to distend it. Other incisions are made to accommodate surgical instruments that may be needed to cut, shave, remove particles, or repair tissue.

TREATMENT OPTIONS

The physician will examine your knee for motion and stability. If the knee is very swollen and painful, your doctor may remove fluid from the joint with a needle. The presence of blood in the fluid may indicate a torn ligament. For some people, a knee brace may provide enough stability, but many people require surgery.

The anterior cruciate ligament can be reconstructed by taking a tendon from another site near the knee and creating a new ligament. The operation is usually performed using an arthroscope (see Arthroscopic Surgery, p.634). Recovery from any ligament surgery is a long process. You will be on crutches for several weeks and will need to undergo several months of physical therapy to improve your knee's range of motion and to regain muscle strength.

Home treatment is generally recommended for minor ligament strains and sprains. Rest your knee, elevate it, and apply ice to minimize swelling and pain (see RICE for Sprains, p.636). A ligament strain or sprain may not fully heal for 4 to 6 weeks; avoid sports and other strenuous activities.

Torn Cartilage

Two small disks of protective cartilage, the medial meniscus and the lateral meniscus, are sandwiched between the femur (thighbone) and the tibia (shinbone). A torn cartilage usually refers to these structures, which may be damaged if the knee is twisted while it is bearing weight—for example, when turning to hit a tennis ball or dribbling a basketball around an opponent.

SYMPTOMS

Symptoms of a torn meniscus include pain (especially when the knee is straightened), buckling, swelling, clicking, and locking of the knee.

TREATMENT OPTIONS

Your physician may take x-rays of your knee and may use magnetic resonance imaging (see p.150) or arthroscopy (a type of endoscopy, see p.142) to confirm the diagnosis. In the past, surgeons removed all of the injured meniscus through a large incision. It was later discovered that this treatment caused some people to develop arthritis and deformities. Today, surgeons repair and preserve as much of the meniscus as possible during arthroscopic surgery (see p.634). This technique allows surgeons to remove only the torn segments of the meniscus, leaving unharmed portions in place. Recovery takes about a month.

A promising, experimental procedure involves taking samples of a person's cartilage-growing cells, making them reproduce in the test tube, and then transplanting them back into the joint to grow new cartilage. Time will tell whether this technique will improve outcomes.

Shin Splints

A shin splint is inflammation of and pain in the fibrous tissues that connect muscles to the front and side of the shins. Shin splints occur most often in people who perform high-impact sports (such as running, tennis, and basketball) in which constant pounding on a hard surface damages the shin. This injury is more common in active, athletic young people who exercise without stretching beforehand.

Symptoms include pain on the front of the shin, swelling, and redness. Treatment for shin splints includes RICE therapy (see p.636), nonsteroidal anti-inflammatory drugs, and using a shoe insert to help absorb impact. You can help prevent shin splints by stretching before exercising. If pain persists, your doctor will examine your leg and may take an x-ray to rule out a stress fracture (see Types of Fractures, p.595).

Ankle Fracture

Broken ankles frequently occur in young people during sports. Symptoms include sudden, severe pain (which is made worse with pressure), swelling, bruising, and sometimes deformity around the injured area. A minor fracture may be mistaken for a sprain (see next article). If pain in your apparently sprained ankle has not subsided within 3 days, the ankle may be fractured and you should see your doctor.

He or she will realign the bone ends and your foot will be immobilized with a cast or removable boot. Swelling may persist for some time even after the bones have healed. Use a support bandage to help reduce swelling once healing has occurred and during your rehabilitation exercises. Nonsteroidal anti-inflammatory drugs will help relieve pain. (See also Fractures, p.594.)

Ankle Sprain

A sprain is a stretched or torn ligament, tendon, or muscle. The ankle's anatomically vulnerable position leaves it susceptible to stress and injury; it is the most commonly sprained joint in the body. A sprained ankle usually occurs when you roll over onto the outside of your foot, thereby placing the full weight of your body on the ligaments supporting the ankle.

Symptoms, which vary in intensity depending on the severity of the injury, include pain, tenderness, redness, bruising, swelling, or loss of mobility of the ankle. Apply RICE therapy (see below) and do not put weight on the ankle. Take aspirin or ibuprofen for pain and to help reduce swelling. If you have any doubt about whether your ankle has been broken, see your doctor so that he or she can rule out a fracture (see previous article).

Ruptured Achilles Tendon

A ruptured Achilles tendon is a complete tear of the tendon (see What Do Tendons and Ligaments Do? p.612) that connects the calf muscle to the heelbone. As a result, the muscle is no longer joined to the bone, making it impossible for you to raise your heel off the ground. A torn or ruptured Achilles tendon causes sudden, severe pain, tenderness, and swelling. Sometimes, the break in the tendon is visible under the skin.

If you suspect that you have this injury, get medical help immediately. Surgery, in which the ends of the tendon are brought together and stitched, may be performed while you are under general anesthesia. In some cases, an extra piece of tendon taken from another muscle in the calf is stitched around the reattached ends as a reinforcement. The incision is stitched closed and the leg is immobilized in a cast that extends from foot to knee, with your foot positioned so that it points downward to facilitate healing of the tendon. Complete recovery takes at least 3 months, including an exercise rehabilitation program to help you regain full range of movement and to reduce stiffness.

Achilles Tendonitis

Achilles tendonitis is inflammation in the Achilles tendon. Without treatment, this condition can become chronic, increasing the risk of a rupture (see previous article). The Achilles tendon connects the calf muscles to the heel. It is the largest tendon in the body, and is also the strongest, withstanding great force each time the body's weight is raised on the forefoot and toes. Achilles tendonitis is usually an overuse injury that predominately occurs in runners and other athletes who run. It occasionally is a sign of a body-wide joint condition such as ankylosing spondylitis (see p.602).

The pain is most severe just above the back of the heel. At first it occurs only with sprinting or prolonged running. In advanced cases, however, even climbing stairs produces pain, and the tendon may become stiff

RICE for Sprains

RICE is a mnemonic device to help you remember the treatment for a sprain—rest, ice, compression, and elevation. If you have any doubt about whether your injury may be a fracture (see p.594), see your doctor. Otherwise, be vigilant about following these steps:

Rest is vital to the recovery of injured tissue. Do not use the affected area for several days.

Ice the affected joint during the first 24 hours after the injury. It helps reduce inflammation and pain. If you do not have an ice pack, put ice in a plastic bag and wrap it with a thin towel or use a bag of frozen vegetables. Apply the ice constantly or in intervals for 24 hours.

Compression of the injured area with an elastic bandage helps reduce swelling, but do not wrap the bandage too tightly.

Elevation of the sprained joint for the first 24 hours, including during sleep, helps drain fluid and reduce swelling.

Calf Stretch to Prevent Achilles Tendonitis

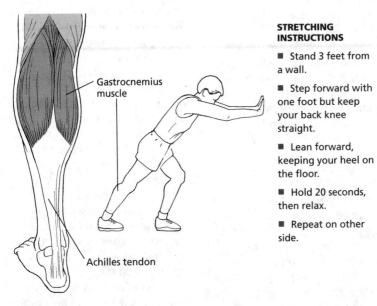

STRETCHING INSTRUCTIONS

- Stand 3 feet from a wall.

- Step forward with one foot but keep your back knee straight.

- Lean forward, keeping your heel on the floor.

- Hold 20 seconds, then relax.

- Repeat on other side.

Achilles tendonitis is caused by sudden and strenuous stretching of the Achilles tendon during exertion. To prevent this injury, stretch your calf muscle and Achilles tendon before exercising.

and swollen. Achilles tendonitis should be treated as early as possible.

If you have a mild case, your doctor may recommend stretching your Achilles tendon before you run (see Calf Stretch to Prevent Achilles Tendonitis, above), applying ice afterward, and using nonsteroidal anti-inflammatory drugs for pain. For severe or persistent tendonitis, some athletes wear a splint or cast to immobilize their aching tendons.

Broken Bones in the Foot

Foot fractures usually occur on the metatarsals, the bones that make up the middle of the foot. Pounding the foot against the ground (as in jogging) or falling are the most common causes of bone fractures in the foot, but simply stepping off a curb in an awkward manner can break a foot bone.

Symptoms include swelling and bruising around the injured area, sometimes with deformity, accompanied by severe pain and loss of function. Putting pressure on your foot or moving it will make pain worse.

Small fractures can be mistaken for a sprain (see p.635). If an apparent sprain has not healed within 3 days, see your doctor. He or she will take an x-ray to see if there has been a fracture.

Broken metatarsal bones are usually treated with a cast; broken toes are usually treated by "buddy taping" (taping the broken toe to a healthy adjacent toe). Your doctor may recommend nonsteroidal anti-inflammatory drugs to relieve pain.

Bunions

A bunion is a firm bump that forms at the base of the big toe joint due to a deformity or enlargement of the bones of the big toe, causing them to push out. As this bony protrusion rubs against your shoe, the skin may redden and the underlying bursa swells and becomes painfully inflamed. The resulting bursitis (inflammation of the bursa) may be severe enough to cause you to limp.

Women develop bunions about ten times more often than men, probably because they are more likely to wear shoes that are narrow, pointed, and high-heeled; pressure from the shoe causes the deformity of the toe joint. The prevalence of bunions increases with age, both because older people are more likely to have arthritis-related deformities of their feet and because many people do not wear shoes that accommodate the shape of their feet. Once a bunion arises, soft leather shoes that are wide enough, have low heels, and lace up can reduce pressure and pain. Other good footwear choices include athletic shoes with soft toe boxes or open sandals with straps that do not touch the irritated area.

You can also protect the bunion with a thick, doughnut-shaped moleskin pad, which relieves pressure from your shoe. Custom-made shoe inserts that help redistribute your weight and take pressure off the bunion can also help. Nonsteroidal anti-inflammatory drugs can ease pain and swelling.

When bunions make wearing shoes difficult and all other remedies have failed, your physician may recommend a bunionectomy, surgery in which the bunion is reduced by cutting or straightening the bone so that the toe points directly ahead. A special walking shoe, splint, or cast, as well as crutches, are needed for several weeks after surgery.

Fallen Arches

Fallen arches are feet that have little or no arch between the heel and toes, resulting in a sole that rests flat on the ground. Nearly everyone has flat feet at birth; the arches do not develop fully until about age 6, after the ligaments and muscles in the soles are completely formed.

Some people never develop arches in their feet; others get flatter feet over time as the ligaments that normally support the arches loosen or stretch (or, in rare cases, after a tendon on the inner side of the foot ruptures), usually due to weight gain.

Many people with fallen arches have no symptoms, but others experience fatigue, pain, or stiffness in the feet, legs, and lower back. If you have painful fallen arches, your doctor may prescribe custom-designed arch supports for your shoes to help redistribute your weight over your feet. Exercises can help strengthen ligaments and muscles that have become weak.

Foot and Heel Pain

The human foot is an engineering marvel. It must provide stability, yet it must also be flexible enough to accommodate uneven surfaces. It must be strong in order to act as a rigid lever that propels your body forward with each stride, yet it must be supple enough to absorb the impact of each step. To do all this, the foot has 26 bones, more than 100 ligaments, and 19 muscles—not counting the 12 leg muscles that connect it to the rest of the body. Over the course of an average day, the feet are subjected to weight loads equivalent to several hundred tons.

As you age, your feet may widen. Many foot and heel problems are aggravated by ill-fitting shoes. Foot pain can also be a

---

Swollen Legs, Ankles, or Feet

Swelling, or edema, of the legs, ankles, and feet causes them to feel bloated and heavy. Throughout the body, fluids normally pass back and forth between the blood and the tissues. When there is extra pressure in the veins of the legs, fluid is forced out of the blood and into the tissues.

The most common cause of such excess pressure in the leg veins is gravity due to long periods of standing, or age-related changes in the leg veins. Leg swelling is also often a premenstrual sign, probably because the small blood vessels become "leaky" for unknown reasons.

Leg swelling also occurs during pregnancy, mainly because the pressure of the enlarged uterus slows the return of blood from the leg veins to the heart. If you are pregnant, excessive, persistent swelling of your feet can indicate preeclampsia (see p.932), and should be reported to your doctor immediately.

Another common cause is varicose veins (see p.706),

which also slow the return of blood from leg veins to the heart.

Although swollen legs are seldom an emergency, they can sometimes signal a medical problem such as a blood clot, infection, or heart failure (see p.683). Swelling can also be a sign of malnutrition or serious disorders of the liver, kidneys, or intestine.

Several simple, effective measures can help relieve swelling. In a reclining position, elevate your feet. Wearing support hose can also help. Walking can help improve swelling from varicose veins. For those who are overweight, weight loss is beneficial because it reduces pressure on the veins of the legs.

Swollen legs can also be helped by dietary changes, especially by cutting down on the sodium (salt) in your diet. If these approaches fail, your doctor may prescribe a diuretic drug to increase the rate at which your body excretes fluids. Your doctor should check your potassium level if you are taking a diuretic.

complication of medical conditions such as diabetes (see p.832), poor circulation, arthritis (see p.605), gout (see p.604), and obesity (see p.853).

Foot and heel pain can usually be treated successfully, but resolution is often slow. Wear well-fitting shoes with soft, shock-absorbent soles. Orthotic devices, such as shoe inserts that help redistribute your weight over the foot, may absorb some of the impact on the feet and heels. Your doctor may recommend nonsteroidal anti-inflammatory drugs to relieve pain and inflammation or suggest alternating heat and cold applications on the affected area. Foot and heel pain almost always disappears with time. Read the articles in this section to find out if your pain is related to a specific structure of the foot.

Foot Ulcers

Foot ulcers are open sores on the surface of the foot. Foot ulcers can be caused by poor circulation; because of this, people with diabetes (see p.832) are more prone to them. When there is insufficient arterial blood to the foot, tissues are starved for nutrition, and when there is impaired return of blood in the leg veins to the heart, tissue in the foot can break down.

Foot ulcers can also be caused by nerve damage that prevents the sensation of pain, by constant pressure on the foot (such as the pressure that often occurs on the heels of people who are bedridden), or by poorly fitting shoes. The ulcer may or may not be painful. If the ulcer is infected, it will produce pus.

Burning Feet

A continual burning or stinging sensation in the feet is relatively common, especially in people over age 65. This condition may be caused by nerve damage called polyneuropathy, by athlete's foot (see p.530), or by allergic reactions to socks or chemicals in shoes.

Diagnosis, cause, and treatment of polyneuropathy require your doctor's attention. However, if burning feet are caused by something less serious, you may get relief from the following home remedies:

- Place your feet in cool water twice a day for 15 minutes.

- Reduce the amount of time you stand.

- Wear shoes that do not cramp your feet (make sure your shoes are made of a material that allows your feet to breathe).

- Wear socks made of cotton.

If you have a foot ulcer, see your physician. Although most ulcers can be treated without surgery, an infected ulcer can lead to gangrene (see p.878). In severe cases, surgery to increase the blood supply to the feet, or even amputation, may be necessary.

Your physician may recommend preventive measures such as the use of support stockings to aid in circulation, as well as keeping your feet elevated above your heart. This will also reduce swelling and help the ulcer drain.

Hammer Toe

Hammer toe is a deformity in which the bones of one or more of the smaller toes curl downward into a clawlike position. This disorder is usually caused by ill-fitting shoes, although it may be set in motion by a tight tendon (which prevents the toe from resting flat on the ground), muscle weakness, or arthritis (see p.604). The second toe is most

often affected, and it often has a corn on it (see p.555) from the pressure of being in contact with a shoe.

Discomfort can be relieved by using a toe pad, sold in drugstores. Your doctor may also suggest a splint, exercises, or a shoe insert that helps redistribute your weight on the foot. In addition, wearing shoes with roomier, extra-depth toe boxes will keep your toes from bunching. Hammer toe becomes harder to treat if the toes stiffen. In severe cases, a small piece of bone may be surgically removed so that the toe can resume a normal position.

Morton Neuroma

Morton neuroma is an irritation of a nerve in the foot caused by two metatarsal bones (the bones that make up the central arch of the foot) rubbing together. The resulting enlargement of the nerve can produce an array of troubling sensations, including severe pain, burning, cramping, and numbness, which may be felt not only between the toes but also in the balls of the feet. People who have a Morton neuroma sometimes compare the pain to the discomfort of stepping repeatedly on a pebble, marble, or nail.

Roomier shoes, pads that relieve pressure on the neuroma, and an injection of corticosteroids (see p.895) into the painful area can all bring relief. If these treatments fail, the growth may need to be surgically removed. Although surgery is usually successful, the nerve tissue may grow back and form another neuroma.

Plantar Fasciitis

Plantar fasciitis, inflammation of the fibrous tissue on the bottom of the heel and underneath the foot, is a common cause of heel pain. In some people, poor footwear provokes the condition; in many others, plantar fasciitis occurs without any apparent reason.

SYMPTOMS

Plantar fasciitis produces pain that is most severe on the inner portion of the sole just in front of the heel. The area is tender when pressure is applied, and the pain increases when the foot is flexed upward. The pain is most severe with the very first step in the morning. It usually subsides as the tissues warm up and stretch out with walking, only to recur after periods of inactivity.

TREATMENT OPTIONS

The first step to recovery is to rest the inflamed tissues, but you

Common Foot Problems

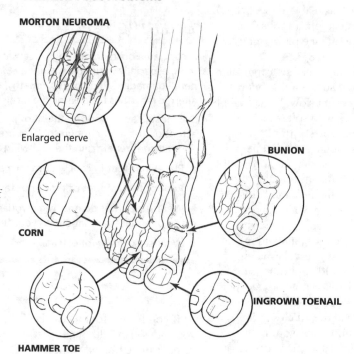

MORTON NEUROMA

Enlarged nerve

CORN

HAMMER TOE

BUNION

INGROWN TOENAIL

Morton neuroma is a noncancerous tumor. It may be caused by the rubbing together of two metatarsal bones (the bones that make up the central arch of the foot). Severe pain, burning, cramping, and numbness are common symptoms.

Corns are small areas of thickened skin that develop on the top or side of the foot due to excessive rubbing, often from poorly fitting shoes.

Bunions are characterized by hard, fluid-filled sacs that form on the outside of the big toe due to irritation; the toe may also be deformed.

Hammer toe is a deformity in which the bones of one or more of the smaller toes, usually the second toe, curl downward into a clawlike position. Ill-fitting shoes are the primary culprits, although muscle weakness and arthritis can also cause it.

Ingrown toenails usually occur from cutting your nails improperly. If nails are not cut straight across, the skin presses against the nail of the toe; irritation, pain, and infection may result.

do not have to stay off your feet. Instead, cushion your aching heel by placing a simple quarter-inch foam pad in the heel of your shoes. If this does not help, try wearing a heel cup. The next option is an over-the-counter shoe insert. Wear the cushion in all your shoes, including street shoes and athletic footwear.

To reduce inflammation, apply ice to your heel for 10 to 15 minutes after you have been active. Nonsteroidal anti-inflammatory drugs can relieve pain and swelling. Stretching exercises are important. Before you get out of bed in the morning, move your foot up and down, then left and right, to warm up your tissues. Repeat the maneuvers before you walk.

Since a tight Achilles tendon places stress on the heel, stretch it every day as described in Calf Stretch to Prevent Achilles Tendonitis (see p.637). Your doctor may refer you to a podiatrist for custom-fitted orthotic devices or for the most effective exercises for your condition. If your pain persists, consider ultrasound (see p.148) treatments. If these treatments do not provide relief, your physician may suggest an injection of corticosteroid medicine (see p.895).

Heel Spurs

Heel spurs are bony projections that develop on the surface of the calcaneus—the heel bone. They look sharp and often are blamed for severe heel pain. However, in most cases, plantar fasciitis (see previous article) causes the pain in a heel that also happens to have a spur. Usually, treatment for plantar fasciitis relieves the pain, even though nothing has been done to remove the spur. Try the remedies for plantar fasciitis before considering an operation for heel spurs.

Leg Cramps

Cramps, or contraction of the muscles, in the calves and lower legs are very common, especially after exercise and, for some people, at night. Cramps that occur with exercise may be caused by poor circulation and can indicate peripheral vascular disease (see p.701). Most cramps that occur with exercise are not caused by problems with the circulation but by muscle injury; they can be avoided by stretching your calves (see p.637) before and after working out.

You may be able to stop a cramp from progressing by flexing your calf when you feel the first twinge. If this fails, press your foot firmly against the floor and walk around. Some doctors believe that quinine supplements, available in tonic water or in over-the-counter formulas, can reduce the frequency of leg cramps. Do not take quinine if you are pregnant, have quinine hypersensitivity, or have a glucose-6-phosphate dehydrogenase deficiency (see Hemolytic Anemia, p.719).

Taking vitamin E (in the daily dose of 400 international units) seems to work for some people. Your body's potassium level could be low, particularly if you are taking diuretic medicines. Eating several bananas can help restore your potassium level. Taking a magnesium supplement on a daily basis has also helped people avoid leg cramps.

Heart, Blood Vessels, and Circulation

THE HEART AND THE BLOOD

Your blood carries nutrients to every cell in your body and, at the same time, carries away waste material produced by the cells. To accomplish this task, blood must constantly circulate (see How You Circulate Blood, p.108). The heart and blood vessels are responsible for moving the blood throughout the body.

Pumping the blood The heart is a pump and, although it is only the size of a fist, it has remarkable strength and endurance. The heart is a muscle made up of four chambers. Oxygen-depleted blood returning from the veins of the body enters the upper chamber on the right side of the heart (the right atrium) and drops into the lower chamber (the right ventricle), where it is pumped through the pulmonary artery into the lungs.

As it passes through the lungs, blood takes up new oxygen and gives off the waste product carbon dioxide. The blood then returns from the lungs through the pulmonary veins, enters the upper chamber on the left side of the heart (the left atrium), drops into the lower chamber (left ventricle), and is pumped out to the body through the aorta, the largest artery.

Your Heart

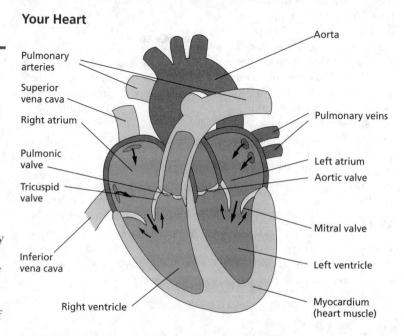

- Aorta
- Pulmonary arteries
- Superior vena cava
- Right atrium
- Pulmonic valve
- Tricuspid valve
- Inferior vena cava
- Right ventricle
- Pulmonary veins
- Left atrium
- Aortic valve
- Mitral valve
- Left ventricle
- Myocardium (heart muscle)

Oxygen-rich blood enters the left atrium from the pulmonary vein. The atrium conducts blood to the left ventricle, which pumps the blood through the aorta, the body's main artery. The aorta divides into smaller arteries that then divide and redivide like branches of a tree until they become microscopically thin capillaries that reach virtually every tissue in the body. The body tissues extract oxygen and nutrients from the blood and deposit waste material (including carbon dioxide) into the blood. On the return trip, the oxygen-depleted blood is propelled into the right atrium. From there, blood empties into the right ventricle, which pumps the blood into the pulmonary artery and then into the lungs, where carbon dioxide leaves and oxygen enters the blood.

Every minute, the pumping of the ventricles circulates 5 quarts of blood through your body. The blood travels through 60,000 miles of blood vessels to reach all tissues. Your heart beats all the time, whether you are asleep or awake, and will have beat about 2 to 3 billion times by the time you are 80 years old.

The rhythm of the heart The pumping rhythm of the heart is started by a small group of pacemaker cells in the heart muscle called the sinoatrial (SA) node.

The SA node is located in the right atrium. It beats automatically but also takes orders from the brain. The brain is constantly monitoring the level of physical exertion, the amount of oxygen in the blood, and the pressure in the arteries. If the brain senses a need to increase or decrease heart rate, it can send a signal over nerves that lead to the SA node.

For example, if you stand up from a resting position too abruptly, your blood pressure can quickly drop, making you feel dizzy. This reduction in blood pressure is detected by nerve endings in the arteries, which relay the information to the brain. The brain then sends a message over nerves to the SA node, which tells the heart to speed up.

To get the heart to beat, the SA node first sends an electrical signal that causes the two atria to contract, which pumps blood down into the ventricles below them. Then the signal reaches a second group of specialized cells called the atrioventricular (AV) node.

From there, special bundles of fibers (called bundle branches) carry the signal into the left and right ventricles, telling them to contract and pump blood out of the heart.

A wide variety of abnormalities can affect the rhythm of the heart. Some of these can be very serious; others are harmless and may not require treatment.

The heart valves The heart contains four important valves that direct blood to flow correctly through the heart. Between the left atrium and left ventricle is the mitral valve, and between the

right atrium and right ventricle is the tricuspid valve.

These valves act like gates between the atria and ventricles—opening to allow blood to be pumped from the atria to the ventricles and closing to prevent blood from flowing backward into the atria when the ventricles pump.

Between the left ventricle and the aorta is the aortic valve, and between the right ventricle and the pulmonary artery is the pulmonic valve. These valves allow blood to be pumped out of the heart and keep the blood from flowing backward into the heart. When these valves are injured, the heart can malfunction.

The covering of the heart The heart is covered by a thin lining called the pericardium. The pericardial sack protects and contains the heart. When inflamed, it can interfere with the pumping action of the heart and cause chest pain.

THE CIRCULATION: ARTERIES AND VEINS

Arteries are blood vessels that carry blood from the heart to the lungs and throughout your body. The walls of arteries are composed of three layers: an inner lining, middle membranes and muscle, and outer connective tissue.

Arteries divide and redivide like the branches of a tree until, finally, the tubes become microscopically thin blood vessels called capillaries, which feed nearly every tissue in the body.

When arteries pass through the liver and kidneys, the blood gets rid of some waste material. When it passes through the in-

testines, it picks up nutrients. As it travels through the body, blood picks up and drops off many different substances (such as hormones and nutrients). See How You Circulate Blood, p.108.

Like any tissue, the heart muscle requires a constant blood supply in order to survive. The coronary arteries provide blood to the heart muscle. Coronary artery disease (see p.652) occurs when these arteries become damaged by fat deposits (such as in atherosclerosis, see p.653) that block the flow of blood to the heart muscle.

The coronary arteries wrap around the surface of the heart. The aorta, the largest artery, sends blood to the left main coronary artery. This vessel divides into two more branches: the left anterior descending artery and the circumflex artery.

These branches carry blood to the front, side, and back of the heart. The right coronary artery is another vessel that branches off the aorta; it feeds the right side and bottom of the heart.

The arteries through which oxygen-rich blood passes become progressively narrower. The smaller tubes are called arterioles; the smallest blood vessels are the capillaries.

Only one cell thick and finer than a human hair, the very thin capillaries allow passage of oxygen and nutrients from the blood to the tissues and of carbon dioxide and wastes from tissues to the blood. This transfer of substances between the blood and the tissues could never take place in the arteries because the walls are too thick.

After blood has passed

through the capillaries, it enters the venules, the smallest and narrowest veins. It then flows through veins that grow progressively wider and larger until it reaches the body's largest vein, the vena cava, and then enters the right atrium of the heart.

On its return trip from the body through the veins, heading to the heart, blood moves at a much slower pace than it does when it is pumped through the arteries to the body. It is propelled less by the pumping heart and more by contracting muscles (which compress the walls of veins).

One-way valves in the veins prevent blood from being pulled backward and away from the heart by gravity.

BLOOD PRESSURE

Blood Pressure

Blood pressure is essential for life. Everyone needs to have a certain amount of blood pressure to keep the circulation going.

Without adequate blood pressure, blood would not be able to reach the cells in your body to supply them with the oxygen and nutrients they need for life. Think of the water pressure in the pipes of your home. The water pressure must be high enough to get hot water from the heater in the basement to a shower on the second floor.

Similarly, normal blood pressure allows the heart and the circulation to get enough blood from the heart to all cells of the body.

When the heart pumps, pressure in the arteries temporarily increases (systolic pressure). When the heart relaxes between beats, pressure in the arteries temporarily decreases (diastolic pressure).

Each beat creates a wave of pressure that starts in the left ventricle, then moves outward through all the arteries of the body.

High, Normal, and Low Blood Pressure

The level of your blood pressure profoundly affects your health. High blood pressure greatly increases your risk for heart disease, stroke, and other serious illnesses.

To classify your blood pressure, the doctor or other health professional averages two or more readings taken after you have been seated quietly for at least 5 minutes. For example, if you have a blood pressure of 135/85 mm Hg on one occasion

How Blood Pressure Is Measured

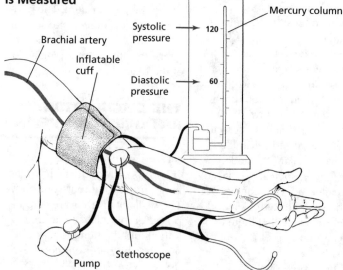

To measure blood pressure, a cuff is wrapped around your arm and a stethoscope is placed below the cuff to listen for the heartbeat in the brachial artery. The cuff is pumped up to exert increasing pressure and is attached to a column of mercury, which measures the pressure. The pressure in the cuff is pumped up to a level higher than your systolic pressure. The cuff's pressure keeps any blood from flowing through the artery, so no heartbeat is heard. Slowly the pressure in the cuff is lowered; when it reaches your systolic pressure, the heartbeat can suddenly be heard. In this example, the sounds began to appear at a systolic pressure of 120 millimeters of mercury (mm Hg). When cuff pressure is reduced below the diastolic pressure in the artery, the heartbeat sound disappears. In this example, it occurs at a diastolic pressure of 60 mm Hg.

and 145/95 mm Hg on another, you have an average blood pressure of 140/90 mm Hg.

As shown in the table below, a blood pressure of less than 120/80 is considered "normal"—unless it is too low, as we discuss later. People with normal blood pressure have the lowest risk of developing heart disease and stroke problems. People in the "prehypertension" category have a greatly increased risk of developing hypertension, and require lifestyle changes to reduce the risk. People with Stage 1 hypertension generally require medication, although aggressive changes in lifestyle can sometimes eliminate the need for medication. People with Stage 2 hypertension require medications along with lifestyle changes.

Blood pressure that is below 80/50 mm Hg is very unusual in a person who feels healthy; usually such a low blood pressure is a sign of illness. A blood pressure this low may not be able to pump adequate amounts of blood, oxygen, and nutrients to the brain and other parts of the body.

The brain is the organ that is most quickly damaged when the circulation is slowed or stops. Low blood pressure in someone who is feeling ill may indicate significant dehydration, bleeding, poor heart function, or an infection that needs to be treated. Immediate medical treatment is required.

A reading in the range of 130 to 139 over 85 to 89 mm Hg is considered "high/normal" and should be rechecked yearly, sometimes more often.

Shock

When there is not enough blood flowing through the body to supply the oxygen and nutrients your cells need for survival, it creates a life-threatening condition known as shock. People who develop shock can die if the condition is not treated promptly.

Shock results from extremely low blood pressure. Sometimes this lack of pressure in the arteries is brought on by a heart problem that prevents the heart muscle from pumping out enough blood to supply the body.

The most common examples are a heart attack (see p.663) and serious rhythm abnormalities (see Abnormal Heart Rate and Rhythm, p.672) that keep the left ventricle of the heart from pumping adequately.

Sometimes low blood pressure results from inadequate amounts of blood. One common cause is severe dehydration, which diminishes the amount of fluid in the blood. Dehydration caused by prolonged vomiting, diarrhea, or inadequate intake of fluids can cause low blood pressure.

Another cause is heavy bleeding that results in the loss of more than 20% of the body's blood. Blood loss of this magnitude can follow a severe injury or be the result of bleeding from the stomach or intestines. The rupture of a thoracic aortic aneurysm or abdominal aortic aneurysm can also quickly lead to shock.

Shock can also quickly develop from the toxins produced by severe infections. A form of shock called anaphylaxis is brought on by a severe allergic reaction, which causes vessels to dilate (open up) and leak fluid.

SYMPTOMS

Shock is defined by the combination of low blood pressure (particularly compared to your normal blood pressure) and symptoms that indicate there is not enough blood flowing through the body to supply the brain and other organs. Symptoms can include mental confusion; cool, clammy skin; and reduced urine production.

Blood tests may indicate that certain organs, particularly the liver and kidneys, are not functioning normally. Rapid pulse, shallow breathing, and loss of consciousness can also accompany shock.

TREATMENT OPTIONS

Shock requires emergency medical treatment. Medical care for shock includes restoring blood volume by administering fluid and blood, using medicines to

CATEGORY	SYSTOLIC BLOOD PRESSURE (MM HG)		DIASTOLIC BLOOD PRESSURE (MM HG)
Normal	Less than 120	and	Less than 80
Prehypertension	120–139	or	80–89
Stage 1 hypertension	140–159	or	90–99
Stage 2 hypertension	Over 160	or	Over 100

Lifestyle Changes to Prevent and Treat High Blood Pressure

There are steps you can take to help prevent the development of high blood pressure, and to help treat it without using drugs.

■ **Load up on fruits and vegetables.** A diet containing lots of fruits and vegetables appears to be the single best dietary approach to preventing high blood pressure. Such a diet contains fiber, potassium, magnesium, and calcium, all of which seem to protect against high blood pressure.

■ **Eat potassium-rich foods.** A diet rich in potassium protects against high blood pressure and strokes. Potassium-rich foods include oranges, bananas, raisins, figs, baked potatoes with skin, baked beans, low-fat yogurt, and bran cereal.

■ **Skip the salt.** If you have high blood pressure, avoid salty foods and do not add salt to foods. If you do not have high blood pressure, there is controversy as to whether avoiding salty foods will protect you against getting it. Some people seem to be more sensitive to salt and benefit from cutting down on salty foods. More recent studies indicate that salt reduction may be especially beneficial for people over age 60 and for African Americans.

■ **Trim down and shape up.** The bigger you are, the harder the heart has to work to pump blood to all parts of your body. Reducing your weight to a normal level can be all that is necessary to prevent or cure high blood pressure. Losing extra pounds has a big impact on your blood pressure even if you do not get down to your ideal weight. This is especially true for people who carry their extra bulk around the waist—those who are apple-shaped rather than pear-shaped (see p.48). The relationship between high blood pressure and being overweight is especially pronounced for young to middle-aged adults.

■ **Exercise.** Even if you are not overweight, exercise can reduce high blood pressure. Aerobic exercise, such as jogging, biking, or brisk walking, three to five times a week for at least 30 minutes has been shown to be effective in preventing high blood pressure. It is not entirely clear how this happens, but a reasonable theory is that exercise widens the millions of arterioles in your body, thereby reducing resistance to blood flow. Exercise also conditions the heart to pump more efficiently, reducing its workload.

■ **Reduce excessive alcohol consumption.** Drinking more than two alcoholic beverages a day—two glasses of wine, two beers, or two shots of hard liquor (see How Much Alcohol in Your Drink? p.64)—significantly raises your risk of having high blood pressure. However, there is some evidence that one alcoholic drink a day can lower blood pressure. Reducing your alcohol intake can sometimes diminish your need for antihypertensive medicine.

■ **Stop smoking.** If you have high blood pressure, smoking increases your risk of having a heart attack.

■ **Practice relaxation techniques.** Various kinds of behavioral therapy, including biofeedback, yoga, and tai chi, may have some beneficial effect on high blood pressure. Studies indicate that the effect is not great—and not enough for people who have a serious degree of high blood pressure. However, for some people, it may be enough to reduce the need for drugs. See The Relaxation Response: Dr Benson's Advice (p.90).

increase blood pressure by narrowing the small arteries, or using medicines to strengthen the pumping action of the heart.

Emergency personnel also use medical antishock trousers that compress the veins in the legs, squeezing blood from the legs into the heart. Giving extra oxygen through a mask or plastic tubes (nasal prongs) into the nose increases the body's supply of oxygen. Once the blood pressure is in the normal range, treatment is directed at the cause of the shock.

High Blood Pressure

High blood pressure, or hypertension, is a condition in which the pressure of the blood in the arteries is too high. It is one of the greatest threats to public health in the developed nations of the world, both because it is so common and because, unchecked, it leads to a host of devastating complications, including heart attacks and strokes.

High blood pressure often causes no symptoms until it has already caused a significant amount of damage to the body, which is why it is known as "the silent killer." One of the most important things you can do is to have your blood pressure checked during regular visits to your doctor.

Blood pressure goes up when the heart pumps blood with more force or the arterioles narrow, creating more resistance to the circulating blood.

To understand how the narrowing of the arterioles can affect blood pressure, imagine squeezing a tube of toothpaste. If the tube has a normal-sized opening, you only have to squeeze the tube with normal pressure; the toothpaste can flow through the opening easily and controllably.

However, if the opening were the size of a pinhole, you would have to squeeze a lot harder to push toothpaste through the hole.

High blood pressure can be a normal response of the body when there is an increased demand for blood and its nutrients. When you exercise, your heart rate increases and your heart contracts more forcefully. At peak exercise, your blood pressure is at its highest level.

The brain constantly senses your blood pressure. When your brain determines that your body needs to increase or decrease blood pressure, it sends messages through the nerves of the autonomic nervous system (see Your Vital Functions and the Autonomic Nervous System, p.106).

These messages tell the muscles in the walls of the arterioles to clamp down or to relax, and also tell the heart to slow down or speed up. Several hormones also influence the blood pressure by affecting the amount of blood in the body and the resistance caused by the arterioles.

Your blood pressure normally goes up and down during the day, as your level of stress or physical exertion changes. For this reason, doctors generally take the average of several measurements to determine your average blood pressure.

Some people become very anxious in a doctor's office or hospital, and their blood pressure rises above their typical level during their visit. Doctors call this "white coat hypertension" because the person's blood pressure has been raised by anxiety brought on by being in a medical situation.

It is difficult to diagnose and follow up on the condition of a person who experiences this kind of stress. Doctors may ask a person whose blood pressure appears high during an office visit to take multiple readings with a home blood pressure machine (see p.85).

The decision to start treatment for high blood pressure is never made after just a single blood pressure reading in the doctor's office or hospital (unless blood pressure is dangerously high).

Contrary to its name, "hypertension" does not mean you are too tense in the usual sense of the word. While it is true that blood pressure tends to rise with anxiety and other strong emotions, many people with high blood pressure are not excessively stressed.

The vast majority of cases of high blood pressure (about 95%) have no known cause. This condition is called primary high blood pressure or essential high blood pressure.

High blood pressure may start at any age, but usually begins during middle age. Intensive research is underway to uncover the causes of primary high blood pressure, in the hope that the information will lead to new and better treatment for the disease.

Primary high blood pressure may run in families. There are racial differences as well. African Americans tend to get high blood pressure at an earlier age than white Americans. Also, high blood pressure tends to be more severe in African Americans.

The remaining 5% of cases of high blood pressure stem from an underlying medical condition; this is called secondary high blood pressure.

If your doctor has determined that you have high blood pressure, he or she usually will ask questions, perform a physical examination, and conduct laboratory tests to determine if another disease is responsible for the elevation in your blood pressure. See Causes of Secondary High Blood Pressure (p.648).

HOW HIGH BLOOD PRESSURE DAMAGES THE BODY

Heart damage High blood pressure leads to diseases of the heart and blood vessels in a number of ways. First, the heart must work harder because it is pumping the blood against a consistently higher-than-normal level of pressure. Just as the muscles in your

Causes of Secondary High Blood Pressure

Secondary high blood pressure is caused by an underlying medical condition. You can find out more about the diseases below by looking them up in the index of this book.

Kidney diseases The kidneys play a critical role in controlling blood pressure. Many different diseases affecting the kidneys can raise blood pressure, including diabetes, nephritis, and narrowing of the major arteries into the kidneys. High blood pressure itself can damage the kidneys, making the high blood pressure worse.

Drugs The drugs that most commonly cause an increase in blood pressure are birth-control pills, estrogen, thyroid hormone pills, corticosteroid drugs, amphetamines, cocaine, and nasal decongestant drops or sprays. Caffeine and the regular use of excessive amounts (more than two drinks a day) of alcohol can also raise blood pressure.

Pheochromocytoma This is a rare type of tumor that causes the adrenal glands to produce an excess of norepinephrine and similar hormones that raise blood pressure.

Cushing syndrome This condition results in excessive production (usually by the adrenal glands) of corticosteroid hormones, which increase blood pressure.

Conn syndrome This condition produces an excess of the hormone aldosterone, which increases blood pressure; it is usually caused by another rare type of benign (noncancerous) tumor of the adrenal glands.

Coarctation of the aorta In this condition, the aorta has a constriction shortly after leaving the heart. The heart must generate high blood pressure to push blood through the constriction.

---

arm get bulkier when you lift weights, the muscular wall of the heart, particularly the left ventricle, grows thicker from more strenuous pumping.

Unlike the muscles of your arm, however, the thicker heart muscle is not necessarily stronger. Indeed, since the heart's blood supply often does not increase to the same degree as the muscle, the heart may actually become weaker after many years of high blood pressure. Eventually, this can lead to heart failure (see p.683).

Atherosclerosis High blood pressure is one cause of the initial damage of the inner walls of the arteries that leads to atherosclerosis (see p.653). The increased blood pressure causes microscopic cracks in the inner lining of the arteries. These cracks provide fertile ground for the buildup of fat deposits. Even-

tually, these blockages interfere with the ability of the blood to carry oxygen and nutrients to the muscles they serve.

In this way, high blood pressure poses a double threat to the heart. First, it increases the heart muscle's workload, which increases the heart's need for oxygen and nutrients. Second, it reduces the heart muscle's supply of oxygen and nutrients by promoting atherosclerosis of the coronary arteries. This combination increases the chance of a heart attack and the development of heart failure.

Kidney damage High blood pressure also promotes atherosclerosis of the arteries that serve other organs. Serious consequences can result if these organs are starved of the oxygen and nutrients they need.

Narrowing of the arteries feeding the kidneys can cause the

kidneys to malfunction. When the blood supply to the kidneys is reduced, the body produces a hormone called renin, which initiates a series of chemical reactions that cause the arterioles to clamp down further. The result is high blood pressure that leads to kidney damage, which leads to more high blood pressure.

Aneurysms Another way high blood pressure damages arteries is by weakening and stretching vessel walls. This can lead to the formation of balloonlike projections called aneurysms (see p.698).

Like balloons, aneurysms burst when exposed to too much pressure. They commonly develop in the small arteries of the brain, eyes, or kidneys or in larger blood vessels such as the aorta. A burst aneurysm in the small arteries of the eyes can lead to visual impairment or even blindness.

Strokes Untreated high blood pressure can also lead to strokes by causing atherosclerosis of the arteries that feed blood to the brain. The narrowing that results can limit blood flow and starve a part of the brain of the oxygen and nutrients it needs. This is called an ischemic stroke (see p.345).

High blood pressure can also cause rupture of blood vessels in the brain, causing a brain hemorrhage (see p.350). A hemorrhage occurs when high blood pressure has weakened the walls of the arteries in the brain.

Ischemic strokes and brain hemorrhages can both produce devastating and permanent loss of speech, strength, comprehension, and sensation. They can also result in coma and death.

Chronic high blood pressure has also been shown to shrink brain tissue in people over age 65.

Other diseases that worsen damage from high blood pressure Damage to the heart, brain, and other organs caused by high blood pressure is even more likely if you have other conditions that affect the cardiovascular system. These risk factors include diabetes, smoking, elevated levels of cholesterol, or a family history of heart disease.

Diagnosing and treating high blood pressure is especially crucial if you also have one or more of these other conditions.

SYMPTOMS

Like many serious diseases, high blood pressure does not produce symptoms until it has slowly and silently produced damage to various organs, which then begin to malfunction.

Many people live with high blood pressure for years without experiencing any symptoms. In these people, the only way of knowing that they have high blood pressure is to have their blood pressure measured.

About one third of an estimated 50 million people with high blood pressure in the United States do not know they have it; consequently, they are not treated and risk serious illness.

The most common symptoms caused by high blood pressure are headaches (usually in the back of the head, particularly when you awaken in the morning), dizziness, or light-headedness. However, the headaches are often so mild that they are ignored.

When high blood pressure becomes severe, it may produce symptoms. The most severe symptoms are caused by a hypertensive crisis, in which blood pressure is often greater than 210/120 millimeters of mercury (mm Hg).

Symptoms of this crisis include severe headache, double vision, nosebleed, rapid heartbeat, ringing in the ears, and twitching muscles. Nausea, vomiting, and mental confusion can also occur.

TREATMENT OPTIONS

Since high blood pressure is a chronic (ongoing) condition, your blood pressure needs to be checked regularly, even if it is being treated. It should be checked each time you visit your doctor.

People are increasingly checking their own blood pressure at home. You can learn to take your blood pressure the way the doctor does, using a blood pressure

cuff and stethoscope (see p.644), or you can use a home blood pressure machine (see p.85).

These machines are generally accurate, but they need to be checked periodically. Take the machine to your doctor's office and have the reading on the machine compared to your blood pressure reading taken in the usual way. Machines that measure blood pressure in your finger are more comfortable but less accurate than machines that measure pressure in your arm.

Your doctor will recommend a course of treatment for you based on the severity of your high blood pressure. For milder cases (stage 1), lifestyle changes may be enough to keep the problem in check.

If your blood pressure level is in one of the more severe categories, you will probably need to take medications. Also, if you have any other conditions that increase the risk of damage to the heart and blood vessels (cardiovascular risk factors), your doctor will probably treat your high blood pressure more aggressively and earlier.

Even if you take medicine for your high blood pressure, nonpharmacological measures, such as exercise and a diet rich in fruits and vegetables and low in salt, can still be useful. Making these lifestyle changes (see p.646) can allow you to reduce the amount of medicine you will need.

When drugs are necessary, the choice of drug is often determined by your age, your racial and genetic background, the presence or absence of damage to your kidneys and other organs,

Choosing the Right Drug for High Blood Pressure

Since high blood pressure medicine generally needs to be taken indefinitely, cost, convenience, and tolerance are extremely important in deciding on the best regimen. Every drug works better when accompanied by lifestyle changes (see p.646). There are many classes of drugs for high blood pressure and there are many different drugs within each class. Some of the more commonly used drugs are listed here.

CATEGORY	MOST COMMONLY USED DRUGS	DEMONSTRATED BENEFITS	PRECAUTIONS/SIDE EFFECTS
Thiazide diuretics	Hydrochlorothiazide, chlorthalidone	Can reduce risk of strokes and heart attacks; is relatively inexpensive; is convenient (you can take just once a day)	Causes increased urination; can deplete potassium in the body; occasionally causes sexual dysfunction in men
Beta blockers	Atenolol, propranolol, nadolol, metoprolol, labetalol, acebutolol	Can reduce risk of strokes and heart attacks; protects the heart in people who also have coronary artery disease; relatively inexpensive; convenient (you take just once a day)	Can cause sleep disturbances, fatigue, and/or depression; may cause problems in people with heart block, heart failure, or asthma; may cause sexual dysfunction in men
Angiotensin-converting enzyme (ACE) inhibitors	Captopril, enalapril, lisinopril, ramipril	Protects the kidneys in people who also have diabetes and kidney insufficiency; protects the heart in people after a major heart attack or congestive heart failure	Can sometimes cause deterioration in kidney function, dizziness, or a dry tickling cough; should not be taken by pregnant women; may cause sexual dysfunction in men
Angiotensin-receptor antagonists	Losartan, irbesartan	Probably have same benefits as ACE inhibitors (above)	May cause sexual dysfunction in men; works like ACE inhibitors, but less likely to cause cough
Calcium channel blockers	Verapamil, diltiazem, nifedipine, felodipine, amlodipine	Useful for people with deteriorating kidney function; useful for people with angina	May cause headache, dizziness, weakness, constipation, edema, or rapid or slow heartbeat; generally not recommended for people with congestive heart failure; may cause sexual dysfunction in men
Methyldopa	Methyldopa	Useful during pregnancy	May cause difficulty thinking in older people; can cause illnesses such as lupus; may cause sexual dysfunction in men
Hydralazine	Hydralazine	Relatively inexpensive	Can cause high fevers; may cause sexual dysfunction in men
Alpha blockers	Prazosin, terazosin, doxazosin	May improve blood levels of fats	Can cause light-headedness, dizziness, headache, or drowsiness
Reserpine	Reserpine	Convenient (you can take just once a day); least expensive	Can cause nasal stuffiness and depression; may cause sexual dysfunction in men

Which Drugs Should I Try First for High Blood Pressure?

Most people with high blood pressure that requires drug treatment have no other medical conditions that affect drug choice. If you are among this group, you should first try thiazide-type diuretics such as hydrochlorothiazide or chlorthalidone. If you have one of the medical conditions listed at left, look for the recommended blood pressure–lowering medications in the right-hand column.

OTHER CONDITIONS	RECOMMENDED (OR NOT RECOMMENDED) MEDICINES
None	Thiazide diuretics and beta blockers are recommended first for most people with high blood pressure (because they are the only treatments that have been proven to lower blood pressure and prevent heart attacks and strokes, they are no more likely than other medicines to cause side effects, and they are much less expensive than most other high blood pressure drugs)
Heart attack	Beta blockers or angiotensin-converting enzyme (ACE) inhibitors
Angina	Beta blockers, or longer-acting calcium channel blockers if you also have asthma, chronic bronchitis, or emphysema
Congestive heart failure	ACE inhibitors and diuretics
Diabetes	ACE inhibitors (avoid diuretics because they can raise blood sugar)
Gout	No particular drug is recommended for people with gout, but diuretics should be avoided because they can aggravate gout
Over age 65	Diuretics and beta blockers (because they are the best studied treatments and are very effective unless you have a condition, such as the ones listed on this chart, that would make them less favorable to use)
Impotence	ACE inhibitors, calcium channel blockers, and alpha blockers (because they are least likely to aggravate this problem)
Asthma or chronic emphysema or bronchitis	No particular drug is recommended for people with these conditions, but beta blockers should be avoided because they can aggravate both conditions
Pregnancy	Methyldopa

the risk of side effects, and the presence of other diseases.

No single medicine is ideal for all people, and each person's program of blood-pressure control needs to be individually tailored. Drugs differ in the way they lower blood pressure and, depending on each person's characteristics, in their potential for unwanted side effects.

For stage 1 or 2 high blood pressure, doctors usually start treatment with a single medicine. For more severe cases, treatment may start with two or three drugs.

If the initial strategy does not achieve the desired effect, dosages can be increased or different drugs can be substituted. If your blood pressure is severely elevated (stage 4), you may be hospitalized and given continuous intravenous medicine. Monitoring is also required.

Doctors once believed that it was of no benefit, and might even be harmful, to treat high blood pressure in people over age 60. The theory was that older people needed a higher blood pressure because their arteries

were stiffer. Some doctors feared that lowering the blood pressure of older people to levels that were normal in younger people might cause strokes or kidney failure.

A wealth of research now has shown that people over age 60 get just as much benefit, if not more, from treating high blood pressure. With proper treatment, they are much less likely to develop heart failure, strokes, and heart attacks.

DISEASE OF THE HEART'S ARTERIES: CORONARY ARTERY DISEASE

Coronary Arteries

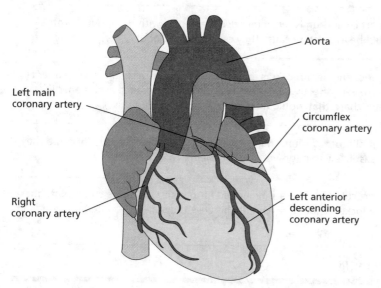

The right and left main coronary arteries branch off from the aorta and wrap around the heart. The left main coronary artery further divides into the left anterior descending and circumflex arteries, which feed the front, back, and side of the heart. The right coronary artery supplies blood to the right, front side of the heart and also to the undersurface of the heart.

Coronary artery disease is disease of the heart's arteries, the coronary arteries. It is the most common cause of death in the United States and in the developed nations of the world. Even in developing countries, coronary artery disease is a major and increasing problem.

Coronary artery disease is present in many people who have no symptoms from it (but may have symptoms in the future). When it causes symptoms, they can be mild and subtle or sudden and devastating.

Coronary artery disease can cause the chest pain called angina (see p.657), abnormal heart rhythms (see p.671), heart attack (see p.663), congestive heart failure (see p.683), and cardiac arrest (see p.678).

Almost all coronary artery disease comes from a condition called atherosclerosis (see p.653), which can affect not only the arteries of the heart but also all of the arteries of the body.

The Wall of an Artery

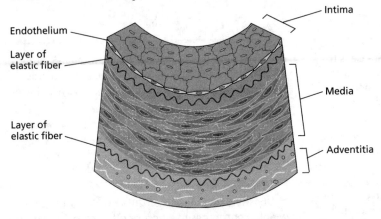

A normal artery is a tube composed of several layers. Blood flows through the open channel inside the artery. The innermost layer is called the intima; it is lined with a single layer of cells called the endothelium. It is in the intima that atherosclerosis mainly develops. Under the intima is a layer of elastic fiber, followed by a layer called the media, in which there are mainly smooth muscle cells. This layer is primarily responsible for the strength of the artery wall. Then comes another layer of elastic fiber and a final layer called the adventitia.

WHO GETS CORONARY ARTERY DISEASE?

While some people are born with genetically determined conditions that make them more likely to get coronary artery disease, lifestyle is a far more important factor than genetics.

Smoking, physical inactivity, elevated levels of cholesterol, high blood pressure, and being overweight all greatly increase your risk. The presence of more than one of these factors multiplies the threat of coronary artery disease.

Although it is difficult to prove, there is evidence that emotional states such as depression and suppressed anger are associated with a greater risk of coronary artery disease. Depressed people also have a lower chance of recovery from a heart attack and a greater risk of dying prematurely after a heart attack.

Some people erroneously believe that coronary artery disease affects only men. Menstruating women are protected to some degree, probably because they have higher blood levels of the hormone estrogen.

However, after menopause, a woman's risk of coronary artery disease rapidly increases. More women die of coronary artery disease than any other condition. Many more postmenopausal women die of coronary artery disease than breast cancer and lung cancer combined.

The symptoms of coronary artery disease can be harder to recognize in women. When a diagnosis of coronary artery disease is first made in a woman, the disease tends to be more severe than when the diagnosis is made in a man. Women are also less likely to survive a heart attack than men.

Also, treatments such as angioplasty (see p.661), coronary bypass surgery (see p.662), and reperfusion therapy (see Heart Attack, p.663) may result in more complications for women than men, and women may not be offered these treatments as early as men in the course of their disease.

Atherosclerosis

Atherosclerosis is a buildup of fatty deposits on the inside of the arteries that narrows the vessels and slows down blood flow. It is the most common form of coronary artery disease.

Every organ and tissue in the body needs a supply of fresh, oxygen-rich blood. That blood is pumped to all parts of the body through tubes called arteries. It is crucial that these vessels stay in good working order for you to survive.

A healthy artery is like a clean pipe. It has smooth lining and is free of blockages that interfere with blood flow.

Atherosclerosis begins as microscopic damage to the inner lining of the artery walls. Many forces can cause this damage, including high blood pressure, cigarette smoke, diabetes, elevated levels of cholesterol and triglyceride, possibly elevated levels of a substance called homocysteine, conditions that cause blood to clot more easily, drugs such as cocaine and androgens, and possibly infections of the inner linings of the arteries.

The first signs of damage are fatty streaks called plaque in the wall of the arteries. These fatty streaks begin early in life and even occur in young adults.

Whatever causes the initial

Preventing Heart Disease

The first strategy in preventing heart disease is to reduce your chances of developing coronary artery disease as much as you can. Here is an overview of the known and potential risk factors, and what you can do about them.

■ **Tobacco abuse** Smoking more than doubles your chance of developing coronary artery disease and it makes you up to six times more likely to have a heart attack. Smoking can be directly linked to 20% of coronary artery disease deaths, and each cigarette you smoke raises your risk. The solution is to quit. Your risk decreases rapidly after quitting and returns to almost that of nonsmokers within 3 years. (For ways to quit smoking, see p.59.)

■ **High cholesterol level** The higher your blood cholesterol level, the greater your risk of developing coronary artery disease. If your cholesterol is high (see p.669), your risk of coronary artery disease drops 2% to 3% for each percent you lower your cholesterol. The first step in reducing your blood cholesterol level is to eat a low-fat diet that limits foods from animal sources. Your doctor will tell you how low you need to go, and if taking cholesterol-lowering drugs is advisable in your case.

■ **High blood pressure** The higher your blood pressure, the greater your risk of coronary artery disease. Lowering high blood pressure protects you against coronary artery disease and protects you even more against stroke. For details on what high blood pressure is, and various natural and medical ways to lower it, see p.644.

■ **Physical inactivity** Regular exercise can decrease your risk of heart attack by a third to a half. If you have been inactive for a long time, and are overweight and out of shape, talk to your doctor before starting an exercise program.

■ **Obesity** Being more than 20% over your ideal body weight contributes to a host of other coronary artery disease risk factors, including high blood pressure, diabetes, high levels of blood lipids, and a sedentary lifestyle.

■ **Diabetes** You are three to seven times more likely to die of cardiovascular disease if you have diabetes. An aggressive approach to controlling diabetes and other risk factors may reduce your chances of cardiovascular complications.

■ **Gender** See Who Gets Coronary Artery Disease? (p.652).

■ **Aspirin** In men over 50, there is reasonable evidence that taking a regular-strength (325 milligrams) aspirin every other day or taking 81 milligrams of aspirin every day reduces the chance of developing coronary artery disease. In women, there currently is

Benefits of Physical Fitness in Reducing the Risk of Cardiovascular Death in Men

Men who exercise moderately, such as by walking briskly, two or three times a week for at least 30 minutes each time have a decreased risk of heart disease and death. The effect of exercise on reducing the risk of heart disease in women is not clearly established, but most experts expect that it is similar to reducing the risk in men.

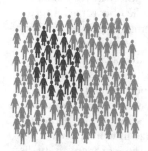

20 OF 100 MEN IN THE GENERAL POPULATION WHO ARE 65 TO 85 YEARS OLD WILL DIE OF CARDIOVASCULAR DISEASE WITHIN 10 YEARS

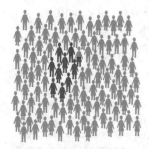

9.4 OF 100 MEN WHO EXERCISE TWO TO THREE TIMES A WEEK WHO ARE 65 TO 85 YEARS OLD WILL DIE OF CARDIOVASCULAR DISEASE WITHIN 10 YEARS

less evidence of benefit. On the other hand, aspirin can cause side effects, including bleeding, so talk to your doctor before starting on a regular dose of aspirin.

■ **Excessive alcohol intake** The key here is moderation. Moderate drinking, one to two drinks a day, seems to decrease your chances of developing heart disease. However, more than that raises your risk. This advice is generally given to both men and women, although there is some evidence that more than one drink of alcohol per day may slightly increase the risk of breast cancer in women.

■ **High homocysteine level** People who have high levels of this natural substance in their blood may have an increased risk of developing coronary artery disease. The level of homocysteine in your blood can be measured by a blood test. You can inherit a tendency to have a high homocysteine level, but it seems that the cause in most people who have moderately high levels is a dietary deficiency of folic acid (folate) and vitamins B_6 and B_{12}. There is no consensus yet among doctors about whether people in general, or people with known coronary artery disease, should have their homocysteine level measured. For people with high homocysteine levels, there also is no proof that lowering the level is beneficial. Nevertheless, it is

prudent to take folic acid (400 micrograms) and vitamins B_6 (100 milligrams) and B_{12} (100 micrograms) in pill form if your level is high, particularly in people who have had a parent or sibling develop coronary artery disease before age 55.

■ **High triglyceride level** A high level of this fat—especially in association with a low level of high-density lipoprotein (HDL)—in the blood appears to predict heart disease, although not as strongly as a high cholesterol level. Your triglyceride level is best determined by fasting for 12 hours before the blood test. The main steps in reducing an excessive blood triglyceride level is to cut down on the amount of sugar and refined starches in your diet, lose weight if you are obese, limit your alcohol intake, and control diabetes.

■ **Infection** A microorganism called *Chlamydia pneumoniae*—which is a common cause of pneumonia, bronchitis, and throat and sinus infections—can cause an infection of the lining of the arteries. Research indicates that such an infection may be a significant first step in developing atherosclerosis, at least in some people. It has not been shown that testing for this infection, or giving antibiotic treatments if it is present, is beneficial in preventing atherosclerosis. However, this possibility is being studied.

damage, the result is that platelets from the bloodstream gather at the site, soon to be joined by a gruel-like mixture of fats, calcium deposits, and cell debris.

Gradually, cells from the wall of the artery surround the mixture. There is inflammation in the wall of the artery; immune system white blood cells become activated, race to the injured area, and try, unsuccessfully, to heal it.

A fibrous cap forms over the fatty deposit. The deposit can grow, progressively blocking

blood flow and ultimately causing chest pain (angina). The fibrous cap can also rupture, causing a heart attack.

SYMPTOMS

As more material is deposited, an atherosclerotic plaque continues to grow, eventually interfering with blood flow through the artery. When the blood flow is obstructed beyond a certain critical point, symptoms develop.

If atherosclerosis develops in the coronary arteries, you may develop chest pain (angina) or

have a heart attack. Blockages in the arteries that feed blood to the brain can cause a stroke (see p.342). Blockages in the arteries that serve the legs result in a painful condition called intermittent claudication (see Atherosclerosis of the Arteries to the Legs, p.701).

The heart, too, requires a steady supply of oxygen and other nutrients. The vessels that feed the heart are the coronary arteries. Except in the most unusual circumstances, healthy coronary arteries are able to meet the heart's demand for oxygen-rich blood. These arteries can accommodate up to five times their usual flow of blood during periods of extreme exertion, such as a marathon run.

When the heart muscle gets the blood it needs to respond to the exertion required, the body works as it should; the muscle is working harder and burning more energy but is getting a constant supply of new energy (such as sugar or oxygen) from the blood.

When the blood supply cannot provide enough energy to meet the needs of the heart muscle, however, bad things can happen. The heart muscle may strain (causing chest pain), start to pump less effectively, develop abnormal heart rhythms, and even suddenly stop pumping blood; this is cardiac arrest.

How Atherosclerosis Develops

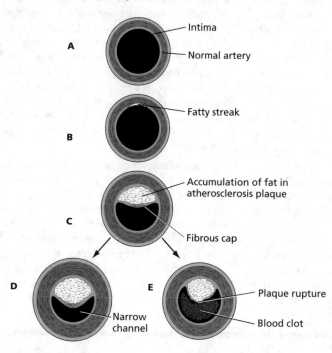

A This is a normal artery with a smooth, even intima—the innermost layer of an artery. Smoking, high blood pressure, and (possibly) infection inflict microscopic injury to the intima, which can make it susceptible to penetration by fatty particles in the blood.

B In this stage, which begins in the late teenage years and in early adulthood, fatty particles from the blood penetrate and settle in the intima, forming a fatty streak (plaque).

C Over the years, the accumulation of fat continues, and the plaque of atherosclerosis grows larger. The fatty deposit in the plaque is covered by a tissue called a fibrous cap. The plaque begins to bulge into the open channel through which blood flows. The wall of the artery thickens.

D This process can continue, progressively narrowing the channel. At some point, blood flow is obstructed enough so that you will develop angina if the part of the heart served by that artery must work too hard.

E Sometimes, the fibrous cap ruptures, and blood cells traveling through the channel are exposed to the fatty inside of the plaque. This causes a blood clot to form at the site of the rupture. This change can occur quite suddenly, and accounts for many heart attacks.

TREATMENT OPTIONS

The first step in fighting atherosclerosis is to limit the progression of the disease. You can do this through lifestyle changes such as eating a low-fat diet, quitting smoking, controlling high blood pressure, treating diabetes, and getting regular exercise.

Also, taking an aspirin a day (because it makes the blood less likely to clot) can greatly reduce the chances of a heart attack for men and women with coronary artery disease, and even for people who have not already developed coronary artery disease but have significant cardiac risk factors.

Ask your physician if taking a daily aspirin is a good idea for you. If you have already had a heart attack, all of these measures become even more important; they can reduce your chance of having another heart attack and of dying prematurely.

If the blockage in your arteries has advanced to the point where you have debilitating symptoms despite taking medicine—or if you are in serious danger of having a heart attack—you may need angioplasty or surgery.

Coronary artery bypass surgery (see Bypass Surgery, p.662) restores blood flow to deprived areas of the heart by grafting a vessel onto the heart to carry blood around the obstruction in the diseased arteries.

Angina

Angina (or angina pectoris) is pain in the chest caused by coronary artery disease. Pain in the chest is an extremely common symptom. Many things besides heart disease can cause chest pain, including tension in the muscles of the chest wall, gastroesophageal reflux (see p.747), pericarditis (see p.697), and pleurisy (see p.502).

It is important to distinguish angina from other causes of chest pain because it is treated differently and has a different prognosis (outlook). Knowing that your chest pain is not angina can be very reassuring.

Many people who have chest pain worry that they may have a heart condition, but only a minority of people with chest pain do.

SYMPTOMS

Angina is a sensation of pressure, aching, or burning in the middle

---

Angina: *When You Visit Your Doctor*

QUESTIONS TO DISCUSS WITH YOUR DOCTOR:

■ Have you had chest pain? What brings it on? How long does it last? Does it stay in your chest? Does the pain go anywhere else in your body?

■ How frequently do you get chest pain? Is there a change in your usual pattern?

■ Do you ever get chest pain at rest?

■ What relieves the chest pain? If you take nitroglycerin, how long does it take for the pain to go away? How many doses of nitroglycerin do you usually need to take before the pain resolves? How often do you take nitroglycerin?

■ Do you get short of breath when you lie down or exert yourself? Do you awaken in the middle of the night short of breath? Do your ankles swell?

■ Do you ever feel like you are going to faint? Have you fainted?

■ Do you get a rapid or pounding heartbeat for no reason?

■ Do you get pain in your calves when you walk?

■ Do you have sudden brief episodes of weakness in an arm or leg, loss of vision (like a shade being pulled over your eyes), or difficulty speaking? These could be warning symptoms of stroke (see p.342). People with coronary artery disease are at increased risk of stroke.

■ Do you know what each of the medications you are taking does? Do you know the side effects of each medication?

■ Are you doing everything you can to modify the risk factors (such as smoking, high blood pressure, high cholesterol, or diabetes) that can worsen your coronary artery disease?

YOUR DOCTOR MIGHT EXAMINE THE FOLLOWING BODY STRUCTURES OR FUNCTIONS:

■ Heart rate, blood pressure, and weight

■ Pulses

■ Major arteries (for abnormal noises)

■ Veins in the neck

■ Heart and lungs

■ Ankles and legs (for swelling)

YOUR DOCTOR MIGHT ORDER THE FOLLOWING LAB TESTS OR STUDIES:

■ Electrocardiogram (see p.135)

■ Echocardiogram (see p.665)

■ Exercise stress test (see p.660)

Angina Pain

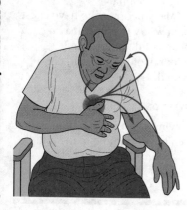

Burning, pressure, or aching in the chest can signal an attack of angina. The pain most often concentrates beneath the breastbone or in the upper abdomen, but often is also felt in the neck, jaw, shoulder, elbow, wrist, and back.

of the chest. It commonly occurs during physical exercise, emotional stress, and exposure to cold temperatures, or after big meals.

When arteries are severely narrowed (more than 80%), angina can also occur at rest. The discomfort typically starts underneath the breastbone (sternum); it may spread up into the neck, jaw, and shoulders (usually the left shoulder) and even down the arm. Often, it is accompanied by a sense of anxiety or uneasiness.

The pain of angina is usually not sharp. Rather, it is more a sense of pressure or squeezing. Sometimes, it is just an uncomfortable sensation, not really a pain. Angina is not affected by the position of your body or by taking a deep breath, whereas

other causes of chest pain, such as pleurisy or pericarditis, often are.

Usually an attack of angina lasts just a few minutes. If it has been triggered by exertion, it usually subsides within a few minutes when you rest. When such pain lasts more than 20 minutes, it could indicate a heart attack.

If you have this type of pain and it lasts more than 20 minutes, call an ambulance.

TREATMENT OPTIONS

When angina is suspected, the doctor usually performs an electrocardiogram (ECG) (see p.135) and an exercise stress test (see p.660). These tests, particularly the stress test, help detect coronary artery disease.

The ECG is completely safe.

Tests for "Silent" Coronary Artery Disease

Coronary artery disease (CAD) begins years before it causes symptoms. Although it is beneficial for everyone to try to prevent CAD, it is especially important for people who already have early signs of disease to try to slow its progress.

It is neither practical nor of any proven value for people who seem healthy to have an exercise stress test (see p.660) or riskier tests such as an angiogram (see p.659) to try to diagnose CAD. For this reason, doctors are developing simple and risk-free tests to try to detect CAD in its earliest stages. One simple blood test—testing cholesterol levels—definitely signals an increased risk of CAD.

Homocysteine level tests (see Risk of Cardiovascular Disease With Elevated Homocysteine Level, p.675) and tests for infection with *Chlamydia pneumoniae* (see

p.655) may also indicate an increased risk. A test called a supersensitive C-reactive protein test, which indicates inflammation in artery walls, may also signal an increased risk.

Other more expensive but low-risk tests that take pictures of the coronary arteries are being developed. One example is an electron-beam computed tomography (CT) scan, with or without the injection into the blood of a contrast agent (see p.147). Another is a special magnetic resonance imaging (MRI) scan. Thickening of the inner wall of the carotid arteries in the neck, revealed through ultrasound (p.148) pictures, seems to indicate an increased risk of CAD. Using CT, MRI, and ultrasound for this purpose is still experimental, and of unproven value.

Coronary Angiogram

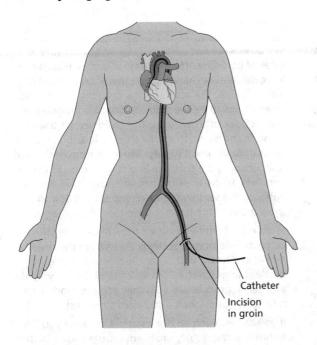

Catheter

Incision
in groin

A long, narrow, plastic tube (the catheter) is inserted into an artery in the leg through a small incision in the groin. It is advanced over a guidewire through the circulatory system until it reaches the heart. From there it is threaded into the coronary arteries and a contrast dye is released, outlining all the coronary arteries on an x-ray.

Angiogram of Narrowed Artery

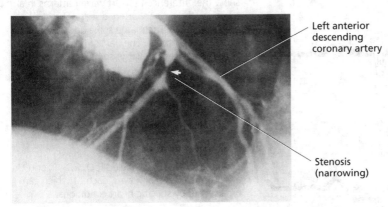

Left anterior
descending
coronary artery

Stenosis
(narrowing)

This angiogram shows several of the major coronary arteries outlined by the contrast dye. The arrow indicates the point of severe narrowing, or stenosis, from coronary artery disease.

The chance of having a heart attack during a stress test is 1 of 10,000.

A cardiac catheterization with a coronary angiogram (see p.659) carries a slightly higher risk of a heart attack (about 1 of 5,000), but is more accurate in making the diagnosis of coronary artery disease.

A coronary angiogram is used to diagnose coronary artery disease when the ECG or stress test is inconclusive or when treatment with angioplasty or surgery is needed. However, the angiogram is less accurate in detecting the "vulnerable plaques" that can cause heart attack (see p.663).

Treatment for angina depends on how severe it is, whether it has recently become more severe (even if it is still mild), how much it interferes with your life, and your expectations and goals.

Some of the following may help your angina:

■ **Reduce risk factors.** Work on eliminating any risk factors that make coronary artery disease and angina worse (such as smoking, excessive weight, high blood pressure, and elevated cholesterol) and make lifestyle changes to reduce your chance of getting diabetes (see p.832).

■ **Adjust your daily activities.** If certain kinds of activity regularly cause angina, try performing the activity more slowly. Your heart is under more stress in the mornings and after meals, so try reducing physical activity at those times.

■ **Reduce stress and anger.** If anger and stress regularly bring on your angina, consider entering a stress-reduction program.

Exercise Stress Test

An electrocardiogram (ECG) (see p.135) cannot detect all cases of coronary artery disease, in part because you are resting and not challenging your heart at the time that the ECG is performed.

An exercise stress test challenges your heart to work harder by seeing how well the arteries can handle the demands of exercise. This stress test is used to diagnose coronary artery disease and, if it is known you have coronary artery disease, to determine how well your medicines are working to treat it.

The test requires you to walk on a treadmill or peddle a stationary bike while attached to a machine. Your heart rate and blood pressure are measured periodically throughout the test.

Healthy arteries can accommodate the increased blood flow that is generated during exertion. If your arteries cannot meet this demand because of plaque buildup and blockages, the heart will not get enough oxygen and you may experience chest pain.

Lack of oxygen to the heart may also produce abnormal ECG wave patterns.

The test is graded by the presence of symptoms, by ECG changes during the test, by the duration of exercise when the symptoms or changes occur, and by your blood pressure and heart rate at your peak exercise level.

Stress tests are not perfect. They do not identify all cases of coronary artery disease and their results can indicate an abnormality when there is no coronary artery disease. The accuracy of a stress test can be somewhat improved by injecting a radioactive isotope into a vein at peak exercise level. The radioisotope travels through the blood to the heart muscle and detects areas of poor blood supply. The most frequently used radioisotopes are thallium and technetium. PET scanners, which also use isotopes, are now being used to enhance the sensitivity of exercise testing and to show areas of the heart muscle that are damaged.

More recent studies indicate that an exercise stress test with additional readings taken from the right side of the heart, with a special device to measure subtle changes in the T waves of the ECG, or with an echocardiogram (see p.665) may provide more accurate information than a standard stress test.

If you cannot exercise (for example, because you have arthritis or respiratory problems), drugs such as dobutamine, adenosine, or dipyridamole can be given to make the heart work harder even though you are not exercising. As in an exercise stress test, radioisotopes or echocardiography are often used to detect areas of the heart that have a poor blood supply.

Electrocardiographic Changes During Exercise Stress Test

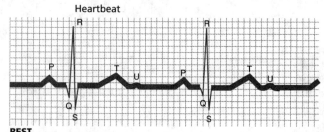

REST

EXERCISE — Depressed ST segment

These tracings from an electrocardiogram (ECG) show the difference in heart wave patterns in a person with coronary artery disease at rest and during exercise. Each large spike upward represents one heartbeat. The part of the wave pattern just after the large spike is called the ST segment. At rest, the level of the ST segment is the same as the level of the wave just before the spike (the pattern is normal despite the presence of coronary artery disease). However, during exercise, the level of the ST segment has become depressed. This indicates the presence of coronary artery disease.

The parts of the ECG labeled P, Q, R, S, T, and U are specific electrical waves, each of which can be affected by specific heart conditions.

Angioplasty with Balloons or Stents

Angioplasty is a technique for widening an artery narrowed by atherosclerosis or another condition.

One type of angioplasty is called percutaneous transluminal coronary angioplasty, or balloon angioplasty. In this procedure, a catheter is inserted into an artery through the skin of the groin. Using guidewires that can be steered, and with x-rays to guide its path, the catheter is pushed to the site of the blockage in the coronary artery.

Once in position, a tiny balloon at the tip of the catheter is inflated repeatedly. The balloon squashes and fractures the atherosclerotic plaque against the wall of the artery, opening up the blocked channel and restoring blood flow. Angioplasty usually requires a brief (1 day) hospital stay.

A newer angioplasty technique is used in up to 80% of cases. After opening up the narrowed part of the artery by temporarily inflating a tiny balloon, a small circular wire mesh called a stent is left in place to keep the narrowed part open.

When it is released from the tip of the catheter, the stent expands to become as wide as the artery, flattening the plaque. In many people, stents produce longer-lasting results than balloon angioplasty alone. New types of stents have chemicals embedded in the wire mesh that keep the artery open longer than regular wire mesh stents.

Angioplasty is more effective than drugs at relieving angina and improving exercise tolerance. However, it has not been proven to reduce the subsequent risk of heart attack or death in comparison to drugs.

Plaques in the left main coronary artery cannot be treated with angioplasty because there is an unacceptably high risk of complications from the procedure. When three or more coronary arteries need treatment, bypass surgery is often preferred to angioplasty.

Angioplasty is successful in opening an artery in about 90% of people. But the blockage returns within 6 months in about 40% of those treated and angina returns within 1 year in about 25% of those treated.

If blockage and angina have not recurred after 1 year, the odds are good that they will not recur. Risks of angioplasty include damage and weakening of the wall of the coronary artery, and heart attack.

Still newer techniques involve using tiny metal blades or lasers to chew up the atherosclerotic plaque (not just to push the plaque against the wall of the artery).

Another newer technique called transmyocardial laser surgery drills tiny holes through the coronary arteries and into heart muscle in an attempt to improve blood supply. It is being tried in people with angina who are not getting relief from medicines, and in whom angioplasty or bypass surgery is either not possible or has been ineffective.

Balloon Angioplasty

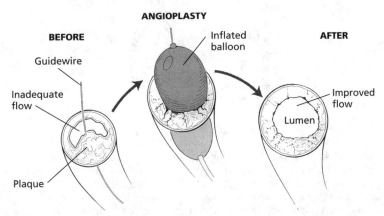

ANGIOPLASTY

BEFORE

Guidewire

Inadequate flow

Plaque

Inflated balloon

AFTER

Improved flow

Lumen

In balloon angioplasty, the cardiologist threads a thin guidewire through the coronary artery to the point of blockage. A deflated balloon catheter is then passed over the guidewire. The balloon is inflated and squeezes the plaque. After the balloon and guidewire are removed, the vessel's interior space (lumen) is enlarged. Increasingly, wire mesh devices called stents (not shown) are inserted by the catheter (and often expanded by the balloon) at the site of the obstruction to keep the channel open.

■ **Exercise.** Even though exercise can bring on angina, a supervised program of exercise can safely strengthen the heart and eventually reduce angina. Start slowly, and gradually build up your level of exercise during optimal times of the day. Your physician can tell you what you can and cannot do.

Medication also plays an important role in treatment:

■ **Nitrates** come in several forms. One kind (nitroglycerin) is a pill that you place under your tongue when you first feel pain or discomfort. Nitroglycerin should relieve angina within 5 minutes; it works by causing the coronary arteries to widen, increasing blood flow to the heart. Another kind of nitrate is a long-acting nitrate in pill form that you take every day to try to prevent angina attacks. There are also nitrate sprays and skin patches.

■ **Beta blockers** are used to slow the heart rate so the heart does not have to work as hard. They reduce the risk of abnormal heart rhythms and lower blood pressure.

■ **Calcium channel blockers** are often used instead of beta blockers if you have asthma or chronic obstructive lung disease, heart block (see p.680) and related conduction system abnormalities, or symptoms from peripheral arterial disease (see Atherosclerosis of the Arteries to the Legs, p.701). They lower blood pressure and widen coronary arteries.

■ **Aspirin** is used to help prevent the formation of new blood clots in diseased blood vessels by affecting platelet function.

■ **Angiotensin-converting enzyme (ACE) inhibitors** are

often started within a few days of a heart attack to help your heart work more efficiently, primarily by lowering blood pressure, which your heart must work against.

If all these treatments fail to give you adequate relief from your angina—or if the angina is new, severe, recently increased in severity, or is occurring at rest—more aggressive (and risky) treatments may be necessary, such as angioplasty (see p.661) or coronary artery bypass surgery (see below). Hospitalization for diagnosis and treatment may be required.

■ **Gene therapy** In an experimental treatment for angina, genes

injected into heart muscle cause small blood vessels to grow into parts of the heart that are starved of a sufficient blood supply.

Bypass Surgery

Coronary artery bypass graft surgery restores blood flow to deprived areas of the heart by grafting a vessel onto the heart to carry blood around the obstruction in the diseased arteries.

Approximately half a million Americans undergo coronary artery bypass graft (CABG) surgery each year. This operation can dramatically improve the quality of life and boost life expectancy

Coronary Artery Bypass Operation

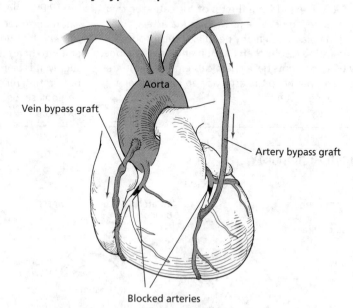

Aorta

Vein bypass graft

Artery bypass graft

Blocked arteries

In coronary artery bypass graft operations, an artery or piece of vein from another part of the body is used to bypass the blocked coronary arteries. Here one bypass graft (a vein) is used to bypass one blocked artery, and a second bypass graft (the left internal mammary artery) is used to bypass a second blocked artery. Blood flow through a graft delivers blood to the heart muscle by bypassing the blocked artery.

for some (but not all) people with coronary artery disease.

For bypass surgery, you are under general anesthesia. The surgeon cuts through your breastbone to gain access to the heart. In traditional open heart surgery, the beating of your heart is stopped to enable the surgeon to operate on a heart that isn't constantly moving. However, stopping the heart requires you to be on a heart-lung machine that pumps oxygen-rich blood through your body, temporarily substituting for the pumping heart. After the operation is completed, your heart is started again, you are taken off the heart-lung machine, and your chest is sewn closed.

Because the heart-lung machine can cause some complications, many centers are now operating with the heart still beating, thus eliminating the need for the machine. Outcomes of this less invasive approach seem quite acceptable, although it is not yet clear if they are superior.

Whether a heart-lung machine is used or not, the operation requires the surgeon to take a vein or artery from another part of your body and use the vessel to reroute blood flow around the blocked heart vessel so that the heart muscle can get the nourishment it needs.

When the replacement vessel is an artery, it typically is an internal mammary artery taken from your chest; when it is a vein, it typically is a saphenous vein taken from your leg. In either case, the artery or vein is a "spare" vessel; blood flow to that part of the body does not suffer when the spare vessel is removed.

If the grafted vessel is a vein from a leg, one end is attached to the aorta and the other is sewn onto the diseased coronary artery, below the blockage.

When a chest wall artery is used, the upper end is usually left in place and the lower open end is attached to the diseased coronary artery, below the blockage.

After surgery is completed, your heart is started again, you are taken off the heart-lung machine, and your chest is sewn closed. Most people stay in the hospital for 4 to 5 days after an uncomplicated operation, although your doctor will probably ask you to get up and walk 1 to 2 days after surgery.

While you are in the hospital, you may be scheduled for a cardiac rehabilitation program, which you will attend after leaving the hospital. Cardiac rehabilitation helps you and your heart gain strength, and teaches you "heart-healthy" practices that will protect you from future heart disease.

If your job does not require much exertion, you can usually return to work within 6 weeks after the operation. People who do heavy labor, however, need to wait longer or, in some cases, need to find another type of work.

Bypass surgery is very effective in controlling symptoms of cardiovascular disease. People often feel as if they have been given a new lease on life after the surgery.

Bypass surgery prolongs life only in people who have obstruction of the left main coronary artery or obstruction of three or more arteries with some degree of heart failure.

The surgery is also not a cure for coronary artery disease. After surgery, angina can recur, either from the buildup of plaque in arteries that were not bypassed or because blockages have formed in the grafts. To combat this effect, dietary and lifestyle changes in addition to aggressive control of cholesterol with drugs are extremely important after surgery.

CABG surgery also is more risky than angioplasty or treatment of angina with medicine. Possible complications of the surgery include heart attack, bleeding, and stroke. Stroke may occur if blood clots develop and travel to the brain, or if bleeding or periods of low blood pressure deprive the brain of oxygen during the surgery.

The risk of death from bypass surgery is about 1% to 2% with a very experienced surgical team.

Heart Attack

A heart attack, also known as a myocardial infarction, occurs when a portion of the heart muscle dies.

Heart attacks are a serious cause of illness and the most common cause of death in the United States and other developed nations. Each year, about 1.5 million people in the United States have a heart attack, and about half a million die, more than half of them before they can reach a hospital.

An increased understanding of the causes of heart attacks has lead to greatly improved prevention and treatment strategies, and to a falling death rate. More than 90% of the people who make it to the hospital in time to receive treatment survive their hospital stay.

A similar percentage makes it through the following year. In all, 600,000 people die of a heart attack each year—the equivalent

How Vulnerable Plaques Cause Sudden Heart Attacks

A heart attack occurs suddenly but the coronary artery disease that causes it has been present for many years. The coronary artery disease may not even have caused any symptoms. What changes occur suddenly that can cause a heart attack?

For many years, it was thought that a large plaque in the wall of the coronary artery—the kind that causes angina whenever a heart is made to work too hard and that a doctor can see with a coronary angiogram—was blocking most of the artery.

It was believed that a small blood clot became wedged at the site of the plaque and suddenly blocked blood flow completely. In this theory, large plaques caused both angina and heart attacks.

It was a reasonable theory, but it was wrong. Research has shown that most heart attacks are caused by rupture of the plaque, and that small plaques are often responsible.

It is now known that what makes a plaque prone to cause a heart attack is not how big it is, but how it is built. Every plaque has a fatty core and a top composed of a meshwork of fibers.

If the top is thick and the core is small, dry, and hard, the plaque is unlikely to rupture—it is "stable." Big plaques often fit this description.

However, if the top is thin and the core is filled with lots of soft, fatty material, the plaque can rupture—it is "unstable." When the blood in the artery comes in contact with this fatty material, it forms a big clot at the site of the rupture that can suddenly stop blood flow in the artery, causing a heart attack.

Vulnerable plaques with thin tops and soft fatty cores may be small and may not block blood flow or cause symptoms. They may even be so small that they cannot be seen on a coronary angiogram.

Doctors are trying to develop tests to detect vulnerable plaques. At this time, no tests are of proven value. But, in the near future, doctors may have blood tests—probably tests that reveal inflammation—that may be able to tell if you are at increased risk for having vulnerable plaques.

If so, pictures of your coronary arteries, possibly using special kinds of magnetic resonance imaging (see p.150), may be taken. Alternatively, your doctor may prescribe medicines, such as statin drugs (see p.671), that will make the plaques less vulnerable.

Stable and Unstable (Vulnerable) Plaques

STABLE **UNSTABLE**

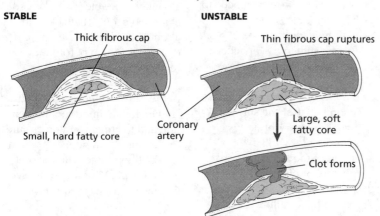

Thick fibrous cap

Small, hard fatty core

Coronary artery

Thin fibrous cap ruptures

Large, soft fatty core

Clot forms

Plaques with thick fibrous caps and small, hard fatty cores are unlikely to rupture. Unstable plaques have a large, soft fatty core and a thin fibrous cap. When they rupture, a clot can form and cause a heart attack.

of the entire population in a medium-sized city.

Almost all heart attacks occur in people who have coronary artery disease from atherosclerosis (see p.653). When the narrowed arteries are blocked and blood cannot feed a part of the heart, it usually causes severe pain, and can also cause congestive heart failure (see p.683).

It also can cause abnormal heart rhythms (see p.671) that can lead, in turn, to cardiac arrest (see p.678). If the blockage is not opened within 3 hours, 90% of the part of the heart that is starved of blood is likely to die.

The death of a part of the heart muscle is called a heart attack. During that 3-hour window of time, the heart muscle is not yet dead. It can be brought back to normal function, over time, if the obstruction to its blood supply can be removed.

There are various techniques for trying to open up a blocked coronary artery. They are called "reperfusion" techniques ("perfusion" means blood flow, and "reperfusion" means restoring blood flow), and they can be lifesaving.

For this reason, it is extremely important to seek medical care at the first signs of a heart attack.

SYMPTOMS

The typical symptoms of a heart attack are similar to those of angina, but more severe and longer lasting. You feel a pain that is usually squeezing or burning or feel a terrible pressure in the middle of your chest. This pain may also travel up to your neck, jaw, or shoulder or down the arm and into your back.

Sweating, dizziness, weakness, and shortness of breath often

Echocardiogram

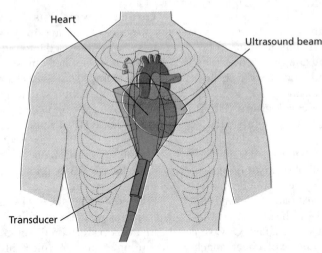

A device called a transducer sends ultrasound waves and receives the waves when they bounce off and echo back from the heart. The transducer sits lightly on the skin, which is covered by warm gel. By placing the transducer on various areas of the chest, the ultrasound waves bounce off different parts of the heart. These pictures allow examination of the heart's structures from all angles. The four parts of the chest where the transducer is placed most often are midway up and just left of the breastbone (sternum), over the left breast, just below the bottom of the breastbone, and just above the top of the breastbone, at the bottom of the neck.

accompany the pain of a heart attack. If you have chest pain that lasts longer than 20 minutes and is not relieved by rest (or by a dose of nitroglycerin), get immediate medical attention by calling 911 or the emergency telephone number in your area.

Immediately after you place the call, chew and swallow an aspirin and drink a glass of water. This thins the blood, which helps the heart get more blood if you are, indeed, having a heart attack.

Less commonly, a heart attack may cause a sensation that feels more like indigestion—you get a sick, aching feeling high in the middle of your abdomen. It can cause a feeling of great weakness, or a sense that you are about to faint.

Heart attacks can even occur without causing symptoms. Such silent heart attacks, as well as heart attacks with unusual symptoms—including heartburn, nausea, or sudden light-headedness and sweating—are more common in women, diabetics, and people older than 65.

Some studies have found that heart attacks are more likely to occur in the early morning, between about 5 and 9 AM. Other studies have found that, at least in northern regions, heart attacks may occur more often in the winter months.

DIAGNOSTIC TESTS

When a heart attack is suspected, the doctor will first take your blood pressure and heart rate, and listen to your heart and lungs to get a sense of how effectively your heart is working. The diagnosis of a heart attack is based on your symptoms, your physical exam, an electrocardiogram, and blood tests for heart muscle enzymes.

Electrocardiograms (ECGs) (see p.135) show injury to the heart muscle and can differentiate injury that goes through the entire wall of one part of the heart (Q-wave heart attack) from injury of just part of the wall (non-Q–wave heart attack). An ECG that shows a new Q-wave is strong evidence of a heart attack. An ECG pattern in a non-Q–wave heart attack is harder to interpret.

The ECG can also spot potentially dangerous abnormal heart rhythms and heart block (see p.680), which can occur during a heart attack.

Cardiac enzyme tests detect the presence of certain cardiac enzymes that are released into the bloodstream when heart muscle tissue is injured. Two enzymes looked for most often to detect heart damage are troponin and creatine kinase MB. Troponin is detectable in the blood as early as 4 hours after a heart attack; creatine kinase MB peaks at 12 to 24 hours afterward.

For people who already have chest pain and a new Q-wave heart attack pattern on the ECG, measuring cardiac enzymes only provides more information for an already certain diagnosis. The cardiac enzymes become very important in making the diagnosis, however, when the ECG pattern is of the non-Q–wave type. Creatine kinase MB enzyme measurements are also useful in determining how much of the heart muscle has been damaged, since more damage often leads to higher levels of the enzyme.

Echocardiograms (see p.665) are sometimes helpful in showing parts of the wall of the heart that are not pumping effectively, which occurs in a heart attack. When the heart attack has caused congestive heart failure, echocardiograms can also help determine how badly the heart attack is affecting the overall ability of the heart to pump, and whether any of the heart valves are malfunctioning.

Chest x-rays to look for an enlarged heart or other indications of congestive heart failure are another diagnostic tool. They are also helpful when the diagnosis is uncertain and other possible explanations for chest pain, such as pneumonia, exist.

The diagnosis of a heart attack is often not clear when you are first seen by the doctor. The doctor may therefore decide to keep you in the hospital overnight, to better diagnose a heart attack and to be immediately prepared to treat any serious complications that might develop if you are having a heart attack. Most people who are admitted to a hospital for a possible heart attack turn out not to have had one.

TREATMENT OPTIONS

You will probably be placed in an intensive care unit (or coronary care unit), where there are more nurses and doctors, and more equipment to monitor your condition and to treat emergencies.

For the first few days after a

Heart Muscle Damage From Heart Attack

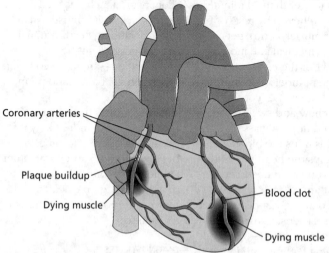

Coronary arteries

Plaque buildup

Dying muscle

Blood clot

Dying muscle

A clot in an already narrowed coronary artery can completely cut off blood flow to the heart. If blood flow is not restored quickly, 90% of the tissue fed by the blocked artery will die within 3 hours.

heart attack, you might need to rest in bed and have your heartbeat continuously monitored to make sure that dangerous rhythms do not develop. You may also need supplementary oxygen to provide more nutrition to the injured heart muscle and an intravenous line put in your hand or arm so that medicines can be given to you immediately in case of an emergency.

If you are in shock (see p.645) or have congestive heart failure, you may require a catheter placed into an artery in your arm to measure blood pressure continuously. You may need to have a catheter inserted into your bladder to measure the amount of urine you are producing or perhaps have a catheter inserted in your neck to measure how effectively your heart is pumping.

You may also need:

- **Oxygen**

- **Intravenous nitroglycerin** This drug may be used to ease the pain of angina and improve blood flow to the injured heart muscle.

- **Narcotics** Drugs such as morphine can help treat recurring pain.

- **Heparin and aspirin** These blood-thinning drugs are used to help prevent the formation of new blood clots in diseased blood vessels. A newer blood-thinning medicine called tirofiban, when added to heparin and aspirin, may bring further benefits. In people who have had a non-Q–wave heart attack (see Electrocardiograms, p.666), a new blood-thinning medicine called enoxaparin may be superior to heparin.

- **Beta blockers** These drugs are used to slow the heart rate so

Clot-Busting Thrombolytic Treatments

Thrombolytic therapy involves treatment with "clot-buster" medicines that can dissolve a blood clot in a coronary artery that has caused the heart attack.

The therapy can improve your chance of survival by as much as 30%. It is most effective if it is started within 90 minutes of the first sign of chest pain. However, thrombolytic therapy is still highly beneficial if performed within 6 hours after a heart attack and continues to show positive effects up to 12 hours after symptoms begin.

Clot-busting drugs include tissue-type plasminogen activator (tPA) and its variants, as well as streptokinase and urokinase, and drugs called GpIIb/IIIa inhibitors, such as abciximab.

Thrombolytic therapy is not right for everyone. People who have recently had active bleeding (such as from a stomach ulcer) are not good candidates, since the bleeding can worsen.

People who have pericarditis (see p.697) or those who have recently had a transient ischemic attack (see p.342), a stroke, surgery, dissection of an aortic aneurysm, or cardiopulmonary resuscitation (see p.1201) also are not good candidates because bleeding can occur in the injured tissue.

People with excessively high blood pressure are also at increased risk of developing complications from thrombolytic therapy.

Coronary angiography (see p.659) followed by angioplasty (see p.661) or coronary bypass graft surgery (see p.662) is sometimes used in the early hours of a heart attack as another way of trying to open up the obstructed artery and restore blood flow to the heart.

Coronary angioplasty is often performed when drugs have failed to dissolve the clot or to treat people who are not good candidates for thrombolytic therapy. However, it can only be performed if the institution has the capability to perform emergency surgery if a complication occurs.

Even though balloon angioplasty is highly effective in opening the arteries, it is often not available because less than 20% of hospitals in the United States have the facilities to perform the procedure on an emergency basis.

Also, in people who are having a heart attack, it has not been proven to be more effective than medicines in reducing the risk of having another heart attack or of dying.

the heart does not have to work as hard, and to prevent abnormal heart rhythms. They reduce the risk of dying of heart disease in the months after a heart attack.

- **Angiotensin-converting enzyme inhibitors** If these drugs are started within the first 36 hours after a heart attack, they help your heart work less hard, and reduce your risk of dying over the next 30 days, especially if you have had a major heart attack.

■ **Thrombolytic therapy** (see right)

After a heart attack, you generally need to stay in the hospital from 4 to 7 days. The exact length of time depends on the severity of the attack, and whether or not you have any complications.

During your hospitalization, doctors will perform tests to evaluate how well your heart is functioning and to assess your risk for having another heart attack. The strength and function of your heart can be measured with an echocardiogram to determine where the heart muscle has been injured.

You will be monitored to check for any abnormal heart rhythms. You will also undergo a less strenuous form of the usual treadmill stress test (see p.660) to see if it is safe for you to leave the hospital without any further invasive tests.

If the stress test indicates a problem, or if you have periods of angina after the heart attack, the next step is cardiac catheterization to measure the pressures in the heart chambers and major blood vessels to gauge the severity of your coronary artery disease.

If the problem is stenosis (narrowing) in one artery that is cutting off a significant amount of blood flow, angioplasty (see p.661) with a balloon and possibly a stent might be used to open the vessel. When two or three vessels are involved or if the blood supply to a large portion of the heart muscle is in danger, bypass surgery (see p.662) will

Aspirin

Most people know aspirin as a humble painkiller. It has been the mainstay of every home medicine cabinet for more than 100 years. More recently, this simple medicine has proved to be a powerful tool in the treatment of cardiovascular disease.

Aspirin has an anticlotting effect in the blood. When a blood vessel is injured, more and more platelet cells clump around the damaged area until a clot forms on the vessel wall. Aspirin counteracts the platelets' clotting action by making them less able to stick to one another, and it may also fight inflammation in a plaque caused by atherosclerosis.

If you have coronary artery disease, but have not had a heart attack, regular use of aspirin can reduce your overall risk of heart attack or stroke by 25%. If you have just had a heart attack, taking 162 milligrams a day of aspirin (the equivalent of half a standard-sized tablet) within 24 hours of the first heart attack cuts your chances of dying by more than 20%.

Aspirin may also benefit people who have not been diagnosed with coronary artery disease. Findings from two large studies indicate that aspirin may prevent a first heart attack even if you have not been diagnosed with heart disease, particularly in men over age 50. Many doctors recommend that men over age 50 take 81 milligrams of aspirin a day. The largest randomized controlled studies (see p.33) of aspirin were conducted first in men, because men are more likely to have heart attacks. Most doctors are not yet willing to routinely recommend aspirin for women, because large studies in women have not been completed.

Do not begin taking aspirin on a regular, daily basis for any reason without first talking to your doctor. Aspirin can cause serious bleeding, may increase your risk for brain hemorrhage (see p.350), and, like all drugs, has side effects that make it intolerable to some people.

Do not take aspirin if you have a liver or kidney disease, a peptic ulcer or other gastrointestinal bleeding disorder, or an allergy to aspirin or other nonsteroidal anti-inflammatory drugs, or if you are taking the blood-thinner warfarin.

probably be recommended to restore blood flow to the area.

Medicines can also help increase your chances of survival after a heart attack. Primary among these is aspirin, which decreases the chance of having another heart attack by 31%. Another powerful blood-thinner called warfarin shows similar results, but is used infrequently because of the inconvenience of monitoring and the risk of bleeding.

If your cholesterol level is above average, potent cholesterol-lowering drugs (see p.671) can help prevent another heart attack. Beta blockers have also been shown to increase survival, as have ACE inhibitors, especially in cases where the heart's pumping ability has been compromised. These drugs are discussed in Choosing the Right Drug for High Blood Pressure (see p.650).

If you have had one heart attack, you are at greater risk for having another, and of dying prematurely. However, if you take charge of your life and your lifestyle, you can greatly improve the odds of recovery after release from the hospital.

LIFE AFTER A HEART ATTACK

Recovering from a heart attack requires making physical, emotional, and lifestyle adjustments. The first step is to help your injured heart muscle heal. Doctors once thought that 6 to 8 weeks of complete bed rest was the ideal prescription. It is now known that the opposite is true.

Physical activity enhances the recovery process for damaged heart muscle by helping to recondition it. But you must introduce exercise slowly, and with supervision. Most people start walking a few minutes a day in the hospital as early as 1 or 2 days after a heart attack.

When you are able to walk 30 minutes at a time and climb stairs, you will be able to participate in most activities of daily living. Before you go home, your doctors may administer a less strenuous type of treadmill stress test to evaluate your heart's performance at different levels of exertion. This information will provide the basis for determining how much activity you can safely do.

You can safely resume sexual relations if you can climb a flight of stairs without experiencing pain or shortness of breath, or have done well on the less strenuous type of treadmill stress test performed after the heart attack. Participating in a medically

supervised cardiac rehabilitation program can help you make the necessary lifestyle changes. A good program lasts at least 12 weeks and includes three 20- to 40-minute aerobic exercise sessions a week.

A rehabilitation program can also help you cope with the psychological changes and lifestyle adjustments that follow a heart attack. The first step in long-term recovery is to reduce the risk factors that lead to cardiovascular disease in the first place.

At the top of the list is smoking. Most hospitals run organized smoking cessation programs that can help you quit. Research shows that people with coronary artery disease can safely use the nicotine patch (see p.60).

You can benefit from restricting the amount of saturated and transunsaturated fat (see p.39) in your diet and from eating more fruits, vegetables, and high-fiber foods. If dietary changes alone are not sufficient to lower your cholesterol level, medicines may be necessary.

Other known contributors to heart disease are a high stress level and an "angry" personality type. You will need to learn how to slow down and enjoy life more after a heart attack. The stress management and relaxation training component of many cardiac rehabilitation programs can help you learn to handle stressful emotions.

In addition, many people become depressed and anxious after a heart attack and worry that they will never be able to return to good health. These feelings can slow the healing process, so it is important to address these issues with a qualified counselor.

You will probably leave the hospital with new drugs to lower blood pressure and cholesterol, control angina, reduce the chance of blood clots, and prevent abnormal heart rhythms and heart failure. Make sure you know how and when to take each of these. Also, be familiar with any potential side effects.

Finally, your biggest asset in your recovery period is a support network of your family, friends, and medical team. Rely on them for the emotional and physical help you need as you get back to good health.

Elevated Cholesterol

Elevated cholesterol means that you have more cholesterol in your blood than your body needs. Cholesterol is one of a group of fats (lipids) that serve either as material for building cells or as an energy source for the body. Your liver can manufacture most of the cholesterol your body needs.

In addition to knowing the level of total cholesterol in your blood, it is important to know the levels of different kinds of fats. High levels of low-density lipoprotein (LDL, the "bad" cholesterol) worsen atherosclerosis, whereas high levels of high-density lipoprotein (HDL, the "good" cholesterol) protect you against atherosclerosis: HDL cholesterol actually removes cholesterol from the lining of your arteries. High levels of a third type of fat, triglycerides, also worsen atherosclerosis.

Diets that are rich in saturated fats and trans-fats raise levels of LDL cholesterol, and trans-fats also lower HDL cholesterol—a

Current LDL Cholesterol Targets

If you are at . . .

VERY HIGH RISK

You have a history of heart disease (heart attack, unstable or stable angina, a heart procedure such as angioplasty or bypass) or other vascular disease (narrowing of the arteries to your brain or in your legs, aortic aneurysm) *and* also have at least one of the following:

- Multiple major risk factors for cardiovascular disease, including cigarette smoking, high blood pressure, a family history of premature heart disease, age over 50 in men (60 in women), and, especially, diabetes

- Severe and poorly controlled risk factors, such as smoking

- Multiple risk factors for metabolic syndrome, especially high triglycerides (200 or over) and low HDL (below 40)

- A history of heart attack or unstable angina

THE LATEST GUIDELINES SAY . . .

An LDL of less than 70 is a reasonable goal, and usually requires the use of cholesterol-lowering drugs

HIGH RISK

You have a history of heart disease or other vascular disease, as defined just above, *or* one of the following:

Diabetes

Vascular disease (as defined above)

Two or more risk factors for heart disease (as defined just above)

An LDL of less than 100 is a reasonable goal, including cholesterol-lowering medicines if lifestyle changes alone do not achieve the goal.

MODERATELY HIGH RISK

You have two or more risk factors for heart disease that create a 10% to 20% chance of having a heart attack in the next 10 years. You can find a heart attack risk calculator at www.nhlbi.nih.gov/health/index.html#tools.

An LDL of less than 130 is a reasonable goal, but a lower target of less than 100 is also reasonable.

MODERATE RISK

You have two or more risk factors for heart disease that create a chance of 10% or less of your having a heart attack in the next 10 years (see risk calculator, just above).

An LDL of less than 130 is a reasonable goal.

LOW RISK

Having no more than one risk factor for heart disease

An LDL of less than 160 is a reasonable goal.

double whammy. Replacing foods that are rich in saturated fats and trans-fats with foods rich in monounsaturated and polyunsaturated fats greatly improves the cholesterol profile. That can be achieved by replacing red and processed meats with a combination of fish, nuts, legumes, and poultry.

There is no doubt that lowering levels of total cholesterol, LDL cholesterol, and triglycerides—plus raising levels of HDL cholesterol—is good for your health. And as new studies are reported, the target levels for each of these types of blood fat levels have changed (see Current Blood Cholesterol Targets, on this page).

SYMPTOMS

A high level of cholesterol causes no symptoms, although a very high level can cause fatty patches called xanthomas (see p.541) on the skin or along the membrane that covers a tendon, such as the Achilles tendon. When high cholesterol leads to atherosclerosis (see p.653), the atherosclerosis can cause symptoms.

TREATMENT OPTIONS

Most people with high cholesterol are diagnosed when their physician performs a cholesterol test as part of a routine examination (see p.80 for recommendations on frequency of cholesterol testing). If you have high cholesterol, you may need to be tested more frequently.

If you have a problem with high cholesterol, the first step is to change your diet. In general, limit all foods that are high in saturated fat and cholesterol (such as red meat, butter, and foods containing butter).

Instead, choose foods such as fruits, vegetables, and whole-grain products that are naturally low in fat and high in complex carbohydrates and fiber.

If you smoke, ask your doctor for help in quitting (see p.59). The risks of smoking are even greater if your cholesterol is high.

Regular exercise for a minimum of 30 minutes a day at least three times a week can raise the levels of HDL in your blood. If diet and exercise do

---

Current Blood Cholesterol Targets

Over the past 20 years, studies have indicated that there are clear health benefits if the levels of different types of cholesterol are kept at target levels. Those recommendations have changed as new studies have been reported, and may change again. The current recommendations are:

Total Cholesterol Level	Total Cholesterol Category
Less than 200 mg/dL	Desirable
200–239 mg/dL	Borderline high
240 mg/dL and above	High
HDL Cholesterol Level	**HDL Cholesterol Category**
Less than 40 mg/dL	Low (representing risk)
60 mg/dL and above	High (heart-protective)
Trigylceride Level	**Triglyceride Category**
Less than 150 mg/dL	Normal
150–199 mg/dL	Borderline high
200–499 mg/dL	High
500 mg/dL and above	Very high

Adapted from the Third Report of the National Cholesterol Education Program of the National Heart, Lung, and Blood Institute.

---

not lower your cholesterol enough, your doctor may prescribe drugs, particularly if you have other risk factors for atherosclerosis.

DRUGS USED TO LOWER CHOLESTEROL

Research shows that aggressively lowering cholesterol levels can dramatically increase the life expectancy for people who are at high risk or already have coronary artery disease—even if their cholesterol levels are in the normal range.

There are several types of medicines used to lower cholesterol:

■ **Statins** are a group of similar medicines that are very effective in lowering both total and LDL cholesterol, and slightly raising

HDL cholesterol. They are generally free of side effects, although occasionally they cause liver or muscle damage. Some have more recently been shown to prevent stroke and heart attack.

■ **Niacin** is a vitamin that is effective in lowering total and LDL cholesterol, and more effective in raising HDL cholesterol. Shortly after swallowing a niacin pill, you may have a flushed sensation (heat and redness of the skin); this can be prevented by taking 81 milligrams of aspirin shortly before taking the niacin.

■ **Bile acid–binding resins** are powders or pills that cause the liver to take LDL cholesterol out of the blood, lowering both total and LDL cholesterol levels. These drugs are not as strong as statins and niacin. Also, they tend to increase levels of triglycerides (making them a problem for people whose triglyceride levels already are high). They often cause constipation, bloating, and gas, and are less popular than the first two kinds of treatment.

■ **Gemfibrozil** is a pill that is very effective at lowering triglycerides and raising HDL cholesterol, but only moderately effective at lowering total cholesterol and LDL cholesterol. It can cause abdominal pain and liver and muscle injury.

■ **Ezetimibe** is a pill that reduces the amount of dietary cholesterol that is absorbed. When used in combination with other cholesterol-lowering drugs, particularly statins, it can further lower blood cholesterol levels.

ABNORMAL HEART RATE AND RHYTHM

Normal Heart Rhythm

A heartbeat involves the contraction of the two ventricles, which pump blood to the rest of the body. The contraction of the two ventricles is preceded by contraction of the two atria, which fill the ventricles with blood. Normally, the heart beats at a rate of 60 to 100 times per minute in a regular and orderly fashion.

Each normal heartbeat is started by an electrical impulse that begins in a small group of specialized muscle cells called the sinoatrial (SA) node. The SA node, a natural pacemaker, is located in the wall of the right atrium.

The signal from the SA node spreads quickly to the two small, upper chambers of the heart (atria), causing them to contract. The signal then travels to another specialized bundle of cells, the atrioventricular (AV) node, and on to the ventricles through special pathways called bundle branches.

When the signal reaches the ventricles a fraction of a second later (after the ventricles have had time to fill with blood), it causes them to contract.

It is normal for the heart to speed up during periods of exercise or emotional anxiety, answering the body's need for more oxygen and to get rid of more waste products. Fever, anemia, an overactive thyroid gland, and some drugs (such as decongestants, caffeine, amphetamines, and cocaine) can also cause the heart to pump faster than normal.

Heart rhythm abnormalities develop when there is a malfunction in the heart's electrical system. The rhythm abnormalities, which range from mild to life-threatening, can change the regular contraction of either the atria or the ventricles.

Conduction Pathways of the Heart

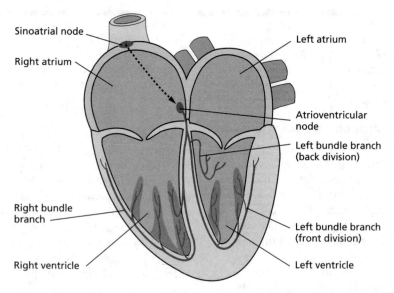

The conduction pathways are specialized tissues that carry electrical signals and coordinate the beating of the heart. The signal triggering a contraction of the heart begins in the sinoatrial node located in the wall of the right atrium. From there, the signal travels to the atrioventricular node and then on to the ventricles through the right and left bundle branches.

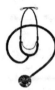

Atrial Fibrillation: *When You Visit Your Doctor*

QUESTIONS TO DISCUSS WITH YOUR DOCTOR:

■ Are you fatigued? Do you become short of breath with exertion or when you lie down?

■ Do you get chest pain or pressure with exertion or at rest? Is there a change in your usual pattern?

■ Do you have swelling in your ankles?

■ Do you ever feel like you are going to faint? Have you fainted?

■ Do you have sudden brief episodes of weakness in an arm or leg, loss of vision (like a shade being pulled over your eyes), or difficulty speaking? These could be warning symptoms of stroke (see p.342). People with atrial fibrillation are at increased risk of stroke.

■ Do you drink alcohol or caffeine-containing beverages? These can cause atrial fibrillation.

■ Is there a chance that cardioversion (shocking the heart to put it back into its normal rhythm) would be helpful (if you have had atrial fibrillation for less than a year)?

■ Do you need to take blood-thinning medication (such as warfarin or aspirin) if you are not already taking it?

YOUR DOCTOR MIGHT EXAMINE THE FOLLOWING BODY STRUCTURES OR FUNCTIONS:

■ Heart rate, blood pressure, and weight

■ Heart and lungs

■ Pulse

■ Veins in the neck

■ Ankles and legs (for swelling)

YOUR DOCTOR MIGHT ORDER THE FOLLOWING LAB TESTS OR STUDIES:

■ Thyroid function tests (blood tests) at least once because thyroid abnormalities can cause atrial fibrillation

■ Blood levels of digoxin

■ Blood levels of minerals (such as potassium and magnesium) regularly

■ Tests of kidney function regularly

■ Prothrombin time (time it takes blood to clot) if you are taking warfarin to thin your blood

■ Electrocardiogram (see p.135)

■ Holter monitor (see p.680) or an event monitor if you may be going in and out of atrial fibrillation

Abnormal Rhythms of the Atria

Atrial tachycardia results when electrical impulses are generated from somewhere in the atria other than the sinoatrial (SA) node. The heart beats faster than usual, but in a very regular fashion.

When the condition comes on suddenly and lasts between a few seconds to several hours, it is called paroxysmal atrial tachycardia (PAT) or paroxysmal supraventricular tachycardia.

PAT is often the result of a disruption in the heart's triggering signal as it travels through the atrioventricular node. The condition can occur in people who have no underlying heart disease, often during emotional stress. It is aggravating, but is usually not a serious problem. It also can occur if you are born with unusual electrical pathways in your heart, in which case it can be a more serious problem.

Atrial fibrillation is a common heart rhythm disturbance experienced by more than 2 million Americans. Instead of forcefully contracting in a coordinated manner, the walls of the left and right atria quiver and do not effectively pump blood into the ventricles.

Sometimes the atrial fibrillation comes and goes, and sometimes it stays constant. It can occur in people who have otherwise healthy hearts. However, it is more common in those who have heart valve disorders, overactive thyroid glands, lung disease, pulmonary embolus, and inflammation of the heart's lining.

Home Remedies for Paroxysmal Atrial Tachycardia

You can use various procedures to interrupt an attack of paroxysmal atrial tachycardia. The first of these is to arch your head as far backward as possible. Another is to blow as hard as you can into a difficult-to-inflate toy balloon.

A third option is a technique called the Valsalva maneuver. This is accomplished by trying to exhale forcefully with your mouth closed and while you pinch your nose shut. If these techniques are not effective or if you have frequent attacks, call your doctor.

As with many heart rhythm abnormalities, it is often caused by coronary artery disease.

Atrial fibrillation is important for three reasons. First, it can signal the presence of another disorder. Second, since the heartbeat is often more rapid than is normal or healthy, the heart pumps blood less efficiently. Third, in atrial fibrillation, the blood can pool in the atria, forming clots that can travel from the heart and lodge in an artery in another part of the body.

If one of these clots blocks a vessel in the brain, it can cause a stroke (see p.342). Atrial fibrillation causes about 15% of all strokes.

Atrial flutter is another type of rhythm disturbance related to the atrial chambers. Compared to atrial fibrillation, the contractions of the atria are more regular, but they are still inefficient in moving blood from the atria into the ventricles.

Also, in atrial flutter, the heart can be forced to beat at a dangerously fast rate. Although they are two different rhythm abnormalities, atrial fibrillation can develop and coexist in people who have atrial flutter.

Wandering atrial pacemaker and multifocal atrial tachycardia are examples of atrial

rhythm disturbances in which frequent, unpredictable beats arise from different areas of the atria. These disturbances are usually an indication of lung or heart disease, serious metabolic disturbances, or toxicity of certain medicines.

SYMPTOMS

Abnormal rhythms of the atria may cause no symptoms at all. You may feel palpitations—the sensation that your heart is racing at a fast pace, fluttering, or "flip-flopping."

It is very common for people to feel palpitations. Palpitations alone are no cause for alarm. However, if the abnormal rhythm is making the heart pump less efficiently, you may feel fatigue, breathlessness, dizziness, chest pressure, or tightness along with the palpitations. If you have these associated symptoms, call your doctor.

TREATMENT OPTIONS

An electrocardiogram (see p.135) can detect an abnormal rhythm of the atria. If the rhythm comes and goes, a Holter monitor or event monitor (see Monitoring Heart Rhythm, p.681) may be needed.

Wandering atrial pacemaker and multifocal atrial tachycardia usually do not cause serious symptoms or require treatment.

Atrial tachycardia or PAT attacks can often be stopped by various maneuvers you can perform yourself (see Home Remedies for Paroxysmal Atrial Tachycardia, above). If these don't work, drugs such as beta blockers or calcium channel blockers can prevent or abort an attack.

Atrial fibrillation or atrial flutter requires immediate hospitalization if you are having chest pain or heart failure or your heartbeat is very fast. The ideal treatment for atrial fibrillation is to reestablish a normal heart rhythm and then maintain it with the use of medicines.

There are several methods for reestablishing a normal rhythm. One of the most effective is cardioversion. This is a synchronized electrical shock to the heart that interrupts the abnormal heart rhythm, allowing the SA node to take over and conduct a normal rhythm.

If your heart is only mildly diseased, beta blockers or amiodarone can bring the heart rate back to normal. When the abnormal rhythms are caused by abnormal electrical pathways in the heart and cannot be successfully treated with drugs, your doctor may recommend a treatment called radiofrequency ablation.

In this procedure, a small

Risk of Cardiovascular Disease With Elevated Homocysteine Level

Homocysteine is a normal product of protein metabolism in the body. People who have elevated levels appear to have an increased risk of cardiovascular disease. In general, if a person has high levels of homocysteine, he or she is two times more likely to suffer a heart attack or stroke. The risks for women are half those for men.

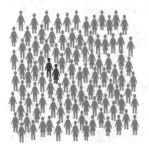

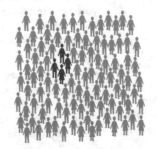

2 OF 100 MEN IN THE GENERAL POPULATION WHO ARE 65 TO 74 YEARS OLD WILL HAVE A HEART ATTACK WITHIN A YEAR

4 OF 100 MEN WITH ELEVATED HOMOCYSTEINE LEVELS WHO ARE 65 TO 74 YEARS OLD WILL HAVE A HEART ATTACK WITHIN A YEAR

catheter is threaded into the heart, as in cardiac catheterization; radio waves from the tip of the catheter destroy the abnormal pathways.

An implantable device can be used to detect recurring atrial fibrillation and deliver a small shock to the heart to make the rhythm regular again. This is similar to the implantable defibrillator (see below) used to correct abnormal rhythms of the ventricles.

If it is not possible for your heart to maintain a normal rhythm, drugs such as beta blockers, digitalis, and calcium channel blockers can at least help keep your heart rate from going too fast. Your symptoms should disappear once the drugs begin to control your heart rate.

In addition, your doctor will probably recommend that you take the blood-thinning medicine warfarin to prevent formation of blood clots in your atria and to prevent the possibility of a stroke or another complication from blood clots in the future.

Abnormal Rhythms of the Ventricles

Since the ventricles are primarily responsible for pumping blood out of the heart and into the body, abnormal rhythms of the ventricles often have more serious consequences than abnormal rhythms of the atria.

"Extra heartbeats" (premature ventricular contractions) are beats that start in the ventricles, rather than in the sinoatrial (SA) node, as in the normal heartbeat. They often occur in healthy people and can be caused by stimulants such as asthma medicines or decongestants.

They can also be brought on by the caffeine in coffee, tea, and cola drinks, by alcohol, or by the nicotine in cigarettes. When they occur in people with heart disease, they indicate an increased risk of more serious abnormal rhythms.

Ventricular tachycardia (VT) involves a rapid, coordinated, rhythm that begins from an abnormal trigger in the ventricles. Unlike the normal heartbeat, it does not start in the SA node. Often, the heart rate is between 140 and 300 beats per minute.

VT can last for just a few seconds, in which case it often does not cause symptoms. This can happen in people whose hearts

Implantable Defibrillators

An implantable defibrillator is similar to a pacemaker. It can detect the heart's rhythm and send an electrical impulse to the heart muscle. However, whereas a pacemaker detects a missing natural heartbeat and sends a tiny electrical signal to stimulate the heart to beat, a defibrillator detects potentially lethal abnormal heart rhythms and sends a large electrical signal to shock the heart muscle to try to restore its normal rhythm.

The electric shock is strong enough to cause some discomfort, but can be lifesaving. Some devices detect abnormal rhythms that could lead to ventricular fibrillation and deliver small electrical impulses (like a pacemaker) to try to pace the heart out of the abnormal rhythm.

If this fails to restore the rhythm to normal, the device then delivers the strong electric shock needed to end the abnormal rhythm.

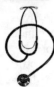

Fainting: When You Visit Your Doctor

QUESTIONS TO DISCUSS WITH YOUR DOCTOR:

■ Did you feel light-headed, like you were going to faint, just before you fainted? This often occurs with vasovagal syncope (see Nonserious Causes of Fainting, p.677).

■ Did you faint shortly after a heavy meal or after drinking a lot of alcohol? This often occurs with vasovagal syncope (see Nonserious Causes of Fainting, p.677).

■ Did you faint just after you had sudden, unexpected pain or another sudden unexpected sensation? This could be vasovagal syncope (see Nonserious Causes of Fainting, p.677).

■ Did you faint while standing with your knees locked and legs straight for some time, such as in church? This could be vasovagal syncope (see Nonserious Causes of Fainting, p.677).

■ Did you faint just after you coughed, laughed hard, urinated, or passed a bowel movement? This could be situational syncope (see Nonserious Causes of Fainting, p.677).

■ Did you faint just after you stood up suddenly from a lying or sitting position? This could be caused by medicines that affect blood pressure or by dehydration.

■ Did you faint while you were exercising strenuously? This is a danger sign that could indicate a variety of heart abnormalities.

■ Did you feel pain in your chest or palpitations around the time you fainted? This is a danger sign that could indicate a variety of heart abnormalities.

■ Did you faint while you were lying or sitting, not changing your body position, and without any warning? This could indicate a potentially dangerous abnormal heart rhythm.

■ Did you injure yourself when you fainted? This indicates that you fainted without any warning, which points to possible serious heart disease or a seizure.

■ Did people who saw you faint say that you were unconscious for more than 1 minute? This is a danger sign. Most nonserious episodes of fainting last less than 1 minute.

■ Did people who saw you faint say that your body jerked uncontrollably for more than 5 seconds while you were unconscious? You may have had a seizure. With nonserious kinds of fainting, a person may have a few jerking movements that last less than 3 to 5 seconds.

■ Did you soil yourself with urine or feces, was your tongue sore or bleeding after you regained consciousness, or were you confused or "out of it" for more than 5 minutes after you regained consciousness? You may have had a seizure.

YOUR DOCTOR MIGHT EXAMINE THE FOLLOWING BODY STRUCTURES OR FUNCTIONS:

■ Pulse and blood pressure lying down, sitting, and/or standing

■ Heart

■ Brain and nervous system

YOUR DOCTOR MIGHT ORDER THE FOLLOWING LAB TESTS OR STUDIES:

■ Electrocardiogram (see p.135), Holter monitor (see p.680), or event monitor (see p.681) if a heart problem is suspected.

■ Electroencephalography (see p.136) and computed tomography (see p.149) or magnetic resonance imaging (see p.150) of the brain if a seizure is suspected.

■ Test for fecal occult blood (see p.791) to check if there is bleeding in your digestive system.

■ Tilt-table testing is occasionally performed if vasovagal syncope (see Nonserious Causes of Fainting, p.677) is suspected. In this test you are strapped to a table (to prevent you from falling) and your heart rate and blood pressure are monitored as the table is tilted to rapidly change your body position from lying flat on your back to standing upright. This sudden change, particularly the effect of gravity pulling blood into your legs and away from your heart, can cause your blood pressure to temporarily drop and, in turn, can cause you to faint. Sometimes you are also given an intravenous drug to bring out the tendency for your blood pressure to drop.

beat normally or in those who have a more unusual inherited condition of the conducting system called the prolonged QT interval syndrome, or long QT syndrome.

When VT lasts for minutes or hours, it often (but not always) leads to more serious symptoms because the heart is unable to pump blood efficiently. Sometimes, VT turns into ventricular fibrillation (see below), which can be fatal.

Most of the time, VT that lasts more than a few seconds is an indication of a serious underlying heart condition, usually cardiomyopathy (see p.682) or advanced coronary artery disease.

Ventricular fibrillation (VF) is a condition in which the electrical impulses governing the beating heart are completely disorganized. As a result, the muscle of the ventricles quivers rather than beats. The ventricles no longer can pump blood out into the body, which leads to cardiac arrest, in which circulation stops.

Death follows within minutes if the heart cannot be restarted. VF most often occurs in people with coronary artery disease. It is the most common cause of death after a heart attack. Electrical shock or anesthesia can also bring on VF.

SYMPTOMS

If you have occasional extra heartbeats, you may feel a sudden thump in the middle of your chest, or you may have no symptoms. VT often produces palpitations (a rapid, forceful heartbeat).

If the pumping efficiency of your heart is reduced, you can have chest pressure and feel weak, light-headed, and breath-

less; you may faint. VF rapidly causes loss of consciousness and sudden death if it is not corrected.

TREATMENT OPTIONS

An electrocardiogram (see p.135) can detect an abnormal rhythm of the ventricles. If this rhythm comes and goes, a Holter monitor or event monitor (see Monitoring Heart Rhythm, p.681) may be needed to detect it.

Extra heartbeats (premature ventricular contractions) require no treatment if you are healthy. If the symptoms bother you, avoid caffeine, decongestants, cigarettes, and alcohol—all of which can contribute to the problem. In a person with a healthy heart, medicines are usually not advised unless the palpitations are very bothersome. Even when they are vexing, they are usually not serious.

When treatment is prescribed, it usually involves low doses of beta blockers. If you have known heart disease, your doctor may prescribe an antiarrhythmic medicine to diminish the number of extra beats.

VT that lasts for more than a few seconds and causes symptoms is often treated with antiarrhythmic drugs such as quinidine, procainamide, and disopyramide. These medicines, however, also have the paradoxical potential to cause abnormal heart rhythms, so they require careful monitoring.

Monitoring is done by assessing the effect of each drug while using a 24-hour cardiac monitor (Holter monitor). Sometimes, it is necessary to evaluate the effects of several medicines before you find a drug that works best for you. Some cardiologists recommend electrophysiologic testing

(see p.680) to see if the medicine is working or is able to cure the arrhythmia.

VT that lasts for several minutes can be an emergency because it can degenerate into VF. For this reason, if the rhythm occurs in a medical setting, it often is treated by a machine that delivers a shock to your heart to try to restore normal heart rhythm.

If you have repeated episodes of VT that cannot be controlled with drugs, a cardiologist may put a small machine called an implantable defibrillator (see p.675) into your body; it gives the heart a shock whenever your heart develops VT.

VF leads to cardiac arrest and is an emergency requiring immediate cardiopulmonary resuscitation (see p.1201).

Fainting

Fainting involves a temporary loss of consciousness. It is very common. In one survey, nearly half of the people interviewed said they had fainted at least once in their lives.

Sometimes people fall when they faint, striking and injuring themselves. Most of the time, fainting is caused by a minor abnormality, but occasionally it can be caused by a serious condition. Because of this, talk to your doctor about any fainting spell.

You may or may not remember what was happening just before you fainted or immediately after you awakened. It is important to talk to those who may have seen you faint to find out what they noticed just before, during, and after the event.

Nonserious causes of fainting
The most common cause of faint-

ing, particularly in someone younger than age 50, is a condition called vasovagal syncope (syncope is the medical term for fainting). It is caused by abnormal reflexes that make the heart temporarily beat slowly and make the arterioles widen, causing blood pressure to drop. You usually feel like you are going to faint and have time to sit or lie down before you faint.

Other common and nonserious causes are dehydration or a recent viral illness. Fainting can occur after anything that raises pressure in your chest, such as coughing, laughing hard, urinating, or straining to have a bowel movement (called situational syncope).

Certain medicines that affect blood pressure—such as antihypertension medicines, heterocyclic antidepressants, and tranquilizers—may increase the tendency to faint. Excessive consumption of alcohol can also cause fainting.

Serious causes of fainting

Sometimes, a loss of consciousness is caused by a seizure (see p.374). The period of unconsciousness is often longer than 1 to 2 minutes and the body jerks uncontrollably for at least 30 seconds and often longer. People who have a seizure may soil themselves with urine or feces. They may bite their tongue and are often confused and extremely weak for some hours after regaining consciousness.

A loss of consciousness can also be caused by abnormal heart rhythms, including the kind that can cause sudden death. Also, heart conditions that block the outflow of blood, such as aortic stenosis (see p.690), can cause fainting.

Cardiac Arrest

Cardiac arrest occurs when the heart suddenly stops pumping. Each year, a quarter of a million people in the United States die of cardiac arrest.

Abnormal rhythms of the ventricles—ventricular tachycardia (see p.675) and ventricular fibrillation (see p.677)—are responsible for 90% of cases of cardiac arrest.

The other 10% are caused by heart block (see p.680), in which the heart simply stops pumping frequently enough to sustain life, or abnormal rhythms of the atria (see p.672) in which the heart is beating too rapidly to pump blood efficiently.

In most people, cardiac arrest is caused by coronary artery disease (see p.652). Cocaine can trigger cardiac arrest by causing the coronary arteries to spasm, which also deprives the heart muscle of oxygen.

Viral infections of the heart muscle can also cause the abnormal heart rhythms that lead to cardiac arrest. Less commonly, an accidental electric shock, excessive intake of alcohol, or, in rare cases, hereditary conditions of the heart muscle cause cardiac arrest.

The immediate use of cardiopulmonary resuscitation (CPR) (see p.1201) after a person goes into cardiac arrest can partially maintain blood flow while you are waiting for emergency help to arrive.

For this reason, it is a good idea to be trained in CPR. Classes are widely available at local hospitals and Red Cross chapters. If emergency medical crews arrive on the scene in time, they can sometimes restart the heart using defibrillation equipment that administers an electric shock to the heart muscle. If the person recovers from cardiac arrest, it is crucial to identify and treat the underlying cause of the problem to avoid a recurrence.

Alternative Medicine: Eating Fish Reduces Risk of Sudden Death

Around 1980, researchers found that natives of Greenland, even though they eat a lot of fatty foods, die less frequently of coronary artery disease. Greenlanders also eat a lot of fish of many kinds.

Researchers speculate that a substance in fish oils called n-3 polyunsaturated fatty acid might be a protective factor.

There is strong evidence (from many large studies) that men who eat any kind of fish at least once a week have a risk of sudden death that is about half that of men who eat less fish. This has not been studied as well in women, because heart disease is less common in women under age 65. Whether n-3 polyunsaturated fatty acid is the cause of this benefit in men is unclear.

Some doctors now recommend that people who have known heart disease eat two meals of fish a week.

Pacemakers

Pacemakers are used when your heart will not beat fast enough. Pacemakers consist of a small box called an impulse generator that sends a tiny electrical signal down a wire that travels through the veins and into the heart.

The tip of the wire rests against the heart muscle. The electrical signals travel down the wire, stimulate the heart muscle, and cause the heart to pump. Each electrical signal causes one heartbeat. You cannot feel the electrical impulses, although people with pacemakers occasionally feel a slight flutter when their heart rate changes.

Temporary pacemakers, whose impulse generator is outside the body, are used in emergencies, when your heart first starts beating too slowly, and can be left in place for several days. Using them for longer periods increases the risk of infection or the formation of blood clots.

Permanent pacemakers are needed when your slow heart rate is not due to a temporary condition. They run on batteries that typically last for 7 to 12 years. The generators for permanent pacemakers are implanted just beneath the skin, under the collarbone, and the wires are passed into the heart through a large vein that runs under the collarbone.

Some pacemakers stimulate only one heart chamber, while others have electrodes that trigger both the atrium and the ventricle. The operation to insert a permanent pacemaker takes only an hour or two and can be done using local anesthesia.

Most pacemakers have the capacity to monitor the heart's natural rhythm and release an electrical impulse only if your heart rate dips below a certain level, usually 60 beats per minute. The most sophisticated devices sense when there is an increase or decrease of the body's demand on the heart and raise or lower your heart rate accordingly.

There are very few limitations to living with a pacemaker. Because the pacemakers are metal, going through airport security can sometimes require special arrangements. Also, magnetic resonance imaging (see p.150) cannot be performed, because the magnet pulls on the metal.

The newer devices have improved shielding so that you do not have to worry about interference from household electronics. Pacemakers tend to slow down as the batteries run low, so you need to have the device checked every few months. It can be checked in your doctor's office, or even over the phone using a special device.

If your pacemaker needs to be reprogrammed, your doctor can use a radio transmitter to change the pacemaker's instructions without any invasive measures. When the battery needs to be changed after about 7 to 10 years, another operation is necessary.

Permanent Pacemaker

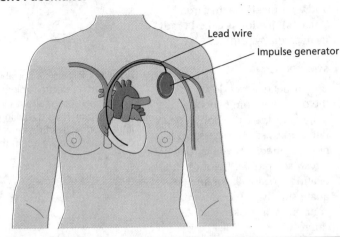

Lead wire

Impulse generator

A pacemaker sends tiny electrical signals to the heart chambers to keep the heart beating in a normal rhythm. The impulse generator is implanted beneath the skin near the collarbone. Wires lead from the impulse generator through the blood vessels below the neck and down into the heart, where the tips of the wires press against the heart muscle.

Electrophysiologic Testing of the Heart

Electrophysiologic testing is used to diagnose and treat problems in your heart's rhythm, or in its ability to conduct electrical impulses. It is usually performed at a hospital. You are given local anesthesia, and a doctor threads tiny electrodes through an artery in your groin up into the heart (as with cardiac catheterization).

The electrodes can detect some electrical abnormalities in your heart more accurately than a conventional electrocardiogram. They can also stimulate the

heart and determine if the stimulation provokes an abnormality of your heart's rate or rhythm.

If the testing does provoke an abnormality, the doctor will give you one or more medications to eliminate it; then your heart will be stimulated again to see if the drugs work.

The electrodes can also deliver a shock to your heart to stop an abnormal heart rhythm or to eliminate an abnormal pathway in the heart that causes abnormal heart rhythms.

Slow Heartbeat, Heart Block, and Sick Sinus Syndrome

A slow heart rate is fewer than 60 beats per minute. People who are physically fit can have a slower-than-average heart rate because their cardiovascular system works extremely efficiently. As a result, it takes the heart fewer contractions to deliver an adequate supply of fresh blood to the body.

The heart also beats more slowly during sleep. However, heart damage or illness can also lead to abnormal slowing of the heart. The three most common causes are excessive doses of heart-slowing drugs, heart block, and sick sinus syndrome.

Heart-slowing drugs—such as digitalis, quinidine, beta blockers, or calcium channel blockers—cause the heart to beat too slowly. Your doctor will monitor for this effect on every visit and can adjust the dose to prevent it.

Heart block occurs when the electrical impulse that triggers a contraction slows down as it travels from the heart's upper cham-

bers (atria) to its lower chambers (ventricles). In some cases, the signal does not get through at all, resulting in a very slow heart rate.

Heart block can come and go or become permanent. Heart block is usually caused by coronary artery disease (see p.652) or cardiomyopathy (see p.682).

Sick sinus syndrome is a condition in which the heart's natural pacemaker—the sinoatrial (SA) node—does not send its signal regularly. Usually the signal is too infrequent, and therefore the heart rate is too slow. Sometimes, the heart rate alternates between beating too slowly (bradycardia) and too quickly (tachycardia). The combination is called brady-tachycardia syndrome.

SYMPTOMS

If your heart slows down mildly, the only symptom may be fatigue. A dramatic drop in heart rate can cause weakness, dizziness, fainting, or even cardiac arrest (see p.677). If your heart is beating too slowly for an adequate supply of blood to reach your brain, a stroke (see p.342) can result.

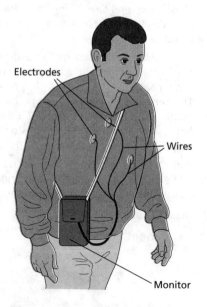

Holter Monitor

Electrodes

Wires

Monitor

A Holter monitor is a portable device for recording electrocardiogram readings as you go about your daily life. The monitor is useful in uncovering abnormal heart rhythms that occur when you are not in the doctor's office.

TREATMENT OPTIONS

Your doctor may need to administer emergency medication to bring your heartbeat back up to normal. Another solution is to insert an artificial pacemaker (see p.679) to keep your heart rhythm stable. A temporary pacemaker can be threaded through a vein to your heart and kept in place until your heart returns to normal.

If your heart block is permanent, it is necessary to surgically implant a permanent pacemaker. If a medication you are taking is causing the slowing, your doctor will have you decrease the dose or discontinue that drug.

Monitoring Heart Rhythm

If you have an abnormal heart rhythm that occurs intermittently, your doctor may ask you to wear a portable electrocardiogram (ECG) (see p.135) device called a Holter monitor.

Holter monitor The Holter monitor, also called an ambulatory ECG, is a recording device that monitors your heart rhythm over a 24- to 48-hour period, while you go about your day-to-day activities and while you sleep.

The monitor records your heart function through small metal discs called electrodes, which are temporarily affixed to your chest. The electrodes detect the electrical signal created by each heartbeat. The signal is transmitted to and stored in a small box (the recorder) that is small enough to fit into the pocket of a jacket or in a pouch hung around your neck.

Using a Holter monitor does not require any special preparation other than, if you are a man, possibly shaving your chest. You will receive instructions on how to make entries in your symptom diary and how to reattach the leads if they become loose. You will also need to keep the device dry.

During the test period, you will be asked to keep a diary of your symptoms and of your daily activities. Write down any time you feel fatigue, dizziness, chest pain, palpitations, or other indications that your heartbeat may be disturbed. Many devices also have a button you can use to mark the tracing when your symptoms occur.

At the end of the test period, the doctor will compare your diary with the information in the recorder. In particular, your physician will look for any rhythm abnormalities that occurred while you were having symptoms.

A drawback to the Holter monitor is that the recording period may not be long enough to identify abnormalities if your symptoms occur infrequently. In this case, your doctor may recommend you use an event monitor (see below).

Sometimes, the monitor detects the presence of heart rhythm disturbances that could indicate the potential for a serious problem in the future, even if those disturbances do not cause you symptoms at the time they are detected by the Holter monitor. Your doctor will discuss with you if any further testing is necessary.

Event monitor An event monitor is a small, portable device for recording ECG readings. The battery-operated instrument is about the size of a deck of cards and fits easily into a pocket. Like a Holter monitor, an event monitor takes ECG readings while you go about your day-to-day activities (and while you sleep) to determine if you are having abnormal heart rhythms.

An event monitor is particularly useful if you are having symptoms that could be caused by an abnormal heart rhythm, but the symptoms occur infrequently (perhaps once or twice a week) rather than many times in an average 24-hour period.

While a Holter monitor takes an ECG reading continuously for up to 24 hours, the event monitor can be used for weeks or months and records the ECG reading periodically.

When you have symptoms that might be caused by an abnormal heart rhythm—such as palpitations, chest pain, or dizziness—you activate the event monitor and it keeps a record of your ECG reading at that moment.

There are two kinds of event monitors:

■ Nonlooping monitors are small devices that you carry in your pocket or purse. When you feel you may be having an abnormal heart rhythm, you press the monitor against your chest just over your heart. It records your heart rhythm for about 30 seconds. Most nonlooping monitors can store several 30-second periods. These devices are very useful if your symptoms tend to last for a few minutes.

■ Looping monitors have electrodes that strap to your chest. They take a continuous ECG reading, just like a Holter monitor, but the monitor does not store the information unless you tell it to.

When you press a button, the monitor permanently stores your ECG reading, starting with the pattern that occurred a few seconds before you pressed the button, and for some time after. The looping monitor is useful if your symptoms last only a few seconds because it records your heart rhythm for some time before you feel the symptoms, which a nonlooping monitor cannot do.

Whichever event monitor you use, keep a diary indicating precisely how you were feeling and what you were doing at the time you activated the device.

DISEASES OF THE HEART MUSCLE AND LINING

Cardiomyopathy

Any heart disease involving weakening of the heart muscle (myocardium) can be known as cardiomyopathy. This is a broad term covering many conditions, all of which result in injury to the heart muscle and impaired heart function.

In some forms of cardiomyopathy, the weakened heart muscle becomes thinned; in other forms it becomes abnormally thickened. In any event, the ventricles of the heart often can no longer pump blood as effectively. Blood stagnates in the heart, making it more likely to form clots. These can break free and cause an arterial embolism (see p.701).

In addition, the beleaguered heart muscle becomes more prone to potentially dangerous abnormal heart rhythms (see p.672). Congestive heart failure (see p.683) often develops.

Cardiomyopathy is sometimes caused by myocarditis, which is inflammation of the heart muscle. An underlying infection is often the source of the problem. The human coxsackievirus B and human echovirus are the most commonly implicated causes of myocarditis.

More recent research indicates that a mutant strain of the human coxsackievirus B may be more likely to cause myocarditis and cardiomyopathy. The human immunodeficiency virus, Lyme disease, and a tropical parasite called *Trypanosoma cruzi* can also be responsible.

Chronic inflammatory conditions such as lupus and transplant rejection reactions after a heart transplant can also result in myocarditis.

Coronary artery disease can also lead to permanent weakness of the heart muscle by causing a state of reduced blood flow to much of the heart (ischemic cardiomyopathy); this can occur even if it has not caused the death of any heart muscle from a heart attack.

In other people, injury to the heart muscle occurs due to the toxic effects of drinking too much alcohol (alcoholic cardiomyopathy). This can result from a lifetime of binge drinking or the cumulative effects of four or five drinks a day over 5 to 10 years.

Vitamin deficiencies caused by the poor diet that often accompanies alcoholism also weaken the heart. In its early stages, alcoholic cardiomyopathy can be reversed by abstaining from alcohol. As the disease progresses, however, heart muscle damage becomes permanent.

Restrictive cardiomyopathy is another type. The heart muscle is either thickened or is invaded by abnormal cells or other material. The most common form is the enlargement that can be seen in response to high blood pressure, aortic stenosis, or other conditions that create increased resistance (against which the heart has to pump).

An unusual inherited condition called hypertrophic cardiomyopathy causes the heart muscle to thicken, particularly the wall between the two ventricles. In severe cases, the overgrowth of muscle obstructs the passage of blood out of the heart and may cause fainting or even sudden death.

This disease usually occurs before the age of 40 and can affect children as young as age 10. It has been responsible for the deaths of several young athletes.

SYMPTOMS

In its earlier stages, cardiomyopathy may cause no symptoms. It may be discovered by accident, when a chest x-ray performed to diagnose another condition shows an enlarged heart.

When cardiomyopathy causes symptoms, they are the symptoms of a failing heart: fatigue, weakness, and unusual breath-lessness with even mild exertion or when lying down.

When cardiomyopathy causes abnormal heart rhythms (see p.672), symptoms can include palpitations, light-headedness, fainting, and even sudden death. People with hypertrophic car-diomyopathy can also develop chest pain.

TREATMENT OPTIONS

The diagnosis of cardiomyopathy is often clear from your symp-toms, the results of a physical examination (particularly signs of heart failure), and the results of a chest x-ray, echocardiogram, and electrocardiogram.

Occasionally, a test called an endomyocardial biopsy is neces-sary. In this test, a catheter is inserted into a vein in the neck and passed down into the heart. A small piece of the inner heart wall is removed using a tiny metal device at the tip of the catheter. The biopsy sample of heart tissue is then examined under the microscope.

There are treatments for all forms of cardiomyopathy, includ-ing the two most common causes of symptoms: heart failure and abnormal heart rhythms.

People who have alcoholic cardiomyopathy seem to be par-ticularly sensitive to the effects of alcohol; giving up drinking alco-hol is the most important step in treating the condition. After that, the symptoms of heart failure can be controlled with drugs and dietary changes.

Treatment for hypertrophic cardiomyopathy can help control symptoms of chest pain and shortness of breath. More impor-tantly, it can decrease your risk

Cardiomyopathies

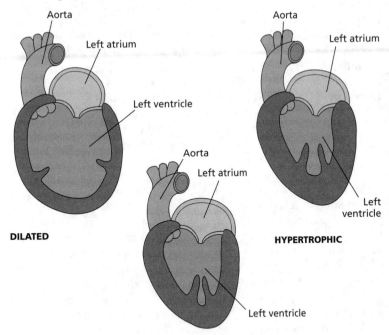

Heart muscle damage can be classified into three major categories. Dilated cardiomyopathy is a condition in which the heart muscle fibers have stretched to the point where the heart can no longer contract forcefully. Hypertrophic cardiomyopathy results from a thickening of the heart muscle that limits the capacity of the ventricles and may interfere with the functioning of the aortic valve. In restrictive cardiomyopathy, the heart muscle becomes so stiff that the ventricles cannot expand to fill with blood.

for sudden cardiac death. Usually this requires taking beta blockers or calcium channel blockers. You may also need to take medi-cation to prevent abnormal heart rhythms. Avoid strenuous exercise because it can bring on sudden cardiac death.

Sometimes it is necessary to implant a pacemaker (see p.679) or implantable defibrillator to keep heart rhythms regular. If blood flow in the heart is severely hampered by the thick-ened heart muscle, you may need to have a portion of the heart muscle surgically removed to alleviate the problem.

If other members of your fam-ily have hypertrophic cardiomy-opathy, you should be examined to determine if you have it, even if you are not experiencing any symptoms.

Congestive Heart Failure

Congestive heart failure (CHF) is the inability of the heart to pump enough blood to meet the body's needs. It is one of the major causes of illness and disability in the United States, is the leading cause of hospitalization in people over age 65, and kills more than

40,000 people each year. CHF affects nearly 5 million people in the United States and the numbers are growing, especially among elderly adults.

Although deaths from heart attacks are decreasing in the United States, deaths from heart failure are increasing. However, treatments have improved over the past decade.

In heart failure, the left ventricle (and sometimes the right ventricle) of the heart begins failing as a pump. The left ventricle's job is to pump oxygen-rich blood to all of the body (except the lungs); the right ventricle's job is to pump oxygen-poor blood into the lungs to make it oxygen-rich. The failure of this pump leads to a variety of symptoms.

CHF can be caused by many different diseases that affect the heart muscle, the most common being coronary artery disease (see p.652), cardiomyopathy (see p.682), high blood pressure (see p.644), and diseases of the heart valves (see p.689).

Some doctors do not diagnose CHF accurately or do not treat it aggressively enough. If you have symptoms of CHF and have been diagnosed with it but you are not getting better after treatment, get a second opinion. You may not be getting the most modern and effective treatment. With proper treatment, most people's symptoms improve.

SYMPTOMS

Because the left ventricle is unable to pump enough blood out of the heart to meet all the body's needs, many organs start to malfunction. Insufficient blood flow through the brain, kidneys, and muscles, for example, can cause weakness and fatigue.

Also, failure of the left ventricle causes blood to back up in the circulation that leads into the left ventricle: first in the lungs and then in the right ventricle. If the right ventricle is also failing, this causes blood to back up into the veins of the body, which empty blood into the right ventricle.

When blood backs up into the lungs, breathing becomes difficult. At worst, you become very short of breath, even at rest. When blood backs up in the veins, fluid starts to leak out of the veins into the tissues, causing swelling. You can see the swelling in some places, such as your legs.

The swelling also often occurs in other places: in the space around the lungs (see Pleural Effusion, p.515), in the abdomen, and in the liver. When fluid builds up in your body, you gain weight.

The symptoms of congestive heart failure can be mild or severe and can develop gradually or suddenly; it all depends on how suddenly and how badly the heart is failing.

The symptoms of heart failure can also be compounded by the response of other organs to the heart failure. For example, the kidneys respond to a low blood flow by retaining salt and water. This increases the heart's workload and adds to the swelling and weight gain.

CHF falls into four categories based on how much your activity is limited. In class 1 CHF, you can participate in ordinary physical activity without noticing any symptoms. Class 2 CHF causes shortness of breath or other discomfort during moderate activity but no symptoms during light activity or rest. Class 3 CHF means that any physical activity will bring on symptoms.

The most advanced form of heart failure, class 4, means you suffer from shortness of breath and fatigue even while resting and may have trouble breathing while lying down.

TREATMENT OPTIONS

Your doctor can often detect CHF through physical examination, particularly when the condition is severe. A chest x-ray may show the backup of blood in the lungs, even when the doctor cannot detect it through physical examination.

An echocardiogram can give a more precise measure of how effectively the heart is pumping. The amount (fraction) of blood in the ventricles that is pumped out (ejected) into the circulation is called the ejection fraction. When the ejection fraction is less than 50%, it is considered abnormal.

Taking care of yourself is very important in fighting heart failure. The three most important things you can do are:

Avoid salty foods. Salt causes you to retain fluid, and fluid retention can worsen heart failure. Avoid foods that are obviously salty as well as most canned and prepared foods. Also, do not add salt to food.

Weigh yourself regularly. The retention of fluid from heart failure causes you to gain weight. It is very important for you to weigh yourself regularly and keep a written record of your weight. Try to weigh yourself at

Echocardiogram

Echocardiography, or cardiac ultrasound, is a way of taking pictures of the shape and functioning of your heart. Like all kinds of ultrasound (see p.148), it is noninvasive; no objects or substances enter your body and there is no risk from having the test.

An image of the beating heart is made by sending sound waves through the chest wall and into the heart muscle; the waves bounce back off of the various parts of the heart, and the echocardiogram machine creates a picture of the heart from these reflected sound waves.

An echocardiogram can be easily conducted in the doctor's office, as well as in a hospital, and is an excellent way to see:

■ Abnormalities in the covering of the heart (pericardium)

■ Abnormalities in the thickness or function of the heart wall

■ Increased or decreased size of the four chambers of the heart

■ Abnormalities of the heart valves

■ Direction and velocity of blood flow

■ Effectiveness of the heart as a pump

Although the echocardiogram is usually done while you are lying down and at rest, it also can be performed like an electrocardiogram as part of an exercise stress test (see p.660).

A related technique, transesophageal echocardiography (TEE), plays a role in the diagnosis of many conditions of the heart and aorta. In TEE, a probe is passed through the mouth and down the throat into the esophagus, the passageway to the stomach.

Because it is an invasive procedure that requires sedation, TEE is more expensive and slightly riskier than traditional echocardiography. However, it is better at detecting infections of some heart valves and at looking for blood clots in certain heart chambers. It is also useful for diagnosing and examining the severity of an aneurysm in the aorta.

Drugs for Treating Heart Failure

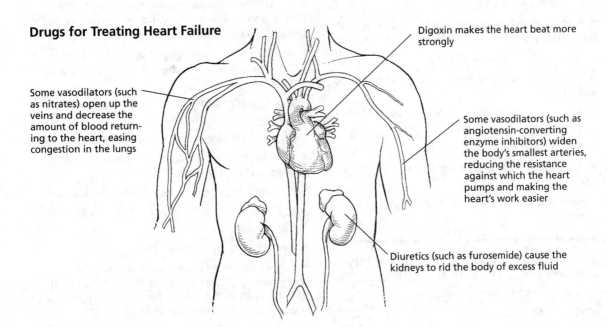

Digoxin makes the heart beat more strongly

Some vasodilators (such as nitrates) open up the veins and decrease the amount of blood returning to the heart, easing congestion in the lungs

Some vasodilators (such as angiotensin-converting enzyme inhibitors) widen the body's smallest arteries, reducing the resistance against which the heart pumps and making the heart's work easier

Diuretics (such as furosemide) cause the kidneys to rid the body of excess fluid

Different drugs ease the symptoms of congestive heart failure in different ways. Drugs are often used in combination.

Newer Treatments for Congestive Heart Failure

Research may be implicating immune system substances called cytokines as playing an important role in causing the heart muscle cell abnormalities that lead to heart failure. Experimental treatments aimed at blocking the effects of one such cytokine, called tumor necrosis factor (TNF), show some promise. Other promising experimental treatments block the effects of adrenaline on the heart in a similar but more potent way than beta blockers.

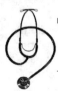

Congestive Heart Failure: When You Visit Your Doctor

QUESTIONS TO DISCUSS WITH YOUR DOCTOR:

- Are you short of breath when you exert yourself? How many flights of stairs or how many blocks can you walk before getting short of breath?

- Do you ever feel short of breath without exerting yourself?

- Are you short of breath when you lie flat? Do you ever feel the need to get up suddenly to catch your breath in the middle of the night?

- How many pillows do you use to sleep? Has this increased recently?

- Do you have a chronic cough?

- Do your legs become weak or fatigued when you exercise?

- Are your ankles swollen or do you have an increase in the size of your abdomen?

- Are you following a low-salt diet?

- Are you ever light-headed or dizzy or do you have palpitations?

- Have you been taking your medications as directed?

YOUR DOCTOR MIGHT EXAMINE THE FOLLOWING BODY STRUCTURES OR FUNCTIONS:

- Heart rate and blood pressure
- Veins in the neck
- Pulse
- Heart and lungs
- Ankles and legs (for swelling)
- Abdomen (for fluid or an enlarged liver)

YOUR DOCTOR MIGHT ORDER THE FOLLOWING LAB TESTS OR STUDIES:

- Finger probe blood test (to estimate oxygen saturation of blood at rest and with exercise) if you are short of breath. An oximeter finger probe softly clamps onto the fingertip and measures oxygen in the blood; the skin is not broken.

- Blood tests for minerals and salts (such as sodium, potassium, chloride, bicarbonate, calcium, and magnesium)

- Blood tests of kidney function (such as blood urea nitrogen and creatinine)

- Blood levels of some medications (such as digoxin)

- Prothrombin time (time it takes blood to clot) if you are on blood thinners

- Complete blood cell count (to check for anemia)

- Chest x-ray (to look for excess fluid in or around the lungs)

- Electrocardiogram (see p.135)

- Echocardiogram (see p.665) to estimate the strength of the heart and to evaluate the function of the heart valves. Ask for the results of the ejection fraction; see Congestive Heart Failure, p.683.

- Exercise stress test (see p.660)

the same time each day, such as the first thing in the morning, and when you are lightly dressed and not wearing shoes. Ask your doctor when to call him or her because you have gained too much weight.

Stay off your feet and sit with your feet elevated. Fluid retention is greatest in the legs because gravity pulls the fluid in your body down. When possible, reduce the amount of time you are upright. When you are sitting down, keep your legs propped up on a footstool or chair. This helps move fluid out of the tissues of the legs and into the blood, and then into the kidneys and out of the body, as urine.

There are powerful medicines available for heart failure. Here are some of the most commonly used drugs:

Diuretics encourage your kidneys to make more urine, which keeps you from retaining too much fluid (with all its complications). Diuretics come in varying strengths. Milder diuretics, called thiazides, are often all that is necessary. A commonly used and more powerful diuretic is furosemide. If your dose of diuretics is too strong, you will pass too much urine and become dehydrated. Also, both the thiazides and furosemide cause your body to become depleted in potassium by passing potassium in your urine. To counter this, eat and drink foods rich in potassium (such as bananas and orange juice), take potassium pills or liquid medicine, or take a medicine that counteracts the tendency of your kidneys to lose potassium. Your doctor will work with you on a plan for making sure you are

taking just the right amount of diuretic and that the potassium level in your blood is normal.

Angiotensin-converting enzyme (ACE) inhibitors reduce the workload of the heart. They are an important part of the treatment of heart failure. ACE inhibitors can cause an increase in the level of potassium in the blood, which is the opposite of the effect of diuretics. In some people, particularly those with narrowed arteries in the kidneys, ACE inhibitors can cause some degree of kidney failure. For these reasons, your doctor will perform regular blood tests. A newer class of medicines, the angiotensin-receptor antagonists, acts similarly to ACE inhibitors and are being evaluated for CHF.

Vasodilators are one of several other medicines that work like ACE inhibitors to decrease the workload of the heart. They include hydralazine, long-acting nitrates, and prazosin and may be used if you cannot tolerate ACE inhibitors.

Digitalis is a natural medicine that comes from plants and has been used for hundreds of years. It strengthens the contraction of the heart. The level of digitalis in your blood must be measured regularly because abnormally high levels can cause heart block (see p.680) and abnormal heart rhythms (see p.672).

Beta blockers reduce the effects of adrenaline and related substances that cause the heart to beat more rapidly. For many years, beta blockers were avoided when treating congestive heart failure because of concern that they could further weaken the pumping strength of the heart. More recently, it has been found

that many beta blockers do more good than harm. The evidence is strongest for a new beta blocker called carvedilol.

Cor Pulmonale

In cor pulmonale, the heart's right pumping chamber (right ventricle) becomes dilated and weakened and is unable to force blood effectively into the lungs. The left ventricle—the ventricle that fails most often—remains normal.

Most cases of cor pulmonale in this country are caused by the chronic lung diseases chronic bronchitis and emphysema (see p.517).

Cor pulmonale stems from high blood pressure in the arteries of the lungs. It occurs because, over time, emphysema or chronic bronchitis destroys the small air sacs and blood vessels in the lungs, making it harder for oxygen to get into the blood.

Lower blood oxygen levels cause the arteries in the lungs to clamp down, raising the pressure in the pulmonary arteries (pulmonary hypertension). The right ventricle must work harder to pump against the increased pressure.

A less common cause of pulmonary hypertension and cor pulmonale is multiple, recurring blood clots that lodge in the blood vessels of the lungs (pulmonary emboli).

In a small number of people, mostly young women, a disease of unknown cause called primary pulmonary hypertension causes cor pulmonale. The diet drugs fenfluramine and dexfenfluramine have also caused pulmonary hypertension.

SYMPTOMS

When the right ventricle fails, blood backs up in the veins leading into the right ventricle. Pressure in the veins rises, causing fluid to leak out of the veins and into the tissues. The legs become swollen first.

The liver swells and scarring develops—a condition called cirrhosis (see p.765). Fluid then backs up into the abdomen, which can become swollen with fluid (a condition called ascites).

TREATMENT OPTIONS

Cor pulmonale is easily diagnosed through physical examination. The extent to which the function of the right ventricle is impaired can be determined by an echocardiogram (see p.665).

Cor pulmonale cannot be treated without treating the underlying chronic lung disease; this is achieved with drugs to open the airways and reduce inflammation in the lungs.

The most important step is to ensure that your blood has an adequate concentration of oxygen by using a small plastic tube to deliver extra oxygen to your nose through nasal prongs. Raising the blood's oxygen level causes the arteries in the lungs to relax, lowering the pressure in the pulmonary artery and reducing the work of the right ventricle.

Diuretic drugs and sometimes digitalis (see left) may be helpful. However, these drugs must be carefully monitored by your doctor to avoid side effects.

Heart Transplant

If you have a severely damaged heart but are otherwise healthy, you may be a candidate for a heart transplant.

This option is explored when the heart muscle is impaired to the point where it can no longer function adequately, such as in severe heart muscle disease (cardiomyopathy). It is considered only after all forms of medical treatment have failed, and it is reserved for people who are not expected to live longer than 2 years without the intervention.

Although the first human heart transplant operations were performed in the late 1960s, the procedure was largely discontinued for the next decade because of insurmountable complications that limited the recipient's chance of survival.

In the early 1980s, however, a powerful new drug called cyclosporine was introduced. Cyclosporine greatly extended survival rates by keeping the body from rejecting the foreign organ. You must take the drug for the rest of your life, and it can cause serious side effects.

Today, 83% of heart transplant recipients survive the first year; 72% are alive for at least 4 years after the operation. The most common cause of death following transplant surgery is the body's rejection of the new organ.

More people need heart transplants than get them, because there are not enough donor hearts available. In 1997, just 2290 heart transplants were performed in the United States. It is estimated, however, that at any given time there are at least 20,000 people on the waiting list for a new heart in this country alone. A large portion of them die before a donor heart becomes available.

Organs generally come from organ donors under 40 who have died from a vehicle crash, gunshot wound, or severe head injury and whose bodies are being kept alive by machines.

HEART TRANSPLANT SURGERY AND RECOVERY

In a heart transplant operation, your diseased heart is replaced by a healthy heart from a donor. The operation requires general anesthesia, and takes approximately 4 to 12 hours to perform.

Your chest is opened by cutting the breastbone, and a heart-lung machine is used, as it is in coronary artery bypass graft surgery (see p.662), to pump oxygen-rich blood through your body. All but the right atrium of your heart is removed; the donor heart is then put in its place and attached to the major blood vessels.

After surgery, you usually stay in the hospital about a week, spending most of the time in an intensive care unit. However, complications can keep you in the hospital much longer.

During your hospital stay, special precautions will be taken by everyone entering your hospital room to prevent transmitting infections to you, because the immunosuppressive drugs used to prevent your new heart from being rejected by your immune system reduce your ability to fight infection.

After you leave the hospital, you will be encouraged to begin an exercise program as soon as you are able (usually about 6 weeks after surgery); the only restriction is to avoid any activities, including sexual activity, that cause pain in the breastbone.

The drugs used to prevent

rejection of the transplanted organ make you vulnerable to infections and cancers. They can also cause kidney damage, high blood pressure, tremors, and excessive hair growth. Nearly all people lose bone mass and have swollen gums.

You will need to have frequent heart tissue biopsies during your recovery period to determine if the immunosuppressive drugs are working. You will have coronary angio-graphy every year after the transplant.

A heart transplant operation is not for everyone. People who are elderly or have other diseases are likely to have complications during the long and difficult operation. The ideal recipient is under 55 years old and does not have other chronic conditions such as lung disease, diabetes, cancer, kidney or liver failure, or peripheral vascular disease.

Also, you need to be physically and mentally able to adhere to the strict program of monitoring and treatment that follows the operation.

Heart transplantation is expensive—the average cost ranges from $57,000 to $110,000. Most health insurance companies pay for the operation. However, Medicaid covers the procedure in just 33 states, and Medicare will cover the surgery only if it is performed at approved centers.

DISEASES OF THE HEART VALVES

Blood moves continuously through the four chambers of the heart: into the right atrium, into the right ventricle, out the pulmonary artery into the lungs and back into the left atrium, into the left ventricle, and out the aorta to the rest of the body.

Four one-way valves (see illustration on p.690) in the heart keep the blood moving through the pumping chambers in the proper direction.

Properly functioning valves open at the right moment to permit the blood to move forward from one chamber to the next, then close tightly to prevent blood from flowing backward. Damaged or diseased heart valves can disrupt this process.

When the opening of a heart valve is narrowed, the heart must exert extra force to propel the blood through the valve. A valve that is too wide or does not close efficiently allows blood to regurgitate back into the heart. This also forces the heart to work harder, since it must keep pumping blood it has already pumped.

Although defects can involve all four heart valves, by far the most common problems are defects of the aortic valve and the mitral valve.

Heart Murmurs

A heart murmur is a whooshing sound related to your heartbeats, created by blood being pumped inside the heart. It can be heard when a stethoscope is placed on your chest.

Many heart murmurs are "innocent," meaning that they do not stem from an underlying heart problem. Children's hearts are closer to the chest wall, and doctors frequently hear murmurs in children that are not caused by any kind of heart disease. Sometimes conditions that place stress on the heart—such as anemia, pregnancy, or a fever—also create an innocent murmur.

A heart murmur can indicate an abnormality of some structure inside the heart. Heart valve abnormalities are the most common causes of "noninnocent" heart murmurs.

Some murmurs are caused by valves that become stiff and do not open enough to allow blood to flow easily through them. When a heart valve is narrowed (stenotic), for example, the stream of blood being pumped through the narrowed valve makes noise. It is the same as if you were to pinch the tip of a garden hose with the water running at full pressure—the narrowing causes an increased noise.

Other murmurs are caused by blood falling backward through a leaky valve that does not close completely. The valves of the heart are built to keep blood traveling in one direction only. When the valves leak, pressure differences push blood backward through the valve, causing a murmur.

Sometimes people are born with heart valves that are an unusual shape, which can also cause a heart murmur. Some people are born with holes in the walls between either the atrial chambers (atrial septal defect) or the ventricle chambers (ventricular septal defect) of the

Blood Flow Through Normal Heart Valves

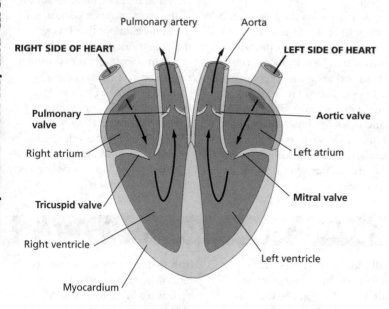

Four one-way valves govern the blood flow through the heart. The valves open to let blood out of the heart chambers, then close tightly to prevent blood from moving backward in the wrong direction. If a valve is stenotic—that is, it is too narrow and stiff—the heart may not be able to pump enough blood past the restricted opening. If a valve is insufficient, it does not shut properly and thus allows blood to flow backward in the wrong direction. Arrows show the normal direction of blood flow. See also How You Circulate Blood (p.108).

heart. Blood pushing through these small holes can cause murmurs.

SYMPTOMS

Heart murmurs do not themselves cause symptoms. However, the conditions that cause the murmurs can also cause symptoms including fatigue, weakness, shortness of breath, swelling in the legs and abdomen, chest pain, and fainting spells.

TREATMENT OPTIONS

The presence of a heart murmur may be detected through physical examination. Just by listening to the murmur with a stethoscope, your doctor can often make a diagnosis as to whether the murmur is innocent or indicates a heart abnormality. The examination often gives your doctor an idea of what the abnormality is and how severe it may be.

A heart murmur is described as systolic if it occurs in the heart's contracting phase or diastolic if it occurs during the resting phase of the heartbeat.

Murmurs are also graded on a scale of 1 (barely audible) to 6 (very loud), depending on how well they can be heard with the stethoscope and whether the tur-

bulence they create can be felt when the doctor's hand rests on your chest.

The chamber where the sound originates and its pitch and duration are also important factors. The doctor takes all these elements into account when determining if a heart murmur indicates an underlying problem.

If your doctor's examination reveals a murmur that probably represents an abnormality in the heart, further tests are performed, most commonly an echocardiogram (see p.665).

The treatments for noninnocent heart murmurs depend on the condition that is causing the murmur. Many are heart valve abnormalities (see next article).

Aortic Stenosis and Insufficiency

The aortic valve sits at the junction between the left ventricle and the body's major artery, the aorta. Normally, the aortic valve is composed of three leaflets. The left ventricle pumps oxygen-rich blood through the aortic valve to the aorta, and ultimately to all organs in the body.

The aortic valve normally keeps blood from falling back into the left ventricle, and normally provides little resistance to the flow of blood.

Aortic stenosis is a condition in which the aortic valve becomes stiff, its opening becomes narrowed, and the valve impedes the flow of blood.

One kind of aortic stenosis is inherited: some people are born with only two, not three, leaflets in their aortic valve. This usually does not pose a problem in childhood. However, later in life,

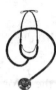

Aortic Stenosis: When You Visit Your Doctor

QUESTIONS TO DISCUSS WITH YOUR DOCTOR:

- Are you fatigued?

- Do you become short of breath with exertion or when you lie down?

- Do you have chest pain or pressure with exertion or at rest?

- Do you have swollen ankles?

- Do you ever feel like you are going to faint? Have you fainted?

- Do you know how severe your condition is?

- Do you know the reasons to have surgery to fix the stenosis and what the risks are from not having surgery when it is needed?

- Do you need to take antibiotics before certain dental and medical procedures?

YOUR DOCTOR MIGHT EXAMINE THE FOLLOWING BODY STRUCTURES OR FUNCTIONS:

- Heart rate, blood pressure, and weight

- Heart and lungs

- Pulse

- Veins in the neck

- Ankles and legs (for swelling)

YOUR DOCTOR MIGHT ORDER THE FOLLOWING LAB TESTS OR STUDIES:

- Electrocardiogram (see p.135)

- Echocardiogram (see p.665)

---

these leaflets can stiffen to the point where the valve cannot open fully.

Another cause of aortic stenosis is degeneration of the aortic valves, for unknown reasons, later in life. A third cause is rheumatic fever (see p.697), which was once common in the United States and other developed countries; today it has become rare in developed countries due to improved sanitation and living conditions. However, it is still a common disease in developing countries.

In each type of aortic stenosis, more and more scar tissue builds up on the valve, making the valve less able to open. Because the left ventricle is pumping against increasing resistance, it must work harder. As a consequence, the muscle of the left ventricle becomes progressively thicker.

Aortic insufficiency (also

Aortic Valve Insufficiency

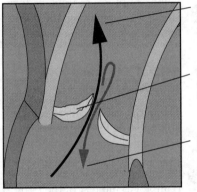

Proper direction of blood flow

Diseased valve does not close completely

Blood regurgitating back into chamber

Heart valves should open to allow blood to flow in the proper direction and then close, not allowing blood to flow backward. Valve insufficiency occurs when damage to a heart valve prevents the valve from closing tightly and allows blood to flow backward through it. In aortic valve insufficiency, the left ventricle is pumping blood through the leaky aortic valve. The ventricle must work harder because it must pump extra blood—not only the blood that has entered the chamber normally, but also the blood that has leaked backward through the insufficient valve.

called aortic regurgitation or aortic incompetence) is a condition in which the aortic valve does not close completely. This allows blood to leak back into the left ventricle from the aorta during the relaxed (diastolic) phase of the heart's contraction.

There are many causes of aortic insufficiency. In the past, the most common cause in the United States was rheumatic fever (see p.697). Today a significant cause is infectious endocarditis (see p.695), a bacterial infection of the heart valve.

Several conditions cause the beginning of the aorta, just above the aortic valve, to widen. This, in turn, pulls apart the valve leaflets and can cause aortic insufficiency. Conditions that can widen the aorta include aneurysms (see p.698) of the aorta, a disease of the wall of the aorta called Marfan syndrome, connective tissue diseases such as lupus (see p.898) and rheumatoid arthritis (see p.606), and infection with syphilis (see p.893).

Sometimes a deformity is present at birth that worsens over time due to the wear and tear of the heart's constant pumping. While aortic insufficiency often develops slowly, it can come on suddenly, such as when it is caused by a dissecting aortic aneurysm (see p.698) or bacterial infection of the aortic valve.

SYMPTOMS

Aortic stenosis does not cause symptoms for many years. When it does, you may feel breathless and develop other symptoms caused by congestive heart failure (see p.683). The left ventricle of the heart has been overworking for many years, and finally tires.

Even without the presence of coronary artery disease, the coronary arteries may become compressed by the thickened left ventricle, and you may develop chest pain (see Angina, p.657).

If the valve is small, the heart muscle may not be able to provide enough blood to the brain; you could have fainting spells and even die suddenly. Once symptoms develop, the outlook for aortic stenosis is not good; 75% of people with the condition die within 3 years if they do not get proper treatment.

Aortic insufficiency often develops slowly and without symptoms for many years. The first symptoms are often prominent palpitations; you can feel your heart pounding forcefully (though not rapidly), particularly when you lie down. You may also feel a pounding in your head.

The left ventricle gradually stretches to accommodate the extra blood that flows back from the aorta. Eventually, the heart muscle becomes weakened to the point where you become breathless and develop symptoms of heart failure (see p.683).

Chest pain can also develop, along with excessive sweating (particularly with the chest pain). When aortic insufficiency develops suddenly, it leads to congestive heart failure and is a medical emergency.

TREATMENT OPTIONS

Your doctor can usually hear the murmurs caused by aortic stenosis and insufficiency years before symptoms develop. An echocardiogram (see p.665) is very helpful in making the diagnosis and in determining how severe the condition is.

In aortic stenosis, when an echocardiogram shows that the condition is becoming severe, even if you do not yet have symptoms, surgery to replace the valve is often recommended. In people who are old and frail, but who need treatment of aortic stenosis, a balloon catheter that widens the aortic valve is sometimes used instead of surgery, but it does not produce permanent results.

In aortic insufficiency, drugs can be used to decrease the pressure in the arteries. This makes it less likely that blood will be pushed backward and down into the left ventricle and reduces the effort the heart must expend. Drugs may delay the need for surgery for many years.

Your doctor will monitor your condition with regular echocardiograms. When your left ventricle shows signs of enlarging or when your heart is no longer pumping with full force, it is time to consider surgery even if you have no symptoms. When aortic insufficiency develops suddenly, it requires emergency surgery to replace the valve.

With an experienced surgical team, the risks of surgery are low and the development of future symptoms is prevented. If you put off the surgery until you develop symptoms or until the heart shows signs of failing, the results of surgery may not be as good.

Mitral Stenosis and Insufficiency

The mitral valve connects the left atrium to the left ventricle and normally allows oxygen-rich blood from the lungs to pass into the left ventricle, where it is pumped to the rest of the body.

Mitral stenosis involves a stiffening of the valve and a narrowing of the mitral valve opening. The most common cause of mitral stenosis is rheumatic fever (see p.697), which ultimately causes the left atrium to widen and blood to back up into the lungs.

Mitral stenosis develops slowly and does not cause symptoms for many years. In the past, when rheumatic fever and mitral stenosis were more common, women often discovered they had this problem during pregnancy, when the extra workload on the heart brought on symptoms.

Mitral insufficiency (also called mitral regurgitation or mitral incompetence) is much more common than mitral stenosis. It is caused by a condition that deforms the shape of the mitral valve and allows blood to be pumped back up into the left atrium when the left ventricle contracts, instead of the blood exiting the aorta.

The most common cause of severe mitral insufficiency was once rheumatic fever (see p.697). Now it is congestive heart failure, which causes the left ventricle and left atrium to stretch, widening the mitral valve and allowing blood from the ventricle to leak into the left atrium.

Mitral valve prolapse (see p.694) also is a common cause of mild mitral insufficiency.

SYMPTOMS

In mitral stenosis, you may have no symptoms for several years. Ultimately, congestive heart failure develops as blood backs up into the lungs. When this happens, you experience shortness of breath during exertion or when lying down. You may also have white frothy or bloody phlegm (sputum).

When mitral stenosis is severe, the high pressure in the atrium leads to stretching and enlargement, which makes this chamber more susceptible to atrial fibrillation (see p.673). This abnormal heart rhythm is characterized by rapid, irregular heartbeat and fatigue.

In mitral insufficiency, symptoms also develop slowly. In many people, symptoms never develop. When they do, the most prominent are fatigue, breathlessness, and other symptoms of congestive heart failure. Atrial fibrillation also occurs more often in people with long-standing mitral insufficiency.

TREATMENT OPTIONS

Your doctor may suspect a diagnosis of mitral stenosis or mitral insufficiency after listening to your heart; each condition causes a characteristic heart murmur.

Echocardiography (see p.665) is helpful in confirming the diagnosis and in estimating the severity of the problem.

Mitral Valve Prolapse

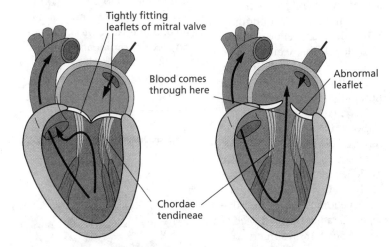

Tightly fitting leaflets of mitral valve

Blood comes through here

Abnormal leaflet

Chordae tendineae

NORMALLY CLOSED MITRAL VALVE   **PROLAPSED MITRAL VALVE**

The left side of the heart is shown. A normal mitral valve has two tightly fitting leaflets that close completely when the left ventricle contracts, allowing no blood to be pumped back up into the left atrium. Instead, all the blood is pumped out the aorta. The leaflets are held tightly to the wall of the ventricle by structures called chordae tendineae.

In mitral valve prolapse, the mitral valve leaflets are too large and too loosely attached by the chordae tendineae. When the left ventricle contracts, the valve leaflets are pushed up into the left atrium (they prolapse into the left atrium), leaving a space between them through which blood leaks into the atrium. Thus, some of the blood is pumped backward up into the left atrium; normally all the blood is pumped out the aorta. As the leaflets are pushed up into the atrium, they often become taut and, like a sail catching a gust of wind, they cause a snapping sound, or click, that can be heard through a stethoscope. When blood leaks through them, in a type of mitral insufficiency, it also creates a murmur that can often be heard through a stethoscope.

In mitral stenosis, some treatment must be started if you have symptoms. Drugs may help control the symptoms. Blood thinners may be necessary to prevent emboli (clots) from causing strokes and other complications.

When your valve narrows to a particular point, heart function goes rapidly downhill. It is best to perform surgery before the heart starts to fail. Since it is frequently not possible to reconstruct the scarred valves surgically, it is often necessary to replace the valve (see below). The risk of death for this type of operation is 2% to 3%.

In mitral regurgitation, mild symptoms of congestive heart failure are treated with drugs. When this treatment does not provide adequate relief or when an echocardiogram shows that your left ventricle is enlarging or pumping poorly, you need surgery.

Sometimes the valve can be repaired during surgery and does not need to be replaced. There is evidence that people are more likely to survive the operation and live longer when the valve is repaired rather than replaced. The risk of death from surgery to repair the valve is 5% if your heart is still functioning adequately.

When mitral insufficiency is caused by congestive heart failure that stretches the mitral valve, surgery on the valve will not help. The goal of treatment is to improve heart muscle function with medication, which aims to reduce the size of the chambers of the left side of the heart, reducing mitral insufficiency.

Mitral Valve Prolapse

Mitral valve prolapse is a condition in which the two leaflets of the mitral valve are somewhat enlarged. They push back into the left atrium when the left ventricle contracts and sometimes allow leakage of blood back into the atrium (this is a type of mitral insufficiency). Sometimes, the cords that attach the leaflet to the valve are too long, making the valves floppy.

Echocardiograms (see p.665), which are performed to determine the shape of the mitral valve in healthy young adults, have revealed some slight abnormalities in up to 20% of young women. However, most of the time, mitral valve prolapse causes no medical problems.

Mitral valve prolapse often causes no symptoms. Occasionally, irregular heartbeats, fatigue, stabbing chest pain not brought on by exercise, and dizziness or blackouts may result.

In extremely rare cases, mitral valve prolapse can cause sudden death.

Your doctor may suspect mitral valve prolapse if he or she hears a clicking sound, often followed by a brief heart murmur. The click is probably caused by sudden tension on the oversized, floppy valve—the way a sail on a sailboat can snap when it gets hit by a gust of wind. The click and the murmur can come and go in mild cases.

An echocardiogram is sometimes used to diagnosis mitral valve prolapse and to determine its severity.

Mitral valve prolapse almost never requires surgical correction. In fact, usually no treatment

Replacement Heart Valves

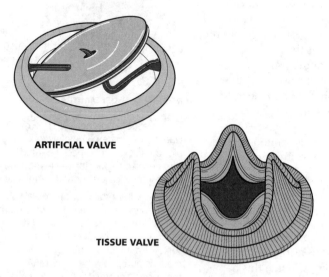

ARTIFICIAL VALVE

TISSUE VALVE

Malfunctioning heart valves can be surgically replaced with substitutes. Artificial valves are made of metal and synthetic materials. Tissue (or bioprosthetic) valves are built from animal tissue, which often comes from pigs.

at all is necessary. If you find you have troublesome symptoms such as palpitations or chest pain, your doctor may recommend that you control them with beta blockers (see p.650).

If you have oversized and floppy valve leaflets and some degree of mitral insufficiency, you have a somewhat higher risk of developing a valve infection (see Infectious Endocarditis, below) after having dental work or other procedures.

For this reason, your doctor may recommend that you take antibiotics before such procedures (see p.481).

Valvotomy and Valve Repair and Replacement

Valvotomy In people who have aortic stenosis or mitral stenosis, a procedure called valvotomy is sometimes performed. A catheter with a balloon at the tip of it is inserted into a blood vessel in your groin or arm. The tip is passed so that it touches the stiff valve and the balloon is inflated. The balloon can pop open the stiff, tight valve and reduce the degree of obstruction.

This technique usually offers some immediate relief, but the stenosis (narrowing) of the valve may return within months. The virtue of valvotomy is that it does not require open-heart surgery. The concept and technique of valvotomy is much like that of angioplasty (see p.661).

Surgical valve repair Valve repair or replacement requires open-heart surgery. The operation involves temporarily stopping the heart so the surgeon can work on heart tissue when it is

not moving. During surgery, the body is supported by a cardiopulmonary bypass machine. The chance of death during surgery generally ranges from 1% to 5%, depending on which valves are replaced and on how many valves need to be operated on during the surgery. In people who are very sick and require emergency surgery, the risk of death during surgery is higher.

Because valve repair preserves the body's own structures, you do not risk the complications that sometimes accompany inserting artificial valves. Valve repair is being used successfully to remedy mitral insufficiency. Although it is preferred to replacement, it is not always possible to perform, depending on the nature of the valve problem.

Surgical valve replacement

When a diseased valve is replaced, the replacement valve can be crafted from synthetic material (an artificial valve), can be taken from a pig (pig's heart valves are similar in size and shape to human valves), or can be constructed from your own tissue. Both tissue and synthetic valves are equally good at restoring the normal flow of blood through the chambers of the heart. The advantages of each type of valve can be simply summarized:

■ Artificial valves last longer before requiring replacement. Most people who have artificial valves live out their lives without requiring valve replacement, while 50% of people with tissue valves need to have them replaced within 15 years.

■ Tissue valves are much less

likely than artificial valves to form blood clots.

Because artificial valves are more likely to cause blood clots, people with artificial valves must take blood thinners. However, this raises the risk of serious bleeding.

In people under age 55, artificial valves tend to be favored because they last longer and because the risk of bleeding (in those who take warfarin) is less than in older people.

Artificial valves may not be advisable for women who plan to bear children because warfarin cannot be taken during pregnancy. However, newer blood thinners may be used as alternatives. Because bleeding from warfarin is more likely in people older than 55, tissue valves tend to be favored in this age group.

All types of valves are susceptible to infection (endocarditis). For this reason, if you have valve replacement, you need to take antibiotics anytime there is a risk that bacteria might be released into your bloodstream. This can happen during dental work or other medical procedures.

Infectious Endocarditis

Endocarditis is an infection of the heart valves or lining. Although it is most often a bacterial infection, endocarditis can also be caused by other microorganisms.

Infection may develop in a healthy heart when a particularly aggressive form of bacteria enters the bloodstream and settles on the valves. More often, the infection occurs in heart valves that have been damaged

Endocarditis

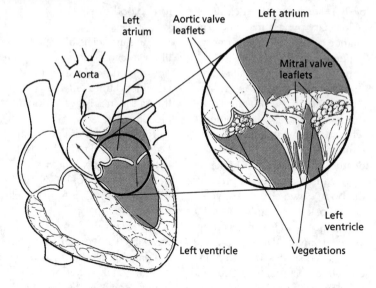

In endocarditis, clumps of bacteria and blood clots (vegetations) can accumulate on the surface of the heart's valves and interfere with their function. Vegetations often develop on leaflets of the mitral valve (through which blood enters the left ventricle) and the aortic valve (through which blood flows to the rest of the body). Destruction caused by the bacteria usually leads to leaking of the heart valves, which can cause severe heart failure. Vegetations can also break off and travel to other organs of the body, causing embolisms.

by a previous bout of rheumatic fever or other form of heart disease.

Infections can also settle on artificial valves used to surgically replace damaged valves. The microorganism causing the infection often enters the bloodstream when small blood vessels are injured during dental work, examination of the intestinal tract, or genital and urinary procedures. Intravenous drug users are especially at risk for this infection.

As the infection develops, the infecting organisms and the blood cells trying to fight the infection mix to form growths called vegetations

that stick to the surface of the valves.

Endocarditis can be either acute or subacute. Symptoms depend largely on the type of organism causing the infection.

In the acute form, the heart is attacked by especially aggressive bacteria, such as staphylococcus (see p.878). The bacteria settle on the valve and grow rapidly.

More often, as in the subacute form, the endocarditis is caused by less aggressive bacteria that settle on a valve and that more slowly multiply and cause vegetations. *Streptococcus viridans* is the most common bacteria causing subacute endocarditis.

SYMPTOMS

Acute endocarditis typically causes significant symptoms such as high fever, shaking chills, profound weakness, and fatigue. The infection can cause serious damage to the heart valve, resulting in heart failure and death.

Subacute endocarditis produces more subtle symptoms such as mild weakness and fatigue, intermittent low-grade fevers, and aching muscles.

Both kinds of endocarditis can lead to septic embolism, in which clumps of the infected vegetations break off and travel to other parts of the body, including the lungs, brain, skin, and kidneys or other organs.

Depending on the size of these clumps and where they lodge, they can cause all the usual problems of an arterial embolism (see p.701), compounded by the fact that the particles are infected and can cause infections in organs where they lodge.

TREATMENT OPTIONS

The two best ways to diagnose endocarditis are blood cultures (see p.159), which are usually abnormal, and an echocardiogram, especially a transesophageal echocardiogram, which is best at showing the vegetations on the heart valves.

Infective endocarditis is treated with an intravenous antibiotic for 4 to 6 weeks; the antibiotic used depends on the organism involved. In an effort to prevent serious heart damage, antibiotic treatment is sometimes started even before laboratory tests confirming the disease are complete.

If the infection is particularly aggressive or has spread deeply into the heart tissue, emergency surgery may be necessary to replace the infected valve with an artificial valve (see p.694).

People with diseased or artificial heart valves should take a preventive dose of antibiotics before undergoing any medical procedure that could introduce bacteria into the bloodstream. If you have a heart valve problem or a heart murmur, ask your doctor if you need to take this precaution.

Pericarditis

The heart is surrounded by a smooth, thin, two-layer sac called the pericardium that looks somewhat like a cellophane bag. Pericarditis occurs when this membrane becomes inflamed.

Most often the inflammation is caused by a viral infection, but other microorganisms (such as tuberculosis bacteria) can also infect the pericardium. Inflammation from a connective tissue disease such as lupus (see p.898) can also cause pericarditis.

Pericarditis may also be a complication of a heart attack or of chronic kidney failure, heart surgery, or chest surgery. Finally, pericardial inflammation can occur if the pericardium is invaded by tumors—particularly lymphomas (see p.727) and breast or lung cancer—and from radiation therapy for tumors.

Once inflamed, the pericardial layers rub against each other, creating friction. Sometimes the inflammation leads to an accumulation of excess fluid in the pericardium, a condition called pericardial effusion.

In constrictive pericarditis, which is a chronic form of the disease, prolonged inflammation leads to the buildup of scar tissue on the pericardium.

SYMPTOMS

The primary symptom of pericarditis is sharp chest pain, which is caused by the inflamed tissue rubbing against the heart or lungs. The ache may radiate to the neck and shoulder as well.

The pain is usually distinguished from angina or a heart attack because it is aggravated by coughing or breathing. Also, unlike angina, the discomfort can be relieved by changing your posture, such as sitting up or leaning forward.

Fever, chills, and fatigue are also common. Your doctor may be able to hear a "friction rub" when listening to your chest with a stethoscope. A large pericardial effusion or constrictive pericarditis can prevent the heart chambers from filling with blood normally, leading to heart failure or shock.

Viral pericarditis or pericarditis associated with a heart attack or heart surgery usually resolves in a week or two.

When pericarditis is caused by a bacterial infection (particularly tuberculosis) or by tumors, the symptoms often become increasingly severe. Pericarditis from an inflammatory disease such as lupus can come and go, causing recurring chest pain.

TREATMENT OPTIONS

Your symptoms and the results of a physical examination may provide strong clues to the diagnosis. An electrocardiogram (see p.135)

can show changes that suggest pericarditis, but the best diagnostic test is an echocardiogram (see p.665).

If the source of the condition is not obvious, you may need to undergo more extensive testing. In rare circumstances, your doctor may need to use a needle to draw a sample of fluid from around your heart; the fluid is sent to the laboratory for analysis.

Treatment for pericarditis depends on the underlying cause. If a viral infection is to blame, the only therapy may be anti-inflammatory drugs to control pain. Bacterial infections require antibiotics. If kidney failure is responsible, immediate dialysis is necessary.

When the fluid volume in the pericardial sac builds up to the point where it interferes with heart function, it is an urgent situation. The pressure can be temporarily relieved by drawing out fluid with a needle. Heart surgery may be necessary to drain fluid or to cut away scar tissue.

Rheumatic Fever

Rheumatic fever is an inflammatory disease that can attack the body's connective tissue, particularly the tissue of the heart, joints, skin, and, sometimes, the brain.

The heart is virtually always affected, at least temporarily. There can be lasting damage to the heart valves (rheumatic heart disease), which develops after an untreated streptococcal infection such as strep throat or scarlet fever.

It is thought that the reaction of the immune system to the

streptococcal bacteria causes the immune system to damage the heart and other organs, as in other autoimmune diseases (see p.870).

Rheumatic fever most often affects children between the ages of 5 and 15, although younger children and adults can be affected. In the past 50 years, in the United States and other developed nations, rheumatic fever has become rare because the strains of streptococcal bacteria that cause it are much less common.

However, in developing nations, rheumatic fever is still a common and serious problem. Once a person develops rheumatic fever, he or she is vulnerable to getting it again with subsequent streptococcal infections.

SYMPTOMS

Rheumatic fever develops several weeks after a streptococcal infection. The main symptoms of rheumatic fever, not all of which are present in every case, are arthritis, small bumps (nodules) over bones, sudden irregular and uncontrollable jerking movements, a rash, and symptoms of heart inflammation.

Heart symptoms are not always present, even when the heart is diseased. However, symptoms of pericarditis (see p.697), heart block (see p.680), and heart failure (see p.683) can occur. These initial symptoms of rheumatic fever can last months.

When rheumatic fever was common in the United States, it caused a great many children to be absent from school. Some cases of rheumatic fever can be very mild; many people who have rheumatic heart disease do not remember having had a serious, prolonged illness resembling rheumatic fever when they were young.

For some people, acute rheumatic fever goes away without causing serious damage. However, others have permanent damage to the heart valves. The most common heart valve abnormalities are aortic stenosis and insufficiency (see p.690) and mitral stenosis and insufficiency (see p.692).

These conditions can produce breathlessness, palpitations, fainting, chest pain, and sudden death.

TREATMENT OPTIONS

Rheumatic fever is diagnosed mainly by your symptoms and a physical examination. A blood test to detect streptococcal infection can help in the diagnosis.

The main treatment for the symptoms of rheumatic fever is taking anti-inflammatory drugs, most often aspirin. In severe cases, corticosteroid drugs (see p.895) are used to reduce inflammation.

Once rheumatic fever has developed, antibiotics do not help. If you have had rheumatic fever in the past, you need to take antibiotics regularly to prevent future streptococcal infections because recurring infections can cause another attack of rheumatic fever.

DISEASE OF THE ARTERIES AND VEINS

Aneurysms

Normally, an artery is a straight tube of a constant diameter. In an aneurysm, a section of the artery balloons out, widening its diameter. The wall of an artery that has an aneurysm is weaker than the wall of a normal artery and can burst, creating serious internal bleeding.

Aneurysms most often occur in the body's largest artery, the aorta; the next most common site are the smaller arteries of the brain. Rupture of these aneurysms causes brain hemorrhage (see p.350). Aneurysms also occur in the arteries of the legs, but are less likely to cause serious problems than aortic or brain aneurysms.

Aortic aneurysms are classified by their location and characteristics. Aneurysms that occur in the portion of the aorta that comes out of the heart and travels through the chest cavity (thorax) are called thoracic aortic aneurysms.

Aneurysms that occur in the part of the aorta that lies in the abdomen are abdominal aortic aneurysms.

Aortic aneurysms usually form at a spot on the artery wall weakened by atherosclerosis and long-standing high blood pressure. Blood vessel walls are constructed out of multiple layers of muscle and connective tissue. When plaque deposits form on the inside of the artery, oxygen and other nutrients cannot penetrate the plaque to get to

Common Sites for Aortic Aneurysms

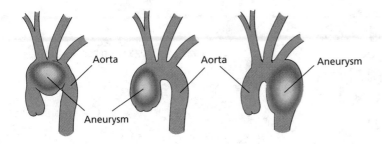

THORACIC AORTIC ANEURYSMS

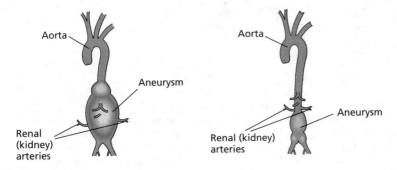

ABDOMINAL AORTIC ANEURYSMS

Aneurysms most frequently form on the major arteries of the trunk and legs. Common sites are the upper and lower sections of the aorta and the arteries of the legs. Thoracic aortic aneurysms form on the portion of the aorta in the chest cavity near the heart (top). Abdominal aortic aneurysms commonly develop on the lower part of the aorta near the junction with the arteries that supply the kidneys (bottom).

the middle layer of tissue. The lack of nourishment weakens this tissue.

Eventually, the force of the pounding blood stretches the damaged vessel wall. Aneurysms are more common in people with severe chronic bronchitis and emphysema caused by smoking. About 3% of people between ages 65 and 80 have an abdominal aortic aneurysm.

There is also a clear genetic component to aneurysms, de-monstrated by the fact that they are far more common in men and in people who have close relatives with the same problem. Infections such as advanced syphilis can also damage the aorta, leading to an aneurysm.

A small number of people suffer from an inherited connective tissue disorder called Marfan syndrome, which increases their susceptibility to developing aneurysms (even if they do not have atherosclerosis).

A problem related to aneurysms is aortic dissection, in which blood pushes its way into the middle of the wall of the aorta. The blood separates the inner wall from the outer wall and can push its way down the whole length in a matter of seconds. It, too, stems from the degeneration of the wall of arteries.

Aortic dissection almost always occurs in people who have long-standing high blood pressure. The area of dissection is weak and can rupture, leading to catastrophic internal bleeding.

SYMPTOMS

Aortic aneurysms frequently cause no symptoms, unless they rupture. They are often discovered when the doctor examines your abdomen or during an imaging procedure—such as an ultrasound (see p.148), computed tomography (see p.149), magnetic resonance imaging (see p.150), or x-ray (see p.145)—for an unrelated problem.

However, large thoracic aneurysms may cause chest or back pain, shortness of breath, hoarseness, coughing, or a feeling that you are full after eating just a little.

When an aortic aneurysm ruptures, it may cause severe stabbing pain, often followed by loss of consciousness. The loss of blood into the chest or abdomen results in shock (see p.644). About 80% of people who have ruptured aneurysms die, half of them before reaching the hospital.

Symptoms of a dissecting aortic aneurysm vary, depending upon the location of the tear. When it is in the upper aorta,

Repairing an Aortic Aneurysm With a Stent Graft

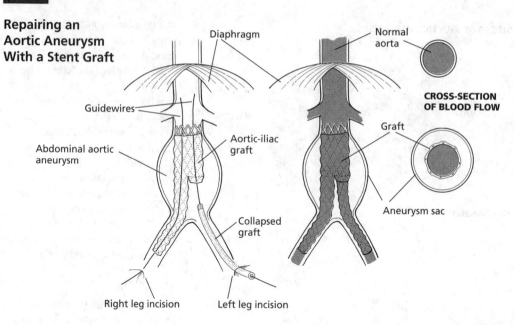

A thin, flexible guidewire is inserted into the blood vessels, usually through a small incision in the artery of one of the legs. The wire is threaded up to the site of the aortic aneurysm. A catheter containing the stent graft is pushed over the guidewire until the stent graft is in the correct position. Then the graft is released from the catheter. The stent graft is built to expand until its walls touch the walls of the healthy part of the aorta. A second stent graft can be inserted through the left leg if the aneurysm is very large. The two stent grafts form a new channel for blood to flow into the legs, taking pressure off the weakened and stretched walls of the aneurysm.

---

you may experience severe, tearing chest pain, shortness of breath, or pain between the shoulder blades.

A dissecting aneurysm in the lower aorta results in abdominal or bowel pain, and leg or flank pain if the tears extend into adjoining leg or kidney arteries.

TREATMENT OPTIONS

The treatment for aortic aneurysms is surgery, which involves replacing the damaged part of the aorta with a tube of synthetic material. Because most candidates for aneurysm surgery already have extensive cardiovascular disease, there is a 4% rate of heart complications from the operation. This is double the rate for most other kinds of surgery.

For this reason, and because aortic aneurysms of smaller diameter are much less likely to rupture, doctors usually wait until the aneurysm is 5 centimeters in diameter, about the diameter of a peach, before recommending an operation.

For a smaller aneurysm, the strategy is to undergo periodic radiologic imaging to gauge how fast it is expanding. If it is growing rapidly, you may need to have it repaired immediately.

A promising new procedure to repair aortic aneurysms without the trauma of surgery involves inserting a synthetic tube, called a stent, inside the aorta, at the point of disease. All of the pressure in the blood pushes against the walls of this tube, and not against the weakened natural walls of the aorta, reducing the chance of a rupture.

To position the stent-graft, doctors insert a small catheter into an artery in the groin and pass the catheter up into the aorta. Using x-ray imaging, the stent is then guided over the catheter, to the location of the aneurysm, where the stent is then made to expand to the size of a normal aorta. The stent essentially becomes the wall of the aorta, replacing the normal wall.

Arterial Embolism

An embolism is a solid particle that travels in the bloodstream to another location, where it lodges in a narrower vessel, blocking the blood supply to an organ. The solid particle is usually a blood clot, a cholesterol particle, or a combination of the two.

An embolism can block arteries to any body part or organ, but most commonly affects the legs, kidneys, and brain (see Stroke, p.342, for a discussion of brain embolism).

More than 95% of the time, a large embolism is a blood clot that originates in the heart. This can occur when the heart's chambers are not pumping normally—such as in atrial fibrillation (see p.673) or cardiomyopathy (see p.682) or after a heart attack.

It also can occur when the inner wall of the heart has been damaged, such as after a heart attack or with heart valve disease (see p.689).

Occasionally, if the heart's atria or ventricles have a hole in them, a clot that starts in a major vein such as in the legs can pass through the hole, enter the arterial system, and cause an embolism.

Minute emboli, known as microemboli, can also come from the heart but more frequently are the result of cholesterol particles given off by plaques (caused by atherosclerosis) in the aorta or arteries leading into the brain.

Sometimes microemboli come from material on a malfunctioning cardiac valve or a tumor in the heart called a myxoma.

Microemboli can occur during procedures such as angioplasty (see p.661) or coronary atherec-

tomy (see p.702), which attempt to clear blockages in the coronary arteries; this can cause a heart attack.

SYMPTOMS

Symptoms depend on the location of the embolus and the extent to which it blocks the flow of blood. An embolism in the brain that causes a stroke can result in some degree of brain damage.

When circulation to an arm or leg is blocked, the part of the limb below the blockage becomes cold, pale, weak, numb, and painful, and there is no pulse. Without treatment to restore circulation, the tissue dies and gangrene may set in. Amputation is necessary in about a quarter of cases.

Blockages of arteries leading to the kidneys can cause kidney damage, high blood pressure, and blood in the urine. In some situations, however, the effects of the blockage are less severe because there are other vessels (called collaterals) that can supply the tissue with blood.

TREATMENT OPTIONS

The first step is to pinpoint the location of the blockage and take steps to remove it. Angiography (see p.659), a procedure that involves injecting dye into the arteries so that they can be examined under x-ray, is the diagnostic tool most commonly used to find the embolism.

Emboli can be treated medically or surgically. Low doses of clot-dissolving agents such as streptokinase, urokinase, and tissue plasminogen activator can be administered directly to the clot

by passing a catheter to the site of the blockage and releasing the clot-busting drug right at that point. This method results in fewer complications than when the drug is given by injection through a vein to travel to all parts of the body.

Blood-thinning drugs that prevent more clots from forming (such as heparin or aspirin) are also part of medical treatment. Sometimes angioplasty (see p.661) can physically squash the clot and reduce the obstruction in blood flow.

If all else fails, an embolectomy is also an option to remove the clot or to replace or bypass the blocked vessel.

Atherosclerosis of the Arteries to the Legs

The buildup of fat-laden plaque (atherosclerosis) on the inside of the arteries limits the amount of blood that can get through to the muscles. When this happens in the arteries that supply blood to the legs, the leg muscles can be deprived of oxygen during exercise, a condition called peripheral arterial disease or peripheral vascular disease.

The main symptom of vascular disease of the legs is intermittent claudication, which causes the symptoms described below.

The risk factors for atherosclerosis of the leg arteries are the same as those for coronary artery disease: smoking, high blood pressure, high cholesterol, diabetes, sedentary lifestyle, and family history of heart disease.

The disease is more likely to progress rapidly in people who smoke or have diabetes.

Uncontrolled peripheral vascular disease can lead to gangrene and the need for amputation of the affected limb.

SYMPTOMS

You feel a cramping, aching, or heaviness in the muscles below the blockage. These sensations are brought on by exercising and subside after a few minutes of rest. The pain is usually felt in the calf muscles or the back of the thigh, above or below the knee. Coolness in the leg, skin ulcers, and impotence are other signs of vascular disease.

Symptoms of intermittent claudication develop gradually over a period of years. The problem usually begins as mild pain in one leg during exercise. If there is atherosclerosis in the arteries to the other leg, both legs may develop claudication.

When the blockage severely limits blood flow, the foot and toes often ache, even while resting. This sensation can be painful enough to awaken you from sleep and may be relieved by

Bypassing Leg Blockages

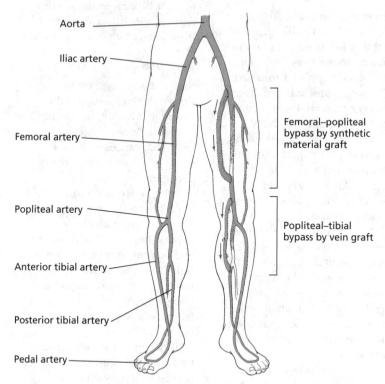

Aorta

Iliac artery

Femoral artery

Popliteal artery

Anterior tibial artery

Posterior tibial artery

Pedal artery

Femoral–popliteal bypass by synthetic material graft

Popliteal–tibial bypass by vein graft

The large arteries that supply the legs with blood are common locations for atherosclerosis, particularly at points where the arteries branch to form other, narrower arteries. When a major blockage occurs, restoring blood flow may require bypass surgery. This rerouting of blood can be accomplished with synthetic materials or by using one of your own veins. Bypassing blockages in arteries of the legs is like bypassing blockages in coronary arteries (see p.662).

Atherectomy Devices

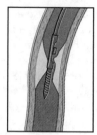

DIRECTIONAL CORONARY ATHERECTOMY

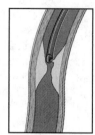

EXTRACTION ATHERECTOMY

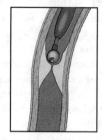

ROTATIONAL ATHERECTOMY

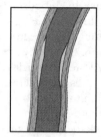

AFTER ATHERECTOMY

Blood flow can be restored to narrowed arteries (such as those in the heart or legs) by cutting away the plaque deposits that line the vessels. This technique, called atherectomy, is performed using any of several tools that are threaded into the artery over a guidewire. Directional and extraction atherectomy use blades to cut away the plaque and remove it. In rotational atherectomy, a rotating blade trims the plaque from the artery walls.

dangling your feet over the side of the bed.

TREATMENT OPTIONS

To diagnose peripheral vascular disease, your doctor will take your medical history and perform a physical exam, including measuring the blood pressure in your arms and legs.

An angiogram (see p.659), in which dye is infused into the main artery leading to the legs and an x-ray taken, is necessary to determine both the exact location and the severity of the blockage if bypass surgery is planned (see Bypassing Leg Blockages, right).

Unless your symptoms are extremely severe, the first step in treatment is to try to reduce the risk factors that have led to the atherosclerosis. Lowering your cholesterol level if it is too high can help slow progression of the disease. Quitting smoking and taking a daily aspirin tablet can reduce your chances of serious complications.

Give your foot extra care (see Complications of Diabetes, p.836, for advice on foot care) to avoid infection in the affected leg; this can also help lower your risk for amputation.

Regular, supervised exercise can dramatically increase the distance you are able to walk without symptoms. Some people benefit from the drugs pentoxifylline and cilostazol, which help blood cells flow more smoothly.

For people who have disabling claudication, surgery may be a reasonable option. One method is to graft a vessel onto the artery, to bypass the blockage. This is similar to coronary

How Deep Vein Thrombosis Leads to Pulmonary Embolism

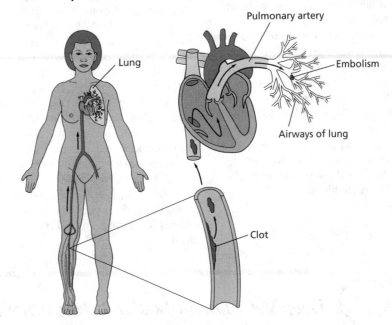

Stagnant blood in the deep veins of the legs is prone to forming clots. If one of these clots breaks free, there is a danger that it will travel up the veins into the right side of the heart and then out into the lungs, where it can lodge in an artery. This is called pulmonary embolism (see p.512). It is a potentially life-threatening condition that can cause sharp chest pain, shortness of breath, rapid heartbeat, fainting, and even death.

artery bypass surgery performed on the heart.

A less invasive procedure is atherectomy (see illustration on p.702), in which a small tool on the end of a catheter is used to cut away the plaque from the inside of the artery.

Angioplasty (see p.661) can also be used to open peripheral arteries. To prevent the vessel from narrowing again after a balloon angioplasty procedure, a small metal mesh tube called a stent is sometimes placed in the artery.

Deep Vein Thrombosis

Deep vein thrombosis (DVT) is a condition in which clots form in the large veins of the legs.

Two main factors contribute to the formation of clots in the deep veins. The first is stagnation of the blood in the lower veins. The contraction of the calf muscles as you walk helps propel blood in the leg veins back to the heart. An extended period of bed rest, prolonged surgery, or even a lengthy airplane flight prevents this action from taking place.

Other factors that slow blood flow in the leg veins are a

decrease in the heart's pumping ability (due to congestive heart failure).

DVT can also occur if your blood has a greater-than-normal tendency to form clots. This can be an inherited condition or can stem from infection, cancer, or connective tissue disorders. It can also be caused by taking oral contraceptives. In addition, injury or surgery tends to dramatically increase the level of clotting factor in the blood.

SYMPTOMS

DVT can develop without causing symptoms. If DVT involves the larger leg veins in the thigh, the leg begins to swell. When DVT occurs in the legs of the calf, it can cause pain in the calf.

DVT clots in the leg veins can occur without any symptoms at all. If one of the clots in the deep veins breaks free, it can travel to the lungs and block a pulmonary artery. This is called a pulmonary embolism (see p.512) and can cause sharp chest pain, shortness of breath, fainting, and even death.

TREATMENT OPTIONS

It is difficult for your doctor to diagnose DVT simply by examining your leg. If there is swelling or tenderness, your doctor may send you for various diagnostic tests. Most often, the first test is an ultrasound (see p.148) of your leg veins, which can visualize the clots and measure the speed of the blood flow in your veins.

If ultrasound is inconclusive, you may need to have a venogram or magnetic resonance imaging (MRI) (see p.150). A venogram involves injecting dye

Deep Vein Thrombosis/Pulmonary Embolism: *When You Visit Your Doctor*

QUESTIONS TO DISCUSS WITH YOUR DOCTOR:

- Do you still have pain, warmth, or swelling in the affected area?

- Do you have chest pain or shortness of breath?

- Has anyone else in your family had a blood clot? If so, have they (and you) been tested for blood-clotting abnormalities?

- Do you know if your blood relatives have a tendency to form blood clots? If so (and even if not), should your relatives be tested?

- Are you taking the birth-control pill? You should never take oral contraceptives if you have had a blood clot.

- Could you be pregnant? If you have had a blood clot, you may need to take medication to thin your blood during pregnancy?

- If you are pregnant, are there medications you can safely take to prevent a clot during pregnancy?

- Do you know how long you will have to remain on anticoagulation therapy?

- While on anticoagulation therapy, do you know what foods to avoid and what medication interactions to watch out for?

YOUR DOCTOR MIGHT EXAMINE THE FOLLOWING BODY STRUCTURES OR FUNCTIONS:

- Heart rate and blood pressure

- Heart and lungs

- Affected arm or leg (to be sure the swelling, redness, and warmth are resolving)

YOUR DOCTOR MIGHT ORDER THE FOLLOWING LAB TESTS OR STUDIES:

- Prothrombin time (see p.156) if you are on anticoagulant medicines such as warfarin

- Ultrasound (see p.148) of affected area, if blood clot may have recurred

- Blood tests (for various blood-clotting abnormalities; see p.709) if you have a family history of blood clots or if this is your second episode

into the veins to look for blockages.

The MRI carries no risk and has the advantage of showing veins high in the leg and in the pelvis, where clots can form. It will soon replace venography. However, it is more expensive and more difficult to schedule on an emergency basis than ultrasound.

If the diagnostic tests show that DVT is confined only to the veins in the calf, the tests may be repeated several times over the following few weeks to ensure that the condition has not spread into the veins above the knee, where the chance of developing a pulmonary embolus is greater. Alternatively, your doctor may decide to treat the DVT of the calf.

Treating DVT traditionally required 5 to 7 days of hospitalization, continuous intravenous treatment with a blood-thinner called unfractionated heparin, and repeated blood tests to be certain the dose of heparin was correct.

A new form of the drug, known as low molecular weight heparin, administered in once- or twice-a-day injections under the skin, without the need for frequent blood tests, now makes it possible for you to be treated at home. (If you have also had a pulmonary embolus from the DVT, most doctors still recommend hospitalization for a few days.)

Along with the heparin, which thins the blood immediately, you will be given another blood-thinning drug, warfarin. This pill takes several days to become effective, and is usually pre-scribed for 12 weeks to 6 months, depending on how severe your condition is, whether you have had DVT before, and whether you have an underlying condition that makes you especially vulnerable to developing DVT again.

In severe cases of DVT, "clot-busting" thrombolytic drugs (see p.667) can be delivered directly to the site of the problem via catheter. However, this procedure is effective only if it is performed within 2 weeks of the formation of the clot.

After treatment for DVT, your doctor will prescribe specially fitted elastic stockings that you wear every day. Although these garments are somewhat uncomfortable, it is important to wear them. They reduce by half the incidence of pain when walking that often follows DVT. These stockings also help prevent leg swelling, skin breakdown, and infection.

Phlebitis

Phlebitis means inflammation of a vein. It usually occurs in veins that are just beneath the surface of the skin rather than in deeper veins. However, if phlebitis is not treated, it can spread into the deeper veins, causing deep vein thrombosis (see p.703) and its associated problems.

Phlebitis is more likely to develop when circulation through the veins is slower than normal, such as in varicose veins, or when your blood has an increased tendency to form clots.

Phlebitis sometimes follows injury to a vein, especially in people with poor circulation. For example, the condition often

How Phlebitis Can Cause Deep Vein Thrombosis

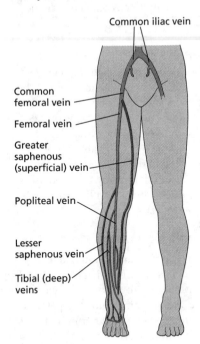

Common iliac vein

Common femoral vein

Femoral vein

Greater saphenous (superficial) vein

Popliteal vein

Lesser saphenous vein

Tibial (deep) veins

Phlebitis poses a particular risk when it affects the greater saphenous vein in the upper leg because this vein connects directly with the deep venous system. A clot in the greater saphenous vein has the potential to grow into the common femoral vein, resulting in deep vein thrombosis (DVT). A clot in the lesser saphenous vein can grow into the popliteal vein, resulting in DVT.

develops in the legs after some minor injury to a varicose vein in that area.

An intravenous catheter that is left in a vein for an extended period of time, or the use of illicit intravenous drugs, can also damage a vein and bring on inflammation.

Phlebitis commonly occurs in people with pancreatic cancer. Less frequently, it develops in people with breast and ovarian cancers. It can also occur in people who have connective tissue disorders such as lupus.

SYMPTOMS

Phlebitis is characterized by warmth, redness, and pain of the skin and tissues underneath the skin. The outward signs of the condition can occasionally be confused with inflammation of the skin (cellulitis) or the lymph system (lymphangitis), both of which cause warmth and redness in the extremities.

TREATMENT OPTIONS

Physical examination usually makes clear the diagnosis of phlebitis. Your doctor may perform an ultrasound (see p.148) of the leg veins to determine if the phlebitis has spread into the deep veins and caused deep vein thrombosis, which occurs about 30% of the time.

Spread to the deep veins is most likely when phlebitis affects two particular leg veins—the greater and lesser saphenous veins. If spread to the deep veins has not occurred, treatment includes applying warm compresses, taking anti-inflammatory drugs such as ibuprofen or indomethacin, and wearing elastic compression stockings. Sometimes ultrasound is performed every few days to evaluate the progression of clotting.

Raynaud Disease

Raynaud disease is a condition in which the small arteries (capillaries) in the skin constrict (narrow), cutting off blood flow to the extremities. Your hands and feet are the most common places for

this to occur, but your ears and nose may be affected as well.

Episodes are generally triggered by exposure to cold air or by emotional distress. Raynaud disease often occurs in people with a connective tissue disease such as scleroderma, lupus, and rheumatoid arthritis. It also can occur in people who regularly use jackhammers or chain saws, which can damage the blood vessels in the hands. It is also more likely to occur in smokers.

The condition is called Raynaud disease when it occurs without any associated illness. It is called Raynaud phenomenon when it occurs in association with other medical conditions. Raynaud disease first shows up in a person's late teens or early 20s and affects women much more frequently than men.

SYMPTOMS

When the arteries constrict, the skin of your fingers or toes turns white and then blue as the oxygen in the blood is used up. There is often a sharp line of demarcation between the abnormal (white or blue) portion at the end of the fingers or toes and the more normal tissue next to it.

The affected extremity also usually feels numb or prickly. Within 5 to 10 minutes after getting into warmer air, the capillaries dilate (open) and blood flow resumes.

TREATMENT OPTIONS

Raynaud disease or phenomenon is usually diagnosed by the description you give to your doctor. Tests are not usually necessary to diagnose the condition, but they are often performed to see if you

have any of the underlying diseases associated with the condition, such as lupus and other connective tissue diseases, or previous injury to your hands.

In general, treatment involves preventing an attack by protecting yourself from the cold with a hat, warm socks, and gloves. You may even want to wear mittens when removing food from the refrigerator. Quitting smoking is imperative. Vasodilator medicines, such as nifedipine, and biofeedback techniques can also ease symptoms.

Varicose Veins

Varicose veins are twisted, rope-like blood vessels that run just beneath the surface of the legs. Half of all women have varicose veins to some degree as they grow older.

Varicose veins develop because of the failure of a series of small, one-way valves in the veins. These valves prevent blood from being pulled by gravity back down to the feet. As the heart pumps, the valves open to let blood through and then shut to prevent flow from falling backward. If one of these valves starts to malfunction, blood leaks through it and pools above the valve below it. This causes the vein above the lower valve to bulge.

The vein eventually becomes so large that it is visible through the surface of the skin. A leg in which there are many varicose veins also becomes somewhat swollen because fluid from the blood in the bulging veins starts to leak into the tissues around the veins.

A common cause of varicose veins in women is pregnancy.

The weight and size of the fetus presses on the veins in the pelvis, increasing the pressure in the veins of the legs. This can cause the valves in the leg veins to weaken.

A tendency toward developing varicose veins can result from a genetic defect in the valves or in the wall of the vein. Damage to the valves from deep vein thrombosis (see p.703) can also lead to varicose veins.

SYMPTOMS

Symptoms of varicose veins are often described as dull aching, heaviness, cramping, and swelling in the lower part of the leg. The discomfort is often worse after a day of standing.

Other complications are discoloration, inflammation, and bleeding sores that can develop on the skin covering the vein. Clots can also form in the distended veins.

TREATMENT OPTIONS

Self-care measures Treatment for varicose veins begins with conservative measures to control the accumulation of blood in the lower extremities. You will be measured for elastic support stockings, which stretch from your ankle to just above your knee. These stockings compress the veins and help push blood back toward the heart. To be most effective, put on the stockings every morning as soon as you wake up. Putting on a nylon stocking underneath the elastic support stocking can sometimes help the elastic stocking slide on more easily.

If you have considerable leg swelling, elevate your ankles so

Effect of Exercise on Leg Circulation

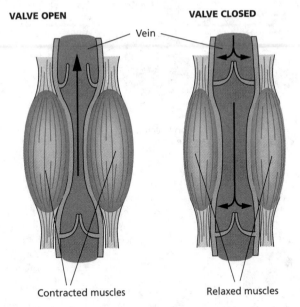

VALVE OPEN   **VALVE CLOSED**

Vein

Contracted muscles   Relaxed muscles

Exercise is crucial in preventing the pooling of blood in the lower extremities. When leg muscles contract, they squeeze blood up through the veins toward the heart, forcing open the valves of the veins. After the muscles relax, blood is kept from falling back down into the legs by the valves of the veins.

Formation of Varicose Veins

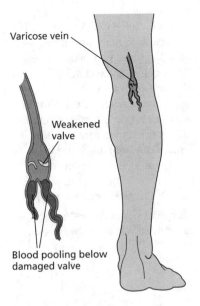

Varicose vein

Weakened valve

Blood pooling below damaged valve

A series of one-way valves prevents blood in the veins from flowing back down the legs toward the feet. When these valves are weakened, blood leaks through and moves back down to where it came from, pooling on top of the valve below. This pooling of blood causes the veins to stretch and bulge toward the surface of the skin, forming varicose veins.

Sclerotherapy for Varicose Veins

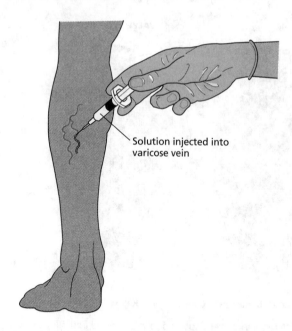

Solution injected into
varicose vein

Varicose veins can sometimes be eliminated by injecting a substance into the
vein that intentionally damages the inner lining of the vessel. Scar tissue
develops that eventually causes the vein to disappear. Sclerotherapy is primarily
a cosmetic procedure that can be used on small veins.

they are higher than the level of your heart for two 30-minute periods each day. This will reduce the swelling dramatically. Do this in addition to wearing the elastic stockings.

Exercise is also important in controlling varicose vein symptoms. The action of the calf and thigh muscles helps to pump the blood upward toward the heart. Swimming is an ideal activity since the pressure of the water can compress the veins the same way the elastic stockings do. Losing weight will also help relieve

symptoms by reducing pressure on the legs.

If you have varicose veins, be especially vigilant about proper skin hygiene. Your skin can easily become dry and itchy in areas that are stretched from the swelling. Scratching can lead to sores or a skin infection (cellulitis). A good moisturizing skin cream can help alleviate this problem. Use lanolin or hand cream; avoid petroleum jelly, which is less effective.

Surgical procedures Several treatments are available to elimi-

nate varicose veins. Sclerotherapy is a process in which a substance is injected into small veins to them. It is primarily a cosmetic procedure. Small, dilated vessels can also be treated with lasers (see p.582), although the cosmetic result is sometimes not as good.

For larger varicose veins causing serious symptoms, the best long-term treatment is surgical removal of the vein, sometimes called "stripping." Once the vein is removed, you should have relief from your symptoms. Since a varicose vein has already lost its ability to function, blood flow in the leg does not get worse when the affected vein is removed.

Before removing a varicose vein, however, your surgeon will want to make sure there are no clots in the deep vein system. If there are clots in the deep veins, the superficial veins could be providing circulation around the clot, and stripping them could worsen the swelling in your legs.

People sometimes worry that having a varicose vein removed could be a problem if they ever need to have coronary bypass surgery because leg veins are often used for the graft. However, a varicose vein would never be used for this purpose since the damaged vessel walls make it more likely to expand and form an aneurysm if it were grafted onto the heart.

Blood Disorders

The body is composed of trillions of cells. They all need a constant supply of nutrients (especially oxygen and sugars) to survive, and they all produce waste matter that must be eliminated. The heart and blood vessels bring blood to every cell. The blood brings nutrition and carries away waste. Without circulating blood, the body would quickly die.

There are about 5 to 6 quarts of blood in your body. About half of the volume of blood is a salt-water liquid called plasma; the other half is composed of blood cells that perform critical functions. The plasma carries sugars and other nutrients to the cells and carries away most of the waste. The blood cells are produced in the marrow of the bones and then enter the blood (see How You Make Blood, p.109).

Red blood cells There are more red blood cells (called erythrocytes) in your body than any other type of cell. Each of them lives about 120 days and is constantly being replaced by younger red blood cells.

Red blood cells transport oxygen from your lungs to the cells throughout your body. A protein called hemoglobin inside each red blood cell carries the oxygen and then releases it.

Anemia (see p.713) is a common condition in which there are not enough red blood cells. There are also some uncommon conditions in which there are too many red blood cells, causing the blood to get thick, which can make circulation less efficient.

White blood cells White blood cells (called leukocytes) defend your body against invading microorganisms and other foreign substances. Some white blood cells directly attack and engulf germs, killing them. At the same time, these white blood cells alert other types of white blood cells to initiate an attack on other similar germs. This cascade of reactions is part of the immune system response.

The immune response recruits several other types of killer white blood cells and stimulates the production of antibodies. Some white cells make toxic substances that directly injure invading parasites such as worms.

The role of white blood cells in the immune system response is described in more detail in Infections and Immune System Diseases (see p.863). Most cancers of blood cells involve the white blood cells. There is also a condition called leukopenia in which there are not enough white blood cells.

Platelets Platelets (called thrombocytes) are small pieces of blood cells that help the blood clot. When you cut yourself, you bleed because the walls of the tiny blood vessels at the site of the cut have been injured, allowing blood to escape.

Platelets move to the site of injury, stick to each other and to the injured edges of the blood vessel, and form a plug (clot) that seals the leak and keeps more blood from escaping. Chemicals in plasma make the clot strong and permanent.

Platelets also help repair injury to larger blood vessels, such as arteries, by releasing several substances that cause the artery to constrict (narrow) to a smaller diameter. This limits how much blood is lost from the injured vessel and slows the flow of blood in the area of the cut. Without this constriction of the vessel, the clot would be washed away by force of blood pressure.

While this action of platelets can be very helpful, the same capability of platelets to form clots and cause arteries to constrict can contribute to heart attacks, strokes, and insufficient blood flow in the legs. The action of platelets can also lead to blood clots in veins.

A variety of diseases can decrease the number of platelets in the blood to dangerously low levels, causing risk for serious bleeding. Other diseases increase the risk of bleeding by causing platelets to malfunction. There also is a condition in which there are too many platelets, causing an increased tendency to form blood clots (and, paradoxically, sometimes to bleed because the platelets do not work well).

Birth of Blood Cells

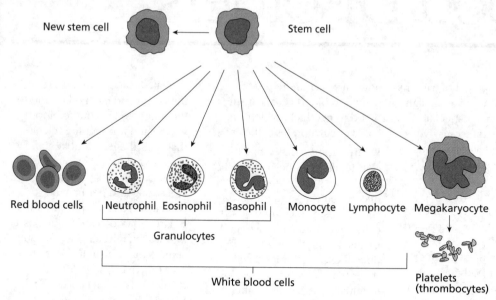

New stem cell · Stem cell

Red blood cells · Neutrophil · Eosinophil · Basophil · Monocyte · Lymphocyte · Megakaryocyte

Granulocytes

White blood cells

Platelets (thrombocytes)

Blood is composed of the cells shown here, plus plasma. The stem cell is the "mother cell." Stem cells divide to reproduce themselves and divide to give birth to all the different types of blood cells. Stem cells live in the bone marrow but sometimes travel in the bloodstream. Stem cells harvested from the bone marrow or bloodstream are essential for successful stem cell transplantation.

Red blood cells are born in the bone marrow; there are more of them in the body than any other type of cell.

White blood cells protect you against infection and foreign substances. There are three types of white blood cells: granulocytes, monocytes, and lymphocytes.

Granulocytes are made in the bone marrow. There are three different types of granulocytes: neutrophils, eosinophils, and basophils.

Neutrophils are the most abundant type of granulocyte and play a key role in killing bacteria. Eosinophils are important in killing parasitic infections such as amebae or worms. Basophils are involved in allergic reactions.

Monocytes are made in the bone marrow. Some monocytes travel into organs such as the lungs, where they turn into another white blood cell (called a macrophage) and help eradicate both bacterial and viral infections.

There are many kinds of lymphocytes, which are also made in the lymph glands, spleen, and thymus.

Megakaryocytes are very large cells that live in the bone marrow and spin off many little pieces of themselves called platelets (thrombocytes), which are important in the clotting of blood.

Blood clotting is a complicated business. You need your blood to clot at the right time, and in the right place, such as when the skin is cut. Blood is able to clot not only because of platelets but also because of a large number of different enzymes in the blood. Inside the body, blood vessels are injured frequently either by minor bumps or falls or from high pressures inside blood vessels that can cause small tears. Without the ability of the blood to clot, serious internal bleeding would occur.

One of the wonders of nature (in healthy people) is the ability of the blood to clot just enough to seal dangerous leaks, but not to clot too easily. The body makes some substances that encourage blood clots, and other substances that eliminate blood clots. There is a delicate balance between the action of these substances. This section describes diseases in which the balance is disrupted.

BLOOD DONATION AND TRANSFUSION

If your blood is deficient in red blood cells, platelets, or clotting factors, you may require a transfusion, in which blood from another person (or people) is infused into your bloodstream through a catheter in your vein.

Every year in the United States, 14 million units of donor blood are transfused into people who are ill, have been injured, and/or are deficient in some or all of the different components of blood.

The need for donated blood is constant. A single pint can benefit several people, and can be lifesaving. When you give blood, the red blood cells may go to one person, and other components (see below) may go to others.

Giving blood is completely safe. Receiving blood still has some risks, but they are very small and are almost always outweighed by the benefits.

BLOOD COMPONENTS

Blood has many different components, and most people who need a blood transfusion need only certain components. The use of different parts of blood, and the length of time each component can be stored, varies:

Red blood cells, which carry oxygen and are commonly used to treat anemia, can be refrigerated for a maximum of 42 days; they can be frozen for up to 10 years.

Platelets are essential for controlling bleeding and are given to people with leukemia and other forms of cancer or who are undergoing chemotherapy. Platelets can be stored for a maximum of 5 days.

Plasma, used to control bleeding, can be frozen for up to 1 year. Different useful products can be extracted from plasma. Albumin is extracted from plasma and used to treat shock.

Gamma globulin from plasma is used to augment low levels of antibodies that occur in some diseases, thereby helping to prevent infection. Gamma globulin also is used to block other antibodies that are causing disease, such as in the neurologic disease Guillain-Barré syndrome (see p.377).

Cryoprecipitated antihemophilic factor, which contains clotting factors, is made from fresh-frozen plasma and may be stored frozen for 1 year. It is occasionally given to people with hemophilia or von Willebrand disease, but has largely been replaced by more highly processed clotting factors or genetically engineered factors.

White blood cells were once given as transfusions to people who had very low numbers of them. However, doctors now use natural substances called growth factors, which encourage your own white blood cells to grow, making the transfusion of someone else's white blood cells into your body unnecessary.

AUTOLOGOUS BLOOD DONATION: GIVING BLOOD TO YOURSELF

Having several pints of your own blood removed and stored before surgery is called autologous transfusion. About 10% of all blood transfusions in the United States are autologous transfusions.

Usually, you give 1 pint at a

Safety of Blood Transfusions: Dr Churchill's Advice

I'm surprised by how many people are concerned about the safety of receiving a blood transfusion. The nation's blood supply is safer today than it has ever been. Any unit of blood that you get as a transfusion has been tested for hepatitis B virus, hepatitis C virus, human immunodeficiency virus (HIV), human T-cell lymphotrophic virus type 1, and syphilis. Nothing is perfect; there is still a tiny risk of an infectious agent in blood. But the risk is much less than it is for other medical treatments that people accept without thinking.

For example, the chance of catching HIV in a blood transfusion is approximately 1 in every 676,000 units of blood, whereas the chance of a serious, potentially fatal adverse reaction to penicillin is 1 in every 30,000 people. When your doctor says you need a blood transfusion and explains to you why the need exists, you should not hesitate.

W. HALLOWELL CHURCHILL, MD
BRIGHAM AND WOMEN'S HOSPITAL
HARVARD MEDICAL SCHOOL

Safety of Giving Blood

The average adult body contains 10 to 12 pints of blood, a supply that is continuously replaced. Donating 1 or 2 pints (units) of blood does not cause any problems for your body. Occasionally, people faint when they give blood, not because the loss of blood caused them to faint, but because they are frightened.

Donating blood is easy and safe. You cannot get any disease, including the acquired immunodeficiency syndrome (AIDS), by donating blood. To donate, contact your local branch of the American Red Cross or a hospital. In general, you must be at least 17 years old, in good health, and weigh at least 110 pounds to donate. When you donate blood, you will be asked a number of questions required by the Food and Drug Administration about your health and factors that affect your health. They are asked to help ensure the safety of the blood supply.

The most common reasons for being excluded from donating blood are being anemic (having a low blood count); having elevated temperature, pulse, or blood pressure; having traveled to a country where malaria is prevalent (malaria can be passed to someone receiving a blood donation); and being at risk for infection with the human immunodeficiency virus (HIV). If you are healthy, you can donate blood regularly throughout the year; however, wait 56 days between donations.

time for several weeks in advance of scheduled surgery. This process ensures a perfect match, since you will be transfused with your own blood if it is necessary.

If you donate your own blood and do not need it, it is generally not available for use by other people because the strict safeguards to prevent infection are not applied to blood you donate to yourself.

SYNTHETIC BLOOD

Research into synthetic blood substitutes has been a subject of intense interest for many years. An ideal synthetic blood product would permit transfusion to a person of any blood type, would be composed of compounds that are free of infectious agents or substances that could cause an immune system reaction, would not deteriorate during storage or require refrigeration, and would be made of readily available materials. Although several products have appeared promising, all have had serious side effects.

Compatibility of Blood Types

There are four major blood types: A, B, AB, and O. Each of the groups is further divided into Rh types: Rh positive or Rh negative. The blood type is determined by antigens on the surface of the cell. In the United States, the most common blood type is O positive, and the least common is AB negative.

People with type O blood are called "universal donors"; in an emergency, their blood can be given to anyone. People with type AB blood are "universal recipients"; in an emergency, they can receive blood from anyone.

As the chart shows, if you have type A or type B blood, your blood is compatible only with certain other blood types. If the blood type of the donor is not compatible with the blood type of the recipient, a potentially severe transfusion reaction will occur, characterized by fever, chills, back pain, and shortness of breath. In severe cases, shock or

IF THIS IS YOUR BLOOD TYPE	YOU CAN RECEIVE BLOOD OF THE FOLLOWING BLOOD TYPES
A	A, O
B	B, O
AB	A, B, AB, O
O	O

organ failure occurs. This is why your blood type is carefully determined before you receive a transfusion. Because there are other "minor" blood types that may be incompatible, there is still a possibility of a transfusion reaction, even if the major blood types match. However, the reactions caused by these types of transfusions are easily treated.

ANEMIA

Anemia is a condition in which the blood has too few red blood cells, causing low levels of hemoglobin, the protein inside red blood cells that delivers oxygen from the lungs to all tissues of the body. Anemia has many causes and is broadly divided into two categories: anemias that are caused by a decreased or defective production of red blood cells and anemias that are caused by increased destruction of red cells in the blood.

The symptoms of all forms of anemia occur because the oxygen-carrying capacity of the red blood cells is reduced, although symptoms vary depending on how low the level of hemoglobin drops. Anemia is very common. Perhaps 10% to 15% of women in the United States have at least mild anemia, mostly from iron deficiency. Mild anemia may not produce any symptoms. It is most often detected through a routine blood test, such as a complete blood cell count (see p.154).

In more severe cases, anemia can cause headaches, tiredness, shortness of breath, and light-headedness. It can also cause your heart and breathing rate to increase to compensate for the lack of oxygen in the bloodstream.

NORMAL PRODUCTION OF RED BLOOD CELLS

The production of red blood cells starts in the bone marrow, where immature cells called stem cells begin to develop into mature red blood cells. As the red blood cells develop, they make hemoglobin, essential for transporting oxygen throughout the body. After about 5 days in the bone marrow, red blood cells (called reticulocytes at this stage) are released into the bloodstream, where they complete their maturation and circulate for about 4 months.

REDUCED PRODUCTION OF RED BLOOD CELLS

Several conditions hinder the production of red blood cells in the bone marrow. Poor diet, chronic blood loss, or gastrointestinal problems that inhibit absorption can create a deficiency of minerals and nutrients—such as iron, vitamin B_{12} (as in pernicious anemia), or folic acid—which are essential to produce red blood cells.

Aplastic anemia (see p.720), in which the formation of all cells in the bone marrow is compromised, reduces the number of red blood cells, as well as white blood cells and platelets. Chronic illnesses such as cancer, some infections, and kidney failure can also reduce red blood cell production.

BLOOD LOSS

Anemia can be caused by bleeding, most commonly due to heavy menstrual flow in women. Anemia also can be caused by bleeding in the digestive system,

What Causes Different Types of Anemia?

Anemia can be caused by reduced or defective production of red blood cells or by a high rate of destruction of red blood cells, which carry vital oxygen to the body's tissues. Four types of anemia are shown here.

IRON-DEFICIENCY ANEMIA	APLASTIC ANEMIA	HEMOLYTIC ANEMIA	PERNICIOUS ANEMIA

In iron-deficiency anemia, a lack of iron prevents the bone marrow from making enough hemoglobin for the red cells. The red cells are small and have a reduced oxygen-carrying capacity.

In aplastic anemia, defective formation and division of stem (infant) cells in the bone marrow cause fewer red and other blood cells.

In hemolytic anemia, the rate of red blood cell production is normal or high, but the cells are destroyed at a much faster rate than normal.

A deficiency in vitamin B_{12} causes the bone marrow to produce red blood cells that are larger than normal and fewer in number.

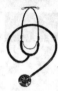

Anemia: *When You Visit Your Doctor*

Anemia is not a disease but can be a warning sign of several serious diseases. It is therefore vital that its cause be accurately diagnosed and treated. If your doctor suspects anemia, he or she may ask you the following questions:

■ Do you have nosebleeds or do you bruise easily? Do you have more gum bleeding than usual when you brush your teeth? Have you ever seen bright red blood in your bowel movements or on toilet paper? Have you ever had black tarry bowel movements? Have you noticed that your urine is dark in color?

■ If you are a woman, are your menstrual periods very heavy or frequent?

■ Do you have ulcers (see p.752) or fibroids of the uterus (see p.1074)?

■ Do you take aspirin or other nonsteroidal anti-inflammatory drugs? These and other medicines can cause erosion of and bleeding from the stomach lining.

■ Do you drink a lot of alcohol? Alcohol can irritate the stomach and increase the likelihood of bleeding. It can also interfere with blood production.

■ Do you get heartburn or an upset stomach? This may be a sign of gastroesophageal reflux (see p.747), which can cause blood loss.

■ Do you have frequent diarrhea? Diarrhea can interfere with the absorption of important nutrients such as iron and vitamins.

■ How is your diet? Important vitamins like folic acid can be found in fresh fruits and vegetables.

■ Do you donate blood regularly? Donating blood without replacing the iron you lose can make you deficient in iron.

■ Have you engaged in high-risk sexual activity or do you use intravenous drugs? These situations can put you at risk for infection with the human immunodeficiency virus (HIV), which is often accompanied by anemia.

■ Are you pregnant? Pregnant women are more prone to iron deficiency.

Your doctor will perform a physical examination, look for any abnormalities, and check your bowel movement for blood. Rarely, iron deficiency can cause brittle, spoon-shaped nails; dry, coarse skin; cracks at the corners of your mouth; and inflammation of the tongue. Your physician may follow up with laboratory tests to confirm a suspected diagnosis of anemia.

Common tests include:

Complete blood cell count (see p.154) to determine the quantity of red blood cells and hemoglobin. This test usually includes a measurement of red blood cell size, which can often distinguish iron deficiency from vitamin B_{12} and folic acid deficiency; it also measures the amount and types of white blood cells and platelets.

Fecal occult blood test (see p.791) to detect hidden blood in the bowel movements.

Peripheral blood smear to observe the shape of red blood cells and look for abnormalities of white blood cells and platelets.

Reticulocyte count to see whether your bone marrow is producing enough new blood cells. Reticulocytes are immature red blood cells.

Blood levels of nutrients such as vitamin B_{12}, folic acid, and iron.

Other tests to determine kidney function or the function of other organs (such as the thyroid or liver).

If these tests fail to reveal the reason for anemia, a bone marrow biopsy (see p.720) may be required.

Testing for Anemia: Dr Goldberg's Advice

If the doctor finds that you are anemic, the next question is whether you need extensive tests to determine why you are anemic. If you are a menstruating woman, the three most common causes of anemia are (1) iron deficiency, (2) iron deficiency, and (3) iron deficiency caused by a loss of iron in the menstrual blood. You usually don't require extensive testing, and can replace the iron by taking a supplement.

On the other hand, if you are a woman who has entered menopause, or if you are a man, the cause of your anemia is not loss of menstrual blood, and the doctor needs to do further tests. If your anemia is caused by iron deficiency, you could be losing blood somewhere else in your body. For example, you may need to have tests of your intestinal tract to make sure you do not have a hidden cancer that is bleeding. Or your anemia may be caused by some other condition besides iron deficiency, which requires additional testing for a diagnosis.

JOAN HELPERN GOLDBERG, MD
HARVARD VANGUARD MEDICAL ASSOCIATES
HARVARD MEDICAL SCHOOL

such as from a stomach ulcer or intestinal cancer; bleeding in other organ systems, such as the urinary system; or bleeding from a severe injury. When a person has thrombocytopenia (see p.736), in which low levels of platelets (which help blood clot) cause the person to have a tendency to bleed, anemia from blood loss is more likely.

DESTRUCTION OF RED BLOOD CELLS

In a condition called hemolytic anemia (see p.719), red blood cells are destroyed faster than they are produced. This can be caused by an unusual reaction to some medicines or infections. It also can occur for no clear reason.

Iron-Deficiency Anemia

An insufficient amount of iron in the body leads to iron-deficiency anemia, the most common type of anemia. About 10% to 15% of menstruating women in the United States have iron-deficiency anemia.

One of the most important roles of iron is as part of hemoglobin, the protein in red blood cells that carries oxygen to the body's tissues. Iron deficiency occurs when the blood's iron supplies are depleted because of excessive blood loss, the body cannot absorb iron from the diet, or the diet lacks iron-rich foods.

Iron-deficiency anemia due to bleeding can be caused by the regular use of nonsteroidal anti-inflammatory drugs such as aspirin or ibuprofen, which can cause bleeding in the gastrointestinal tract. Severe injury, in which there is great loss of blood, can also cause anemia. Women who have heavy menstrual periods are frequently at risk, as are pregnant women, whose developing fetus increases the requirement for iron.

Diseases that can cause blood loss include peptic ulcer (see p.752), hemorrhoids (see p.795), gastroesophageal reflux (see p.747), inflammatory bowel disease (see p.787), and cancer of the stomach (see p.756) or the intestines (see Colon Cancer, p.791).

Rapid bleeding from the lower part of the gastrointestinal tract (such as the large intestine and rectum) appears bright red in the stools or on toilet paper. Slow bleeding may not be obvious. For example, bleeding from the upper intestine or the stomach is usually not visible unless it is excessive, in which case it makes your bowel movements look black and tarry. This is why your doctor performs a fecal occult blood test (see p.791)—to check for hidden blood loss from your gastrointestinal tract.

Less frequently, bleeding can occur with disorders of the urinary tract, including bladder or kidney cancer. You may see blood or blood clots in your urine, or your urine may simply appear pink. However, blood loss is not always apparent.

Some people have a medical condition that interferes with their ability to absorb iron, often because they have had part of the stomach removed through

Gender Differences and Iron Levels

Low iron levels and iron-deficiency anemia are much more common in menstruating women than in men, because of the iron that is lost from the body during menstrual bleeding.

WOMEN

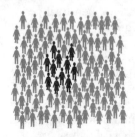

11 OF 100 MENSTRUATING AND NONMENSTRUATING WOMEN HAVE LOW IRON LEVELS

MEN

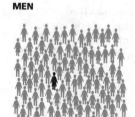

1 OF 100 MEN HAS A LOW IRON LEVEL

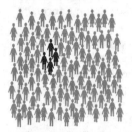

4 OF 100 MENSTRUATING AND NONMENSTRUATING WOMEN HAVE IRON-DEFICIENCY ANEMIA

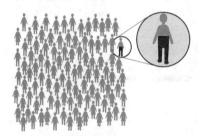

0.5 OF 100 MEN HAVE IRON-DEFICIENCY ANEMIA

taste), and a craving for ice or unusual foods.

More obvious signs in very severe, long-standing iron deficiency include spoon-shaped or brittle, flattened nails; inflammation of the tongue (see Tongue Variations, p.490); mouth sores (see p.487); and, in rare cases, difficulty swallowing.

TREATMENT OPTIONS

If you suspect that you have an iron deficiency, see your physician. He or she will perform a complete blood cell count (see p.154) and may then measure the level of iron in your blood. It is extremely important to determine why you are low in iron. Your doctor may investigate potential sources of blood loss by performing one or more of the tests described in Anemia: When You Visit Your Doctor (see p.714), and may also perform a colonoscopy and upper endoscopy (see p.744).

The most critical step in correcting an iron deficiency is to investigate and treat the cause. While treating the underlying condition, your doctor will replenish your body's store of iron by prescribing iron supplements, which are available in tablet form and are most effective when taken before meals.

Upset stomach is a common side effect of iron supplements. Coated forms of iron are easier on the stomach; absorption of iron from coated pills is adequate but absorption from uncoated pills is better. If you cannot take the tablet form, your doctor may give you injections of iron. Iron may make you constipated but this is easily treated; your doctor

surgery, or because of conditions affecting the intestinal lining, such as celiac disease (see p.774) or inflammatory bowel disease (see p.787). Infants and young children with immature digestive systems may also have difficulty absorbing iron and may require an iron supplement.

A diet lacking in iron is the least likely cause of iron-deficiency anemia; people who take a daily general vitamin and mineral supplement get adequate iron. Iron-fortified foods, such as cereals, also provide iron, as do many beans, vegetables, and grains. Iron deficiency is more common among the impoverished and the elderly (who are more likely to have poor diets) and in infants.

SYMPTOMS

Many people with iron-deficiency anemia have no symptoms. Some report feeling tired, having difficulty breathing, and, less often, having headaches, ringing in the ears (see Tinnitus, p.459), abnormalities in the taste of food (either diminished taste or unpleasant

Preventing Anemia: Pumping Up Iron-Deficient Blood

The best way to prevent iron deficiency is to eat iron-rich foods. The recommended daily allowance (RDA) of iron is 10 milligrams for men and 15 milligrams for women. If you are pregnant or breast-feeding, your doctor may prescribe supplements containing 30 to 60 milligrams of iron (your prescription might give a different dosage of milligrams because of the other minerals in the tablet).

Food is the best source of iron, which is found in red meat and eggs. Green leafy vegetables such as spinach, kale, and Swiss chard are also rich in iron, as are whole grains, and fortified breads and cereals. Other foods that contain iron include clams, oysters, avocados, beets, dates, kidney and lima beans, lentils, peaches, pears, dried prunes, pumpkin, raisins, and soybeans.

Excessive amounts of iron (more than 100 milligrams a day) can hinder the absorption of calcium and zinc. Over many months to years, too much iron can cause diabetes and liver and heart disease. Disease from excessive iron usually results from a genetic tendency to absorb too much iron, known as hemochromatosis, or from having frequent blood transfusions. Taking iron supplements for many years to treat an anemia that was not caused by an iron deficiency also can lead to problems.

---

can recommend a stool softener or laxative.

Tell your physician if you are taking antacids, drink tea, or use medicines such as proton pump inhibitors or H_2-receptor antagonists, all of which can interfere with iron absorption. Vitamin E and zinc can also reduce iron absorption. If you know that you are prone to iron deficiency, eat plenty of iron-rich foods (see Preventing Anemia: Pumping Up Iron-Deficient Blood, above) or take an iron supplement.

Breast-feeding offers infants a more readily absorbed source of iron than formula or cow's milk. Adding apple juice to iron-fortified infant cereals also helps increase iron absorption.

Vitamin B_{12}–Deficiency Anemia

Vitamin B_{12}–deficiency anemia is caused by a lack of vitamin B_{12} in the diet or an inability to absorb the vitamin from the diet. This interferes with the production of red blood cells in the bone marrow. Enlarged red blood cells called macrocytes are formed in this disease.

Vitamin B_{12} is found only in meat and dairy products, which most Americans consume in ample supply. Vitamin B_{12} is stored in the liver, where the average healthy adult holds enough to last up to 5 years.

Except for vegetarians who exclude all dairy products, eggs,

meat, and fish from their diet, the main reason for this vitamin deficiency is a problem absorbing the vitamin from the small intestine into the bloodstream.

To be absorbed, vitamin B_{12} must first combine with a protein called intrinsic factor, which is produced in the lining of the stomach. Some people do not make enough intrinsic factor and, as a consequence, cannot absorb enough vitamin B_{12} from their diet. This condition is called pernicious anemia. In pernicious anemia, which is an autoimmune disease (see p.870), antibodies are produced that block the production of intrinsic factor. Without treatment with intrinsic factor, pernicious anemia can be fatal.

Other problems with absorption develop because only one small section of your small intestine absorbs vitamin B_{12}. When there is damage to the intestinal lining, significant vitamin B_{12} deficiency occurs. This can occur in celiac disease (see p.774), in an inflammatory disease of the digestive tract such as Crohn disease (see Inflammatory Bowel Disease, p.787), or following surgical removal of the stomach (the stomach produces intrinsic factor) or part of the small intestine (where vitamin B_{12} is absorbed).

Pernicious anemia seems to run in families and usually affects people over 40. Because of its role in the health of the nervous system, severe vitamin B_{12} deficiency can cause serious damage to the brain, spinal cord, and nerves.

SYMPTOMS

As with other anemias, you feel tired and short of breath and have headaches with vitamin

B_{12}–deficiency anemia. Pernicious anemia may cause your skin to look yellow. It may also cause your heart and breathing rate to speed up to compensate for the lack of oxygen in your blood-stream.

Symptoms from nervous system damage are common. You may feel numbness or tingling in your hands and feet and have difficulty keeping your balance. Confusion, depression, and memory loss are other symptoms. In addition, your tongue may hurt.

A vitamin B_{12} deficiency can also affect levels of other components of the blood, causing lower-than-normal levels of white blood cells, which help fight infection, and of platelets (see Thrombocytopenia, p.736), which help blood clot. In severe cases, vitamin B_{12}–deficiency anemia may cause sterility.

TREATMENT OPTIONS

If you experience symptoms of a vitamin B_{12} deficiency, see your doctor. Make sure you tell your physician if a close family member has pernicious anemia. Your physician will perform a complete blood cell count (see p.154) and may look at a smear of your blood cells under a microscope. This will reveal low levels of hemoglobin and the presence of the large red blood cells that form in the disease. Often, white blood cells also look abnormal.

Your doctor will also check your vitamin B_{12} level, and perform other tests to look for the underlying cause of the vitamin B_{12} deficiency.

Most people with pernicious anemia who cannot absorb vitamin B_{12} do not ever regain the ability to absorb it and must take

vitamin B_{12} injections for the rest of their lives. These shots are required only once a month.

In most cases, you can prevent a vitamin B_{12} deficiency by ensuring that the vitamin is included in your diet (see p.44), and by having regular checkups to test for vitamin B_{12} levels if you are at risk. Vegetarians who develop a vitamin B_{12} deficiency can take vitamin B_{12} pills instead of shots, since they have no basic deficiency in their ability to absorb the vitamin.

Folic Acid–Deficiency Anemia

This anemia, caused by a deficiency in folic acid, is similar to vitamin B_{12} deficiency—the red blood cells are enlarged and there are fewer of them. The white blood cells often look abnormal, and there may be a decreased number of both white blood cells and platelets.

Unlike vitamin B_{12}, folic acid is not stored in large amounts or for long periods by the body. A continuing supply of the vitamin is required. The body can be depleted of folic acid by an increased production of red blood cells for a long duration, such as in chronic hemolytic anemia (see p.719).

The most common cause of deficiency is a diet that does not contain enough folic acid. Deficiency can also be caused by any condition that interferes with your ability to absorb folic acid from the small intestine, primarily celiac disease (see p.774) or Crohn disease (see Inflammatory Bowel Disease, p.787), by any surgery that removes part of the small intestine, or by alcoholism.

Folic acid is readily available in liver, leafy green vegetables, and whole grains, but cooking can easily destroy it. Various intestinal diseases lead to poor absorption of folic acid. Alcoholics often have a folic acid deficiency due to eating a poor diet; the alcohol also interferes with folic acid metabolism, even when the vitamin is absorbed.

In one of the most important medical discoveries of recent years, taking a folic acid vitamin pill or getting folic acid in adequate amounts through diet was found to reduce the most common birth defect, neural tube defects (see p.985), by 70%.

Folic acid also appears to help normalize the body's levels of homocysteine, a natural substance that, when elevated, contributes to heart disease and stroke.

In 1998, the government mandated that folic acid be added to grain products such as bread and flour. Women who are planning a pregnancy should take folic acid supplements in the months leading up to pregnancy to protect against anemia and birth defects. Folic acid supplements should be taken by all pregnant women; the vitamin is present in prenatal vitamins.

SYMPTOMS

In its early stages, folic acid deficiency may not cause symptoms. In more severe cases, it causes headaches, tiredness, an inflamed tongue, pallor, breathlessness, and chest pain. Sometimes tingling in the feet occurs due to the effect of deficiency on the nervous system.

TREATMENT OPTIONS

If you think that you could be deficient in folic acid, see your doctor. He or she will perform a complete blood cell count, which can reveal the presence of the large red blood cells the disease produces and low levels of hemoglobin and folic acid. Your doctor will look for an underlying cause of deficiency by using laboratory tests and, possibly, by evaluating your gastrointestinal tract if your diet is not the cause.

Treatment depends on the underlying cause. If you have a persistent, incurable condition such as chronic hemolytic anemia (see right) or have undergone intestinal surgery that interferes with your ability to absorb folic acid, your doctor may recommend that you take folic acid supplements.

In addition, if you take any drugs that interfere with folic acid—such as some seizure medicines, anticancer drugs, or methotrexate—your doctor may prescribe folic acid pills to prevent deficiency. If you are otherwise healthy, the recommended daily allowance is 400 micrograms.

For the vast majority of people, it is safe to take folic acid supplements. However, some studies show that taking more than 400 micrograms of folic acid daily may mask symptoms of a vitamin B_{12} deficiency, a condition that is more common in older people. If you are in this group, talk to your physician before taking supplements.

Hemolytic Anemia

Hemolytic anemia is distinguished by hemolysis, the premature destruction of red blood cells. There are many inherited and acquired hemolytic anemias (see Sickle Cell Anemia and Sickle Cell Trait, p.721, and Thalassemia and Thalassemia Trait, p.723).

As in other anemias, the end result of hemolytic anemia is a reduction in hemoglobin, the oxygen-carrying protein inside red blood cells. When cells are destroyed prematurely, the body produces new blood cells to compensate. Anemia occurs when destruction of cells outpaces the bone marrow's ability to produce new blood cells.

There are many causes of hemolytic anemia. Some inherited forms are characterized by an abnormal red blood cell membrane that is rigid and fragile, which causes the red cells to be trapped and destroyed in small blood vessels in the spleen. In spherocytosis (an inherited problem with the red blood cell membrane), there are numerous small, spherical, and fragile red blood cells.

In other inherited forms, there is a deficiency of a certain enzyme needed by red blood cells: glucose-6-phosphate dehydrogenase (G6PD). This deficiency causes the cells to rupture and die in the presence of certain substances, resulting in anemia. G6PD deficiency affects about 15% of black men in the United States. Medications such as some antibiotics or quinine-based drugs for malaria cause hemolysis of red blood cells in people with G6PD deficiency.

A small number of people of Mediterranean descent who have G6PD deficiency react to a substance in the fava bean and develop a condition called favism.

Acquired hemolytic anemia is not caused by inherited abnormalities in the cells themselves, but rather by outside forces. Malaria (see p.887), in which normal red blood cells are destroyed by microorganisms that infect the cells, is one example. Another example is the result of physical injury that can occur when blood flows over an artificial heart valve. Healthy red blood cells take a literal beating in these cases, and some are destroyed.

In some people, an autoimmune disease (see p.870) causes the body to mistakenly perceive its own red blood cells as foreign and kill them. Hemolytic anemia caused by an immune reaction can also occur when incompatible blood (see Compatibility of Blood Types, p.712) is transfused into the bloodstream.

In hemolytic disease of the newborn, the mother's immune system destroys the red blood cells of her fetus.

SYMPTOMS

The symptoms of hemolytic anemia are often similar to those of other types of anemia, including pallor, fatigue, headache, shortness of breath, and rapid heartbeat. Yellowing of the skin and the whites of the eyes (called jaundice), however, is a more specific sign of hemolytic anemia; it reflects a high concentration of yellow-brown pigments released into the blood when red cells are destroyed. Dark urine can also occur due to these pigments in the urine.

TREATMENT OPTIONS

Hemolytic anemia can be evaluated by inspecting a blood smear (see p.714). The blood smear often reveals large numbers of immature red blood cells and, in some forms of hemolytic anemia, abnormally shaped cells. Other specialized blood tests are necessary to confirm the diagnosis and to determine the cause.

Your doctor will treat the underlying condition as the first step in correcting it. For example, autoimmune disorders can be controlled by immunosuppressive drugs. People with G6PD deficiency should alert their doctor so that they are not prescribed medicines that could cause red blood cell destruction. Some inherited forms of hemolytic anemia are treated by surgical removal of the spleen, where the red blood cells are being destroyed.

Aplastic Anemia

Aplastic anemia is a rare but serious condition caused by the failure of the bone marrow to produce enough red blood cells, white blood cells, and platelets. Adequate production relies on the health of bone marrow stem cells, which are the most immature form of all blood cells.

In aplastic anemia, the stem cells or the environment that nurtures them is damaged. This can occur with long-term exposure to toxins (such as insecticides or benzene-containing substances such as gasoline) or nuclear radiation.

Some people acquire aplastic anemia from a virus, others through cancer treatment with radiation therapy or chemotherapy. A wide range of drugs can cause aplastic anemia and a susceptibility to it may be inherited by some people. However, the cause is unknown in over half the people with this condition.

SYMPTOMS

In many cases, the only sign of aplastic anemia is a reduction in blood levels of platelets, red blood cells, and white blood cells, which can be detected by a blood test called a complete blood cell count (see p.154).

A reduction in platelets (which help blood clot) can cause nosebleeds, bleeding gums, or bruising of the skin. Low levels of red blood cells cause the symptoms of anemia (pallor, fatigue, headaches, and increased heartbeat). When the level of white blood cells is low, there is an increased risk of infection.

TREATMENT OPTIONS

A diagnosis of aplastic anemia is confirmed by a bone marrow biopsy (above right). People who are undergoing treatment for cancer and who have low blood counts are given transfusions of red blood cells or platelets to replace the depleted blood cells. A platelet donor may be sought from family or friends.

Since white blood cells cannot be transfused, you will be extremely vulnerable to infection until your white blood cells are replenished. For this reason, if you have a fever, you may need intravenous antibiotics and should be isolated from visitors.

For severe aplastic anemia, a bone marrow transplant (see p.732), which can cure the dis-

Bone Marrow Biopsy

A bone marrow biopsy is removal of some bone marrow from the inside of bone. It is performed to diagnose or evaluate the progress of treatment of diseases such as anemia and leukemia. Using a local anesthetic (see p.168), a sturdy hollow needle is guided into the pelvic bone and a sample of marrow is removed. You will feel some pressure from insertion of the biopsy needle, followed by a dull pain as the marrow is taken up into the needle. The marrow is then examined under a microscope for signs of disease.

ease in more than half the people under age 40, may be performed. While awaiting a bone marrow donor, or if you are not a candidate for a bone marrow transplant, your doctor may prescribe medicines (including immunosuppressive drugs such as antithymocyte globulin, antilymphocyte globulin, or cyclosporine in combination with androgens) that stimulate the bone marrow to produce more cells. Genetically engineered growth factors, substances that induce the growth of blood cells, sometimes are helpful.

Anemia of Chronic Disease

Anemia can occur with some chronic diseases. The symptoms are similar to other forms of anemia, including pallor, fatigue, headache, rapid heartbeat, and weakness. Anemia of chronic disease can be a complication of cancer (see p.738); organ damage; persistent infections such as tuberculosis (see p.504) or human immunodeficiency virus (HIV) (see p.872); and rheumatoid arthritis (see p.606), systemic lupus erythematosus (see p.898), or inflammatory bowel disease (see p.787).

People with long-term kidney failure often become anemic because their kidneys can no longer make erythropoietin, the hormone that regulates the bone marrow's production of red blood cells. A genetically engineered form of erythropoietin is used to treat people who cannot produce it themselves.

If the anemia is very severe, blood transfusions (see Blood Donation and Transfusion, p.711) can help improve symptoms in people whose anemia is caused by other medical conditions.

Sickle Cell Anemia and Sickle Cell Trait

Sickle cell anemia is a hereditary blood disease that causes episodes of intense pain, vulnerability to infections, chronic hemolytic anemia (see p.719), organ damage, and, in some cases, death. It is caused by inheriting a sickle cell gene from both parents.

Sickle cell trait, which usually does not cause symptoms, occurs when a person inherits a sickle cell gene from only one parent.

People with sickle cell anemia make an abnormal form of hemoglobin in their red blood cells called hemoglobin S. Low levels of oxygen cause the hemo-globin S to form tiny rigid rods that bend the cells into their sickle shape. Instead of being oval, the cell is curved like a sickle (or hook). As a result, the cells become very rigid and are easily destroyed, leading to hemolytic anemia.

Also, because of their shape, the cells do not flow easily through the body's small blood vessels, causing them to clog the passages and reduce blood flow (and thus oxygen) to the body's tissues. This causes further deformity of the cells and can cut off the blood supply to nearby tissues.

Without oxygen, the area starts to hurt; this is the source of the pain caused by sickle cell anemia, called a sickle cell crisis. An affected person may experience bone pain, kidney damage, blood in the urine, and sometimes damage to the intestines and lungs. A sickle cell crisis that affects the brain can cause stroke (see p.342), seizures, or unconsciousness.

Early on, sickle-shaped cells tend to become trapped and destroyed in the liver and spleen, resulting in a shortage of red blood cells. The resulting anemia, when severe, can cause the affected person to be short of breath and easily tired.

Sickle cell anemia and trait mainly affect blacks and Hispanics of Caribbean ancestry. Due to its toll on the organs and the individual's ability to thrive, sickle cell anemia lowers life expectancy to about 40 years.

A blood test called hemoglobin electrophoresis can identify people who have either sickle

Appearance of Sickle Cells

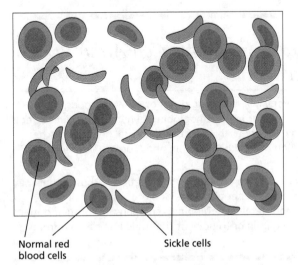

Normal red blood cells   Sickle cells

In sickle cell anemia, normally round and flexible red blood cells become sickle shaped and rigid. The sickle-shaped cells are fragile and break up, resulting in anemia, and tend to block small blood vessels, leading to severe pain.

cell trait or sickle cell anemia. It is recommended that all newborns be tested for sickle cell anemia.

There is also a prenatal test to determine whether the fetus will have sickle cell anemia, will carry sickle cell trait, or will be unaffected. In 3 of 4 cases, if both parents carry the gene, the prenatal test will reveal that the fetus will not have sickle cell anemia.

If only one parent has sickle cell trait, there is no chance that their children will have sickle cell anemia. A child whose parents both have the sickle cell trait has a 25% chance of inheriting sickle cell anemia. Women with sickle cell anemia are at higher risk of having a miscarriage and having a child with a low birthweight.

SYMPTOMS

Symptoms usually do not occur until 6 months of age. Sickle cell anemia affects people in different ways. Some people feel very few effects and can manage them well on their own, while others have severe pain from sickle cell crises and require treatment in the hospital.

Periods of severe pain in the joints, back, abdomen, and chest are the most common symptoms of sickle cell anemia. If crises are not treated, tissues may become permanently damaged. Crises are more common during an infection or after an injury.

Any infection can make the anemia worse. Bacterial infections, such as meningitis and pneumonia, are more common among infants and young children with sickle cell anemia and are the leading cause of their death.

Other symptoms include nerve damage, delayed growth and development, and skin ulcers on the legs. In addition, men may experience painful, prolonged erections (see Priapism, p.1096), infants may have painfully swollen fingers and toes, and adults may be more prone to gallstones. Symptoms may be made worse or more frequent by pregnancy, high altitudes, surgery, anesthesia, or infection.

TREATMENT OPTIONS

There are many treatments that prevent complications and relieve suffering, but there is no cure for most people with sickle cell anemia. Some people may be cured with bone marrow transplantation. For most people, the goal of treatment is to prevent the crises.

An effective medicine called hydroxyurea is now available to reduce the number of crises. Crises that cause severe pain are treated with pain relievers, intravenous fluids, and oxygen. Antibiotics are given if infection is suspected, and blood transfusions are given if the anemia becomes very severe.

Preventing infection begins at 2 months of age with immunizations against the *Haemophilus influenzae* bacteria, hepatitis B, and pneumonia. At 4 months, babies should start receiving daily doses of the antibiotic penicillin and should continue to receive these doses until adulthood. Later in life, flu shots are also important.

To help keep red blood cells from clumping, drink at least 2 quarts of water a day and avoid strenuous exercise, which increases your requirement for oxygen. Pay special attention to your dental hygiene to prevent gum infections, and see your doctor immediately for treatment of illness, infection, or injury. Wearing a medical identification medallion (see p.1190) could save your life in a sickle cell crisis.

Gene Therapy for Sickle Cell Anemia and Thalassemia

A form of gene therapy involves using drugs or other methods to activate the person's genes for fetal hemoglobin. All humans produce a fetal form of hemoglobin before birth; after birth, natural genetic switches "turn off" production of fetal hemoglobin and "turn on" production of adult hemoglobin.

Scientists are seeking ways to activate these genetic switches so that they can make the blood cells of people with sickle cell anemia and thalassemia produce more fetal hemoglobin to compensate for their deficiency of adult hemoglobin or to prevent the sickle hemoglobin from crystallizing.

Thalassemia and Thalassemia Trait

Thalassemia is an inherited disorder of red blood cells caused by a defect in the production of hemoglobin, the oxygen-carrying protein in red blood cells. In severe forms, the red blood cells produced by the bone marrow are fragile and quickly destroyed, which causes hemolytic anemia (see p.719).

Thalassemia, one form of which is often called Mediterranean anemia, occurs most frequently in people of Italian, Greek, Middle Eastern, Southern Asian, and African ancestry. The disease is transmitted by parents who carry the thalassemia gene. A carrier has one or more normal genes, a condition known as thalassemia trait. Most people with thalassemia trait lead completely normal, healthy lives.

When two carriers become parents, there is a one-in-four chance that any child they have will inherit a thalassemia gene from each parent and have a severe form of the disease. There is a two-in-four chance that the child will inherit one normal and one abnormal gene and become a carrier like his or her parents. There is a one-in-four chance that the child will inherit two normal genes from his or her parents and be completely free of the disease or carrier state.

Parents may choose to have genetic counseling (see p.130) to determine if they carry the gene for thalassemia; prenatal testing using chorionic villus sampling (see p.918) or amniocentesis (see p.917) can detect thalassemia in a fetus.

The two main forms of thalassemia are called alpha- and beta-thalassemia, depending on which part of the hemoglobin is affected in red blood cells.

Alpha-thalassemia is rare. A total lack of alpha-hemoglobin always causes death of the fetus or newborn. The alpha trait is fairly common, yet rarely leads to serious problems. It can lead to a mild anemia in which the red blood cells are slightly smaller than normal.

Beta-thalassemia, also called Mediterranean anemia, can range from very severe to having no effect on health. Your doctor can diagnose beta-thalassemia by blood smears that reveal the characteristic pale, small red blood cells and by the hemoglobin electrophoresis blood test.

Early diagnosis of the severe form (thalassemia major) is essential to prevent as many complications as possible. The spleen, liver, and heart soon become greatly enlarged in thalassemia major without treatment. Bones become thin and brittle and bones of the face become distorted. Heart failure and infection are the leading causes of death among children with untreated thalassemia major.

Most children with beta-thalassemia appear healthy at birth but, during the first 6 months, they lack energy and are fussy, have a poor appetite, and have an enlarged spleen due to the increased destruction of red blood cells. Bones grow abnormally as the bone marrow expands to make up for the short life of the red blood cells. Yellowing of the skin (called jaundice) often develops.

When children with thalassemia are treated with frequent transfusions (generally every 3 to 4 weeks) aimed at keeping their hemoglobin level near normal, many complications can be prevented. However, repeated blood transfusions lead to a buildup of iron in the body, which can damage the heart, liver, and other organs. An iron-chelating medicine can help rid the body of excess iron, preventing or delaying problems related to iron overload. The drug is usually administered via a mechanical pump that pumps the drug underneath the skin while the child is sleeping.

Children with thalassemia major who are treated with frequent blood transfusions and iron chelation can live 20 to 30 years or longer. Thalassemia has been cured using a bone marrow transplant (see p.732). However, this form of treatment is possible only for a minority of people who have a suitable bone marrow donor. In addition, the transplant procedure is risky and can result in death.

CANCERS OF THE BLOOD CELLS (LEUKEMIAS)

Leukemia is a broad term used to describe an increased production of malignant (cancerous) white blood cells, which inhibits the body's ability to manufacture red blood cells, platelets, and healthy white blood cells.

More than 25,000 people are diagnosed with leukemia every year. Leukemia is 10 times more prevalent among adults than children; most cases occur in people over age 65.

There are four major types of leukemia: acute lymphocytic, acute granulocytic, chronic granulocytic, and chronic lymphocytic.

In the acute forms, the malignant cells take over the bone marrow quickly, crowding out normal cells, and progression of the disease is rapid. The chronic forms of leukemia progress more slowly and do not cause severe deficiencies of functioning blood cells until later in the course of the disease. The treatments for acute and chronic leukemias are different.

If your doctor suspects that you have leukemia, he or she will refer you to a hematologist, a physician who specializes in treating blood cancer.

Acute Lymphocytic Leukemia and Acute Granulocytic Leukemia

Acute lymphocytic leukemia (ALL) occurs when a type of white blood cell called a lymphocyte reproduces uncontrollably in the bone marrow and blood. Lymphocytes fight viruses, bacteria, and other infections.

Acute granulocytic leukemia (AGL) develops when another type of white blood cell called a granulocyte turns malignant and reproduces unchecked. This disease is also called acute myelogenous leukemia.

Granulocytes are produced in the bone marrow, and lymphocytes are produced in the lymph glands and bone marrow. Normally, these white blood cells start out as immature cells called blasts, and develop into mature infection-fighting white blood cells.

In ALL and AGL, these new cells fail to mature and begin to overpopulate the bone marrow, blood, and lymph glands. As a result, the bone marrow becomes impaired and may not produce enough healthy white blood cells, red blood cells, or platelets.

ALL is more common in children; AGL is more likely to affect adults. In most cases, the cause of these leukemias is not known; they are not inherited. They may occur more often in people who have received radiation therapy or chemotherapy for another kind of cancer, and in people exposed to certain industrial toxins such as benzene.

The chances for recovery

Leukemia's Effect on Blood

In leukemia, abnormal white blood cells, which live much longer than normal white blood cells, are produced in the bone marrow. The abnormal cells accumulate in the marrow, the blood, and various organs, and prevent the marrow from making enough normal blood cells.

MICROSCOPIC VIEW OF NORMAL BLOOD

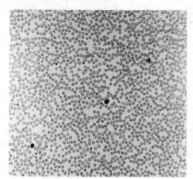

The most frequently occurring cells are the small, oval-shaped red blood cells. A few normal white blood cells (the larger, darker cells) are also present.

MICROSCOPIC VIEW OF THE BLOOD IN A PERSON WITH LEUKEMIA

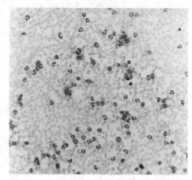

Compared to the normal blood at left, there are many more white blood cells (the larger, darker cells).

depend on the aggressiveness of the disease (how many immature cells are being produced and at what rate), and your general health. Without treatment, death can occur within weeks or months.

SYMPTOMS

Early in the course of ALL or AGL, you may feel as if you have a flu that will not go away. Fever, fatigue, aching joints, and swollen lymph glands are common.

If the disease has progressed to the point where your bone marrow is not producing enough red blood cells, you may have symptoms of anemia (see p.713). In addition, failure of the bone marrow to produce platelets creates clotting problems, and you may find that you bruise or bleed more easily than usual. You may develop infections due to low numbers of normal white blood cells.

TREATMENT OPTIONS

Your doctor will conduct a number of tests to determine the type of leukemia you have and the best course of treatment. Blood tests can reveal the levels of white blood cells, red blood cells, and platelets, and the presence of the immature blast cells. If the results of the blood tests are abnormal, a bone marrow biopsy (see p.720) may be necessary.

You may also need a lumbar puncture (p.161), in which a sample of the fluid that surrounds your brain and spinal cord is removed from your lower back and examined for the presence of the blast cells of leukemia.

Treatment is based on your general health and on how you would respond to chemotherapy (see p.741) and radiation therapy (see p.741). Chemotherapy, which is given to almost everyone with ALL and AGL, is administered by tablet, injected into a vein, and sometimes also injected into the cerebrospinal fluid that surrounds your brain and spinal cord.

Treatment proceeds in two stages: induction therapy and consolidation therapy. In the first induction phase, you receive chemotherapy for as long as it takes to bring about a remission, which is the elimination of any evidence of leukemia. This can take several weeks.

Consolidation therapy, which may include chemotherapy and radiation therapy, aims to destroy any remaining cancer cells. Sometimes a bone marrow transplant (see p.732) is also performed.

ALL is a curable kind of cancer, especially in children. More than half of children and a sizable fraction of adults with ALL can be cured by chemotherapy.

AGL can be cured by chemotherapy in 20% to 30% of people; bone marrow transplantation may cure more than half of those who are in their first remission from chemotherapy.

Chronic Granulocytic Leukemia

Chronic granulocytic leukemia (CGL), also called chronic myelogenous or chronic myelocytic leukemia, is the uncontrolled proliferation of white blood cells called granulocytes in the bone marrow. The leukemic cells are more mature than in acute granulocytic leukemia (see previous article). As a consequence, the

levels of granulocytes in your bloodstream rise dramatically.

CGL affects about 5,000 people each year, usually those over 50; the risk is slightly greater among people who have had exposure to radiation, such as survivors of nuclear radiation.

Most people with the disease have an acquired chromosomal abnormality, known as the Philadelphia chromosome, in which portions of two different chromosomes are switched. This rearrangement causes the uncontrolled production of white blood cells.

SYMPTOMS

There are two phases of CGL. In the milder phase, you may have no symptoms. Some people have flulike symptoms, feel generally tired (especially after physical exertion), and have shortness of breath. You may also have pain or a feeling of pressure in the upper left side of your abdomen caused by an enlarged spleen. Sweating at night, weight loss, and anemia (see p.713) are other common symptoms.

Most people with the disease eventually enter a more severe phase after 3 to 5 years (called a "blast transformation" because the blood is filled with blast cells, which are immature white blood cells), the symptoms of which parallel acute granulocytic leukemia (see previous article).

TREATMENT OPTIONS

Your doctor can diagnose CGL by performing blood tests and sometimes a bone marrow biopsy (see p.720). An increased number of granulocytes in the blood and bone marrow, and the presence

Risks and Benefits of Fludarabine for Chronic Lymphocytic Leukemia

Chronic lymphocytic leukemia (CLL) usually does not require treatment unless it causes severe fatigue, weakness, swollen glands, or anemia. Fludarabine, a newer treatment for advanced CLL, is both more potent and less toxic than older treatments used to treat CLL, such as chlorambucil. Fludarabine improved the symptoms of CLL better than the earlier treatments, although it is not yet known if it improves survival compared with the older treatments.

FLUDARABINE

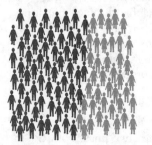

60 OF 100 PEOPLE WHO HAVE CLL AND TOOK FLUDARABINE HAD SYMPTOMS IMPROVE

OLDER TREATMENTS

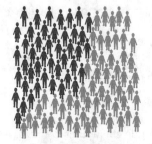

44 OF 100 PEOPLE WHO HAVE CLL AND TOOK THE OLDER TREATMENTS HAD SYMPTOMS IMPROVE

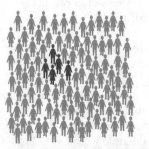

5 OF 100 PEOPLE WHO HAVE CLL AND TOOK FLUDARABINE EXPERIENCED NAUSEA AND VOMITING

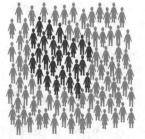

25 OF 100 PEOPLE WHO HAVE CLL AND TOOK THE OLDER TREATMENTS EXPERIENCED NAUSEA AND VOMITING

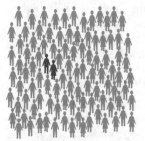

2 OF 100 PEOPLE WHO HAVE CLL AND TOOK FLUDARABINE EXPERIENCED HAIR LOSS

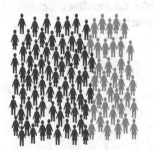

65 OF 100 PEOPLE WHO HAVE CLL AND TOOK THE OLDER TREATMENTS EXPERIENCED HAIR LOSS

of the Philadelphia chromosome, confirm the diagnosis.

Chemotherapy (see p.741) taken as tablets or injections is given on an outpatient basis. Chemotherapy alleviates symptoms and permits the bone marrow to begin producing normal amounts of healthy cells again. Your physician will monitor your blood and adjust your medicine to ensure that the drug is having the desired effect on your blood count.

Overall, a person with CGL lives an average of 3 to 4 years after the diagnosis is made. If a blast transformation occurs, the prognosis is not good.

It is important to have regular and frequent checkups of your blood cell count. High doses of chemotherapy and radiation may be used to destroy all your blood cells in preparation for a bone marrow transplant (see p.732), ideally from a brother or sister but sometimes from an unrelated donor whose tissue type matches yours.

This can produce a cure in at least half of the people with this disease and is the only treatment that offers the possibility of a cure. The transplant should be performed as soon as possible after the diagnosis; it is not successful if attempted during a blast transformation.

Chronic Lymphocytic Leukemia

In chronic lymphocytic leukemia (CLL), there is an excessive number of white blood cells called lymphocytes in the blood, lymph glands, spleen, and bone marrow. As the disease advances, the cancerous lymphocytes spread to other tissues, replacing normal infection-fighting white blood cells and causing swelling of the lymph glands, liver, and spleen and reducing the ability to fight infection.

The large number of cancerous white blood cells interferes with the bone marrow's ability to produce a normal amount of red blood cells and platelets, which can cause anemia (see p.713) and bleeding.

CLL is the most common leukemia in the United States. It mainly affects people over 50.

SYMPTOMS

An estimated 60% to 80% of people with CLL have no symptoms and are found to have the disease during a blood test performed for another reason. Many people in this group do not require treatment, and their disease may not get worse for 10 to 15 years.

For others, subtle, flulike symptoms may occur, including dizziness, fatigue, and general malaise. Some people experience fever, swollen glands, infections, and/or excessive sweating. As the spleen grows, the upper left portion of the abdomen may feel full and your appetite may wane; weight loss may also occur. There may also be bruising and excessive bleeding due to a reduction in the number of platelets in the blood.

A person with CLL lives an average of 6 years after the diagnosis is made, but 25% of people live for more than 10 years and die of other diseases.

On the other hand, people who reach an advanced stage of the disease, on average, live less than 2 years. If the disease is at an early stage when first diagnosed, the prognosis is better.

TREATMENT OPTIONS

Treatment depends on the aggressiveness of the disease and is required only when the leukemia advances. If your disease is stable, your doctor may recommend only periodic blood tests.

In people who have anemia, a low platelet count, or other symptoms, treatment usually begins with chemotherapy in pill form and, sometimes, corticosteroid drugs (see p.895). The treatment has few side effects and you do not need to be hospitalized.

This treatment course is usually effective in reducing or eliminating symptoms, and many people see significant improvement for a while. If symptoms recur, treatment with other anticancer drugs may be recommended. A bone marrow transplant (see p.732) is a possibility for some younger people, but its use is still very experimental.

CANCERS OF LYMPH GLANDS (LYMPHOMAS)

Lymphoma is a broad term for cancer of the lymph glands. The lymphatic system includes the lymph glands (also called lymph nodes); tiny vessels called lymphatics that link the glands; and your spleen, thymus, tonsils, and adenoids.

Lymph glands produce and house disease-fighting immune cells (white blood cells called lymphocytes) and trap infectious agents when you are sick, which causes your glands to swell.

The lymphatics form a network that extends into all parts of the body. Their job is to transport lymph, a watery fluid that contains lymphocytes. Clusters of lymph glands are found in this network, mostly in the underarm, groin, neck, and abdominal areas.

Lymphomas can originate in virtually any part of your body, and they can spread by way of the far-reaching channels of the lymph system to almost any tissue or organ. When lymphomas develop, the lymph glands become swollen.

More than 80% of people diagnosed with lymphoma have one or more enlarged lymph glands that do not hurt but are persistently swollen. The swelling that occurs with lymphoma is not the same as the swollen glands you develop in response to infection, when swelling is temporary and the glands are usually tender to the touch. If you experience swollen glands without any other sign of infection for more than 2 weeks, see your doctor.

Lymphomas are divided into Hodgkin disease and non-Hodgkin lymphoma. Most physicians view Hodgkin disease as the most treatable and curable lymphoma. There are more than a dozen subtypes of non-Hodgkin lymphoma, some with more favorable outlooks than others.

Diagnosing Lymphomas

To diagnose cancer of the lymph glands, your physician will first perform a physical examination to look for enlarged lymph glands and enlargement of other organs connected to the lymph system, such as the liver and spleen.

Next, your doctor may perform blood and urine tests. Sometimes, a lymphoma causes swelling of lymph glands inside the body, rather than under the skin where they can be easily seen and felt. For this reason, your doctor may take a chest x-ray (see p.145) and sometimes a computed tomography (see p.149) scan of your chest, abdomen, and pelvis to locate affected glands.

He or she will also arrange for a surgical biopsy of a lymph gland. If the gland is situated near the surface, the biopsy may require only a local anesthetic and take half an hour; if the gland is less accessible, you may need to have a brief operation and spend a day or two in the hospital.

A pathologist then examines the specimen under the microscope to see if the swollen lymph gland is filled with cancerous cells or if it is swollen with normal cells, which happens when the immune system fights an infection. Additional information is gained from analysis of bone marrow taken during a biopsy (see p.720).

Hodgkin Disease

Hodgkin disease is one kind of lymphoma (cancer of the lymph glands). Every year, Hodgkin disease is diagnosed in more than 7,000 people in the United States. It occurs most often in people 15 to 34 years old, and in people over 55. It can also occur in children. Hodgkin disease typically originates in one lymph gland and spreads through the lymphatic vessels in an orderly pattern to adjacent glands. It is more easily cured than non-Hodgkin lymphoma (see p.730).

Hodgkin disease is classified by type and is staged to determine treatment and outlook. There are four types of Hodgkin disease, which are classified by how the biopsy specimen looks under the microscope.

Nodular sclerosis This type occurs in up to 80% of people with the disease and usually affects young women. It most often affects the neck and chest area (including the thymus, lymph glands, and connective tissues in the area between the lungs near the heart). The prognosis is generally quite good.

Lymphocyte predominance The majority of the cells seen in the biopsy specimen are normal-appearing lymphocytes. It is the least common type but has the best prognosis.

Mixed cellularity A widespread lymphoma that occurs mostly in older men and is the third most

Outlook for Curing Hodgkin Disease With Radiation and Chemotherapy

Hodgkin disease is usually curable with radiation and chemotherapy; treatment dramatically improves the prognosis. The outlook is best in people who are in the early stages of the disease.

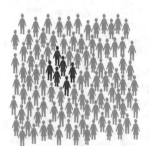

6 OF 100 PEOPLE WHO HAVE HODGKIN DISEASE AND DO NOT UNDERGO TREATMENT ARE STILL ALIVE 5 YEARS AFTER DIAGNOSIS

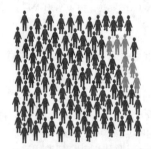

93 OF 100 PEOPLE WHO HAVE EARLY-STAGE HODGKIN DISEASE AND UNDERGO TREATMENT ARE STILL ALIVE 5 YEARS AFTER DIAGNOSIS

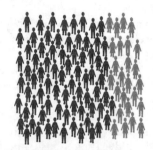

75 OF 100 PEOPLE WHO HAVE ADVANCED HODGKIN DISEASE AND UNDERGO TREATMENT ARE STILL ALIVE 5 YEARS AFTER DIAGNOSIS

Risk of Other Cancers After Hodgkin Disease Treatment

People who undergo treatment for Hodgkin disease are more likely than people of the same age without Hodgkin disease to develop another form of cancer in the future.

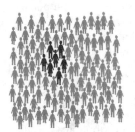

7 OF 100 PEOPLE WHO HAVE HODGKIN DISEASE AND WERE TREATED WITH RADIATION AND CHEMOTHERAPY DEVELOP ANOTHER FORM OF CANCER WITHIN 15 YEARS

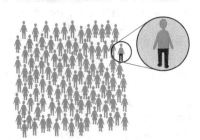

0.3 OF 100 PEOPLE WHO DO NOT HAVE HODGKIN DISEASE DEVELOP CANCER (OTHER THAN HODGKIN DISEASE) OVER THE NEXT 15 YEARS

common type of Hodgkin disease. The prognosis is fairly good.

Lymphocyte depleted This rare type is characterized by a lack of normal white blood cells in the gland and the presence of many abnormal cells. The prognosis is the poorest of the group. Usually the disease is widespread at the time of diagnosis.

SYMPTOMS

The outlook for Hodgkin disease improves greatly with early diagnosis and treatment. See your doctor immediately if you have any of the following symptoms: painless, swollen glands in the armpit, neck, or groin; persistent fever; night sweats; persistent itchy skin without a rash; weight loss without dieting; or persistent fatigue. Your doctor will evaluate the need for further tests.

STAGES

Once you have been diagnosed with Hodgkin disease, your hematologist will study your x-rays and computed tomography (see p.149) scans, and will often order a test called a gallium scan, which identifies the lymph glands that contain cancer cells.

In some cases, surgery is necessary to evaluate the presence of the cancer cells in the abdominal lymph glands and the spleen. This information is necessary to determine the stage of your disease, which dictates the type of treatment, different chemotherapy combinations, and the need for radiation therapy. These tests are repeated periodically to assess the progress of your treatment.

Stage I Cancer limited to one lymph node area.

Stage II Cancer occurs in two or more lymph node areas on the same side of the diaphragm (the sheet of muscle that separates the chest from the abdomen).

Stage III Cancer occurs in lymph glands on both sides of the diaphragm, such as in the chest and in the abdomen, and may have spread to the spleen.

Stage IV Cancer has spread to an organ beyond the lymphatic system, such as the bone marrow or liver, and may or may not be found in nearby lymph glands.

These stages are subdivided by capital letters after the Roman numerals (for example, stage IA or stage IB). The "B" category means that there are associated symptoms, such as fever, weight loss, and heavy sweating during the night. In stage IIIA, cancer is found above and below the diaphragm, but there are no symptoms. In stage IIIB, cancer is also found above and below the diaphragm and the person has symptoms, such as fever, weight loss, and night sweats.

TREATMENT OPTIONS

The treatment and chances of recovery depend on how far the disease has spread and on your general health. All stages of Hodgkin disease can be treated, either by radiation therapy (see p.741) for early stages or chemotherapy (see p.741) or both. Bone marrow transplantation (see p.732) is increasingly being used for people who have a relapse after chemotherapy or radiation therapy.

The type of treatment you receive will be tailored to your condition. Hematologists are very careful in staging the disease, sometimes using surgery to most accurately determine the stage.

It is important to give the most powerful treatment for your stage but to limit, if possible, the extent of treatment since there is an increased risk for the development of other cancers from the therapy itself.

From 80% to 90% of people are completely cured of the disease with stage I or II detection and treatment. Even people who have advanced cancer have a good prognosis. Ten years after treatment, from 50% to 80% remain completely cured.

Radiation therapy alone may be given at earlier, less advanced stages of the disease, or when the cancer affects the upper body. Chemotherapy may be used alone or with radiation therapy. It is usually prescribed in more advanced cases when the cancer has spread to several parts of the body.

After either form of treatment, a relapse can occur, which may be treated with a different type of chemotherapy. If this fails, a bone marrow or a stem cell transplant may be performed.

Non-Hodgkin Lymphoma

Non-Hodgkin lymphoma is cancer of the lymph glands that occurs when some lymphocytes (white blood cells manufactured in the bone marrow and lymph glands) turn into cancerous cells.

The different types of non-Hodgkin lymphoma are classified as low grade, intermediate, and high grade according to the size, type, and pattern of the abnormal cells, which can be observed under a microscope, and by tests that identify and stain chemicals on the surface of the cells.

Low-grade non-Hodgkin lymphoma has a longer survival rate (75% of people live 5 years after diagnosis) than high-grade non-Hodgkin lymphoma. The low-grade type is slow growing and may not produce symptoms. Initially, your physician may check you periodically but not treat the disease until symptoms develop.

Intermediate non-Hodgkin lymphoma is the most common form, representing 65% of all cases; it affects all age groups and its incidence is rising rapidly, largely because it is common in people with acquired immunodeficiency syndrome (AIDS).

Almost half of those with the intermediate form can be cured with treatment. However, if treatment does not produce a complete remission, average survival drops to less than 18 months.

High-grade non-Hodgkin lymphoma is rare (affecting fewer than 5% of people with the disease), and usually affects children and young adults. The three subtypes include lymphoblastic lymphoma, which usually targets young males; Burkitt lymphoma, which affects young adults of both genders; and a type of high-grade non-Hodgkin lymphoma that is more common in people with AIDS.

Non-Hodgkin lymphoma is more common and more serious than Hodgkin disease (see p.728). Although teenagers and young adults are prone to some rare types of non-Hodgkin lymphoma, this cancer is most common after age 45, and the likelihood of having it increases late in life.

The risk of non-Hodgkin lymphoma also increases appreciably in people whose immunity has been lowered, such as people who take immunosuppressive drugs following an organ transplant or people with the human immunodeficiency virus (HIV).

SYMPTOMS

In addition to persistent, painless swollen glands (usually in the armpit, neck, or groin), people with non-Hodgkin lymphoma may have general symptoms, including unexplained fever without infection, drenching night sweats, significant weight loss without dieting, or gastrointestinal discomfort. If you have any of these symptoms, see your doctor. Some people who have advanced non-Hodgkin lymphoma feel fine.

TREATMENT OPTIONS

Your physician or hematologist will conduct a thorough examination. If he or she suspects non-Hodgkin lymphoma, the next step is to obtain a lymph gland sample to learn as much as possible about any malignant cells that are found. Further radiology testing will identify which lymph glands are affected.

The work of the pathologist is crucial. The course of the disease can be predicted by examining the size and type of cancer cells through a microscope and determining the extent to which they have altered a lymph gland's normal architecture.

The outlook is usually better when the cells are small and the glands' internal structures are intact than when the cells are large and have obliterated normal landmarks. When the cancerous lymphocytes are small, the cancer is generally slow growing and the disease can wax and wane, with signs disappearing and reappearing over 15 years.

When the lymphocytes are large, the cancer is more aggressive, and people usually die within a few years if treatment is not successful.

As with Hodgkin disease, the swollen lymph glands may be inside the body. They can be viewed by imaging techniques such as x-rays and a computed tomography (see p.149) scan.

The number of lymph glands affected is not a reliable indicator of the severity of the disease. Because the lymph glands constitute a single organ system, the disease becomes more serious when it travels to other structures, such as the liver, skin, or lungs.

Your overall health and resilience affect the choice of treatment; an older person in good physical condition may be able to withstand the rigors of treatment.

Treatment is similar to that of Hodgkin disease. Chemotherapy (see p.741) is the standard treatment, and it often produces a remission. If this approach fails, or the disease recurs, the dose or type of chemotherapy may be increased. A person with a low-grade non-Hodgkin lymphoma lives an average of 6 to 8 years after the diagnosis.

Paradoxically, the aggressive intermediate lymphoma, although it can lead to an early death, also is more likely to be completely cured than some of the less aggressive kinds of lymphoma. A bone marrow transplant (see p.732) may be attempted.

Multiple Myeloma

Multiple myeloma is a rare type of cancer caused by a type of white blood cell called a plasma cell that multiplies uncontrollably in the bone marrow. Plasma cells are responsible for the production of antibodies that fight infectious agents and for-

eign substances that enter the body. An excessive number of plasma cells in the bone marrow interferes with and impedes the production of red blood cells, platelets, and other white blood cells, leading to anemia (see p.713) and a greater susceptibility to bleeding.

In addition, the plasma cells produce substances that cause the progressive weakening of bone, leading to pain and fractures. Multiple myeloma can increase the risk of infection because healthy plasma cells become less efficient at producing antibodies. Sometimes, the antibodies produced by the cancerous plasma cells slowly damage the function of the kidneys.

Multiple myeloma more commonly affects people over 50 and occurs twice as frequently in blacks as in whites. Although a person with multiple myeloma lives an average of 3 years after the diagnosis, many people live

much longer and some die of other causes.

SYMPTOMS

The main feature of multiple myeloma is pain in the bones, particularly the back and ribs, that gets worse when you move. Progressive weakening of the bones may lead to fractures. Symptoms of anemia may occur as production of red blood cells is reduced due to the myeloma itself or kidney failure.

TREATMENT OPTIONS

The condition is diagnosed based on blood tests, x-rays of your bones to reveal deterioration, and a bone marrow biopsy (see p.720). In addition to excess plasma cells in the bone marrow and reduced numbers of other blood cells in your blood, your doctor will measure the levels of antibodies produced by cancerous plasma cells; very high levels of antibodies are present in mul-

Outlook for Surviving Multiple Myeloma With Chemotherapy

Chemotherapy can prolong life and improve the symptoms of multiple myeloma, but cannot cure it. Bone marrow transplantation offers the only hope for a cure, but is generally reserved for people who are younger than 60 and in good health except for the multiple myeloma, since the chance of success is greater in these people.

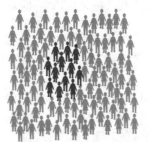

12 OF 100 PEOPLE WHO HAVE MULTIPLE MYELOMA AND UNDERGO CHEMOTHERAPY ARE STILL ALIVE 5 YEARS AFTER DIAGNOSIS

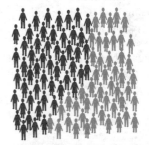

52 OF 100 PEOPLE WHO HAVE MULTIPLE MYELOMA AND HAVE A BONE MARROW TRANSPLANT ARE STILL ALIVE 5 YEARS AFTER DIAGNOSIS

tiple myeloma. One antibody, called B_2-microglobulin, is particularly useful in helping determine the progress of the disease.

Symptoms of multiple myeloma can be relieved and people can live long, productive lives with the disease. If you are not anemic and have no symptoms, your physician may recommend no treatment at all. In the early stages of the disease, treatment aims at maintaining bone strength, which includes exercising, eating calcium-rich foods, and taking bone-strengthening medicines called bisphosphonates. Depending on the extent of the damage to your bones, your doctor may recommend that you avoid lifting heavy objects or engaging in strenuous activity.

You may need to take antibiotics because of your increased risk of infection from the lack of infection-fighting cells. For more advanced forms of the disease, chemotherapy (see p.741) may be used to destroy the plasma cells; this can cause a temporary remission but frequently must be repeated.

Radiation therapy and/or painkilling medicines can help relieve severe bone pain. Radiation therapy is helpful in relieving pain because it kills some of the cancer cells in the bone that are causing pain due to rapid growth, expansion, and pressure on the surrounding bone. High-dose chemotherapy regimens and stem cell transplant may also be used (see next article).

Bone Marrow Transplantation

Bone marrow transplantation first involves obtaining healthy bone marrow stem cells, the primitive cells that form all of the blood cells (see p.710), either from the sick person or from a donor.

These stem cells are then given to the person whose own bone marrow has been destroyed by high doses of chemotherapy and/or radiation therapy. This is done to create new bone marrow, thereby restoring blood cell production and immune system function.

Most often, a bone marrow transplant is performed after massive doses of chemotherapy and/or radiation therapy are administered to eradicate cancer cells from the blood in a person who has a cancer of the blood cells, such as leukemia.

It may also be used in people who have other nonblood cancers (such as breast cancer) that are very sensitive to chemotherapy. Because the very high doses of chemotherapy and radiation that might kill and cure the cancer also kill the bone marrow, the marrow must be replaced afterward.

Occasionally, a bone marrow transplant is performed to try to cure a noncancerous blood disorder, such as aplastic anemia or sickle cell anemia. The old, diseased bone marrow is killed and replaced with healthy bone marrow stem cells that will make healthy blood cells.

Bone marrow transplantation is a rigorous and potentially dangerous treatment. It is typically used in people who are younger than 60 years old because they are more likely to tolerate the procedure.

ALLOGENEIC (DONOR) BONE MARROW TRANSPLANT

In this type of transplant, a healthy donor gives stem cells to a sick recipient (the host). The immune system cells of the donor recognize the cells of the host as foreign (and vice versa), and the immune system does not like foreigners.

This can cause two serious problems. The first is graft rejection; residual immune system cells in the host that were not killed by chemotherapy and radiation can attack and reject the graft (the donor cells).

The second potential problem is graft versus host disease, in which the graft cells from the donor perceive the host's tissues as foreign, and attack those tissues. Graft versus host disease is the major complication of allogeneic bone marrow transplants, and can be fatal. In 1999, Harvard researchers discovered a method that may prevent many cases of graft versus host disease.

Since the development of bone marrow transplants, the ideal donor has been a healthy identical twin, because an identical twin's blood cells are genetically identical to the recipient's. Therefore, the host cells will not reject the graft cells, and the graft cells will not attack the host.

The next best donor is a brother or sister whose immune system is very closely matched to that of the recipient. The more closely matched two people are, the more similar are the proteins—called human lymphocyte

What Happens During an Allogeneic Bone Marrow Transplant?

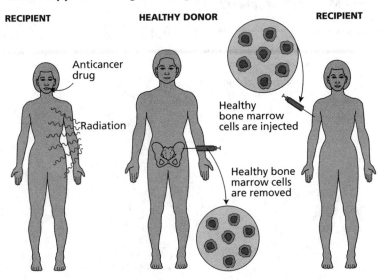

RECIPIENT

Anticancer drug

Radiation

HEALTHY DONOR

Healthy bone marrow cells are injected

Healthy bone marrow cells are removed

RECIPIENT

First, the recipient has radiation therapy and chemotherapy to kill the cancerous cells in the bone marrow and elsewhere in the body.

Second, a donor (usually a sibling) whose tissue type matches that of the recipient is located and a sample of his or her bone marrow is extracted from the pelvic bone or the blood. When donor cells are obtained directly from the bone marrow, a needle is inserted into the bone marrow (usually in a hipbone) and about 1 to 2 quarts of healthy marrow is sucked out.

When donor cells are obtained from the blood, the donor's blood is circulated through a machine that filters out the stem cells. This is called a peripheral stem cell transplant. The donor cells are then frozen and made ready to give to the recipient.

Third, the healthy donor cells are injected into the recipient's bloodstream as in a blood transfusion. The primitive stem cells travel to the bone marrow, where they reproduce and replace all the destroyed blood elements.

Genetically engineered growth-stimulating factors are often given to help speed the regeneration of bone marrow cells once the transplanted stem cells have reached the marrow.

---

antigens (HLAs)—that are found on the surface of their cells.

The odds of a good HLA match are about 25% when two siblings are tested; this increases to 75% if six siblings are tested. Occasionally (less than 10% of the time), a donor who is not a blood relative is a very close match.

Improved techniques for matching HLAs—by analyzing the DNA that makes the HLA proteins—have led to greater success in transplantation.

More recently, matched, unrelated donors have become available through the National Marrow Donor Program. This is a very useful source of marrow for those without matched family members, but it carries a somewhat higher risk of graft rejection and of graft versus host disease.

Another risk of allogeneic bone marrow transplant is suppression of the immune system. With most transplants, drugs that suppress the immune system are given so that any immune system cells that were not killed by the chemotherapy and radiation therapy will not attack and reject the graft cells. These drugs can damage various organs (particularly the liver and kidney) or can lead to infections such as viral infections of the lungs.

Finally, recipients are at serious risk until the transplanted stem cells have created enough new red blood cells, white blood cells, and platelets. In particular, low levels of white blood cells make the person vulnerable to infection, and low numbers of platelets make the person vulnerable to bleeding.

AUTOLOGOUS (SELF) BONE MARROW TRANSPLANT

This type of transplant, the most common method of bone marrow transplantation, gives people back their own stem cells. The problem of matching tissues is eliminated if the healthy stem cells given are that person's own stem cells, taken from his or her own marrow or blood.

Stem cells in a person with cancer are almost always healthy and are not cancerous (even though they come from a person who has cancer).

Autologous transplants have two obvious advantages over allogeneic transplants. Since the patient's own cells are being used, there is no risk of graft rejection (and, hence, no need to use medicines to suppress the immune system) and there is no risk of graft versus host disease.

Like allogeneic (donor) bone marrow transplants, autologous bone marrow transplants carry the risk of infection and bleeding because of inadequate numbers of white blood cells and platelets.

Unlike allogeneic bone marrow transplants, autologous bone marrow transplants carry the risk of putting some of the patient's cancerous cells back into his or her body, in addition to the healthy stem cells.

New techniques are being developed that purge all cancer cells from the marrow and blood before the stem cells are infused back into the body.

What Happens During an Autologous Bone Marrow Transplant?

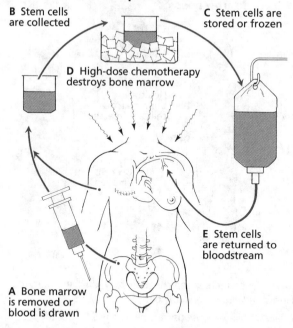

B Stem cells are collected

C Stem cells are stored or frozen

D High-dose chemotherapy destroys bone marrow

E Stem cells are returned to bloodstream

A Bone marrow is removed or blood is drawn

In autologous bone marrow transplantation, people provide their own stem cells—they donate the cells to themselves. First, stem cells are obtained either from the bone marrow or from the blood (A). These stem cells are collected (B) and then stored or frozen (C) for safekeeping. The person undergoes high-dose chemotherapy (D) and sometimes radiation therapy to destroy the bone marrow. The frozen cells are thawed and returned to the bloodstream through an intravenous catheter (E). The stem cells find their way to the bone marrow, where they begin to produce healthy new blood cells.

OTHER BLOOD DISORDERS

Agranulocytosis

Agranulocytosis is a rare condition in which there is a dramatic decline in the number of neutrophils, white blood cells that fight infection, in the bloodstream. This condition arises either because the neutrophils are not being produced in the bone marrow or because they are not being released to the bloodstream. Without the protection of neutrophils, the body is left virtually defenseless against some types of infection.

Agranulocytosis can be caused by treatment with chemotherapy (see p.741), which destroys many helpful blood cells at the same time it destroys cancer cells. It can also occur due to an autoimmune reaction, in which your body mistakenly perceives the helpful white blood cells as invaders and destroys them. More rarely, it occurs as a reaction to medicines such as penicillin or anti-inflammatory agents, or upon exposure to environmental chemicals, solvents, or other irritants.

SYMPTOMS

Symptoms of various infections—such as sore throats, mouth ulcers, or pneumonia—are common. If you experience any of these symptoms, especially if you are taking any prescription medicines, see your doctor. In some people, infections progress quickly and are more severe. Occasionally, infection can be fatal in a person with agranulocytosis.

TREATMENT OPTIONS

Your physician uses blood tests to look for a decreased number of white blood cells. He or she may confirm a suspected diagnosis with a bone marrow biopsy (see p.720). Your bone marrow will recover its neutrophil-producing ability once the causative substance is eliminated. In the meantime, your doctor may prescribe antibiotics, which are given intravenously (through your vein) to treat or prevent infections.

Hemophilia

Hemophilia is a bleeding disorder. There are several forms. In the most common type, called hemophilia A or classic hemophilia, the blood lacks sufficient amounts of a clotting factor called factor VIII, which causes a tendency to bleed.

Hemophilia B, or Christmas disease, is characterized by a deficiency in factor IX, another clotting factor.

Both conditions are inherited and are caused by an abnormal gene on the X chromosome. Females are rarely affected. Because they have two X chromosomes, even if one carries the abnormal gene, the normal gene on the other X chromosome compensates.

Males have only one X chromosome (along with one Y chromosome). Therefore, if a male inherits an abnormal X chromosome from his mother, he will make very little of the clotting factor and will have hemophilia. In rare cases, the disease arises without any family history, probably due to genetic mutation of one of the mother's X chromosomes.

SYMPTOMS

Symptoms vary depending on the severity of the disease. In severe cases, bleeding may first become apparent when an infant scratches himself or herself and bleeds profusely and for a long time. Infants who are circumcised may have severe bleeding. The bleeding tendency can cause serious bruises and bleeding into the joints that cause the joints to become swollen, painful, and stiff.

In mild cases, bleeding may not be severe. However, severe bleeding (for example, into the brain) can occur and can be fatal. If you suspect that your bleeding is not normal or that your baby has a tendency to bleed, see your physician.

TREATMENT OPTIONS

Regardless of the extent of your hemophilia, your doctor will recommend that you avoid activities that can cause internal or external bleeding, such as contact sports. However, exercise is important and you should pursue activities such as swimming and walking. Medicines are available to correct the deficiency of clotting factor.

In mild cases of hemophilia, slow infusions of desmopressin acetate into a vein may stop a bleeding episode. More severe conditions may require transfusions of special clotting factors.

These factors were once obtained from donated blood but can now be made by genetic engineering. In the 1980s, many hemophiliacs received clotting factors that were contaminated by the viruses that cause hepatitis and acquired immunodeficiency syndrome (AIDS). There is no risk of acquiring these infections with genetically engineered clotting factor medicines.

Polycythemia

Polycythemia is the excessive production of red blood cells in the bone marrow, causing the blood to thicken and clot in the veins. There are several forms of this disorder. In polycythemia vera (the most serious form), red blood cells, granulocytes (to a lesser extent), and platelets are overproduced. The cause is not known.

In secondary polycythemia, other conditions that deprive the body of oxygen (such as lung disease or living at high altitudes) cause red blood cells to be produced in excess to compensate for the reduction in oxygen.

In stress polycythemia, there is a normal number of blood

cells but a reduced amount of plasma (the waterlike substance in blood). This also makes the blood somewhat thicker. Mild dehydration caused by smoking and/or diuretic drugs can produce this type of mild polycythemia.

SYMPTOMS

Polycythemia vera produces dizziness, headaches, a feeling of fullness in the head, and a reddish complexion. Some people have intense itching. The increased numbers of platelets can lead to blood clots that cause serious complications, including stroke (see p.342). Secondary polycythemia and stress polycythemia rarely produce symptoms.

TREATMENT OPTIONS

Treatment of polycythemia vera aims to reduce the number of red blood cells, lower the viscosity (thickness) of the blood, and minimize your risk of blood clots and stroke. To achieve this, your doctor may regularly withdraw a pint of blood on a schedule determined by how quickly the number of red blood cells rises. This treatment continues as long as the overabundance of red blood cells persists.

Medicines are also available in tablet and injectable form to control the production of blood cells; many people with polycythemia can control the disease by taking medicine. Secondary polycythemia and stress polycythemia are treated by resolving the underlying cause or, if mild, may require no treatment.

Porphyria

The porphyrias are a rare group of hereditary diseases characterized by an abnormality in the production of hemoglobin (the oxygen-carrying protein in red blood cells) in which the body has difficulty making heme, the oxygen-carrying portion of hemoglobin.

Heme is normally manufactured by the bone marrow and liver. However, in the porphyrias, the process is defective. As a result, proteins called porphyrins are deposited in the skin, brain and nervous system, liver, and digestive system, damaging and sometimes destroying these structures. A genetic test is available to determine if you have a gene for porphyria, or whether or not a fetus is affected.

SYMPTOMS

There are many types of porphyria, and symptoms vary. They can include nausea and vomiting, abdominal pain, muscle weakness and cramping, blistering or itching of the skin that leads to permanent scarring in areas exposed to light, and psychological disorders such as depression (see p.395) or psychosis (see p.409).

Some people have excessive growth of hair on their arms, hands, face, or legs. Fingernails and toenails may become deformed. Symptoms may be activated by sunlight, taking certain drugs (such as barbiturates), drinking alcohol, or the fluctuating hormone levels that occur during pregnancy or when using birth-control pills.

TREATMENT OPTIONS

Your physician can detect porphyria by blood test and by testing your bowel movements and urine. There is no cure for porphyria; symptoms can start in childhood and, if severe, can kill the child within a few years.

When the disease starts in adulthood, it is usually milder. Symptoms can be controlled by avoiding offending substances.

Thrombocytopenia

Thrombocytopenia is a deficiency of platelets, the pieces of cells that help blood clot and arrest bleeding. There are two categories of thrombocytopenia: idiopathic and secondary.

Idiopathic thrombocytopenia is also called idiopathic thrombocytopenic purpura or autoimmune or immune thrombocytopenia.

Idiopathic means that the cause is unknown; purpura is the term for a rash of red-purple spots on the skin caused by tiny areas of bleeding.

Idiopathic thrombocytopenia is often caused by an autoimmune response (see p.870) in which the body mistakenly attacks and destroys the platelets. Children sometimes experience this after a viral illness. It is more often temporary and is not as serious in children as it is in adults.

Women are more susceptible than men to this condition, and it tends to be persistent—waxing and waning over time. People infected with the human immunodeficiency virus (HIV), the virus that causes acquired immunodeficiency syndrome (AIDS), frequently have low platelets, also due to an attack by antibodies.

Secondary thrombocytopenia occurs as a symptom or complication of another disorder, such as leukemia (see p.724), when platelets are overwhelmed by the malignant production of other blood cells and are not produced in appropriate numbers.

In other people, secondary thrombocytopenia is brought on by a reaction to certain medicines, such as anticancer drugs, sulfonamides, heparin, and quinidine. Heavy alcohol use can also lead to a decrease in the production of platelets, resulting in thrombocytopenia.

SYMPTOMS

Most people with thrombocytopenia have no symptoms. When the platelet count becomes very low, the main symptom is a characteristic rash of tiny red-purple spots on your skin, often on your ankles and feet. Thrombocytopenia can also cause nosebleeds, easy bruising, and heavy periods in women. Bleeding may be excessive and difficult to control.

Serious internal bleeding, such as into your brain or hemorrhaging from your stomach, can also occur if your platelet count is very low—below 10,000. A normal platelet count is between 150,000 and 400,000.

TREATMENT OPTIONS

If you notice any abnormal bleeding or you have the rash of red-purple spots on your skin, see your doctor. He or she may conduct blood tests to measure your level of platelets and the level of other blood cells in your bloodstream. Because many different drugs can cause the condition, your physician may recommend that you stop taking certain prescription drugs.

If your immune system appears to be causing the disease, your doctor may prescribe corticosteroid drugs (see p.895) to suppress the autoimmune response. If your condition is serious and drugs do not help, you may require a splenectomy (removal of the spleen) to prevent your spleen from destroying platelets.

Treatment for secondary thrombocytopenia begins with resolving the underlying condition or stopping medicines.

Treatment may not be necessary if there are no symptoms, which is often the case in children. However, if your platelet count falls below a certain level, the risk of bleeding is so great that you will need transfusions of platelets. A newer natural substance called thrombopoietin makes the platelet count rise and may replace platelet transfusions.

Von Willebrand Disease

Von Willebrand disease is the most common inherited bleeding disorder. The disease arises as a result of a defect in von Willebrand factor, a clotting factor that is important in order for platelets to work well.

The defect in von Willebrand factor also affects factor VIII (the clotting factor that is missing in hemophilia A; see p.735). As a result, the mechanism responsible for clotting blood is damaged, and bleeding can be difficult to control.

Like hemophilia, von Willebrand disease is inherited; unlike hemophilia, it affects men and women equally. People who know the disease runs in their family may want to have genetic testing (see p.132) before having a child to determine the risk of a child receiving the gene for the disease.

The bleeding tendency is less than in hemophilia. Von Willebrand disease may first be noticed due to severe nosebleeds and/or excessive menstrual bleeding. Easy bruising, blood in the urine or bowel movement, and abundant bleeding after surgery are other indicators of von Willebrand disease.

Your doctor diagnoses von Willebrand disease by blood tests, tests of bleeding times, and shortages of clotting factors. Treatment is similar to that of hemophilia—infusions of desmopressin acetate, which stimulates the blood vessels to release von Willebrand factor; transfusions of von Willebrand factor; and avoidance of contact sports or other situations in which you could injure yourself and bleed. You should also avoid medicines that increase a tendency to bleed, such as aspirin and other nonsteroidal anti-inflammatory drugs.

CANCER

For articles on specific cancers, look up the name of the cancer in the index on p.1251.

WHAT IS CANCER?

Each of us begins as a single cell. The fertilized egg begins dividing and, for a while, there is just a ball of cells, all of which look the same. Slowly, the ball of cells begins to take a human shape.

In some places, cells keep dividing and multiplying (for example, tiny fingers form and grow longer). In other places, cells stop multiplying. A series of signals tells some cells to multiply and others to stop multiply-ing. If this process were not very carefully controlled, our organs would not form properly, and we would come out shaped rather strangely.

Cancer also begins as a single cell—a cell that should not multiply but begins to do so. What should have been a single cell—for example, a cell in the lining of your large intestine—becomes a growing ball of cells, called a primary (original) tumor.

First, the ball of cancer cells pushes against and squashes the normal cells around it. Then it starts to burrow through the normal cells, a process called invasion. The invading cancer cells then reach a blood vessel or lymph vessel, enter the circulation, and spread to other parts of the body in a process called metastasis. After taking up residence in other parts of the body, cancer cells begin to form new growths, called metastatic tumors, causing damage in areas of the body that are sometimes far away from where the cancer started.

Every cell in the body has genes that, if activated, tell the cell to multiply. And every cell has other genes that, if activated, tell the cell to stop multiplying. These genes are required for normal growth, which starts in the uterus and continues in childhood.

Most Common Causes of Death Due to Cancer in the United States

Several types of cancer are the biggest killers of both men and women in the United States. In particular, lung cancer (caused predominantly by cigarette smoking) is responsible for the most deaths of both men and women. Other major cancers are shown in the table. (Due to rounding of percentages, women's total exceeds 100%.)

MEN	% OF DEATHS	WOMEN	% OF DEATHS
Lung	32	Lung	25
Prostate	14	Breast	17
Colon/rectum	9	Colon/rectum	10
Leukemias/lymphomas	9	Leukemias/lymphomas	8
Kidney/bladder	5	Ovary	6
Pancreas	5	Pancreas	5
Stomach	3	Uterus/cervix	5
Melanoma	2	Kidney/bladder	3
Mouth	2	Melanoma	1
All others	19	Mouth	1
		All others	20

Risk Factors and Cancer Deaths

The chart shows that dietary factors are the leading cause of cancer, followed closely by tobacco.

RISK FACTORS	% OF DEATHS FROM CANCER
Diet	35
Tobacco	30
Infections	10
Sexual behavior	7
Occupation	4
Excessive use of alcohol	3
Ultraviolet light and radiation from outer space	3
Cancer-causing toxins in the environment	2
Medicines and medical procedures	1
All other risk factors	5

In cancer, one of two things happens. A gene that causes the cell to multiply (called an onco-gene, or cancer gene) is turned on or a gene that keeps the cell from multiplying (called a tumor-suppressor gene) is turned off.

One or more oncogenes must be turned on and one or more tumor-suppressor genes must be turned off for the cancer process to occur in most people. Occa-sionally, a person is born with a defective tumor-suppressor gene; this person is more vulnerable to getting cancer (but may not inevitably get cancer). Usually, the genetic changes that lead to a cancer occur not because of a genetic error a person is born with, but because something in the environment (such as ciga-rette smoke or a cancer-causing virus) has caused the genetic changes.

One characteristic of most cancer cells is the presence of a substance called telomerase. This enzyme constantly repairs dam-age that leads to shortening of a spindle (the telomere) that holds the chromosomes of the cell together. This spindle shortens each time a normal cell divides and, when the spindle becomes very short, the cell dies. How-ever, if telomerase is keeping the spindle from shortening, the cell becomes "immortal"—an essen-tial property of a cancer cell.

After a cancerous tumor starts, the immune system sometimes tries to attack and kill it. How-ever, at the same time, tiny blood vessels begin to grow into the cancer and provide it with nour-ishment. Without those blood vessels, the cancer would starve and die. Most cancers start years before they cause symptoms.

PREVENTING CANCER

You can do more to prevent can-cer by following a healthy life-style (see Taking Charge of Your Health, p.29) than by doing any-thing else. You can also help prevent cancer by seeing your doctor regularly and having cer-tain cancer screening tests—such as Pap smears (see p.1066) and mammograms (see p.1056), although a healthy lifestyle accomplishes the most.

Taking some vitamins or some medicines, such as nonsteroidal anti-inflammatory drugs, may protect against getting certain cancers, but this has not been proven. Various substances in your diet, as well as tobacco, account for the largest number of deaths from cancer.

Scientists do not know what all the dietary risks are, but do know that people who change their diet when they move from one part of the world to another can also alter their risk of cancer dramatically.

DIAGNOSING CANCER

Your doctor may suspect cancer based on your symptoms, a physical examination, and the results of blood tests or x-rays. Newer types of blood tests that can detect small numbers of can-cer cells are very promising. However, the only way to be cer-tain is to take a sample of tissue that is thought to contain cancer, such as a growth on the lining of your intestine, and examine it under a microscope. The appear-ance of the tissue not only can confirm the presence of cancer, but also can tell something about

Stages in Cancer Development

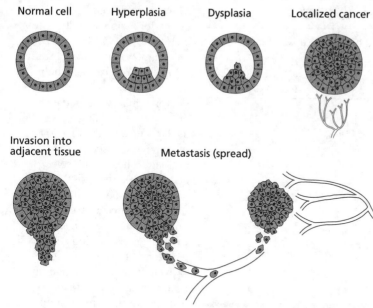

Normal cell   Hyperplasia   Dysplasia   Localized cancer

Invasion into adjacent tissue   Metastasis (spread)

Cancer cells develop out of normal cells. Most cancers are solid balls of abnormal tissue (with the exception of blood cancers). The first abnormal growth of a normal cell results in hyperplasia, which is an excess number of normal-appearing cells. Next, some of the excess cells begin to appear abnormal; this is called dysplasia. These abnormal cells then multiply into a localized cancer, a ball of abnormal cells.

Each of these steps is caused by the activation of an oncogene (cancer-causing gene), as well as the inactivation of a tumor-suppressor gene, which protects against cancer.

Although some cancers remain localized, many begin to invade adjacent tissue. The cells of the growing cancer then invade the lymph vessels and spread to nearby lymph glands, and/or they invade the blood vessels and spread through the bloodstream to other organs. Most cancers grow quite large, and some have already spread before they are detected.

whether it is likely to be a slow-growing or fast-growing cancer.

Under a microscope, cancer cells look wild and disorderly compared to the normal cells around them—in other words, cancer looks ugly.

Along with making the diagnosis of cancer, the doctor needs to determine how far the cancer may have spread; this process is called staging. If the cancer is in an early stage, the chance for cure is greater. Knowing the stage also may dictate the best treatment, since different stages often require different treatments.

TREATING CANCER

There are many different kinds of cancer, and not all of them behave the same or respond to the same treatment. The goal of cancer treatment is to kill the cancerous cells but spare healthy cells from injury, but this is rare.

Most treatments that kill cancer also injure healthy cells and tissue. In general, the more cancer cells there are in the body, the worse the outlook for survival. Therefore, treatments try to remove or kill as many cancer cells as possible.

Traditional cancer treatments involve cutting out many of the cancer cells (surgery), radiation aimed at cancer cells (radiation therapy), medicines that kill cancer cells (chemotherapy), and, for some cancers, hormones or hormone-blocking medicines.

Cancer Surgery

Surgery is used when a large number of cancer cells are together in one place (usually the primary tumor) and when the surgeon can reach that place without causing serious harm. Surgery is used to treat about half of all cancers.

To determine the degree to which the cancer may have spread, the surgeon removes not only the obvious cancer, but a portion of what appears to be healthy tissue around the cancer.

Surgeons also often remove lymph glands near the cancer to see if the cancer cells have spread to them. If the cancer has spread to the lymph glands, there is a greater chance that the cancer has metastasized (spread) to other parts of the body as well.

Radiation Therapy

Radiation is useful in treating many types of cancer when the cancer is localized to one or a few spots in the body. Cancer cells are killed by levels of radiation that do not kill normal cells.

There are different ways of using radiation to kill cancer cells. Most often, a machine is used to point a beam of radiation at the cancer. Usually, there is some damage to the normal cells that lie between the cancer and the skin since they are right in the line of fire. Newer machines are better able to focus radiation on cancer deep in the body, sparing the normal tissues above the cancer.

Some cancers are killed by radioactive substances (called radionuclides) injected into the blood; these substances stick to the cancers but not to healthy tissues.

Finally, it is sometimes possible to place small radioactive particles into an organ, right next to or inside a cancer. By placing a source of ongoing radiation close to or inside a cancer, the cancer cells get a much higher dose of radiation than do the surrounding normal cells (see p.1109 for an example of how this technique is used to treat prostate cancer).

Chemotherapy

Chemotherapy is anticancer medicine. It is most often used when a cancer is not isolated to one place but has metastasized (spread) throughout the body.

It is not always possible to perform surgery on cancer that has spread, or for radiation therapy to find and kill cancer cells in all parts of the body. Chemotherapy delivered to every tissue in the body via the bloodstream, however, can reach cancer cells wherever they are. For many cancers, combinations of chemotherapy medicines are given because they are more effective than if given alone.

A complete response to chemotherapy is defined as the disappearance of all detectable cancer. However, there often is some cancer left that cannot be detected, and this cancer can grow back and spread further.

A partial response is defined as a decrease (by more than half) in the amount of tumor. Many cancers develop a resistance to chemotherapy over time.

A major advance that has reduced the risks from chemotherapy is colony-stimulating growth factors. These natural substances help the bone marrow recover from the injury it sustains during chemotherapy, leading to a more rapid production of healthy blood cells.

Hormone Therapy

The growth of some types of cancer cells is affected by hormones. These cancers can be effectively treated by using hormones or hormone-blocking medicines to slow the growth of the cancer. (See Breast Cancer, p.1055.)

Newer Treatments

Newer treatments that are potentially more powerful and less injurious than chemotherapy or radiation therapy are under development. Techniques are being developed to strengthen the immune system's ability to fight cancer, including the development of vaccines against cer-

---

Believe It or Not: Arsenic May Help Treat One Kind of Leukemia

Research from China, confirmed in the United States, has shown that low doses of arsenic (low enough to cause only mild side effects) are able to cause remission in most people with acute promyelocytic leukemia— even those whose disease did not improve with conventional treatments.

In acute promyelocytic leukemia, young white blood cells called promyelocytes build up in large numbers in the blood because they become "immortalized"—that is, they do not go on to develop into more mature cells and then die, like the promyelocytes in most people do.

Although research is still preliminary, doctors are cautiously optimistic. It remains to be seen if remission of acute promyelocytic leukemia will last for a long time and if recurring treatments with arsenic will be required and can be given without serious side effects.

tain kinds of cancer. Combinations of antibodies (to target cancer cells) and toxins (to kill cancer cells) are being created and tested.

Still newer treatments are under development, based on the recent major discoveries about how cancer starts and progresses, and how the body tries to fight it. For example, scientists are trying to use genetic engineering to turn tumor-suppressor genes (which keep a cancer cell from growing) back on and to turn off the genes that allow a cancer cell to invade the tissue around it.

Scientists are also using genetic engineering to try to turn off the telomerase enzyme (found in most cancer cells) that appears to be necessary for the cancer cell to continue to live and divide.

Finally, various techniques are being used to turn off the growth of the blood vessels that nourish the cancer. In animal cancer studies, some of these techniques have produced encouraging results.

KEEPING CANCER IN PERSPECTIVE

It is terrifying to be told you have cancer. Cancer causes more fear and hopelessness than any other disease. Yet the prognosis for many kinds of cancer is very good compared to other diseases. For example, a person who has just been diagnosed with a severe case of the lung disease emphysema (see p.517) is less likely to be alive in 5 years than a person just diagnosed with most types of cancer. Yet the diagnosis of cancer—any cancer—leads many people to believe that they will soon die, and that the death will be painful. Indeed, many people are afraid even to discuss cancer.

If you or someone you love has a terminal form of cancer (or any other disease), ask the doctors for information about the cancer, its treatment, and its probable outcome. Advances have been made to control pain and other symptoms, and there are many support services available. Final days can usually be lived with comfort and dignity, and with loved ones nearby. See also Hospice, p.1141.

Digestive System

The digestive system transforms what you eat into the substances you need to survive. The system is made up of a tube that is 30 feet long and includes the mouth, throat, esophagus, stomach, small intestine (duodenum, jejunum, and ileum), large intestine (also called the colon), rectum, and anus.

Attached to that tube are three essential organs: the liver, gallbladder, and pancreas.

Together, over the course of 12 to 24 hours, this system takes what you eat, extracts the nutrients, and eliminates the wastes.

To extract nutrients, food must be physically and chemically chopped up into microscopically small pieces. A carrot stick you eat turns into a huge number of different substances—vitamins, minerals, proteins, sugars, and fiber—that move around in your stomach and intestines. The body uses these substances in many different ways.

Some of the sugars may be stored in the liver to give you energy when you need it 3 days later. Some of the calcium in the carrot is added to your bones to give them strength. Some of the vitamins travel to a cell in the lining of your intestine and protect against mutations that could lead to cancer.

The fiber stays in the intestine as bulky waste. But it is essential waste, critical in eliminating other material (including excess fats and sugars) that can damage the

Gastrointestinal Tract

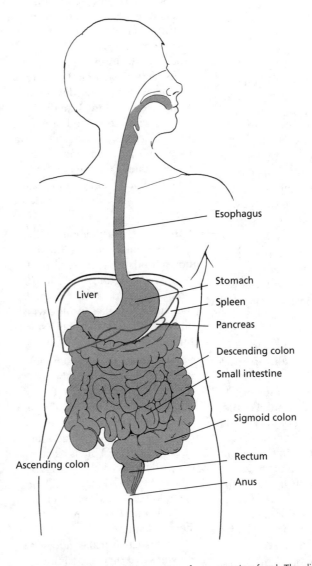

The gastrointestinal tract is a system for processing food. The digestive system starts at the mouth and includes the throat, esophagus, stomach, small intestine, colon (large intestine), rectum, and anus. The liver, gallbladder, and pancreas are also part of the digestive system. The spleen is located in the abdomen, but is not part of the digestive system.

body. Waste is eliminated in a bowel movement.

DIGESTIVE PROCESS

Mouth The first step in the digestive process can begin even before food makes a physical appearance. The aroma or even the thought of food can set off the chemical processes that initiate digestion. Salivary glands produce saliva, a combination of water and enzymes. When food enters the mouth, it is physically chopped up by the teeth and chemically broken down by the enzyme amylase, which is made by the salivary glands. Water in saliva helps dissolve the food and the tongue shapes the softened matter into an easily swallowed ball called a bolus.

Esophagus The bolus then enters a foot-long tube called the esophagus. As food enters the esophagus, the windpipe closes off to prevent you from inhaling the food. The esophagus pushes the food down into the stomach using powerful, muscular, wavelike contractions (called peristalsis) controlled by the action of involuntary muscles (see p.593) in its wall. At the bottom of the esophagus, a ring of muscle (the lower esophageal sphincter) relaxes to let food into the stomach. When this sphincter does not function normally, juices full of acid from the stomach splash back up into the esophagus, producing the common and painful condition heartburn.

Stomach Your stomach can hold a quart of food. The muscles in the wall of the stomach spend 3 to 6 hours churning the food around, and a powerful digestive juice filled with acid and enzymes chemically breaks down food (especially proteins) into smaller pieces. The stomach acid also kills most microorganisms that may have contaminated the food.

Liver In addition to its role in breaking foods down, the liver has several other essential functions. It processes nearly every nutrient to make the nutrients usable by other parts of the body. It is a storehouse of vitamins (such as vitamin B_{12}) and of sugars, which are used when the body needs energy. Like the kidney, it cleans the blood of impurities. The liver also creates many essential substances, including some proteins that keep the volume of blood from dropping and others that are essential for blood clotting.

Pancreas In addition to making digestive chemicals that break down food, the pancreas makes hormones that allow cells to use circulating nutrients. For example, the pancreas makes insulin, which allows body cells to use the sugar brought to them by the blood.

Small intestine Stomach muscles send the food into the first part of the small intestine (the duodenum), where it is subjected to enzymes and bile salts that are primarily designed to digest fats. The enzymes and bile salts are made in the liver, sent through a tube to be stored in the gallbladder, and sent via another tube (the bile duct) to be emptied into the duodenum.

The pancreas makes additional enzymes that digest food further; it sends the enzymes to the duodenum through the pancreatic duct. Once food has been broken down into millions of pieces, the pieces can be absorbed into the bloodstream and carried, where needed, to different parts of the body.

Large intestine What remains after this exodus of nutrients is undigestible waste matter, which is propelled from the small intestine into the large intestine (colon). The walls of the large intestine absorb water, leaving waste in the form of feces. The feces are expelled from the body by way of the rectum and the anus.

Upper Endoscopy

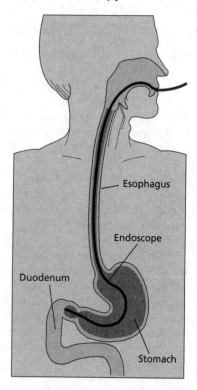

In upper endoscopy, an endoscope is passed through the mouth to view the esophagus, stomach, and duodenum, revealing bleeding or other abnormalities. It can also be used to take a biopsy sample.

Viewing the Upper Gastrointestinal Tract

When your medical history and a physical examination indicate that you may have a disorder of the upper gastrointestinal tract (including the esophagus, stomach, and duodenum—the upper portion of the small intestine), your doctor may take a closer look with one of the following tests.

You will be asked to fast for up to 6 hours before a test. The test may be performed in a hospital, clinic, or doctor's office, usually by a radiologist, who is an expert in performing diagnostic imaging procedures and interpreting the results. Upper endoscopy is performed by a gastroenterologist.

PROCEDURE	WHY IT IS PERFORMED	WHAT TO EXPECT
Upper endoscopy	To take a sample of tissue for biopsy; find sites of gastrointestinal bleeding or peptic ulcers or irritated areas in the lining of the upper intestinal tract; remove foreign bodies; treat esophageal varices (swollen veins); and treat blockages, precancerous diseases, and some cancers.	A local anesthetic will be sprayed into the back of your throat and a sedative will be given intravenously. A lighted flexible endoscope will be passed through your mouth into the esophagus, stomach, and duodenum (air may be passed into the digestive tract to open the area to provide a better view). Small instruments may be passed through the endoscope to take a tissue sample, repair injured tissue, inject drugs, remove tumors, or perform other procedures.
Barium swallow (upper gastrointestinal tract series)	To create an indirect picture of the lining of the upper intestine and a moving picture of food and liquids traveling through the upper gastrointestinal tract. Used to detect swallowing disorders, polyps, tumors, duodenal and stomach ulcers, and narrowing of the esophagus and other areas.	Standing or sitting in front of an x-ray table, you will drink a mixture of water and barium (through which x-rays cannot pass) or eat a barium-coated cookie. As you swallow, the radiologist will make a series of x-rays (a camera may rotate around you) or a videotape as the barium moves through your throat, esophagus, stomach, and duodenum.
Computed tomography (see p.149)	To obtain detailed pictures of the inside of your body in order to detect pockets of infection (abscesses), tumors, inflammation of the intestines, enlargement of organs (such as the liver and pancreas), fluid in the abdomen, and enlarged lymph glands in the abdomen.	You may drink a solution that will enhance the image made by the scanner. You will lie very still on a table in a large, metal, tunnel-like device (a camera will rotate around you as you move through the tunnel).

ESOPHAGUS

Heartburn and Indigestion

Heartburn and indigestion are common but imprecise terms used to describe recurring, burning pain in the upper abdomen or lower chest. The pain is often accompanied by a bitter taste in the mouth and a bloated sensation. The term indigestion is also sometimes used to refer to a similar pain that occurs after eating.

Heartburn and indigestion affect 20% to 30% of Americans, and are more common among people who are overweight and who smoke. They tend to become more common as people grow older, although they can affect people of all ages. The symptoms may be caused by many different conditions, including gastro-esophageal reflux disease (see p.747), gastritis (see p.752), peptic ulcer (see p.752), and gallstones (see p.770).

Angina (see p.657), a pain usually felt in the chest due to a lack of oxygen to the heart, can also cause pain in the upper part of the abdomen, especially if it is the lower part of the heart that lacks oxygen.

You can often treat heartburn or indigestion without seeing your doctor. Antacid medicines and H$_2$-blockers (see p.1161), available without a prescription, reduce the amount of stomach acid and may eliminate symptoms. Stopping smoking and reducing your consumption of alcohol can also be helpful. Some people report relief with various alternative medicine treatments (see right).

Heartburn: Dr Van Dam's Advice

Doctors, particularly gastroenterologists like me, see lots of patients who seek care for heartburn. But there are many more people who regularly suffer from heartburn and don't do anything about it. "It's just heartburn," they say.

However, the damage caused by acid reflux can lead to scar formation in the esophagus (which can make it difficult to swallow) or to a condition called Barrett's esophagus, which is a precancerous condition.

Therefore, it is important that individuals report symptoms of even "simple" heartburn to their doctors. There often is no need for tests, and the remedy may be as easy and inexpensive as regularly using a nonprescription medicine. But you should tell your doctor about heartburn.

JACQUES VAN DAM, MD, PHD
BRIGHAM AND WOMEN'S HOSPITAL
HARVARD MEDICAL SCHOOL

Alternative Medicine: Heartburn

Try one of the following alternative remedies to help your heartburn:

■ Ginger root taken in capsules after eating (may help absorb acid)

■ Licorice extract taken in tablets or powders before meals and at bedtime (may help suppress acid production but use only for 1 to 2 weeks because some kinds of licorice can raise blood pressure)

■ 1 teaspoon baking soda in 1 cup water

■ Bitters such as gentian root, wormwood, and goldenseal in capsules or as a liquid extract before meals

■ Aromatic herbs such as catnip and fennel (brew in teas)

■ Chamomile with marshmallow root

■ Acupuncture

■ Stress-reduction techniques such as the relaxation response (see p.90), biofeedback (see p.395), hypnotherapy (see p.394), and certain yoga movements

Indigestion: Dr Welker's Advice

Q I have indigestion that comes and goes. It's not really bad but it's annoying. Is there anything I can do to prevent it?

A Yes. There are several simple steps you can take to prevent indigestion. Don't eat too much at one meal. Avoid irritants such as alcohol, cigarettes, and drugs including aspirin, ibuprofen, and naproxen. You might also benefit from reducing your intake of acidic foods (such as fruit juices and tomatoes), fatty foods, and caffeine.

Eat at a leisurely pace, relax after eating, don't lie down right after eating (wait 2 to 3 hours), and don't exercise right after eating (since exercise draws blood away from the stomach and impairs digestion). If your indigestion worsens or becomes painful, see your doctor.

ROY D. WELKER, MD
BRIGHAM AND WOMEN'S HOSPITAL
HARVARD MEDICAL SCHOOL

Hiatal Hernia

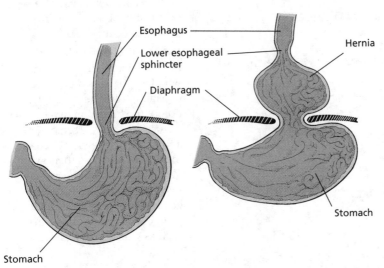

NORMAL STOMACH

STOMACH WITH HIATAL HERNIA

Esophagus

Lower esophageal sphincter

Diaphragm

Hernia

Stomach

Stomach

A normal stomach is shown at left. The stomach with a hiatal hernia (right) shows part of the stomach protruding upward into the chest through an opening in the diaphragm (the band of muscle that separates the chest from the abdomen and helps you breathe).

If your indigestion does not get better with these treatments, if it promptly comes back after you have stopped treatment, if you lose your appetite and lose weight, or if you have other symptoms that worry you, contact your doctor.

Inflammation of the Esophagus

Inflammation of the esophagus, also called esophagitis, is a symptom of several common conditions.

SYMPTOMS

Gastroesophageal reflux disease (GERD) is caused by an intermittent weakness of the lower esophageal sphincter, a circular group of muscles that normally tightens to protect the esophagus from backflow of acid from the stomach. Normally, the sphincter opens to let a mouthful of swallowed food into the stomach, and then shuts.

In GERD, the sphincter relaxes spontaneously without a swallow. This allows the backflow (reflux) of stomach acid up into the esophagus, causing irritation and a burning, uncomfortable sensation (heartburn) that radiates up the middle of the chest.

Heartburn often occurs after eating (when there is more acid in the stomach) or at bedtime, when the sphincter may be more relaxed and, because you are lying down, gravity is not keeping stomach acid down. In some cases, the pain extends to the neck and arms, mimicking the symptoms of a heart attack. GERD can also cause a sore throat, a

Gastroesophageal Reflux Disease

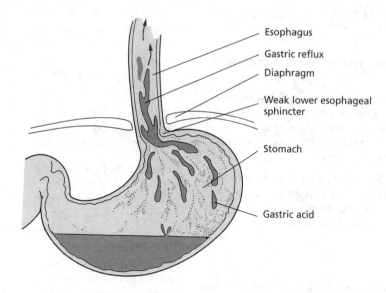

Esophagus
Gastric reflux
Diaphragm
Weak lower esophageal sphincter
Stomach
Gastric acid

Gastroesophageal reflux disease occurs when the lower esophageal sphincter, a high-pressure zone designed to keep digestive juices in the stomach, relaxes more than it should. When this happens, stomach acid flows back up into the esophagus, causing heartburn.

Surgery for Gastroesophageal Reflux Disease

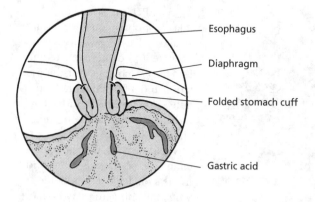

Esophagus
Diaphragm
Folded stomach cuff
Gastric acid

In a procedure called fundoplication, which is used to treat gastroesophageal reflux disease, the surgeon folds the top of the stomach around itself to create a high-pressure zone that functions as a lower esophageal sphincter. This allows food to pass through to the stomach but prevents acid from backing up into the esophagus.

chronic cough, and a feeling of a lump in the throat.

Overweight people and pregnant women may experience GERD because they have more pressure in their abdomens. Taking certain medicines (see p.749), smoking, drinking alcohol or coffee, and eating chocolate or high-fat foods may also increase the chance of reflux.

People who have recurring GERD over many years have an increased risk of cancer of the esophagus; there is no proof that treating GERD reduces this risk.

Hiatal hernia is a common condition in which part of the stomach protrudes upward into the chest through an opening in the diaphragm, the muscle that separates the chest and abdomen and helps with breathing. The herniation impairs the efficiency of the lower esophageal sphincter and can cause acid reflux, which may be worse at night. Hiatal hernia occurs more often in overweight people and smokers.

Esophagitis due to infection is more common among people who have damaged immune systems; it is a frequent complication of the human immunodeficiency virus (HIV) (see p.872) and in those receiving chemotherapy or radiation therapy to treat cancer. When the immune system is impaired, the esophagus is much more easily attacked by infectious microorganisms such as viruses, bacteria, and fungi.

TREATMENT OPTIONS

If your symptoms are mild, try one of the home remedies for GERD listed on p.749. Antacids

Home Remedies for GERD

Changes in diet and lifestyle are the foundation of treatment for GERD. Take the following steps to reduce the frequency of flare-ups:

■ Avoid eating large meals, which stay in the stomach longer and increase chances for reflux. Eat smaller portions more often.

■ Do not consume food or drink that increases acid secretions, decreases the pressure of the lower esophageal sphincter, or slows stomach emptying. Offenders include greasy, high-fat foods, tomato products, carbonated drinks, citrus fruits, chocolate, beverages with caffeine (such as coffee, tea, or colas), peppermint, spearmint, or alcohol. However, not every person with GERD has a bad reaction to all these substances.

■ Do not smoke; nicotine stimulates stomach acid and impairs the function of the sphincter.

■ If you are overweight, lose weight.

■ At the first sign of heartburn, drink a large glass of water.

■ Talk to your doctor about limiting medicines that contribute to GERD (see below).

■ Do not eat 2 hours before going to bed.

■ Do not wear tight belts, waistbands, or other clothing that puts pressure on your stomach.

■ If you have heartburn at night, elevate the head of your bed by placing 6-inch blocks under the bed's feet at the head of the bed, or use a wedge-shaped pillow to angle your upper body.

■ Stay upright after eating and avoid bending down or straining to lift heavy objects.

Medicines That Can Cause GERD

The following medicines can cause the heartburn of GERD:

■ Bronchodilators such as theophylline

■ Calcium channel blockers such as diltiazem, nifedipine, and verapamil

■ Nonsteroidal anti-inflammatory drugs such as aspirin, ibuprofen, and naproxen

■ Progestins such as medroxyprogesterone acetate and norethindrone acetate

■ Tricyclic antidepressants such as amitriptyline, nortriptyline, and protriptyline

can also help. If these simple measures do not work, you need to see your doctor.

Several kinds of medicines are useful. Medicines called H_2-blockers or proton pump inhibitors can decrease the amount of acid in the stomach and therefore the amount of acid that is refluxed into the esophagus.

Medicines called prokinetic agents such as metoclopramide can increase the tightness of the sphincter and keep acid from refluxing. Cisapride can cause serious heart rhythm abnormalities, particularly if you take it with certain other drugs (see p.1176).

If your symptoms recur (which happens in up to 80% of people), you may need to continue taking medication or, as a last resort, have surgery (see p.748) to tighten the lower esophageal sphincter. Esophagitis caused by infection is treated with antiviral, antibiotic, or antifungal medicines.

Cancer of the Esophagus

Cancer of the esophagus affects men more often than women, and blacks more frequently than whites. Since the 1970s, there has been a rise in the frequency of cancer of the esophagus in white men.

Smoking and drinking alcohol increase the risk of esophageal cancer, and together they increase risk even further. Radiation therapy (see p.741) to the neck area, and disorders that chronically irritate the esophagus, such as gastroesophageal reflux disease (see p.747), also increase the risk of esophageal cancer.

Tumor in the Esophagus

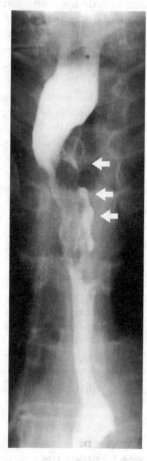

This x-ray of the upper gastrointestinal tract shows a cancerous tumor in the esophagus. The swallowed barium drink, which shows up as white on x-rays, cannot move through the space in the middle of the esophagus because a tumor (arrows) has grown into the space.

SYMPTOMS

Symptoms often do not appear until a tumor is in an advanced stage. The most common symptom is difficulty swallowing (first solid food but eventually liquids as well), which is accompanied by weight loss. As the tumor grows, regurgitating becomes fre-quent, and the risk of aspiration pneumonia (see p.498) increases as food and liquids are inhaled into the lungs.

TREATMENT OPTIONS

See your doctor immediately if you have difficulty swallowing. He or she will perform tests—such as those described in Viewing the Upper Gastrointestinal Tract (see p.745)—to see if there is a blockage in the esophagus and to take a sample for biopsy of any blockage that looks like a tumor.

Regardless of the treatment approach, the outlook for esophageal cancer is poor because it is often detected late. Your choice of treatment will be based in part on how much discomfort you are willing to tolerate. Most cancers of the esophagus are treated with a combination of surgery, radiation therapy (see p.741), and chemotherapy (see p.741).

Esophagectomy (removal of most of the esophagus) may be performed if it can remove all or most of the cancer. The upper portion of the esophagus is then attached to the stomach. Sometimes, a portion of the large intestine is used to replace the section of the esophagus that has been removed.

When a tumor of the esophagus cannot be removed by surgery, something must be done to overcome the blockage caused by the tumor. Sometimes the tumor shrinks for a while from radiation therapy and chemotherapy. Sometimes a new esophageal pathway (bypass) can be created (so that the person can continue to eat).

In other people, the esophagus can be widened using a

Cancer of the Esophagus

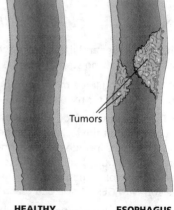

HEALTHY ESOPHAGUS

ESOPHAGUS WITH CANCEROUS TUMORS

A normal esophagus (left) has thin, even walls. An esophagus with cancerous tumors (right and in the x-ray at far left) causes difficulty swallowing because the tumor growing out of the walls of the esophagus has narrowed the space in the middle.

series of rods or a balloon that widens the opening. Then a stiff tube called a stent is inserted to keep the esophagus open.

Esophageal Spasm and Achalasia

The muscles of the esophagus push swallowed food down into the stomach. Esophageal spasm and esophageal achalasia are disorders of these muscles.

In esophageal spasm, the muscles contract in an uncoordinated way, causing severe chest pain and difficulty swallowing food and liquids.

In esophageal achalasia, the normal wavelike movements of the lower portion of the esophagus do not occur, causing food that ordinarily would pass into the stomach to build up in the lower esophagus. This can cause undigested food to come up into the throat, bad breath, and a foul taste in your mouth.

In most people, the causes of esophageal spasm and achalasia are unknown. Women are more commonly affected by achalasia than men, but esophageal spasm affects men and women equally.

If you experience difficult or painful swallowing, see your doctor immediately. A barium swallow (see p.745) can reveal any abnormalities in the structure of the esophagus and in the pattern of swallowing. Another test (esophageal manometry) uses a small instrument that measures the pressures in the esophagus at various locations.

The most useful treatments for esophageal spasm are medicines that relax the muscles of the esophagus, such as calcium channel blockers and nitrates. These pills can be swallowed or dissolved under the tongue at the time of pain.

Esophageal achalasia can be treated with prescription medicines that relax the constricted lower segment of the esophagus or with mechanical devices (such as a balloon inserted and inflated) designed to widen the esophagus.

As a last resort, a laparoscopic or conventional surgical procedure called a myotomy, in which the muscle at the lower end of the esophagus is cut to release the stricture, is sometimes performed.

Esophageal Stricture

An esophageal stricture is a narrowing of the esophagus that makes swallowing difficult. Other symptoms include pain when swallowing, weight loss, and regurgitation of food.

A stricture can be caused by a congenital (from birth) narrowing of the esophagus (called a ring or web), cancer of the esophagus (see p.749), inflammation of the esophagus (see p.747), or scar tissue that forms after ingesting caustic substances.

Esophageal dilatation (widening the esophagus) is the most common method for relieving esophageal stricture, rings, and webs. For dilatation, a series of rods or balloons is inserted into the esophagus to widen its channel. Surgery to remove the narrowed portion is sometimes necessary.

Esophageal Varices

Esophageal varices are swollen veins in the lining of the walls of the lower esophagus; they may rupture and cause dangerous bleeding. The swelling of the veins is caused by increased pressure (called portal hypertension) in the portal vein, a blood vessel that moves blood from the stomach and intestines to the liver.

Portal hypertension is often caused by cirrhosis of the liver (see p.765). The scarring caused by cirrhosis raises the pressure of the portal vein. Symptoms include having black bowel movements (the blood in the bowel movement comes from the upper part of the digestive tract) and vomiting blood.

In recent years, several treatments have been shown to reduce portal vein pressure and therefore to reduce the chance of bleeding from esophageal varices. These treatments include regular daily use of beta blockers and nitrates.

If an esophageal vein ruptures, it is a medical emergency. You may need a blood transfusion to restore normal blood count, heart rate, and blood pressure and you will need treatment if the bleeding does not stop on its own.

About half of all episodes of bleeding from esophageal varices get better on their own, although the risk of recurrence is high. For people who require treatment, intravenous drugs can be given that cause blood vessels to clamp down and reduce the pressure in the portal vein and the esophageal veins.

If these medicines fail to stop bleeding, a thin wire with a balloon attached can be guided through the mouth and down into the esophagus and stomach; the balloon is inflated to open up against the wall of the veins and stop the bleeding.

Another treatment, endoscopic sclerotherapy, involves injecting a solution into the bulging esophageal veins, causing them to shrink. This method is effective in 90% of cases but can cause ulcers of the esophagus, more bleeding, or narrowing of the esophageal opening (strictures).

Endoscopic ligation is a newer technique in which the veins are tied off with small, elastic rubber bands. This method is safer than sclerotherapy and just as effective.

STOMACH

Gastritis

Gastritis is inflammation of the stomach lining. It can be caused by overuse of alcohol, smoking, long-term use of aspirin or other nonsteroidal anti-inflammatory drugs (NSAIDs), infection with the bacterium *Helicobacter pylori* (see p.754), or severe injury or shock.

Occasionally, gastritis is caused by an autoimmune condition (see p.870) in which the immune system mistakenly attacks the cells that line the stomach.

The symptoms of gastritis can include nausea, vomiting, and pain or discomfort in your abdomen that is made worse by eating. Erosion of the stomach lining may cause blood in your stools (turning them black when significant bleeding comes from the stomach).

Anemia (see p.713), which causes you to look pale and be fatigued, can result from chronic gastritis due to a slow loss of blood.

Your doctor will advise you to stop the causes of gastritis you have control over to see if symptoms go away. If you need to continue taking an NSAID but you are experiencing stomach irritation, you may be able to switch to another drug called misoprostol, which lessens stomach irritation.

Your doctor may also test for *H pylori*. If the test result is positive, you will be prescribed treatment to kill the bacterium. If the test result is negative, or it is positive but you do not benefit from treatment, the doctor may prescribe a medicine to reduce stomach acid.

The only certain way to make a diagnosis of gastritis is for your doctor to view the lining of your stomach using upper endoscopy (see p.745), although this is usually not necessary.

Peptic Ulcers

Peptic ulcers are sores in the lining of the stomach and duodenum (the first part of the small intestine). They affect about 4 million people in the United States and can occur at any age.

Duodenal ulcers usually appear between ages 30 and 50 and are more common in men. Stomach ulcers usually occur later in life, after age 60, and affect women more often.

The cause of most stomach and duodenal ulcers is the bacterium *Helicobacter pylori* (see p.754). Irritants include aspirin and other nonsteroidal anti-inflammatory drugs (NSAIDs), alcohol, coffee with or without caffeine, and smoking.

A rare cause of ulcers is a condition in which stomach acid is produced in much higher-than-normal amounts (see Zollinger-Ellison syndrome, p.758).

Studies show that peptic ulcers often run in families and occur more often in people with type O blood. Despite the popular belief that ulcers are a side effect of living a high-pressure life, experts no longer believe that stress causes ulcers, although stress may make a person more sensitive to the pain of an ulcer.

Stomach Ulcer

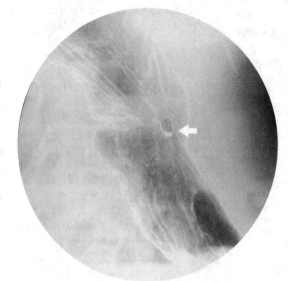

This photograph (taken from an upper gastrointestinal tract series) shows a stomach ulcer. The arrow points to the ulcer, outlined in white by the barium that has been swallowed.

Peptic Ulcers

PEPTIC ULCER VIEWED THROUGH ENDOSCOPE

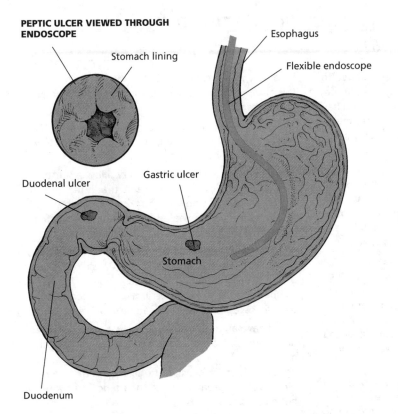

Stomach lining

Esophagus

Flexible endoscope

Duodenal ulcer

Gastric ulcer

Stomach

Duodenum

Peptic ulcers can form in the stomach (gastric ulcers) or duodenum (duodenal ulcers). A bacterium called *Helicobacter pylori*, which invades the stomach lining, causes almost all duodenal ulcers and about 80% of gastric ulcers. *H pylori* infection inflames the stomach lining and may increase the stomach's secretion of acid, which can lead to ulcers. Using a flexible endoscope, your doctor can view your stomach and duodenal lining and check for ulcers.

SYMPTOMS

Some people have no symptoms of peptic ulcer. The most common symptom is a burning pain in the upper abdomen. The pain usually occurs 2 to 3 hours after eating or very late at night. It can last minutes or several hours.

When the ulcer occurs on the back wall of the duodenum, the pain is sometimes also felt in the back. Eating or taking an antacid often brings temporary relief of the pain caused by duodenal ulcers.

Belching, a bloated feeling, nausea, vomiting, and loss of appetite are less common symptoms. With a duodenal ulcer, nausea, vomiting, or pain that is worsened by eating usually indicate obstruction of the stomach outlet caused by inflammation and swelling of the tissues around the narrow channel that connects the stomach to the duo-

denum. Food does not easily get from the stomach to the duodenum through the obstruction.

Ulcers can cause bleeding, which can cause vomiting of bloody material (the partially digested blood looks like coffee grounds), or passage of black bowel movements. The anemia from bleeding can cause weakness and faintness or fainting.

In some people, the bleeding is slow and detectable only by tests for blood in the bowel movement (see p.791) and by blood counts that reveal anemia and iron deficiency.

Ulcers can get progressively deeper and penetrate through the wall of the stomach or duodenum, producing sudden and severe pain and shock (see p.645). This is a medical emergency.

TREATMENT OPTIONS

If your symptoms persist, or if you are taking antacids or nonprescription H_2-blockers frequently, see your doctor. He or she will ask about your symptoms and may perform several tests to confirm a diagnosis and to help determine treatment.

Your doctor may perform a barium swallow or upper gastrointestinal tract series, upper endoscopy, and biopsy to establish the location and size of any erosion. These tests are described on p.745. You may also have blood tests for anemia and *H pylori* and a stool sample test to look for blood.

If your tests reveal ulcers and *H pylori*, your doctor will prescribe one of several different regimens, including antibiotics to kill *H pylori* (see p.754). In addition, your doctor may prescribe

Helicobacter pylori *and Antibiotic Treatment for Ulcers: A Medical Breakthrough*

Before 1994, people with recurring ulcers needed to take acid-reducing treatments for many years. Today you can undergo 1 to 2 weeks of treatment and have a good chance of never needing to take ulcer medicines again because of a medical breakthrough: the discovery that many ulcers are caused by bacteria.

Most bacteria find the acid environment of the human stomach extremely inhospitable. But the spiral-shaped bacterium *Helicobacter pylori* is able to thrive in human stomachs and the stomachs of other warm-blooded animals because *H pylori* is uniquely equipped to protect itself against stomach acid.

H pylori produces large quantities of urease, an enzyme that generates ammonia, to neutralize the stomach acid. The bacterium surrounds itself with "walls" made of ammonia that protect it from the stomach acid that could kill it. Then, like a corkscrew, the bacterium twists itself into the mucous layer that protects the stomach lining from corrosive gastric juices.

Scientists believe that *H pylori* contributes to ulcers in several ways, including thinning the protective mucous layer and poisoning nearby cells with ammonia and other toxins.

In the United States, about 10% of people under age 30 and 60% of people over age 60 are infected; infection is more common in poor people. It is also more common in developing countries and in people who move to the United States from developing countries.

Although infection with *H pylori* does not cause problems in most people, in some it can lead to gastritis (see p.752) and ulcers. In rare cases, it can lead to a kind of lymphoma (see p.727) of the stomach lining. It is also probably involved in many cases of stomach cancer (see p.756).

There are three ways to diagnose infection with *H pylori*. The first is a blood test that measures antibodies against the bacterium in your blood.

The second is a test in which you swallow a substance that is broken down by the urease that is made by *H pylori*. The broken-down substance is then absorbed into the blood and exhaled (if you have an infection with *H pylori*, testing your breath will detect it).

A slightly more accurate test of infection is endoscopy (see p.745), which involves taking a sample (for biopsy) of the stomach lining. If the urease made by *H pylori* can be found and the bacterium can be seen under the microscope, a diagnosis can be confirmed.

If you have an ulcer and infection with *H pylori*, your doctor will prescribe a course of antibiotics and other medicines. Several very effective medicines must be used together. They will not only help your current ulcer heal but greatly reduce the chance that you will get more ulcers.

Many different drug regimens are used to eradicate *H pylori*. Three of the most widely used are outlined at right. Each is called a triple-therapy regimen because it includes three different kinds of medicines, and each is about 90% effective in eliminating the infection.

Regimens that involve two kinds of medicines (double-therapy regimens) are somewhat more convenient but less effective. The main differences among the three different triple-therapy regimens are expense, side effects, and convenience.

TREATMENT	HOW OFTEN TAKEN	SIDE EFFECTS	ADVANTAGES AND DISADVANTAGES
Treatment 1 Two antibiotics (either clarithromycin and metronidazole <u>or</u> clarithromycin and amoxicillin) plus a proton pump inhibitor (such as omeprazole)	Twice a day for 10 to 14 days	Infrequent; occur in 5% of people	Can take fewer pills less often than in treatment 3; more expensive than treatments 2 or 3
Treatment 2 Two antibiotics (either clarithromycin and metronidazole <u>or</u> clarithromycin and amoxicillin) plus a single pill of ranitidine and bismuth citrate	Twice a day for 2 weeks	Infrequent	Can take medicine less often than in treatment 3; less expensive than treatment 1
Treatment 3 Two antibiotics (either metronidazole and amoxicillin <u>or</u> metronidazole and tetracycline) plus an H_2-blocker and bismuth subsalicylate	Four times a day for 2 weeks	More frequent; include diarrhea, nausea, and vomiting; occur in about 10% of people	Least expensive and as effective as treatments 1 and 2 if taken as prescribed; need to take more pills more often

Helicobacter pylori

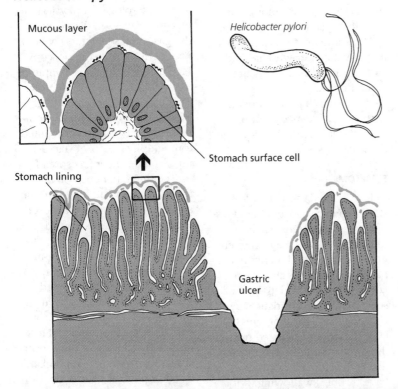

Mucous layer

Helicobacter pylori

Stomach surface cell

Stomach lining

Gastric ulcer

The corkscrew-shaped bacterium *Helicobacter pylori* thrives in the stomach because it can produce large quantities of urease, an enzyme that generates ammonia to neutralize the acid that quickly kills other bacteria. *H pylori* attaches itself to the surface of stomach cells after twisting through the mucus that protects the lining from corrosive gastric juices.

Benefits of Antibiotics for Stomach and Duodenal Ulcers

Treatment with antibiotics in people with ulcers greatly reduces the chance of an ulcer coming back.

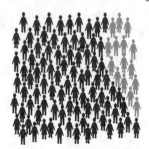

85 OF 100 PEOPLE WHO HAVE HAD ULCERS IN THE PAST AND DO NOT TAKE ANTIBIOTICS DEVELOP ANOTHER ULCER WITHIN 1 YEAR

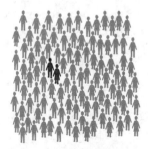

2 OF 100 PEOPLE WHO HAVE HAD ULCERS IN THE PAST AND TAKE ANTIBIOTICS DEVELOP ANOTHER ULCER WITHIN 1 YEAR

medication—such as antacids, H_2-blockers, proton pump inhibitors, or ulcer-coating agents—to reduce the amount of stomach acid.

The antibiotic eradicates the bacteria, while the acid-reducing and ulcer-coating medicines improve the stomach's ability to heal the damage that has already occurred.

If your ulcer is caused by NSAIDs, the drug misoprostol can be effective.

You will also be advised to avoid aspirin and other NSAIDs, caffeine-containing beverages, decaffeinated coffee, alcohol, smoking, and chewing tobacco, all of which can interfere with the healing of an ulcer.

Stomach Cancer

Cancer of the lining of the stomach is more common in men and rarely occurs before age 50. The causes of stomach cancer are not clear, but the bacterium *Helicobacter pylori* (see p.754), which causes peptic ulcers (see p.752), may be an important factor.

A diet that includes a large amount of salted, smoked, or pickled food is also thought to contribute. Having gastritis (see p.752) for many years and having a family member who has had stomach cancer also appear to raise the risk.

The outlook for most people with stomach cancer is poor; only about 7% are alive 5 years after diagnosis.

SYMPTOMS

In its early and most curable stage, stomach cancer often does not cause symptoms. As the tumor grows, you may experience upper abdominal discomfort and bloating or fullness after meals. Loss of appetite, weight loss, nausea, vomiting, and fatigue may occur as the disease progresses.

If the tumor is located near the point where the esophagus meets the stomach, you may have trouble swallowing. If it is located in the lower portion of your stomach, it can block the movement of stomach contents out of the stomach and cause you to vomit.

TREATMENT OPTIONS

If you experience abdominal pain, discomfort, and bloating that is not relieved by simple remedies, or if you start to lose your appetite and lose weight, see your doctor. He or she will take your medical history and perform a physical examination, usually including an examination of your rectum and stools for signs of bleeding.

If your doctor thinks diagnostic studies are necessary, he or she may order a series of x-rays of your upper gastrointestinal tract (see p.745). Alternatively, your doctor may refer you to a gastroenterologist (a physician who specializes in disorders of the gastrointestinal tract), who may perform upper endoscopy (see p.745) and take a sample of tissue for laboratory evaluation.

If cancer is confirmed by biopsy, your doctor may recommend blood tests and computed tomography (see p.745) to determine if the cancer has spread.

Treatment depends on the type of cancer you have and the stage at which it was diagnosed. If the cancer has not spread beyond the stomach, surgery to remove all or part of the stomach, along with chemotherapy (see p.741), is recommended. Nearby lymph glands may also be removed to determine if cancer has spread to them and to reduce the chance of the cancer spreading from the lymph glands to other parts of your body.

Preventing Stomach Cancer

By the time it is diagnosed, stomach cancer is usually incurable. Follow these prevention guidelines:

■ Eat fresh food. Avoid eating too many smoked, cured, fermented, or pickled foods.

■ Avoid foods—such as sausage or bacon—that have been cured with the preservative nitrate.

■ Do not smoke cigarettes, pipes, or cigars or chew tobacco.

■ Limit your alcohol intake.

■ Eat at least five servings of fruits and vegetables each day (one serving is ½ cup).

■ If you have a stomach infection caused by *Helicobacter pylori* (see p.754), take the antibiotics your doctor prescribes to eradicate the bacterium. Some experts have recommended that every person, regardless of symptoms, be tested for *H pylori* and, if the test result is positive, be treated for the infection as a way of preventing stomach cancer. This recommendation is controversial.

If all of the stomach must be removed, the surgeon attaches the bottom of the esophagus to the top portion of the small intestine. If the tumor is blocking the place where the stomach and esophagus meet, only a portion of the stomach is removed and the remaining part of the stomach is connected to the esophagus.

If the cancer obstructs the lower portion of the stomach, that portion is removed and the remaining section is attached to the duodenum (the top part of the small intestine).

If the cancer has spread, surgery may not be recommended; chemotherapy and radiation therapy (see p.741) can help shrink the tumor and relieve pain.

Vomiting Blood

Vomiting blood, known medically as hematemesis, is a frightening and serious condition that always requires immediate medical attention. The bleeding can be caused by gastritis (see p.752), a bleeding ulcer (see p.752), bleeding veins in your esophagus (see Esophageal Varices, p.751), or a tear in the lower portion of your esophagus.

Blood in vomit may appear as red streaks or larger amounts of red or brown blood. Partially digested blood may look like coffee grounds in vomit. Your doctor will use upper endoscopy (see p.745) to view your esopha-

NSAID Use and the Risk of Stomach and Intestinal Bleeding

Nonsteroidal anti-inflammatory drugs (NSAIDs), such as aspirin and ibuprofen, can damage the lining of the stomach and intestine. The injured lining can easily bleed, and bleeding can be significant enough to require hospitalization. The risk of bleeding increases with increasing doses.

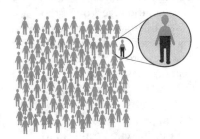

0.5 OF 100 PEOPLE WHO ARE OVER AGE 65 AND DO NOT USE NSAIDS WILL BE HOSPITALIZED FOR SEVERE STOMACH AND INTESTINAL BLEEDING WITHIN 1 YEAR

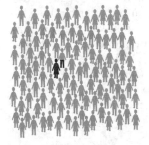

1.4 OF 100 PEOPLE WHO ARE OVER AGE 65 AND TAKE HALF THE STANDARD DOSE OF AN NSAID EVERY DAY WILL BE HOSPITALIZED FOR SEVERE STOMACH AND INTESTINAL BLEEDING WITHIN 1 YEAR

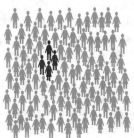

4 OF 100 PEOPLE WHO ARE OVER AGE 65 AND TAKE THREE TIMES THE STANDARD DOSE OF AN NSAID EVERY DAY WILL BE HOSPITALIZED FOR SEVERE STOMACH AND INTESTINAL BLEEDING WITHIN 1 YEAR

gus, stomach, and duodenum. Treatment depends on the cause; in severe cases, a blood transfusion may be required.

Zollinger-Ellison Syndrome

Zollinger-Ellison syndrome is a rare disorder that causes severe peptic ulcers (see p.752). The main symptoms are abdominal pain, diarrhea, yellow fat in the stools, and bleeding. The condition is caused by production of high levels of the hormone gastrin, which stimulates greatly increased acid production in the stomach. In most people, the high levels of gastrin are caused by a gastrinoma, a tumor that is often located in the pancreas or in the wall of the duodenum.

A blood test to measure your levels of gastrin and another hormone called secretin (which is also high in people with Zollinger-Ellison syndrome) can help make the diagnosis. Treatment includes acid-lowering medicines such as proton pump inhibitors and H_2-blockers, both of which decrease acid production. Surgery is performed to remove the tumor or tumors. If cancer has spread, you may also need chemotherapy (see p.741).

LIVER

Hepatitis From Drugs or Toxins

Hepatitis, or inflammation of the liver, can be caused by drugs that have direct toxic effects on the liver. The most common example is the nonprescription painkiller acetaminophen. High doses of acetaminophen, especially if mixed with three to four alcoholic drinks, can cause serious liver injury.

Other medicines that can injure the liver are methyldopa (used to lower blood pressure), isoniazid (used to treat tuberculosis), valproate (used to treat seizures), and amiodarone (used to treat irregular heart rhythms). Symptoms of toxic liver damage from drugs include nausea, vomiting, sweating, and general discomfort.

Your symptoms will determine if you need to take an antidote to the drug or will need to have your stomach pumped to rid your body of any drug that still remains in your stomach (but has not yet been absorbed into your bloodstream).

Sometimes medicines damage the liver through an unusual allergic reaction that can produce symptoms such as fever, rash, and muscle aches. In addition to the drugs listed above, the following drugs also cause allergic damage to the liver: phenytoin (used to treat seizures), chlorpromazine (used to treat psychosis), erythromycin and trimethoprim-sulfamethoxazole (antibiotics), and halothane (an anesthetic that is no longer widely used).

Acute Hepatitis

Hepatitis means inflammation of the liver. In acute hepatitis, the inflammation occurs abruptly and can cause severe symptoms. There are numerous causes, including alcohol abuse and medications (see Hepatitis From Drugs or Toxins, left), but most acute hepatitis is caused by the hepatitis viruses discussed below.

Hepatitis B or C can lead to more chronic liver disease and sometimes liver failure. Otherwise, acute viral hepatitis usually goes away on its own.

Hepatitis A is the most common of the hepatitis viruses and the least serious. An estimated 50% of Americans have been infected with hepatitis A at some time and, as a result, are immune to it and carry antibodies to it. The virus is more common in areas where standards of sanitation and hygiene are poor. Infected people temporarily carry the virus in their blood and shed it in their bowel movements.

During the brief infectious period (which usually lasts 6 days to 6 weeks), the virus can spread. Transmission is usually through the ingestion of food or water that has been contaminated by infected fecal material. It can also be spread by eating shellfish that has not been properly cooked. Recovery usually takes 1 or 2 months. In rare cases (usually in people over 40), hepatitis A virus infection can lead to acute liver failure (see p.764) and even death. However, in most people, recovery is complete.

Hepatitis B is transmitted by infected blood (usually through blood transfusions and needles shared by intravenous drug abusers), sexual contact with infected semen, and, possibly, contact with infected saliva. Babies can become infected at birth if the mother is infected. Health care workers and people who work in institutions that house high-risk individuals are also vulnerable to the virus.

Some people who become infected with the virus never develop hepatitis and never become ill from it. Others develop mild to severe cases. On occasion, hepatitis B infection can cause acute liver failure (see p.764). It usually takes 1 to 4 months to recover from the initial attack of hepatitis. A substantial number of people become carriers or develop chronic hepatitis (see p.762), and some of these people develop cirrhosis and chronic liver failure.

When infants become infected with the hepatitis B virus at birth, there is a 90% chance that they will develop chronic hepatitis later in life. In contrast, if healthy young adults become infected with the hepatitis B virus, there is only about a 1% chance that they will develop chronic hepatitis.

Hepatitis C, once referred to as non-A, non-B hepatitis, is spread in the same way as hepatitis B, although there is controversy over how easily it can be spread by sexual contact. Many people infected with the hepatitis C virus do not develop acute hepatitis. Others develop hepatitis that can be very severe but that rarely leads to acute liver failure (see p.764). People with the acute form of the illness recover within 3 to 4 months.

More than 50% of people with a hepatitis C virus infection develop chronic hepatitis (see p.762) and some develop cirrhosis and chronic liver failure and/or liver cancer. An estimated 3.9 million Americans have chronic hepatitis from the hepatitis C virus (worldwide, 70 million people are infected).

In the United States, 10,000 people each year die of chronic liver disease from the hepatitis C virus. Some are or were intravenous drug users. Others were infected from blood transfusions they received before 1990 (before the virus was discovered and blood was tested for the virus).

The risk of hepatitis C seems to be higher among those with immune deficiencies, such as people who have had organ transplants and who have acquired immunodeficiency syndrome (AIDS).

Hepatitis D is a virus that by itself cannot cause hepatitis or other diseases. But when someone is infected with both the hepatitis B virus and the hepatitis D virus, a severe form of acute hepatitis usually develops. Hepatitis D appears to be transmitted through close personal contact rather than exposure to blood.

Hepatitis E is a virus similar to hepatitis A but is very rare in the United States. It can be very dangerous to pregnant women, about 20% of whom develop life-threatening destruction of the liver with hepatitis E.

SYMPTOMS

There is an incubation period between the time you become infected with a hepatitis virus

---

Interferon in the Treatment of Hepatitis B Virus Infection

Some people who are infected with the hepatitis B virus cannot eliminate the virus from the liver on their own. These people are at increased risk of cirrhosis and liver cancer. Interferon is a medication that stimulates the immune system to fight the virus. Several studies have examined the effectiveness of interferon in the treatment of hepatitis B. Although interferon may successfully treat the infection in some people, it is unclear if interferon will decrease the risk of developing cirrhosis or liver cancer.

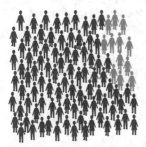

88 OF 100 PEOPLE WHO HAVE CHRONIC HEPATITIS B AND DO NOT TAKE INTERFERON CONTINUE TO HAVE DETECTABLE INFECTION AFTER 1 YEAR

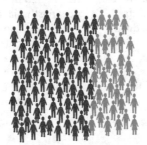

67 OF 100 PEOPLE WHO HAVE CHRONIC HEPATITIS B AND TAKE INTERFERON FOR 3 MONTHS CONTINUE TO HAVE DETECTABLE INFECTION AFTER 1 YEAR

Viewing the Liver, Pancreas, Gallbladder, and Bile Ducts

Physicians use a number of techniques to help diagnose and treat diseases of the liver, pancreas, gallbladder, and bile ducts. This chart describes the procedures that enable a clear view of these internal structures. Tests are performed in a hospital, clinic, or doctor's office, usually by a radiologist, who is an expert in performing diagnostic imaging procedures and interpreting the results.

PROCEDURE	WHY IT IS PERFORMED	WHAT TO EXPECT
Ultrasound (see p.148)	To see obstructions of the bile ducts (such as stones or tumors) and view the gallbladder and its contents.	After fasting, you will lie down on a table and a clear gel will be smoothed over your abdomen to improve contact with the probe. The probe (which gives off high-frequency, echo-producing sound waves) will be passed over your abdomen while the images made by the echoes are viewed on a video screen.
Computed tomography (CT) (see p.149)	To see tumors of the bile ducts, liver, or pancreas and inflammation of the pancreas and to view the liver and spleen.	After (usually) fasting for 12 hours, you may be asked to drink a solution that will enhance the image made by the scanner. You will lie very still on a table in a tunnel-like device as a camera rotates around you.
Magnetic resonance (see p.151) cholangio-pancreatography	To provide pictures of the bile ducts and ducts of the pancreas and to view the liver, bile ducts, and pancreas.	You will lie inside a tunnel-like device, surrounded by a large magnet. A camera will take pictures of the inside of your body.
Percutaneous transhepatic cholangiography	To provide pictures of the bile ducts, to view the bile duct system, and to perform biopsies and surgical procedures (such as removing stones stuck in a bile duct).	After fasting, you will lie down on a slanted x-ray table and a needle will be placed into a vein in your hand or arm to deliver a sedative and other medicine. Guided by ultrasound (see p.140) and using local anesthesia, a flexible needle will be inserted through the skin over your liver and placed into a bile duct. A contrast medium (see p.139) will be injected into the bile duct and x-rays taken. You may have a feeling of fullness. You will need to stay in bed for at least 6 hours after the procedure so your doctor can ensure there has been no bleeding or infection caused by the procedure.

PROCEDURE	WHY IT IS PERFORMED	WHAT TO EXPECT
Endoscopic retrograde cholangio-pancreatography	To see obstructions (such as stones or tumors) and inflammation of the bile ducts and pancreatic ducts, to view the opening into the intestines of the bile duct and pancreatic duct, and to perform biopsies and surgical procedures (such as removing stones stuck in a bile duct).	After fasting for up to 12 hours, an intravenous tube will be placed into a vein in your hand or arm to deliver medicines. An anesthetic spray will be used to numb the back of your throat and an endoscope will be inserted through your mouth and down into your esophagus, stomach, and duodenum. Air will be pumped in to inflate the intestines so the doctor can locate the opening of the main bile duct and pancreatic duct. A small hollow tube (catheter) will be inserted into the opening of the ducts and a dye will be injected so that the ducts show up on x-rays; instruments may be passed into the ducts.
Liver biopsy	To obtain a sample of liver tissue for microscopic examination to look for evidence of hepatitis, cirrhosis, liver cancer, abscesses, or Kaposi sarcoma.	Using local anesthesia, a needle will be inserted through the skin and into the liver. The needle tip may be guided to the diseased part by ultrasound or CT. Alternately, a small incision will be made near the navel and an endoscope (see p.142) will be placed inside the abdomen to view the surface of the liver.

Ultrasound of the Gallbladder

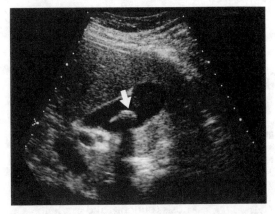

This ultrasound scan shows the gallbladder as a clear, black, oval space with a large, round, white area (arrow), indicating a gallstone.

Cancer of the Pancreas

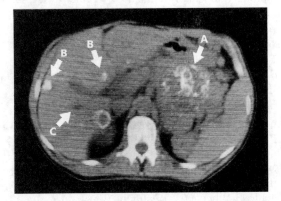

In this computed tomography scan, there is a large tumor in the pancreas (A). The tumor has irregular edges and contains calcium (white area). The tumor has spread to the liver, which is on the left. Small white spots (B) and the clear spot (C) are areas in the liver to which the pancreatic cancer has spread.

and the time you first develop symptoms of acute hepatitis. This incubation period varies depending on the virus: hepatitis A, 6 days to 6 weeks; hepatitis B, 4 to 12 weeks; and hepatitis C, on average, 7 weeks.

Symptoms of acute hepatitis are general and easy to confuse with other conditions; they include loss of energy and appetite, nausea, vomiting, itchy skin, abdominal pain (in the upper right portion of the abdomen), fever, and tea-colored urine.

These symptoms are followed by jaundice (yellowing of the whites of the eyes and skin) and sometimes weight loss. In rare cases, symptoms are very severe and life-threatening (see Acute Liver Failure, p.764).

Some people with hepatitis B or hepatitis C virus infection have no symptoms or very mild symptoms of acute hepatitis at first, but then, years later, develop symptoms of chronic hepatitis (see right).

TREATMENT OPTIONS

Symptoms (particularly sudden jaundice) make a diagnosis of hepatitis very likely, but blood tests are necessary to establish it. Blood tests of liver enzymes can reveal the widespread death of liver cells, a central feature of any kind of hepatitis. Other blood tests can detect known hepatitis-causing viruses and can help your doctor determine the prognosis (outlook).

There is no specific treatment of acute viral hepatitis. Treatment is aimed at helping you feel more comfortable. Although it is not necessary for recovery, you may feel better if you rest in bed. A

high-calorie diet may be prescribed, with the majority of food eaten in the morning to prevent nausea later in the day. If you have recurring vomiting, you may need to be fed intravenously. (See also Chronic Hepatitis, below.)

Chronic Hepatitis

Chronic hepatitis (inflammation of the liver) can follow infection with the hepatitis B, C, and D viruses (see p.759). It can also occur as an autoimmune disease (see p.870).

Chronic viral hepatitis infection can be very serious, leading to cirrhosis (see p.765). In some people, it leads to liver cancer. Chronic hepatitis C is almost as common as alcoholism in causing cirrhosis of the liver. Chronic hepatitis B accounts for about 10% of all cases of liver disease and cirrhosis.

Autoimmune hepatitis is an autoimmune disease in which the immune system mistakenly attacks its own liver cells. It is primarily a disease of young women, although it affects men and people of all ages.

SYMPTOMS

The symptoms of chronic hepatitis are like those of cirrhosis (see p.765).

DETERMINING THE SEVERITY OF CHRONIC HEPATITIS

Because hepatitis may cause no symptoms in the early stages, chronic hepatitis is often discovered accidentally through a blood test for another reason. To confirm suspicions of hepatitis and help direct the course of treat-

ment, your doctor will perform blood tests, some of which may reveal that the liver is functioning poorly. Others can show that scarring is gradually obstructing the small bile ducts. Still other blood tests can reveal the virus that may be causing the chronic hepatitis.

In the case of hepatitis B virus, blood tests can make an important distinction. If people have antibodies against the virus in their blood, they are not contagious and are unlikely to have chronic hepatitis. However, if they have parts of the virus circulating in their blood (substances called surface antigen and E antigen, or the actual DNA of the virus), they are contagious.

Some people who have parts of the virus circulating in their blood have chronic hepatitis and are contagious. Others carry the surface antigen and E antigen in their blood but do not yet have hepatitis. These people are hepatitis B carriers and, although they are not ill, they can still transmit the virus to others. Knowing the results of different tests is important when making decisions about your treatment and in preventing the spread of the infection.

The severity of chronic hepatitis is best determined by a liver biopsy (see p.761). A microscopic view reveals the extent of the damage to liver cells and the amount of scarring and can help estimate how active the hepatitis B virus is. A liver biopsy is often needed to get an accurate prognosis (outlook) and can help determine your treatment. Biopsies may need to be repeated over time to detect changes in

Preventing Hepatitis A and B

You can prevent infection with hepatitis A virus and hepatitis B virus. Effective vaccines are available that, within a few weeks, produce long-lasting immunity to hepatitis viruses A and B.

If you have been exposed to someone who has had an active infection of either hepatitis A or B, you need immediate protection. A blood product called immune globulin has antibodies that will temporarily provide protection. Specific recommendations are as follows:

HEPATITIS A

VACCINE SHOULD BE GIVEN TO:

- Anyone traveling to parts of the world where hepatitis A virus is common (the vaccine must be started several months in advance)

- Anyone often exposed to the virus or stool specimens (such as day care workers or medical laboratory workers)

IMMUNE GLOBULIN SHOULD BE GIVEN TO:

- Anyone in close contact with someone who has been diagnosed within the past 2 weeks (close contact includes kissing, sexual relations, sharing food preparation tasks, eating from the same plates or utensils, or sharing the same bathroom)

LIFESTYLE CHANGES

- Avoid sharing plates, utensils, or bathrooms with someone who has an active infection

- If you are traveling to parts of the world where the virus is prevalent, do not eat any uncooked or partially cooked food or drink possibly contaminated water

HEPATITIS B

VACCINE SHOULD BE GIVEN TO:

- All infants
- All unvaccinated children under age 18
- Anyone whose skin has been pierced by a needle, razor, or other possibly contaminated instrument
- Anyone who has had sexual contact with someone who has had hepatitis B
- Any baby born to a woman who has had hepatitis B (the baby can be immunized immediately after birth)
- Anyone whose work, travel, or status increases their exposure to the hepatitis B virus, such as health care workers exposed to

blood; residents (including prison inmates) and staff of custodial institutions; intravenous drug abusers; hemophiliacs or others who frequently need blood products; household or sexual contacts of people who have had hepatitis B or come from parts of the world where it is prevalent; or travelers to parts of the world where the virus is prevalent (the vaccine must be started several months in advance)

IMMUNE GLOBULIN SHOULD BE GIVEN TO:

- Any baby born to a woman who has had hepatitis B (the baby can be immunized immediately after birth)

- Anyone who has had his or her skin pierced by a needle, razor, or other possibly contaminated instrument

- Anyone who has sexual contact with someone who has had hepatitis

LIFESTYLE CHANGES

- Do not share any possibly contaminated object that could penetrate the skin and/or could have come in contact with blood such as a needle, razor, or toothbrush

- If you are having sexual relations with an infected person, be sure to use a condom

Risks of Hepatitis C Infection

Most people infected with the hepatitis C virus eventually develop chronic liver diseases.

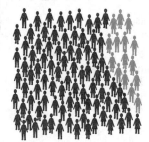 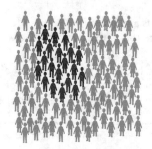 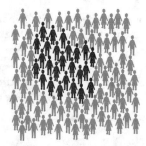

85 OF 100 PEOPLE WHO HAVE HEPATITIS C DEVELOP CHRONIC HEPATITIS

20 OF 100 PEOPLE WHO HAVE CHRONIC HEPATITIS DEVELOP CIRRHOSIS WITHIN 20 YEARS

25 OF 100 PEOPLE WHO HAVE CIRRHOSIS DEVELOP LIVER CANCER WITHIN 20 YEARS

---

your liver and therefore in your prognosis and treatment.

TREATMENT OPTIONS

The most often used treatment for chronic hepatitis from hepatitis B or C infection is interferon alfa plus ribavirin. One of two kinds of interferon (called "pegylated and nonpegylated") is used. About half the people who take interferon alfa receive some benefit. It can cause a variety of side effects, including fatigue, fevers, autoimmune thyroiditis (see p.850), difficulty concentrating, and emotional disturbances.

In people with hepatitis B infection, interferon is most helpful in those with chronic hepatitis that has been verified by a liver biopsy, very abnormal liver enzymes (called aminotransferases), and low levels of the virus in the blood. Adding lamivudine to the interferon appears to be beneficial.

Interferon alfa is recommended for many people with chronic

hepatitis C infection, although success in eradicating the infection is not as great as with hepatitis B infection.

A lower dose of interferon is effective for treating hepatitis C (a higher dose is needed to treat hepatitis B), which means that adverse effects from treatment are less severe. The antiviral agent ribavirin may help improve the outlook in chronic hepatitis C infection.

In people with hepatitis C infection, those under the age of 45 who have had the disease for less than 5 years and do not yet show evidence of cirrhosis are most likely to respond to interferon alfa. As many as 50% of people can benefit from interferon treatment.

Autoimmune hepatitis is difficult to diagnose and is usually diagnosed by excluding other possible diagnoses. Blood tests may help make the diagnosis. When injury to the liver is severe, the disease can be life-

threatening. Corticosteroid drugs are the main treatment, although immunosuppressive agents may be used as well.

Acute Liver Failure

Acute liver failure strikes previously healthy people suddenly. In both acute and chronic liver failure (see Cirrhosis, next article), there is injury to or death of the liver cells, which make necessary proteins and remove toxins from the circulation.

The causes of acute liver failure include:

■ Hepatitis A, B, D, and E and possibly C

■ Hepatitis from the herpes simplex virus, which can occur with chemotherapy and with immunosuppressive therapy (during a transplant) because these treatments make the immune system more vulnerable to infection with the herpes simplex virus

- Toxicity from normal doses of acetaminophen when it is taken with another medicine or with large amounts of alcohol or taken while fasting

- Acetaminophen overdose

- Allergic reactions to some medicines, most commonly: halothane (an anesthetic); sulfonamide, tetracycline, and amoxicillin-clavulanic acid (antibiotics); quinidine and procainamide (heart rhythm–normalizing drugs); phenytoin (used to treat seizures); isoniazid (used to treat tuberculosis); estradiol (used to treat menopausal symptoms); methyldopa (used to treat hypertension); and disulfiram (used to treat alcohol abuse)

- Poisoning from herbs, solvents, and some mushrooms (specifically *Amanita phalloides*)

- Heatstroke

- Wilson disease (from the excessive accumulation of copper in the liver)

- Pregnancy

- Reye syndrome (see p.1017)

SYMPTOMS

In acute liver failure, the changes are sudden and dramatic. Within 2 to 10 days, the affected person can go from feeling healthy to being comatose. The initial symptoms are general discomfort and nausea, soon followed by jaundice (yellowing of the whites of the eyes and skin) and change in mental status (encephalopathy) such as agitation or delusions.

If liver function recovers, brain function also usually returns to normal, although some people suffer permanent damage. Other symptoms include sweating, a feeling of faintness, a tendency to bleed or bruise easily, and excessive thirst.

TREATMENT OPTIONS

The diagnosis of acute liver failure often is obvious from the person's symptoms. Blood tests reveal that the liver is failing to make essential substances (such as albumin and blood-clotting factors) and that toxins are building up in the blood.

Treatment depends on the cause. When acute liver failure is caused by a viral infection, antiviral treatments are of little use. When it is caused by an acetaminophen overdose or poisoning from mushrooms, antidotes can be given. Ulcer-preventing drugs are given to reduce stress-related ulcers that can occur with liver failure.

Coma may be treated with blood or plasma transfusions to detoxify the blood. Liver transplantation (see p.767) may be the only option for people at risk of dying.

Cirrhosis

In cirrhosis, or chronic liver failure, there is irreversible injury to and scarring of the liver. Chronic liver failure proceeds more slowly than acute liver failure but has a worse outlook.

Liver cells are slowly damaged and therefore the function of the liver becomes slowly impaired. Essential substances made by the liver such as albumin and blood-clotting factors slowly drop, and toxic substances that normally are rendered nontoxic by the liver slowly build up.

Scarring obstructs the flow of blood through the liver, which causes portal hypertension (increased pressure in the main vein of the liver) and bleeding into the digestive tract.

Cirrhosis of the liver can result from many conditions. In the United States and Europe, the most common cause is heavy alcohol use. Liver disease caused by alcohol starts with a buildup of fat inside liver cells. It progresses to the death of many liver cells through repeated periods of alcoholic hepatitis and, finally, leads to scarring.

The amount of alcohol needed to induce liver damage differs among people. In general, it takes a lower daily intake of alcohol to produce cirrhosis in a woman than it does in a man.

A variety of other diseases that cause ongoing injury to and inflammation of the liver can also lead to cirrhosis. Examples include chronic viral hepatitis (see p.762); chronic liver infection from microorganisms (other than viruses) usually found in the tropics, such as bacteria or parasites; and several inherited diseases, including cystic fibrosis (see p.1003), antitrypsin deficiency, hemochromatosis (excess iron accumulation), and Wilson disease (excess copper accumulation).

More rarely, autoimmune diseases (see p.870)—in which the immune system attacks the bile ducts, liver cells, or the channels that transport bile from the liver to the intestines—cause cirrhosis.

Rare allergic reactions to certain medicines—including oral

contraceptives, isoniazid, and methyldopa—can also lead to cirrhosis. In some people, the cause is never determined.

SYMPTOMS

In chronic liver failure, you may not feel any symptoms for many years as the liver becomes slowly but increasingly disabled from progressive injury to the liver cells, and becomes deformed from scarring.

The initial symptoms are usually fatigue, weakness, and exhaustion followed by a loss of appetite and weight. You may have mild jaundice (yellowing of the whites of the eyes and skin). Easy bleeding and bruising occur because the proteins needed to clot blood are not being produced in sufficient quantities.

Your skin may itch due to the buildup of toxins. You become more sensitive to the effects of certain drugs that are normally cleared by the liver. Toxins start to build up, causing brain changes (see Acute Liver Failure, p.764).

In advanced stages of the disease, the skin may become yellow due to jaundice, and gallstones may form. In addition, because of increased pressure in the main vein of the liver (the portal vein) caused by scarring, veins in the stomach and esophagus become swollen. These swollen veins, called varices, are fragile and are prone to bursting (see Esophageal Varices, p.751), which can cause life-threatening bleeding.

Low blood levels of albumin, an essential protein made by a healthy liver, cause fluid to leak from the blood into the body's tissues, causing swelling, particu-larly in the legs. Because of the low albumin and increased portal vein pressure, fluid starts to pool in the abdomen, which becomes enlarged.

This pool of fluid (called ascites) in the abdomen also can become infected from bacteria circulating in the bloodstream, which can be life-threatening. Muscles begin to shrink and the arms and thighs become progressively thinner.

TREATMENT OPTIONS

Doctors often suspect a diagnosis of chronic liver failure based on symptoms and physical examination. The symptoms include some degree of confusion, poor appetite, and nausea. In the early stages of cirrhosis, the liver is enlarged; in later stages, it is shrunken and bumpy. The doctor can detect these changes in the size and shape of the liver by physical examination.

The examination can reveal other clues that can indicate underlying liver failure, including jaundice (yellowing of the whites of the eyes and the skin), tiny blood vessels that look like spiders on the surface of the skin, and an uncontrollable tremor of the hands.

Blood tests may show that the liver is not making adequate amounts of certain essential substances (such as albumin and blood-clotting factors), that toxins (such as ammonia) are building up in the blood, or that the bile ducts are being blocked by scarring. This provides additional strong evidence of a diagnosis of chronic liver failure.

Cirrhosis can also be indicated by various tests that take pictures of the liver—including computed tomography (see p.760), ultrasound (see p.760), and radionuclide scanning (see p.137). Diagnosing cirrhosis may require a liver biopsy (see p.761), which reveals both damage to liver cells and scarring throughout the liver.

The damage to the liver cannot be reversed, but further injury can be prevented. Treatment aims at correcting the conditions that cause the disease, such as eliminating alcohol.

Other treatments are directed at relieving symptoms and reducing complications. Your doctor may prescribe diuretics to help relieve water retention and laxatives to hasten the removal of toxic substances from the large intestine. Liver transplantation (see p.767) may be necessary if other options are not helpful.

Liver Cancer

Cancers that have started in other organs—particularly the gastrointestinal tract, breasts, and lungs—often spread (metastasize) to the liver, where they start to grow. The liver is vulnerable to metastatic cancer because of its large size and the large amount of blood that flows through it.

Cancer that originates in the liver, called primary liver cancer, is becoming more frequent in the United States. There are two types of primary liver cancer—hepatoma and cholangiocarcinoma.

Hepatoma develops in the liver cells and is more common in men who have long-term liver disease (see Cirrhosis, p.765; Hepatitis B, p.759; Hepatitis C, p.759) and who are older than 50.

Cholangiocarcinoma develops

Liver Transplantation

Advances in surgical technique and follow-up care, as well as more sophisticated methods of preserving donor organs, have made liver transplantation feasible in the past 15 years.

However, a scarcity of donor livers means that many people die waiting for a transplant (see Organ and Whole Body Donation, p.1143).

Livers for transplantation are usually obtained from people who have died of a head injury, are younger than 60, have healthy livers, and have a compatible blood type and liver size.

Today, liver transplantation prolongs life for longer than 5 years in 70% of recipients. It is a delicate and arduous surgery that is recommended only for children and adults with severe liver disease that would otherwise be fatal, seriously life-limiting, or progress to cause irreversible brain damage.

At the same time, the individual must be healthy enough to survive the physically taxing surgery and recovery period. Children who receive transplants often have been born with a defective liver.

Conditions that warrant liver transplantation in adults include:

- Cirrhosis of the liver (see p.765)
- Sclerosing cholangitis (a rare form of inflammation of the bile ducts)
- Hepatic vein thrombosis (blockage)
- Severe, acute, life-threatening hepatitis (see p.758)
- Chronic viral hepatitis (see p.762)
- Cancers that originate in the liver (see p.766)

The procedure usually takes place in a major medical center and can take up to 10 hours. For a transplant, you receive a general anesthetic (see p.168), your abdomen is opened, and all or part of the liver is removed and replaced with the necessary parts of the donor organ. Recovery can take up to 4 months. The support of family and health care aides is vital.

Transplant recipients must take immunosuppressive drugs for the rest of their lives to inhibit the body's natural propensity to reject the foreign tissue from the transplanted liver. The repertoire of immunosuppressive agents, and medicines to prevent infection, is expanding, contributing to a brighter outlook.

in the bile ducts and tends to affect young adults without chronic liver disease; it is more common in people with ulcerative colitis (see Inflammatory Bowel Disease, p.787).

SYMPTOMS

In its early stages, liver cancer often causes no symptoms. Pain in the upper right portion of the abdomen is among the first specific symptoms, along with fatigue, weight loss, and loss of appetite. Jaundice (yellowing of the whites of the eyes and skin)

and the development of fluid that swells the abdomen are symptoms of more advanced disease.

TREATMENT OPTIONS

Suspicions of liver cancer are confirmed or ruled out by tests to examine the liver, such as ultrasound (see p.760), computed tomography (see p.760), magnetic resonance imaging (see p.151), magnetic resonance angiography (see p.147) of the hepatic artery, and a liver biopsy (see p.761).

Blood tests to see how well the liver is functioning may also be performed. Other blood tests to look for proteins that are made by primary liver cancers, or by cancers that start in the large intestine and often spread to the liver, may also be performed. Sometimes, to determine the stage of the cancer, you may need to have conventional or laparoscopic surgery so your doctor can evaluate how far the cancer has spread.

With primary liver tumors that have not yet spread outside the liver, it is sometimes possible for surgery to remove all of the tumor, offering a hope of cure. More often with primary liver tumors, and nearly always with secondary liver tumors, surgical removal of the tumor is performed only when the tumor is blocking a vital structure such as the bile duct. Liver transplantation (see p.767) is rarely an option and only then if the cancer has not spread outside the liver, which is not usually the case.

Chemotherapy (see p.741) can be injected (through a catheter) directly into the artery that provides the blood supply to the tumor. In this way, higher concentrations of the toxic medicine can be applied to the tumor, and lower concentrations circulate elsewhere in the body. Radiation and other newer procedures are also available to reduce pain.

Gilbert Syndrome

Gilbert syndrome is an inherited disorder in which bilirubin, the yellowish-orange pigment in bile, is not processed correctly. A type of bilirubin called unconjugated bilirubin builds up in the blood because the liver has a diminished ability to process it into conjugated bilirubin. The raised levels of unconjugated bilirubin can be detected on blood tests.

From 3% to 10% of the general population has Gilbert syndrome. Most people with this condition have no symptoms, rarely have visible jaundice (yellowing of the whites of the eyes and skin), and have nothing to worry about.

Gilbert syndrome has no adverse effects on health. In the few people whose jaundice is visible, the drug phenobarbital can reduce the bilirubin level and eliminate the visible jaundice.

Liver Abscess

An abscess is a collection of pus encased in a thin membrane. An abscess of the liver is usually caused either by bacteria that travel from infection in the intestines (a consequence of appendicitis or diverticulitis) or by amebiasis, an infection with a parasite. The abscess can cause a high fever, chills, nausea, vomiting, pain in the upper right portion of the abdomen (where the liver is), and weight loss.

Suspicions of a liver abscess can usually be confirmed by ultrasound (see p.760) or computed tomography (see p.760) of the liver. Blood tests may reveal the infecting bacteria, or samples of the pus may be collected by using ultrasound to guide a needle to the site of the abscess to remove a sample. A similar procedure is used to drain the abscess. Intravenous antibiotics are given to treat the infection.

PANCREAS

Acute Pancreatitis

Pancreatitis is inflammation of the pancreas, the large gland behind the stomach. Between 50,000 and 80,000 people have acute pancreatitis each year.

The pancreas serves two vital functions: it secretes digestive enzymes that break down food and it secretes hormones (primarily insulin and glucagon) that regulate the amount of glucose (sugar) in your blood. In pancreatitis, the digestive enzymes that the pancreas normally secretes into the intestine start to attack and digest the pancreas itself.

The most common causes of pancreatitis are gallstones (see p.770) that get stuck in the pancreatic ducts and alcohol. Less often, pancreatitis is caused by medicines, including acetaminophen, sulfonamides, or thiazide and furosemide diuretics.

A severe blow to the abdomen or any kind of diagnostic or surgical procedure in the abdomen can also cause pancreatitis, as can viral infections such as mumps and hepatitis. Rarely, a person is born with an abnormally shaped duct leading out of the pancreas, which can lead to pancreatitis.

A first attack of pancreatitis is often followed by complete recovery but can lead to severe complications and death. Repeated attacks (or a very severe first attack) can lead to chronic pancreatitis (see p.769), scarring of the pancreas, and reduced production of digestive enzymes and hormones.

Sometimes repeated attacks cause the formation of large cysts (pseudocysts) that contain digestive enzymes. If these pseudocysts rupture and spill their contents into the abdomen, serious consequences, such as peritonitis (see p.801), can result.

SYMPTOMS

Most acute attacks last only a few days, but severe bouts may last longer. The primary symptom is sudden severe pain in the upper portion of the abdomen, often accompanied by nausea and vomiting. However, the nature of the pain varies from person to person. In many people, the pain is severe, radiates to the back, and is constant.

The pain may grow in severity and is made worse by eating. You may notice that your abdomen is swollen and tender. You may also feel nauseated and vomit. In severe cases, you become dehydrated and your blood pressure may drop so precipitously that you feel faint.

Multiple organ failure (such as of the heart, lungs, or kidneys) may occur and, if bleeding or infection develops, you may go into shock.

TREATMENT OPTIONS

While you are having an attack, your doctor may take blood to monitor the level of pancreatic enzymes, which are released into the bloodstream during an attack. Concentrations of magnesium, calcium, sodium, potassium, and bicarbonate may be abnormal during an attack of pancreatitis. Your blood sugar and lipid levels (cholesterol and other fats) will also rise. Your doctor may also perform ultrasound (see p.760) or computed tomography (see p.760) to help diagnose the problem.

Treatment depends on the severity of your attack. Although acute pancreatitis usually heals on its own, you may be admitted to the hospital to receive intravenous fluids and painkillers. You will not be permitted to eat because food causes the pancreas to produce digestive enzymes, which worsens pancreatitis.

If your attack is caused by gallstones, the stones often get stuck in the duct of the pancreas only temporarily and then pass into the stools. If this does not occur, you may need to have your bile duct opened and the stone removed using endoscopic retrograde cholangiopancreatography (see p.761). The gallbladder may need to be removed at a later time.

If your pancreatitis is caused by drinking alcohol, you must stop immediately to allow the pancreas to heal; you should stop permanently. You will have recurring attacks of pancreatitis if you continue drinking, which, in turn, can lead to chronic pancreatitis (see below) and permanent damage.

Chronic Pancreatitis

In chronic pancreatitis, severe or recurring inflammation of the pancreas has caused permanent damage to the pancreas. Alcohol abuse is responsible for about 90% of cases of chronic pancreatitis.

Other causes include gallstones, some medicines, inherited abnormalities in the shape of the ducts (tubes) of the pancreas, and mutations in a particular gene.

In chronic pancreatitis, inadequate digestive enzymes are produced, leading to impaired digestion and slowly progressive nutritional deficiencies. Deficient production of hormones, particularly insulin, can lead to diabetes mellitus (see p.832).

SYMPTOMS

It may take many years of alcohol abuse before symptoms of chronic pancreatitis surface. There is often constant abdominal pain. Recurring attacks of acute pancreatitis (see p.768), with severe pain and other symptoms, may also occur, though they become progressively less frequent and less severe as each attack permanently damages more of the pancreas.

Nutritional deficiencies and diabetes can lead to weight loss and symptoms of vitamin deficiency (particularly of vitamin B_{12}). Bowel movements become yellow, foul-smelling, and float because they contain undigested fat.

TREATMENT OPTIONS

Report any persistent abdominal pain to your doctor. To identify abnormalities in your pancreas, he or she may perform one or more imaging tests, including ultrasound (see p.760), endoscopic retrograde cholangiopancreatography (see p.761), and computed tomography (see p.760).

Treatment includes analgesics to relieve pain, insulin if needed, and pancreatic enzymes taken as a medicine to help you digest food normally. If you drink alcohol, you must stop (see p.65). Sometimes repeated attacks of acute pancreatitis cause the formation of large cysts (pseudocysts) that contain digestive enzymes. Surgery or endoscopy (see p.142) may be needed to drain a pancreatic pseudocyst or to remove part or all of the pancreas.

Cancer of the Pancreas

Cancer that starts in the pancreas is of two types. Cancers of the pancreatic ducts (adenocarcinomas) constitute more than 90% of cases; the remaining cancers are tumors of cells (most commonly the insulin-producing cells) that make hormones. Pancreatic cancer is almost exclusively a disease of older people, and the incidence of this disease is rising as people live longer.

Cigarette smoking and chronic pancreatitis (see p.769) may be contributing factors. Because the initial symptoms are subtle, pancreatic cancer often spreads significantly before it is diagnosed. The outlook is poor.

SYMPTOMS

Vague abdominal discomfort is often the only symptom of pancreatic cancer as the tumor develops. Another symptom is gnawing pain, radiating from the abdomen to the back, that improves when you bend forward. Your appetite becomes poor, and you begin to lose weight.

Most pancreatic tumors affect the head of the pancreas. When they grow larger, they can block the outflow of bile from the liver and bile ducts into the intestine. This causes bilirubin, an orange-yellow pigment, to build up in the body. Jaundice (yellowing of the whites of the eyes and skin), itching, brown urine, and very light, clay-colored bowel movements follow. By the time you become jaundiced, the tumor usually has grown very large.

In people with tumors of hormone-producing cells, the symptoms depend on the hormone that is overproduced. Most often, excessive amounts of insulin are produced, leading to low blood sugar levels and faintness, confusion, trembling, and sweating.

TREATMENT OPTIONS

If your doctor suspects pancreatic cancer, he or she will perform a number of tests, including blood tests for tumor markers (proteins produced by tumors that circulate in the blood).

Although ultrasound (see p.760) and computed tomography (CT) (see p.760) are the mainstays for identifying pancreatic cancer and determining how advanced the tumor is, both methods can miss cancers.

Other tests include endoscopic retrograde cholangiopancreatography (ERCP) (see p.761), which also permits biopsy of the tumor and relief of any blockage. Doctors sometimes use CT to guide a delicate needle to the pancreas to collect cells, which are then examined under a microscope to determine if they are cancerous.

Removal of all or part of the pancreas is the only treatment; it is beneficial only in the few people who have been diagnosed before the cancer spreads. The likelihood of recurrence is high and is more likely to occur if cancer cells are found in nearby lymph nodes or if the tumor has spread to adjacent tissue.

Radiation therapy and chemotherapy may be used to shrink the tumors or treat them after surgery, but these treatments do not extend a person's life. Placing stiff tubes (stents) in the bile duct using ERCP can significantly improve the quality of life without surgery.

GALLBLADDER AND BILE DUCTS

Gallbladder Disease

The gallbladder normally is a way station that receives bile from the liver and then contracts during meals to eject the bile into the intestines to aid in digestion.

Sometimes the liquid bile crystallizes as it sits in the gallbladder, forming small stones that grow larger. Most stones develop when the amount of cholesterol is disproportionately greater than the other components of bile. About 10% of adult Americans have gallstones, although many never have problems or symptoms.

Symptoms develop when a gallstone, chemicals in the bile, or bacterial infection irritate the wall of the gallbladder, causing inflammation (a condition called cholecystitis), or when stones leave the gallbladder and travel into and block the cystic duct, the main bile duct, or the pancreatic duct.

Several conditions appear to increase the risk of gallstones:

Being female Estrogen increases cholesterol in the bile. Normal levels of estrogens, sometimes augmented by the estrogens in oral contraceptives or hormone replacement therapy, make women more likely to form gallstones.

Being pregnant Women who have had several pregnancies are especially susceptible.

Being obese Being extremely overweight increases the risk for women but not for men.

Undergoing rapid weight loss Diets with an intake of fewer than 500 calories daily raise the risk of gallstones by 20%.

Having gallstones slightly increases the risk of gallbladder cancer (see p.773), especially if the gallstones are large.

Chronic cholecystitis is long-standing irritation and inflammation of the gallbladder wall from the presence of gallstones and low-grade infections. It may produce no symptoms or minimal symptoms for many years, but, ultimately, people who have chronic cholecystitis will have an attack of acute cholecystitis, in which pain is sudden and severe.

Acalculous cholecystitis is a less common subtype (10% of cases) of acute inflammation in which the gallbladder becomes inflamed in the absence of gallstones. It seems to happen more often in people who are seriously ill from some other cause such as an injury, a major operation, severe burns, or diabetes and in women who have had a long labor before childbirth.

SYMPTOMS

Pain in the upper right portion of the abdomen is the most common symptom of cholecystitis. In acute cholecystitis, the pain is sudden and intense and may become more noticeable when you inhale deeply or when you move abruptly. The pain often radiates to the back of the right shoulder, but it can remain isolated to the abdomen.

You may also feel nauseated and vomit, lose your appetite, and have a fever. Many people who have acute attacks report that they felt the same type of pain before, but that it disappeared on its own. Possibly these previous attacks involved passing small stones that caused only temporary blockage.

Jaundice (yellowing of the whites of the eyes and skin), dark urine, and pale bowel movements can occur, particularly when a stone blocks the bile duct. High

Symptoms and Frequency of Gallstones

Gallstones are very common and usually do not cause symptoms. However, once a person with gallstones develops abdominal pain, nausea, or vomiting, these symptoms often continue to recur.

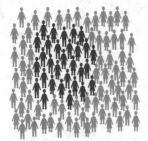

30 OF 100 WOMEN DEVELOP GALLSTONES BY AGE 75

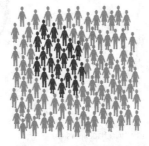

20 OF 100 PEOPLE WHO HAVE GALLSTONES DEVELOP SYMPTOMS WITHIN 20 YEARS

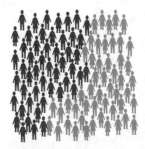

50 OF 100 PEOPLE WHO HAVE ONE EPISODE OF GALLSTONE-RELATED ABDOMINAL PAIN HAVE ANOTHER EPISODE WITHIN 1 YEAR

fever and shaking chills can indicate infection or perforation of the gallbladder; they constitute a medical emergency. When a gallstone blocks the pancreatic duct, it causes the symptoms of pancreatitis (see p.768).

TREATMENT OPTIONS

If you have symptoms of acute cholecystitis, call your doctor immediately. He or she will draw blood to measure levels of white blood cells (high levels indicate infection) and will test your liver function. Ultrasound (see p.760) can help your doctor see the gall-

stones and any thickening of the gallbladder wall from inflammation.

A nuclear medicine scan (see p.137) can show that the gallbladder is not functioning normally. If you have signs of infection, you may be admitted to the hospital, where you will be observed closely and receive painkillers and intravenous antibiotics.

When you are not having an attack of acute cholecystitis but have had intermittent symptoms that make your doctor suspect you have gallstones, blood tests

of liver function may be performed. Your doctor may also want to see a picture of your gallbladder, usually using ultrasound.

The symptoms caused by gallstones can be similar to the symptoms caused by several other abdominal conditions, including peptic ulcer (see p.752) or pancreatitis. For this reason, other tests may be necessary to diagnose or rule out these conditions. If your doctor is concerned that a stone might be stuck in a bile duct, endoscopic retrograde cholangiopan-

Laparoscopic Gallbladder Removal

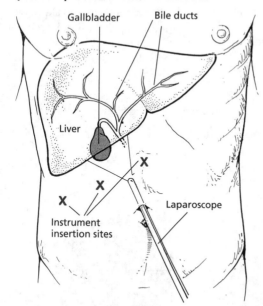

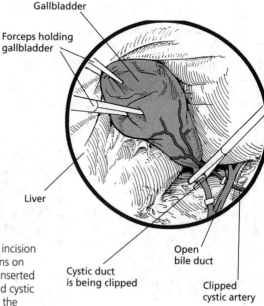

VIEW THROUGH LAPAROSCOPE

For gallbladder removal, a laparoscope is inserted through a small incision just above or below the navel. Forceps placed through two incisions on the right side are used to position the gallbladder. An instrument inserted through the third incision is used to clip and cut the cystic duct and cystic artery and to detach the gallbladder from the liver. The organ and the stones it contains are then removed through the laparoscope.

creatography (ERCP) may be performed (see p.761) to view the duct.

After an attack of acute cholecystitis, or with recurring milder symptoms from gallstones, surgery to remove the gallbladder and gallstones is often recommended. Some doctors also recommend surgery in people who have diabetes (see p.832) or a chronic infection of the gallbladder with the bacteria salmonella, even if they have not yet had symptoms.

Usually the surgery is performed using a laparoscope (see p.772). Bile duct stones can be removed during ERCP; the bile duct opening is cut and the stone removed. If you have a bile duct stone, your doctor may perform this surgery before removing your gallbladder or instead of removing your gallbladder.

For people who do not want surgery, or are too frail to undergo it, there are several alternatives. One is taking the drug ursodiol, which can dissolve gallstones over a period of 1 to 2 years. Once treatment ends, however, the chance of recurrence is 50% within 5 years.

Lithotripsy (the use of shock waves to pulverize stones) can break gallstones into fragments that are small enough to pass through the bile ducts and be eliminated, or to be dissolved with ursodiol. With lithotripsy, there is a 50% chance that the stones will recur within 5 years.

Laparoscopic Gallbladder Removal

Until the 1990s, a cholecystectomy (removal of the gallbladder) was performed by open surgery, in which the surgeon makes a 5-inch long incision in the abdomen to gain access to the gallbladder.

Today, more than 90% of cholecystectomies are performed using a type of endoscope called a laparoscope that requires only four small keyhole incisions in the abdomen to allow for insertion of the laparoscope and surgical instruments. Because the laparoscopic technique involves less cutting of tissue, people recover more quickly than they did from the traditional open surgical technique; they have less pain and can return to normal activities more rapidly.

Before laparoscopic surgery, you will receive general anesthesia. Four small incisions are made; one for the laparoscope, two for the instruments that are used to position the gallbladder, and one for insertion of an instrument to cut and withdraw the gallbladder.

If complications such as bleeding occur (which is rare), the surgeon can convert the procedure to open surgery by making an abdominal incision. People report less pain after laparoscopy than with the open method; many spend only a single night in the hospital and can go back to work within a week or two.

Occasional diarrhea is the most common side effect of living without a gallbladder; this can usually be relieved by taking cholestyramine, a powder that absorbs bile.

Lithotripsy is rarely advised, since it is often not completely effective.

Cancer of the Gallbladder and Bile Ducts

Cancerous tumors of the gallbladder and bile ducts are rare. People with gallstones are at slightly higher risk.

Cancer of the gallbladder or bile ducts may not cause any symptoms at first, or it may cause tenderness in the upper right portion of the abdomen. You may also have jaundice (yellowing of the whites of the eyes and skin), itchy skin, and weight loss.

If your doctor believes that you have cancer, he or she will perform an ultrasound (see p.760). If the cancer has not spread, the gallbladder and bile ducts may be removed. If the cancer has spread to the liver or other organs, survival rates are poor.

SMALL INTESTINE

Carcinoid Tumors

Carcinoid tumors are a rare type of cancer that usually forms in the appendix, intestine, or lungs. As they grow, the tumors release large quantities of the hormone serotonin as well as other active substances.

Usually there are no symptoms unless the tumors spread. In that case, the serotonin, which is released into the bloodstream, may cause recurring diarrhea and flushing of the face and neck, along with abdominal cramps, wheezing, and puffy eyes. Some carcinoid tumors that spread are fatal. There are also rare forms that do not release hormones and are usually not a problem.

Blood and urine tests are usually performed to confirm the presence of excess serotonin. You may also have ultrasound (see p.148) or computed tomography (see p.149) to verify the presence of tumors. Tumors that are diagnosed early can be surgically removed. Chemotherapy (see p.741) can also help reduce the size of tumors. Your doctor can prescribe medicines that ease the effects of the excess serotonin and relieve the wheezing, flushing, and diarrhea.

Celiac Disease

Also known as celiac sprue, nontropical sprue, and gluten-sensitive enteropathy, celiac disease is sensitivity of the small intestine to gluten, a protein found in rye, wheat, and barley. The sensitivity causes an inability to absorb nutrients due to inflammation and damage to the intestinal lining.

Oats also contain gluten, but

Celiac Disease

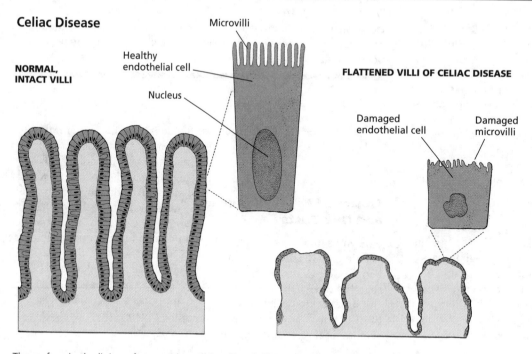

NORMAL, INTACT VILLI

Microvilli

Healthy endothelial cell

Nucleus

FLATTENED VILLI OF CELIAC DISEASE

Damaged endothelial cell

Damaged microvilli

The surface in the lining of a normal small intestine (left) is covered with fingerlike projections called villi that extend into the space within the bowel. Each villus is about 0.5 mm long and covered with endothelial cells. To maximize contact with nutrients, the surfaces of these cells are covered with tiny hairlike microvilli. In the bowel of a person with celiac disease (right), the villi flatten out or disappear. The absorptive endothelial cells become distorted and lose their microvilli. As a result, the intestine cannot absorb food properly.

of a different type. Research indicates that people with celiac disease can eat oats. People who have celiac disease may become anemic due to poor absorption of iron, folic acid, or both. Failure to absorb calcium and vitamin D can lead to osteoporosis (see p.596). Celiac disease can affect children (see p.774).

SYMPTOMS

Symptoms of celiac disease can begin at any age. If you have celiac disease, you are likely to develop diarrhea when you eat any food that contains gluten. The diarrhea can be so severe that extreme and life-threatening dehydration develops. Bowel movements are typically bulky, light tan or gray, frothy, rancid smelling, and tend to adhere to the toilet bowl. The stickiness is due to the high fat content.

Not everyone who has celiac disease has diarrhea; some people only have symptoms of malabsorption (see next article), which can have multiple consequences. Weight loss is common. If protein levels are too low, legs may swell. The gums may bleed due to a vitamin K deficiency. Lack of other vitamins can produce neurological impairment (nerve and thought-process disorders), dry skin, and soreness of the lips or tongue.

TREATMENT OPTIONS

Celiac disease is difficult to diagnose in its early stages. Results from a number of diagnostic studies, including blood tests, bowel movement examinations, and intestinal x-rays after barium is swallowed (see p.745), may raise the suspicion of celiac disease. Celiac disease is suspected when

results of a biopsy of the small intestine show microscopic abnormalities.

Consuming a gluten-free diet is the main course of treatment. Gluten is found not only in cereal and wheat but is a hidden ingredient in many prepared foods (see p.776). People who are sensitive to gluten must scrutinize food labels carefully and be wary of unlabeled processed food.

Malabsorption

Malabsorption is an impaired ability of the lining of the small intestine to absorb nutrients, vitamins, and minerals and make them available to the bloodstream. Unabsorbed food leaves the body in bowel movements.

Many conditions can cause malabsorption, including chronic pancreatitis (see p.769), removal of part of the small intestine or stomach, lactose intolerance (see p.798), Crohn disease (see Inflammatory Bowel Disease, p.787), diverticulosis (see p.783), and celiac disease (see p.774).

Heart failure (see p.683) and inflammation of the blood vessels are cardiovascular disorders that can impede absorption of nutrients by causing swelling of the intestinal lining.

SYMPTOMS

If you have malabsorption, you may experience diarrhea and weight loss. You may also have vitamin deficiencies, mineral deficiencies, or anemia.

TREATMENT OPTIONS

To diagnose malabsorption, your doctor will take a medical history, evaluate your symptoms, and perform blood tests to look for ane-

mia (see p.713). He or she may also evaluate your stools for the presence of fat that has not been absorbed by the body and take a biopsy sample of tissue from your small intestine. This is done by inserting a flexible viewing tube through the mouth to the intestines and extracting the tissue. Treatment is based on the underlying cause.

Meckel Diverticulum

Meckel diverticulum is a small sac (diverticulum) that opens from the last portion of the small intestine (the ileum) and sometimes is lined with stomach tissue. In some people, it is present from birth; it usually causes no problems.

Symptoms occur only if the diverticulum bleeds or becomes obstructed or infected. Obstruction can produce sudden, severe pain in the upper right side of your abdomen. Because this symptom is more often caused by other conditions such as appendicitis (see p.782) and gallbladder disease (see p.770), Meckel diverticulum can be difficult to diagnose.

The best diagnostic test involves injecting a radioactive dye into the bloodstream, which travels to the diverticulum and causes it to light up on a nuclear medicine scan (see p.137) if there is stomach tissue present. When the diverticulum causes an obstruction of the intestine called intussusception (see p.1010), x-rays usually show the blockage.

Infections are treated with antibiotics. Transfusions may be needed if bleeding is extensive. If necessary, the diverticulum can be removed by surgery.

Hidden Sources of Gluten

If you have celiac disease, you must not eat foods or take medicines containing gluten. Certain fresh foods are gluten-free, including fresh meat, poultry, fish, vegetables, fruit, and milk. A major problem for people with celiac disease is that commercially processed foods that come in containers are not required to state on their labels whether or not the food contains gluten.

Therefore, you need to follow some general rules and then do some homework on any food item that may contain gluten. For any commercially processed food, always read the label. If the label contains any of the words found in the "Do Not Eat" column below, avoid those foods.

For foods in the "May be OK to Eat" column, you must verify that the food is gluten-free. You need to contact the manufacturer or review lists of food items maintained by celiac disease organizations.

You also can obtain some of this information on the Web site affiliated with this book (see bottom of any index page for Web site address). This site will also direct you to advice on how to shop for gluten-free foods, how to avoid gluten when eating out or traveling, how to avoid medicines that contain gluten, and links to Web sites of various celiac disease organizations.

Many doctors also recommend that you avoid eating anything made from oats, but studies have led some doctors to approve of oats in a gluten-free diet. Ask your doctor for advice.

FOODS	DO NOT EAT	MAY BE OK TO EAT
Grains and cereals	Wheat, rye, or barley in any form, including white or whole-grain flour, bread, bread crumbs, malt, unidentified starches or fillers, spelt, semolina, kamut, triticale, couscous	Rice, corn, potato, soybeans, any other beans, nuts, including: white or brown rice, rice flour, corn, cornmeal, cornstarch, popcorn, potato, sweet potato, potato starch, soy flour, arrowroot, tapioca, plain beans, plain nuts
	Oats (consult your doctor)	Oats (consult your doctor)
	Pasta and noodles containing wheat, rye, or barley	Gluten-free* pasta made from cornmeal, rice flour, bean flour, potato starch, or polenta
	Breads that contain wheat, rye, or barley in any form	Gluten-free* breads made from gluten-free ingredients including gluten-free yeast, baking powder, baking soda, xanthan gum, rice flour, tapioca, bean flours, cornstarch, potato starch
	Most commercial cereals	Gluten-free* cereals made from cornmeal, puffed corn, or rice

*"Gluten-free" means that you have verified (by contacting the manufacturer, a celiac disease organization, or an authoritative Web site) that the product is gluten-free.

FOODS	DO NOT EAT	MAY BE OK TO EAT
Dairy products	Processed cheese, cheese mixes, blue cheese	Plain natural cheese
	Yogurt that is unlabeled or contains fillers or additives	Plain yogurt, or other yogurts that are gluten-free*
	Ice cream that is unlabeled or contains fillers or additives	Gluten-free* ice cream without fillers or additives
	Low-fat or fat-free cottage cheese, sour cream, or cheese spreads	Whole, low-fat, and fat-free milk; full-fat cottage cheese and sour cream
Meats	Commercially prepared (such as marinated) fresh or frozen meat; prepared meals; processed meat such as lunch meat or sausage	Fresh fish, meat, or poultry
Vegetables	Creamed vegetables	Fresh, frozen, or canned vegetables without sauces
	Canned soups, soup mixes, bouillon cubes	Homemade soups with allowed ingredients
	Most salad dressings	Gluten-free* salad dressings
	Rice mixes; some converted rice	Plain white, brown, or wild rices
	French fries fried in oil that has already fried breaded foods	French fries fried alone
	Hydrolyzed vegetable protein	. . .
Miscellaneous	Modified food starches, food starch	Cornstarch, potato starch, tapioca, arrowroot
	Natural flavors, additives, or stabilizers	Lecithin, carrageenan, methylcellulose
	Unidentified gums, fat replacers	Gums such as xanthan gum, locust bean (carob bean), cellulose, tragacanth
	Grain vinegar	Rice, wine, or apple cider vinegars
	Malt or rice syrup	Sugar
	Most candy; some candy bars	Gluten-free* candy bars
	Imported soy sauce made from wheat	Gluten-free* soy sauce
Alcohol	Beer, whiskey, grain alcohol	Wine, light rum, potato vodka

DIARRHEAL DISEASES AND DISORDERS

(See also Diarrhea in Children, p.320; Food Safety, p.87; Food Poisoning, p.881)

Mild, Temporary Diarrhea

Diarrhea is an extremely common symptom of viral illness and, in the United States, usually resolves on its own without treatment. However, diarrhea occasionally is severe and life-threatening. Worldwide, diarrhea and dehydration are a leading cause of death among infants.

Mild, temporary diarrhea usually lasts 1 to 7 days. You may have two to eight loose to watery bowel movements per day. This type of diarrhea is very common and usually does not require a visit to the doctor. The most common causes of mild diarrhea are viral infections of the small intestine and food poisoning. See Home Remedies for Diarrhea, right.

Viral gastroenteritis Gastroenteritis means inflammation of the stomach and small intestine. The usual cause is a viral infection. Two viruses—rotavirus and the Norwalk virus—are the main culprits in gastroenteritis, which most often affects children between 6 months and 2 years old and can be severe. Gastroenteritis can also occur in older children and adults, but the symptoms are usually milder.

The Norwalk virus, often found in shellfish or contaminated water, can cause outbreaks in schools, in camps, on cruise ships, or in other places where people live closely. It occurs mainly in spring and winter; symptoms usually last 24 to 48 hours. Infections caused by either rotavirus or the Norwalk virus are contagious, and people develop symptoms within 1 to 2 days after exposure.

Along with diarrhea, people with viral gastroenteritis commonly have fever; mild, cramping stomach pains; and usually mild nausea (which sometimes leads to vomiting). In adults, the diarrhea usually produces only mild dehydration.

However, in infants, the dehydration can be severe and even life-threatening; viral gastroenteritis with dehydration is the most common cause of hospitalization in children under age 3.

Food poisoning (See also p.881.) Most cases of food poisoning are mild and temporary and are caused by bacteria growing on a food you have eaten. Either the bacteria themselves or the toxic substances they produce cause the symptoms of the disease.

If you develop diarrhea and other related symptoms (such as abdominal pain or nausea) and someone who shared a meal with you in the past several days also has similar symptoms, you may be suffering from food poisoning. Food poisoning can also cause severe diarrhea. See Food

Home Remedies for Diarrhea

Diarrhea is a common problem with a wide variety of causes—from flu to food poisoning. While you are deciding whether it is serious enough to call the doctor (see Diarrhea: When to Call Your Doctor, p.779), try these home remedies to keep comfortable and avoid more serious health problems.

Drink liquids To prevent dehydration, take frequent sips of room-temperature water or any fluid that tastes good to you (except milk and caffeine-containing beverages). Drink as much as you can to replace lost fluids. Better still, drink a homemade oral rehydration solution (see Traveler's Diarrhea, p.780) or sports drink. Give infants with diarrhea (see p.299) a commercially prepared electrolyte solution, available at any drugstore.

Do not eat until you feel better Then consume rice or rice cereal, clear soups, flavored gelatin, or broth. Avoid bread, pasta, and other wheat products, as well as fresh fruits, corn, and processed bran. Also avoid milk products; you may not tolerate them easily for several days.

Do not take antidiarrheal medicines unless prescribed by your doctor They can mask symptoms and, in the case of infection with salmonella bacteria or shigella bacteria or of antibiotic-caused diarrhea, can actually make symptoms worse by preventing the intestine from expelling the bacteria from the body.

Rest at home in bed This will not only help you regain strength but will help limit the spread of viral or bacterial organisms to others.

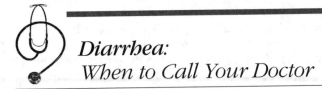

Diarrhea:
When to Call Your Doctor

Call your doctor if you have diarrhea and any of the following apply:

- You have black or bloody bowel movements.

- You have pus in your bowel movements.

- You have abdominal pain and cramps that are not relieved by having a bowel movement.

- You are dehydrated (your mouth feels dry and you are thirsty and weak).

- You have a fever above 101°F with chills and vomiting.

- You have traveled to a foreign country recently and the diarrhea started while you were there or within a week of returning.

- You are taking medicine for another condition and your diarrhea has persisted for more than 4 weeks (diarrhea may be a side effect of the medicine).

- Your diarrhea lasts more than 1 week.

- You are taking immune-suppressing medicine.

Poisoning with salmonella and campylobacter, p.780.

Severe Diarrhea

Severe diarrhea is defined as more than 10 watery bowel movements each day. If you have difficulty drinking enough fluids to make up for the fluids that have been lost, you can become dehydrated. Severe diarrhea is often accompanied by blood or pus in the bowel movements (dysentery).

The usual causes of severe diarrhea are the infections listed here, although inflammatory bowel disease (see p.787), some tumors, and pancreatic insufficiency (in which the pancreas does not make enough digestive enzymes) are occasional causes.

If you have severe diarrhea, your doctor is likely to take a stool sample to test for infection with bacteria or parasites. If you are dehydrated, you will receive oral

How Antibiotics Cause Diarrhea

The bowel, like many parts of the body, is naturally populated by beneficial bacteria, along with some bad ones. The two types compete for food, and the beneficial bacteria are usually successful in out-competing and therefore minimizing the number of bad bacteria.

When you take certain antibiotics in order to kill a bacterial infection, many beneficial bacteria in the bowel are also killed, leaving gaps in the natural assortment of bacteria and giving some types—particularly *Clostridium difficile*—room to proliferate.

C difficile releases a toxin that irritates and inflames the large intestine, causing diarrhea. *C difficile* is not naturally found in everyone; it is more common in people who are hospitalized. Ampicillin and other penicillins, cephalosporin drugs, and aminoglycosides most often cause antibiotic-induced diarrhea.

Symptoms include profuse, watery, and foul-smelling stools, abdominal cramps, and fever. Symptoms can occur within 4 to 9 days after starting the antibiotic, although they may start as early as 24 hours after taking the antibiotic or may not occur until up to 6 weeks after you stop taking it.

See your doctor if you think an antibiotic is causing your diarrhea. He or she may prescribe the drugs metronidazole or vancomycin. The drug cholestyramine, which carries the inflammation-causing toxin produced by *C difficile* out of the gastrointestinal tract, may also be prescribed.

Make sure you drink plenty of water to replace the fluids lost in diarrhea and do not take antidiarrheal medicines, which can be dangerous (especially in infants) because they encourage your body to retain the toxin.

rehydration solutions (see Traveler's Diarrhea, below right) or intravenous solutions of salt water.

Shigellosis Infection with the shigella bacteria usually causes severe diarrhea. Shigellosis usually starts suddenly and causes watery diarrhea. In many people, after 1 to 2 days, the bowel movements become less voluminous, more frequent, and bloody. Severe cramping and straining with production of little or no feces is another symptom.

Shigellosis is acquired by ingesting contaminated food or water, which occurs more often in places where sanitary conditions are poor. It is a very common and significant problem in the developing nations of the world, including countries in South and Central America, Africa, the Middle East, and the Far East. However, it is even a problem in developed countries such as the United States.

Food poisoning with salmonella and campylobacter

These are two types of bacteria that contaminate a large portion (up to 50%) of chickens and eggs. Both can cause diarrhea that ranges from mild to severe, and both can ultimately heal without antibiotics. However, elderly people, children less than 1 year of age, and people with compromised immune systems should be treated with antibiotics. Campylobacter infections should be treated with antibiotics if the diarrhea is severe or symptoms are worsening.

Amebic dysentery Amebic dysentery is caused by a parasite called *Entamoeba histolytica*. It usually develops gradually and may persist for weeks or months

if not treated. It is common in developing nations but unusual in developed countries.

Cholera Cholera is an infection of the small intestine caused by the bacterium *Vibrio cholerae*. The bacterium releases a toxin that causes severe watery diarrhea. Cholera always causes severe dehydration and can be life-threatening. It is spread by ingesting water or food that is contaminated with the bacterium.

Food poisoning with *Escherichia coli* 0157:H7

E coli can contaminate any food but most often contaminates meat. It releases a toxin like the shigella toxin (see left), causing severe and often bloody diarrhea. It can damage small blood vessels throughout the body (especially in the brain and kidneys) and can be fatal. The very young and elderly are most susceptible. The best way to prevent this infection is to cook meat thoroughly (see p.88).

Chronic Diarrhea

People who have diarrhea for more than 4 weeks have chronic diarrhea and should see their doctor. Many medicines can cause diarrhea, as can caffeine. Acute diverticulitis (see p.783) and inflammatory bowel disease (see p.787) can also cause watery bowel movements.

Traveler's Diarrhea

Traveler's diarrhea is an intestinal infection acquired when you consume water or food contaminated with fecal matter that contains bacteria, parasites, or viruses. If you have any doubts

about the safety of food or water in a place you are visiting, follow the precautions on p.96.

When diarrhea is watery and copious, it can lead to dehydration. Children and elderly people are especially vulnerable, but dehydration is dangerous at any age. If a member of your traveling party has severe diarrhea, get medical help; the doctor may want to give fluids intravenously if the dehydration is serious.

It is a good idea to pack commercially prepared rehydration solutions to sip in case you have diarrhea on your vacation. You can make your own solution by adding to 1 liter (or 1 quart) of boiled, bottled water, 3/4 teaspoon of salt, 4 tablespoons of sugar, and 1 teaspoon of baking soda. Let the mixture cool, add 1 cup of orange juice, and sip about 3 pints per day until the diarrhea stops.

You can prevent traveler's diarrhea by taking two tablets or 2 tablespoons of a common, over-the-counter bismuth preparation four times a day, starting 2 days before leaving and while on your trip. This can reduce the risk of diarrhea by 50%. Your bowel movements and tongue may be temporarily stained black with this treatment. Doxycycline has been used for prevention but makes your skin sensitive to the sun and is less desirable to use.

Taking certain antibiotics every day (particularly trimethoprim-sulfamethoxazole and fluoroquinolones) can also reduce the chance of infection, but bismuth is preferred because it is equally effective, and using antibiotics increases the development of antibiotic-resistant bacteria (see p.880).

LARGE INTESTINE

Constipation

Constipation is a general description of bowel movements that are small, hard, and/or infrequent. There is wide variation in how frequently individuals have bowel movements so it is difficult to say what is normal.

It is most important to contact your doctor about any change (after it has persisted for several weeks or more) in the pattern of bowel movements that has been normal for you. Such changes from your normal pattern can indicate a problem. Your doctor will ask you questions about your bowel movements and about other symptoms of digestive tract problems. He or she will examine your abdomen and rectum and will usually check to see if there are signs of blood in the bowel movement.

Depending on what the doctor discovers, various blood tests, along with a barium enema (see p.784), plain x-rays (see p.145) of the abdomen, or endoscopy (see p.142), may be required.

Most of the time, constipation is caused by lifestyle factors rather than by a medical condition. Lack of fiber in the diet, too little exercise, and inadequate intake of fluids are the primary causes of constipation, but any alteration in your customary diet or routine can cause it. Menstruation, stress, and travel are also factors. Overuse of laxatives may have the paradoxical effect of causing constipation with time.

Sometimes constipation is caused by medical conditions or their treatment. Constipation can occur as a side effect of some medicines, including sedatives and calcium channel blockers. When it is caused by an underlying medical condition—such as irritable bowel syndrome (see p.789) or an underactive thyroid gland (see Hypothyroidism, p.848)—the condition is usually mild and easily treated.

Constipation can also be caused by a more serious condi-

Laxatives

Laxatives are stimulants that irritate the intestines and promote bowel movements. Examples of laxatives are bisacodyl, anthraquinone, cascara, castor oil, phenolphthalein, and senna. Used once or twice for occasional constipation, they are effective. However, laxatives can lead to dependency and have diminished effects with daily use for months or years. They can also cause changes in the bowel over time. If you think you need a laxative, ask your physician for advice.

How the Colon Works

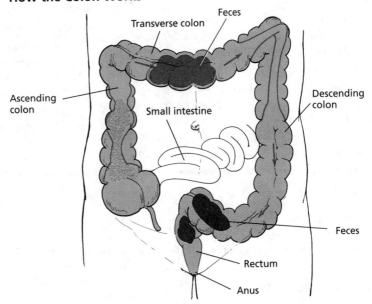

Fluid and indigestible particles pass from the small intestine to the large intestine (colon) at the junction in the lower right corner of the abdomen. Slow, churning motions move this material (called feces) along the ascending segment of the colon, and fluids and minerals are absorbed. Feces solidify in the transverse colon and are propelled down the descending colon toward the rectum.

Alternative Medicine: Constipation and Hemorrhoid Treatment

Constipation and hemorrhoids often occur simultaneously. Inactivity promotes both, and straining to defecate can set the stage for hemorrhoids. Here are some alternative remedies:

■ Press out constipation with acupressure. Place all fingertips three finger widths below the navel and,

applying gentle but firm pressure, press 1 inch until you sense a firmness. Keep pressing for 3 minutes as you breathe slowly and deeply from your diaphragm.

■ Apply aloe vera gel to your anal area regularly.

■ Chinese medicine recommends three oranges a day or two bananas in the morning.

Preventing Constipation

Preventing constipation is easier than treating it. Follow these steps to avoid constipation:

■ Eat a well-balanced diet that is high in fiber (beans, bran, whole grains, and fresh fruits and vegetables) to give bulk to bowel movements and ease their passage. Limit foods that produce gas. Keep meals small and more frequent.

■ Take bulk-forming agents—such as psyllium, methylcellulose, and pectin—which are available without a prescription at the drugstore.

■ Drink at least eight glasses of water a day.

■ Exercise regularly to keep your system in good working order. Walking 20 to 30 minutes a day is particularly helpful.

■ Set a schedule and train your system to expect to have a bowel movement at a certain hour or after

meals. Start by sitting on the toilet for 10 minutes at the designated time until your body begins to respond; do not strain.

■ Respond to the urge to defecate without delay.

■ Do not strain, which can cause other health problems, including hemorrhoids (see p.795) and blood pressure problems.

■ Use stool softeners such as docusate.

■ If stool softeners are not effective, try osmotic agents (sometimes called mild laxatives) such as milk of magnesia, Epsom salts, lactulose, and sorbitol, which promote more fluid in your feces.

■ Avoid laxatives, but if you feel you must use them, see p.781 for guidelines.

---

tion, such as cancer of the colon, that is producing an obstruction in the flow of bowel movements.

Appendicitis

Appendicitis is inflammation of the appendix, a small fingerlike appendage that sticks out from the top portion of the colon (large intestine). The purpose of

the appendix is not known.

Appendicitis most often affects otherwise healthy people between the ages of 10 and 30; it is rare under the age of 2 and in older adults.

Appendicitis can occur when the appendix becomes obstructed by feces. The portion of the appendix beyond the blockage becomes tender and inflamed

and sometimes infected. In most people who have an acutely inflamed appendix, the painful symptoms come on suddenly and do not go away; the solution is surgery to remove the appendix (appendectomy).

Occasionally, the symptoms of appendicitis come and go or produce recurring abdominal pain, but this is thought to be rare.

SYMPTOMS

When you get appendicitis, the pain usually starts in the area around your navel. It becomes steadier and more severe over several hours and moves to the lower right portion of the abdomen. The pain is made worse by coughing, sneezing, and other sudden movements. You may feel nauseated and vomit, lose your appetite, or have diarrhea.

You might also have a low-grade fever of 100°F to 101°F. The symptoms often depend on the location of your appendix, which can vary from person to person. When a woman gets appendicitis during pregnancy, the pain may be focused in the upper right side or the lower left part of the abdomen because the fetus has pushed the appendix out of its normal position.

TREATMENT OPTIONS

If you have pain in your abdomen, the things that you do (such as what you eat or the position of your body) that make it better or worse can be of great help to your doctor in trying to diagnose the problem. If you have symptoms of appendicitis and the pain gets worse, do not take laxatives or pain medicine; call your doctor.

Your physician will ask about your symptoms and examine your abdomen by gently pressing on different areas. You may need several tests. The white blood cell count (see p.158), as shown by a blood test, is often elevated in appendicitis. Other blood tests may be performed to look for other causes of sudden and severe abdominal pain, such as pancreatitis (see p.768) and gallbladder disease (see p.770).

A variety of imaging tests may also be used. Computed tomography (see p.784) can accurately detect appendicitis. Ultrasound (see p.148) can detect other causes of abdominal pain such as an ovarian cyst (see p.1080) or ectopic pregnancy (see p.929). Pregnant women and people over the age of 60 often have unusual symptoms and may require more extensive testing.

The death rate for untreated appendicitis can be as high as 15%. Serious consequences usually result when an infected appendix bursts and releases its contents into the abdominal cavity, causing peritonitis (see p.801). This is more likely to occur if appendectomy is delayed.

Appendectomy is performed using general anesthesia. An incision is made in the lower right portion of your abdomen. The appendix is lifted up, clamped at its base, and then cut away from the cecum (to which it is attached). The remaining stump is stitched to the cecum. Recovery time is usually 3 or 4 days.

Alternately, appendectomy can be performed using laparoscopic surgery. Several keyhole incisions are made in the abdomen, and a viewing instrument and surgical instruments are inserted to aid in removal of the appendix.

Although its use is growing, laparoscopic surgery has not yet become the clear choice for most people who require appendectomy—as it has for people who require gallbladder removal (see p.772).

Diverticulosis and Diverticulitis

Diverticula are small balloonlike pouches that push out from the wall of the large intestine (colon). A person who has one or more of these pouches has diverticulosis, a condition that may cause no problems. If a diverticulum becomes blocked, infection and inflammation can develop, resulting in diverticulitis. Perforation of the diverticulum may also cause problems.

Diverticulosis is one of the most common afflictions of the colon, affecting about 10% of Americans and up to 50% of those over age 60. A person may have a single diverticulum or as many as several hundred. Most people have few or no symptoms.

Diverticulosis

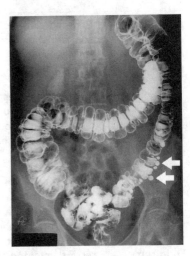

This x-ray shows the presence of diverticula. Barium (white area) outlines the shape of the entire large intestine. The small, white pouches (arrows) coming out of the bowel wall are the diverticula.

Viewing the Colon

Doctors use a number of diagnostic imaging tools to gain a better view of the colon (large intestine). For most tests, you will be asked to fast for up to 6 hours beforehand and take laxatives or enemas or both to help clear the colon. Tests are performed in a hospital, clinic, or doctor's office, usually by a radiologist, who is an expert in performing diagnostic imaging procedures and interpreting the results.

PROCEDURE	WHY IT IS PERFORMED	WHAT TO EXPECT
Barium enema	To detect colon cancer, inflammatory bowel disease, polyps, obstructions, and diverticulosis.	You will take a laxative 1 day before and have a cleansing enema just prior to the procedure. A barium solution (through which x-rays cannot pass) will be instilled into your rectum, producing an urge to defecate. While you hold in the barium and assume different positions, the radiologist will gently press on your abdomen to direct the barium to your colon and take x-rays (air may be injected into the colon during filming). Your bowel movements may be white or a lighter color than usual for several days after the procedure.
Computed tomography (see p.149)	To detect cancer, causes of abdominal discomfort, inflammatory bowel disease, and obstructions.	You may drink a solution that will enhance the image made by the scanner. You will lie very still on a table in a large, metal, tunnel-like device (a camera will rotate around you as you move through the tunnel). A barium solution may be instilled into your rectum to enhance the x-ray image made by the scanner.
Anoscopy (see Endoscopy, p.142)	To detect causes of bleeding and anal pain, hemorrhoids, fissures, and fistulas.	As you lie on your side with knees bent, your doctor will insert a slim, flexible, plastic viewing tube into your rectum, using slow, gentle pressure.
Sigmoidoscopy (see Endoscopy, p.142)	To view the lower third of the large intestine (colon) in order to detect cancer, proctitis, or inflammatory bowel disease or to take a biopsy.	After taking a laxative, drinking a cleansing solution, and perhaps taking an oral or intravenous sedative, you will lie down on your side with your knees bent. The doctor will gently insert a lubricated, flexible, lighted endoscope (see p.150) through the anus into the rectum (air is pumped into the bowel to allow the tube to be positioned properly). You may feel some cramping, which can be relieved by breathing deeply.
Colonoscopy (see Endoscopy, p.142)	To view the large intestine (colon) in order to detect bleeding, cancer, inflammatory bowel disease, fissures, or abscesses; remove polyps; or take a biopsy.	Same as sigmoidoscopy.

Colonoscopy and Sigmoidoscopy

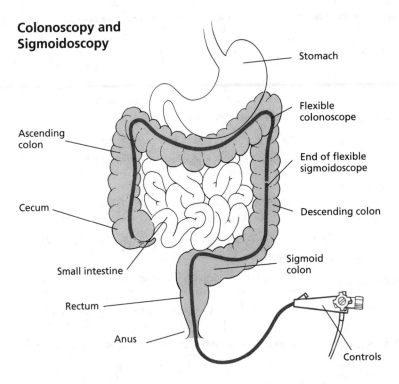

Scientists are uncertain about what causes diverticulosis. They speculate that pressure inside the intestine may increase when a person's diet contains very little fiber, leading to a slower transit time of stools down the intestine, less frequent bowel movements, and more straining with defecation. These factors make diverticulosis more likely. Physical activity may lower the risk.

In diverticulitis, most infections are small and heal themselves. However, they can lead to an abscess on the bowel wall, which may destroy surrounding tissue and create a fistula (see p.794). Complications can include obstruction of the intestine due to scarring. If a perforation of the diverticulum causes spillage of feces into the peritoneal cavity in the abdomen, peritonitis (see p.801) can develop and surgery is required.

A flexible sigmoidoscope allows your doctor to visually examine the rectum, sigmoid colon, and part of the descending colon. A flexible colonoscope is a longer tube that allows a view of the entire bowel from rectum to cecum.

Diverticulitis

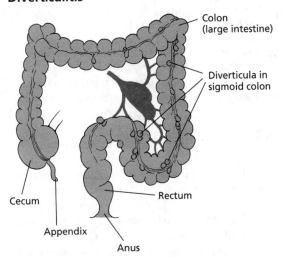

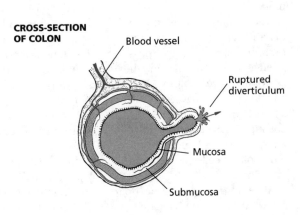

In diverticulosis, small pouches (diverticula) may form in the colon, usually in the sigmoid colon (left). Diverticula commonly form from a ballooning of the two inner layers of the colon wall, the mucosa and submucosa. In diverticu-litis, they become blocked and infected. The diverticula can rupture (right), allowing fluid to leak into the abdominal cavity, which causes peritonitis.

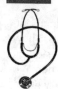

Diverticulitis: When You Visit Your Doctor

QUESTIONS TO DISCUSS WITH YOUR DOCTOR:

■ What is your current diet? How much fiber (from fruits, vegetables, or bran) do you eat?

■ Have you had any recurrence of abdominal pain? Where was it located? How severe was it on a scale of 1 to 10 (10 being the worst)? How long did it last? Was it relieved by having a bowel movement?

■ Have you had constipation, diarrhea, or both?

■ Do you take stool softeners?

■ Have you recently had unexplained fevers or chills?

■ Have you noticed blood in your bowel movements?

YOUR DOCTOR MIGHT EXAMINE THE FOLLOWING BODY STRUCTURES OR FUNCTIONS:

■ Temperature, blood pressure, pulse

■ Thorough examination of the abdomen and rectum (if you have had symptoms)

YOUR DOCTOR MIGHT ORDER THE FOLLOWING LAB TESTS OR STUDIES:

■ Complete blood cell count (if you have had blood in your bowel movements)

■ Test for blood in your bowel movements (if you have had symptoms)

■ Barium enema or computed tomography (see p.784) (if you have had recurrent pain)

SYMPTOMS

Diverticulitis can cause sudden intense abdominal pain that can be triggered when a seed or a piece of stool becomes trapped in a diverticulum. As debris accumulates, the diverticulum distends, closing off its blood supply and causing a microscopic perforation. Sometimes a pus-filled abscess forms around the perforated diverticulum. The affected person may become feverish and nauseated, have constipation or diarrhea, and have an elevated number of white blood cells, indicating infection.

Bleeding can also occur (up to 30% of people who have diverticulitis have rectal bleeding), usually when a pouch becomes irritated and, in the process, a blood vessel alongside it ruptures or is injured.

TREATMENT OPTIONS

If your doctor suspects that you have diverticulitis, he or she will perform an abdominal, rectal, and pelvic exam. Your physician might also order x-rays or computed tomography (see p.149) of the abdomen. A barium enema (see p.784) may also be required. Intravenous antibiotics may be given and food restricted. At least 85% of people recover with this therapy.

If you have no relief, your doctor may recommend surgery to remove the inflamed segment of colon. The ends of the healthy colon are rejoined by stitching or stapling them together.

If you do not require surgery, once the inflammation has subsided you may be able to prevent attacks by gradually increasing the amount of fiber in your diet; your doctor may recommend that you take unprocessed bran or psyllium-containing bulk laxatives. Avoiding foods with seeds is usually recommended.

Ileus

Ileus is a temporary failure of the ability of the muscles of the intestine to contract. As a result, gas and stools build up in the intestine. Ileus is most often caused by abdominal surgery, injury, inflammation of the abdominal lining (see Peritonitis, p.801), pancreatitis (see p.768), loss of blood supply to the intestine, or drugs such as narcotics.

The main symptoms of ileus are a bloated and uncomfortable abdomen. Vomiting in small amounts may occur. Hiccups are also common. The diagnosis is usually clear from your doctor's physical examination but x-rays of the abdomen may show the condition.

When ileus is causing obstruction, it is treated by inserting a tube through the nose or mouth into the intestine to relieve any pressure that is building up.

Inflammatory Bowel Disease

Inflammatory bowel disease is a term for several chronic (long-term) conditions that cause inflammation or ulceration of the small and large intestines. Ulcerative colitis and Crohn disease are the two major forms of inflammatory bowel disease, which together affect up to 2 million Americans. Men and women are equally affected, and most people first develop inflammatory bowel disease between the ages of 15 and 40.

In ulcerative colitis, the inflammation and ulceration affects the

---

Ulcerative Colitis

CUT-AWAY VIEW OF COLON (LARGE INTESTINE)

Inflamed mucosa

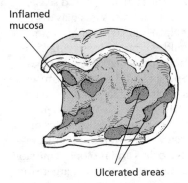

Ulcerated areas

Ulcerative colitis usually affects the innermost layer (mucosa) of the rectum and colon, where it leads to inflammation and erosive ulcers.

---

lining of the colon and rectum. In Crohn disease, the inflammation can affect any part of the gastrointestinal tract, but the most common site is the end of the small intestine or large intestine, which develops ulcers following repeated inflammation.

Inflammatory bowel disease can sometimes mimic other conditions such as irritable bowel syndrome (see p.789), a more common and less serious ailment. Unlike inflammatory bowel disease, there is no apparent anatomical damage or inflammation with irritable bowel syndrome.

Researchers are not sure what causes inflammatory bowel disease. An environmental stimulus, such as a virus or bacterium, may play a role. In genetically vulnerable people (inflammatory bowel disease seems to run in families), it might disrupt the bowel lining and trigger an inflammatory reaction.

SYMPTOMS

Ulcerative colitis causes bloody diarrhea, and stools may contain mucus and pus. You may also have fever and abdominal pain. Periods of ulcerative colitis can occur every few months but in some people occur all the time or rarely.

Crohn disease can cause abdominal pain, bloody diarrhea, and loss of appetite. Malabsorption (see p.775) can occur, leading to anemia and weight loss. In other people, symptoms include rectal bleeding, rectal abscess, and rectal fissures and fistulas (see p.794). In advanced cases, intestinal obstruction can occur. Other parts of the body may be affected as well, causing arthritis,

skin diseases, and eye inflammation.

TREATMENT OPTIONS

Inflammatory bowel disease is suspected when laboratory tests indicate anemia (see p.713), an elevated white blood cell count, and blood in the feces. Since bacterial infections produce the same symptoms, tests on a stool sample can often detect these pathogens. Your physician may also perform sigmoidoscopy or colonoscopy (see p.784) or take x-rays.

Suppositories or enemas containing aminosalicylates or corticosteroid drugs (see p.895) may be used to treat the inflammation directly when only the rectum or lower part of the large intestine is affected. However, when diseased tissue extends farther away from the anal opening, oral medicines may be necessary. The first treatment is usually sulfasalazine. Although it can safely be taken as long as needed, some people experience headaches, nausea, and loss of appetite.

A related group of medicines, the aminosalicylates, tend to have fewer side effects. Mesalamine is the most often prescribed drug from this group. For people who do not respond to these drugs, corticosteroids (see p.895) often produce remission, but also produce many side effects and are undesirable to take for long periods. Budesonide, a new corticosteroid, is given as an enema, and is quite effective, with fewer side effects than corticosteroid pills.

Another treatment using nicotine patches is being investigated for ulcerative colitis, which develops less frequently in smokers. Drugs that modulate the immune

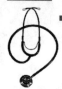

Ulcerative Colitis:
When You Visit Your Doctor

QUESTIONS TO DISCUSS WITH YOUR DOCTOR:

- Has your bowel movement frequency increased or decreased since your last visit?

- Have you noticed blood or mucus in your stool at any time?

- How is your abdominal pain?

- Do you think your medicines are helping you?

- How is your appetite?

- Has your weight changed since your last visit?

- How is your mood?

YOUR DOCTOR MIGHT EXAMINE THE FOLLOWING BODY STRUCTURES OR FUNCTIONS:

- Temperature, blood pressure, pulse, weight

- Thorough examination of the abdomen and rectum

- Examination of any parts of the body where you have symptoms (such as your joints or eyes)

YOUR DOCTOR MIGHT ORDER THE FOLLOWING LAB TESTS OR STUDIES:

- Complete blood cell count (possibly every year, or more often if you are having symptoms)

- Blood albumin level (possibly every year, or more often if you are having symptoms)

- Erythrocyte sedimentation rate (see p.157) or C-reactive protein (see p.155)

- Sigmoidoscopy or colonoscopy (if you are having new or worse symptoms)

- Barium enema, colonoscopy, or abdominal computed tomography (if you are having new or worse symptoms)

system, such as mercaptopurine and azathioprine, are also recommended for people who cannot take corticosteroids.

Surgery to remove the large intestine is the last resort for people who do not respond to medication. The risk of colon cancer begins to rise after 8 years of having inflammatory bowel disease. In people who have colitis of all parts of the large intestine, the risk of cancer can be as high as 30% to 40% after 20 to 25 years. For this reason, surgery to remove the colon is recommended to prevent cancer in those with the most severe disease.

In people who do not have colon cancer, most surgeons remove the colon and create a pouch for feces from the small intestine, leaving the anus intact.

After surgery, you will have about six liquid bowel movements per day. A small number of people need to have an opening made in the abdominal wall; it is connected to an external bag that collects waste (see Colostomy and Ileostomy, p.793).

When the colon is removed, ulcerative colitis is cured, but there is a remaining risk of cancer in the pouch made of small intestine.

In contrast, surgery does not generally cure Crohn disease. Nonetheless, many people who suffer from Crohn disease require surgery to remove large sections of the bowel, drain abscesses, remove dead tissue, or widen narrowed portions of the intestine. Despite these efforts, Crohn disease often recurs. A combination of three medicines—azathioprine, mercaptopurine, and metronidazole—can help prevent a recurrence of Crohn disease.

Dietary measures may also help. You may be able to control mild symptoms by staying away from foods that cause diarrhea. Special liquid diets may cause the symptoms of Crohn disease to abate. There is some evidence that taking fish oil capsules may relieve the symptoms of ulcerative colitis and prolong remission in Crohn disease, but larger studies are needed to confirm these early results.

There are new drugs on the horizon for Crohn disease. One example is a genetically engi-

neered antibody, called inflix-
imab, that neutralizes a substance
that causes inflammation and
helps the fistulas of Crohn disease heal.

Intestinal Obstruction

Intestinal obstruction is a blockage of the small or large intestine
that may be complete or partial.
Obstruction can be caused by
conditions that physically block
the inside of the intestine, such
as inflammation from inflammatory bowel disease (see p.787),
diverticulitis (see p.783), or cancer (see p.791).

Obstruction also can be caused
by conditions that twist or press
down on the outside of the intestine, such as a hernia (see p.800)
or scar tissue (adhesions) that
can develop after abdominal
surgery. Sometimes the obstruction cuts off the blood supply to
part of the intestine (strangulation); this is an emergency that
requires surgery.

Swelling of the abdomen and
constipation occur with obstruction of the large intestine. With
partial blockage, you may pass
some diarrhea around the blockage, which eases pain. In the
small intestine, symptoms include
cramping and sometimes severe
pain in the middle portion of
your abdomen, as well as nausea
and vomiting.

Your doctor will take x-rays
of your abdomen, which usually
reveal the problem. Intestinal
obstruction can reverse itself
without any treatment, especially
if it is from ileus (see p.786).
However, if it does not improve
after 6 to 24 hours, or if there
are signs of strangulation,
surgery usually is required to

remove whatever is causing
the obstruction and to cut away
any part of the intestine that has
died because of the strangulation.

Irritable Bowel Syndrome

Also called spastic colon or irritable colon, irritable bowel syndrome is a constellation of symptoms that includes abdominal
cramping, diarrhea, and bloating.
Irritable bowel syndrome affects
10% to 22% of otherwise healthy
adults, primarily women, and
usually starts in early adulthood.

Gastroenterologists see more
people with irritable bowel syndrome than any other condition,
although most people with the
condition do not see a doctor.

The causes of irritable bowel
syndrome are unclear. There is
some evidence of disturbances in
the function of the nerves or
muscles in the gastrointestinal
system, and of abnormal processing of gastrointestinal sensations
by the brain.

SYMPTOMS

You may have intermittent lower
abdominal cramps and bloating,
accompanied by spells of diarrhea and/or constipation. You
may have excessive mucus (but
not blood) in your bowel movements, and the feeling that you
have not fully emptied your rectum after a bowel movement.

Pain can range from mild to
intense and can interfere with
normal eating or sleeping patterns; it may temporarily subside
after having a bowel movement
or passing gas. Nausea, dizziness,
and fainting can occur.

TREATMENT OPTIONS

Since there are no tests for irritable bowel syndrome and the
bowels appear to be normal,
doctors have established a specific set of criteria to identify the
condition.

■ There must be abdominal pain
or discomfort and a varying pattern of defecation (which must
occur 25% of the time for it to be
considered a symptom) on a
continuous or recurring basis for
at least 3 months. The pain or

Alternative Medicine: Irritable Bowel Syndrome

In addition to gradually increasing the amount of fiber-rich foods in your diet, you may be able to stem the symptoms of irritable bowel syndrome with herbal remedies. Preparations of peppermint oil (coated to prevent heartburn) have a history of success in Europe. Ginger is widely used in Asian countries to ease gastrointestinal discomfort.

Other herbs known to have an antispasmodic effect include chamomile, valerian, and rosemary. Try these herbs in tea preparations.

Many people with irritable bowel syndrome have used hypnosis (see p.394), relaxation therapy (see p.90), and biofeedback (see p.395) to gain comfort, relaxation, and control over their symptoms.

discomfort is relieved with a bowel movement or is accompanied by a change in the frequency or consistency of bowel movements.

■ The varying defecation pattern must fit at least three of the following characteristics: altered bowel movement frequency; a change in bowel movement form (hard, or loose and watery); altered passage of bowel movement (straining, urgency, or feeling of incomplete evacuation); passage of mucus; and/or bloating or the sensation of having a distended abdomen.

Your doctor will take an extensive medical history and ask you specific questions about possible dietary, emotional, and psychological triggers. He or she may also order blood tests and examine your stool for infectious agents, especially parasites. Sigmoidoscopy (see p.784) may be performed to exclude tumors, and barium x-ray or colonoscopy (see p.784) may help rule out cancer in people with a strong family history.

Once irritable bowel syndrome is diagnosed, you may feel a mixture of relief (because your symptoms have a nonthreatening cause) and distress (because there is no cure). Each person with irritable bowel syndrome is different, and treatment should be tailored to your specific symptoms and needs.

The first treatment step is usually dietary. If you notice that certain foods or liquids trigger your symptoms, avoid them. Common triggers are caffeine, sorbitol-containing gums and beverages, gas-producing vegetables (such as beans, cabbage, or broccoli),

dairy products, alcohol, raw fruits, and fatty foods.

Adding fiber to increase the stool's bulk and speed its transit may help relieve constipation and abdominal pain. Fiber should be introduced gradually because it can aggravate symptoms before starting to relieve them. Methylcellulose may produce less gas than psyllium.

If fiber does not relieve constipation, your doctor may prescribe tegaserod. Tegaserod is approved only for women, but it seems to help women with irritable bowel syndrome who have mainly constipation rather than diarrhea. The nonprescription antidiarrheal agent loperamide or bismuth is often recommended to relieve diarrhea.

If your symptoms persist, your doctor may prescribe medicines to relieve cramping, including anticholinergic drugs or tricyclic antidepressants such as amitriptyline and desipramine. If these measures fail, many people turn to alternative therapies (see p.789) for help.

Intestinal Polyps

Polyps are small, mushroom-shaped growths on the lining of the large intestine (colon). Although they are usually noncancerous, one type of polyp called an adenomatous polyp can develop into colon cancer (see p.791). Adenomatous polyps occur primarily in people over 50.

The cause of polyps is unknown, though some people inherit a tendency to have multiple polyps and therefore an increased risk of cancer. Up to 50% of the population has polyps.

The risk of cancer is related to the size of the polyp; the larger it grows, the greater the chance of colon cancer. The stages in the development of a cancer, such as a colon cancer from a polyp, are described below.

SYMPTOMS

Most people never know they have polyps. The most frequent symptom is rectal bleeding. Anemia (see p.713) and its symptoms of fatigue, pallor, and light-headedness may result from bleeding polyps. Large polyps sometimes cause intestinal blockage or, in rare cases, profuse, watery diarrhea.

TREATMENT OPTIONS

To diagnose polyps, your doctor will conduct a thorough medical

---

Polyps in Colon

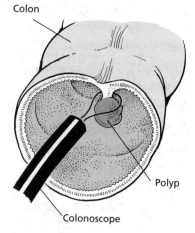

Colon

Polyp

Colonoscope

Polyps are tumors that are often harmless, but some can develop into cancer. They are diagnosed using a colonoscope, a type of flexible endoscope that includes a tiny camera, light, and surgical instruments (such as the loop shown) for taking a biopsy or removing a polyp.

history and physical examination, order blood tests, and test your bowel movements for blood (see below). He or she may also conduct one or more of the procedures described in Viewing the Colon (see p.784), including barium enema, sigmoidoscopy, or colonoscopy.

Polyps are usually removed during colonoscopy. The doctor can see and thereby diagnose the polyp through the colonoscope and, at the same time, remove it with a heated loop that cuts it off. If you have a large number of polyps or if the structure of the polyps appears suspicious to your doctor, he or she will have the tissue examined under a microscope to determine the type of polyp and to look for cancer cells.

Since polyps tend to recur, you should have colonoscopic examinations every 3 years if you have had one polyp diagnosed, particularly if it was an adenomatous polyp.

Cancerous polyps are removed, sometimes along with surrounding tissue. Removal of all or part of the colon may be required if the cancerous polyps are growing very quickly.

Colon Cancer

Colon cancer is cancer of the large intestine. It is also called colorectal cancer. Most colon cancer starts from adenomatous polyps (see Intestinal Polyps, p.790). Only a small percentage of all the different types of polyps that develop in the colon (about 1%) ultimately become cancerous.

Preventing Colon Cancer

Lifestyle changes can help prevent colon cancer. The following appear to reduce risk:

■ **Diet** Low-fat, high-fiber diets with several daily servings of fruits, vegetables, and cereals may reduce your risk, although a 1999 study did not find that a higher-fiber diet protected US women against colon cancer. A diet rich in calcium and folate (which is a micronutrient in leafy green and yellow vegetables) may also reduce risk.

■ **Nonsteroidal anti-inflammatory drugs (NSAIDs)** Although researchers do not know why, people who take these medicines for several years seem to have lower rates of intestinal cancer. However, regular use of aspirin, which is one kind of NSAID, does not reduce the risk of colon cancer.

■ **Stopping smoking** Cigarette smoking increases risk.

■ **Hormone replacement therapy** A 30% to 40% reduction in the risk of colon cancer occurs in women who have taken estrogen after menopause.

■ **Removal of polyps** Removing adenomatous polyps (see Intestinal Polyps, p.790) eliminates a potential site of malignancy.

The following screening schedule is appropriate for most people. However, talk to your doctor about risk factors that can make a more frequent screening schedule advisable for you. If you have a first-degree relative (such as a parent or sibling) who has had colon cancer, for example, you are two to three times more likely to get the disease than the rest of the population.

EXAMINATION	HOW IT IS PERFORMED	WHEN TO HAVE IT
Fecal occult blood test	Stool is examined for presence of hidden (occult) blood.	Annually after age 50 or before age 50 if you have a parent or sibling who has had colon cancer or an adenomatous polyp.
Sigmoidoscopy or colonoscopy (see p.785)	Rectum and lower colon, or the whole colon, are examined through a lighted, flexible tube.	Every 3 to 5 years after age 50 or before age 50 if you have a parent or sibling who has had colon cancer or an adenomatous polyp.

Colon Cancer

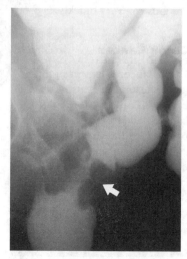

This x-ray of the colon shows a cancerous tumor growing into and greatly narrowing space in the middle of the colon (arrow). As a result, only a little of the barium (white) is seen.

The change from an adenomatous polyp to colon cancer occurs slowly, over about 5 to 10 years, because of a series of genetic changes. If you have a polyp removed before it becomes malignant, that polyp cannot develop into colon cancer.

Colon cancer is the second leading cause of cancer deaths in the United States. It is believed to arise, to some degree, from lifestyle habits such as a high-fat, low-fiber diet and smoking cigarettes. Heredity also plays a role; up to 25% of people with colon cancer have family members who have had the disease. Diseases that increase the chance of colon cancer include inflammatory bowel disease (especially ulcerative colitis, see p.787) and possibly diabetes.

Because there are no symptoms in the early stages, you should be screened for colon cancer if you are over 50 (see Preventing Colon Cancer, p.791).

SYMPTOMS

Both noncancerous and cancerous polyps usually cause no symptoms. Even after polyps evolve into cancer, symptoms are rare until the growth is large, when it may block the large intestine or bleed into the stools. By then, the cancer may have penetrated the wall of the intestine and spread to the lymph glands in the abdomen or to other organs.

TREATMENT OPTIONS

If you have rectal bleeding, your physician may perform one or more diagnostic tests. Flexible sigmoidoscopy (see p.785) is

Stages of Colon Cancer

Colon cancer is classified into stages by how advanced it is. Colon cancer is highly treatable in its early stages. The stages, treatment, and survival after 5 years are outlined below:

STAGE/LOCATION OF SPREAD	TREATMENT	CHANCE OF SURVIVAL 5 YEARS AFTER DIAGNOSIS
I / Cancer is confined to colon wall.	Removal of the bowel	85% to 100%
II / Cancer has spread through colon wall.	Removal of the bowel and sometimes radiation therapy (see p.741)	60% to 70%
III / Cancer has spread through colon wall and to the lymph nodes.	Removal of the bowel, radiation therapy, chemotherapy (see p.741), and immunotherapy to boost the immune system	30% to 60%
IV / Cancer has metastasized (spread) to other parts of the body.	Removal of the bowel, radiation therapy, chemotherapy, immunotherapy, and sometimes surgery to remove tumors that have spread to the liver	3%

Benefits of Combination Therapy for Colon Cancer

If colon cancer partially invades the bowel wall and spreads to the lymph nodes, affected people have a better outlook with a combination of surgery and chemotherapy than with surgery alone. The most effective chemotherapy is a combination of the drugs leucovorin and fluorouracil.

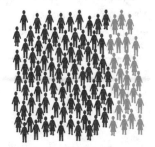

77 OF 100 PEOPLE WHO HAVE INVASIVE COLON CANCER AND ARE TREATED WITH SURGERY ALONE ARE ALIVE 4 YEARS LATER

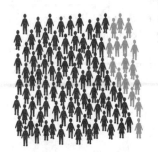

84 OF 100 PEOPLE WHO HAVE INVASIVE COLON CANCER AND ARE TREATED WITH A COMBINATION OF SURGERY AND CHEMOTHERAPY ARE ALIVE 4 YEARS LATER

---

often the first approach when bright red blood is the symptom, since it is likely that the bleeding is coming from the far end of the colon.

If the blood shows up on a test for occult (hidden) blood (see p.791), a barium enema (see p.784) or colonoscopy (see p.784) may be performed. They can both reveal colon cancer, as well as other causes of bleeding, including hemorrhoids (see p.795), proctitis (see p.797), noncancerous polyps, or cancerous polyps, which become colon cancer when they grow into and through the wall of the large intestine.

Colonoscopy is generally preferred because it is slightly better at detecting cancer, and because biopsies of a possible cancerous tumor or removal of bleeding polyps can be performed during the colonoscopy. The doctor may remove a small piece of any abnormal-looking tissue to test it for cancer. Regular colonoscopies are recommended for people at high risk for colon cancer.

Colon cancer is classified by stages (see Stages of Colon Cancer, p.792) and treatment depends on the stage. Surgery to remove

all or part of the bowel is recommended for every stage; this involves cutting the abdomen and removing the affected portion of the intestine (colectomy).

The surgery can also be done using an endoscope (see p.142) after the surgeon makes several keyhole incisions in the abdomen. This procedure is controversial and the subject of a national study.

Surgery is sometimes followed by radiation therapy and/or chemotherapy. Most people with colon cancer do not need a colostomy (see next article); surgical procedures that spare the anal sphincter allow the majority of people to retain control of their bowels.

Colostomy and Ileostomy

Colostomy and ileostomy are operations in which portions of the intestine are removed and an opening called a stoma is made in the abdominal wall to allow passage of feces. Bowel movements are routed through the stoma and into a pouch that is attached to the stoma on the outside of the abdomen.

The surgery is usually per-

formed when it is necessary to remove damaged sections of the intestines but when it is not possible to reconnect the two ends.

In colostomy, which can be temporary or permanent, part of the large intestine (colon) is removed and the end of the colon is brought to the surface of the abdomen and stitched. In ileostomy, the colon and rectum are usually removed completely and the lower end of the small intestine is attached to the opening in the abdomen. This procedure is permanent.

Before surgery, you will take antibiotics to reduce the level of bacteria in your body. During the procedure, which is performed using general anesthesia (see p.168), your doctor makes an incision in the abdomen and removes the damaged part of the intestine. After surgery, you will be fed intravenously for several days, and introduced gradually to a diet of solid foods that minimizes gas and eases the passage of bowel movements.

After surgery, your doctor may suggest dietary changes to restrict gas-forming and odor-causing foods, including beans, eggs, fish, and carbonated drinks. A nurse will instruct you in the proper care and hygiene of the stoma and in the cleaning and emptying of the pouch. Eventually, many people need to wear only a pad over the stoma (except when defecating).

People with ileostomies usu-ally cannot remove the pouch except to empty it. In some cases, the surgeon can create a reservoir inside the abdominal wall to collect feces; the reservoir can be emptied periodically during the day.

The challenges of adapting to a colostomy or ileostomy can be great but can be eased by taking measures that help improve your physical and mental well-being. See Ostomies (p.1235) for support information.

RECTAL AND ANAL DISORDERS

Anal Fissure and Fistula

Anal fissures are tears in the delicate lining of the anal canal; they occur near its opening. An anal fissure may be superficial or deep and may extend up the anal canal. Fissures are thought to occur when a hard stool tears the lining of the anal canal.

An anal fistula is a channel that connects the inside of the anus to the skin outside the anus. A fistula usually develops when a rectal abscess (a pus-filled sac) (see p.797) spreads in canal-like fashion from the inside of the rectum to the outer skin.

Fistulas can occur with conditions such as inflammatory bowel disease (see p.787) or colon cancer (see p.791).

SYMPTOMS

Anal fissures cause pain during bowel movements that can persist for several hours after the bowel movement; the pain then subsides until the next bowel movement. Fissures can also bleed, producing red blood on toilet paper. An abscess, which most often causes a fistula, can cause pain and tenderness and can discharge pus and feces onto the outer surface of the skin.

TREATMENT OPTIONS

A visual examination is usually enough for a doctor to diagnose an anal fissure. A fistula may require more in-depth observation using anoscopy (see p.784) to differentiate it from other conditions and to determine the extent and direction of the fistula's channel.

Fissures often heal on their own, and many respond well to simple measures, including stool softeners and glycerin suppositories that lubricate the lower rectum. Taking a warm bath for 10 to 15 minutes after each bowel movement may relieve pain temporarily.

Fistulas are treated by draining the abscess of pus and cleaning out the channel of the fistula after using a local anesthetic to dull the pain.

Fecal Impaction

Fecal impaction is a condition in which bowel movements become dry, hard, and cannot be passed from the rectum. It is most common among very young children, elderly people, and anyone who is bedridden.

You may feel like you need to have a bowel movement, and have pain in your abdomen, rectum, and anus. Diarrhea can occur when loose stool squeezes around hard, impacted feces.

Your doctor will insert a gloved finger into your rectum to identify the impaction. It can be removed manually or by having an enema (injecting fluid into the rectum through a tube).

Fecal Incontinence

Fecal incontinence is the inability to control bowel movements, resulting in evacuation of the bowels at unpredictable times and socially unacceptable places. Severe diarrhea and fecal impaction (see previous article) can produce temporary fecal incontinence.

Fecal incontinence can produce minor soiling between bowel movements or seepage of feces when expelling gas. It can also occur with a temporary bout of diarrhea. A woman may experience fecal incontinence after vaginal childbirth, sometimes due to tearing of tissues or a surgical incision (see Episiotomy, p.938). Fecal incontinence can also be so severe that you can no longer control even solid bowel movements. This is most likely to occur in people who are immobile or weak.

Causes include an anal sphinc-

Muscles of Fecal Continence

CONTINENCE

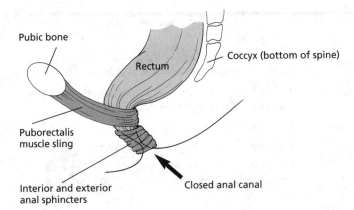

Pubic bone

Coccyx (bottom of spine)

Rectum

Puborectalis muscle sling

Interior and exterior anal sphincters

Closed anal canal

DEFECATION

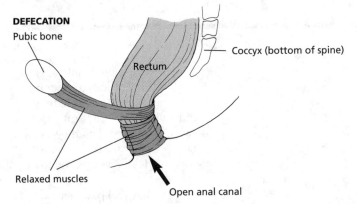

Pubic bone

Coccyx (bottom of spine)

Rectum

Relaxed muscles

Open anal canal

The puborectalis muscle forms a sling that holds the rectum at a 90-degree angle, which, along with the internal and external sphincters, prevents the passage of stool (top). As feces fill the rectum, it distends and the puborectalis muscle relaxes, allowing the rectum to straighten. At the same time, the internal sphincter relaxes and the stool moves toward the anus (bottom).

ter or rectum that has abnormal nerve or muscle function, spinal cord injury or nerve damage, inflammatory bowel disease (see p.787), and surgery that involves the anus.

SYMPTOMS

Depending on the cause, you may or may not feel the urge to defecate; the degree to which you can control defecation may vary.

TREATMENT OPTIONS

Fecal incontinence can almost always be treated. Do not be embarrassed to discuss it with your doctor, who will perform a digital rectal exam (see p.1103). He or she may also test the reflexes of your anus, which should contract when touched. If the anus does not respond as it should, the nerves that control continence may be damaged. Sigmoidoscopy (see p.784) may also be used to look for inflammation, sores, or growths.

Taking fiber supplements such as psyllium can help you have bulkier stools and decrease incontinence. Decreasing your intake of several sugars—lactose (in milk), fructose (in fruit), and sorbitol (in berries and other fruit)—can decrease diarrhea. Performing Kegel exercises (see p.1051) every day can also help strengthen the anal sphincter and pelvic floor muscles.

Your doctor may prescribe antidiarrheal agents such as loperamide. A daily enema with tap water may help prevent the condition.

Hemorrhoids

A hemorrhoid is a swollen vein in the rectum and anus. The majority of hemorrhoids (and those responsible for most symptoms) are located inside the anus. In some people, they occur outside the anus (prolapsed hemorrhoids). External hemorrhoids occur near the opening of the anus.

Hemorrhoids are caused by increased pressure in the veins of the anus, often from straining during a bowel movement to expel dry, hard feces. They also often occur during pregnancy and after giving birth.

SYMPTOMS

Bright red blood on stools or toilet paper is often the first symptom of internal hemorrhoids,

Home Remedies for Anal Itching

Anal itching is a common and annoying problem. Although it is usually harmless, it is a good idea to have a persistent problem checked by your doctor. Anal itching can be a symptom of conditions that require treatment, including psoriasis, allergy, pinworms, hemorrhoids, or an anal fissure or more serious disorder.

In most people, anal itching is caused by minor irritation, often due to use of scented soaps or scented toilet paper. The aim of the following home remedies is to minimize irritation to the sensitive tissues:

- Keep the anal area clean by washing daily with unscented soap and warm water. Dry gently but completely with a towel or even a blow dryer.

- Wear loose cotton underwear to improve air circulation.

- Apply an over-the-counter cleansing lotion designed specifically for the region around the anus.

- Avoid scented and colored toilet paper; use lubricated cleansing pads instead.

- Apply chilled witch hazel to the irritated area.

- Apply an over-the-counter hydrocortisone cream.

- Do not scratch. Scratching can irritate the area more and cause swelling that can cause further itching.

Hemorrhoids

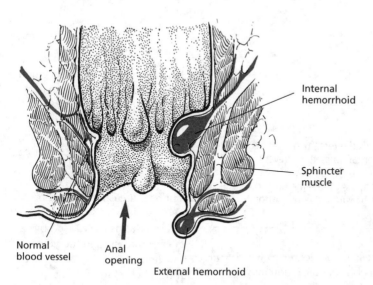

External hemorrhoids are located on the edge of the anus. Internal hemorrhoids develop inside the anus; they are sometimes pushed out during a bowel movement or childbirth.

Labels: Internal hemorrhoid; Sphincter muscle; Normal blood vessel; Anal opening; External hemorrhoid

which are usually painless. Hemorrhoids near the anal opening may not be noticed until they fill with blood and form a clot, which can vary from the size of a pea to the size of a walnut, forming a blue lump around the anus.

You may feel pain that increases for a day or two but usually dissipates within a week as the clot dissolves. After the clot disappears, small, empty pouches of skin often remain.

Prolapsed hemorrhoids are unmistakable; you can sense a mass protruding from your anus that may be painful with friction and may itch. They can move back into the anal canal on their own or in response to gentle pressure from your fingertips. When internal hemorrhoids are permanently prolapsed, they can become inflamed and may issue a watery discharge.

TREATMENT OPTIONS

If you have rectal bleeding, see your doctor. He or she will perform a rectal exam (see p.1103) to feel for abnormalities and may look for internal hemorrhoids through a lighted tube called an anoscope (see p.784). To rule out colon cancer (see p.791) and other sources of bleeding, your doctor may perform a sigmoidoscopy or colonoscopy (see p.784).

To prevent hemorrhoids, gradually increase the fiber (see p.38) in your diet to 25 to 30 grams a day and drink eight glasses of water daily. Also, respond quickly to the urge to defecate and avoid straining on the toilet. Finally, performing Kegel exercises (see p.1051) can help strengthen the muscles of the anus.

To relieve the symptoms of most hemorrhoids, your doctor may recommend sitting in plain, warm water for 10 to 15 minutes several times a day and applying cold packs to the affected area while resting in bed with your buttocks on a pillow.

Over-the-counter aids include petroleum jelly or hemorrhoid creams that contain lidocaine to temporarily relieve pain, hydrocortisone preparations to cool inflammation, or cotton pads soaked in witch hazel to ease itching.

Surgery may be recommended for internal hemorrhoids. In surgery, rubber bands are placed around the distended hemorrhoid, which causes it to lose its blood supply, shrivel, and fall off.

Pilonidal Sinus

A pilonidal sinus is a recurring abscess (pus-filled sac) in the small pit in the skin above the cleft between the buttocks. Caused by ingrown hair, a pilonidal sinus usually occurs in young men who have a lot of hair.

A pilonidal sinus starts out as a painful swelling and progresses to an ulcer that leaks fluid or pus. See your doctor at the first sign of swelling; he or she may be able to drain the abscess of fluid. Otherwise, the infection and the skin around it will be surgically removed. Keep the area clean and dry to prevent a recurrence.

Proctitis

Proctitis is inflammation of the rectum. It may be accompanied by bleeding, pain, and a discharge of mucus or pus. Proctitis often accompanies conditions that cause inflammation of the colon, such as inflammatory bowel disease (see p.787), dysentery (see p.780), or sexually transmitted diseases such as gonorrhea (see p.891).

Your doctor can definitively diagnose proctitis by proctoscopy (examination of the rectum with a viewing tube). He or she may also perform a biopsy (removal of rectal tissue for microscopic evaluation). Proctitis is cured by treating the underlying cause. Symptoms may be relieved by using prescribed enemas or suppositories that contain a corticosteroid drug, which reduces inflammation.

Rectal Abscess

A rectal abscess is an infected sac of tissue encased in pus that can occur high in the rectum, in the lower rectal area, or around the anus.

Rectal abscesses most often occur in men; people who receive anal intercourse are most susceptible. People who have inflammatory bowel disease (see p.787) or diabetes mellitus (see p.832) are also more often affected. If a rectal abscess is not treated, an anal fistula (an abnormal channel) (see p.794) may develop, which can lead to further infection that spreads.

An abscess can cause serious pain in the rectal area, especially during defecation. Bleeding and discharge of mucus and pus may also occur. Your doctor will perform a rectal examination or insert a flexible viewing tube to identify an abscess. If an abscess is found, you will receive a local anesthetic to numb the area and the abscess will be drained. This procedure can be performed in the doctor's office.

OTHER GASTROINTESTINAL TRACT DISORDERS

Lactase Deficiency and Lactose Intolerance

Lactose is the main sugar in milk and milk-based foods. You need an enzyme called lactase, made in the small intestine, to digest lactose. When too little lactase is produced, lactose is not digested. Instead, it passes intact through the small intestine and into the colon, where it is fermented by bacteria, producing hydrogen and other gases.

Undigested lactose also draws water into the colon, resulting in diarrhea. These symptoms are distressing, but they do not interfere with the digestion of other nutrients or cause long-term damage to the intestines.

Some degree of lactase deficiency is extremely common; from 5% to 15% of the white population and more than 80% of people of African and of Asian descent are affected.

Lactase deficiency can arise for several reasons. In rare cases, infants are born without the ability to produce lactose. For reasons that are not understood, lactase production in people of African, Asian, and Native Ameri-

Lactose Intolerance

NORMAL LACTOSE ABSORPTION AND DIGESTION IN SMALL INTESTINE

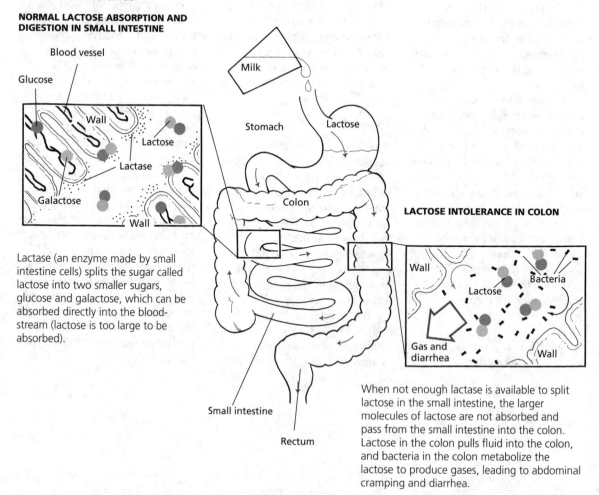

Lactase (an enzyme made by small intestine cells) splits the sugar called lactose into two smaller sugars, glucose and galactose, which can be absorbed directly into the bloodstream (lactose is too large to be absorbed).

LACTOSE INTOLERANCE IN COLON

When not enough lactase is available to split lactose in the small intestine, the larger molecules of lactose are not absorbed and pass from the small intestine into the colon. Lactose in the colon pulls fluid into the colon, and bacteria in the colon metabolize the lactose to produce gases, leading to abdominal cramping and diarrhea.

can descent wanes significantly with age.

In addition, the enzyme deficiency can be acquired with certain gastrointestinal conditions such as inflammatory bowel disease (see p.787), celiac disease (see p.774), and, briefly, after viral gastroenteritis (see p.778).

SYMPTOMS

If you have lactose intolerance, you may experience abdominal pain, bloating, gas, or diarrhea after you consume dairy products.

TREATMENT OPTIONS

If you believe that you are lactose intolerant, you should try a lactose-free diet for 1 to 2 weeks. If symptoms persist, see your doctor. There are several ways to diagnose lactose intolerance. Your doctor may recommend that you eliminate dairy products from your diet to see if the symptoms disappear.

Other tests include a lactose-tolerance test, in which you drink lactose dissolved in water and then have a blood test to measure the amount of lactose that has been absorbed into your blood.

A hydrogen breath test measures the amount of hydrogen in your breath every half hour for 5 hours after you consume a solution of lactose and water. In lactose-intolerant people, fermenting lactose in the colon yields a detectable amount of hydrogen. Tests of acid in the feces are used for infants and young children.

If you are lactose intolerant, you can help eliminate symptoms and still consume dairy products by taking the following measures:

■ Consume small quantities of dairy products. You may be able to tolerate small amounts if you cannot tolerate normal amounts.

■ Eat yogurt or aged cheeses instead of drinking milk.

■ Space your consumption of dairy products throughout the day; frequent, small meals may help the bacteria in your colon adjust to the presence of lactose.

■ Eat lactose-containing foods with other foods.

■ Use enzyme supplements (available in tablet form at many drugstores) to convert lactose to glucose, or drink lactose-free dairy products.

Food Allergies and Intolerance

Much confusion surrounds the difference between food intolerance and food allergy. Food intolerance is an adverse reaction to foods because the foods cannot be properly digested. Lactose intolerance, for example, is a food intolerance caused by a deficiency in the enzyme needed to digest the milk sugar lactose.

Foods may be poorly tolerated for a variety of reasons. However, many people who have difficulty tolerating certain foods appear

---

Home Remedies for Gas

Excess gas in the form of flatulence or burping can sometimes be resolved by making some minor adjustments in your diet and lifestyle. Try these home remedies:

■ Chew more slowly and thoroughly; gas can be a sign of undigested food. The physical act of chewing produces salivary enzymes in your mouth that are the first stage of digestion.

■ Eat in a calm environment; stress can cause flatulence and burping.

■ Avoid foods that are known to cause indigestion, such as milk products, beans, cabbage, carbonated beverages, and alcohol. Some foods are more difficult to digest than others.

■ Take a short walk after meals to prevent gas through regular exercise.

■ Take simethicone, activated charcoal, or bismuth.

■ Try an herbal remedy. Follow meals by chewing fennel seeds, or sipping teas of peppermint, anise, or chamomile.

■ Lie flat on your back and bring your left knee to your chest. Hold for 10 seconds, then repeat with the other knee.

If these home remedies do not help, see your doctor.

Eight Foods Cause Most Food Allergies

Although 33% of the U.S. population believe they are allergic to foods, only about 1% actually are. Reactions can be mild or severe. Eight foods cause about 90% of all allergies: cow's milk (primarily in infants), eggs, wheat, peanuts, soy, tree nuts, fish, and shellfish. As little as half a peanut can cause a severely allergic person to have a fatal reaction and severe reactions can even be caused by kissing someone who has recently eaten peanuts.

to have no underlying physical problems.

Food allergy is an abnormal response of the immune system to a food, even a very small quantity. It occurs when the body produces antibodies to a food and these antibodies react with the food to start an allergic reaction. Symptoms can include itching and swelling of the mouth, lips, or airways, sometimes causing extreme breathing problems, itchy skin or a rash, wheezing, and loss of consciousness.

Symptoms can appear within minutes to an hour after ingesting the offending food. Anaphylaxis (see p.894) is a sudden, severe, and life-threatening reaction that occurs in rare cases as part of a food allergy.

Whether significant food allergies are caused by additives in food, such as sulfites, is controversial. Sulfite-containing foods and beverages definitely can provoke serious symptoms in some people, but it remains unclear if it is the sulfites that are causing the adverse reaction.

If your doctor thinks you have food allergies, you may be referred to an allergist, who will first take a medical history (which may be all that is required to diagnose the problem) and possibly

perform a skin or blood test. As part of the skin test, food extracts and placebo (inactive) substances are inserted into the skin by a needle prick or puncture. A positive reaction to a food, indicated by a raised bump, means there is more than a 50% chance that you are allergic. The test is very useful in ruling out allergy.

Blood tests include a radioallergosorbent test and the enzyme-linked immunosorbent assay, which are used to indicate the presence of IgE antibodies in the blood. However, these tests are not foolproof.

An elimination diet is the most reliable test. In it, you eliminate all suspicious foods (such as dairy products, caffeine, alcohol, grains, red meat, and sugar) one at a time for 2 weeks and then gradually reintroduce them one at a time. If the symptoms get better with eliminating the food from your diet, and return with reintroduction of a food, an allergy to the food is likely.

There are no treatments for food allergies except to avoid the offending food. Those at risk for severe reactions should carry portable injections of epinephrine for use at the first sign of an anaphylactic reaction.

Hernias

A hernia is the protrusion of a portion of the intestine through a weak point in the intestinal or abdominal wall. Most often, hernias occur through a weak point in the groin, but they also occur through a natural weak point elsewhere in the abdomen, such as around the navel.

Hernias in the groin, called inguinal hernias, account for 75% of all hernias. A second type of hernia near the groin, called a femoral hernia, occurs most frequently in overweight women.

Hernias sometimes develop at weak points in the abdomen caused by previous surgery; these are called incisional hernias.

SYMPTOMS

A bulge is a symptom of all hernias. If the hernia becomes strangulated by twisting, it may cut off the supply of blood to the bowel, causing pain and tissue death, a life-threatening condition preceded by vomiting and nausea.

TREATMENT OPTIONS

If you suspect that you have a hernia, see your doctor, who will diagnose the problem by physical examination. Some hernias can be managed by wearing a device (truss) that puts pressure on the hernia and holds it in. Living with some kinds of hernias can be risky because it can eventually be impossible to push the swelling back into place, which can lead to intestinal obstruction (see p.789). Talk to your doctor about the risks you face with your hernia.

Hernias can be repaired by open surgery, in which an inci-

Inguinal Hernia

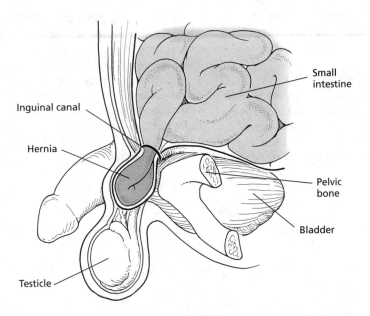

Inguinal canal

Hernia

Testicle

Small intestine

Pelvic bone

Bladder

An inguinal hernia is the protrusion of the intestine or fatty tissue into the groin through a weakness in the abdominal wall. Here a loop of intestine pushes through the inguinal canal above a testicle.

sion is made and the herniated tissue is pushed back into position and stitched there. Sometimes a small patch of synthetic material is placed over the gap to serve as scaffolding on which scar tissue will grow. This helps fortify the weakened muscle so that the hernia will not recur.

For laparoscopic hernia repair, the surgeon makes three small keyhole incisions in the abdomen, which is then inflated with carbon dioxide to help the surgeon view the inside of the abdomen. Surgical instruments and a small video camera are inserted via the laparoscope and, while watching a monitor, the instruments are inserted through the other openings.

The surgeon pushes the distended organ back into place and staples a patch over the opening. A newer laparoscopic technique involves blowing up a balloon in the abdominal space to provide an open area in which the surgeon can work, reducing the possibility of injury to the intestines and blood vessels.

After laparoscopic hernia surgery you are usually able to return to work in 1 to 2 weeks and to lift heavy objects in 4 to 6 weeks.

Ischemia of the Bowel

Ischemia of the bowel is a deficiency in the supply of blood, oxygen, and other nutrients to the bowel. The most common cause is atherosclerosis (see p.653), an accumulation of cholesterol in the lining of the blood vessels serving the bowel. Ischemia can also be caused by a blood clot. The condition usually affects older people.

Depending on the extent of blockage, you may have mild discomfort or sudden, severe, cramping abdominal pain (focused around the navel) that is made worse by eating. If a blood clot causes total obstruction of the arteries supplying the bowel, you will have sudden, severe pain, sometimes accompanied by blood in the stool.

Report any sudden, severe abdominal pain to your doctor. To diagnose blocked blood vessels, you may need to have magnetic resonance angiography (see p.150) to identify the location of the blockage. Surgery is the only treatment, either to remove the clot and repair the damaged area or to remove the affected portion of the intestine.

Peritonitis

Peritonitis is inflammation of the peritoneum, the membrane that lines the abdomen. It is usually caused by infection with bacteria due to an underlying abdominal disorder, such as a ruptured appendix. It also occurs commonly in people with fluid (ascites) in their abdomen.

Appendicitis is the most common cause of bacterial peritonitis, but it can also occur when perforations in the abdomen result from diverticulitis (see p.783), a peptic ulcer (see p.752), a gangrenous gallbladder (see p.878), or a strangulated hernia (see p.800). Chemical peritonitis arises from pancreatic enzymes, gastric acid, and bile that penetrate the peritoneum due to injury to the intestine or biliary tract.

SYMPTOMS

Intense abdominal pain and tenderness are the most common features of peritonitis. The location and severity of pain depend on the underlying cause. You may feel wavelike cramps at first, and your abdomen may become rigid. Your blood pressure may drop (making you feel dizzy and weak) and you may vomit. You may also have a fever.

TREATMENT OPTIONS

Peritonitis is an emergency that requires hospitalization. Your doctor will ask you to describe your symptoms to determine the cause. You may also need to have x-rays and blood tests to identify the source of your symptoms.

Treatment includes surgery to remove infected tissue (such as a burst appendix) or to repair perforations, such as a peptic ulcer. Your doctor will prescribe antibiotics (taken either orally or by intravenous infusion) and you may need to receive nutrients and fluids intravenously until your condition stabilizes.

Urinary System

The urinary system is an elaborate recycling and waste removal system. It filters the equivalent of about 45 gallons of blood every day in order to clean the fluid of waste material and reclaim important minerals (such as sodium and potassium) so they do not leave the body in the urine.

The kidneys also regulate and maintain the correct acid level of the blood by retaining acid or releasing it into the urine. Urine contains the waste products and a small fraction of the fluid filtered from the blood.

The urinary system also plays an important part in maintaining the right volume of blood in your body. Any fluid you drink is absorbed into the blood and increases the total volume of blood in the circulation. When the blood volume is higher than normal, the kidneys respond by eliminating more fluid in the urine.

If you drink too little fluid, or lose a great deal by sweating during exercise or a fever, the kidneys respond by eliminating less fluid in the urine, which helps you from becoming dehydrated.

The urinary tract is composed of two kidneys, two ureters, the bladder, the prostate (in men), and the urethra.

Kidneys Each of the two kidneys is about the size of your fist. They lie on either side of your spine in the upper abdominal cavity. Blood flows into each kidney through its renal artery (renal is the medical term used when referring to kidneys), and then flows through an extensive network of smaller arteries inside each kidney.

Each kidney contains about 1 million microscopic filtering units called nephrons. Nephrons begin with the glomerulus, a tuft of capillaries that filter fluid and waste from the blood. The cells and proteins in the blood stay inside the blood vessels and do not get filtered out.

The rate at which blood is filtered is called the glomerular filtration rate; it is a way for doctors to measure how well the kidneys are functioning.

The fluid and waste filtered out in the glomeruli then travel through an intricate set of microscopic tubes (called tubules) before leaving the kidneys as urine. It is in the tubules that the kidneys regulate the fluid, electrolyte, and acid balance of the body. If the tubules receive signals saying the body needs more of a substance (such as fluid, minerals, or acid), they absorb these substances from the urine back into the blood.

Urinary Tract

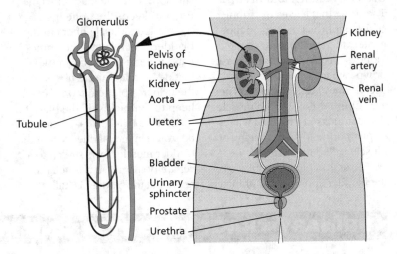

The urinary tract is composed of two kidneys, two ureters, the bladder, the prostate (in men), and the urethra. The kidneys (each about the size of your fist) flank the spine in the back upper part of the abdominal cavity. They filter waste material out of the blood and eliminate it from the body in the urine. The kidneys also regulate the amount of water, minerals, and acid in the body.

Urine and Your Health

The appearance and composition of urine offers important clues about your body's health. Urine is composed mainly of water (about 95%), waste products, and salts. Normally, it is clear and yellow.

Cloudy urine may indicate the presence of bacteria and white blood cells from a urinary tract infection (see Cystitis, below), although this is not always the case.

A reddish hue can indicate bleeding due to infection or inflammation of the glomerulus, but can also be caused by certain foods containing red pigments, such as beets. If you have ever wondered what causes the pungent smell of your urine after eating asparagus, it is a substance called asparagine, an amino acid found in many plants, but especially present in asparagus.

Urine tests (see p.805) can detect excess amounts of glucose (sugar) in the urine, which may suggest diabetes. Small amounts of glucose in the urine are a normal occurrence during pregnancy.

Protein in the urine can be found in a number of diseases of the kidneys, including inflammation of the kidneys or a defect in kidney filtration called nephrotic syndrome (see p.820). Protein in the urine also occurs when kidney function is declining because of diabetes or high blood pressure.

Ketones are small molecules that accumulate in the blood and urine when you have not had a meal for many hours, or in diabetes when the body does not have enough insulin.

Doctors sometimes measure the amount of uric acid, calcium, oxalate, sodium, and other substances in the urine of people who form kidney stones, which are often composed of these substances.

Kidney function is often checked by measuring levels of blood urea nitrogen (BUN) and creatinine in the blood. As kidney function declines, not enough BUN and creatinine are filtered into the urine, and higher levels are measured in the blood. Occasionally, a urine specimen collected over 24 hours is measured for urea and creatinine.

Ureters, bladder, and urethra
The urine that leaves the tubules of the nephrons collects in the center (the renal pelvis) of the kidneys. From there, urine passes down two long tubes (one from each kidney) called ureters. They are composed of smooth muscle that contracts in rhythmic waves to push urine toward a bag of muscle called the bladder.

The action of muscle fibers of the bladder and urinary sphincter (the exit from the bladder to the urethra) keeps the urine inside the bladder. Muscle fibers in the bladder wall relax to accommodate urine as it collects in the bladder, while muscle fibers of the urinary sphincter contract to keep the urine inside the bladder.

Up to 400 milliliters of urine can be stored in the bladder. When the bladder muscle fibers stretch to a certain point, nerve cells tell the brain that the bladder is full.

When you urinate, you relax your pelvic muscles and the opening of the urethra to allow urine to pass. At the same time, nerves tell the bladder muscles to contract and the urinary sphincter to relax, which helps the bladder to empty.

In women, the urethra empties just above the vagina. In men, the urethra passes through the middle of the penis and empties at the tip of the penis.

URINARY TRACT INFECTION AND INFLAMMATION

Cystitis

Most infections of the urinary tract involve the lower portion of the tract—the bladder and urethra. Cystitis is infection of the bladder; urethritis (see p.808) is infection of the urethra. They usually occur together, although some kinds of infections cause only urethritis.

Most urinary infections in women start because bacteria from the digestive tract that live on the skin around the anus get pushed up toward the vagina

Common Tests for Kidney and Urinary Tract Disorders

Your doctor may perform one or more of the following tests to evaluate the health of your kidneys and urinary tract:

URINE TEST

Urine tests (see p.158) look for the presence of many different substances, such as glucose, protein, white blood cells, or red blood cells, which can indicate an infection or disease of the kidneys or bladder.

KIDNEY BIOPSY

A kidney biopsy is an examination of a tissue sample from a kidney. It may be needed to make a diagnosis when it is unclear what has caused a disease of the kidneys such as acute or chronic kidney failure, glomerulonephritis (see p.810), or nephrotic syndrome (see p.820). The tissue is sent to a laboratory for a pathologist to examine under a microscope.

A kidney biopsy is either percutaneous (through the skin) or open (surgical). In a percutaneous biopsy, a local anesthetic is injected into the area over the tissues to numb them. Using ultrasound (see p.148) for guidance, the doctor inserts a hollow needle through the skin and into a kidney, and a tiny sample of tissue is extracted.

This procedure is less painful than an open biopsy, and is often done in an outpatient setting. You can resume normal activity within a week.

In an open biopsy, you must receive general anesthesia (see p.168). The surgeon makes a small incision over a kidney, removes a piece of kidney tissue, and stitches the incision closed. You may need to stay overnight in the hospital and may have some pain in your back after the biopsy.

However, this procedure has a lower risk of bleeding than a percutaneous biopsy and is performed if the risk of bleeding is very high.

RADIONUCLIDE SCAN

Radionuclide scans are discussed on p.145. In this procedure, substances that emit small amounts of radiation (radionuclides) are injected into a vein and collected in the kidneys. Using single photon emission computed tomography (see p.149), a scanning machine revolves around you to record cross-sectional images, which can be constructed into a whole image of a kidney.

One type of radionuclide binds specifically to kidney tubules to provide an image of their function. Serial scans track the course of the dye through the urinary system, providing detailed images of anatomical structure.

INTRAVENOUS PYELOGRAM (IVP)

This x-ray procedure provides images of the urinary system by injecting into a vein a small amount of contrast medium (see p.147), which is filtered into the urinary system. This makes the urinary system visible on an x-ray.

Your doctor may use it to look for an obstruction in the urinary system, for kidney stones or tumors, for causes of recurring kidney or urinary tract infections, or for the cause of blood in the urine.

You will be asked to avoid food and fluids for 12 hours before the procedure, and to empty your bowel with a laxative. The radiologist will first take x-rays of your abdomen while you are lying down. Then you will receive an injection of contrast medium, usually into the vein of an arm.

Periodically, x-rays are taken to follow the course of the dye from the blood into your kidneys and then to your ureters. Once your bladder is full, you will be asked to urinate. A final x-ray is made of the bladder to see how empty it is.

COMPUTED TOMOGRAPHY (CT) SCAN

A CT scan (see p.149) is a faster and perhaps more complete way of looking at most abnormalities of the kidneys. It also has the advantage of taking images of structures near a kidney, in case the problem turns out not to be with a kidney but with a nearby organ.

CYSTOURETHROGRAM

A cystourethrogram is an x-ray test done primarily to diagnose disorders in children. It helps evaluate the function of the bladder during urination. After injecting a contrast medium (see p.147) directly into the bladder through a catheter, you will urinate while x-rays are taken.

This procedure helps pinpoint anatomical problems that cause conditions such as vesicoureteral reflux (see p.821), which causes urine to move back up the ureters (the tubes that empty the kidneys) instead of into the bladder.

Female and Male Urethras

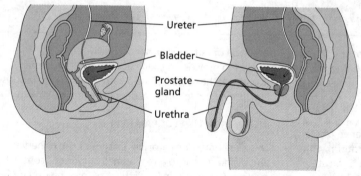

The urethra is a tube that conducts urine from the bladder to the outside of the body. A woman's urethra (left) is about 1½ inches long. Women are more vulnerable to bladder infections because bacteria have a shorter distance to travel to get to the bladder. A man's urethra (right) is approximately 9 inches long.

and the opening of the urethra. This often happens during sexual intercourse. Then, the bacteria travel up the urethra and into the bladder. Nutrients in the urine give them nourishment.

The bacterium *Escherichia coli* (commonly known as *E coli*), which lives in the digestive tract, causes 80% of the cases of cystitis that occur in women. However, other bacteria and sexually transmitted organisms can also cause infection in both men and women.

Women are especially susceptible to cystitis because of the short length of their urethras and the proximity of the urethral opening to the anus, where bacteria thrive.

Some women are more susceptible to having cystitis after menopause. A drop in estrogen levels shifts the balance of microbes in the vagina and can encourage the growth of bacteria, which can spread to the urethra and cause infection in the bladder.

Women who use a diaphragm for birth control are at higher risk for cystitis, although the risk is still low. Older women who have prolapse of the bladder or uterus are also at risk for cystitis. In these conditions, bacteria may not be adequately flushed out because the bladder may not empty completely. Instead, the bacteria stay and multiply inside the bladder.

Cystitis also can affect older men whose prostate glands are enlarged, which can prevent complete emptying of the bladder.

Any condition that reduces the flow of urine out of your body—and thus permits bacteria to stay in the bladder and urinary tract—can increase your risk of cystitis. Pregnant women may be more susceptible to urinary infections because of the pressure of the enlarging uterus on the ureters. People with kidney stones (see p.818) or bladder tumors (see Cancer of the Bladder, p.822) are more likely to get urinary infections. Conditions that weaken the immune system, such as diabetes, may also lead to urinary tract infections.

SYMPTOMS

Cystitis sometimes produces severe burning pain during urination and causes a frequent, urgent need to urinate, often in only small amounts. The urge may wake you in the middle of the night. The urine of a person

Cranberry Juice for Cystitis

Long used by women to prevent bladder infections, cranberry juice earned a measure of clinical respect in a small study conducted at Harvard in 1994. Women at risk of cystitis drank either 10 ounces of cranberry juice a day or a placebo that looked and tasted identical to cranberry juice. Women who drank the juice were somewhat less likely to have urinary tract infections.

How does this apply to you? Cranberry juice may help prevent symptoms of cystitis. However, it should not be used in place of medical care. A 3-day course of antibiotics is likely to be more effective and is often less expensive than cranberry juice. A stronger recommendation will be possible if other studies confirm the value of drinking cranberry juice.

In this study, cranberry juice was not used (and should not be used) to treat the symptoms of pyelonephritis, women with urinary tract diseases, people with diabetes or impaired immune systems, or men.

with cystitis is usually cloudy and often pink or bloody.

Blood in the urine is common but temporary in cystitis. If you see blood (in any amount) in your urine and you do not have the other symptoms of cystitis, see your doctor.

If you also have back pain, chills, fever, nausea, and vomiting, you may not have cystitis; the infection may have spread up into the kidney (see Pyelonephritis, p.808).

TREATMENT OPTIONS

If you are a man with symptoms of cystitis, call your doctor. Urinary infections are unusual in men younger than 50. In older men, a urinary tract infection can indicate another urinary tract condition such as an enlarged prostate (see p.1098) or prostatitis (see p.1096).

If you are a woman with symptoms of cystitis for the first time, or if you have symptoms and are pregnant, call your doctor. If you have symptoms of pyelonephritis, you should call your doctor immediately.

If you have had frequent recurrences of cystitis, discuss these three approaches with your doctor:

■ Keeping a supply of antibiotics at home to take at the first sign of a lower urinary tract infection. Despite the risks of side effects (such as stomach upset and diarrhea) and the possibility of promoting the growth of antibiotic-resistant organisms (see Hospital-Acquired Infections and Antibiotic-Resistant Bacteria, p.880), self-treatment of recurring cystitis has generally been proven to be safe and effective.

Preventing Cystitis in Women

These measures can help reduce your risk of cystitis (bladder infection) caused by bacteria:

■ Urinate when you feel the urge and try to empty your bladder completely each time. Delaying urination or retaining urine gives bacteria a chance to multiply.

■ Wipe genitals from front to back after using the toilet. This makes it less likely that bacteria from the rectum will contaminate the urethra or vagina.

■ Urinate and drink a glass of water after intercourse. This helps flush out any bacteria that have been pushed into the urethra.

■ Drink plenty of water every day (at least eight 8-ounce glasses) to dilute your urine.

■ Drinking cranberry juice may have some value (see p.806). If you use it, start as soon as you have symptoms of an infection.

■ If you use a diaphragm, spermicides, and/or cervical cap and have recurring cystitis, consider switching to another form of birth control. Spermicides kill helpful bacteria that ordinarily limit the growth of *Escherichia coli* (*E coli*) in the vaginal area.

Antibiotics After Sex for Cystitis

Some women encounter cystitis (bladder infection) for the first time shortly after they become sexually active, developing so-called "honeymoon cystitis." During intercourse, bacteria in and around the vagina are pushed up into the urethra, the tube that carries urine from the bladder out of the body.

Because the female urethra is short, the bacteria do not have to travel far to reach the bladder. Eight of 10 times the infecting organism is *Escherichia coli* (commonly known as *E coli*), a bacterium that thrives in the digestive tract.

To help prevent cystitis, try to urinate before and after sexual intercourse. This is sometimes enough to discourage the growth of bacteria in the urine and flushes out bacteria that may have been introduced into the urethra during intercourse.

If you repeatedly have cystitis after sexual activity, your doctor may recommend you take a single dose of antibiotic right after sexual intercourse. A single dose is often enough to prevent cystitis by killing the small numbers of bacteria that have just entered the bladder but have not had enough time to multiply and cause infection.

- Taking low doses of antibiotics every day for several months.

- Taking an antibiotic right after having sex (see Antibiotics After Sex for Cystitis, p.807) if your recurring infections regularly occur after sexual intercourse.

If you have symptoms of cystitis, your doctor may want to examine a sample of your urine under a microscope to look for bacteria and white blood cells (which indicate infection).

He or she may also use a chemical strip to test for white blood cells or perform a culture. The culture can identify the exact type of bacteria that are causing the infection so that your doctor can choose an antibiotic that will kill them.

To test your urine, your physician will first ask you for a "clean-catch" urine specimen. This means a sample that is free from contamination by bacteria that is normally present on the skin of your genitals. You provide a clean-catch specimen by using a cleansing wipe around the urinary opening before starting to urinate and then using a sterile container to catch the flow of urine a few seconds after you begin urinating.

If bacteria are found in the urine sample, your physician will prescribe antibiotics. An excellent drug regimen to follow for most people (unless you are allergic to it) is 3 days of a combination of trimethoprim and sulfamethoxazole.

This 3-day course is easier to take and causes fewer side effects than 10 days of ampicillin, a regimen that was once widely used. One third of all *E coli* strains that cause cystitis are now resistant to ampicillin because of widespread use.

Drink plenty of water and avoid coffee and alcohol, which can irritate the bladder. With treatment, symptoms usually disappear within a day or two. However, take the drugs for as long as your doctor recommends.

If you have a relapse within 2 weeks of completing treatment, you may have a kidney infection or cystitis caused by an organism that is resistant to the antibiotic prescribed; either way, see your doctor so that a different treatment can be started.

Urethritis

Any kind of inflammation of the urethra, including infection, is called urethritis. Bacterial infections of the bladder (see Cystitis, p.804) also usually involve the urethra, the tube that transports urine from your bladder to the outside of your body.

There are several other infections that primarily or exclusively cause urethritis. The sexually transmitted diseases gonorrhea (see p.891) and infection with *Chlamydia trachomatis* (see p.892) are the most significant, because they can lead to serious complications. With a sexually transmitted bacterial infection, you should notify all sex partners so they can be treated as well.

It is important to treat urethritis because it can progress to cause more serious conditions such as stricture (narrowing) of the urethra, arthritis, and pelvic inflammatory disease (see p.1077).

Urethritis is not caused only by infection. It can also be caused by vigorous sexual activity that irritates the urethra, or by irritation from spermicides, condoms, or a diaphragm. In both sexes, it can occur due to bruising from insertion of a catheter into the urethra.

Pyelonephritis

Pyelonephritis is an infection of the kidney, usually from bacteria that spread from the bladder up the ureters to the kidneys. It is more likely to develop if there is some obstruction of the urinary tract that impairs the free flow of urine.

It also is more common in people who have had a catheter inserted into the urethra to drain urine from the bladder, which can occur during general anesthesia for surgery, in people who are critically ill, or in people with urinary incontinence.

Pyelonephritis also is more common in those who have had cystoscopy (see p.825) or surgery on the urinary tract. It can occasionally lead to a serious blood infection (see Bacteremia, p.878) and therefore always requires the attention of your doctor.

Pyelonephritis can be a recurring problem, often because of some problem in the way the urinary tract is built. In children, an important cause of recurring pyelonephritis is vesicoureteral reflux (see p.821), which is a backwash of urine from the bladder into the ureters and up into the kidneys.

This is caused by an abnormality of a valve where the ureter joins the bladder. Normally, the valve allows the urine to pass only from the ureter to the bladder.

If the urine contains enough bacteria, the reflux permits infection to reach the kidneys. Repeated infection and inflammation of the kidneys, which commonly starts in childhood, can lead to scarring of the kidney tissue and irreversible kidney damage later in life.

SYMPTOMS

If you have pyelonephritis, you may have burning when you urinate and you may feel the need to urinate frequently and urgently; these symptoms are the same as those of cystitis and urethritis.

Unlike cystitis and urethritis, however, you may also have pain in your back (usually on one side), a high fever, chills, nausea, and/or vomiting.

TREATMENT OPTIONS

If you have the symptoms of pyelonephritis, see your doctor as soon as possible. Your urine will be examined under the microscope to see if there are bacteria and white blood cells (which indicate infection).

Your doctor will also perform a urine culture to determine what kind of bacteria are causing the infection, and what antibiotics will kill them.

Most acute cases of pyelonephritis are easily cured with antibiotics, rest, and plenty of fluids. In more serious cases, hospitalization is recommended, but usually for only a few days.

Since pyelonephritis can be caused by conditions that produce obstruction of the urinary tract, your doctor may recommend that you have an intravenous pyelogram (see p.805), kidney ultrasound, or cystoscopy (see p.825).

Interstitial Cystitis

Interstitial cystitis is chronic (long-term) inflammation of the wall of the bladder. It affects approximately 1 of every 1,000 to 2,000 adult women in the United States.

The causes of interstitial cystitis are not known. Some researchers believe that viruses or other microorganisms that have not yet been discovered may be responsible for the condition. Other possible causes include allergic reaction, autoimmune disease (see p.870), hormone disturbance, or the presence of toxic substances in the urine.

SYMPTOMS

Symptoms can include a stabbing pelvic pain and a frequent, intense urge to urinate. In extreme cases, you may need to urinate more than 50 times a day and 10 times a night.

TREATMENT OPTIONS

Interstitial cystitis is more difficult to diagnose than bacterial cystitis because, unlike bacterial cystitis, the urine samples of people with interstitial cystitis rarely reveal any bacteria.

Your primary care doctor may refer you to a urologist or obstetrician/gynecologist, who will first take a thorough medical history to rule out other possible explanations for symptoms, such as infection, bladder cancer (see p.822), or spasms of the bladder wall (see Incontinence, p.826).

Next, the doctor usually performs cystoscopy (see p.825), which permits direct viewing of the wall of the bladder. After you drink fluid to distend your bladder, a fiberoptic probe is inserted through the urethra. A diagnosis of interstitial cystitis is confirmed by seeing tiny hemorrhages or sores on the bladder wall.

A variety of treatments have been tried, but each seems to help only some people. Your doctor may recommend one or a combination of the following:

Bladder distension This involves stretching the bladder by filling it with fluid to relieve symptoms.

Instilled medicines A catheter is used to deliver drugs (such as

Alternative Medicine: Interstitial Cystitis

Some people have found relief from the symptoms of interstitial cystitis by using:

■ Acupuncture to relieve pain

■ Biofeedback (see p.395) to learn to relax the muscles of the pelvic floor

dimethyl sulfoxide, which inhibits inflammation and pain) directly into the bladder.

Oral medicines Drugs such as amitriptyline (a heterocyclic antidepressant; see p.400) block pain. Other drugs that strengthen the bladder's protective lining,

which many researchers believe is compromised in interstitial cystitis, may also be used. A natural substance called arginine has been found to reduce symptoms.

Self-care Some people find relief by following a low-acid diet that excludes citrus foods,

coffee, tea, spicy foods, alcohol, and chocolate.

Surgery Surgery to expand the bladder is still a controversial approach. It has been used to help some people whose bladders have shrunk due to the condition.

KIDNEY DISEASE AND KIDNEY FAILURE

Glomerulonephritis

Glomerulonephritis (sometimes called "nephritis" for short) is inflammation of the glomeruli, the tiny tufts of capillaries that filter blood in the kidneys by removing fluid and waste products from the blood.

When the filters are not working effectively, protein and red blood cells pass into the urine. Loss of protein from the bloodstream can lead to fluid buildup (edema) in all parts of the body, including the legs, face, and hands. This is called nephrotic syndrome (see p.820); it occurs more commonly in children than in adults.

There are two forms of glomerulonephritis—acute and chronic. Acute glomerulonephritis produces sudden and severe symptoms and requires urgent treatment.

The chronic form comes on slowly over a period of months. Chronic glomerulonephritis can come and go, or progressively get worse, ultimately causing chronic kidney failure (see p.812).

There are many different causes of glomerulonephritis. A streptococcal infection (see p.879), particularly of the skin (but also of the throat), can trigger an immune reaction that leads to glomerulonephritis.

Certain diseases that involve immune system abnormalities—such as lupus (see p.898) or bacterial endocarditis (see p.695)—can cause glomerulonephritis. Hepatitis B and C may also cause glomerulonephritis.

In addition, there are several conditions that cause both glomerulonephritis and hemorrhaging in the lung. Some kinds of glomerulonephritis occur without a known cause or another disease being present.

SYMPTOMS

Severe, acute glomerulonephritis can cause smoky or red urine (due to red blood cells leaked into the urine by the damaged glomeruli), a flulike feeling, nausea and vomiting, and limited ability to produce urine. You may retain fluid, first in your lower legs and ankles, and, in more severe cases, throughout the body (nephrotic syndrome).

Chronic glomerulonephritis that is mild may cause no symptoms. Your physician may find protein in your urine from glomerulonephritis when performing urine testing for another reason. Other people are diag-

nosed during an investigation of smoky or red urine caused by blood in the urine.

TREATMENT OPTIONS

See your doctor if you have any of the symptoms above. Your physician will test a sample of your urine to look for protein and red blood cells.

If your doctor suspects glomerulonephritis, he or she may perform tests such as a kidney ultrasound, computed tomography scan (see p.805), or intravenous pyelogram (see p.805). In most cases, a kidney biopsy (see p.805) is necessary in order to make a diagnosis.

Treatment of acute glomerulonephritis depends upon the cause. Sometimes the only treatment necessary is to not eat salty foods, avoid adding salt to your food, and take diuretic medicines to increase urination.

More severe disease may require treatment with corticosteroids (see p.895) to reduce inflammation, diuretics, and other medicines for complications such as high blood pressure and anemia. More potent immunosuppressive drugs may also be prescribed.

The treatment for chronic

glomerulonephritis starts with diagnosing and treating any underlying disease. Medicines are used to reduce accompanying high blood pressure and loss of protein in the urine.

You may receive antihypertensive drugs for high blood pressure, diuretics to reduce fluid accumulation and swelling, and corticosteroids or immunosuppressive drugs to reduce inflammation.

Polycystic Kidney Disease

Polycystic kidney disease is an inherited disorder that produces multiple clusters of fluid-filled, noncancerous cysts on the kidneys. This causes enlargement of the kidneys and can interfere with their function.

Polycystic kidney disease may affect as many as half a million adults in the United States, usually people over the age of 30. A rare form of the disease affects children and is usually apparent in infancy. Many children with polycystic kidney disease go on to have chronic kidney failure.

Many adults have mild disease and experience only minor problems with kidney function. In adults who have cysts that are numerous and large, the cysts may damage enough of the kidney to cause high blood pressure and chronic kidney failure (see p.812).

People with polycystic kidney disease may have a higher incidence of kidney stones (see p.818) and may also have liver cysts. For some people with polycystic kidney disease, end-

Simple Kidney Cysts

Simple, usually solitary kidney cysts are soft, fluid-filled pouches in one or both kidneys. They are common—about 50% of people over 50 are thought to have at least one.

Simple kidney cysts rarely produce symptoms, and are almost always noncancerous (benign). Your doctor may find a cyst when performing an imaging procedure such as magnetic resonance imaging or ultrasound on your abdomen for another purpose.

Unless the cyst is extremely large and compressing other organs, or is causing pain in your back or abdomen, doctors usually recommend no treatment.

Occasionally, a cyst is drained by inserting a needle into it to relieve pressure. Although these cysts are rarely cancerous, the fluid may be examined for cancerous cells.

After drainage, cysts may recur. Laparoscopic surgery (see p.142) can be more effective in removing cysts permanently.

---

stage kidney failure can result as early as their 30s or 40s.

SYMPTOMS

Many people with polycystic kidney disease have no symptoms, but some have high blood pressure (see p.644). Occasionally, the disease causes pain in the back and upper side, frequent nighttime urination, kidney stones, and blood in the urine.

TREATMENT OPTIONS

If you have a family history of polycystic kidney disease, your doctor may perform an ultrasound, magnetic resonance imaging, or a computed tomography scan to examine your kidneys. Sometimes a diagnosis of polycystic kidney disease is made when one of these studies is performed for other reasons.

There is no way to prevent polycystic kidney disease, but your doctor will recommend a

regimen to prevent complications and ease symptoms.

If the disease has progressed, the cysts may be drained to prevent the enlarged kidneys from interfering with the function of other organs. High blood pressure is treated with medicine.

When the disease progresses to chronic kidney failure and end-stage kidney disease, dialysis (see p.815) or a kidney transplant (see p.814) is required.

Acute Kidney Failure

Acute kidney failure (also called acute renal failure) is the abrupt loss of kidney function. It affects about 3 of 10,000 people in the United States each year.

Acute kidney failure can cause a life-threatening accumulation of fluids and wastes in the body, and a consequent imbalance of chemicals that are well regulated by healthy kidneys.

What Is Kidney Failure?

Also called renal failure (renal is the word doctors use when referring to the kidneys), kidney failure describes a diseased kidney's impaired ability to filter impurities from the blood.

Kidney failure takes two forms—acute and chronic. The last stage of kidney disease is called end-stage kidney disease. It is discussed in Chronic Kidney Failure (below right).

Acute kidney failure is a sudden loss of kidney function. Although acute kidney failure can be very serious, most people recover and have normally functioning kidneys once the underlying condition is treated.

Chronic kidney failure is a progressive loss of kidney function that develops over many years. Chronic kidney failure can lead to end-stage kidney failure, which requires dialysis (see p.815) or a kidney transplant (see p.814).

The most common causes of acute kidney failure are a sudden drop in the blood flowing through the kidneys, caused by excessive bleeding (including during surgery), shock, or severe dehydration.

Acute kidney failure can also be caused by medicines that cause interstitial nephritis (see Medicine-Induced Interstitial Nephritis, p.817); by renal artery stenosis (see p.821); by obstruction of the outflow of urine from both kidneys, which can occur with prostate enlargement (see p.1098) or tumors of the bladder; and by diseases that start in the kidney such as glomerulonephritis (see p.810).

Acute kidney failure can be life-threatening if you are not treated. Dialysis, which is sometimes done on a temporary basis, may be required. Acute kidney failure usually can be reversed when the underlying cause is treated.

The risk of death is higher among the elderly, people who are taking immunosuppressive drugs, and people who have other serious chronic diseases, such as liver, heart, or lung disease.

SYMPTOMS

Symptoms of acute kidney failure may include drastically decreased urine production, nausea, vomiting, and loss of appetite. Your legs may swell as fluid accumulates.

You may notice mental changes, such as fatigue, agitation, confusion, and fluctuating moods. Confusion and drowsiness precede coma in people who are not treated.

Other symptoms depend on the condition that is causing the kidney failure. In some people there may be no symptoms at all; the change in kidney function may be diagnosed when the person has blood tests for another reason.

TREATMENT OPTIONS

If you believe that you have acute kidney failure, call your doctor or go to a hospital. Your doctor will perform tests of your blood and urine, which will reveal whether you have kidney failure (but not, necessarily, what has caused it) and evaluate your condition for imbalances caused by impaired kidney function.

You may also require a kidney biopsy (see p.805), ultrasound testing (see p.148) of your kidneys and abdomen, an abdominal x-ray, or computed tomography or magnetic resonance imaging scans (see p.151).

The goal of treatment is to stop the progression of kidney failure by treating the underlying condition; this often reverses the disease in a few days, weeks, or months, depending on the cause.

It is also necessary to prevent the accumulation of excess fluids and wastes. Your intake of protein may be restricted to prevent your kidneys from having to process it. Diuretics may be given to increase fluid excretion.

Other drugs may be used to control the level of potassium in your blood. You may need kidney dialysis (see p.815) if your kidney damage is severe.

Chronic Kidney Failure

Chronic kidney failure (also called chronic renal failure) is a serious, long-term condition of the kidneys that causes a progressive loss of kidney function and, ultimately, end-stage kidney failure.

In this disorder, which occurs over a period of years, the kidneys gradually lose their ability to filter body wastes from the blood and dispose of them in the urine. As a result, there is a buildup of toxins and fluid in the blood, which produces few symptoms at first. Indeed, you may not have symptoms until most of the kidneys' function is lost.

The diseases that most often cause chronic kidney failure are diabetes (see p.832) and high blood pressure (see p.644), particularly if they are not well-controlled by treatment.

Other conditions that cause chronic kidney failure are glomerulonephritis (see p.810), polycystic kidney disease (see p.811), vesicoureteral reflux (see p.821), and recurring pyelonephritis (see p.808). Some medicines taken in excess over many years can damage the kidneys (see p.817), as may exposure to mercury or lead.

The changes in the chemical and fluid balance of the blood due to kidney failure can cause complications in virtually every body system, including the heart and nervous system. For example, if levels of potassium build up in the blood (because the kidneys cannot get rid of extra potassium), it can cause cardiac arrest (see p.677).

The kidneys also normally produce important hormones; if these hormones cannot be pro-

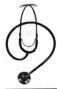

Chronic Kidney Failure: *When You Visit Your Doctor*

QUESTIONS TO DISCUSS WITH YOUR DOCTOR:

■ Are you following the proper diet? Has your diet been properly explained to you?

■ What is your energy level? Has it changed from the last visit?

■ Do you have a decrease in your appetite, weight loss, or nausea or vomiting?

■ Do you have difficulty sleeping at night?

■ Do you have difficulty concentrating or with your memory?

■ Do you have chest pain or shortness of breath?

■ Is your skin itchy?

■ Do you feel cold?

■ Are you urinating more or less frequently?

■ Are you taking your medications or any over-the-counter medications?

■ Is your kidney disease hereditary? Should your family members be tested?

■ Can you do anything to slow the progression of your disease?

■ Will you need dialysis?

■ Do you need (and could you qualify for) a kidney transplant? How do you get on a transplant list? Can a family member donate a kidney to you? Can your spouse or a friend donate a kidney to you?

YOUR DOCTOR MIGHT EXAMINE THE FOLLOWING BODY PARTS OR FUNCTIONS:

■ Heart rate, blood pressure, and weight

■ Eyes

■ Veins in the neck

■ Pulse

■ Heart and lungs

■ Abdomen (to see if it is tender when pressed gently)

■ Ankles and legs (for swelling)

■ Attention span and memory

YOUR DOCTOR MIGHT ORDER THE FOLLOWING LAB TESTS OR STUDIES:

■ Blood levels of minerals and salts (such as sodium, potassium, chloride, bicarbonate, calcium, magnesium, and phosphorus)

■ Tests of kidney function (such as blood urea nitrogen and creatinine)

■ Complete blood cell count (to check for anemia)

■ 24-hour urine collection for creatinine and protein (but only periodically)

duced, complications arise. For example, kidneys produce a hormone called erythropoietin that stimulates the production of red blood cells. In chronic kidney failure, fewer red blood cells are produced and anemia (see p.713) develops.

Kidneys also produce hormones that affect blood pressure and the strength of bones. In chronic kidney failure, you may have high blood pressure and osteomalacia (see p.595).

END-STAGE KIDNEY FAILURE

End-stage kidney failure occurs when the kidneys' function has been reduced to less than 10% of normal and they can no longer perform life-sustaining removal of waste and water from the body. The function of the kidneys must be taken over by dialysis (see p.815) or by a new kidney through a transplant (see right).

End-stage kidney failure and the symptoms it causes are called uremia.

People with diabetes represent the majority of those who have end-stage kidney failure.

SYMPTOMS

A symptom of chronic kidney failure is a decrease in the amount of urine you produce in a day (even if frequency of urination has increased). This may not occur until the disease is far advanced.

Other symptoms emerge gradually over time. You may feel tired and nauseated and have no appetite.

End-stage kidney failure is characterized by more severe symptoms because the kidneys can no longer filter enough toxins

and fluid from the body. You may have fatigue, itchy skin, headache, vomiting, confusion, seizures, shortness of breath due to accumulation of fluid, and anemia.

TREATMENT OPTIONS

Depending on the degree of kidney failure, your doctor will recommend treatments to minimize progression of the disease and delay the onset of end-stage kidney failure.

If possible, it is important to treat the underlying medical condition that is causing kidney damage.

Other treatments focus on problems caused by the damaged kidneys. If you have anemia, you may receive injections of the hormone erythropoietin to stimulate blood cell production.

Vitamin D and calcium help to prevent osteomalacia as well as control levels of phosphate in the blood, which build up because of the kidneys' inability to excrete phosphate.

Proper nutrition is essential to ensure you take in enough calories. You may be advised to restrict the amount of protein you eat to reduce the workload the kidneys have in processing it. Your doctor will prescribe a diet that is high in carbohydrates and balanced in salt and fluids.

Do not take any medicines without asking your doctor first. Many medicines can easily accumulate to high or toxic levels in your blood because of your poorly functioning kidneys.

A team of clinicians may be involved in your care, including a nephrologist (doctor who specializes in kidney problems), nurses, and a dietitian to help you plan

meals. You may be asked to keep a daily record of how much liquid you drink and how much you urinate.

People who have end-stage kidney disease usually have been monitored closely by their physicians over 10 to 20 years for chronic kidney failure and have received the treatments described.

End-stage kidney disease is fatal unless dialysis is performed regularly or you have a kidney transplant. Dialysis and/or kidney transplantation offer many people with end-stage disease the opportunity to live a relatively normal life.

Kidney Transplantation

In a kidney transplant, a healthy kidney is placed beneath the skin in the abdomen. The kidney may be from a living person or a cadaver.

About a third of kidneys are donated by living relatives; this is possible because you can live with only one kidney. A kidney from a cadaver must be removed within 30 minutes of death; it can be maintained for only a few hours before transplantation.

Kidney transplantation is one of the most commonly performed transplant procedures and is successful in more than 80% of cases. The most significant problem is locating a donor who matches your blood and tissue type. Even with blood and tissue matching, the greatest risk of transplant failure is rejection. Only an identical twin can be a perfect match.

The immune system may respond to the new kidney as if it were a foreign invader, and reject it. This usually occurs in

Surgery for Kidney Donation

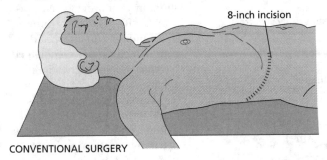

CONVENTIONAL SURGERY

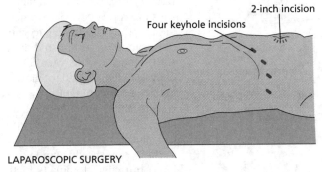

LAPAROSCOPIC SURGERY

People wishing to donate a kidney usually undergo major surgery, in which a large incision is made and the 10th and 11th ribs are spread to remove the kidney (top). In laparoscopic surgery (bottom), a newer technique that is still under study, surgeons use a laparoscope to remove a kidney through a 2-inch-long incision near the navel. Surgical instruments and a camera are inserted through four smaller incisions.

the first 8 weeks after surgery. To prevent rejection, powerful drugs are given to suppress the immune system. If a transplant fails, you will need to resume dialysis treatments (see above right).

To be considered for transplant surgery, you must be healthy enough to survive the physical rigors of surgery and lifelong treatment with immunosuppressive drugs. Because these drugs also decrease your body's response to infection, they increase your risk of infection.

Kidney transplantation is performed in a hospital, and usually requires a hospital stay of 5 to 10 days. While you are under general anesthesia, the surgeon makes an incision in your abdomen and clamps the blood vessels and ureters of the diseased kidney. The blood vessels and ureters of the donor kidney are then stitched to your blood vessels and bladder. The clamps are removed and blood flows through the donor kidney, which then produces urine that collects in your bladder.

The diseased kidney is left in place because it usually causes no harm and removing it requires a major operation. In addition, even if the diseased kidney

works poorly, its small capacity to clean toxins from the blood may be of some use.

The donor kidney is sewn into the inner part of your abdominal wall, where it can be felt by you and your doctor much more easily than the original kidney could be. The new kidney is placed close to the surface so that it can be more easily accessed for biopsy. A biopsy of the transplant is often needed to determine if rejection is occurring so that further treatment can be given.

Dialysis

Your kidneys filter body wastes from the blood and dispose of them in the urine. As a result, they maintain the right amount of fluid, acid, and minerals in your blood and body.

When your kidneys fail, your blood can be run through a machine called a dialyzer, or dialysis machine. This machine performs the same function as a healthy kidney.

Dialysis may be temporary or permanent. For example, some people with acute kidney failure require it for a period of time, until their kidneys heal. Other people, primarily those with end-stage kidney failure, must undergo dialysis for life, or until a donor kidney becomes available for transplantation (see p.814).

There are two types of dialysis: hemodialysis and peritoneal dialysis. Hemodialysis is usually performed in a hospital or outpatient center, though it can be performed at home if someone who lives with the patient can learn the techniques that are required.

Kidney Dialysis

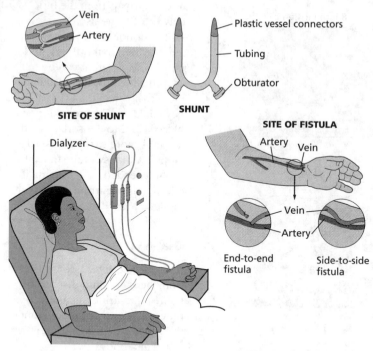

SITE OF SHUNT

- Vein
- Artery

SHUNT

- Plastic vessel connectors
- Tubing
- Obturator

SITE OF FISTULA

- Artery
- Vein
- Vein
- Artery

End-to-end fistula

Side-to-side fistula

Dialyzer

Kidney dialysis removes blood through an arm or leg artery, cleanses the blood of impurities (as a healthy kidney does), and returns the blood to the body. Ongoing dialysis requires that large amounts of blood be removed and replaced several times a week. To permit you to be repeatedly connected to the dialysis machine, a shunt or fistula is created.

Shunts are plastic tubes that are surgically connected to the blood supply beneath your skin. The device shown uses plastic connectors to connect an artery at one end and a vein at the other. It has two spots, called obturators, into which needles are placed. One removes blood from the body and the other returns cleansed blood to the body.

Fistulas are large natural blood vessels that are joined surgically by connecting an artery to a vein. Often this is done just above the wrist. The artery and vein are connected either side-to-side or end-to-end. In either case, a large blood vessel forms and bulges under your skin. Two needles are inserted into the blood vessel; one removes blood and the other returns it.

Since peritoneal dialysis is a simpler procedure, it is performed at home.

HEMODIALYSIS

In hemodialysis, your blood is run through a small filter that cleans it. Because dialysis must be performed frequently and repeatedly, a reliable and relatively comfortable way of connecting the filter to your bloodstream is needed. (If emergency dialysis is required, a special intravenous catheter that can be used for many weeks is placed in one of your large veins.)

If long-term dialysis is re-quired, doctors create a fistula or shunt in your arm (see illustration at left). A fistula is formed by connecting an artery and a vein, which creates an enlarged blood vessel just beneath the skin.

Alternately, a shunt can be made from a piece of artificial material and surgically connected between the artery and vein. Both a fistula and a shunt make it easier to repeatedly place a needle into the bloodstream to withdraw blood for testing and dialysis, to return blood from the dialysis machine, and to inject medicines and minerals.

After the fistula is formed, it takes about a month before you can start using it for dialysis. With a fistula, you should avoid wearing constrictive clothing (which could press on the fistula) and avoid heavy lifting.

Both the catheter used for emergency dialysis and the shunt used for long-term dialysis can become infected. Though infection can usually be treated with antibiotics, if treatment is unsuccessful or if a clot blocks the catheter or shunt, the device must be replaced.

Before hemodialysis, the access area in your arm or leg is cleaned and two needles are inserted, one that will carry your blood to the dialysis machine and one that will carry the cleansed blood back to your body.

As your blood travels through the dialysis machine, membranes in the machine remove excess fluid and minerals and various toxins. The cleansed blood is then put back into your body. Most people undergo dialysis three times a week for about 4 hours each session.

Some people have an inaccurate idea of the experience, which causes them to reject dialysis. They may imagine they would be in a coma and a machine would be breathing for them. Or they would not be allowed to talk. Or they would die immediately if the machine were turned off.

These ideas are incorrect. It is true that if you do not get regular dialysis treatments, you may eventually die of kidney failure (though it would take weeks or months). Getting disconnected from the dialysis machine does not suddenly endanger you in any way.

When you undergo dialysis, you must sit still while your bloodstream is connected temporarily to the machine, but you are fully conscious and can read, watch TV, or listen to the radio. After dialysis, the machine is disconnected and you are free to go home.

PERITONEAL DIALYSIS

In peritoneal dialysis, the peritoneal space—formed by the inner lining of the abdominal wall—is filled with a cleansing solution called dialysate. The solution enters the peritoneal space via a catheter that is placed through your abdominal wall into the space.

To position a catheter, a small incision is made in the abdomen using local anesthesia, and the catheter is inserted by a surgeon.

To perform peritoneal dialysis, a bag containing dialysate is attached to the catheter, and the fluid is allowed to drain into the space with the help of gravity.

The bag is then disconnected and you can go about your usual activities while the fluid remains in your abdomen.

The fluid remains there for about 4 hours while the dialysate absorbs toxins directly from the tiny blood vessels in the abdominal lining. Some excess fluid may also seep through the peritoneal lining into the dialysate.

During the next exchange, the fluid is drained by release of a clamp, and empties through the catheter back into the bag. Each exchange takes about an hour and is performed four times a day, 7 days a week. This type of dialysis is called continuous peritoneal dialysis.

Another method of peritoneal dialysis is known as continuous cycling peritoneal dialysis. Each night, you connect yourself to a machine that automatically performs multiple exchanges while you sleep. You must stay connected to the dialysis machine for 9 to 10 hours every night of the week, but you are free from having to perform any dialysis during the day.

ADVANTAGES AND DISADVANTAGES

There are advantages and disadvantages to both types of dialysis.

Hemodialysis usually requires you to go to an outpatient center for treatment, which can be inconvenient. On the other hand, it involves only 12 hours of dialysis per week. Hemodialysis can also be performed at home, if someone you live with is able to assist you.

Peritoneal dialysis is performed at home, but is much more time-consuming (approximately 28 hours per week) than hemodialysis and requires your active participation. You need to be well-coordinated and have good vision.

Your doctor may strongly recommend one type of dialysis for you, despite your preferences. For example, people with heart disease tend to do better on peritoneal dialysis while very large people may be more adequately dialyzed with hemodialysis.

Still, you can live a full life—even traveling all over the country (and world)—on either form of dialysis with just a bit of advanced planning.

Medicine-Induced Interstitial Nephritis

Whereas inflammation of the glomerulus (see p.810) is called glomerulonephritis, inflammation of the area around the kidney tubules is called interstitial nephritis. This condition is often caused by an adverse reaction to medicines.

Medicines circulating in the blood are eventually broken down by the liver or eliminated through the kidneys in the urine. Some drugs damage the kidneys as they are filtered from the blood.

Sometimes it is the accumulation of a drug in the kidneys over time that causes a toxic response and kidney damage.

Other times, a drug stimulates an allergic response when the immune system perceives the drug as foreign and attacks it. Lymphocytes (see p.710) may attack kidney tissues containing the drug and cause interstitial nephritis.

Symptoms vary according to the severity of the body's response. Low-grade interstitial nephritis may cause no symptoms as it slowly damages the kidneys. More severe inflammation of the kidneys can lead to painful urination, fever, and pain on one side of your back.

Your doctor can diagnose interstitial nephritis by looking for white blood cells, including eosinophils (see p.710), in your urine. A blood test may also reveal increased eosinophils in the blood.

Kidney damage from medicine-induced interstitial nephritis can often be reversed if the drug causing it is stopped immediately. Some people need to undergo a period of dialysis (see p.815) while their kidneys heal.

Your doctor may restrict your intake of fluids and salt to reduce fluid retention. Protein may also be restricted to ease the kidneys' work.

The high blood pressure that may result when the kidneys are not functioning properly can be treated with medicines. If the disorder is not diagnosed early enough, irreversible kidney damage that has been caused by chronic kidney failure (see p.812) can develop.

Drugs that can cause interstitial nephritis (although they do so only rarely) include ampicillin, penicillin, and some nonsteroidal anti-inflammatory drugs, including ibuprofen, indomethacin, and naproxen.

Some drugs that cause no damage by themselves can cause interstitial nephritis when used in combination (although this occurs only rarely). These drug combinations include diuretics plus prostaglandin inhibitors such as ibuprofen, as well as diuretics plus calcium supplements.

When you see a doctor, always give him or her a list of all the medicines you are taking—including nonprescription medicines—so that potentially dangerous combinations can be avoided.

Kidney Stones

A kidney stone starts as a fleck of solid material in the kidney onto which minerals (such as calcium salts or uric acid) bind and develop into a stonelike structure.

The most common kidney stones are made up of calcium combined with oxalate, another mineral. They affect men more often than women.

Other kidney stones are made up of uric acid, cystine, or methionine. If you have had one kidney stone, you are at higher risk of having another.

Kidney stones usually start to develop in the middle of the kidney. If they are small, they may cause no problems. You may pass a tiny stone through the ureter, and then out with urine, and not even know it.

However, stones that are larger than about 1/5 inch may impede the flow of urine out of a kidney and cause the kidney to swell painfully. If a stone moves into a ureter or into the urethra and causes blockage, it can cause severe pain (renal colic).

Doctors do not know why

Kidney Stones

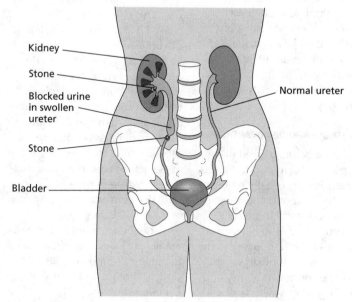

Kidney stones can occur in the kidney itself or in a ureter (the tube that connects the kidney to the bladder). Stones lying in the kidney often cause no symptoms. However, when they enter the ureters (unless they are tiny and pass quickly through the ureter), they can cause severe pain. If a kidney stone blocks the flow of urine, cystoscopy may be required to prevent urine from backing up into the kidney.

Methods of Kidney Stone Removal

If a kidney stone does not pass on its own with your normal urine flow, it may be treated by one of the methods described below.

METHOD	HOW IT WORKS
Extracorporeal shock wave lithotripsy	On an outpatient basis in a hospital or lithotripsy center, this procedure takes 1 hour and requires no anesthesia. While you are on a special table, shock waves are directed through water pouches placed on the skin near the stone. The shock waves break up the stone into smaller pieces that can be passed out the ureter.
Cystoscopy (see p.825)	If a stone is lodged in a ureter near the bladder, cystoscopy may be used. Using local or general anesthesia, a narrow viewing tube is inserted into the urethra and guided to the bladder and up into the ureter. An instrument can be inserted into the cystoscope to grasp and pull out the stone. Electrical or laser energy may be used to break up the stone.
Percutaneous (through the skin) lithotripsy	This outpatient procedure is used to break up stones larger than 1 inch. It requires a sedative. A viewing tube is inserted through a small incision in your side and the stone is broken up with ultrasound or electric energy.
Surgery	Surgery is used for stones that are large or hard to reach. While you are under general anesthesia, the surgeon makes an incision in your side. Another incision is made into the ureter or kidney to reach and remove the stone; the incision is then stitched closed. This method is used only for unusual cases when simpler methods have not worked.

some kidney stones form. They seem to run in families. They also affect people living in hot climates more often, probably due to dehydration caused by perspiration, which, in turn, causes the urine to be more concentrated.

When the material that causes a kidney stone is more concentrated, it is more likely to start or enlarge a stone.

People who have one of several disorders, including gout (see p.604), hyperparathyroidism (see p.852), malabsorption (see p.775), or inflammatory bowel disease (see p.787) may be at higher risk for kidney stones.

Researchers have also discovered extremely small bacteria that may live in some people's kidneys and may start the process of forming stones. Further study could one day lead to new approaches to preventing kidney stones.

SYMPTOMS

The chief symptom is pain, which may become severe. The pain usually starts in the lower side of the back and moves down to the groin area, following the path of the ureter. Pain is usually intermittent.

Other symptoms include nausea and vomiting, blood in the urine, blocked urine flow, and reduced urine output. Infection may produce fever, chills, and weakness, and cloudy or unpleasant-smelling urine.

TREATMENT OPTIONS

See your doctor if you experience the pain described above. He or she will prescribe a painkiller to ease discomfort, perform urine and blood tests, and arrange for imaging tests such as intravenous pyelography (see p.805).

If a stone is identified, your doctor may order metabolic tests to help determine the cause. These tests include a complete evaluation of your blood, a 24-hour urine sample (collecting your urine for a day), and, if you pass a stone, analysis of its contents.

Treatment can take several forms. If you are like 90% of sufferers, your stone will pass on its own within 6 weeks. Drinking lots of water (twelve 8-ounce glasses a day) may help flush it out. Your doctor may ask you to strain your urine and save any tiny pebbles or specks.

Calcium stones, caused by excreting too much calcium in your urine, can be prevented by taking thiazide diuretics.

For stones containing uric acid, your doctor may prescribe a drug that maintains the alkaline state of your urine. He or she may also prescribe allopurinol, a drug that decreases the production of uric acid. Allopurinol is often prescribed for gout.

Some kidney stones are caused by the lack of a potent inhibitor to stone formation that is called citrate. Citrate can be taken either in pill form or mixed in water.

To prevent recurrences, drink plenty of fluids (enough to keep your urine almost colorless) and follow your doctor's dietary recommendations, which may include decreasing protein intake and limiting salt.

Nephrotic Syndrome

Nephrotic syndrome is a group of symptoms and laboratory signs that are caused by injury to the kidney's tiny filters (glomeruli).

The injury causes protein (particularly albumin) to leak out of the blood and into the urine. This lowers the amount of albumin in your blood, which causes fluid to leak out of your blood vessels and into your tissues and makes your body swell. Though the kidneys may otherwise function normally, they cannot excrete excess salt in the urine, which exacerbates the retention of fluids.

The cause of nephrotic syndrome in about 85% of children and 20% of adults is a condition called minimal-change disease (so-named because only very mild abnormalities are found during a kidney biopsy). The condition is usually not associated with high blood pressure or kidney failure.

The most common cause of nephrotic syndrome in adults is diabetes. Various other diseases of the glomerulus that are more severe than minimal-change disease (including diseases such as glomerulosclerosis, membranous glomerulopathy, membranoproliferative glomerulonephritis, and mesangial proliferative glomerulonephritis) can also cause nephrotic syndrome.

Other less common causes of nephrotic syndrome include lupus, multiple myeloma, the human immunodeficiency virus, and a side effect to medicines.

SYMPTOMS

Symptoms include swelling of the legs, feet, abdomen, and face. You may feel tired, have no appetite, and have diarrhea.

TREATMENT OPTIONS

In addition to a complete medical history and physical examination, your doctor will test your blood and urine. You may also require a kidney biopsy (see p.805).

The condition called minimal-change disease can usually be cured by taking corticosteroids (see p.895) and diuretics to promote fluid loss. However, remission and relapses of the excessive protein in the urine are common.

If your kidney biopsy shows that nephrotic syndrome is caused by other, more serious diseases of the glomerulus other than minimal-change disease, you may need to take powerful immunosuppressive drugs. Your doctor will instruct you to stay on a diet that restricts salt and fluid.

Vesicoureteral Reflux

Vesicoureteral reflux is the back-wash (reflux) of urine from the bladder up into the ureters and the kidneys.

You are born with a valve at the junction of the bladder and the ureter. This valve prevents the urine from going backwards from the bladder to the ureter during urination, when pressure in the bladder is high.

In vesicoureteral reflux, the valve does not function well, and urine can flow back up to the kidneys, introducing bacteria from the bladder into the kidneys and/or increasing the pressure inside the kidneys, either of which can damage the kidneys.

Vesicoureteral reflux is more common among children, in whom it can cause severe high blood pressure (because the kidneys can greatly influence blood pressure). If severe reflux is not corrected, it may lead to end-stage kidney failure (see p.814).

In many children with mild reflux, the condition gets better over time.

SYMPTOMS

Reflux often causes no symptoms at all, but it can cause pain in your side and (when it occurs due to recurring urinary tract infections) fever, pain when you urinate, and other symptoms of infection.

If the reflux causes kidney damage, your blood pressure may be high. If damage is extensive, you may have symptoms of chronic kidney failure (see p.812).

TREATMENT OPTIONS

If you have symptoms of vesi-coureteral reflux, see your doctor. Tests may include intravenous pyelography (see p.805). If this test suggests reflux, a confirmatory procedure called a voiding cystourethrogram (see p.805) may be performed. The tests can help show whether or not the kidneys have been damaged.

Treatment depends on the severity of the condition, but often includes taking low doses of antibiotics to keep urine free of infection.

Surgery may be recommended when the reflux is severe or does not respond to treatment. In surgery, the ureters are first cut from the bladder and then stitched back into the bladder at a more oblique angle, which helps prevent urine from refluxing back up. In most people, surgery is effective.

Renal Artery Stenosis

Renal artery stenosis involves narrowing and/or obstruction of the main blood vessel (artery) that supplies blood to the kidney.

The impaired blood supply causes a chemical and hormonal chain reaction that can lead to high blood pressure (see p.644) or chronic kidney failure (see p.812).

Renal artery stenosis may be caused by a thickening of the artery wall (fibromuscular dysplasia) or by blockages inside the artery caused by plaques from atherosclerosis (see p.653).

Fibromuscular dysplasia occurs more often in women and younger adults. Atherosclerosis occurs primarily in older adults.

SYMPTOMS

There are usually no symptoms. Renal artery stenosis may be discovered while investigating high blood pressure or a decline in kidney function.

TREATMENT OPTIONS

Your doctor may suspect renal artery stenosis if you have high blood pressure and if a noisy sound (called a bruit) can be heard through a stethoscope with every heartbeat as blood is pushed past the area of obstruction.

A magnetic resonance imaging scan (see p.151) of the kidney may be performed to view the flow of blood through the artery and to look for the narrowed area. An ultrasound (see p.148) can reveal the size of the kidney, which is often smaller due to decreased blood flow. An angiogram (see p.147) may be performed to more accurately locate blockage or narrowing.

Treatment aims to control blood pressure and restore blood flow to the kidney. Medicines can control high blood pressure. Surgery to widen the narrowed artery lowers blood pressure and restores the flow of blood to the kidney.

Your doctor may recommend angioplasty (see p.661), in which a balloon-tipped catheter is guided through an artery in your leg and into the narrowed renal artery. The balloon is then expanded, which presses the narrowed artery walls outward, opening the channel.

Alternately, bypass surgery (see p.662) may be performed to remove the damaged segment of artery and rejoin the healthy ends. In rare cases, it is necessary to remove one kidney to control high blood pressure.

Renal Vein Thrombosis

The renal veins are the veins that carry blood out of the kidneys. In renal vein thrombosis, one of the veins becomes partially or completely obstructed by a blood clot.

Renal vein thrombosis can result from blockage of the vein by a tumor or by serious injury to the back or abdomen. It can also occur with nephrotic syndrome (see p.820) and (very rarely) can affect infants who are extremely dehydrated.

Symptoms include extreme pain in your back on one side of the spine or in the lower back. However, most often, renal vein thrombosis does not cause symptoms.

Report symptoms to your doctor, who will test your urine for the protein and red blood cells that are signs of kidney damage. Blood tests will look for any changes in kidney function. A Doppler ultrasound (see p.139), which looks at blood flow through blood vessels, may detect renal vein thrombosis by showing areas where a blockage is slowing the flow of blood.

Your doctor may also order a special x-ray involving the injection of a contrast medium (see p.147) into a blood vessel via the groin. The contrast dye makes its way into the renal vein, and a sequence of x-ray pictures shows where the clot blockage is. The use of a contrast dye can cause side effects. For this reason, a test without potential side effects (usually magnetic resonance imaging of the renal veins) may be performed.

Treatment involves taking anticoagulant drugs to reduce blood clotting. If a kidney tumor is blocking the vein, it is treated as described in Cancer of the Kidneys (see p.823).

CANCER

Cancer of the Bladder

Bladder cancer is a malignancy that usually starts in the inner lining of the bladder. The disease usually occurs in people over 50. Men are three times more likely than women to develop it, probably because men have a higher rate of smoking, which is a major risk factor for bladder cancer.

The outlook for most people is very good if the disease is diagnosed and treated early. About 80% of people with bladder cancer live more than 5 years after treatment.

About 75% of all bladder cancers are confined to the inner lining of the bladder (the epithelium) and are easily removed by surgery. In some cases, an electric probe is used to destroy cancer cells. Cancers confined to the lining rarely spread to other parts of the body.

Bladder Cancer

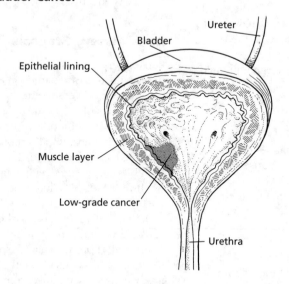

About 75% of all bladder cancers are confined to the epithelium (inner lining) of the bladder and can be surgically removed.

Bladder cancer is often a result of exposure to a cancer-causing chemical, but usually occurs many years after the person was exposed. About half of all cases occur in people who smoked cigarettes at some time in their lives.

The cancer also develops more frequently in people who work with leather, rubber, dye, aluminum, and certain paints because they have been exposed to substances called aromatic amines.

SYMPTOMS

In its early stages, bladder cancer may cause no symptoms. Most people are diagnosed when they see blood in their urine. Less often, there is frequent and/or painful urination.

TREATMENT OPTIONS

See your doctor if you see blood or blood clots in your urine or if your urine is pink, orange, or the color of red wine. Your doctor will test your urine to rule out infection and may also send urine to the lab to look for cancerous cells.

The surest way to diagnose bladder tumors is by cystoscopy (see p.825), which permits the doctor to look directly at the bladder lining and locate any tumors or irregularities in the lining. At the same time, a biopsy sample may be taken and sent to the pathology lab for diagnosis.

Occasionally, a tumor may be so small that it cannot be seen during cystoscopy. Instead, it is diagnosed by finding cancerous cells in the urine or by performing multiple small biopsies of all parts of the bladder wall.

Treatment depends on the stage of the cancer. The most common early form, which has not spread from the inner lining, is curable with surgery. However, since the cancer often recurs, cystoscopy may be recommended every 3 to 6 months for several years to ensure that there are no new cancerous tumors.

After surgery, chemotherapy (see p.741) or immunotherapy may be used. In immunotherapy, the bacterium bacille Calmette-Guérin is applied directly to the bladder to stimulate the body's natural immune response, causing it to kill any remaining cancer cells.

When cancer has spread to the bladder's muscle layer, removal of the bladder (and any other affected organs) may be required. In men, the seminal vesicles, pelvic lymph nodes, and prostate are also removed. Almost all men experience impotence (see p.1092) after this surgery.

In women, the ovaries, ureters, urethra, and part of the vaginal wall are removed, in addition to the bladder. A course of chemotherapy and radiation therapy may be recommended after surgery. More than half the people live for more than 5 years after surgery.

When the bladder is removed, an artificial bladder must be created. The traditional approach is to move the ureters to empty into an isolated piece of the intestine. The piece goes through the wall of the abdomen and empties into a plastic bag worn on the outside of the body. This is called an ostomy and is similar to the ostomies that are formed after

surgical removal of the intestine (see p.793).

A newer approach is a "bag-less" urinary reservoir. This is a pouch made of intestine just inside the abdominal wall. You can insert a catheter through a small hole in the abdominal wall and empty the urine. Sometimes the internal pouch can be connected to the urethra so that you can urinate normally.

Cancer of the Kidneys

Kidney cancer is a malignant growth of kidney tissue. In general, kidney cancers spread to other parts of the body less quickly than some other cancers.

However, they are difficult to identify early because they usually do not cause symptoms in their early stages. A cancerous tumor of the kidney usually does not interfere with kidney function until it is large.

Between 60% and 75% of people who are treated in the early stages of kidney cancer survive for at least 5 years after treatment.

Renal cell carcinoma accounts for about 75% of all kidney cancers. It affects men twice as often as women, usually those over age 50. Your risk for having this type of kidney cancer increases if a relative has had this type of cancer, if you have ever smoked cigarettes, or if you have been exposed to asbestos, cadmium, or gasoline.

Transitional cell cancer, the same kind of cancer that affects the bladder, can also be located in a ureter or the kidney, and represents about 10% of kidney cancers. This form occurs more often in people who have used painkillers containing phenacetin for a long time.

Wilms tumor (see p.999), another type of kidney cancer, occurs almost exclusively in children.

SYMPTOMS

Blood in the urine due to bleeding from the tumor is the most common symptom, but a dull, aching, flank pain or abdominal lump may also be present.

Other possible symptoms include weight loss, fever, and swelling of the lower extremities. If the cancer has spread, symptoms can occur in the organs to which it has spread; for instance, you may have pain in your bones.

TREATMENT OPTIONS

See your doctor if you have blood in your urine. He or she will test your urine and, if cancer is suspected, may perform imaging tests, such as x-rays of the kidneys, ureters, and bladder; intravenous pyelography; ultrasound (see p.148); or a computed tomography or magnetic resonance imaging scan of your kidney.

A bone scan or chest x-ray may also be performed to make sure the cancer has not spread.

Renal cell carcinoma is usually treated by removing the diseased kidney (you can function normally with one healthy kidney). When the tumor is small, only the tumor is removed and the kidney is left in place. Sometimes, nearby lymph glands are also removed and tested for cancer cells. There is currently no effective chemotherapy treatment, and radiation therapy is not usually effective.

If you have transitional cell cancer, the standard treatment is to remove the kidney along with the ureter and part of the bladder.

Researchers are investigating new approaches. These include immunotherapy, which boosts the body's own cancer-fighting cells in the immune system.

OTHER URINARY TRACT DISORDERS

Bladder Stones

Bladder stones are crystallized stonelike structures in the bladder. They are often a consequence of another urinary tract condition, such as urinary tract infection or an enlarged prostate (see p.1098).

The stones can develop when urine becomes concentrated and its contents crystallize. The majority of bladder stones occur in men.

A bladder stone that is too large to pass through the urethra (which connects the bladder to the outside of your body) may cause frequent, painful, or difficult urination. You may see blood in your urine and have discomfort in the lower abdomen and/or penis.

Your doctor will examine you and test a sample of urine for blood and infection; x-rays of the bladder may be performed.

The first line of treatment for bladder stones is consuming plenty of fluids in an attempt to flush out the stone. If this fails, other types of therapies can be used, depending on the location and size of the stone.

Nonsurgical approaches try to break up the stone inside the bladder so that smaller pieces pass through the urethra in the urine. These approaches are the same as those used for kidney stones (see Methods of Kidney Stone Removal, p.819).

Injury to the Bladder and Urethra

The bladder is not highly susceptible to injury because of its location; it is tucked low in the abdomen. Injury most often occurs when a severe force breaks a pelvic bone, which in turn punctures the bladder, or when a serious motor vehicle collision or other injury places enough pressure on a full bladder to burst it.

In either case, the bladder may leak urine into the abdominal cavity, which can lead to serious infection.

Injury to the urethra in women is rare because a woman's urethra is short and well-protected. In men, the urethra may be injured by a sharp blow to the penis. These injuries are usually not serious but can cause a narrowing of the urethral channel if scar tissue forms during the healing process.

If you have been severely injured and your doctor suspects

Cystoscopy

Cystoscopy is a procedure that allows a doctor to look directly at the urethra and bladder. In cystoscopy, a narrow tube with a light and camera is inserted through the urethra and into the bladder. The physician can look at all the structures and at any stones, tumors, or other conditions of the urinary tract.

The procedure is usually performed on an outpatient basis using a flexible cystoscope and local anesthesia, although sometimes a rigid cystoscope and spinal or general anesthesia are required. Flexible cystoscopic examinations are usually performed in the doctor's office; rigid cystoscopic examinations are usually performed in a hospital. While you are lying on your back, your doctor will gently insert the cystoscope into your urethra and your bladder. You may be able to view the images on a monitor.

Depending on the reason for the test, your doctor may pass water into your bladder to see how much it retains. He or she may also insert a small instrument to remove a tiny sample of tissue for examination under a microscope.

After cystoscopy, you will probably be advised to avoid exercise and sexual intercourse for a week or two and to drink lots of fluids.

Most cystoscopic examinations are completed without complications. However, there is a small risk of bladder infection or injury to the urethra or bladder. A small amount of blood in your urine is normal during the first day after the examination, but should be reported to your doctor if it persists. Similarly, report any difficulty urinating or fever, which can signal injury or bladder infection.

Cystoscopy

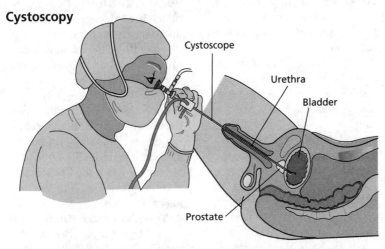

Cystoscopy permits a doctor to view the urethra, bladder, and prostate gland. The cystoscope, which is inserted through the urethra, contains a light and forceps at one end. If a rigid cystoscope (like the one shown here) is used, you are usually given spinal or general anesthesia. If a flexible cystoscope is used, no anesthesia is required, and the procedure can be done in a doctor's office.

that you have a punctured bladder, draining the fluid with a catheter is usually all that is necessary. If there is urine leakage directly into the abdomen, emergency surgery will be performed to repair the bladder and remove any urine that has spilled into the abdomen. Antibiotics are given to prevent infection.

Most injuries of the urethra heal on their own. You may need a catheter to drain urine for several days during the healing process.

Urethral Stricture

Urethral stricture is a narrowing of the urethra, the channel through which urine passes out of the bladder. A rare condition, it is most often caused by scar tissue that develops after injury to the urethra or by untreated sexually transmitted diseases such as gonorrhea (see p.891) or nongonococcal urethritis (see p.893).

Symptoms include painful and/or difficult urination, as well as a slow or intermittent urine stream. You may notice that you urinate more often, but with less volume, or that you dribble urine. Urethral stricture may also be responsible for recurring urinary tract infections.

Report your symptoms to your physician. He or she will perform urine tests to look for infection and may test you for sexually transmitted diseases. If your doctor suspects a urethral stricture, he or she may arrange for cystoscopy (see left) to make the diagnosis.

If necessary, treatment consists of gently stretching the channel of the urethra using local anesthesia to insert a series of rods that gradually dilate (open) the stricture. The dilation may need to be performed several times.

Surgery may be necessary if the channel does not remain open. This involves using tools inserted through a cystoscope to remove the scar tissue that is causing the narrowing.

Urinary Obstruction

Urinary obstruction is blockage of urine flow anywhere in the urinary tract. The blockage prevents urine produced by the kidney from draining out of the body. Eventually, the urine may back up and damage the kidneys.

In men, the most common causes of urinary obstruction are prostate enlargement (see p.1098), bladder cancer (see p.822), a stone in the ureter (see Kidney Stones, p.818), or prostate cancer (see p.1102). In women, it may occur as a result of severe urinary tract infection, stones, or bladder cancer.

Common symptoms include difficulty starting urine flow, prolonged urination with a weaker stream of urine, frequent urination of small amounts, or dribbling urine after urination. Some people experience symptoms of urge incontinence and overflow incontinence (see next article).

In severe cases, you may be unable to urinate at all, you may feel pain in your lower abdomen, or you may notice distension or a mass in your lower abdomen from the distended bladder. You may also have symptoms of a urinary tract infection (see p.804) or a kidney infection (see p.808).

Diagnostic tests may include an ultrasound of the bladder and kidneys or a cystourethrogram (see p.805) to look for the cause of the obstruction. Cystoscopy (see p.825) is sometimes used to look directly at the urinary system for the cause.

In severe cases of obstruction, a catheter may be temporarily required to drain urine from the bladder. Otherwise, treatment with medicines or surgery is directed at the underlying cause.

Incontinence

Incontinence is the involuntary leakage of urine. More than 10 million Americans regularly experience it. While treatment can eliminate or improve the problem in 90% of those who have it, only 1 of 4 people seek help from a doctor.

Many people resign themselves to wearing adult diapers or pads because they mistakenly believe that urinary incontinence is a normal part of aging. Aging does not cause incontinence but can contribute to it. As you age, bladder spasms become more common.

Other people do not raise the problem with their doctors because they are embarrassed or they fear invasive tests or surgery.

Understanding the urinary tract, and the normal process of urination, can help you understand incontinence. In men, an enlarged prostate (see p.1098) may obstruct the flow of urine, causing the accumulation of larger amounts of urine in the bladder that may then leak involuntarily.

In women, the urinary sphincter muscle may become weaker because of damage during childbirth, or because of lower levels of estrogen after menopause.

Many common drugs, including some sedatives, diuretics, antidepressants, narcotic painkillers, alpha blockers, and over-the-counter sleep and cold tablets, also can cause urine retention and/or leakage.

MAJOR TYPES OF INCONTINENCE

Stress incontinence is characterized by leaking a small amount of urine when you cough, sneeze, lift a heavy object, exercise, or otherwise put pressure on your bladder. Stress incontinence is more common in women after childbirth and in men after prostate surgery. Among women under age 60, this is the most common type of incontinence.

Urge incontinence occurs when the bladder develops a spasm. It suddenly contracts and expels urine with little or no warning. This form of incontinence is more common in men and women over age 60.

Overflow incontinence is much less common but can occur in men who have prostate enlargement or in women after pelvic surgery. As a result of partial obstruction, the bladder cannot empty completely, and urine may dribble frequently. It may also occur when the bladder is severely weakened from neurological problems.

Transient incontinence is caused by a temporary or easily changed condition and occurs most often in people older than 65. The factors that most often cause transient incontinence are low estrogen levels, medicines (such as sedatives and calcium channel blockers), delirium (see p.362), urinary tract infection, drinking large quantities of fluids, drinking diuretic beverages (such as coffee or alcohol), heart failure (see p.683), difficulty getting to a toilet when the urge to urinate occurs, and fecal impaction (see p.794).

TREATMENT OPTIONS

If you have incontinence, see your doctor. Make a journal and record at least 3 days of urination habits. Note when the leaking occurred, what you were doing at the time, what makes the problem worse, and what makes it better.

After conducting a medical history to rule out other potential causes, your doctor will perform a genital examination. He or she may also perform simple tests of your reflexes and muscle strength, and of walking. Your doctor may also check to see if your bladder is unusually full, which may indicate that you are not able to completely empty your bladder.

Some people require more sophisticated tests, including tests that measure the flow of urine and detect bladder spasms.

Treatment of incontinence varies according to the type and cause. Treating any underlying condition is necessary first.

Stress incontinence can be alleviated in 50% to 75% of women by:

■ Performing exercises to strengthen the urinary sphincter (see Kegel exercises, p.1051).

■ Learning biofeedback to help you contract the correct muscles.

Preventing Incontinence

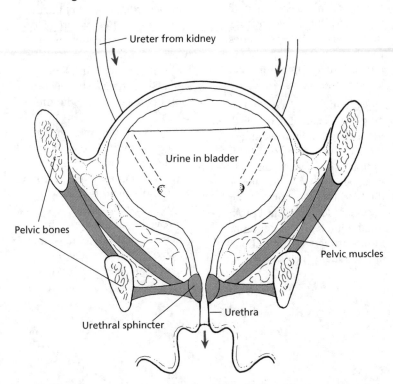

In women, the pelvic muscles around the urethral sphincter contract to retain urine and relax to permit urine to flow. Kegel exercises (see p.1051) strengthen the pelvic muscles and help prevent incontinence.

■ Holding weighted cones in your vagina to strengthen pelvic muscles.

■ Wearing a tampon or pessary while you exercise to prevent leakage; these devices press against the wall of the vagina and compress the urethra.

■ Taking the drugs phenylpropanolamine or pseudoephedrine, which increase the urinary sphincter's ability to contract (this helps 20% to 60% of women). The drugs should not be used without your doctor's advice if you have heart disease or are over age 65.

■ Using a vaginal estrogen cream or taking hormones by mouth (if you have gone through menopause), which can increase the sphincter's ability to stay closed.

■ Having collagen implants. In this procedure, purified collagen from cows is injected around the urinary sphincter. The body breaks down the collagen and forms scar tissue that bolsters the muscles. Injections are given in the doctor's office and usually need to be repeated one or two times. About half the women who have this procedure have improvement of symptoms; it is less successful in men.

■ Having surgery to strengthen the pelvic muscles or to lift the bladder (if the above treatments do not work). Many surgeries require only a small incision in the abdomen. Others are done through the vagina.

Urge incontinence can be helped by retraining the bladder. Retraining can improve urge incontinence in up to 75% of people who have it. It involves increasing the storage capacity of the bladder by learning to suppress sudden urges and prolonging the interval between urination, starting with 1 to 2 hours and gradually increasing to 3 to 4 hours. Another approach is to urinate according to a set timetable.

The most effective drugs for urge incontinence are oxybutynin, propantheline, tolterodine, and some tricyclic antidepressants. Side effects, such as dry mouth, are common with these drugs.

Drugs can improve symptoms of urge incontinence in up to half of affected people; drugs actually cure urge incontinence in up to a third of people affected by it.

Overflow incontinence may improve by taking the alpha blockers prazosin, terazosin, or doxazosin if the problem is an enlarged prostate. These drugs are often used to treat high blood pressure. They can also help relax urethral muscle and the muscle fibers of the prostate, which decreases urinary retention and the tendency to leak urine.

Finally, various implantable devices that help stimulate coordinated activity of the bladder are in use and under development. These devices help some people who have not obtained adequate relief with medicines.

Further information about the causes and treatment of incontinence is available from the Simon Foundation for Continence (1-800-237-4666).

Hormonal Disorders

The explosive physical and emotional changes of adolescence serve as a small but dramatic example of the power of hormones. Hormones affect every stage of our lives—from childhood (when they are essential for growth) to adulthood (when they allow us to reproduce).

HOW HORMONES WORK

A hormone is a chemical signal made by one organ that travels (usually through the blood) to other tissues, causing an effect in those tissues. Hormones are produced by a system of organs or glands (known collectively as the endocrine system) that are scattered throughout the body. Each gland makes specific hormones, which are released when needed to help the body maintain a healthy balance.

Positive and negative feedback The production of a hormone by a gland is triggered by various chemical signals through a process of either positive feedback or negative feedback.

When you eat, sugar is absorbed from the intestines into the blood and carried throughout the body to cells that need the sugar for energy. In order for the sugar to move from the blood into the cells, the hormone insulin also must be present in the blood.

Rising blood sugar levels after a meal cause the pancreas (see p.831) to make insulin. When sugar absorbed from the meal leaves the blood to enter the cells, the dropping blood sugar level causes the pancreas to stop the production of insulin.

Thus, a rising blood sugar level "turns on" the production of insulin and a falling blood sugar level "turns off" the production of insulin. This is an example of positive feedback; the higher the level of a substance in the blood, the more the production of a hormone is turned on.

Here is another example of the feedback system. You need a certain level of thyroid hormone in your blood at all times. The brain center called the hypothalamus detects when the level of thyroid hormone drops below a certain level. The hypothalamus then makes a hormone called thyrotropin-releasing hormone (TRH). TRH travels to the pituitary gland in the brain, causing the pituitary to release another hormone called thyroid-stimulating hormone (TSH), also known as thyrotropin.

TSH travels to the thyroid gland and instructs it to make thyroid hormone. When the level of thy-

Endocrine System

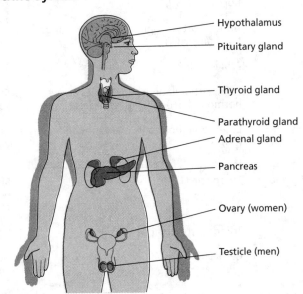

The endocrine system is made up of the glands shown. The hormones they produce and the functions performed are described on p.830.

Glands of the Endocrine System

The glands of the endocrine system, the hormones they produce, the organs the hormones target, and the functions the hormones fulfill are outlined in this chart.

GLAND	HORMONE	TARGET ORGAN OR BODY PART	FUNCTION
Hypothalamus	Antidiuretic hormone (ADH)	Kidneys	Helps regulate reabsorption of water from the kidneys into the blood
	Oxytocin (OXT)	Uterus	Stimulates contraction of the uterus
		Breasts	Stimulates the release of breast milk
	Corticotropin-releasing hormone (CRH)	Pituitary gland	Stimulates the release of ACTH from the pituitary gland
	Thyrotropin-releasing hormone (TRH)	Pituitary gland	Stimulates the release of TSH from the pituitary gland
	Gonadotropin-releasing hormone (GnRH)	Pituitary gland	Stimulates the release of FSH and LH from the pituitary gland
Pituitary gland	Growth hormone (GH)	Many tissues	Causes growth of bones and several organs during childhood and adolescence, improves muscle strength in adults, and increases sugar levels in the blood
	Thyroid-stimulating hormone (TSH)	Thyroid gland	Controls secretion of thyroid hormones by the thyroid gland
	Adrenocorticotropic hormone (ACTH)	Adrenal glands	Controls secretion of cortisol by the adrenal glands
	Prolactin (PRL)	Breasts	Stimulates lactation (milk production)
	Follicle-stimulating hormone (FSH)	Ovaries and testicles	Stimulates growth of eggs in women and sperm in men
	Luteinizing hormone (LH)	Ovaries and testicles	Causes release and maturation of eggs in women and stimulates release of testosterone in men
Thyroid gland	Thyroxine (T_4)	Cells	Stimulates oxygen consumption by cells and regulates metabolism in cells and is essential for normal growth and maturation
	Triiodothyronine (T_3)	Cells	Function is similar to that of T_4
	Calcitonin	Bones	Helps regulate levels of calcium in the blood and build bone strength

GLAND	HORMONE	TARGET ORGAN OR BODY PART	FUNCTION
Parathyroid glands	Parathyroid hormone (PTH)	Bones and kidneys	Regulates levels of calcium and phosphate in the blood and bones
Pancreas	Glucagon	Liver	Raises blood sugar levels to make energy available to the body
	Insulin	Fat cells, liver, and muscles	Increases uptake, storage, and utilization of glucose by cells and increases the making of proteins and the storage of fat
Adrenal glands	Epinephrine	Circulatory system and liver	Increases heart rate and blood pressure and raises blood glucose
	Norepinephrine	Heart, lungs, and blood vessels	Increases blood pressure
	Dehydroepiandrosterone (DHEA)	Most tissues	May have a role in aiding the immune system (main functions are unknown)
	Aldosterone	Kidneys	Regulates exchange of sodium and potassium and regulates blood pressure
	Cortisol	Most tissues	Calms inflammation; helps maintain blood pressure; and affects the metabolism of carbohydrates, protein, and fats
Ovaries	Estrogen	Female reproductive system	Is responsible for the development of female sex characteristics
		Ovaries	Stimulates maturation of eggs
		Uterus	Prepares the uterus for implantation of eggs
		Brain	May protect against degenerative diseases like Alzheimer disease
		Tissues	May help heal wounds
	Progesterone	Uterus	Stimulates growth of vessels in uterine lining to prepare for development into placenta
Testicles	Testosterone	Testicles	Promotes development of male sex characteristics during childhood, promotes growth during childhood, and maintains male sex characteristics (including sperm maturation) during adulthood
	Inhibin	Testicles	Works with testosterone to regulate rate of sperm development

roid hormone goes up above a certain level, the hypothalamus detects it and turns off the production of TRH. This is an example of negative feedback; the higher the level of a substance in the blood, the more the production of a hormone is turned off.

Hormone and hormone receptor: the key and the lock How does a hormone tell a cell to do something? For example, how does insulin tell cells to take in sugar? The hormone is outside the cell. It must get its message to the central nucleus inside the cell, where the nucleus directs the cell to do things like take in and use sugar.

Sticking out from the surface of the cell is a structure called a receptor; the other part of the receptor is located inside the cell. The outside portion of the insulin receptor is built to fit only insulin (and a few other insulinlike hormones).

Insulin attaches to the insulin receptor, like a key into a lock, and activates it. Once the insulin receptor is activated, it sends a cascade of chemical signals into the nucleus of the cell, leading the nucleus to send back signals that tell the cell to take in and metabolize sugar.

Hypothalamus: the master gland The description of how thyroid hormone is made also serves as an example of the key role played by the hypothalamus. The hypothalamus is a gland located deep in the brain that controls the production of many hormones. It is also an example of how the control of hormones sometimes works through a cascade of signals: from the hypothalamus to the pituitary gland and then to some other hormone-making gland. The hypothalamus is part of the limbic system (see p.340) and is closely tied to emotions and to the control of vital body functions such as blood pressure, heart rate, breathing rate, and body temperature.

REPLACING HORMONE DEFICIENCIES

The causes of hormone deficiency diseases, such as diabetes mellitus, have all been discovered in this century. For example, insulin as the treatment for diabetes was discovered in 1921.

For the next 60 years, animal forms of insulin were extracted from the pancreas glands of pigs and cattle and used to treat humans. In the 1970s, scientists

invented genetic engineering or recombinant DNA technology, which allowed them to make human hormones and other proteins.

Insulin to treat diabetes is just one example of lifesaving discoveries used to treat hormone deficiencies. Thyroid hormone has saved the lives of people with severe hormone deficiencies and helped people who have less severe deficiencies return to normal function. Estrogen and progesterone are often prescribed to ease the symptoms of menopause (see p.1047) and to help prevent osteoporosis and coronary artery disease.

Human growth hormone (see p.861) is an agent used in select cases to accelerate growth in children with short stature; its alleged role in preventing or reversing the signs of aging is controversial.

The hormonal problems covered in this section are, for the most part, grouped according to the hormone-producing glands (such as the thyroid). Your primary care doctor can evaluate and treat many hormonal problems. More complex disorders require referral to an endocrinologist, a specialist in treating hormonal disorders.

DIABETES

Diabetes Mellitus

Diabetes mellitus is often called simply "diabetes." This type of diabetes results from a lack of insulin or a lack of body cells to properly respond to insulin. Diabetes insipidus (see p.859) is a

different condition and is much more rare.

Every cell in the body needs sugar—particularly the sugar glucose—as a source of energy. The hormone insulin acts on cells to help them extract glucose from the blood. In the disease diabetes

mellitus, either the pancreas does not make enough insulin or the body's cells develop a resistance to the action of insulin.

In either case, the effect is the same: levels of glucose rise in the blood because the glucose is not getting into the body's cells.

Insulin is made by cells in the pancreas, a soft organ that lies between the stomach and the spinal column. The pancreas releases insulin into the bloodstream after a meal or a snack. As sugar levels rise, the pancreas secretes more and more insulin, which permits larger amounts of sugar to move out of the bloodstream and into the cells. If sugar levels fall too low, insulin secretion stops and four other hormones (cortisol, glucagon, growth hormone, and epinephrine) are released. This causes the liver to release glucose into the bloodstream.

Under normal circumstances, the blood glucose level is kept in balance—between 65 and 120 milligrams per deciliter (mg/dL)—despite long periods without food during the night or sudden surges in sugar intake at mealtime.

However, this delicate balance is disrupted in diabetes mellitus because the abnormalities of insulin cause blood glucose levels to rise too high, or because excessive doses of medicine used to treat diabetes can cause the blood glucose levels to fall too low.

Diabetes produces a group of intermittent and sometimes permanent symptoms. It also can increase the likelihood of several other serious diseases. For example, adults with diabetes have strokes and fatal heart attacks two to four times as often as people who do not have diabetes. Diabetes is also a leading cause of kidney failure and blindness.

Although diabetes occurs most often in older adults, it is one of the most common chronic disorders in American children (see Diabetes Mellitus, p.1004).

TYPES OF DIABETES MELLITUS

There are three types of diabetes mellitus:

- Type 1 diabetes (formerly known as insulin-dependent diabetes mellitus)

- Type 2 diabetes (formerly known as non–insulin-dependent diabetes mellitus)

- Gestational diabetes

Type 1 diabetes is an autoimmune disease (see p.870) in which the immune system attacks the insulin-producing cells (beta cells) of the pancreas. As a result, the pancreas produces progressively less insulin.

For some months or years, the immune system's attack on the pancreas occurs quietly. There is still enough insulin being made; the symptoms of diabetes have not yet developed.

But eventually, the body cannot make enough insulin. Blood sugar (glucose) levels rise to a dangerously high level. The insulin that the pancreas cannot make must be replaced with daily injections of insulin for the body to survive.

Type 1 diabetes usually first occurs before age 35, most often between ages 10 and 16. It affects males and females equally. About 5% to 10% of diabetics have type 1 diabetes.

Researchers believe that type 1 diabetes may be set off by a combination of genetics and viruses. One theory is that people with type 1 diabetes are genetically vulnerable to certain autoimmune diseases that can be triggered by exposure to a virus.

Viruses are suspected because diabetes sometimes begins after an infection with a virus. Cox-sackievirus has been identified as a possible culprit in some cases. Other researchers believe that exposure to certain toxins might be the trigger. Some investigators question whether an infant's exposure to the proteins in cow's milk can provoke diabetes.

Type 2 diabetes is the most common form of diabetes. At least 90% of diabetics have type 2 diabetes. In this form, the body's cells gradually become less responsive to insulin (insulin resistance). Normally, when insulin attaches to a cell, it sends a signal inside the cell that tells chemicals called glucose transporters to take glucose into the cell.

In insulin resistance, that signal is blocked, and the cells do not take in enough glucose from the blood. This causes blood sugar levels to rise, which leads

Type 2 Diabetes at a Glance

Type 2 diabetes:

- Affects about 14 million Americans, about half of whom are not aware that they have the disease (625,000 new cases are diagnosed each year).

- Is three times as common today as it was in 1960.

- Is more likely to develop in people who are over 40, obese, sedentary, have a family member who has diabetes, or are African American, Hispanic, or Native American.

- More than doubles your risk for a stroke or heart disease.

How Sugar Gets Into Cells

IN A HEALTHY PERSON

1

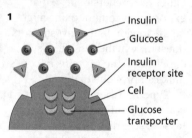

- Insulin
- Glucose
- Insulin receptor site
- Cell
- Glucose transporter

In a healthy person, the hormone insulin and the sugar glucose sit outside cells. Insulin then fits into a specific insulin receptor on the surface of the cells.

2

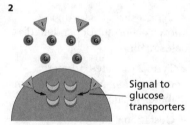

Signal to glucose transporters

When insulin attaches to its receptor, signals are sent (arrows) to chemicals called glucose transporters.

3

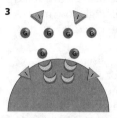

In response to the signal, the glucose transporters move to the surface of the cell, where the glucose molecules are waiting to enter.

4

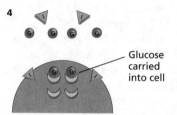

Glucose carried into cell

Glucose is carried into the cell by the glucose transporters; the cell now has the glucose it needs for energy.

IN A PERSON WITH TYPE 1 DIABETES MELLITUS

Glucose builds up in blood

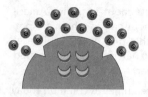

In type 1 diabetes, the pancreas makes little or no insulin. Thus, no insulin is attached to insulin receptors, no signal gets sent to the glucose transporters, and very little glucose gets into the cell (it builds up in the blood instead).

IN A PERSON WITH TYPE 2 DIABETES MELLITUS

Glucose builds up in blood

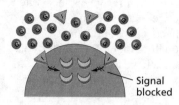

Signal blocked

In type 2 diabetes, the pancreas produces insulin, which attaches to the insulin receptors. The signal sent to the glucose transporters is blocked, however, and they do not go to the surface of the cell to bring in glucose. As a result, very little glucose gets into the cell (as in type 1 diabetes, glucose builds up in the blood instead).

the pancreas to produce even more insulin.

For some months or years, the pancreas can produce enough extra insulin to counteract the effect of insulin resistance. Blood sugar levels remain relatively normal and there are no symptoms. Ultimately, however, the insulin resistance grows stronger and the pancreas becomes exhausted from making extra insulin. At this point, blood sugar levels rise well above normal and symptoms begin.

Type 2 diabetes primarily affects people over 40. Obesity is the single most important cause. Three quarters of type 2 diabetics are or have been overweight. The hereditary link with type 2 diabetes is stronger than it is with type 1 diabetes. African Americans, Hispanics, and Native Americans have the highest risk of developing it.

Gestational diabetes (see p.930) causes blood sugar to rise in some pregnant women. However, blood sugar levels usually return to normal after delivery. Women who have gestational diabetes are at increased risk of developing type 2 diabetes in the future.

SYMPTOMS

There are many different symptoms caused by diabetes. Some symptoms result from the consequences of high blood sugar, while others are caused by the damage that diabetes does to different parts of the body. Symptoms can also occur due to low blood sugar caused by excessive sugar-lowering treatment (with insulin or pills).

The symptoms often develop explosively. Over the course of a few days, a person with type 1

Ø Preventing Type 2 Diabetes

People at risk of type 2 diabetes—especially those over 40 who are overweight and/or have diabetes in the family—can take steps to prevent it by exercising regularly, maintaining a healthy weight, and eating a sensible diet.

Exercise Exercising has several positive effects. It helps reduce your body's need for insulin by keeping excess weight in check and increases the efficiency of insulin's action on the cells of your body. Also, exercised muscles use glucose to make energy, thus naturally lowering the amount of glucose in your bloodstream. Exercise is also good for your heart, blood vessels, and circulation.

Maintain a healthy weight Obesity is a significant risk factor for type 2 diabetes in people over 40. If you weigh 10% or more above what is recommended for your build (see p.51), begin a sensible weight-loss program under your doctor's supervision.

Eat well Consuming 20 to 25 grams of dietary fiber (see p.38) from a wide variety of food sources each day will reduce your chance of getting type 2 diabetes. Eat a variety of foods and keep fats to a minimum. As important as what you eat is how much you eat and when. Avoid eating large meals or skipping meals; either will produce dramatic fluctuations in glucose and stress your metabolic system. Your doctor may recommend a limited calorie diet to help you lose weight and lower your cholesterol.

---

diabetes urinates more, is thirsty, and rapidly becomes dehydrated because of increased urination and vomiting. High levels of acid can accumulate in the blood. The affected person can lose consciousness and die if treatment is not begun quickly.

It is unusual for the symptoms of type 2 diabetes to begin so suddenly or to become so severe. One exception are the symptoms caused by a relatively uncommon condition called hyperosmolar coma (see Diabetic Emergencies, p.1207), which causes weakness and confusion and, unless it is treated promptly, coma.

Increased urination and thirst
When glucose accumulates to

abnormally high levels in the blood, the glucose pulls water out of the body's tissues and into the blood. The kidneys sense the extra water in the blood and transform it into urine, which is eliminated. Your body becomes dehydrated due to increased urination, which is accompanied by increased thirst.

Decreased energy and increased appetite In diabetes, because of insufficient amounts of insulin or resistance to the effects of insulin, the body's cells do not get enough glucose. Simply put, when your cells cannot get enough energy, you feel like you do not have enough energy. And when your cells

cannot get enough food, you feel hungry.

Also, when diabetes produces kidney damage, the inability of the kidneys to rid the body of wastes and toxins causes a loss of energy (and often nausea and a decreased appetite).

Weight loss Despite increased appetite, you may lose weight. Because the body's cells cannot get enough glucose for energy, they use fat for energy instead, which depletes the body's stores of fat. Also, the loss of fluid in diabetes that is not well controlled leads to weight loss (until the dehydration is relieved).

Vision problems Diabetes can temporarily damage the eyes, which can be alleviated with treatment. However, diabetes that remains inadequately treated for a long time can cause permanent eye damage.

Tingling sensations and pain Untreated diabetes damages nerves, which can cause loss of sensation (particularly in the feet and lower legs) or unpleasant sensations, a burning sensation, and pain.

Confusion and loss of consciousness In type 1 diabetes, not only can the profound lack of insulin lead to very high blood sugar and severe dehydration but it also can make the blood more acid and cause other metabolic abnormalities. The combination of all of these abnormalities can lead first to fatigue; then to confusion, nausea, and vomiting; and finally to loss of consciousness and death. Treatment with insulin and intravenous fluids (and sometimes certain minerals) can reverse these symptoms if started soon enough.

Diabetes Symptoms Requiring Urgent Care

Familiarize yourself with the symptoms of diabetes that require immediate attention.

SYMPTOMS	POSSIBLE CAUSES	WHAT TO DO
Excessive urination and thirst	High blood sugar	Check your blood sugar or have your doctor check it.
Fatigue, hunger, weakness (develops gradually)	High blood sugar, especially if accompanied by increased urination and thirst	Check your blood sugar or have your doctor check it. If you checked your blood sugar and it is high, call your doctor.
Rapid breathing, nausea, vomiting, stomach pain, increased urination and thirst	High blood sugar with diabetic ketoacidosis (see Diabetic Emergencies, p.1207)	Check your blood sugar or have your doctor check it. If you checked your blood sugar and it is high, call 911 and your doctor.
Fatigue, hunger, weakness (develops suddenly)	Low blood sugar	Check your blood sugar. If it is low or if you cannot check your sugar, immediately drink a glass of sugared soda or juice to restore your glucose levels to normal. Call your doctor if you do not feel better within 30 minutes.
Trembling, sweating (develops suddenly)	Low blood sugar	Check your blood sugar. If it is low or if you cannot check your sugar, immediately drink a glass of sugared soda or juice to restore your glucose levels to normal. Call your doctor if you do not feel better within 30 minutes.
Headache, double vision (develops suddenly)	Low blood sugar	Check your blood sugar. If it is low or if you cannot check your sugar, immediately drink a glass of sugared soda or juice to restore your glucose levels to normal. Call your doctor if you do not feel better within 30 minutes.
Uncontrollable sleepiness, confusion, fainting	Low blood sugar or high blood sugar	Check your blood sugar. If it is low or if you cannot check your sugar, immediately drink a glass of sugared soda or juice to restore your glucose levels to normal. If your blood sugar is high, immediately call 911 and your doctor. If you are losing consciousness, or have lost consciousness in the past from low blood sugar, have someone give you a shot of glucagon, which raises blood sugar.

In type 2 diabetes, the combination of high blood sugar and severe dehydration can produce the same symptoms. Very low blood sugar from too much medicine (insulin and certain diabetes pills) can also produce these symptoms.

COMPLICATIONS OF DIABETES

Diabetes is one of the leading causes of death and disability in the United States. Complications of diabetes affect the heart, eyes, kidneys, circulatory system, nerves, liver, and skin. However, serious complications are not an inevitable part of diabetes.

For type 1 diabetes, it has been clearly shown that you can decrease your risk of complications by keeping your blood sugar level under tight control (see p.838). Many doctors also believe this is likely to be true for type 2 diabetes as well, although the evidence is not as strong.

Each of the following complications can be detected, treated, and managed with the help of your physician:

Retinopathy is a serious eye problem that can occur when high blood sugar levels damage the tiny blood vessels of the retina, the light-sensitive lining in the back of the eye. You should see an ophthalmologist at least once a year for a diabetic eye exam. The doctor will take regular photographs of your retina and perform a test called fluorescein angiography (which shows even subtle damage) to help detect early retinopathy, which can be controlled by laser therapy (see p.434).

Nephropathy is damage to the delicate filtering system of the kidneys, which reduces their ability to remove waste from your body. Damage to the kidneys from diabetes is made worse if you also have high blood pressure (see p.644). A screening test for small amounts of the protein albumin in your urine can indicate early kidney damage from diabetes. If you have diabetes,

you should have a urine and blood test annually to screen for early signs of kidney disease.

Kidney damage cannot be reversed, but keeping blood sugar and blood pressure under control can reduce the chance of further damage. A type of blood pressure medicine called angiotensin-converting enzyme (ACE) inhibitors (see p.1160) can protect the kidneys even if your blood pressure is not high.

Prompt treatment of urinary tract infections also protects the kidneys. Untreated diabetes often leads to kidney failure, which requires dialysis (see p.815) or kidney transplantation.

Atherosclerosis of the arteries of the heart (see p.653) is more likely to develop in diabetics, leading to angina, heart attack, and heart failure. Keeping your blood sugar in control probably helps prevent atherosclerosis. Keeping your blood pressure and cholesterol in control are even more important if you are diabetic because high blood pressure and high cholesterol seem to be more likely to cause coronary artery disease in diabetics.

Peripheral arterial disease (sometimes called peripheral vascular disease) caused by atherosclerosis is more likely to develop in people with diabetes. Peripheral arterial disease impairs the circulation in arteries, particularly those leading to the brain, legs, and feet. It occurs in many people as a consequence of aging, but is accelerated by high blood sugar levels.

This condition can lead to strokes, injuries (especially to legs and feet) that do not heal, and gangrene, requiring amputation.

Along with the nerve damage of diabetes, it can cause impotence. To prevent peripheral arterial disease, do not smoke, control your blood pressure if it is high, exercise regularly, and keep your blood sugar and cholesterol levels under tight control.

Neuropathy, or nerve damage, occurs in two forms, depending on which nerves are damaged. In peripheral neuropathy, the nerves that control sensation are damaged, leading either to loss of sensation in that part of the body or to pain, numbness, and unsteadiness.

The second type, autonomic neuropathy, damages nerves that control automatic body functions, such as your urinary system and digestive system. Symptoms of autonomic neuropathy include difficulty urinating, impotence, vomiting, diarrhea, or constipation. In severe cases, it can cause severe dizziness when you stand up. You can reduce the chance of getting neuropathy by maintaining strict blood sugar levels.

Foot problems, including foot ulcers and injuries, are common in diabetics for several reasons. Nerve damage can produce loss of sensation, which can make you unaware of a developing sore. Sores that develop heal poorly because blood supply is reduced. Wound infections develop more easily in many diabetics. Sores that become severe may never heal, leading to gangrene and amputation.

Carefully wash and inspect your feet every day for wounds or signs of infection, and consult your doctor if you find anything suspicious. Have a podiatrist clip your nails. Nails should not be cut too short and should be cut

---

Diabetes and Annual Eye Exams

People with diabetes should have an annual checkup by an ophthalmologist to check for three potentially serious conditions that occur more often in people with diabetes: diabetic retinopathy (see p.434), glaucoma (see p.435), and cataracts (see p.430). Glaucoma and cataracts occur twice as often in people with diabetes.

regularly to prevent infection. Always wear shoes, and see your physician about any injuries that do not heal within 2 weeks.

Infections When blood sugar is too high, some white blood cells do not work as effectively in eliminating various infections. Diabetics are particularly prone to yeast infections on the skin or in the vagina, and are also more prone to boils (see p.532) and other bacterial infections.

TREATMENT OPTIONS

If you have any symptoms of diabetes, see your doctor, who will perform a physical examination and test your blood and urine for sugar. If either your blood or urine shows abnormal levels of blood sugar, your doctor may test your blood again. The test may be done after you fast overnight or 2 hours after you eat a meal, or in the form of a glucose tolerance test.

In a glucose tolerance test, you are given sugar water to drink, and your blood sugar levels are measured over the next 5 hours. High glucose levels in the blood will confirm that you have diabetes. Your doctor may also test your urine for the presence of ketones, which are products of fat that often occur in people with type 1 diabetes.

There is no cure for diabetes, but proper treatment can greatly reduce both the symptoms and complications.

Unlike some other conditions, the most important person on the treatment team is the person with diabetes. You will ultimately be the one who is in charge of controlling the disease through careful attention to diet, exercise, and medicine.

What Is "Tight Control" of Blood Sugar?

If you take insulin, your physician will tell you that maintaining tight control of your blood sugar level is essential to decreasing your risk of complications. What exactly is tight control?

It means keeping your blood sugar as close to normal as possible. Your physician may recommend that you check your blood sugar as often as four times a day (using blood for the test) and keep a written record of your glucose level and the amount of insulin you take.

Keeping tight control of your glucose levels can significantly reduce long-term complications, particularly if you have type 1 diabetes. This is probably also true for type 2 diabetes.

Maintaining tight control of blood sugar also raises the risk that you will experience attacks of low blood sugar. Therefore, if you and your doctor decide to try to achieve tight control, you must be very careful about checking your blood sugar and about treating yourself early for symptoms of low blood sugar.

While this can be intimidating at first, most people find that managing their diabetes soon becomes simple and easy.

The most important step to take (and the first one you should take) is to become educated about the disease. Your primary care physician, nurses, and other health professionals will teach you about the disease.

Your physician will organize your treatment plan, perform regular examinations, work with you to regularly monitor your insulin dose and glucose levels, and investigate symptoms that can indicate long-term complications. The American Diabetes Association (see p.1232) can provide useful information.

Other specialists are also involved in caring for diabetes-related problems. An ophthalmologist should perform regular eye examinations to monitor any development of diabetic retinopathy. Podiatrists provide foot care.

Dietitians (nutritional experts) are helpful in planning a diet that suits your medical needs. If kidney function deteriorates, you may need the help of a nephrologist (kidney specialist). The immediate aim of treatment is to normalize levels of glucose in the blood; long-term goals are to prevent complications and extend life.

A small number of people with severe diabetes may benefit from having a pancreas transplant. The transplanted pancreas cells must come from a closely matched donor, and recipients must take powerful antirejection drugs that can have serious side effects.

For type 1 diabetes For people with type 1 diabetes, there are three strategies for normalizing blood glucose levels: daily injections of insulin to replace the hormone that your body is not producing, a nutrition plan, and regular exercise. You will need to

Benefits of Intensive Treatment for Type 1 Diabetes

Intensive therapy with insulin can delay the onset and slow progression of complications in people with type 1 diabetes mellitus in comparison to less intensive "conventional" treatment. This was shown in a randomized, controlled trial (see p.31) of more than 1,400 people who were observed for up to 9 years. Intensive treatment includes monitoring blood sugar at least four times a day and giving insulin at least three times a day—adjusting the dose based on glucose measurements as well as food intake and anticipated exercise.

Conventional treatment involved one or two daily injections of insulin, usually without dosage adjustments. The benefits of intensive therapy were seen in people who had no diabetic complications at the start of the study and in people who already had some complications at the start of the study. However, people treated with intensive therapy were more likely to have severe low blood sugar reactions and to gain weight (10 pounds, on average) than those who had conventional treatment.

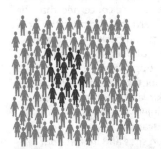

13 OF 100 PEOPLE WHO HAD TYPE 1 DIABETES AND USED INTENSIVE TREATMENT DEVELOPED DIABETIC EYE DISEASE

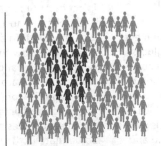

16 OF 100 PEOPLE WHO HAD TYPE 1 DIABETES AND USED INTENSIVE TREATMENT DEVELOPED KIDNEY DISEASE

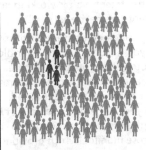

3 OF 100 PEOPLE WHO HAD TYPE 1 DIABETES AND USED INTENSIVE TREATMENT DEVELOPED NERVE DAMAGE

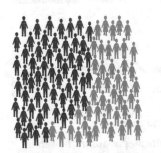

55 OF 100 PEOPLE WHO HAD TYPE 1 DIABETES AND USED CONVENTIONAL TREATMENT DEVELOPED DIABETIC EYE DISEASE

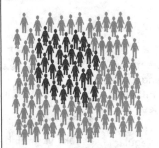

27 OF 100 PEOPLE WHO HAD TYPE 1 DIABETES AND USED CONVENTIONAL TREATMENT DEVELOPED KIDNEY DISEASE

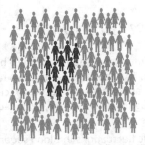

10 OF 100 PEOPLE WHO HAD TYPE 1 DIABETES AND USED CONVENTIONAL TREATMENT DEVELOPED NERVE DAMAGE

monitor your blood glucose levels several times a day (see p.840), and your doctor will also examine you regularly.

Insulin Type 1 diabetics need insulin injections up to several times a day, which they learn to give themselves. In a short time, these subcutaneous (under-the-skin) injections become relatively painless and routine.

Injectable insulin originally was derived from the pancreas glands of either pigs or cattle; increasingly, insulin used today is human insulin produced by genetic engineering. It is available in ultra–short-acting form (insulin lispro), short-acting form (regular insulin), intermediate-acting forms (isophane insulin and insulin zinc), or long-acting form (extended insulin zinc).

The insulin begins to act 30 to 60 minutes (short-acting), 2 to 4 hours (intermediate-acting), or 4 to 8 hours (long-acting) after

Monitoring Glucose and Giving Insulin Injections

Your doctor will tell you how many times a day you need to test your blood for glucose, and when it should be tested. Use a small notebook to write down what time you did the test, the results, what you ate, how you felt, and how much you exercised. This record will tell you and your doctor how well your current treatment plan is working, and whether adjustments are needed.

Your physician or diabetes educator will recommend the kits you need for testing your blood for glucose, which you will do yourself at home. Testing blood (not urine) provides the most accurate indication of the amount of sugar in your blood. The test requires pricking your finger for a sample of blood, which is then applied to a color-coded strip. The strip is placed in a glucose monitor, which provides a reading and helps you gauge the amount of insulin you need.

Some diabetics prefer not to test their blood; they test their urine instead. Although it is second-best, if you choose this form of testing, you should check your urine sugars regularly.

Injecting insulin Your doctor will instruct you on the kind of insulin to use, how much to use, and when to inject it. At first, many people are concerned that the injections will hurt. They learn that, because the needles are very thin and short and because shots are given just below the skin (not deep into muscle), pain is minimal. The abdomen, upper arms, upper legs, waist, and hips are good spots to inject insulin. Stretch an inch or so of skin and insert the needle, releasing the skin as you inject the medicine. Rotate the injection sites so that scar tissue and fat do not accumulate in the injection sites and inhibit your body's absorption of insulin. Use disposable syringes. Dispose of needles in a childproof container.

When Can I Eat?

People who have diabetes need to become creatures of habit. To keep blood sugars in a normal range, the amount and timing of the three factors that influence blood sugar—diet, exercise, and medicine—need to be made regular.

Dramatic fluctuations in blood sugar due to irregular eating or starving the body of glucose, and then suddenly overloading it by eating a big meal, puts stress on your metabolic system and makes it difficult to predict how much medicine you need.

Here are some tips for regulating your blood glucose through food and exercise:

- Eat about the same amount of food each day.
- Eat your meals and snacks at about the same time each day.
- Try not to skip meals and snacks.
- Take your diabetes medicines at about the same time each day.
- Exercise at about the same time each day.
- Talk to your doctor about which times for meals, snacks, medicine, and exercise are best for you. The more you learn about your diabetes, the better equipped you will be to control it.

injection. Most people use a combination of the short-acting and intermediate-acting forms.

The type and amount of insulin you need is based on your blood glucose levels and how much they fluctuate. This varies depending on your weight, diet (the type, quantity, and timing of your meals), level of activity, emotional state, and the presence of infections or other stresses on your body. Your needs may vary from day to day.

Typically, people with type 1 diabetes require injections of short-acting insulin before meals along with a long-acting insulin to cover the time between meals. Alternately, you can carry a battery-operated pump, which auto-

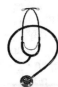

Diabetes: *When You Visit Your Doctor*

QUESTIONS TO DISCUSS WITH YOUR DOCTOR:

■ Are you keeping a diary of your blood sugar levels (a record of the date, time of day, and level of your blood glucose)? How often is your blood sugar under 80 or over 140 milligrams per deciliter?

■ Have you gained or lost weight? Are you excessively thirsty or do you urinate frequently? Are you unusually hungry? Is your vision blurry? These are symptoms of elevated blood glucose.

■ Do you wear shoes at all times to protect your feet? Do you check your feet every day for cuts or sores? Decreased sensation in the feet from diabetes can lead to sores you cannot feel.

■ Do you have chest pain or shortness of breath at rest or with exertion? Diabetes substantially increases your risk of heart attack, and chest pain or shortness of breath may be early warning symptoms.

■ What medications are you taking for your diabetes? Do you ever miss doses?

■ How well are you following your diet to control diabetes?

■ How much do you exercise?

■ Have you ever been shaky, sweaty, light-headed, or confused? These are all symptoms of low blood sugar.

■ Do you know what to do when your blood sugar is low?

■ When did you last see an ophthalmologist? You should have a complete eye exam at least once a year.

■ Do you have burning sensations in your feet? This could be from nerve damage.

■ If you are a woman, are you contemplating getting pregnant? If you are sexually active, are you using birth control? It is very important that your diabetes be well controlled before and during pregnancy.

■ Do you know what you can do to decrease your risk of complications from diabetes?

■ Do you know how pregnancy will affect your diabetes, or what to do to decrease the risk of complications?

YOUR DOCTOR MIGHT EXAMINE THE FOLLOWING BODY PARTS OR FUNCTIONS:

■ Heart rate and blood pressure

■ Eyes

■ Heart and lungs

■ Pulse

■ Feet (for breaks in the skin, for ulcers, and for sensation)

■ Reflexes

YOUR DOCTOR MIGHT ORDER THE FOLLOWING LAB TESTS OR STUDIES:

■ Hemoglobin A_{1c} (a blood test that estimates your average blood sugar for the past 3 months). Be sure you know the results of each test, and what is normal.

■ Urine test once a year. Protein in your urine is a sign that diabetes is affecting your kidneys.

■ Finger stick or blood test to check blood glucose level

■ Cholesterol blood test

matically delivers a continuous supply of short-acting insulin through a needle in your abdomen.

The goal is to inject enough insulin to normalize blood glucose levels—that is, to prevent levels from climbing too high or dropping too low. This is accomplished through frequent glucose testing using a simple test you can perform at home (see p.85).

Doctors are testing the effectiveness and possible side effects of inhaled insulin, instead of insulin injections. The insulin is inhaled before a meal, and rapidly enters the bloodstream just as sugar from the meal is also rising in the blood. The results of the first studies are encouraging. One day, this form of taking insulin could become very popular, especially in people with type II diabetes.

Diet offers double benefits: control of glucose levels and control of weight. A healthy diet for people with diabetes is the same as for people without the disease but is more regimented in its pattern to ensure that the amount of glucose in your blood remains steady. Be sure that you eat a balanced diet while monitoring your intake of carbohydrates. Your dietitian will provide specific guidelines.

A regular meal schedule avoids dramatic ups and downs in blood glucose levels. Eat about the same amount of food each day, consume your meals and snacks at about the same time each day, and never skip meals or snacks. If it has been recommended that you lose weight, eat according to the plan your physician or dietitian recommends.

Exercise is important not only to keep weight in check but also to maintain the health of your blood vessels, which are especially vulnerable to damage. Exercised muscles also use glucose to make energy, thus naturally controlling the overflow of sugar in the bloodstream. In addition, exercise sensitizes the body's cells to insulin, allowing sugar to be used more efficiently.

While exercising, it is important not to overdo it. Too much exercise can cause low blood sugar. Timing is important. Try to exercise 30 minutes after eating a light snack (such as bread, pasta, or a potato) and avoid exercise when you have not eaten for more than 4 hours. Your doctor

can help you coordinate eating, exercise, and insulin injections.

For type 2 diabetes If you have type 2 diabetes, you may be able to control your blood glucose levels with exercise and diet alone.

Weight loss is essential in treating type 2 diabetes, whether you achieve weight loss by reduced calories in your diet, exercise, or both. If you are overweight or even on the high end of normal weight, the first step is to lose weight. This lowers insulin resistance, enabling your body to make more efficient use of what insulin there is.

Exercise lowers insulin resistance, both by increasing muscle activity and by helping you lose weight. Exercise may be even more important for people with type 2 diabetes than it is for those with type 1. It can help you maintain a more constant level of glucose and reduce your risk for heart disease. Talk to your doctor or diabetes educator about an exercise program that is right for you.

Oral hypoglycemic medicines may be needed if your blood sugar remains elevated after weight loss, regular exercise, and a strict diabetic diet. These drugs work by stimulating the pancreas to produce more insulin and to increase the ability of cells to

respond to insulin. They are usually taken once or twice a day before meals. If the oral drugs do not manage your glucose, and you show symptoms of hyperglycemia, you may need to take insulin injections.

Oral hypoglycemic medicines for type 2 diabetes include:

- *Sulfonylureas* These medicines increase the production of insulin by the pancreas and may make tissues more sensitive to insulin. These agents include glyburide, glipizide, glimepiride, and several less potent, older drugs. They are effective in about 65% of people with type 2 diabetes. When the dose of these drugs is too high (compared to the amount of carbohydrate you eat), it can cause low blood sugar.

- *Biguanides* These medicines reduce the production and release of glucose from the liver, and improve the tissue's sensitivity to insulin. Alone, these drugs are about as effective as the sulfonylureas, but they can be combined with sulfonylureas for people who do not do well on either type of drug alone. The main biguanide medicine used today is metformin. Metformin should not be used by people who drink alcohol excessively, have kidney or liver disease, or have signs of congestive heart failure.

Diabetes and Medical Identification

People who have diabetes should always wear medical identification tags or carry a medical identification card that states their illness. Emergency personnel will look for a medallion, bracelet, or wallet card before treating an unconscious person in order to provide the best treatment possible. Medical identification jewelry is widely available. Ask your diabetes educator for more information.

■ *"Glitazones"* This relatively new class of drugs decreases the resistance of cells (particularly muscle cells) to the action of insulin, causing the cells to take in more sugar from the blood. These medicines also cause the liver to decrease the amount of sugar that it produces, thereby lowering sugar levels in the blood. The drugs are usually used in combination with other medicines or with insulin, although they can be used alone. Troglitazone was the first type of "glitazone" medicine on the market. Because this class of drugs can cause liver damage, it is recommended that the drugs be used only when other medicines have failed. Also, people taking these medicines should have frequent liver tests.

■ *Meglitinides* These medicines act like the sulfonylureas, by stimulating the pancreas to produce insulin. They can be used in combination with other pills. The meglitinide medicine in use today is repaglinide.

■ *Acarbose* This medicine acts by inhibiting the intestinal enzymes that are responsible for absorbing sugar from food. It is useful for people who experience an exaggerated rise in glucose immediately after eating, a common problem in those who are in the early stages of type 2 diabetes, as well as for some who have lived with the disease for years.

■ *Heterocyclic drugs* These drugs help relieve the discomfort of diabetic neuropathy, but do not affect blood sugar. Several very promising new medicines are under development and may be even more effective.

INTEGRATING DIABETES INTO YOUR LIFE

Many people find that the steps they take to keep their blood sugar within strict parameters offer immediate benefits—weight loss, increased fitness, higher energy levels, and a better self-image. But balancing food, exercise, and medicine is not always easy. Here are some tips:

■ **Become educated.** Learn as much as you can about your form of diabetes and what you can do to control it.

■ **Know your body.** Learn the signs of ketoacidosis (if you have type 1 diabetes), hyperosmolar coma (if you have type 2 diabetes), and hypoglycemia—and what to do about them (see Diabetic Emergencies, p.1207).

■ **Learn diabetes care skills.** Ensure that checking your own blood sugar is a part of your daily schedule and learn how to give yourself insulin injections.

■ **Exercise daily.** Select an exercise that you like and do it once a day. It is important to get the same amount of exercise every day. Even modest, nonvigorous physical activity improves blood sugar control.

■ **Manage stress.** Emotional and physical stress (such as an infection) can send glucose levels soaring. Find a stress reduction method (see p.90) that suits you, such as yoga, walking, meditation, imagery, or listening to music. Contact your doctor at the first signs of infection.

■ **Get your sex life back on track.** Diabetes can take its toll on sexual function and desire. Due to changes in blood vessels and nerve damage, some men become impotent (see p.1092). For women, sex can be uncomfortable due to yeast infections of the vagina. Discuss these issues with your partner and your doctor, who can recommend solutions, including medicines to treat impotence and yeast infections as well as vaginal lubricants to reduce discomfort.

■ **Plan for an emergency.** Wear a medical identification bracelet (see p.1190).

Low Blood Sugar (Hypoglycemia)

Low blood sugar, or hypoglycemia, is a condition in which the levels of glucose in the bloodstream drop too low to fuel the body's activity.

It most often occurs as a complication of the treatment of diabetes. Your dose of insulin or diabetes pills may be too great or you may have delayed or skipped a meal. Not all diabetes pills cause hypoglycemia; it is mainly a problem with the meglitinides and sulfonylurea drugs.

Less commonly, hypoglycemia occurs in the early months of pregnancy or is caused by prolonged fasting, strenuous exercise (which lowers sugar), or tumors of the pancreas.

SYMPTOMS

The symptoms of hypoglycemia vary significantly among people. Some people may feel weak, hot and sweaty, drowsy, confused, hungry, or dizzy. Other symptoms of low blood sugar include irritability, trembling, rapid heartbeat, blurry vision, and a cold, clammy sensation. Severe hypoglycemia can cause coma.

TREATMENT OPTIONS

If you experience symptoms of hypoglycemia and you are being treated for diabetes, read about tight control of blood sugar on p.838. If you do not have diabetes, see your doctor, who will take a medical history and test your blood for glucose levels at varying times after meals. If you have hypoglycemia, your doctor may perform special diagnostic tests to determine the cause.

Treatment depends on the cause and severity of your condition. For example, if the condition is caused by a drug you are taking, your physician may be able to change the medicine to one that does not cause hypoglycemia.

If you have periodic episodes of hypoglycemia, become aware of the early signs. Immediately eat or drink a sugar-containing food or liquid. If your hypoglycemia is severe and you have lost consciousness due to it in the past, you may require an injection of glucagon, a hormone produced by the pancreas that raises your blood sugar level, or an intravenous infusion of sugar water.

Educate your family and friends about hypoglycemia; they

Diabetic Emergencies

If you or someone you love has diabetes, educate yourself on the following diabetic emergencies:

Ketoacidosis This condition is caused by the body having inadequate amounts of insulin, and therefore occurs primarily in people with type 1 diabetes. Lack of insulin causes high sugar and acid levels in the blood. You become weak, confused, tired, begin breathing fast, and ultimately lapse into a coma unless you get immediate treatment with intravenous fluids and insulin.

Hyperosmolar coma This condition is caused by the body having a partial lack of insulin, and occurs primarily in people with type 2 diabetes. Blood sugar levels slowly climb to extremely high levels, causing you to urinate very large amounts and to become severely dehydrated. Unlike ketoacidosis, the blood does not usually have high acid levels. You become weak and confused, and ultimately can lapse into a coma unless you get prompt treatment with large amounts of intravenous fluids and small amounts of insulin.

Hypoglycemia This condition is caused by taking too much insulin or sulfonylureas, or eating and drinking insufficient amounts of calories. In people taking insulin, hypoglycemia comes on when the insulin effect is at its peak. For those taking a longer-acting form of insulin (the most common form used), the maximum effect is reached 6 to 8 hours after injection.

Symptoms include rapid heartbeat, sweating, trembling, and hunger. If you do not get sugar into your body, you can go into a coma. Carry a piece of candy with you at all times and drink a sugared drink such as orange juice if you feel the symptoms coming on.

should know that you may be so confused or lethargic that you may not think to take a sugar-containing food to alleviate symptoms and they may have to give you the glucagon injection.

THYROID GLAND DISORDERS

In thyroid gland disorders, the function of the thyroid gland in making thyroid hormones is abnormal, the size and shape of the gland is abnormal, or both.

Hyperthyroidism

Hyperthyroidism is overactivity of the thyroid gland, resulting in excess amounts of thyroid hormones in the body.

An overactive thyroid gland produces more thyroid hormone than it should. The thyroid hormone causes the metabolic rate of all the body's organs to increase. Thus, an overactive thyroid makes everything else overactive.

Graves disease is the most common cause of hyperthyroidism in people under age 40. It is an autoimmune disease (see p.870) in which abnormal proteins called thyroid-stimulating antibodies provoke the thyroid to produce too much thyroid hormone.

Graves disease is diagnosed in about 1 of 1,000 people every year, mostly young to middle-

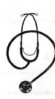

Hyperthyroidism: When You Visit Your Doctor

QUESTIONS TO DISCUSS WITH YOUR DOCTOR:

■ Do you often feel warm, have diarrhea, feel anxious, or have a rapid or pounding heartbeat, or are you losing weight despite having a good appetite? These symptoms could indicate you are not taking enough antithyroid medication.

■ Do you often feel tired or cold, have frequent constipation, or have dry skin, or are you gaining weight for no apparent reason? These symptoms could indicate you are developing an underactive thyroid gland, either because you are taking too much antithyroid medication or because you have had treatments that could cause hypothyroidism.

■ Have you developed a fever, prolonged sore throat, or other signs of infection? In very rare cases, if you are taking antithyroid medications, antithyroid drugs can reduce the number of white blood cells.

■ Could you be having a drug interaction? This can happen if you are taking antithyroid medication along with other medications.

■ Are you pregnant (or planning to get pregnant)? You should not take radioactive iodine or some antithyroid medications if you are (or are planning to become) pregnant. You will need to change the doses of your drugs if you become pregnant.

YOUR DOCTOR MIGHT EXAMINE THE FOLLOWING BODY PARTS OR FUNCTIONS:

■ Heart rate and blood pressure

■ Eyes

■ Hair and skin texture

■ Thyroid gland (for abnormalities in size, consistency, or contour)

■ Heart and lungs

■ Reflexes

YOUR DOCTOR MIGHT ORDER THE FOLLOWING LAB TESTS OR STUDIES:

■ Thyroid function tests (blood tests) approximately once a month until your thyroid function has stabilized (less frequently thereafter)

■ Complete blood cell count (before starting a medication to inhibit your thyroid function)

■ Ultrasound (see p.847) of your thyroid gland or a thyroid uptake scan (see p.846) if your thyroid is abnormal in size or shape

Thyroid Feedback System

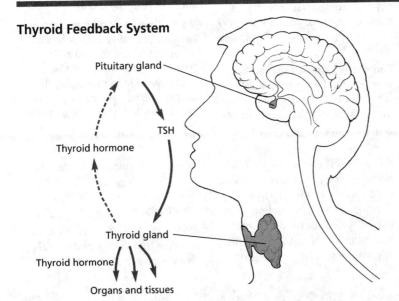

Pituitary gland

TSH

Thyroid hormone

Thyroid gland

Thyroid hormone

Organs and tissues

The thyroid gland produces thyroid hormones in response to a signal from thyroid-stimulating hormone (TSH), which is made in the pituitary gland. The pituitary gland can detect even minute changes in the blood levels of the thyroid hormones. When the levels of the thyroid hormones fall, TSH levels go up; when thyroid hormone levels rise too high, TSH levels fall.

Diagnosing Thyroid Disease

If you have a thyroid disorder, your doctor may order one of the following tests to confirm it or to help determine the course of treatment:

Blood tests The thyroid gland produces hormones called thyroxine (T_4) and triiodothyronine (T_3) in response to a hormone made by the pituitary gland called thyroid-stimulating hormone (TSH). Circulating thyroid hormone then inhibits the release of more TSH from the pituitary, keeping the levels of T_3 and T_4 from going too high. By the same mechanism, when the level of thyroid hormone is low, the TSH level rises, stimulating the production of more T_3 and T_4.

If a thyroid condition causes the gland to make excessive amounts of T_4 and T_3, the TSH level becomes low in response. Likewise, if something happens to the thyroid gland that causes it to make inadequate amounts of T_4 and T_3, the TSH level becomes high in response.

Measuring the amount of TSH in the blood is often the first step in evaluating a suspected thyroid disease. Abnormal levels of TSH may lead your doctor to measure your T_3 and T_4 levels.

Autoimmune diseases (see p.870) are one of the main causes of thy-

Location of Thyroid Gland

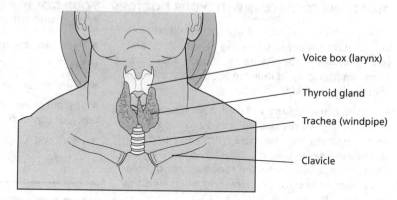

Voice box (larynx)

Thyroid gland

Trachea (windpipe)

Clavicle

The thyroid gland is located at the front of the neck near the trachea.

roid abnormalities. The immune system attacks the thyroid gland in a condition called Hashimoto thyroiditis (see p.850), causing the gland to ultimately become underactive (see Hypothyroidism, p.848).

In Graves disease (see p.844), the opposite happens: different kinds of autoantibodies stimulate the production of T_3 and T_4, causing hyperthyroidism. To investigate these conditions, your doctor may measure thyroid antibodies in your blood.

Radioactive iodine uptake The thyroid gland absorbs iodine, which is used to make thyroid hormone. A radioactive iodine mole-

cule is absorbed in the same way. Within 24 hours of being taken in pill or liquid form, a very small amount of radioactive iodine is absorbed and the radioactivity is measured. For this test, you lie down while a radioactive counter is placed over your neck. The radioactive iodine uptake is the amount of radioactive iodine measured in your thyroid gland.

If your thyroid gland is overactive because of Graves disease, radioactive iodine uptake will be increased. If your thyroid gland is overactive due to thyroiditis, the uptake will be very low. The kind of radioactive iodine you take for this

aged women. The tendency to develop Graves disease can be inherited, though the link is not so strong that every family member will develop the condition.

In about 10% of cases, hyper-

thyroidism is caused by thyroid nodules (see p.850) that produce excessive quantities of thyroid hormones. Sometimes, temporary hyperthyroidism results from inflammation of the thyroid due to a viral infection or the early

stages of Hashimoto thyroiditis (see Thyroiditis, p.850).

SYMPTOMS

Every cell and organ in the body requires thyroid hormone to work normally. Excessive hortest is not damaging to the thyroid gland, unlike the kind used to treat an overactive thyroid gland.

Thyroid scan A thyroid scan is a picture of your thyroid gland taken after radioactive iodine or a different kind of radioactive substance called technetium has been injected into a vein. A thyroid scan can determine which areas of your thyroid gland (usually the thyroid nodules) are making excess thyroid hormone.

Thyroid ultrasound Ultrasound (see p.148) can provide a picture of thyroid nodules. It can determine if a thyroid nodule is solid or partially filled with fluid (cystic). Ultrasound also can help direct the needle used to obtain a thyroid biopsy.

Thyroid fine-needle aspiration biopsy A fine-needle aspiration biopsy is performed to obtain thyroid cells from a thyroid nodule. The cells are examined in a laboratory, usually for the presence of cancer.

A very fine needle is inserted directly into a thyroid nodule and cells are withdrawn for laboratory analysis. The procedure is rapid and almost painless (much like having blood taken), but may cause some bruising or mild pain at the biopsy site.

mone results in more rapid action of many body systems. The intestines respond with frequent bowel movements, the heart rate speeds up, and the sweat glands work overtime, causing sweaty palms and a

moist, smooth-textured skin. An overstimulated nervous system can result in irritability.

You may find your appetite increasing, but lose weight. Your muscles may become very weak. You may also have intolerance to heat, an enlarged thyroid gland (see Goiter, p.850), and tremors.

Anxiety and other nervous symptoms are not uncommon, and you may have difficulty sleeping. Menstrual periods may become irregular, less frequent, and scanty.

About 1 person of 5 with Graves disease has bulging eyes (see p.427), an eye disease that often causes bulging eyes and may cause eyes to be red and swollen and to tear. People with other forms of hyperthyroidism do not have this eye condition.

Elderly people tend to have fewer symptoms of hyperthyroidism. Irritability, apathy, distractibility, unexplained weight loss, or a rapid or irregular heartbeat (even at rest) may be the only symptoms of hyperthyroidism in elderly adults.

TREATMENT OPTIONS

If you experience symptoms, consult your physician, who will examine your thyroid, measure your pulse, look for hand tremors, and ask about other symptoms, including diarrhea and sensitivity to heat.

He or she will also draw blood to measure levels of the hormone thyroxine, which become elevated in hyperthyroidism, and of thyroid-stimulating hormone (TSH), which is very low in hyperthyroidism.

You may also need a radio-

active iodine uptake test (see p.846), in which you swallow a small amount of radioactive iodine. Twenty-four hours later, the concentration in your thyroid gland is measured, and a thyroid scan is performed. Higher levels of radioactive iodine will be apparent if you have Graves disease or a thyroid nodule that is making thyroid hormones.

Treatment of Graves disease aims to reduce the production of thyroid hormones by the thyroid gland and to help reduce the symptoms caused by increased levels of thyroid hormones in the blood. Thyroid hormone production can be reduced by antithyroid medicines, radioactive iodine treatment, or surgery.

Antithyroid medicines These medicines prevent the thyroid from producing hormones. They are usually the first treatment in Graves disease and usually produce results within several weeks. In some people, the drugs produce side effects including rash, itching, or fever. In rare cases, the medicines cause liver inflammation or a deficiency of infection-fighting white blood cells. Call your physician if you have a fever or sore throat or notice any yellowing of your skin.

Though antithyroid medicines are effective while they are being taken, the condition for which they are taken often returns once the drugs are stopped. Your doctor may recommend that you consider a permanent solution (most commonly radioactive iodine) to the overactive thyroid.

Radioactive iodine The radioactive iodine used to treat the thyroid gland is somewhat different from the type used to measure radioactive iodine uptake and used in a thyroid scan (see above left). The type used in treatment injures thyroid cells instead of just temporarily passing through them.

You take a pill containing radioactive iodine, which accumulates in your thyroid gland and kills most of the thyroid cells. It does not injure any other part of your body because it is not absorbed to any significant degree by any organs or tissues other than the thyroid.

After several months, your thyroid gland makes only very small amounts of thyroid hormone. Hyperthyroidism is cured in most people after one dose. In rare cases, a second dose is needed. Your doctor will reevaluate your thyroid function for several months to check for hypothyroidism (underactivity of the thyroid) from the treatment. If your blood tests indicate hypothyroidism, thyroid replacement medicine will be prescribed.

The advantage of radioactive iodine treatment is that it usually fixes the problem for the rest of your life, with one treatment. The disadvantage is that hypothyroidism usually results, and you will have to take thyroid pills for the rest of your life.

Surgery Another way to reduce the amount of thyroid hormone is to surgically remove all or a part of the thyroid gland. This treatment is usually recommended when antithyroid medicine or radioactive iodine are ineffective or cannot be used. However, people with Graves disease under age 20 who do not find relief of symptoms with antithyroid medicine are often treated with surgery.

Surgery is also recommended for people of any age in whom a goiter (see p.850) blocks the windpipe or the passage of food. The operation can often be performed (usually under general anesthesia) with only an overnight stay in the hospital.

The surgeon aims to remove just enough of the gland to relieve the hyperthyroid condition. Usually, however, the gland that is left after surgery cannot make enough thyroid hormone, and you will need to take thyroid pills for the rest of your life.

The bulging eyes that can occur in people with Graves disease sometimes resolve after using one of the measures to reduce production of hormones. However, in some people, the condition persists or worsens. In rare cases (when the eye symptoms are severe or progressive), an ophthalmologist may recommend treatment with corticosteroid medicine (see p.895), radiation (see p.741), or surgery.

Hypothyroidism

Hypothyroidism is a condition in which the thyroid gland does not produce enough thyroid hormone. This slows down the body's metabolism and can cause you to feel lethargic and mentally dull.

Hypothyroidism is the most common type of thyroid disorder. It affects women five to ten times more often than men, and the incidence increases with age.

An estimated 6 of 100 women over age 65 have some degree of hypothyroidism. Even mild forms of the disease, which may not be noticed or diagnosed, can set the stage for severe thyroid problems in the future.

Hashimoto thyroiditis (also called autoimmune thyroiditis) is the most common cause of hypothyroidism in the United States. It is an autoimmune disorder (see p.870) in which the immune system attacks the cells of the thyroid, causing inflammation and destruction of the cells.

Hashimoto thyroiditis often surfaces after childbirth or after treatment with powerful immune system drugs such as interferon alfa or interleukins. It is more common in people who have other autoimmune diseases, such as type 1 diabetes (see p.833), pernicious anemia (see p.717), or Addison disease (see p.856).

Other causes of hypothyroidism are more rare. Surgery to remove part or all of the thyroid gland can result in hypothyroidism. An underactive pituitary gland (see p.860) that produces inadequate levels of TSH will fail to stimulate a normal thyroid gland and can also cause hypothyroidism.

Some children are born without a thyroid gland or with low levels of thyroid hormone, a condition called congenital hypothyroidism. This occurs in about 1 of 4,000 births. Affected children have mental retardation and poor growth unless their condition is recognized and treated, which is usually soon after birth.

SYMPTOMS

If you have mild hypothyroidism, you may not experience any symptoms. When symptoms do appear, they are often vague and progress slowly. Symptoms include a rundown feeling; intellectual dullness; blunted emotions or depression; feeling cold; constipation; muscle aches; dry, scaly, or puffy skin; hair loss;

Hypothyroidism: *When You Visit Your Doctor*

QUESTIONS TO DISCUSS WITH YOUR DOCTOR:

■ Are you taking your thyroid medication? Are you having any side effects?

■ Do you often feel warm, have diarrhea, feel anxious, have a rapid or pounding heartbeat, or are you losing weight despite having a good appetite? These symptoms could indicate you are taking too much thyroid medication.

■ Do you know if any drugs you might be taking interact with your thyroid replacement hormone?

■ Do you often feel tired or cold, have frequent constipation, or have dry skin, or are you gaining weight for no good reason? These symptoms could indicate you are not taking enough thyroid medication.

■ Are you pregnant? You will need to change the doses of your medications if you become pregnant.

■ Do you know how pregnancy will affect your thyroid function?

YOUR DOCTOR MIGHT EXAMINE THE FOLLOWING BODY PARTS OR FUNCTIONS:

■ Heart rate and blood pressure

■ Hair and skin texture

■ Thyroid gland (for abnormalities in size, consistency, or contour)

■ Heart and lungs

■ Reflexes

YOUR DOCTOR MIGHT ORDER THE FOLLOWING LAB TESTS OR STUDIES:

■ Thyroid function tests (blood tests) once a year (more commonly if you have recently changed thyroid medication doses or if you are pregnant)

■ Ultrasound (see p.847) of your thyroid gland if your thyroid is abnormal in size or shape

weight gain; tingling of fingers or toes; decreased tolerance to exercise; joint pain; hoarseness; and irregular menstrual periods.

Hashimoto thyroiditis is a common cause of goiter (see p.850), the physical swelling of the thyroid gland.

A condition called myxedema coma is a serious complication that can occur when hypothyroidism is severe and not treated. In this condition, the affected person feels drowsy, cold, and can become unconscious; emergency medical care is required. You may develop a high cholesterol level or increased blood pressure.

TREATMENT OPTIONS

If you have symptoms of hypothyroidism, consult your doctor, who will ask you about your symptoms, perform an examination, and obtain a blood test of your thyroid-stimulating hormone (TSH) level. An elevated TSH level indicates hypothyroidism.

Because Hashimoto thyroiditis is the most common cause of hypothyroidism, often no further testing is necessary. Sometimes, further tests (such as thyroid antibody levels) are performed.

If your doctor diagnoses hypothyroidism, he or she will most likely prescribe a thyroid hormone replacement medicine, a synthetic copy of the natural thyroid hormones—T_4, T_3, or both—that you lack.

People who are elderly or who have heart disease will take a very low dose initially, since higher levels can place more stress on the heart. Thyroid hormone also has several important drug interactions (see p.1190).

Your doctor will monitor your levels of thyroid hormones (to determine the ideal dose) by measuring your TSH level within about 6 weeks. Once the proper dose is established, your TSH level will be measured less frequently.

Your body may also tell you when your thyroxine dose needs to be modified. If your dose is too low, you will experience some of the same symptoms that brought hypothyroidism to your attention in the first place. Too much thyroxine results in symptoms of hyperthyroidism (see p.844), including rapid heartbeat, nervousness, tremor, and weight loss in spite of a good appetite.

Thyroid Nodules

Thyroid nodules are firm lumps that grow in the thyroid gland. The causes of thyroid nodules are unknown. Most thyroid nodules are not cancerous; in adults, only about 5% of all thyroid nodules are cancerous (see Cancer of the Thyroid, p.851).

If you received radiation therapy to the head or neck as a young person (such as for acne or cancer treatment), your risk of cancer is greater.

Thyroid nodules can be divided into two types based on thyroid scans (see p.847): "cold" nodules, which are not making thyroid hormones, and "hot" nodules, which are.

The majority of nodules are cold and the majority of cold nodules are not cancerous. However, a few cold nodules are cancerous. Hot nodules do not need to be evaluated for cancer since they are virtually never cancerous.

SYMPTOMS

Most thyroid nodules are too small to be noticeable, but your doctor may feel a nodule during a physical examination. Some nodules become painful, and some develop to a size that is large enough to make swallowing difficult.

TREATMENT OPTIONS

Most thyroid nodules are discovered by doctors during routine physical examinations and are

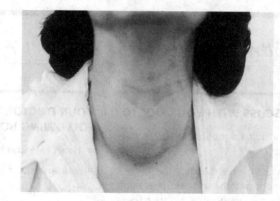

Goiter

A goiter is an enlargement of the thyroid gland, seen here as a balloon-like swelling in the neck.

Goiter

Goiter is a condition in which the thyroid gland becomes enlarged, producing a discernible swelling at the base of the neck. It is usually painless. Although it can appear alarming, most causes of goiter are easily remedied.

Goiter can occur in conditions that cause hyperthyroidism or hypothyroidism—both of which produce their own set of symptoms. A person with a goiter can have normal blood levels of thyroid hormone. In areas of the world where there is a dietary deficiency of iodine, goiters are common.

A goiter can cause symptoms when it presses on structures in the neck. Symptoms are directly related to the size of the goiter. In rare cases, large goiters can interfere with swallowing or breathing by pushing on the esophagus or trachea. Treatment varies depending on the cause.

harmless. To determine whether or not the nodule is cancerous, your physician will perform diagnostic tests to rule out cancer. Usually, a blood test to check your level of TSH and a fine-needle aspiration biopsy (see p.847) are performed first.

Small noncancerous nodules require no treatment. For large cysts, your doctor may extract the fluid with a syringe to collapse the sac. Cancerous nodules require removal of the thyroid gland. A noncancerous nodule that is producing excessive thyroid hormone

and causing hyperthyroidism (see p.844) is usually treated with radioactive iodine (see p.846) and, less often, with surgery.

Thyroiditis

Thyroiditis, or inflammation of the thyroid, can be caused by a variety of conditions. The most common kind of thyroiditis is an autoimmune disease (see p.870) called Hashimoto thyroiditis.

In this condition, immune system cells and antibodies attack the cells in the thyroid. In the first few weeks or months of the condition, there may be a temporary period of hyperthyroidism (thyroid overactivity; see p.844), followed by several months of hypothyroidism (thyroid under-activity; see p.848). In some people, the hypothyroidism phase may be permanent.

Thyroiditis after pregnancy is called postpartum thyroiditis. It occurs in 5% of all women and in 25% of women with type 1 diabetes within the first year after delivery.

Another less common condition is subacute thyroiditis, in which the thyroid gland becomes painful and swollen; both hyper-thyroidism and hypothyroidism may occur temporarily. After a few weeks or months, the condition usually goes away. It may be caused by a viral infection of the thyroid gland and usually follows an upper respiratory infection.

SYMPTOMS

The symptoms of thyroiditis vary with the type of thyroiditis, and change over time. Hashimoto thyroiditis usually causes a swelling of the thyroid gland (see Goiter, p.850) that can cause a visible swelling in your neck or, rarely, trouble with swallowing or breathing.

Subacute thyroiditis can cause pain in the thyroid gland that may also be felt around the jaw, ears, or back of the head. Fever and fatigue are also common in subacute thyroiditis. The symptoms usually last for several months and often disappear on their own.

TREATMENT OPTIONS

Consult your doctor if you have discomfort around your thyroid

gland or have the symptoms of either hyperthyroidism or hypothyroidism. After taking your medical history and performing an examination, your doctor may examine your thyroid gland and measure the blood levels of thyroid hormones (see p.846) and of antibodies if Hashimoto thyroiditis is suspected.

Treatment of Hashimoto thyroiditis is the same as for hypo-thyroidism—a lifelong course of thyroid hormone medicine.

Cancer of the Thyroid

Thyroid cancer is caused by the development of malignant cells in the thyroid gland (see p.846). About 11,000 new cases of thyroid cancer occur each year in the United States. Women are affected about three times more often than men, and the disease usually occurs after age 30.

There are several forms of thyroid cancer. The two most common forms—papillary and follicular cancer—have an excellent long-term prognosis (outlook).

Papillary cancers represent about 70% of all thyroid cancers; they often spread to the lymph glands in the neck but usually do not spread beyond that point. Survival rates over 10 years are between 90% and 100%.

Follicular cancers are the second most common type. They are more likely than the papillary form to spread outside the neck. The outlook is largely dependent on how far the cancer has spread when it is first diagnosed.

Medullary cancers affect about 8% of people with thyroid cancer. Medullary cancers start in cells that make the hormone calcitonin. The amount of calcitonin

in the blood is an indicator of the progression of the cancer before and after surgery.

Anaplastic cancers affect 5% of people with thyroid cancer and have a poor prognosis. They are fast growing and highly malignant. These cancers tend to occur in people over age 60.

Lymphomas (see p.727) can occur in the thyroid gland. This is a rare kind of thyroid cancer.

SYMPTOMS

The main feature of thyroid cancer is one or more lumps or nodules (see p.849) in the thyroid gland. In young people, the growth advances slowly. As the nodule grows, it becomes irregularly shaped and hard. Pain is rare.

Other symptoms, such as hoarseness or difficulty swallowing, sometimes occur when the nodule presses against the nerves of the voice box.

TREATMENT OPTIONS

Contact your doctor if you detect a lump in your thyroid gland. Your doctor may recommend a fine-needle aspiration biopsy, in which a delicate needle is guided into the nodule and a tiny piece of tissue is removed for examination under a microscope.

If the results are inconclusive, your doctor may perform an ultrasound (see p.847) of the nodule or a radioactive iodine uptake scan (see p.846).

Thyroid surgery is the treatment of choice for thyroid cancer; some surgeons remove all of the gland (total thyroidectomy) while others remove only part.

When a cancer has not spread outside of the thyroid gland, surgically removing the thyroid offers a complete cure. When papillary or follicular thyroid cancer has or may have spread, radioactive iodine is sometimes given after surgery. Because thyroid cells are the only cells in the body that can retain iodine, malignant cells that have spread anywhere in the body may absorb the radioactive iodine and be killed by it.

PARATHYROID GLAND DISORDERS

Hyperparathyroidism

Hyperparathyroidism is a disorder in which the parathyroid glands (four pea-sized glands located on, but separate from, the thyroid gland) secrete too much parathyroid hormone (PTH). PTH helps keep a healthy balance of calcium and phosphorus in the body.

Overproduction of PTH results in high blood levels of calcium (primarily because PTH causes calcium to leave the bones) and low levels of phosphorus.

Mild forms of hyperparathyroidism are relatively common; more serious forms, which cause major complications, are uncommon.

Hyperparathyroidism occurs more often in people over age 40 and is twice as common among women. The condition is primarily caused by a (usually) noncancerous tumor of one parathyroid gland or, less often, by a general enlargement of all four parathyroid glands.

SYMPTOMS

Some people with mild disease have no symptoms at all. When symptoms appear, they are often very general, such as a feeling of weakness, depression, abdominal pain, or aches and pains. In some people the condition is detected by chance when high levels of calcium are found in the blood during a test for another disorder.

Other people have fractures due to the loss of calcium from the bones (see Osteoporosis, p.596).

More severe disease can cause loss of appetite, increased thirst and urination, vomiting, nausea, constipation, confusion, and impaired memory. The kidneys respond to the overload of calcium in the blood by excreting high quantities of calcium in the urine, which can set the stage for kidney stones (see p.818).

TREATMENT OPTIONS

Your doctor may perform a blood test to measure levels of calcium, phosphorus, and parathyroid hormone; this provides a definitive diagnosis. He or she may refer you to an endocrinologist (hormone specialist) and/or a nephrologist (kidney specialist) for further evaluation and care.

Other tests may include an ultrasound (see p.847) or radioisotope scan (see p.137) of the parathyroid glands to identify which of the four parathyroid glands has a tumor, or whether all of the glands are enlarged. If surgery is necessary, this information will help the surgeon.

Some people require only periodic monitoring of their kidneys (to ensure that kidney stones are not developing) and bone scans to monitor bone loss.

If there is a tumor or overall enlargement of the parathyroid glands, surgery may be recom-

mended. If too much of one of the glands is removed, you could lack enough parathyroid hormone to keep calcium levels adequate (see Hypoparathyroidism, right). In this case you will require calcium and vitamin D supplements to increase the absorption of calcium for the rest of your life.

Hypoparathyroidism

Hypoparathyroidism is a rare disease in which the parathyroid glands, which regulate the body's use of calcium, do not produce enough parathyroid hormone.

Without enough of the hormone, the level of calcium in your bloodstream is reduced below normal levels and the amount of phosphorus increases.

Children can be born with hypoparathyroidism or the condition can occur without apparent cause.

More often it occurs when the parathyroid glands (four pea-sized glands that are located on the back of the thyroid gland) are accidentally removed during surgery on the thyroid glands or surgery for hyperparathyroidism (see left).

The primary symptoms are painful spasms in the hands, arms, feet, and throat—a condition called tetany. Other symptoms include numbness and tingling in the hands or face, thin hair, vaginal yeast infections (see p.1067), dry skin, and oral thrush (see p.488).

If you have symptoms of hypoparathyroidism, your doctor will perform a blood test to measure parathyroid hormone. Immediate relief of tetany is achieved by injections of calcium. Lifelong use of calcium supplements, with vitamin D to increase absorption, completely eliminates the symptoms.

Your doctor will periodically monitor the amount of calcium in your bloodstream to ensure that you have normal levels.

METABOLIC DISORDERS

Overweight and Obesity

The terms "overweight," "obesity," and "morbid obesity" refer to a weight (in relation to your height) that is in an unhealthy range, increasing your risk of developing a number of serious, chronic diseases and of premature death. The risk of many diseases is greater the heavier you are within these three categories. Nearly half of all people in the United States are overweight or obese. To see if you fall into one of these categories, see Determining Your Body Mass Index, p.51.

Being overweight is the result of an imbalance in the amount of calories taken in and the amount of energy expended; people gain weight when more calories are taken in than are used up by the body.

Your body is constantly using energy, even when you are asleep. Intensive physical exertion increases the amount of energy being used.

CAUSES OF BEING OVERWEIGHT

Why are some people overweight? The honest answer is that scientists are just beginning to figure it out. For many years, people believed that being overweight was generally a failure of willpower—you did not have the discipline to exercise, keep from overeating, or both.

Today, it appears that other physical factors may play an important role in determining body weight. In animals and in humans, genes have been discovered that influence appetite and the efficiency with which the body uses energy. It is currently unclear how many people who are overweight have these physi-

Obesity Genes

The best-known obesity gene (the *ob* gene) was discovered in 1994; this gene makes a hormone called "leptin" (from the Greek leptos, which means "thin"). Leptin is made in the body's fat cells when the cells start to swell with fat after a meal. Leptin then travels in the blood to the brain and signals the appetite center to stop feeling hungry.

Leptin also causes the brain to tell cells to burn more energy. Basically, leptin sends a message saying: "You have eaten enough. Now burn what you have eaten." Conversely, when leptin is at low levels (many hours after a meal), its absence sends the opposite message to the brain: "Eat something. Do not burn much energy until you have new food in you."

For leptin's message to be heard by the brain, certain brain cells need a chemical on their surface called a leptin receptor. The leptin in the blood attaches to this receptor, which is the necessary first step for leptin to send its messages to the cells in the appetite center.

A true deficiency of leptin seems to be a rare cause of obesity in humans. However, defects in the leptin receptor and the other chemicals that participate in sending leptin's message to the cells of the appetite center may play a more important role in human obesity.

Some scientists are optimistic that the discovery of the *ob* gene and other recently discovered obesity genes will lead to fundamental breakthroughs in treating obesity. Perhaps in the same way that taking insulin keeps diabetes under control, treatments for obesity will make up for defective obesity genes and help people lose weight—and keep it off—without serious side effects.

Diet Pills

■ **Dextroamphetamine and methamphetamine** are no longer used as diet pills because they do not promote lasting weight loss, can cause serious side effects, and can cause addiction.

■ **Phentermine** can cause a suppression of appetite, but it is not yet clear if long-term use is safe.

■ **Sibutramine** can cause a suppression of appetite, but it is not yet clear if long-term use is safe.

■ **Orlistat** decreases the absorption of fat (and, hence, calories), but frequently causes more frequent, fatty bowel movements and intestinal gas. Its long-term safety is not clear.

■ **Fenfluramine and dexfenfluramine** causes long-lasting suppression of appetite but also serious side effects (damage to the heart valves and to the arteries in the lungs). They have been taken off the market.

■ **"Herbal phen-fen"** is a combination of herbs containing a potentially dangerous chemical (ephedrine). It has not been proven to be effective.

cal causes, and in how many willpower is the main problem.

Surely, willpower remains important. The way you live your life—the types of foods you eat and the amount of exercise you get—also plays a strong role in determining your weight.

Psychological factors also may affect eating habits. Many people eat in response to emotions such as boredom, sadness, or anger. Binge eating is a factor in about 30% of people who seek help for their weight problem.

CONSEQUENCES OF OBESITY

Whether it has physical or psychological causes, obesity greatly increases your risk of several long-term diseases and early death.

People who are 40% overweight are twice as likely to die prematurely as the average person. Being overweight greatly

raises your risk of getting type 2 diabetes (see p.833). It also raises your risk of developing heart disease (see p.652), high blood pressure (see p.644), and stroke (see p.342). It is also associated with higher rates of certain types of cancer.

Overweight men are more likely to die of cancer of the prostate (see p.1101). Overweight women are more likely to die of cancer of the breast (see p.1054)

and uterus (see Cancer of the Endometrium, p.1071).

Overweight men and women are more likely to develop colon and rectal cancer (see p.791), gallbladder disease and gallstones (see p.770), osteoarthritis (see p.605), and gout (see p.604).

The risks of being overweight are also strongly linked with the distribution of fat on the body. Women typically accumulate fat in their hips and buttocks, giving their figures a pearlike shape. Men usually collect fat around their abdomens, giving them more of an applelike shape. Men or women whose fat is concentrated mostly in the abdomen are more likely to develop many of the health problems associated with obesity. Doctors have developed a simple way to measure whether someone has an apple or pear shape. The measurement is called waist-to-hip ratio (see "Apples" and "Pears," p.48).

The emotional and psychological suffering that can accompany obesity can be significant, especially in a culture that strongly equates being slim with being attractive. People who are obese often experience prejudice and job discrimination. Feelings of

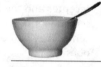

Home Remedies for Weight Loss

Some people find that filling the stomach with a nearly calorie-free food diminishes the appetite and helps with weight loss. One such food is gelatin, which does not contain sugar but may contain flavoring. Dissolving a packet of gelatin in water, stirring it thoroughly, and drinking it 2 to 3 hours after a meal seems to reduce appetite (for the next meal) in some people. This can be done two to three times a day. This home remedy has never been studied scientifically.

How to Evaluate a Commercial Weight-Loss Program

Fad diets and weight-loss programs promising rapid and dramatic results are prevalent but not effective. To be effective, the weight-loss program should meet the following criteria:

Safety Make sure the foods include all of the Recommended Daily Allowances (RDAs) for vitamins, minerals, and protein. The weight-loss diet should be low in calories (energy) only, not in essential foodstuffs.

Slow and steady weight loss Expect to lose only about 1 or 2 pounds a week. Be patient. For you to lose 1 pound of fat you need to burn up (or not take in) 3,500 calories. In order to lose just 1 pound per week, therefore, you need to burn up (or not take in) 500 calories every day.

Doctor approved If you plan to lose more than 20 pounds, if you have other health problems, or if you are taking any medicines, talk to your doctor first. He or she can help you evaluate a program and tailor it to your needs. Always consult your doctor before using any type of liquid formula diet; they can be dangerous.

Maintenance program All good diets should include a maintenance program that helps you keep the weight off. This program should include behavior modification, physical activity, and a reasonable and nutritious dietary plan.

No hidden costs Any commercial weight-loss program should willingly provide a detailed statement of the fees and costs of all services and items, such as dietary supplements or required purchase of foods.

oughly investigate programs that promise instant or dramatic weight loss (see How to Evaluate a Commercial Weight-Loss Program, left).

Very low calorie (fewer than 800 calories a day) diets can help you lose weight but should be attempted only under a doctor's supervision. They can cause imbalances in your body's levels of potassium and other minerals and can cause serious health problems.

Some medicines help diminish appetite (see Diet Pills, p.854). All currently available medicines have only a modest impact; when added to diet and exercise, they can increase the amount of weight you can lose by an additional 5% to 10%.

However, all have side effects, none has been proven safe when used for a year or more, and some have proved so unsafe that they are either no longer prescribed to help weight loss or they have been taken off the market.

In morbidly obese people who have been unable to lose enough weight with any conventional treatment, surgery on the stomach and intestines is sometimes performed to diminish the amount of nutrients and calories that are absorbed. Surgery leads to long-term weight loss but about 1 person of 100 dies from the surgery. Others develop anemia (see p.713) and vitamin and mineral deficiencies, which can usually be corrected with treatment. Some people may feel weak and light-headed and have loose bowel movements after most meals.

rejection, shame, and isolation are common.

TREATMENT OPTIONS

Treatment usually includes a combination of diet, exercise, behavior modification, and sometimes medicine. In severe cases, surgery is used. But the mainstay is diet and exercise.

To lose weight, you must consume less than your body needs for energy. Generally, to lose weight, you should eat between 500 and 1,000 calories less each day than you normally would need for your height and age. Your doctor or a dietitian can help you design a nutritious diet that is low in fat and sugar.

Exercise is also an essential component of a weight-loss program. The most effective calorie-burning form of exercise is aerobic, such as jogging, fast walking, or singles tennis.

Some people benefit from psychological counseling to help cope with the emotional aspects of obesity. Obesity is a chronic condition and weight control must be considered a lifelong effort.

To be safe and effective, any weight-loss program must take the long-term approach. Thor-

ADRENAL GLAND DISORDERS

Addison Disease

Addison disease is a rare hormonal disorder that occurs when the adrenal glands do not make enough of the hormones cortisol and aldosterone. Most cases of Addison disease are caused by an autoimmune disease (see p.870), in which the immune system produces antibodies that attack and destroy the outer layer (cortex) of the adrenal glands, reducing hormone production.

Some cases are caused by cancers that spread (metastasize) to the adrenal glands from other parts of the body, such as the lungs or breasts. Other cases are caused by infections, such as tuberculosis (see p.504), which can affect the adrenal glands.

In rare cases, failure of the pituitary gland to produce the hormone adrenocorticotropic hormone (ACTH) (see p.830)—the hormone that tells the adrenal glands to make cortisol—can cause a dangerous underproduction of cortisol. This is not Addison disease, since the adrenal glands are healthy but are not getting adequate stimulation because the pituitary gland is malfunctioning.

SYMPTOMS

The symptoms of Addison disease develop gradually. You may feel tired and weak and may lose your appetite. Weight loss, nausea, diarrhea, and vomiting are common; dizziness or fainting caused by reduced blood pressure may also occur. Your skin may darken because of increased production by the pituitary gland of the hormone that stimulates the production of skin pigment (melanin). You may also become irritable and depressed, have irregular menstrual periods, and have symptoms of low blood sugar (see Hypoglycemia, p.843).

A stressful event such as an injury or infection can trigger an addisonian crisis, which is characterized by nausea, vomiting, abdominal pain, dehydration, low blood pressure, disorientation, and loss of consciousness.

The crisis occurs because the adrenal glands, which normally increase their production of hormones during times of stress, cannot produce the hormones. An addisonian crisis can be life-threatening.

TREATMENT OPTIONS

If you suspect that you have Addison disease, see your doctor, who will arrange for an adrenocorticotropic hormone (ACTH) stimulation test. ACTH is produced by the pituitary gland and triggers the adrenal glands to release their hormones. If your adrenal glands do not respond to the ACTH injection by making adrenal hormones, the diagnosis is confirmed.

Treatment involves taking replacement hormones in the form of corticosteroid drugs (see p.895). There are two critically important corticosteroids that are deficient in a person with Addison disease (and that need to be replaced): cortisol and aldosterone. The medicine most often

Location of the Adrenal Glands

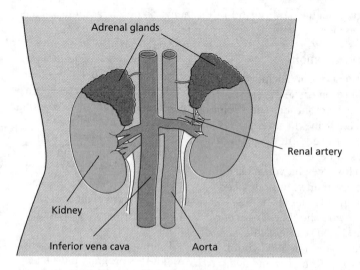

One adrenal gland is located on top of each kidney.

used to replace the missing cortisol is hydrocortisone; fludrocortisone is used to replace the missing aldosterone. Your doctor may also recommend increasing your salt intake.

Whenever you are faced with major stress, such as surgery, you will be given additional, intravenous injections of hydrocortisone, a salty fluid, and glucose. Your doctor will explain to you how to increase your dosage of corticosteroids to maintain your body during times of infection or injury.

All people with Addison disease should wear a medical identification bracelet so that, if they are found unconscious, doctors will know to give them potentially lifesaving corticosteroid treatment.

Aldosteronism

Aldosteronism, also known as hyperaldosteronism, is a condition caused by excess production of aldosterone, a hormone made by the adrenal gland. The surplus causes the body to retain too much salt—which can cause fluid retention and high blood pressure (see p.644)—and too little potassium.

In rare cases, aldosteronism is caused by a tumor or general enlargement of the adrenal gland; this is called primary aldosteronism or Conn syndrome.

More often, aldosteronism is caused by a condition that reduces the flow of blood through the kidneys—such as cirrhosis (see p.765) or heart failure (see p.683). This is called secondary aldosteronism.

SYMPTOMS

The symptoms include high blood pressure (which is caused by a high level of sodium) as well as fatigue and muscle weakness (which is caused by a low level of potassium).

TREATMENT OPTIONS

Report your symptoms to your doctor, who will perform tests to measure levels of sodium and potassium in your blood and urine. If primary aldosteronism is suspected, you will have repeated blood tests of sodium, potassium, aldosterone, and renin (another chemical made by the kidneys), often after altering your diet or taking a pill that can bring out the abnormality.

Your doctor may also arrange for you to have computed tomography (see p.149) to determine if a tumor of the adrenal glands is causing the condition; if there is a tumor, it will be removed.

Treatment for secondary aldosteronism involves restricting your salt intake and increasing foods that are rich in potassium. You will also take the diuretic medicine spironolactone, which interferes with the effect of aldosterone on your kidneys, leading to increased excretion of sodium, decreased excretion of potassium, and, consequently, lower blood pressure.

Cushing Syndrome and Cushing Disease

Cushing syndrome is a rare condition in which there is too much cortisol, the stress hormone, in your blood. Many people develop Cushing syndrome as a result of taking cortisol-like corti-

costeroid drugs (see p.895) for long periods. In healthy people, the adrenal glands produce cortisol in appropriate amounts.

Occasionally, Cushing syndrome is caused by a tumor somewhere in the body that makes adrenocorticotropic hormone (ACTH), a hormone that travels to the adrenal glands and stimulates them to make cortisol.

When the tumor producing ACTH is in the pituitary gland, the disorder is called Cushing disease.

SYMPTOMS

The characteristic symptoms of Cushing syndrome and Cushing disease include a change in body shape and facial features. The upper body accumulates fat (sometimes between the shoulder blades) but the arms and legs become thin because of muscle wasting. The face also accumulates fat and becomes round and red. Skin may be thin and easily bruised, and purple stretch marks may develop on the abdomen, breasts, and thighs.

Women often have excess hair (see Hirsutism, p.558) and men have reduced sexual desire (see Impotence, p.1092). The bones become thin from osteoporosis (see p.596) and are subject to fracture. Fatigue, weak muscles, high blood pressure, and high blood sugar are common. You may also feel irritable, depressed, and anxious.

TREATMENT OPTIONS

Treatment depends on the underlying cause. If your condition is caused by long-term use of corticosteroid drugs, your doctor will slowly reduce your dosage.

Never change your dosage of corticosteroids without consulting your doctor first; if you reduce the dosage below what the body needs, it can cause an addisonian crisis, which can be life-threatening.

Other causes are based on your symptoms and on laboratory tests. Your primary care doctor or a consulting endocrinologist may start with a dexamethasone suppression test. Here is how the test works. Normally, the hypothalamus in the brain makes a hormone called corticotropin-releasing hormone (CRH), which causes the pituitary gland in the brain to release adrenocorticotropic hormone (ACTH). ACTH causes the adrenal glands to make cortisol. This cascade is controlled by negative feedback (see p.829).

For the test, you take a cortisol-like medicine called dexamethasone at night. If you do not have Cushing syndrome, the dexamethasone will, through negative feedback, cause the hypothalamus to produce less CRH, the pituitary gland to produce less ACTH, and the adrenal glands to produce less cortisol. Therefore, the next morning, cortisol levels in your blood will be low.

If you have Cushing syndrome caused by a tumor (in the pituitary gland or in another organ such as a lung) that is making ACTH, the tumor will continue to make ACTH. In the morning, your blood levels of ACTH and cortisol will be high because the tumors do not respond to the negative feedback of dexamethasone; they continue to make ACTH.

If you have a tumor in an adrenal gland that is causing the gland to make too much cortisol, the level of cortisol in the blood will be high but the level of ACTH will be low. This is because the hypothalamus and pituitary gland are responding normally to negative feedback.

If it is established that you have Cushing syndrome that may be due to a tumor, your doctor may take pictures of your pituitary gland, chest, adrenal glands, and other parts of your body using chest x-rays (see p.145), magnetic resonance imaging (see p.150), and computed tomography (see p.149).

If you have a pituitary gland tumor, it will be removed; sometimes radiation therapy (see p.741) is given afterward. If you have a tumor of the adrenal gland, your doctor will also recommend surgery to remove it. If both adrenal glands must be removed, you will need corticosteroid drugs to replace the hormones that your body can no longer produce.

Pheochromocytoma

Pheochromocytoma is a rare type of tumor of the adrenal gland that produces excess adrenaline. The tumor usually starts in the adrenal medulla (the central part of the adrenal gland), which produces adrenaline. In rare cases, the tumor is located in another part of the body.

Your body needs adrenaline to respond to stress (see Fight or Flight Response, p.89) and to maintain healthy blood pressure. When a pheochromocytoma produces too much adrenaline, however, it causes a dangerous rise in blood pressure.

The symptoms of this tumor include sweating, headache, and feeling extremely anxious. You may also have a rapid heartbeat, tremors, nausea (sometimes with vomiting), and weight loss.

Your doctor may perform a urine test to look for the presence of epinephrine, norepinephrine, and dopamine—all forms of adrenaline. He or she may test your blood for higher-than-normal levels of adrenaline; x-rays of the adrenal glands may also be performed.

If you have a tumor, it will need to be removed. This can be accomplished using a laparoscope (see p.142), which minimizes risk.

PITUITARY GLAND DISORDERS

Acromegaly and Gigantism

Acromegaly is a rare condition in which the pituitary gland secretes too much growth hormone, usually as a result of a noncancerous tumor. It results in abnormal growth of the feet, hands, skull, and jaw.

If the tumor develops in a child before about age 10 (which is very rare), it causes overall increased growth. This is called gigantism. Affected children can grow to enormous proportions, some up to 8 feet tall.

Because the internal organs also enlarge, acromegaly and gigantism can cause serious complications, including diabetes (see p.832), high blood pressure (see p.644), heart disease, polyps of the colon, and arthritis. If the pituitary tumor presses on the nerves of the eye, it can cause blindness.

People with acromegaly may first notice that their hands and feet grow large, and that they have soft swellings on their extremities. Later, the condition is distinguished by an enlarging head, hands, and feet. The jaw becomes more prominent, and the voice may deepen.

See your doctor if you have symptoms. He or she will measure the amounts of growth hormone (or another chemical—called somatomedin C, or insulin-like growth factor I—made in the liver in response to growth hormone) in your blood both before and after you take in glucose.

Glucose normally acts by negative feedback (see p.829) to lower growth hormone levels. If glucose does not reduce the amount of growth hormone in the blood, your doctor will suspect that a pituitary gland tumor is releasing large amounts of the hormone (since tumors do not respond to negative feedback signals).

Magnetic resonance imaging (see p.151) and computed tomography (see p.149) can show the tumor, which will be removed by surgery or radiation (see p.741).

If surgery or radiation therapy is not entirely successful, you may need to take medicine to suppress growth hormone production. If the pituitary gland is damaged by surgery or the radiation treatment, you may need to take treatments such as thyroid hormone, sex hormones, and corticosteroids for the rest of your life.

Diabetes Insipidus

Diabetes insipidus is a rare disorder characterized by persistent thirst and frequent and copious urination. The condition is caused by a deficiency of antidiuretic hormone (ADH). ADH is produced in the part of the brain called the hypothalamus and then travels to the pituitary gland, where it is stored and released.

ADH causes the kidneys to retain water. When deficient amounts of ADH are circulating, the kidneys create more urine than they should, and the body becomes dehydrated. Thus, as in diabetes mellitus (see p.832), one feature of diabetes insipidus is excessive urination, which leads to excessive thirst. But the cause of the excessive urination in diabetes insipidus is completely different from the cause in diabetes mellitus.

Most often, diabetes insipidus results from an abnormality (of unknown cause) of the hypothalamus. Occasionally, damage to the pituitary gland—due to injury, a tumor, or surgery—is responsible.

In a small number of people, the hypothalamus and pituitary gland are normal, but the kidneys fail to respond to healthy levels of ADH. This is called nephrogenic diabetes insipidus; it is sometimes present at birth. Sometimes it begins later in life as the result of a disease or disorder that causes kidney damage, or as a result of taking certain medicines, such as lithium, which is used to treat bipolar disorder.

SYMPTOMS

Tremendous thirst and passing enormous quantities of urine (up to 40 pints a day if you continue to take in liquids) are the chief symptoms; some people must urinate every half hour. Infants may wake in the night to drink, or may drink from bath water or even puddles. Older children may wet the bed. Lack of adequate fluid intake results in progressive dehydration and, unless corrected, can lead to coma and death.

TREATMENT OPTIONS

Based on symptoms, your physician will perform blood tests and a water deprivation test. In this

Location of the Pituitary Gland

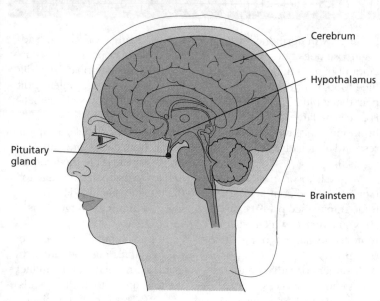

Cerebrum

Hypothalamus

Pituitary gland

Brainstem

The pea-sized pituitary gland, which is controlled by the hypothalamus, is located at the base of the brain.

test, you do not drink anything for several hours. The healthy response to being deprived of water for several hours is for your pituitary gland to release ADH, causing your kidneys to conserve water (so that you do not become dehydrated). Urine is therefore very concentrated.

If you have diabetes insipidus, however, water deprivation will not cause high blood levels of ADH, and you will continue to pass large amounts of dilute urine despite the lack of fluid intake.

If your condition is due to a tumor of the pituitary gland, you may need surgery or radiation therapy. Most people require lifelong treatment with ADH (taken as the drug desmopressin via nasal spray or injection). However, some people whose pituitary gland has been damaged by

injury or through surgery find that normal function returns within a year. People with nephrogenic diabetes insipidus must limit salt intake and take thiazide diuretics to help retain water.

Hypopituitarism

Hypopituitarism occurs when the front lobe of the pituitary gland does not make enough of one or more of the six pituitary hormones it produces. Since all of these pituitary hormones are essential for physical growth, sexual maturation, and many vital functions, hypopituitarism can have serious and even fatal consequences.

In children, it can stunt growth and prevent sexual maturation. In adults, it can cause hypothyroidism (see p.848), low levels of

adrenal steroids such as cortisol and aldosterone, and failure of sexual function and the ability to have children.

The symptoms reflect the combined deficiencies of thyroid, adrenal, and sex hormones: fatigue, weakness, dizziness, intolerance to cold, absent menstrual periods, loss of sexual drive, and impotence.

Hypopituitarism can be present at birth, but more often is caused by a tumor of the pituitary gland (see next article) or by treatment of the tumor, inflammation of the pituitary gland, a head injury, or oxygen deprivation at birth.

Blood and urine tests can usually confirm the diagnosis of hypopituitarism. To find out whether a tumor of the pituitary gland is the cause, computed tomography (see p.149) or magnetic resonance imaging (see p.151) of your pituitary gland are often performed.

Treatment involves lifelong oral medicines or injections to replace the hormones that are not being produced.

Pituitary Tumors

Pituitary tumors are very common growths of the pituitary gland; they are usually located on the front (anterior) lobe.

There are two types: adenomas and craniopharyngiomas. Adenomas are benign (noncancerous) tumors. The most common form is a prolactinoma, which secretes excessive amounts of the pituitary hormone prolactin. In rare cases, these tumors secrete other hormones.

Craniopharyngiomas never secrete hormones but can grow

very large and press on the front or rear lobe of the pituitary.

Pituitary tumors, most of which are tiny, occur in up to 25% of older people in the United States. However, only about 1 of 10,000 people has tumors that cause medical problems.

SYMPTOMS

Small tumors that produce large amounts of the hormone prolactin cause absence of menstrual periods and infertility that can be treated. The tumors also cause production of breast milk in the absence of pregnancy and childbirth in women and impotence in men.

Pituitary tumors that produce other hormones can cause Cushing disease (see p.857), or acromegaly and gigantism (see p.859).

When pituitary tumors are large, they can press on surrounding nerves, causing vision problems and headache. A large craniopharyngioma, because it can destroy much of the hormone production in the pituitary gland, can cause hypopituitarism (see p.860) or diabetes insipidus (see p.859).

TREATMENT OPTIONS

Consult your physician if you have any symptoms suggesting a pituitary tumor. He or she will conduct blood and urine tests to measure levels of pituitary hormones or other hormones. If you have a high level of prolactin, your doctor may want to rule out other potential causes of high prolactin levels, such as various prescription drugs that can raise prolactin levels (including dopamine, haloperidol, metoclopramide, and trifluoperazine).

If your doctor suspects a tumor, you will have magnetic resonance imaging or computed tomography (see p.149) of the brain to identify the size and location of the tumor.

Once diagnosed, prolactinomas can often be treated with the medicines bromocriptine or cabergoline, which lower blood levels of prolactin.

For other tumors, surgery is the most common treatment, and can sometimes be performed via a small incision through the inside of the nose. A portion of the pituitary gland is inevitably removed with the tumor; sometimes, virtually all of the gland is destroyed during surgery. In this case, you will need to take medicines that restore the thyroid, adrenal, and sex hormones that will not be produced naturally because of the injury to the pituitary gland.

Sometimes, radiation therapy can successfully destroy the tumor. The radiation can come from a machine that sends a beam of radiation through the head (to focus on the tumor) or from placing a small radioactive implant into the tumor (this requires minor surgery but delivers the radiation directly to the tumor). Although radiation treatments can often preserve the normal function of the pituitary gland initially, the function often deteriorates with time.

SUPERHORMONES

There has been considerable interest in several "superhormones," to which extraordinary powers have been attributed. In general, these claims are not supported by solid scientific evidence, at least at this time. The current state of knowledge is briefly summarized here.

Growth Hormone

Growth hormone (GH) is produced by the pituitary gland. GH levels are low in childhood but rise dramatically during puberty, falling again as you enter your 30s.

Growth hormone is approved for use in people who cannot make enough of the hormone because of a disease of the pituitary gland. It is also approved to help people with AIDS fight loss of muscle. It is being studied in various other conditions, but has not yet proved to be useful.

Studies have shown that GH can improve muscle strength in older men but does not improve functional capacity or well-being.

More study is needed to identify which people are deficient in GH, whether they would benefit from treatment, and whether there would be risks over the long term. People with naturally high levels of growth hormone in their blood may be at a greater risk for certain cancers.

DHEA

DHEA (dehydroepiandrosterone) is a steroid hormone manufactured by the adrenal glands. Little is known about its role in health or disease, but low levels have been tentatively linked to an increased risk of heart disease in people over 50. In a few very small studies, men reported an increase in well-being and increases in muscle mass and strength after taking DHEA pills.

DHEA may improve survival if given to people with shock (see p.645) or severe infection. One study found that DHEA helped men fight serious infections. However, claims that DHEA can improve memory, boost the function of the immune system, treat diabetes, and reverse Alzheimer disease are unproven.

Although DHEA is available without a prescription and is heavily promoted, few doctors recommend it for people of any age.

Because DHEA is classified as a dietary supplement rather than a drug, the Food and Drug Administration does not regulate how it is made. As a result, there are no standards for quality, purity, or dosage, and its safety cannot be guaranteed.

Melatonin

Melatonin is manufactured by the pineal gland in the brain and is released at night to regulate the timing of the body's sleep-wake cycle. Melatonin levels decline as you age and virtually disappear by old age, possibly explaining why insomnia becomes more common with age.

While there is some preliminary evidence that melatonin can improve the quality of sleep in older people, broad claims that the hormone has antiaging effects are unproven. More investigation is needed to see whether melatonin has any beneficial effect on health.

Limited, cautious use of melatonin to treat insomnia or jet lag is reasonable with the understanding that safe dosage, possible benefits, and potential side effects have not been established. Ask your physician for further advice.

Because melatonin is classified as a dietary supplement rather than a drug, the Food and Drug Administration does not regulate how it is made. As a result, there are no standards for quality, purity, or dosage, and its safety cannot be guaranteed. This raises the possibility that contaminants could be present in the preparations of melatonin available.

In the 1990s, L-tryptophan, another substance used to aid sleep and available without prescription, contained impurities that caused a severe illness called eosinophilia-myalgia syndrome.

Infections and Immune System Diseases

From the moment of birth, we are exposed to a world teeming with a variety of microorganisms (such as bacteria and viruses) and natural and man-made chemicals that can injure us. To survive, the healthy human body comes equipped with a tireless, intricate defense system—the immune system.

The immune system attacks and eliminates most foreign microorganisms and substances that enter your body in a process called the immune response. However, the immune system must first distinguish the invader that it considers to be foreign from the cells and chemicals that make up your own body.

You want your immune system to wage war against what is foreign—not against yourself (see Autoimmune Diseases, p.870). Virtually every cell in your body has markers that identify it as being a part of you, and not something foreign. Early in life, the immune system learns how to recognize these markers of "self."

Throughout your life, your immune system generally succeeds in ridding you of invaders

Lymphatic System

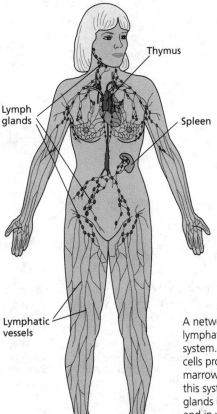

Thymus

Lymph glands

Spleen

Lymphatic vessels

A network of lymph glands (nodes) and lymphatic vessels makes up the lymphatic system. Infection-fighting white blood cells produced by the spleen, bone marrow, and thymus circulate through this system. You can feel your lymph glands in the front and back of your neck and in your armpits and groin, especially if the glands are swollen when you have an infection. There are also many lymph nodes deep inside the body.

and keeping you healthy. However, sometimes it fails, either because the invader overwhelms the immune system or because the war waged by the immune system injures your own tissues as well as attacking and killing the invaders.

What Happens When You Have an Infection?

Microorganisms, commonly called germs, are mindless creatures that have been programmed by nature to do two things—stay alive and reproduce. To accomplish this, they need your body, which is full of nutrition in the form of sugars and other nutrients. Microorganisms can make you very sick—even kill you—as they work at staying alive and reproducing.

STEP 1: ENTERING THE BODY

In order to start an infection, a microorganism must first enter the body. The skin is a strong physical barrier against germs, but they can easily get through if the skin is broken.

Some infections occur when insects penetrate the skin, which permits the germs they are carrying (or those already present on the skin) access to the body. Many microorganisms exist in air; they enter your body when you inhale, though nose hairs help filter out some of them.

Cells on the lining of your throat, windpipe, and bronchial tubes serve as sentries and help trap germs that manage to get past the mouth or nose; these germs are then expelled through coughing or sneezing.

Some germs try to enter through your eyes and are

How Organisms Multiply

Some infectious organisms quietly take up residence in your body and cause no trouble; some even help you, such as bacteria that live in your intestines and help make proteins your body needs. However, some infectious organisms cause symptoms whenever they enter your body, because the immune system immediately attacks them (it is the immune system's attack that causes most symptoms).

In general, the greater the number of organisms, the harder it is for your body to eliminate them, and the sicker you are. It becomes a war, and the number of organisms relative to the number of immune system white blood cells becomes critical in determining the outcome.

If immune system defenses are temporarily weakened, millions of microorganisms can quickly establish a beachhead in their war against the body. That war is going on in your body, to some degree, every minute of every day. The good news is that your immune system cells are usually winning.

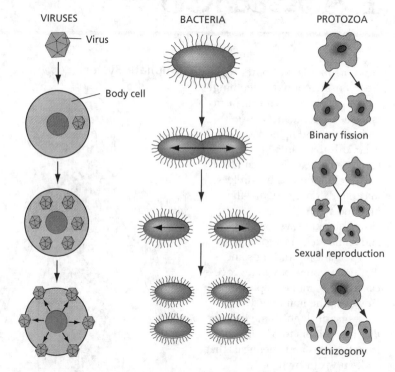

VIRUSES — Virus — Body cell

BACTERIA

PROTOZOA — Binary fission — Sexual reproduction — Schizogony

Viruses can multiply only if they enter your body cells. Once inside your cells, they take over the energy and "machinery" present inside the cell to make thousands of copies of themselves. Often the cell dies as a result.

Bacteria multiply by dividing, and dividing again (and so on). Many common bacteria divide about every 25 minutes. This means that one bacterium can become more than 1 million bacteria in about 8 hours.

Protozoa multiply in a variety of ways. Some divide, like bacteria. Others produce male and female forms. Still others produce small, less mature organisms that can develop into larger adult forms. Some protozoa go through a stage in which they must live inside cells, as parasites, in order to survive.

washed away by tears. Others live in your food or water and enter your body through the mouth, gaining access to the stomach. Your stomach produces acids that kill most infectious microbes. The intestines contain permanent colonies of helpful bacteria that kill invading and potentially harmful germs.

Some microorganisms enter the penis or the vagina during sexual intercourse. The vagina maintains an acidic environment that kills many germs and, like the intestines, contains colonies of helpful bacteria that fight invading germs.

STEP 2: ATTACHING TO YOUR TISSUES

On the unusual occasion when an invader gets past all of the barriers and enters the body, it next must attach itself to your tissues in order to thrive and reproduce. Structures on the surface of the microorganism attach to similar structures on the surface of your cells. These structures, called receptors, serve as "docking stations."

Some microorganisms, such as viruses, can survive only if they take up residence inside the cells. After docking on the surface of the cell, they move through the wall of the cell into its interior.

STEP 3: YOUR IMMUNE SYSTEM REACTS TO THE INVASION

As soon as germs gain entry into the body, the immune system begins to attack them.

The immune system is something like an army. Certain cells serve as commanding officers, issuing orders to start or to stop an attack. They use chemicals called cytokines as signals.

Your Immune System

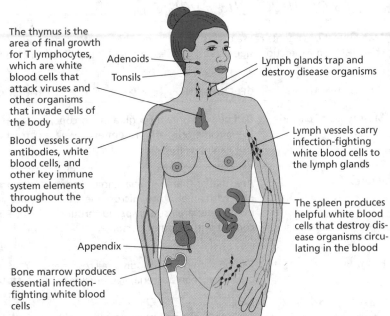

The thymus is the area of final growth for T lymphocytes, which are white blood cells that attack viruses and other organisms that invade cells of the body

Adenoids

Tonsils

Lymph glands trap and destroy disease organisms

Blood vessels carry antibodies, white blood cells, and other key immune system elements throughout the body

Lymph vessels carry infection-fighting white blood cells to the lymph glands

The spleen produces helpful white blood cells that destroy disease organisms circulating in the blood

Appendix

Bone marrow produces essential infection-fighting white blood cells

Many organs play a role in the intricate function of your immune system. The tonsils and adenoids (located in the back of your throat) trap and destroy disease-causing organisms that try to pass through the throat and nasal passages. The appendix also may help kill some organisms, particularly those in your intestines.

Other cells, the troops, take the orders; each troop is assigned a different task. Antigen-presenting cells gobble up a few of the invading germs, chop their proteins into tiny pieces called antigens, and stick the pieces out through their cell walls. The antigens fly like little flags on the cell's surface. It is as if each antigen-presenting cell, flying its flags, is boasting, "I got one." This starts the immune system response.

When other troops (white blood cells called lymphocytes) pass by and see the antigen flags flying on the surface of the antigen-presenting cells, they recognize them as evidence of a foreign invasion, and mobilize to fight that specific invader.

Lymphocytes are found throughout the body—in the lymph glands, spleen, and thymus; in the linings of the throat, lungs, and intestines; and floating in the blood.

There are several classes of lymphocytes. T lymphocytes have several different roles. One kind of T lymphocyte, the kind that is destroyed in people with acquired immunodeficiency syndrome (AIDS), directs the immune response. Other T lymphocytes become memory cells; still others become killer T cells.

Types of Infectious Agents

Many infectious agents cause disease in humans. This chart lists some infectious agents and gives examples of diseases caused by them, as well as the treatment used to eradicate the infectious agent.

INFECTIOUS AGENT	DESCRIPTION	DISEASE	TREATMENT
Most types of bacteria	Can be seen only through a microscope; live outside cells; are present everywhere (for example, in water, food, and air)	Strep throat; urinary tract infections	Antibiotics
Viruses	Are smaller than bacteria; can be seen only with an electron microscope; live inside cells; are usually spread through contact with another person	Common cold; measles; hepatitis; AIDS	Antivirals
Fungi	Can be seen only through a microscope; are larger than bacteria; live outside cells	Yeast vaginitis; histoplasmosis	Antifungals
Chlamydia	Are nearly as small as viruses; live inside cells (like viruses); have some features that are like bacteria	Pelvic infections; pneumonia	Antibiotics
Mycoplasma	Are almost as small as viruses; live outside cells (like bacteria)	Pneumonia	Antibiotics
Rickettsia	Live inside cells (unlike most bacteria)	Rocky Mountain spotted fever; typhus	Antibiotics
Worms	Are small to very large; are passed by contact with contaminated soil, animals, insects, or people; are mainly a health problem in poor, developing countries	Hookworms; filariasis; schistosomiasis	Anthelmintics
Protozoa	Can be seen only through a microscope; are made up of a single cell; are mainly a health problem in poor, developing countries	Malaria; giardiasis	Antiprotozoals
Prions	Are pieces of protein without any nucleic acids (unlike other infectious agents); are passed by eating infected animals (particularly their brains); can cause normally shaped proteins to become deformed, leading to brain cell destruction	Creutzfeldt-Jakob disease; kuru	None

B lymphocytes develop into cells that produce antibodies. Another important kind of lymphocyte is the natural killer cell, which kills in a different way than the killer T cells.

There are two general kinds of immune responses: the development of killer cells and the development of antibodies.

In the first kind of immune response, killer T lymphocytes are mobilized to directly and specifically attack other cells that are infected.

In the second type of response, B lymphocytes make substances called antibodies that specifically lock onto a germ, often immobilizing the germ and allowing it to be destroyed.

One of the many wonders of the immune system is its ability to produce a vast variety of very specific antibodies that are able to lock onto a huge variety of germs.

The killer T cell response protects you most against viral infections. Viruses are hidden inside some of the cells of your body and can survive only if the cell they are living in survives. Killer T cells kill the infected cells and, with them, the viruses they hold.

The antibody response protects you most against bacterial infections, since most bacteria remain exposed outside of your cells. Your body usually actively produces antibodies as a reaction to a new infection.

Antibodies can also be transferred from one person to another. For example, infants (who do not have a fully developed immune system) are protected against many diseases by antibodies from their mother. The mother's body produces these antibodies to protect her from infections to which she was exposed in the past; the antibodies are passed on to protect her baby against the same infections.

Part of the immune response involves the creation of memory cells. These lymphocytes "remember" a past infection and stimulate the immune system to respond even more quickly and aggressively if that same infection recurs.

Many substances in the body play a key role in working with lymphocytes to attack or neutralize foreign microbes. For example, a substance known as complement acts as a kind of sword that punctures the membrane of an infected cell, causing the cell to burst.

Other chemicals help increase the flow of blood (and, hence, the flow of immune system cells) into an infected area. Still others recruit scavenger cells to clean up after the battle is over.

Lymph Glands and Associated Disorders

The lymphatic system is an essential part of your body's ability to fight infection. The lymph glands (nodes) positioned along the lymphatic system act as filters that inhibit the spread of infection. A swollen lymph gland can indicate the presence of infection and also its general location. This chart lists areas where there might be swelling and the disorders that can occur with swelling at that location.

LYMPH GLAND LOCATION	DISORDER
Inside or around the collarbone	Infection of the head or neck; tumor in abdomen or in a breast or lung
Neck or under the jaw	Infection of the mouth; tumor in head or neck; lymphoma
Armpit	Infection of an arm; breast cancer; lymphoma
Groin	Infection of the genital tract or a leg or foot; lymphoma; melanoma; testicular cancer

If the immune system is so efficient, why do people still get infections? Many factors are responsible, including the strength of the infection and the strength of the immune system, and other unknown factors. See How You Fight Viral Infections (p.119) and How You Fight Bacterial Infections (p.118) for illustrations of how the immune system works.

Helping the Immune System Protect Against Infection

ANTIBIOTICS AND OTHER MICROBE-FIGHTING MEDICATIONS

Over the past 50 years, medications have been discovered that kill many types of microorganisms that can cause infections.

First, antibiotics were discovered that could kill bacteria. Subsequently, medications were found that could kill certain viruses, fungi, and other microorganisms and parasites. In developed countries, these advances have diminished the devastation caused by many infectious diseases.

However, these drugs have created their own set of problems. Some produce harmful side effects such as rashes or diarrhea. Also, over time, germs can become resistant to the drugs. One of the most significant causes of this resistance is the overprescribing and overuse of antibiotic and antiviral drugs.

In some countries, people are even permitted to obtain antibiotics without a doctor's prescription. Many minor infections do not require the use of antibiotics; the microorganisms will eventually be conquered by the immune system.

IMMUNIZATIONS

Some infections can be prevented by immunization, a process in which either a part of the microorganism, or a greatly weakened version of it, is introduced into the body. The immune system reacts as if it were being infected with the microorganism, and produces memory cells that are able to recognize certain features of it. When the body is exposed to the microorganism again at a later time, the memory cells respond rapidly and aggressively to eliminate the microorganism before it can establish an infection.

Effective immunizations do not exist for all infections. Those that do exist, however, are among the most valuable tools in medicine. Make certain that each member of your family—adults and children—receives all recommended immunizations.

NEWER APPROACHES TO PREVENTING INFECTIONS

One important approach to some infections is to use a combination of several different drugs, each of

Stress, the Mind, and the Immune System

Your mother or grandmother may have told you that if you let yourself get run down or if you put yourself under too much stress, your immune system would weaken and you could get sick. She was probably right. Studies have shown that stress can make people vulnerable to common, temporary viral infections, like the common cold.

Parts of the immune system (the best-studied examples are natural killer lymphocytes and T lymphocytes) also seem to function less effectively when you are under intense stress. This can occur with the death of a close family member or friend, divorce, job loss, school examinations, anxiety, depression, loneliness, and sleep deprivation.

Whether exhaustion or stress makes a person vulnerable to more serious infections (or to other serious diseases like cancer) is uncertain.

Although scientists are only beginning to understand how it happens, it is clear that the mind can influence the immune system—and vice versa.

The cells of the brain communicate with each other using chemicals called neurotransmitters. Scientists have discovered that the cells of the immune system make and react to neurotransmitters. Likewise, some brain cells make and respond to hormones made by immune system cells. When the immune system is stimulated, electrical activity rises in the hypothalamus (which is located at the base of the brain).

Some studies have found that therapies aimed at reducing stress may boost the functioning of certain immune system cells. However, it has not been proven that this provides significant protection against infections or other diseases. Much exciting research is yet to be done on the connection between the mind and the immune system and on the impact this connection can have on health and disease.

How Vaccines Work

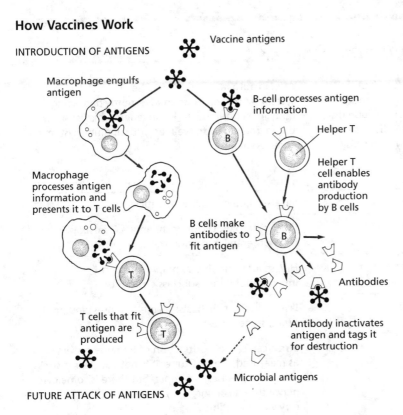

INTRODUCTION OF ANTIGENS

Vaccine antigens

Macrophage engulfs antigen

B-cell processes antigen information

Helper T

Macrophage processes antigen information and presents it to T cells

Helper T cell enables antibody production by B cells

B cells make antibodies to fit antigen

Antibodies

T cells that fit antigen are produced

Antibody inactivates antigen and tags it for destruction

Microbial antigens

FUTURE ATTACK OF ANTIGENS

Vaccines train the immune system to recognize specific viruses or bacteria and to quickly attack them if those viruses or bacteria enter the body in the future. Vaccines usually trigger two major kinds of immune system response: (1) immune system cells (B cells and plasma cells) that make antibodies to molecular pieces of the microorganism (antigens) and (2) immune system cells (T cells) that attack other cells infected by the microorganism.

Sometimes a vaccine consists of live but very weakened microorganisms. More often, antigens from a microorganism are used in the vaccine. Although the antigen itself is a harmless piece of a virus or bacterium, the immune system recognizes it as foreign, and reacts to the antigen as though it was a whole, real virus or bacterium. An attack against the antigen is mounted by white blood cells called macrophages, T cells, and B cells. Certain B cells and T cells "remember" the antigen. If it shows up in the future—this time as part of a real microbe or toxin—the cells eliminate it before it can do any damage.

More recently, new DNA vaccines have been developed. In these vaccines, the DNA gene that instructs the cell to make a particular antigen is injected into your body (instead of the antigen). DNA enters your cells and makes a continuous supply of the antigen. Such DNA vaccines may give longer-lasting immunity and be less expensive.

which injures a germ in a different way. This has proved valuable in treating people with acquired immunodeficiency syndrome (AIDS).

Another experimental approach in treating mild infections (such as most urinary tract infections), as well as serious infections, is to prevent the initial attachment of a microorganism to the body's cells. This strategy is likely to become important in the next decade.

Scientists are also looking at ways to boost the strength of the immune system to fight infection, or to supplement the immune system with manufactured substances (such as antibodies or cytokines), to fight specific infections.

How Your Immune Response Can Harm You

Sometimes while attacking foreign invaders, the immune system also makes the person it is trying to protect feel sicker. A simple example is the common allergy.

The symptoms of an allergy— itchy and runny nose and red and tearing eyes—are not caused directly by the foreign substance (such as pollen) that causes the allergy. Rather, the symptoms are caused by the chemicals used by your immune system to eliminate the pollen.

Another example is "the flu," which occurs when an influenza virus enters the body. The flu virus itself does not damage your tissues or make you feel sick; it is the substances made by your immune system in its battle against the virus that cause you to feel tired and achy and to have a fever.

What Weakens the Immune System?

Several factors can weaken your immune system's ability to perform its normal function of fighting off invading germs or toxins. These factors include diseases you are born with or acquire, medicines you take, and infections of the immune system cells.

Also, in autoimmune diseases (see below), the immune system is "tricked" into inadvertently damaging the body in its attempts to kill invaders. This list shows the factors that can weaken your immune system and gives examples of those factors.

CATEGORY	EXAMPLES
Inherited (congenital) immunodeficiencies	Severe combined immunodeficiency
Medications or treatments	Corticosteroids; cyclophosphamide; azathioprine; chemotherapy; radiation therapy
Illnesses directly affecting the immune system	HIV; severe combined immunodeficiency; immunoglobulin G subclass deficiency
Other systemic illnesses	Liver failure or cirrhosis; severe or long-standing diabetes; some cancers
Stress	Stress can cause malfunction of immune system cells, as measured in a test tube. It is not yet clear if stress can cause diseases in people, but there is some evidence that it can make a person vulnerable to temporary viral infections.
Aging	The possibility of dying of influenza is much higher in the elderly, partly because of impaired immune response and partly because of impaired lung function.

There are more serious examples of damage from your own immune system. In children with bacterial meningitis or in people with lung infections from a parasite called *Pneumocystis carinii,* which is a common infection in people with acquired immunodeficiency syndrome (AIDS), much of the damage to the body comes from the immune system's desperate attempt to kill the invading organism.

Along with drugs that kill the microorganisms, drugs to calm the immune response, such as corticosteroid drugs (see p.895),

are used to improve the outcome of these serious conditions.

Autoimmune Diseases

The body is constantly invaded by substances (such as chemicals or microorganisms) that are foreign—that is, they are not a natural part of the body.

The immune system exists to fight off these foreign invaders. However, sometimes the immune system turns on the very body it normally defends, attacking and injuring normal tissues and causing autoimmune diseases.

Scientists do not yet understand why the immune system malfunctions in this way, but there are two leading theories (both of which may be correct).

The first theory is that a foreign invader, such as a virus, has a chemical structure that is similar to a normal chemical structure on the surface of some of your cells. In attacking the virus, the immune system also inadvertently attacks the structure of your cells, not recognizing that the structure is subtly different.

A second theory maintains that the body's natural tissues

that are attacked by an autoimmune disease are actually infected by invaders, such as viruses, that live inside the cells of the tissue. The immune system sees the invader and attacks it but, at the same time, damages the tissue in which the invader is living.

Sex hormones may play an important role in autoimmune diseases. Women are more often affected by autoimmune diseases. In animals that get autoimmune diseases similar to the diseases that affect people, females are also most often affected. And male animals can become affected when they are given female hormones.

Research into the causes of autoimmune diseases is continuing. Once the causes are determined, more specific treatments for many of these conditions may become available. Until then, the best way to combat these diseases and reduce their effects is with medications such as anti-inflammatory drugs (including nonsteroidal anti-inflammatory drugs and corticosteroids), pain relievers, and drugs that suppress the immune response.

Close monitoring of the condition by your physician, a balance of rest and exercise, and good nutrition may also improve your ability to live with an autoimmune disease.

INFECTIONS

Emerging Infections

Not too long ago, many medical experts believed that all the major infectious diseases of humans were known. While they recognized that we had much more to learn about these diseases, it was thought unlikely that significant new diseases would emerge.

Then came Legionnaires disease, toxic shock syndrome, Lyme disease, and acquired immunodeficiency syndrome (AIDS). It has become clear that, as people of the world become more mobile, diseases that were once isolated to one part of the world are being spread widely.

It also has become clear that there are probably many microorganisms that are still undiscovered, and that were not discoverable until recent technological advances made it possible to find them.

Some experts predict that many diseases not currently considered to be caused by infectious agents—for example, some kinds of arthritis, some diseases of the brain and nervous system, and even atherosclerosis—may indeed be caused by infections.

This proved to be true of stomach ulcers, many of which are now known to be caused by infection with a bacterium (see p.754). It is hard to predict what new infectious diseases will emerge, but most experts agree that there will be more of them.

VIRAL INFECTIONS

Cytomegalovirus Infection

Cytomegalovirus (CMV) is a relative of the herpes virus that causes lip and genital sores, but CMV causes very different symptoms.

Infection with CMV can occur in people of all ages. About 50% of people are permanently infected with the virus. It lives quietly in the body of most healthy people, kept in check by the immune system, causing no symptoms.

When you are first infected with CMV, the symptoms are usually like those of the flu, lasting a few days. Sometimes, CMV causes mononucleosis (see p.877). At other times, it causes no symptoms at all.

After the initial infection, symptoms usually go away; the virus remains in your body for the rest of your life. In healthy people, it causes few symptoms.

When the immune system is weakened, however, such as by organ transplantation or acquired immunodeficiency syndrome (AIDS), the organism begins to multiply. In someone with AIDS, CMV most often affects the colon (causing life-threatening diarrhea) and the retina of the eye (which can ultimately lead to blindness).

However, many other body systems, including the lungs, brain, pancreas, heart, kidneys, and liver, can be affected by CMV.

If you have an active infection, your physician may prescribe the antiviral drug ganciclovir (available as tablets, intravenous infusions, or slow-release pellets inserted in the eye for retinitis) or foscarnet.

HIV and AIDS

The human immunodeficiency virus (HIV) is a type of virus called a retrovirus. It is one of the few viruses that is genuinely new to the human race. The first known human infections occurred in just the past few decades. Even though the virus first began infecting people just a few decades ago, 30 million people worldwide now are infected with HIV, and many have acquired immunodeficiency syndrome (AIDS).

HIV primarily infects white blood cells called CD4 lymphocytes. These cells are critically important in directing the immune system in its battles. They have been called the "generals" that direct an army of other immune system cells.

HIV attaches to a receptor on the outside of the cell, enters the cell, and then uses the cell's energy to multiply. The cell essentially becomes a factory for generating new copies of the virus, and then dies. Thousands of copies of the virus leave the dying cell and go on to infect other cells. These cells are also killed by HIV.

Recognizing that its immune system cells are dying, the body greatly increases its production of the cells, to try to keep up. Without treatment to kill the virus, however, the immune system cells progressively lose the battle against HIV. As the number of CD4 lymphocytes diminishes, susceptibility to infection increases.

HIV usually enters the body during vaginal, anal, or oral intercourse. It is transmitted by direct contact with infected body fluids, including blood (though blood screening has almost completely eliminated transmission by transfusion in the United States), semen, and vaginal secretions; from mother to child in the uterus; or through breast-feeding. It is commonly spread by sharing an infected needle or syringe.

Different body secretions contain varying concentrations of the virus. Generally, the concentrations are highest in semen, blood, and breast milk. They are lower in anal and vaginal fluids and lowest in tears, urine, and saliva. However, under certain circumstances, all can transmit HIV.

Your chance of transmitting or acquiring HIV involves risk factors such as the vulnerability of the tissues exposed to the virus (for example, having another sexually transmitted disease makes you more susceptible to HIV during sexual intercourse with an infected person), the strain of HIV being transmitted, and the length of exposure to the virus.

HIV is more likely to cause infection when it enters the body via certain routes (called routes of transmission). See How Is HIV Transmitted? (below).

There is no evidence that casual touching, kissing, or hugging, or being coughed on by, going to school with, or working with a person who has HIV can spread the virus. You cannot acquire HIV from any insect or by sharing eating utensils, towels, phones, showers, or swimming pools. Items such as toothbrushes and earrings should not be shared because they may be contaminated with blood.

How Is HIV Transmitted?

Unlike many infections, the human immunodeficiency virus (HIV) is not transmitted through the air, by insect bites, or by coughing, sneezing, or other casual contact. HIV can be transmitted by:

- Having unprotected vaginal, anal, or oral sexual intercourse with a person who has the virus.

- Receiving a blood transfusion from a donor who has the virus.

- Sharing needles or syringes with a person who has the virus.

- Exposing an open sore to semen, blood, or vaginal fluids containing the virus.

- Being artificially inseminated with the sperm or semen of a man who has the virus.

- Receiving a puncture wound from a sharp object (such as a needle or scalpel) that is contaminated with the virus.

- Breast-feeding (from an infected woman to the infant).

- Pregnancy (from an infected woman to the fetus).

- Receiving transplanted organs or tissue from a donor who has the virus.

Who Should Get Tested for HIV?

You should be tested for the human immunodeficiency virus (HIV) if you are at particular risk for getting it—for example, if you have had sex without a condom, if you use intravenous drugs and have shared needles with others, or if you are a health worker who has been stuck by a needle that has been used on someone else.

Testing is available from your physician; health clinics; hospitals; and local, state, and federal health departments. You can also perform a test at home (see p.85). Some tests (including the test for HIV that you can take at home) can be taken anonymously; test results will not be placed in a permanent medical record with your name on it.

Some states require that the names of HIV-positive people be reported to health officials. All states require reporting of acquired immunodeficiency syndrome (AIDS) cases to the US Centers for Disease Control and Prevention.

Although discrimination in the workplace and with health insurers is illegal, people who have HIV have experienced discrimination in these and other areas.

The results of two blood tests, considered together, can indicate if you have been infected with HIV. If the result of the enzyme-linked immunosorbent assay (ELISA) is negative, it probably means that you have not been infected. However, it takes an average of 45 days (even as long as 6 months) after you have been infected for the test to show a positive result. If you are concerned that you may have been recently infected (such as through having unprotected sex), the ELISA test may have to be repeated at some future time.

If the ELISA result is positive, it does not mean for certain that you are infected. A second test, the Western blot analysis, is also performed. If that test result is also positive, it means that you are almost certainly infected.

The initial blood test only tells if you have been infected; it cannot determine how serious the infection is. Early diagnosis and treatment offer the best chance for fighting HIV and preventing opportunistic infections. In addition, if you find out you have HIV, take steps to prevent transmitting the disease to others (see How Is HIV Transmitted?, p.872).

Counseling is available before and after testing and is recommended to help you cope with the possibility of being HIV-positive.

EFFECT OF HIV ON THE BODY

HIV, more than any other known microorganism, causes severe damage to the immune system. For this reason, people with HIV become vulnerable to conditions that people with healthy immune systems would fight effectively.

These include opportunistic infections—caused by bacteria, viruses, fungi, and parasites—such as cytomegalovirus (CMV) infection (see p.871) and *Pneumocystis carinii* pneumonia. Various cancers, such as lymphomas (see p.727) and Kaposi sarcoma (see p.547), are also more common in people with HIV.

When the immune system is affected seriously enough—when there are fewer than 200 CD4 cells per microliter (healthy people have more than 800) and when these AIDS-related opportunistic infections and cancers are diagnosed—a person with HIV will develop AIDS.

SYMPTOMS

The symptoms of HIV vary according to the stage of the disease. At the time they are first infected, many people experience fever, fatigue, headaches, muscle pain, and swollen glands. Others have no symptoms. At the time of first infection, there are high levels of the virus in your body, and you can easily spread the infection to someone else.

Treatment with medications against HIV may be particularly important to protect the immune system during this phase of the illness. Symptoms will then go away for months or years, until the immune system has been so weakened that AIDS-related conditions appear.

Oral thrush (a white, curdlike coating on the tongue or mouth caused by a yeast infection; see p.883) is one of the first symptoms that occurs when the immune system has been seriously damaged. Yeast infections may also occur in the vagina.

Preventing HIV and AIDS

Because there is no cure for the human immunodeficiency virus (HIV) infection or acquired immunodeficiency syndrome (AIDS), prevention is essential. Take these steps:

- Always use a latex or polyurethane condom when you have sex.

- Have sex with only one partner whom you know does not have the virus and who has sex only with you.

- Practice safer sex (see p.76).

- Do not use intravenous drugs; if you do, never share needles.

- Get tested if you suspect you may have HIV, to avoid spreading it and to receive early treatment if your test result is positive.

(However, oral thrush and, particularly, vaginal yeast infections are common; they also occur in people who are not infected with HIV.)

You may also have extreme fatigue, headaches, persistent diarrhea, shortness of breath, bruising, night sweats, fever, a dry cough, bleeding from skin growths, pain and numbness in the feet and hands, and swelling of the lymph glands. Mental deterioration and personality changes may occur due to brain infection. The cancer called Kaposi sarcoma may cause purple spots on your skin or on the membranes inside your mouth.

TREATMENT OPTIONS

The blood tests for HIV are described in Who Should Get Tested for HIV? (see p.873). If you have HIV or AIDS, it is vital that you find a physician who is experienced in treating these conditions and that you establish a support system of people who can provide emotional, physical, and spiritual support. See p.1228 of the Appendix for resources.

If you have HIV, other blood tests need to be performed repeatedly to determine how severe the infection is and how successful your treatment is.

The first test (the viral load test) measures the amount of HIV circulating in your blood. The second test (the CD4 count) measures the number of CD4 cells in your blood. It estimates how badly your immune system is affected. The higher the viral load and the lower the CD4 count, the more serious your condition is. Usually, if one test result is bad, so is the other.

Therapy must be individualized and the risks and benefits carefully weighed. As a generalization, highly active, multidrug antiviral treatment is usually given if the CD4 count is less than 200.

Many kinds of treatments are needed for HIV infection:

Antiretroviral therapy involves several drugs (usually given in combination) that limit the ability of HIV to multiply.

The most successful treatments involve taking at least three drugs. Combination therapy can greatly reduce the viral load, increase the CD4 cell count, and improve your prognosis.

Medications to prevent opportunistic infections are needed if your CD4 count is below a certain level.

Vaccination against various microorganisms that can cause opportunistic infections—including hepatitis B, pneumonia, and influenza—is important.

Although there are standards of treatment, drug therapy is often individualized to your personal circumstances. These include your exposure and vulnerability to opportunistic infections, your ability to actively participate in your treatment and comply with the prescribed regimen, whether the virus develops resistance to your medications, and whether you develop side effects.

Over time, HIV can develop a resistance to the drugs, so there is a good chance that you will need to change drugs several times.

A pregnant woman who has an HIV infection can transmit the infection to her fetus. However, if the mother takes antiretroviral drugs and the baby is delivered by cesarean section, it can greatly reduce the chance that the baby will acquire HIV.

If you have HIV, your doctor will explain how to take the drugs and describe their side effects, which are wide-ranging. Managing side effects and the dosage schedule can be a significant challenge. Call your doctor immediately if you have severe side effects or if you stop taking a drug. You will need to see your doctor frequently so that he or she can evaluate your body's response.

Influenza

Influenza (commonly known as "the flu") is a respiratory infection caused by one of the three different types of influenza viruses—A, B, or C. The flu virus enters your body when you breathe in air containing infected droplets, usually generated by someone else's coughing or sneezing. Outbreaks occur nearly every winter, and vary in severity depending on that year's strain of the influenza virus.

If you are like most people, you have had the flu at some point in your life. You may have felt awful for a week or so, but you got over it. However, some people—infants, people over age 60, people with heart or lung disease, or people with chronic diseases that impair the immune system (including diabetes)—are more susceptible to serious complications such as pneumonia and even death.

The virus itself can produce severe pneumonia. It can also weaken the lungs, allowing harmful bacteria to take over and cause a bacterial pneumonia. This can happen even to healthy young adults.

Once exposed to a particular strain of flu, you are immune to that strain for life. Each year there are likely to be new strains to which you have no immunity. Flu shots are tailored to fight the current year's strain; if you need a flu shot, you need one each year.

SYMPTOMS

Symptoms generally occur from 1 to 4 days after being exposed to the virus—the incubation period. You may have a fever, chills, headaches, aching muscles, fatigue, a sore throat, and a cough. However, symptoms vary widely from strain to strain and from person to person.

Usually the fever rises gradually over the first day of illness and then declines. The flu generally runs its course in 5 to 7 days, but you may feel fatigued for several weeks.

TREATMENT OPTIONS

Most cases of the flu are diagnosed based on symptoms; diagnostic tests are rarely necessary. You usually do not need to call your doctor if you get the flu.

You should rest, drink plenty of fluids, and take painkillers to relieve pain and fever. Infants and children under 21 years old should not take aspirin because of the risk of Reye syndrome (see p.1017).

Warm fluids may help soothe a sore throat and humidified air can ease breathing difficulties. Call your doctor if you have trouble breathing or if your fever does not subside after 4 days.

If you are at high risk of complications, your doctor may prescribe the antiviral drugs amantadine, rimantadine, zanamivir, or oseltamivir within 24 hours of the start of your symptoms to lessen the severity of the illness.

Antibiotics (which fight bacteria) are ineffective because flu is caused by a virus. Only if the flu has led to a bacterial infection of your sinuses or lungs is an antibiotic of any value.

Fever: The Early Warning System

Fever is an elevation in temperature above the normal range: 97°F to 99°F. It is one of the body's most effective ways of fighting infection.

Fever is produced when an infection causes infection-fighting white blood cells to become activated, leading to the release of substances that direct the body's temperature-control organ (the hypothalamus) to heat up the body.

The chills you may experience with fever are one way your body creates heat—by forcing you to shiver to stay warm and by signaling you to increase your body temperature by adding more clothing and blankets.

All of these actions effectively raise the body's temperature—and help ward off infection. Fever fights infection by literally killing bacteria; some bacteria cannot survive the heat generated by feverish temperatures.

Higher body temperature also triggers the immune system, which heightens the activity of infection-fighting cells such as phagocytes, neutrophils, and lymphocytes. As a general rule, doctors recommend not giving medication to reduce fever unless a child's temperature is above 102°F or an adult's temperature is above 101°F.

Avian Influenza (Bird Flu)

Different strains of the influenza virus can infect different animals, and these animals can spread some strains of the virus to humans. Strains of the influenza virus that normally infect some birds (such as chickens) can sometimes leap to humans. In recent years, a strain of the virus called H5N1 has done this several times in Asia and in Europe. The H5N1 virus produces a very severe form of flu in humans: Indeed, it has been fatal in some people.

Although the H5N1 virus and other bird flu viruses can cause very serious disease in humans, they do not easily pass from one person to another. The normal human flu viruses produce less severe disease, but are easily passed from one person to another. What experts fear is this: If a bird flu virus like H5N1 were to combine with a normal human flu virus, it could produce a virus that produced very severe disease in humans *and* was easily transmitted among humans. That virus could rapidly spread all over the globe, causing serious illness in a huge number of people.

Unfortunately, this fear is not simply theoretical. In 1917–18 and again in the 1950s, there were worldwide epidemics (called pandemics) of such hybrid viruses. By far the worst was the epidemic of 1917–18—a time before there were flu vaccines or antibiotics. Within weeks after it started, the flu epidemic spread across the entire globe: Twenty million to 40 million people died—as many or more than have died from AIDS in the past 25 years.

Health authorities around the world are constantly on the lookout for outbreaks of bird flu, and have taken action to prevent it from spreading. So far, their efforts have prevented a catastrophic pandemic. Vaccines and drugs are under development to prevent and treat the disease, but as of this writing none has been proven effective.

Hand Washing: Your Best Defense Against Infection

While it is a good idea to wash your hands regularly throughout the day to prevent spreading infection, there are specific times when hand washing can be a particularly potent intervention.

Warm water and soap of any kind are sufficient. Antibacterial soaps are of no value against viruses, which are the most common cause of colds and flu. Also, they offer no additional protection against bacteria and may even enable bacteria to mutate into strains that cannot be killed by antibiotics. Alcohol-based hand-wash products such as Purell are increasingly used in hospitals, and have been proven superior to soap and water.

There is no evidence that wiping a telephone receiver with alcohol is protective.

WASH YOUR HANDS:

Before meals Wash your hands before meals, when your hands are likely to be in contact with your mouth, and more likely to spread infection-causing microorganisms.

Before preparing food For more information, see Safe Food Preparation, p.87.

After using the toilet Fecal matter is a significant source of bacteria and other infection-causing microorganisms, and a significant cause of gastrointestinal infection (see Diarrheal Diseases and Disorders, p.778).

When you have a cold or flu Frequent hand washing after you sneeze, cough, or rub your eyes can help prevent reinfection, and prevent spreading the infection to others.

When you have a skin infection Hand washing helps prevent the spread of skin infections, such as impetigo.

After gardening The soil is rich in bacteria, fungi, and parasites. Wearing gloves is ideal, but thorough hand washing after contact with soil can reduce your risk. You should also have an up-to-date tetanus shot (see p.880).

When people around you have an infection Hand washing decreases the likelihood of acquiring infections that are "going around" your office or home.

Medicine's Triumph Over Smallpox

Smallpox has been eradicated. A life-threatening, contagious viral illness, smallpox was characterized by a fever and body rash that blistered and crusted over, leaving pitted scars, or pock marks.

In 1967, the World Health Organization launched a worldwide eradication campaign with vaccines; in 1979, it declared the world free of smallpox.

Because there is no trace of smallpox left in the human population, vaccinations are no longer required. The virus is still kept at two research laboratories, one in Atlanta and the other in Moscow.

Mononucleosis

Infectious mononucleosis (commonly known as "mono") is an illness usually caused by the Epstein-Barr virus, sometimes by cytomegalovirus (see p.871), and sometimes by a related virus called human herpesvirus 6.

In the United States and other developed countries, infection with the Epstein-Barr virus usually occurs between the ages of 15 and 30. The infection is probably transmitted by saliva. The period between contracting the virus and the emergence of symptoms (the incubation period) is from 7 to 14 days in young adults, but can be longer in older people.

Mononucleosis does not usually cause serious complications. The spleen, which is an organ in the upper left side of the abdomen, swells for several weeks in many people who get mono. The most common serious complication is rupture of an enlarged spleen by injury.

The rupture can cause serious internal bleeding. For this reason, it is important for people with mono to avoid activities—such as contact sports—that could injure the spleen, until their doctor has determined that the spleen has shrunk back to its normal size. Many teenagers with mono feel well enough to return to normal activities before their spleen has returned to normal.

SYMPTOMS

Mono causes extreme fatigue, malaise, fever, headaches, swollen lymph glands in the neck, and a very sore throat. Usually, the symptoms begin suddenly, over 1 to 2 days, but sometimes they develop more gradually.

You feel sick enough to be unable to engage in normal activities for 1 to 2 weeks (sometimes longer). Some people continue to be fatigued for many months after the fever, swollen glands, and other symptoms have subsided.

TREATMENT OPTIONS

Your doctor will conduct a thorough medical history and examination. Two blood tests are very useful in diagnosing mono: a test for an antibody called heterophil (there are various different tests, with different names, for this antibody) and a test that looks for unusually shaped white blood cells called atypical lymphocytes.

Usually, there is no reason to treat mono because it resolves on its own. No antiviral medication has proved to be of value.

It is important that you rest, drink plenty of fluids to prevent dehydration, and take aspirin (if you are over 21) or an aspirin substitute to reduce your fever. Gargle with salt water to relieve the sore throat.

You should not exchange saliva with any other person—by kissing, for example—until you are completely well. Also, if your spleen is enlarged, your doctor may recommend that you not engage in vigorous sports for several months.

BACTERIAL INFECTIONS

Abscesses

An abscess is a thin-walled sac of tissue filled with pus. Pus is composed of infection-causing microorganisms, dead tissue, and white blood cell remnants of the immune system's defenses.

Abscesses can occur in any tissue in the body. They may be caused by an infection that travels through the bloodstream or by infecting organisms that enter a break in the skin.

Abscesses involving the skin cause redness, heat, tenderness, and pain. Abscesses deeper in the body sometimes cause pain, fever, malaise, night sweats, and chills.

Abscesses that are visible are easy to diagnose. Abscesses deep in the body require imaging tests such as computed tomography (see p.149), magnetic resonance imaging (see p.151), ultrasound (see p.148), and nuclear medicine scans (see p.137).

The ideal treatment for every abscess is to open it up to allow the pus to be removed. It can be difficult to remove pus when abscesses are deep in the body; antibiotics alone are sometimes used to slowly heal abscesses.

Bacteremia

Bacteremia is bacteria in the bloodstream. Many people have probably had brief, temporary episodes of bacteremia. In healthy people, the immune system mounts a defense to destroy the bacteria.

Bacteremia is often caused when another infection, such as a urinary tract infection or boil on the skin, spreads to the blood. Bacteria can also be introduced into the bloodstream via surgery, procedures such as cystoscopy (see p.825) or dialysis (see p.815), injury, and intravenous drug use. It can even be caused by having your teeth cleaned.

Bacteremia can become serious if it spreads bacteria to different organs, causing infection. For example, in people who have heart valve disorders, bacteremia can lead to endocarditis (see p.695), which is an infection of the heart valves.

Bacteremia can also lead to life-threatening conditions such as septicemia, in which bacteria multiply and produce toxins. The immune system produces chemicals in large amounts as the body tries to fight the infection.

SYMPTOMS

You may have no symptoms or you may feel weak, tired, and feverish as your body fights the infection. Some types of bacteremia begin abruptly with chills, fever, nausea, vomiting, and diarrhea.

With septicemia, you may develop a high fever, profound weakness, disorientation, rapid breathing, and a low blood pressure. You may even go into shock (see p.645).

TREATMENT OPTIONS

Bacteremia is diagnosed by performing a culture (see p.159) of your blood. Treatment includes antibiotics given intravenously or taken by mouth. Depending on the extent of the infection and the health of your immune system, you may also need treatment in the hospital with intravenous fluids.

Gangrene

Gangrene is the death of tissue (necrosis) due to a blocked blood supply. Causes include frostbite (see p.1211), diabetes mellitus (see p.832), atherosclerosis (see p.653), or a blood clot or embolus.

The condition is called dry gangrene when the tissue dies but does not become infected. When the dying tissue becomes infected, which occurs more often, it is called wet gangrene.

SYMPTOMS

You will feel pain in tissues that are dying due to gangrene. After the tissue dies, it becomes numb and blackened. If the area becomes infected, it will be red and swollen, may ooze pus on the edges of the blackened areas, and may have an odor as infection spreads.

TREATMENT OPTIONS

Your doctor can usually diagnose gangrene just by looking at the affected area; no tests are required. For dry gangrene, you will receive treatment for the underlying disorder that is causing the blockage of blood flow and you may be given antibiotics to prevent infection.

For wet gangrene, powerful antibiotics must be given intravenously immediately to control the infection. You may require surgery to open and drain infected areas and to remove dead tissue.

When there is no hope of saving the tissue, amputation of the affected area is sometimes necessary because dead tissue can easily become infected, and the infection can spread throughout the body.

Staphylococcal Infections

Staphylococcal infections are caused by bacteria called staphylococci ("staph" for short). These bacteria normally live on the skin and in the mucous membranes of the vagina, rectum, mouth, throat, and nose without causing infection.

When the skin is broken due to a scrape or cut, the organisms enter the wound and proliferate. They can spread through the blood to other parts of the body and produce poisons that can damage tissues. Staph infections frequently cause abscesses (see p.877).

Anyone can get a staph infection. However, people whose immune systems are weakened by diseases such as diabetes, acquired immunodeficiency syndrome (AIDS), or cancer are especially vulnerable. Staph infection can occur anywhere bacteria enter the skin or body—including the eyes, where bacteria can cause conjunctivitis (see p.427) or a stye (see p.419); the urinary tract; the digestive tract; and the lungs.

When staph bacteria infect the skin, they can cause boils (see p.532), cellulitis, erysipelas (see p.532), impetigo (see p.531), and folliculitis (see p.532). Staph infections of the nail (see Paronychia, p.569) are often caused by a cut near a fingernail or toenail; the bacteria can infect any open wound.

In rare cases, poisons made by staphylococci enter the bloodstream of menstruating women who use high-absorbency tampons, causing toxic shock syndrome (this page).

A staph infection called scalded skin syndrome most commonly affects newborns, young children, and people whose immune systems are weakened; this condition occurs when poisons produced by the bacteria cause the skin to blister and peel.

Staph can also find its way into the bloodstream through contaminated needles or a skin infection. This can cause bacteremia (see p.878) and life-threatening septicemia, as well as osteomyelitis (see p.595), endocarditis (see p.695), and infec-

tious arthritis (see p.603). Staph bacteria also can cause pneumonia (see p.496) when they congregate in the mucus of the lungs and are not coughed out.

When bacteria are consumed in infected food (usually due to food handling by someone with an infected wound), they can cause staphylococcal food poisoning (see p.881).

While most staphylococcal infections can be treated with antibiotics, some strains have developed a resistance to most antibiotics, and a few are resistant to virtually all antibiotics. This is of particular concern in hospital settings, where the staphylococci can infect medical equipment and gain access to the body through surgical sites.

Toxic Shock Syndrome

Toxic shock syndrome is a rare staphylococcal infection (see previous article) in which the staphylococci bacteria produce poisons that enter the bloodstream and can cause life-threatening illness.

Toxic shock syndrome is often caused by using highly absorbent tampons, which give staph a place to grow and which can create tiny tears in the lining of the vagina. However, it can also occur when an open wound becomes infected.

Symptoms include a sudden high fever (over 102°F), a rash on the soles and palms (which may later peel), vomiting, diarrhea, weakness, muscle aches, and dizziness. In the worst cases, toxic shock causes blood pressure to fall dramatically and can damage the kidneys and liver.

If you suspect toxic shock,

remove any tampon and phone your doctor immediately. Treatment with antibiotics clears the infection in a majority of people; those with a more severe case may require hospitalization to restore fluids and monitor blood pressure.

To reduce the chance of this illness, use a tampon of the lowest possible absorbency and leave it in your vagina for no longer than 4 hours before removing it and inserting a fresh tampon.

Streptococcal Infections

Streptococcal infections are those caused by streptococci ("strep" for short) bacteria. There are many types of streptococci, which can cause a wide range of diseases and disorders.

Strep bacteria normally live on our skin and in the intestines, mouth, and throat. The bacteria cause infection when they gain access to the bloodstream or tissues of the body.

Streptococcus pyogenes is responsible for strep throat (see p.467) and skin infections such as cellulitis (see p.532) and impetigo (see p.531). Strep bacteria also cause infection in open cuts and wounds, including surgical incisions.

Streptococcus pneumoniae (pneumococcus) is the most common cause of pneumonia (see p.496).

When normally occurring strep bacteria move into the bloodstream, they can cause endocarditis (see p.695) in people who have defects of the heart valves.

Strep can cause scarlet fever, rheumatic fever (see p.697), necrotizing fasciitis (a rapidly destructive infection of the skin

Hospital-Acquired Infections and Antibiotic-Resistant Bacteria

Infections acquired in the hospital (also called nosocomial infections) affect about 6% of those who are hospitalized. People whose immune systems are weakened due to disease or chemotherapy are at greatest risk, but nosocomial infections can develop in anyone.

The most common hospital-acquired infections have not changed much over the past three decades. Urinary tract infections, infections of surgical wounds, pneumonia, and bacteremia (see p.878) are the most prevalent.

The bacteria that live in hospitals and other medical settings are becoming resistant to increasing numbers of antibiotics. This is because bacteria that are continuously exposed to antibiotics develop mutations that make them resistant to the drugs. As a result, infections that develop in the hospital tend to be more difficult to treat.

The increasing use of antibiotics in hospitals compounds the problem—more antibiotics are developed and used to help overcome the problem of antibiotic resistance, causing more antibiotic resistance. Science is constantly racing to outwit bacteria.

Doctors attempt to reduce antibiotic resistance by prescribing antibiotics sparingly and only when absolutely necessary. When someone is known to be infected with bacteria that are resistant to most antibiotics, strong measures are taken to isolate him or her from others so that the resistant organisms do not spread.

and deeper tissues), or glomerulonephritis (see p.810). Other types of strep bacteria live normally in the intestines but can cause urinary tract infections if they spread.

TREATMENT OPTIONS

Your doctor makes the diagnosis of a strep infection by taking a culture (see p.159) from the part of your body that is infected—for example, the throat, a sore, phlegm (sputum) from the lung, or the blood. The results of the culture can also help your doctor choose the antibiotic best suited to killing the infection.

People who have rheumatic heart disease (see p.697) and some people with mitral valve prolapse (see p.694) need to take a preventive dose of antibiotics before undergoing dental work (see Antibiotics Before Dental Work, p.481).

Strep that live in the gums can get into the blood and travel to the heart, where the bacteria can infect heart valves damaged by rheumatic fever. Taking antibiotics at the time of dental work prevents the bacteria from growing on the heart valves.

Tetanus

Tetanus is an illness caused by infection with the bacterium *Clostridium tetani*. The bacteria produce a toxin that affects the nervous system. The infection can occur when the bacteria, which live in the soil, contaminate dirt that gets into an opening in the skin.

The diphtheria, pertussis, and tetanus (DPT) vaccination (see p.947), which is given to all children periodically, protects against this infection. Adults should have tetanus booster shots every 10 years.

Symptoms start to appear between 5 and 15 days after exposure. First there are mild spasms and then rigidity of the muscles of the jaw (lockjaw), neck, and face and difficulty swallowing or speaking. Soon after, the chest, back, and abdominal muscles become rigid, which can interfere with breathing and threaten life, especially in children and older adults. Powerful and painful seizures then occur.

If you have any of the symptoms of tetanus, see your doctor immediately. You will be admitted to the hospital, where you will be given an injection to neutralize the tetanus toxin. Intravenous penicillin and removal of infected tissue may also be necessary. Muscle relaxants (to reduce spasms) and sedation are often necessary, as is use of a ventilator (see p.520) to provide breathing support.

If you cut yourself while working in the garden or with soil and you have not been immunized for several years, you should get a tetanus booster shot, which will cause your body to produce antibodies to the bacterium. Antibiotics may also be required.

Typhoid Fever

Typhoid fever is a bacterial infection caused by eating food or drinking water contaminated with feces that contain the bacterium *Salmonella typhi*. The bacteria travel from the small intestine to the bloodstream and then into the liver and spleen, where they reproduce.

They then move via the gallbladder into the intestines. Some people who have no symptoms carry the bacteria in their digestive tract for years and infect others.

The disease is rare in the United States but still occurs in developing countries; typhoid immunization is recommended for travel to some countries (see Immunizations for Travel, p.94). In any country where sanitation is poor, you should avoid eating fresh produce and drinking the local water. Drink only boiled or bottled water and eat only cooked food (see p.96).

Typhoid usually produces symptoms that come on suddenly, including appetite loss, vomiting, headaches, and general malaise. You then have a high fever (which usually occurs at night) with chills, diarrhea, weakness, and extreme fatigue. You may develop a rash typical of typhoid (small, pink, raised spots on the chest and abdomen) and your liver and spleen may be enlarged.

See your doctor immediately if you suspect that you have ty-

phoid; serious complications, including intestinal rupture or bleeding, can occur. Typhoid fever can be confirmed by identifying the bacteria in a sample of your stool or in your blood.

If you have typhoid, you will probably be hospitalized and treated with fluids to prevent dehydration and powerful antibiotics to kill the bacteria. You may be isolated to prevent spreading the infection.

Complete recovery may take several weeks. Your doctor may

test a sample of your stool for several months after you recover to ensure the bacteria have been eradicated.

Food Poisoning

Food poisoning is an adverse reaction to a substance—including bacteria, fungi, viruses, or protozoa—in contaminated food or water. More than 250 different disease-causing organisms can contaminate food and water, usually causing gastrointestinal

---

Transmission of *Escherichia coli* O157:H7

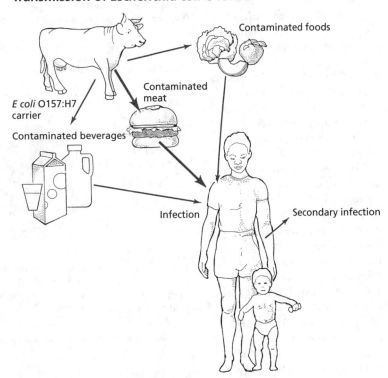

The primary reservoir of *E coli* O157:H7 is cattle, which carry the organism in their digestive tracts and shed it in feces. You can become ill with severe gastroenteritis and potentially fatal kidney disease after contact with the stool of an infected person or animal or from eating contaminated foods (such as meat that has not been adequately cooked, fruits or vegetables contaminated by cattle manure, or contaminated dairy products or water). Elderly adults and children are most vulnerable to serious infection.

symptoms such as vomiting, abdominal cramping, and diarrhea. The organisms cannot be detected by smell or taste in infected food or water.

The most common infections are caused by bacteria, such as salmonella and *Escherichia coli* (commonly known as *E coli)*, or by the Norwalk virus.

Food handling practices that contribute to food poisoning include not washing hands before handling food or after using the toilet; poor personal hygiene; holding or storing food at improper temperatures; cooking food at inadequate temperatures; and using contaminated equipment for food preparation. Read Food Safety (see p.87) for more prevention recommendations.

The symptoms of food poisoning can range from mild diarrhea to life-threatening infections. Some bacteria, such as *Bacillus cereus* and *Staphylococcus aureus* cause symptoms within 24 hours. Others, such as *Clostridium botulinum*, take longer to cause illness but can be lethal if not treated promptly.

The *E coli* O157:H7 bacterium, which can stay alive in undercooked meat, is so powerful that, if only a very small number of organisms—possibly as few as 100—are ingested, it can cause serious infection. The bacterium causes from 10,000 to 20,000 infections in the United States each year and kills about 250 people. It is the main cause of hemolytic uremic syndrome, a potentially fatal kidney disease caused when bacterial toxins escape from the intestines and damage the kidneys and red blood cells.

Heating foods to 160°F kills *E*

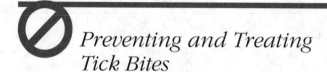

Preventing and Treating Tick Bites

Take these precautions to prevent tick bites:

■ Wear long-sleeved, light-colored shirts; long pants; and closed-toed shoes.

■ Tuck your pants into your socks when hiking.

■ Walk on cleared trails, away from brushy vegetation.

■ Use tick-repellents that contain diethyltoluamide on clothing and skin, but do not apply repellents to the skin of children under 6 years old.

■ Use the tick repellent permethrin, but only on clothing.

After hiking, remove your clothing and perform a thorough tick check (use a mirror or have someone help you). If you see an embedded tick, remove it as shown below. It is important to remove the entire tick; leaving the feeding parts in the skin may transmit infection. Wash the area with soap and water, and do not rub the area until it has been washed.

How to Remove a Tick

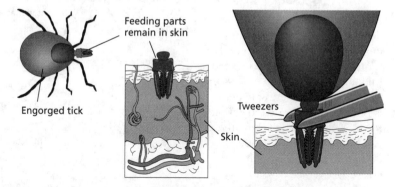

To remove a tick, use tweezers to grip the head firmly, as close to the skin as possible, and pull (straight up) gently and repeatedly. You will feel a small tugging sensation because a tiny piece of skin will remain attached to the tick's feeding parts. If you think the tick's feeding parts were left in the skin, see your doctor. Save the tick in a jar of alcohol so that it can be identified.

coli. Recently, it has been discovered that changes in the way cattle are fed could greatly reduce the amount of contaminated meat that is sold for human consumption.

People who are particularly vulnerable to food-borne pathogens include pregnant or nursing women, elderly adults, infants, and people whose immune systems are weakened, such as those with acquired immunodeficiency syndrome (AIDS) or those who are undergoing cancer treatment.

Cycle of Lyme Disease

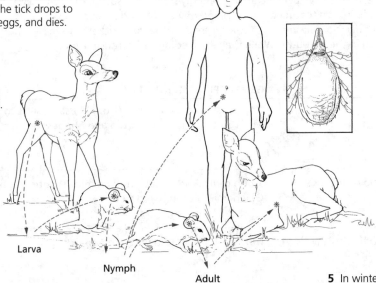

1 An adult tick lives by feeding on the blood of a white-tailed deer. In late fall, the tick drops to the ground, lays eggs, and dies.

2 In late spring, the eggs hatch, producing immature ticks (larvae). Here one attaches to a white-footed mouse. The mouse has Lyme disease bacteria in its blood. When the larva bites the mouse to feed on the mouse's blood, the larva also ingests the Lyme disease bacteria.

Larva

Nymph

Adult

3 The larva drops off the mouse and remains on the ground until the next spring (Lyme disease bacteria will stay alive inside the larva). A year later, the larva turns into a slightly larger kind of immature tick, called a nymph (inset), which is about the size of a poppy seed.

4 The nymph attaches to and feeds on the blood of another animal or a person. When it feeds, it transmits Lyme disease bacteria to the uninfected host. After it feeds, it drops to the ground. In the fall, it molts into an adult (about the size of a sesame seed).

5 In winter, the adult tick seeks a white-tailed deer as its host, and the cycle begins again. Whether or not the adult tick has Lyme disease bacteria inside it, the larvae it produces the next spring will initially be free of bacteria.

Most food poisoning illnesses last from 1 to 3 days and are not life-threatening. If you have severe symptoms, call your doctor, who will try to establish the cause and treat the infection. Home treatment includes drinking plenty of fluids to prevent dehydration. Your physician may recommend a rehydration solution (see Traveler's Diarrhea, p.780) to replace lost nutrients.

FUNGAL AND PROTOZOAL INFECTIONS

Candidiasis

Candidiasis is an infection caused by *Candida albicans*, a fungus that naturally inhabits the skin, bowel movements, mouth, and vagina.

Normally, candida is harmless because its growth is kept in check by bacteria and the body's immune defenses. Conditions that disrupt this balance include tak-

ing antibiotics, which can kill the bacteria that keep candida in check, or having a weakened immune system. These conditions permit the fungus to proliferate, which causes a white discharge that looks like cottage cheese.

In a person whose immune system is weakened, candida can be lethal, traveling through the blood to affect the bones, brain, esophagus, and eyes. Candida also affect the digestive tract, causing bloody diarrhea, cramps, chills, and fever.

Tick-Borne Infections

In the past 20 years, ticks have become an increasingly significant source of serious illness. Ticks are insects that feed on the blood of warm-blooded animals. They carry various microorganisms—bacteria, viruses, protozoa, or rickettsia—in their bodies, often in their mouths. While they are feeding, ticks transmit the

DISEASE	GEOGRAPHIC LOCATION
Lyme disease	Northeastern coastal states (from Massachusetts to Virginia), upper Midwest (especially Wisconsin and Minnesota), and northern California
Human monocytic ehrlichiosis (HME)	South central, southeastern, and mid-Atlantic states (especially Oklahoma, Missouri, and Georgia)
Human granulocytic ehrlichiosis (HGE)	Northeast, upper Midwest, west coast
Colorado tick fever	Mountainous regions of Colorado, Utah, South Dakota, Montana, Wyoming, Idaho, Washington, Oregon, California, New Mexico, and Nevada
Babesiosis	Northeast (especially offshore islands), Maryland, Virginia, Georgia, Wisconsin, Minnesota, California, and Washington
Tularemia	Southeastern, south central, and western states (mostly Arkansas, Missouri, and Oklahoma)
Powassan encephalitis	New York State, Quebec, and sometimes New England
Tick paralysis	Pacific Northwest, Rocky Mountain states, and some southern states
Rocky Mountain spotted fever	Mid- and south Atlantic coasts, western and south central states, and South Dakota and Montana

microorganisms to your blood. To prevent tick bites, follow the guidelines on p.882. If you find a tick on your body, remove it carefully (see p.882). Ticks are responsible for the following infectious diseases in the United States (and many more worldwide):

SYMPTOMS	TREATMENT
Common Flulike symptoms; red "bull's eye" rash at site of bite; arthritis **Less common** Heart block; inflammation of the heart or surrounding tissues; Bell palsy; unusual sensations or weakness of the limbs; meningitis	**Early disease** Antibiotic tablets for 2 to 3 weeks **Advanced disease** Intravenous antibiotics for 2 to 3 weeks
Common High fever; headache; rash of small spots **Less common** Small spots on palms and soles **Complications** Kidney failure; liver failure; confusion; breathing problems; death	Antibiotic tablets
Common Flulike symptoms; nausea; vomiting; cough; confusion **Less common** Rash **Complications** Can be more serious and life-threatening than HME	Antibiotic tablets
Flulike illness with severe headache; inability to tolerate light; short-lived spotted rash (symptoms may persist for 5 to 8 days and then return after 3 days)	Analgesics (painkillers), rest, and fluids
Early symptoms Severe, cyclic fatigue; decreased appetite **Later symptoms** Fever; drenching sweats; muscle aches; joint aches; jaundice **Complications** Anemia; kidney failure	Oral or intravenous antibiotics for 7 to 14 days; blood transfusions in severe cases
Red bump or ulcer at site of bite; swollen lymph nodes near bite, usually in groin or under arm	Antibiotic injections into muscles or veins for 10 to 14 days
Common Headache; confusion; paralysis; often affects children (occurs mainly between May and December)	None
Common Weakness, progressing to paralysis that starts in legs and moves upward to the torso, arms, neck, and head	Removal of embedded tick results in recovery within hours to days
Common Fever; headache; rash of small dots at wrists and ankles that may become patchlike when it spreads to arms and legs; can include palms and soles **Complications** Heart failure; kidney failure; breathing difficulty; death	Intravenous antibiotics or oral antibiotics for 7 to 14 days after temperature has normalized

Candida causes oral thrush (see p.488), which affects both adults and infants. Oral thrush is common in denture wearers and in people with diabetes.

Infants may get the infection on areas of diaper rash (see p.973). Women may have vaginal yeast infections (see p.1066) caused by the fungus. In men it can cause balanitis (see p.1088), which is inflammation of the head of the penis.

People who are overweight may develop candida on the skin in areas that are moist, such as under the breasts or in the genital area.

Your doctor usually diagnoses candidiasis by its appearance; laboratory evaluation of samples of the discharge or cultures of the blood can also be helpful.

Uncomplicated candidiasis is treated with prescription oral antifungal medications (such as fluconazole, nystatin, clotrimazole, or amphotericin B) or vaginal tablets, suppositories, or creams (such as clotrimazole, terconazole, or tioconazole). Some vaginal creams (such as clotrimazole and miconazole) are available without a prescription. More serious infections require powerful antifungal medications, often given intravenously.

If you are prone to recurring vaginal yeast infections, eat yogurt several days a week or drink acidophilus milk—both of which should contain live cultures—to maintain a balance of the helpful bacteria that limit yeast overgrowth. Keep your skin dry and clean to help suppress skin infection.

Cryptosporidiosis

Cryptosporidiosis is a diarrheal infection caused by cryptosporidium, a type of protozoa (single-celled animal). The eggs of this hardy organism can spread by hand-to-hand transmission or by drinking contaminated water.

Cryptosporidium is particularly likely to cause disease in people with acquired immunodeficiency syndrome (AIDS) (see p.872).

Infected people who have healthy immune systems usually have watery diarrhea that lasts up to 2 weeks, sometimes accompanied by abdominal pain, nausea, loss of appetite and weight, and fever.

In immunodeficient people, the diarrhea is profuse and can occur many times daily, causing dramatic weight loss, muscle wasting, severe abdominal pain, and dehydration.

If you have persistent diarrhea, consult your doctor, who will perform stool tests to detect the organisms. The main treatment is to replace fluids lost from diarrhea. In otherwise healthy people, the condition resolves on its own within 2 weeks.

There is no cure for cryptosporidiosis. However, if you have AIDS, your doctor may prescribe paromomycin, which lessens symptoms in some people.

Cyclosporiasis

Infection with the parasite *Cyclospora cayetanensis* occurs by drinking contaminated water or eating food that has been washed with contaminated water. Outbreaks in the United States have occurred from eating contaminated berries imported from other countries.

Infection may produce no symptoms, but it can cause diarrhea, cramps in the abdomen, belching, and gas. In some people the symptoms occur only once; in others the symptoms come and go over many months or years.

People with chronic symptoms also often have fatigue and weight loss. The infection is diagnosed by examining bowel movements and is treated with a combination of the antibiotics trimethoprim and sulfamethoxazole.

Sporotrichosis

Sporotrichosis is an infection caused by the fungus *Sporothrix schenckii*, which is found in soil and vegetation. Infection most often occurs in people who work with plants and arises when this fungus gains entry to the lymphatic system through a cut in the skin.

At first, you may notice a red, painless bump or ulcer near the site of a cut or thorn prick. Over the next several weeks, similar bumps form along nearby lymphatic system channels. In people whose immune systems are weakened, the infection sometimes spreads to the joints.

See your doctor if you have symptoms. The infection is treated with the antifungal drug itraconazole, taken by mouth.

Giardiasis

Giardiasis is an infection of the small intestine caused by the protozoa (single-celled organisms) *Giardia lamblia.* One of the most common parasitic diseases in the world, giardiasis is characterized by diarrhea, abdominal gas, and cramps.

Giardiasis is spread by unsanitary conditions, either by contaminated water or food, person-to-person contact, or sexual contact. The parasite thrives in cold water, including that of mountain lakes and streams that have been contaminated by animals. It resists killing by chlorination; even small numbers of the microorganism in contaminated water can produce disease.

Most people who carry *G lamblia* in their intestinal tracts have no symptoms. When symptoms do occur, they can come on suddenly or gradually.

In acute giardiasis, symptoms arise within 3 weeks of exposure. The first symptoms include watery diarrhea, abdominal pain, and cramps. You may also have a low-grade fever. Diarrhea subsides in most people within about a week, but some affected people have problems for much longer.

In chronic giardiasis, diarrhea may not be the most prominent symptom; instead, you may experience loose bowel movements, flatulence, burping with an unpleasant odor, and weight loss. Symptoms may continue on and off over a period of years.

Report your symptoms to your doctor, who will examine a sample of your bowel movements to make a diagnosis of giardiasis.

Treatment, which is essential to eradicate the infection, may include one of several prescribed drugs, including an antibiotic taken by mouth for up to 10 days. If the first course of treatment fails, which happens in

about 20% of people, you may need further drug treatment.

If treatment repeatedly fails, family members should be tested and treated because they may be symptom-free carriers of the organism.

Malaria

Malaria is a disease caused by four types of protozoa (single-celled organisms) called plasmodia that are spread by the bite of an infected *Anopheles* species mosquito. This disease remains a lethal threat in tropical countries, where the infection-bearing mosquitoes are often resistant to insecticides.

Worldwide, malaria is one of the greatest killers. About 1,000 cases of malaria occur in the United States each year, primarily in people who have returned from other countries with it.

The bite of an infected female mosquito delivers the microscopic parasites to the victim's bloodstream. The parasites move into the liver and reproduce quickly. They then travel in large numbers back to the blood, where they invade and rupture red blood cells, producing repeated chills and fever.

Some parasites remain in the liver, where they remain dormant for months before moving into the bloodstream, causing the cyclical symptoms of malaria.

A strain of malaria-causing protozoa called *Plasmodium falciparum* is responsible for most malaria-related deaths.

People who travel outside the United States should contact the US Centers for Disease Control and Prevention (CDC) for information on steps to take to pre-

vent malaria (CDC's malaria hotline:1–770–488–7788). There is no effective immunization.

SYMPTOMS

You may have no symptoms for up to a month after being bitten by an infected mosquito, or longer if you have been taking antimalaria drugs. Then you will feel flulike symptoms—headache, fatigue, abdominal pain, and muscle aches—followed by alternating fever and chills.

The fever moves through three stages: shivering, a fever of up to 105°F, and profuse sweating with a reduction in temperature. The cycle is repeated as the red blood cells are ruptured by the malaria parasite.

In people with *P falciparum*, the fever may remain constant, and the destroyed blood cells sometimes block blood vessels and cut off blood supply, damaging the kidneys, brain, and spleen. The liver and kidneys may shut down. Death can occur if treatment is not given quickly.

TREATMENT OPTIONS

Your symptoms and recent travel experience may lead your physician to test your blood for malaria. Under a microscope, the microorganisms can be seen inside some red blood cells; their appearance indicates what kind of malaria you have.

Medications are taken either orally or intravenously. You may need to take a combination of several medications. Treatment may also be needed for any complications. For example, kidney damage may require dialysis (see p.815) and severe anemia may require blood transfusions.

Mad Cow Disease

Mad cow disease, medically known as bovine spongiform encephalopathy, is a fatal central nervous system disease of cattle. Affected cattle exhibit changes in behavior, tremors, lack of coordination, and, eventually, death.

This rare condition was first diagnosed in cattle in 1986 and remains isolated to cattle from Great Britain. However, mad cow disease may have been passed on to humans.

Mad cow disease is caused by infection with a prion (see p.866), an unusual kind of infectious agent. British cattle contracted the disease from eating infected material from dead sheep that farmers had put in their meal. Some of the sheep had a similar prion disease called scrapie.

In 1996, 10 people in Great Britain were found to have a variant of Creutzfeldt-Jakob disease (CJD), a fatal central nervous system disease that is also caused by a prion. CJD causes a rapidly progressing dementia (see p.362), muscle spasms, tremor, and rigidity. There is no known treatment and the disease is usually fatal within 1 year.

Strong evidence links the variant CJD in humans to mad cow disease in cattle. Whether the cases were caused by eating the contaminated meat or brains of cattle remains unclear.

Several people with variant CJD were from farms that had cows with BSE. Others were young people who had never worked on farms. Mad cow disease and variant CJD remain rare events. International efforts to quarantine infected cattle and change components of cattle feed, as well as regular surveillance of beef stock, have contained the spread so far.

WORM INFESTATIONS

Ascariasis

Ascariasis is an infection caused by *Ascaris lumbricoides,* the largest and most common roundworm affecting the intestines. The worm can grow up to 10 inches.

Ascariasis is spread by hand-to-mouth contact with soil (or products that have been grown in contaminated soil) that contains human feces that harbor eggs. After the eggs are swallowed, the larvae hatch in the intestines and migrate through the circulation to the lungs. They climb the breathing tubes and are swallowed into the small intestine, where they develop into adult worms that produce eggs (which leave the body in feces). The adult worms live up to 2 years.

Ascariasis can cause a cough soon after infection, as the larvae invade the lungs. Other symptoms include mild pain in the abdomen, vomiting, and, in rare cases, obstruction of the intestines. Ascariasis is a significant cause of malnutrition in many developing countries. Very rarely, people pass the large, cream-colored worm through the mouth or nose or in stool.

Ascariasis can be diagnosed by laboratory evaluation of fecal samples to identify worm eggs. In addition, your doctor may perform x-rays of your gastrointestinal tract.

Taking anthelmintic (antiworm) medication by mouth clears the infection by killing the worms or by paralyzing them so they are swept out of the intestines. They are then passed in bowel movements.

Hookworms

Hookworms are small ($1/2$ inch long) worms that infest people and cause anemia. One of the two species of hookworm infests about a quarter of the world's population. The worms, which thrive in humid, hot regions, are transmitted by contact with infected feces in the soil.

The worms and their larvae enter the body through the skin between the toes of bare feet. Then they move via the blood to the lungs, from where they are coughed up into the mouth and then swallowed into the intestines.

Hookworms attach themselves by their mouth parts to the inner surface of the small intestine, where they grow. They can live in the intestines for up to 5 years, but do not reproduce in humans.

Some people have no symptoms. Others have an itchy skin rash at the site of penetration. You may also experience wheezing or coughing with bloodstained phlegm (sputum), a fever, bloody diarrhea, and abdominal pain. Hookworms can also cause fatigue and anemia.

Hookworms are diagnosed by identifying their eggs in a stool sample. Many cases are not treated, and the worms die and are passed out of the system in bowel movements.

Your doctor may test your blood for iron to ensure that you are not anemic. Hookworms can be eradicated with anthelmintic (antiworm) drugs taken by mouth.

Strongyloidiasis

The tiny worm that causes this infestation, *Strongyloides stercoralis*, is found in tropical regions, primarily outside the United States.

Worms are spread by skin contact with soil that is contaminated with feces containing the larvae of the worm. The larvae penetrate through the skin or mucous membranes and travel through the bloodstream to the lungs and up the airways to the mouth, where they are swallowed into the small intestine.

The worms grow and reproduce in the lining of the intestines, shedding larvae into the feces and bloodstream; those in the blood grow and start the cycle again. In people whose immune systems are weakened, the worms can cause life-threatening pneumonia and other serious disease.

Infested people may experience no symptoms or may have an itchy skin rash. Infestation of the lungs can cause pneumonia or a cough that produces blood-stained phlegm (sputum). You may also feel bloated or have diarrhea if the infestation is heavy.

Your doctor can diagnose the worms by microscopic examination of a stool sample. Treatment is with anthelmintic (antiworm) drugs taken by mouth.

Tapeworms

Tapeworms, also known as cestodes, are ribbon-shaped worms up to 30 feet long that are acquired from eating beef, pork, or fish that has been undercooked.

Several varieties of tapeworms live in the intestines of animals and people, attaching themselves by hooks or suckers to the wall of the intestines.

Ingestion of pork tapeworm eggs can cause infestation of the brain and eye with the tapeworm (in the form of cysts), a condition called cysticercosis. This can lead to seizures, headaches, and visual problems.

Another type of tapeworm, called the dwarf tapeworm because it is about 1 inch long, can be transmitted from person to person when feces are handled and eggs are transferred to the mouth.

Symptoms of tapeworms are usually mild, but may include diarrhea and abdominal pain. Pieces of the larger worms sometimes are shed in the bowel movements or out the anus.

Your doctor may diagnose an infestation by locating eggs or worm pieces in stool. Treatment is with anthelmintic (antiworm) drugs. Tapeworm infestation can be prevented by storing and cooking meat and fish properly and by practicing good personal hygiene.

Trichinosis

Trichinosis is infection with the larvae of a worm that lives in animals, including dogs, bears, and pigs. It is most commonly acquired by eating undercooked pork.

Ingested *Trichinella spiralis* larvae grow in the intestines, where they reproduce and release more larvae, which move into the bloodstream. They are carried into the muscles, where they form cysts.

Trichinosis can be prevented by cooking meat thoroughly or by freezing meat at 0°F for several days.

Most infections are mild and do not cause symptoms. Infections that are severe can cause severe symptoms or, rarely, death. Diarrhea and vomiting may occur within several days of ingesting the worm larvae; about 7 days later, symptoms may recur as the larvae reproduce.

If the larvae move into the muscles, you may experience muscle weakness and pain, facial swelling (particularly around the eyes), conjunctivitis (see p.427), and fever.

Trichinosis is diagnosed based on your symptoms, blood tests, and, sometimes, a biopsy (see p.161) of your muscle tissue to look for larvae. Treatment is with anthelmintic (antiworm) drugs to kill the larvae and worms and corticosteroids (see p.895) to reduce muscle inflammation.

SEXUALLY TRANSMITTED DISEASES

Chancroid

Chancroid is a sexually transmitted disease characterized by enlarged lymph glands in the groin and ulcers on the genitals; it is caused by the bacterium *Haemophilus ducreyi*.

Having chancroid can put you at higher risk for a human immunodeficiency virus (HIV) infection because the open sores provide an entry point for the virus.

Symptoms appear within a week of sexual contact. The first symptom is one or several pimplelike sores surrounded by red skin on the genitals. Within 2 days, the pimple breaks open to become a painful, bleeding ulcer. The lymph nodes in your groin may become swollen and tender.

Because chancroid ulcers can be difficult to distinguish from other infections that cause genital ulcers, such as syphilis (see p.893) and genital herpes (see p.890), your doctor will take a sample from the ulcer for laboratory evaluation.

Treatment is with antibiotics taken by mouth. A latex or polyurethane condom can help decrease the risk of contracting chancroid during sexual intercourse.

Genital Herpes

Genital herpes is a viral infection that produces intermittent periods of painful blisters or sores on the genitals. It is caused by the herpes simplex virus.

Genital herpes is one of the most common sexually transmitted diseases (STDs) in the United States, with an estimated 45 million Americans (1 of 5 adults over age 15) infected. It is transmitted through vaginal, anal, or oral sex.

Like most STDs, it enters the body through a break in the skin. Most people are not aware they have the virus because they never experience symptoms. Moreover, if you have the herpes virus you can infect a sexual partner even if you do not have a current active infection with genital sores.

Once infected, you can harbor the virus without symptoms (latency period) for months or years before an outbreak (active infection period). During latency, the virus lies dormant in the nerve cells, undetected by the immune system's defenses. Emotional or physical stress can activate it.

Having the virus increases the risk that a sexual partner with the human immunodeficiency virus (HIV) might infect you.

If you are pregnant and have an active herpes infection around the time of delivery, your doctor may recommend that you have a cesarean section to prevent transmitting the virus to your newborn, which can cause blindness, brain damage, or even death. Genital herpes can be severe in people with weakened immune systems.

SYMPTOMS

You may first have itchy, painful, or tender skin in your genital area and swollen lymph glands. Some people also feel ill and have a headache or fever.

Painful red blisters filled with a clear fluid burst, ooze, and crust over. The blisters can appear on any part of the penis, scrotum, vagina, or vulva as well as on the inner thighs, buttocks, or anus. Healing of the sores takes about 2 to 3 weeks.

Your first episode (usually the most severe) may also include fever, aches, and fatigue. The frequency of outbreaks varies.

TREATMENT OPTIONS

Report symptoms of genital herpes to your doctor, who may test a sample of the blister fluid or sore for presence of the virus. Every day, wash the sores with soap and water and dry them.

You can reduce the duration, severity, and transmission of infections by taking one of three oral prescription antiviral medications: acyclovir, famciclovir, or valacyclovir.

The best way to prevent transmitting herpes is to not have sex—even with a condom—when you have sores. Even if you do not have sores, you should use a condom every time you have sex. Condoms decrease the likelihood of transmitting infection but do not always prevent transmission.

If you are pregnant, tell your obstetrician if you have had genital herpes so that special care can be taken around the time you deliver your baby.

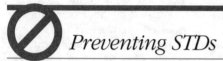

Preventing STDs

A sure (but maybe not very practical) way to prevent sexually transmitted diseases (STDs) is to not have sexual intercourse. The next best choice is to engage in sex only with one uninfected sexual partner who is engaging in sex only with you.

Both you and your partner can be tested for STDs before you have sex for the first time. A latex or polyurethane condom is the best tool for preventing STDs. Follow the recommendations in the article on safer sex (see p.76).

Genital Warts

Genital warts are a sexually transmitted disease caused by the human papillomavirus (HPV). They can occur on the penis, around the anus, in the vagina, and around the cervix (the opening to the uterus). More than 24 million Americans have HPV.

Once you have HPV in your skin or in the membranes of your mouth or genital organs, the virus may stay for life, periodically reactivating to cause the warts and infect sexual partners. HPV also causes warts on other parts of the body.

Having genital warts is the most important risk factor for cancer of the cervix (see p.1068), a cancer that is caused by certain strains of HPV.

SYMPTOMS

Symptoms may not be noticed for months or years after you have had sexual contact with an infected person. The warts look like warts that grow on your hand or arm. When visible, they appear as single warts or cauliflowerlike clusters of raised lumps on the genitals. They may itch and bleed. Rarely, they become infected.

If present in large numbers, the warts may block the anus or birth canal. Warts on the cervix cause no symptoms.

TREATMENT OPTIONS

Warts that are visible can usually be diagnosed based on your symptoms and sexual and medical history. Infected women should have a Pap smear every 6 months. If you have warts on your cervix, your doctor may remove them for laboratory evaluation.

Treatment methods include the application of chemicals by a physician to dissolve the warts. Never use an over-the-counter medication for genital warts—you could seriously damage the delicate skin of your genitals.

Your doctor may also use electricity, freezing, laser treatments, or surgery to remove the warts. Although the warts can be removed, the virus stays in the skin near the site that was infected and can reactivate at any time.

Use a latex or polyurethane condom during sexual intercourse to help prevent spreading the infection.

Gonorrhea

Gonorrhea is caused by the bacterium *Neisseria gonorrhoeae* and is transmitted during sexual intercourse. There are about 600,000 new cases of gonorrhea each year in the United States. Gonorrhea is sometimes transmitted from an infected woman to her infant during childbirth.

Untreated gonorrhea can cause serious complications. If bacteria spread to the fallopian tubes and uterus, they can cause scarring and pelvic inflammatory disease (see p.1077), which can lead to infertility.

Untreated gonorrhea may also lead to urethral stricture (see p.825), which can reduce the flow of urine and lead to urinary tract infection (see p.804).

Gonorrhea can infect the anus and rectum, producing proctitis (see p.797). In men, it can cause epididymitis (see p.1090), inflam-

Facts About STDs

Here are some facts about sexually transmitted diseases (STDs) in the United States. For information on prevention, see Safer Sex, p.76.

- 12 million new cases of STDs occur every year, 3 million of them in teenagers.
- The United States has the highest rates of STDs in the industrialized world.
- STDs play an integral role in transmitting the human immunodeficiency virus (HIV) (see p.872).
- An estimated 45 million Americans have genital herpes (see p.890); most of them do not know it.
- Minorities are disproportionately affected by STDs.
- In women, STDs can cause cancers of the reproductive tract, pelvic inflammatory disease (see p.1077), infertility, and ectopic pregnancy (see p.929).
- STDs can cause mental retardation, blindness, and death in infants who are infected in the uterus or during birth. Other STDs can cause eye infections or pneumonia.
- STDs often occur together. If you have been diagnosed with one, you should be tested for others.

mation of the prostate gland (see Prostatitis, p.1096), and a variety of other serious conditions.

Gonorrhea that is not treated can spread via the bloodstream to cause infections in the bones, skin, or joints.

SYMPTOMS

Most women do not have symptoms and know that they are infected only by being tested for gonorrhea. When symptoms occur, they often develop between 2 and 14 days after being exposed to the bacteria, commonly at the time of a menstrual period.

Women may have a puslike discharge from the urethra or vagina and painful and frequent urination. Others experience pain during sexual intercourse. You may have pain in the lower abdomen and fever if *N gonorrhoeae* has spread to the fallopian tubes.

In men, the most common initial symptom is a discharge from the urethra that is either clear or white, or thick, yellow, and puslike. This discharge appears at the opening of the penis and may stain underwear. Other symptoms include painful urination and burning.

In men or women who have been infected through oral or anal sexual contact, there may be no symptoms or there may be rectal pain during defecation; oral infection may cause sore throat.

TREATMENT OPTIONS

See your doctor immediately if you think you have gonorrhea. Most doctors can diagnose gonorrhea on the basis of symptoms and a physical examination, and

confirm it by laboratory evaluation of the discharge.

In men, discharge from the urethra, at the tip of the penis, is evident. In women, a pelvic examination is usually required to identify and examine the discharge from the cervix or the urethra.

If no discharge is seen (but gonorrhea is still suspected), the first drops of urine passed by either a man or a woman can be tested for bacteria.

Treatment is with antibiotics, which can cure the disease and prevent its spread, though some strains of the bacterium are becoming resistant to the antibiotics that once killed them. It is essential that you inform your sexual partners so that they can also be treated.

Chlamydia

This sexually transmitted disease is caused by the microorganism *Chlamydia trachomatis.* Chlamydia is epidemic in the United States; an estimated 4 million new cases occur every year.

Because symptoms are vague or nonexistent, half of men and 75% of women who have it are unaware of their condition and do not receive treatment.

Infection can lead to serious complications, such as pelvic inflammatory disease (PID) (see p.1077), scarring of the fallopian tubes, which causes ectopic pregnancy (see p.929), and infertility (see p.904). More than 60% of infants born to infected women become infected, often developing eye infections or pneumonia.

In men, chlamydia is a com-

mon cause of nongonococcal urethritis (see p.892). Chlamydia may also cause epididymitis (see p.1089) and pain in the testicles.

Sexually active women are at greatest risk, particularly those who are in their teens or early 20s who have unprotected sex with multiple partners. Men who fit the same profile are also at higher risk.

SYMPTOMS

Chlamydia usually produces no symptoms. If symptoms occur, a woman may have a vaginal discharge, a burning sensation when urinating, or abdominal pain. Men may have a discharge from the penis and burning during urination.

Infection of the rectum (see Proctitis, p.797) due to infection spread by anal intercourse may produce rectal discharge or pain during a bowel movement. A person who performs oral sex can, rarely, get a chlamydial infection of the throat.

TREATMENT OPTIONS

Your physician can test the discharge from your urethra to diagnose the infection. In men, discharge from the urethra, at the tip of the penis, may be evident. In women, a pelvic examination is usually required to identify and examine the discharge from the cervix or the urethra.

The results of an examination are often normal even though the person is infected; therefore, tests should be performed regularly. Newer tests are now available so that the first drops of urine passed by either a man or a woman can be tested for bacteria.

If you have chlamydia, your sexual partners must be informed and treated, or the cycle of infection will begin again. Avoid sexual intercourse until your treatment ends. Infection is treated with an antibiotic taken by mouth.

If the infection is not treated (or is treated inadequately), women can develop PID, which can cause infertility, pelvic pain, and ectopic pregnancy.

To help prevent chlamydial infection, use a condom and a spermicide containing nonoxynol 9, which may have some effect against chlamydia.

In recent years, every gene in the chlamydia microorganism has been identified. This scientific breakthrough is likely to lead to major advances in diagnosis and treatment of (and possibly immunization against) chlamydial infection.

Nongonococcal Urethritis

Nongonococcal urethritis is a sexually transmitted infection and inflammation of the urethra that is caused by organisms other than *Neisseria gonorrhoeae*, which causes gonorrhea.

The nongonococcal form is more prevalent than gonorrhea. Like gonorrhea, this sexually transmitted disease affects both men and women. Most cases are caused by an organism called *Chlamydia trachomatis* (see previous article); other cases are caused by organisms such as genital mycoplasma and trichomonas.

The symptoms are the same as for gonococcal urethritis: pain-

ful and frequent urination and discharge from the urethra. In men, the discharge is much more easily noticed because the tip of the urethra is highly visible. For this reason, nongonococcal urethritis is diagnosed more often in men.

Some men are infected with organisms such as chlamydia or genital mycoplasma and do not have any symptoms. White blood cells may be present in a urine sample or in discharge from the urethra. Specific tests for chlamydia, mycoplasma, or trichomonas can be performed on this discharge.

Treatment is with antibiotics. All sexual partners—including those who have no symptoms—should be treated.

Syphilis

Syphilis is a sexually transmitted infection caused by the bacterium *Treponema pallidum*. Although syphilis is less common than it once was, about 30,000 people every year still are infected with it. In rare cases, syphilis is transmitted from a woman to her fetus.

Unless syphilis is treated, the bacteria remain in your body and can cause serious complications many years after infection. Complications can include vision loss, hearing loss, memory loss, change in personality, and other neurologic or cardiac problems.

SYMPTOMS

Untreated syphilis progresses through several stages:

Primary syphilis Between 3 and 90 days after infection, a chancre (painless ulcer) appears

on the genitals (including the vagina or cervix), rectum, or mouth. It may be accompanied by swollen lymph glands near the site of infection.

Without treatment, the chancre goes away within 6 weeks, but the bacteria stay in the body. In about 15% to 30% of people who get syphilis, the chancre either does not develop or goes unnoticed.

Secondary syphilis Within 2 to 8 weeks after the chancre has gone away, you may get a headache, sore throat, and fever. Your lymph glands may swell again and a rash of nonitchy, tiny red bumps may appear; if you have dark skin, the rash will appear to be darker than the normal color of your skin.

The rash may appear on your palms and soles, which are unusual locations for most rashes.

Highly contagious, painless, silvery patches may occur on the penis, mouth, or vulva. If syphilis is not treated at this stage, symptoms will ultimately subside after 1 to 2 months. However, the bacteria are still in your body.

Tertiary syphilis Many years elapse without any symptoms, but the bacteria remain inside you, causing silent damage. Then, symptoms can develop. This is tertiary syphilis, and it can cause devastating irreversible brain damage (leading to dementia and paralysis) and damage to the heart, bones, skin, and internal organs.

TREATMENT OPTIONS

See your doctor if you have any symptoms, or if you think you have had sexual contact with someone who has syphilis. Do not have sexual intercourse; the sores and patches (which occur during the first and second stages on the mucous membranes) are teeming with bacteria and can easily be transmitted to sexual partners.

Your doctor can confirm a diagnosis of syphilis by testing the fluid from a chancre or by special blood tests. Penicillin given by injection is usually suc-cessful in treating people in the first stage and, often, the second stage. In later stages, some irre-versible damage can be done to organs. Treatment aims to pre-vent the bacteria from causing more damage. The risk of syphilis can be reduced by prac-ticing safer sex (see p.76).

A fetus that is born to a woman with untreated syphilis dies about 40% of the time.

Approximately 10% to 30% of infants who are born to women with untreated syphilis show signs (many of which can be serious) of syphilis infection.

In recent years, every gene in the syphilis bacterium has been identified. This scientific break-through is likely to lead to major advances in diagnosis and treat-ment of (and possibly immuniza-tion against) syphilis.

IMMUNE SYSTEM DISEASES

Anaphylaxis

Anaphylaxis is an immediate and severe, sometimes life-threaten-ing, allergic reaction that occurs within minutes of exposure to an allergy-producing substance (called an allergen).

SYMPTOMS

The most serious consequence of anaphylaxis is a life-threatening narrowing or closing of the air passages, which permit breath-ing. Victims cannot breathe and find it difficult to speak or swal-low; choking and even death may result.

Anaphylaxis may also cause a dramatic and sudden decrease in blood pressure (shock) that can lead to loss of consciousness. Either reaction is a medical emer-gency. Anaphylaxis also often produces an intensely itchy, red, blistery rash or a swelling around the eyes or lips.

TREATMENT OPTIONS

The list of substances that can cause anaphylaxis is extensive. The most common causes are insect venom, injected penicillin, and foods such as shellfish and peanuts. If you have had a previ-ous anaphylactic reaction from penicillin, you may also react to antibiotic drugs that are chemi-cally related, such as those in the cephalosporin family.

If you have had a mild form of anaphylaxis, you are at higher risk of having a severe reaction if you are exposed again to the allergen that produced the first anaphylactic reaction. Therefore, it is important that you wear a medical identification tag (see p.1190) in the form of a bracelet or necklace to inform others that you have had an anaphylactic reaction to a particular substance.

Get immediate emergency help for a person who appears to have anaphylaxis; it can cause death within minutes. Injecting a drug called epinephrine opens the airways and restores blood pressure.

If you have had a previous anaphylactic reaction, your doc-tor will prescribe epinephrine. You will be instructed on how to inject yourself and advised to carry an epinephrine-filled syringe with you at all times in case you have another reaction.

Polymyositis and Dermatomyositis

Polymyositis is a rare, autoim-mune disease (see p.870) that affects about 1 of 200,000 people. Muscle tissue becomes inflamed, which leads to muscle weakness and other symptoms.

When a skin rash appears along with the inflammation of muscles, the disease is called der-matomyositis (dermato = skin; myositis = muscle inflammation). More than two thirds of people with polymyositis or dermato-myositis are women.

Polymyositis and dermato-myositis can last for months or years, but occasionally they go away without treatment. Some adults also have a connective tis-sue disease such as lupus erythe-matosus (see p.898) or sclero-derma (see p.897) in combination with polymyositis.

A small number of people with dermatomyositis also get cancer of the lungs, ovaries, breasts, or other organs.

A very serious form of der-matomyositis in childhood pro-duces inflamed blood vessels, which can result in perforation

About Corticosteroid Drugs

Immune system disorders are often characterized by inflammation, and few drugs are more effective in reducing inflammation than corticosteroids.

Corticosteroid drugs are related to the body's naturally occurring hormone cortisol, which is produced by the adrenal glands. One of the natural actions of cortisol is to reduce inflammation.

Corticosteroids can be injected directly into a painful shoulder or tendon to relieve inflammation, inhaled into the lungs to calm the lung inflammation that occurs with asthma, or applied as creams to inflamed skin. When taken in these ways, they cause few adverse side effects.

When the areas of inflammation that need to be calmed are widespread or located deep inside the body, corticosteroids are given either as intravenous infusions or, more frequently, as pills. The pills used most often are prednisone and prednisolone. Low doses taken for relatively short periods produce few side effects. Many conditions are successfully treated with such doses.

For other conditions, however, it is necessary to take high doses over a long period of time. This can cause mild side effects such as weight gain from increased appetite and fluid retention, excessive hair growth, easy bruising, and slow healing of wounds. It also can cause serious side effects such as osteoporosis, bleeding in the stomach (particularly if used with nonsteroidal anti-inflammatory drugs such as aspirin), mood disturbances, high blood pressure, cataracts, glaucoma, and diabetes.

Another severe side effect from high doses of corticosteroid pills taken for long periods is reduced function of the adrenal glands. This happens when the brain, recognizing the drug circulating in the blood, no longer directs the adrenal glands to make natural cortisol; the adrenal glands then shrink from lack of activity.

Your doctor may recommend that you gradually stop taking the medication. When the medication is stopped, it takes time for the brain and the adrenal glands to resume their natural cortisol production. For this reason, any reduction in your dose of corticosteroids must be tapered off slowly under your doctor's guidance; suddenly stopping the drug can cause serious illness or death.

Your physician will want to see you regularly while you are taking corticosteroid drugs to watch for side effects. He or she may periodically perform blood tests.

With care, corticosteroids can help you live with—and, in some cases, overcome—a chronic inflammatory disease.

---

of the intestines. This childhood disease is extremely rare, affecting fewer than 1 of 1 million children.

SYMPTOMS

Symptoms vary among affected people. Usually, polymyositis comes on slowly, producing fatigue and severe muscle weakness. If it progresses to an advanced stage, heart failure (see p.683) from weakening of the heart muscle can result.

In dermatomyositis, patches of skin take on a reddish or purplish hue, with scaly, itchy areas. The skin of the eyelids, the area just above the eyes, and the skin over the knuckles are most often affected.

TREATMENT OPTIONS

Your doctor may perform electromyography (see p.162), a test that measures the electrical movement of the muscles, and blood tests to look for enzymes that indicate muscle injury. The best test is a muscle biopsy (see p.161), in which a tiny sample of muscle tissue is removed for examination in a laboratory.

The most common treatment is high doses of corticosteroid drugs (see About Corticosteroid Drugs, above) to control muscle and skin inflammation. If corticosteroids fail, immunosuppressive drugs may be prescribed.

Sometimes, intravenous infusions of antibodies called intravenous immunoglobulin are used. Most people respond well to one of these options; however, relapses can occur.

Physical therapy may be recommended to improve muscle strength. Occasionally, the disease does not respond to any treatment. In rare cases, it is fatal.

Reiter Syndrome

Reiter syndrome is characterized by arthritis (see p.605); urethritis (see p.808), which is inflammation of the urethra; and conjunctivitis (see p.427), which is inflammation of the outer covering of the eye.

The condition, which is more common in men, may be caused by a faulty immune system response (see Autoimmune Diseases, p.870) to the bacteria that cause dysentery or those that cause infections of the sexual organs.

There is a genetic component to Reiter syndrome; most people who have it have inherited a particular gene that results in the abnormal immune system response.

SYMPTOMS

Symptoms include burning during urination (from the urethritis), irritation of and discharge from the eyes (from the conjunctivitis), and joint pain and swelling (from the arthritis). These symptoms are often accompanied by weakness, fatigue, fever, and weight loss.

The arthritis usually involves one or two joints, and may last for several days or several months. Low back pain is common. Your ligaments and tendons may also feel hot and inflamed. Mouth ulcers, genital sores, and small crusting sores on the palms and soles may also occur. Many affected people have only the arthritis and no other symptoms.

TREATMENT OPTIONS

Your doctor may prescribe painkillers and nonsteroidal anti-inflammatory drugs to treat the symptoms of arthritis. Corticosteroid drugs, injected directly into an affected joint, can help relieve pain and swelling. Your physician may also prescribe antibiotic drugs.

Treatment is usually effective, although it may not cure the disorder. Reiter syndrome recurs in about one third of people who have it, requiring further treatment, sometimes with slow-acting antirheumatic drugs such as sulfasalazine or methotrexate.

Sarcoidosis

Sarcoidosis is a disease that can cause inflammation in almost any organ, but it most often affects the lungs, eyes, skin, liver, and lymph glands. Immune system cells (particularly one type of immune system cell called a helper-inducer T cell) congregate in various organs to cause inflammation.

Characteristic tiny clumps of cells, called sarcoid granulomas, are formed in the course of the inflammation. Sarcoid granulomas are harmless in themselves but, by virtue of their location (such as in the lining of the lungs and on the eyes) or their size, can cause significant health problems.

The cause of sarcoidosis is not known. The disease affects about 1 of 5,000 to 10,000 people in the United States; women are somewhat more susceptible than men, and blacks are more than 10 times as likely as whites to have the disease.

SYMPTOMS

Many people with sarcoidosis have no symptoms. When symptoms do occur, they usually begin between ages 20 and 40 and may be mild or severe. They also are extremely variable, since so many different organs can be affected.

Like other diseases that produce inflammation throughout the body, sarcoidosis can produce general symptoms such as fatigue, weakness, aching muscles, swollen lymph glands, fever, lack of appetite, and weight loss. In addition, symptoms occur that are specific to the organs that are affected by the disease.

The lungs are affected in about 90% of people with sarcoidosis; shortness of breath, wheezing, and dry cough are common symptoms. The shortness of breath can become so severe that it greatly limits normal activities and can even become life-threatening, requiring a lung transplant.

Some people have joint pain from arthritis. When the disease affects the skin, it can cause painful red nodules (called erythema nodosum), purple patches of scaly skin, acnelike pimples, or cysts.

When sarcoidosis affects the eyes, it can cause blurred vision, tearing, and sensitivity to light. If not treated, blindness can result. Individual nerves, especially nerves of the head, can be affected, leading to a drooping eyelid, weakness on one side of the face, or other symptoms.

TREATMENT OPTIONS

Since many people with sarcoidosis have no symptoms, the disease is sometimes diagnosed by chance. For example, a chest x-ray performed for another reason might show the disease in the lungs or the lymph glands near a lung.

Because the initial symptoms are usually subtle, diagnosis of sarcoidosis can be challenging. It can easily be mistaken for other conditions, including cancer or an infectious disease such as tuberculosis.

Blood tests sometimes reveal higher-than-normal levels of calcium or of angiotensin-converting enzyme. The best test is a biopsy (see p.161) of lung tissue using a bronchoscope (see p.525) or a biopsy of skin or the swollen lymph glands.

Many cases of sarcoidosis are not severe enough to require treatment. Your doctor will want to evaluate your condition periodically to assess whether the disease is progressing. Helpful tests include chest x-rays, lung function tests (see p.494), or eye examinations.

Treatment is often started when the chest x-rays and lung function tests indicate the disease is progressing and interfering with the ability of your lungs to get oxygen. Treatment may also be required if you have ongoing eye inflammation, severe joint disease, painful or disfiguring skin conditions, or impaired nerve function.

When treatment is required, corticosteroid drugs (see p.895) usually control the inflammation. Most people can live successfully with sarcoidosis when they take these drugs. The majority of people with sarcoidosis recover fully within 2 years. There is currently no way to predict who will recover forever, have a recurrence, or become progressively worse (which occurs infrequently with current treatments).

Scleroderma

Scleroderma means hard skin. This autoimmune disease (see

p.870) causes hardness and stiffness of the skin due to overproduction of collagen, the protein that (in normal amounts) gives skin strength and elasticity. In some people, damage to internal organs also occurs.

When skin involvement is widespread as a result of the overproduction of collagen, the disease is called systemic sclerosis or diffuse scleroderma.

Scleroderma affects about 1 of 2,000 people, and women three times more often than men. It occurs more commonly among blacks than whites.

SYMPTOMS

There are two main types of scleroderma: limited and diffuse.

Limited scleroderma causes skin to become shiny and uncomfortably tight on the face and fingers. Sweat glands and hair

follicles are greatly diminished in the affected areas so the skin is dry and hairless. Limited scleroderma sometimes improves on its own. It is almost always accompanied by Raynaud phenomenon (see Raynaud Disease, p.706), a painful condition in which the flow of blood to the hands and feet is constricted, making them abnormally sensitive to heat and cold.

Diffuse scleroderma is the more serious form, affecting one or more major internal organs (such as the arteries, kidneys, and lungs) as well as the skin. Raynaud phenomenon is almost always present. Life-threatening complications can result.

When scleroderma affects the blood vessels in the kidneys, it can cause exceptionally high blood pressure and kidney damage. Respiratory problems, which

Scleroderma

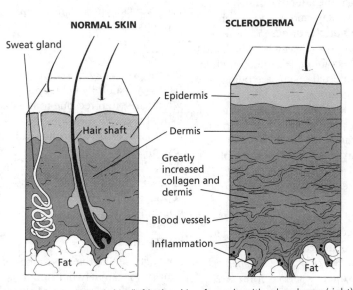

NORMAL SKIN

Sweat gland

Hair shaft

Fat

SCLERODERMA

Epidermis

Dermis

Greatly increased collagen and dermis

Blood vessels

Inflammation

Fat

In contrast to normal skin (left), the skin of people with scleroderma (right) has an overproduction of collagen. This causes a thickening and hardening of the dermis and a thinning of the epidermis. Sweat glands and hair follicles are greatly diminished.

are very common in diffuse scleroderma, cause shortness of breath and increased susceptibility to pneumonia (see p.496).

Gastrointestinal problems, such as severe heartburn, bloating, diarrhea, and constipation, frequently occur. You may also have difficulty swallowing due to stiffness of the esophagus.

TREATMENT OPTIONS

Scleroderma is a potentially serious condition that requires close medical attention. Skin changes, coupled with the characteristic symptoms, often make the diagnosis clear. Sometimes, blood tests and a skin biopsy (see p.161) are used to confirm the diagnosis.

Doctors use specific approaches to manage the milder symptoms of scleroderma; for example, eating small meals helps minimize gastrointestinal problems, and taking drugs to dilate (open) the arteries can help relieve Raynaud phenomenon.

When the disease is more serious—such as when the hands are becoming deformed or when the internal organs are being badly damaged from the progressive thickening of tissue—the drug penicillamine may help prevent further skin thickening and organ damage in some people. Corticosteroid drugs (see p.895) can reduce swelling but do not slow the overall progression of the disease.

People whose internal organs are not affected within the first few years of diagnosis usually have the less serious form. About 3% of people with scleroderma die prematurely.

Sjögren Syndrome

Sjögren syndrome is characterized by dry eyes and dry mouth. Sometimes it occurs in people who have no other disease and sometimes it occurs in people with rheumatoid arthritis (see p.606), scleroderma (see p.897), or systemic lupus erythematosus (see right).

Sjögren syndrome is probably an autoimmune disease (see p.870) in which the immune system attacks the small glands that produce tears, saliva, or both. The cause is unknown, but genetic factors and viruses are thought to play a role. In rare cases, cancers of the lymph glands known as lymphomas (see p.727) develop in people with Sjögren syndrome.

Sjögren syndrome is remarkably common, particularly in older people. About 1 of 100 people over the age of 60 has this illness. It affects women approximately nine times more often than men.

SYMPTOMS

People with Sjögren syndrome have dry, painfully itchy eyes, which are often red due to the lack of tears. Dryness of the mouth can cause difficulty swallowing and speaking. Because of the lack of moisture, people with Sjögren syndrome are more susceptible to eye and throat infections and dental problems.

TREATMENT OPTIONS

To diagnose Sjögren syndrome, your physician may perform tests to evaluate your tear production and blood tests to look for specific abnormal antibodies, which are present in those who have

the disease. The diagnosis may be confirmed by a biopsy (see p.161) of the lip.

Mild cases of dry eye can be treated with tear substitutes in eyedrop form that mimic the natural tear film; eye ointments are available for nighttime use. It is important to report any eye infection to your doctor so that it can be treated. Avoid wind, smoke, air conditioning, and dry indoor air (use a humidifier), and wear goggles while swimming. See your ophthalmologist regularly.

Dry mouth is more difficult to treat. Saliva substitutes can be sprayed into the mouth. Because bacteria thrive when saliva levels are low, it is essential for you to maintain good dental hygiene; use fluoride-containing toothpaste, fluoride gels, or rinses; and have regular dental checkups. Your doctor may prescribe corticosteroid drugs (see p.895) if your symptoms are severe.

Systemic Lupus Erythematosus

Systemic lupus erythematosus (SLE), commonly known as lupus, is a classic example of an autoimmune disease (see p.870). In SLE, the immune system mistakenly makes antibodies to certain components of the cell nuclei, such as DNA. The disease attacks connective tissue in the body as though it were foreign, injuring and sometimes destroying vital organs such as the joints, kidneys, brain, and heart.

Lupus can injure almost any part of the body. If it affects only the skin, the condition is called either subacute cutaneous lupus erythematosus or discoid lupus, depending on the type of rash that is present.

For most people, lupus is mild; about 20% of people recover from it spontaneously. Many others can lead an essentially normal life, even with the chronic symptoms.

Researchers believe that lupus is caused by a combination of factors, including genetic inheritance and possibly an infection or hormonal changes.

It affects about 1 of 3,000 to 4,000 people in the United States. The disease affects blacks almost three times as often as whites; the vast majority of individuals

affected are women in their childbearing years.

SYMPTOMS

Symptoms of lupus vary greatly, depending on which tissues have been attacked and to what degree. The earliest symptoms of lupus are nonspecific, meaning that they could be attributed to a number of conditions.

Fever, fatigue, aches and pains, loss of appetite, weight loss, nausea, and malaise are among the symptoms experienced by most people with lupus. In addition, nearly all affected people have painful, aching joints and muscles. Many develop joint swelling

that causes discomfort and, occasionally, permanent joint damage.

Most people with lupus also have skin problems, and some have an abnormal sensitivity to sunlight, even after limited exposure, with symptoms such as severe rash and fever. (For tips on avoiding sunlight, see Preventing Skin Cancer, p.548.)

Other people with lupus have mouth ulcers, coinlike (discoid) skin sores, hair loss, or a butterfly-shaped rash across the bridge of the nose and upper cheeks on both sides of the face. Lupus symptoms can flare up at any time and are often triggered by ultravi-

Lupus: When You Visit Your Doctor

QUESTIONS YOUR DOCTOR MIGHT ASK:

■ Have you had any of the following symptoms: joint pain; fatigue; difficulty concentrating; depression; headaches; changes in vision; sudden weakness in an arm or leg; swelling of the feet; wide fluctuations in weight; easy bruising; new rashes; fever; hair loss; pains in the chest; or sores in the mouth, nose, or vagina? Any of these symptoms could reflect a worsening of the lupus. Ask your doctor which symptoms should prompt you to call him or her and what organs are affected by your lupus.

■ Are you trying to get pregnant? If so, ask your doctor which medications, if any, you should stop taking.

YOUR DOCTOR MIGHT EXAMINE THE FOLLOWING FUNCTIONS AND BODY SYSTEMS:

■ Blood pressure

■ Mouth, scalp, skin, lungs, heart, lymph glands, and joints. These are the parts of the body most often affected by lupus.

THE FOLLOWING LAB TESTS OR STUDIES MAY BE ORDERED:

■ Tests for antinuclear antibodies, antiphospholipid antibodies, and anti-DNA antibodies. These tests should be done at least once because they help diagnose lupus and its complications.

■ Urine tests, creatinine levels (to check for kidney damage), and a complete blood cell count (to check for anemia and low platelet count). These tests should be done periodically.

■ If you are being treated with nonsteroidal anti-inflammatory drugs, a complete blood cell count and kidney function tests. The tests should be done periodically because these drugs can cause gastrointestinal bleeding and kidney problems.

■ If you are taking corticosteroids, a complete blood cell count and a test of your blood sugar level. These tests should be done periodically because corticosteroids can cause gastrointestinal bleeding and an elevated blood sugar level.

olet light from the sun, emotional stress, fatigue, or other factors.

The most severe complications of lupus involve damage by the immune system to major organs, especially the kidneys. When the lungs are affected, inflammation of the lining of the lungs (see Pleurisy, p.502) can result.

In some people, lupus affects the heart's valves and/or the heart muscle itself, sometimes causing heart failure. Lupus can also cause an inflammation of the membrane around the heart (see Pericarditis, p.697) and heart rhythm disturbances (see p.672).

When lupus affects the brain and nervous system, it can cause headaches, seizures, hallucinations, and loss of movement or sensation. However, milder mental dysfunction such as depression or impaired concentration is more common.

People with lupus are also prone to blood cell abnormalities, due in part to antibodies that attack and destroy specific blood cells, including red blood cells, white blood cells, and platelets (see p.709). Blood clots may form in veins and arteries, causing serious consequences such as stroke (see p.342).

Pregnant women who have lupus are at increased risk of miscarriage. However, most women are able to carry to term with good outcomes for both mother and newborn, especially when the lupus is well-controlled before and during pregnancy.

TREATMENT OPTIONS

The vagueness and intermittence of symptoms combined with the lack of a conclusive diagnostic test make lupus notoriously difficult to diagnose; one study found

that it took an average of 8 years for people with lupus to obtain a definitive diagnosis.

Your doctor may perform several blood tests, including a test for abnormal antibodies called antinuclear antibodies (ANAs). ANAs are present in the majority of people who have lupus but also in people who have several other conditions. In fact, up to 30% of healthy people have low levels of ANA in their blood. Thus, a positive ANA test result does not necessarily mean you have lupus, but a negative test result is strong evidence that you do not.

Two other unusual antibodies are found in some people with lupus: anti-DNA antibodies and anti-Sm antibodies. These antibodies are found essentially only in people with lupus, but not in all people who have lupus. When these antibodies are found, lupus is the likely diagnosis, but the absence of the antibodies does not mean you do not have lupus.

Treatment of lupus is individualized to your circumstances and directed by the symptoms and signs of your illness. Joint pain may be treated with nonsteroidal anti-inflammatory drugs. Pleurisy or severe arthritis may be treated with corticosteroid drugs (see p.895), which often bring rapid and dramatic improvement, although they also can produce side effects.

Immunosuppressive drugs such as azathioprine or cyclophosphamide can help reduce your reliance on corticosteroids and may lessen damage to inflamed organs such as the kidneys.

For people who have milder joint pain, skin symptoms, or

general symptoms (such as fatigue), antimalarial antibiotics, such as hydroxychloroquine, may be effective, though it is not known why.

You can also take self-care measures to reduce flare-ups. Reduce stress, strive for a balance between rest and exercise, eat a healthy diet, and join a support group to help you cope.

For a small percentage of people with lupus, the disease cannot be controlled and its effects are devastating. For about 2% to 3% of affected people, it is fatal, despite all therapeutic efforts.

Polymyalgia Rheumatica and Temporal Arteritis

Polymyalgia rheumatica is a condition in which there is pain and stiffness of the shoulders, upper arms, lower back, hips, and thighs.

A small percentage of people (5% to 15%) with polymyalgia rheumatica develop a type of blood vessel inflammation known as vasculitis that affects medium and large arteries; when this occurs, the condition is called temporal arteritis.

Inflammation can cause the arteries to thicken and narrow, which reduces the amount of blood the artery can carry. In temporal arteritis, the inflammation occurs in branches of the carotid arteries, including the temporal artery, which is located on the upper sides of your face. These arteries provide blood (and with it, oxygen) to the muscles of the face, tongue, jaw, and retina of the eyes.

Both polymyalgia rheumatica and temporal arteritis occur much more often in people older than

Polymyalgia Rheumatica: *Dr Shmerling's Advice*

Most people with polymyalgia rheumatica or temporal arteritis do very well with the recommended treatment. One thing I've found is that some doctors (and patients) become fixated on the erythrocyte sedimentation rate ("sed rate") blood test that we use to monitor how the treatment is working.

The test gives a number, and numbers are easy to understand. Sometimes the blood test number is not quite back down to "normal" and everyone worries about it, even though the patient is clearly much, much better. Sometimes the doctor even tries to drive the test number down to normal by increasing doses of the medicine. That's a mistake.

There may be an innocent explanation: the sed rate rises somewhat above what is called "normal" as part of healthy aging, and the slightly elevated test number may reflect nothing more than that.

If you are under treatment, and feeling much better, but your doctor says your sed rate is still high and you need more medicine, be sure to discuss this explanation of the test with your doctor, before agreeing to take more medication. The doctor should treat the person, not the test result.

ROBERT SHMERLING, MD
BETH ISRAEL DEACONESS MEDICAL CENTER
HARVARD MEDICAL SCHOOL

55, affecting about 1 of 200 in this age group. However, either condition can occur earlier in life. It is not known what causes either disease.

SYMPTOMS

People who have polymyalgia rheumatica often have general symptoms of illness such as malaise, fever, and loss of appetite and weight. Your body may ache, with pain in the muscles of your neck, shoulders, lower back, hips, and thighs, particularly in the morning.

In addition to these symptoms, people with temporal arteritis may experience a throbbing headache on one or both sides of the head, usually above and just in front of the ears. Your scalp may feel sore to the touch, and you may have pain in your jaw and tongue, especially when chewing.

Vision problems, including loss of vision, are the most serious effects of untreated temporal arteritis, but they can almost

always be prevented by early treatment.

Because of the potential for permanent vision loss, a person (especially someone over the age of 55) who starts to feel generally ill, notices the unusual type of headache, and/or has an aching in the shoulders, upper arms, hips, or thighs should contact his or her doctor immediately.

TREATMENT OPTIONS

Although the symptoms of temporal arteritis often are enough to make a diagnosis, your doctor should confirm his or her suspicions by performing a biopsy of the temporal artery.

This involves taking a sample of the artery during a minor surgical procedure that does not require an overnight stay in the hospital. The sample is examined under a microscope for signs of inflammation.

Your doctor may also perform blood tests that measure erythrocyte sedimentation rate (see

p.157) to diagnose polymyalgia rheumatica or temporal arteritis.

Both conditions respond well to treatment with corticosteroid drugs (see p.895). For people with polymyalgia rheumatica, low doses are usually adequate. Treating temporal arteritis, however, requires higher doses, which carries a higher risk of side effects, especially in elderly people. The risk of these side effects is justified not only by how much better people feel with treatment but also because treatment can prevent blindness.

Although, at the start, the corticosteroid pills must be taken every day, after a while your doctor may advise you to take them every other day to reduce the risk of serious side effects.

Your doctor will monitor your condition to determine how well the drug is working to reduce the inflammation of your arteries. Treatment may be necessary for several months or even years. Relapses of temporal arteritis and polymyalgia rheumatica may occur, but most people recover completely from both.

Vasculitis

Vasculitis literally means inflammation of the blood vessels. Vasculitis can occur in any blood vessel, damaging the lining of the vessel and sometimes narrowing or completely blocking it, reducing blood flow or stopping it altogether.

The inflammation causes a cascade of physical problems. Damage to the blood vessel walls results in loss of blood and oxygen to the tissues that the vessels supply, along with damage to the body systems that are supported by the oxygen-deprived tissues. Consequently, the symptoms of vasculitis vary dramatically.

The causes of most types of vasculitis are not known, but an autoimmune disease (see p.870) may be responsible. Researchers also suspect that an allergic reaction, infection with a virus, or even damage to blood vessels from the sun's radiation may cause vasculitis.

Vasculitis may develop in people with chronic rheumatic illnesses such as rheumatoid arthritis (see p.606), may follow an infection, or may develop without any apparent cause.

The following are different types of vasculitis, and are distinguished by the size of the blood vessels involved, the organs involved, and the presence of antibodies called antineutrophil cytoplasmic antibodies (ANCAs):

Takayasu arteritis is a type of vasculitis that affects women under the age of 40 almost exclusively. Inflammation occurs in large blood vessels such as the artery leaving the heart (the aorta). People with this type of arteritis may feel weak, dizzy, and light-headed and have severe muscle pain. The arteries to the arms and legs can become so narrowed from the arteritis that it can be impossible to feel a pulse in the arms or legs, despite normal blood pressure.

Temporal arteritis (see p.900) is a kind of vasculitis that affects medium to large vessels.

Polyarteritis nodosa is a type of vasculitis affecting the small and medium arteries in which the walls of the arteries become inflamed and weakened. Several groups of blood vessels may be affected, including the arteries that serve the kidneys, intestines, and heart. Exposure to the hepatitis B (see p.759) virus has been strongly implicated as a cause of polyarteritis nodosa in some people.

Polyarteritis nodosa is one of the few immune system diseases in which more men are affected than women. Symptoms include aching muscles and joints, fever, loss of appetite, and nerve damage that may cause leg weakness. Other symptoms reflect the area of the body that is served by the damaged blood vessels.

High blood pressure, muscle weakness, skin ulcers, and gangrene may occur. If the blood supply to the intestines is affected, you may have nausea, vomiting, abdominal pain, diarrhea, and blood in the stool. Your doctor can diagnose polyarteritis nodosa by performing a biopsy or by angiography (see p.147), in which dye is injected into blood vessels so that any abnormalities can be seen on x-rays.

Corticosteroid drugs (see p.895) and immunosuppressive drugs may be prescribed to counteract inflammation of the arteries.

Wegener granulomatosis is a very rare form of vasculitis in which inflammation targets the blood vessels in the lungs, sinuses, and kidneys. Symptoms include coughing, a bloody discharge from the nose, breathing difficulty, chest pain, and blood in the urine. The ANCA test result is often positive.

TREATMENT OPTIONS

Treatment depends on the size, extent, and location of the affected blood vessels. The first step is to identify and remove any offending substances, such as a new medication, that may be causing the immune reaction. In some cases, the vasculitis disappears without treatment.

Most types respond very well to corticosteroid drugs (see p.895). Other therapies include immunosuppressive drugs to treat Wegener granulomatosis, antiviral drugs to treat polyarteritis nodosa caused by hepatitis B, surgery to treat advanced forms of Takayasu arteritis, and antibiotic drugs to treat skin vasculitis caused by bacteria.

Infertility, Pregnancy, and Childbirth

Each person begins life as a single cell, after an egg cell from a woman has been fertilized by a sperm cell from a man. That cell then divides and divides again, many times, in a controlled fashion, until there are trillions of cells organized to make a human being.

Although scientists have learned much about this process, a large part of it remains one of life's wonderful mysteries.

Sperm production Each day, a healthy man produces millions of sperm in his testicles. Follicle-stimulating hormone (FSH) initiates sperm production. Testosterone, stimulated by luteinizing hormone (LH), helps sperm mature. Boys become capable of producing sperm at puberty, which usually occurs between ages 10 and 14.

During ejaculation, semen transports between 200 and 500 million sperm into the woman's vagina. Looking like tadpoles under a microscope, the sperm move toward the uterus, in search of an egg. Only about 100 of the sperm succeed in reaching the fallopian tube and contacting an egg. Most of the time, none of them fertilizes an egg.

Egg production A female baby already carries within her about 700,000 immature eggs. Between the time she is born and the time she begins puberty, most of the eggs have already died; only about 300,000 are left. Each egg sits in a little nest in the ovary called a follicle.

When a girl reaches puberty, she begins to have a monthly menstrual cycle, which varies in length, but averages about 28 days. In each menstrual cycle, several eggs begin to mature, but usually one egg matures more than the others.

During the first half of the menstrual cycle, cells in the follicles that surround the maturing eggs produce the hormone estrogen. Estrogen causes the fallopian tubes to contract, and the lining of the uterus (the endometrium) to thicken.

Release of the egg About midway through the menstrual cycle, the ovary releases the most mature egg (ovulation). The follicle in which the egg was resting changes into a structure called the corpus luteum, which starts to produce the hormone progesterone.

Progesterone (produced during the last half of each menstrual cycle) travels in the blood to the uterus, where it stimulates new blood vessels to provide a nourishing, blood-rich lining for the fertilized egg to attach and begin to grow. The corpus luteum stops producing progesterone if a fertilized egg does not attach to the lining of the uterus. As progesterone stimulation to the endometrium decreases, the uterine lining is shed (menstruation).

How does the ovary know when an egg is mature and when it should be released? An area of the brain (hypothalamus) acts as the menstrual clock. It makes gonadotropin-releasing hormone (GnRH), which travels to the pituitary gland (just underneath the brain), causing FSH and LH to be made.

At the beginning of each menstrual cycle, the pituitary gland releases FSH, which travels through the bloodstream to the ovary and helps follicles containing eggs develop and make estrogen.

On about the 11th day of an average menstrual cycle, the pituitary gland increases the production of LH. A surge of LH travels in the blood to the ovary, triggers the release of the egg from the follicle, and stimulates the corpus luteum to produce progesterone. At the end of a menstrual cycle in which no egg has been fertilized, the pituitary gland stops making LH, the ovary stops making progesterone, and menstruation begins again.

How is this cycle controlled so that it starts again every month in which pregnancy has not occurred? The answer again is hormones communicating with hormones.

Just as hormones (FSH and LH) from the pituitary gland travel through the blood, reach the ovary, and cause the ovary to make the hormones estrogen and progesterone, the reverse also occurs. Hormones made by the ovaries—estrogen, progesterone, and inhibin—travel through the blood to the brain and tell the brain when to turn its hormones on and off.

This conversation between the hormones of the brain and of the ovary is what initiates each new menstrual cycle during a woman's reproductive years.

Fertilization and implantation of the egg After an egg is released, it is surrounded by dozens of tiny fingerlike projections (fimbriae) at the end of the fallopian tube. The fimbriae gently guide the egg into the fallop-ian tube, and contractions of the tube carry the egg through the tube toward the uterus.

At the same time, if sexual intercourse has occurred, sperm move up through the uterus and into the fallopian tubes. Sperm are capable of fertilizing an egg up to 40 hours after intercourse.

Sperm and egg usually meet inside the fallopian tube. If a sperm cell successfully enters the egg cell and fertilizes it, the fertilized egg continues to travel through the fallopian tube and into the uterus. It comes to rest in the enriched lining of the uterus (implantation), where it begins to grow.

Conception—the process of fertilization—is a kind of marriage. The egg and sperm each contain half the genes necessary for a complete cell and, ultimately, a complete human being. The union of egg and sperm is finalized within 10 hours of the sperm fertilizing the egg, with the merging of these genes. Within 24 hours, the fertilized egg has started to divide and grow.

By the time 6 days have passed, a 16-celled embryo exists in the uterus. There, if all goes well, it will spend the next 36 to 40 weeks, nourished by the enriched lining of the uterus and then by the placenta, an organ that forms from the embryo and attaches to the uterus.

After 8 weeks, an embryo is called a fetus. During the embryo's development into a fetus, the placenta provides a life-support system—supplying oxygen and nutrients and removing waste. The health and growth of the fetus are directly related to the health and size of the placenta.

When fertilization does not occur If fertilization does not occur—and thus a fertilized egg does not implant in the uterus—the lining of the uterus is shed, leading to the bleeding called menstruation.

This process repeats itself about once every month in most women until a woman, usually in her late 40s to early 50s, goes through menopause.

INFERTILITY

Causes of Infertility

Most couples who want children can have them without difficulty, but some couples have problems conceiving. About one third of fertility problems have to do with male causes and about one third with female causes. The remaining third are either unknown or involve both the man and the woman.

For many couples, a pregnancy does not occur immediately. After 6 months of trying for a pregnancy, only 60% of couples achieve one. Infertility is defined as the inability to conceive after a year of regular intercourse. This happens in an estimated 10% to 15% of couples. However, many couples achieve pregnancy even after having been unable to do so for a year.

Infertility affects more than 6 million American couples. Today, with more knowledge about how lifestyle changes can improve fertility (see Improving Fertility, Naturally: Dr Domar's Advice, p.907), and with improvements in assisted reproductive technology, a pregnancy is achieved by 50% of previously infertile couples.

If you are considering seeking

Critical Events of Female Fertility

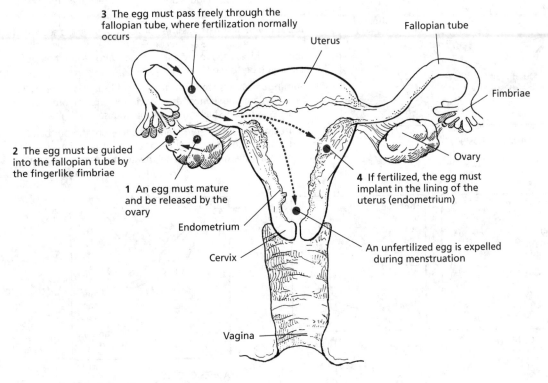

3 The egg must pass freely through the fallopian tube, where fertilization normally occurs

Uterus

Fallopian tube

Fimbriae

Ovary

4 If fertilized, the egg must implant in the lining of the uterus (endometrium)

An unfertilized egg is expelled during menstruation

2 The egg must be guided into the fallopian tube by the fingerlike fimbriae

1 An egg must mature and be released by the ovary

Endometrium

Cervix

Vagina

A woman's ability to become pregnant depends on the function and interaction of several organs.

medical help for infertility, check your medical insurance coverage early in the process. Insurance companies vary dramatically in the amount of fertility testing or treatment they pay for.

IN WOMEN

Age is one of the most important determinants of a woman's ability to conceive. When a woman is between the ages of 30 and 34, about 1 of 7 couples is infertile; between 35 and 39, the rate is about 1 of 5; and between ages 40 and 44, infertility affects 1 of 4 couples.

Other causes of infertility in women include:

■ Problems with the fallopian tubes (which transport the egg from the ovary to the uterus and where sperm and egg meet) represent nearly 30% of infertility problems.

The fallopian tubes can be blocked or pulled away from the ovaries due to scar tissue (adhesions). This damage to the fallopian tubes can be caused by pelvic inflammatory disease (see p.1077), a prior ectopic pregnancy (see p.929), endometriosis (see p.1071), or pelvic surgery.

■ Infrequent ovulation (release of an egg) causes up to 20% of female-related infertility problems. It can result from being extremely underweight or overweight or from having polycystic ovary syndrome (see p.1081). Disturbances of other hormone-producing glands (such as the thyroid, pituitary, or adrenal glands) can also interfere with ovulation.

■ Disorders of the uterus account for about 20% of female infertility. These disorders may prevent an egg from implanting in the uterine wall or may cause a miscarriage. They include noncancerous tu-

Surgery for Infertility

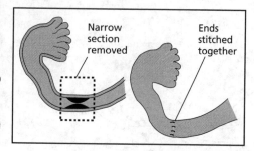

TUBAL REANASTOMOSIS

Several surgical techniques are used to correct anatomic causes of infertility:

Tubal reanastomosis involves surgically removing a section of blocked fallopian tube and reconnecting the two ends with stitches. This is used today only when in vitro fertilization cannot be performed.

Salpingostomy is employed to correct blockages at the end of the fallopian tube. It involves opening the fimbriae outward and, occasionally, stitching down the edges.

Adhesiotomy is surgery to remove adhesions (fibrous bands of tissue that abnormally connect structures) from fallopian tubes by releasing them with a scalpel, heated instrument, or laser.

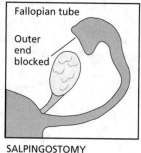

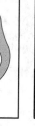

SALPINGOSTOMY

ADHESIOTOMY

mors such as fibroids (see p.1074), an extra fibrous band in the uterus, and scarring of the uterus caused by prior surgery. Endometriosis may cause release of toxic products or an ovarian cyst (see p.1080) that can block the release of eggs from an ovary.

IN MEN

About one third of infertility problems are caused by problems in the man. In order to be fertile, a man must be able to produce enough sperm and most of the sperm must be able to move adequately (this is called motility) in order to travel into the uterus and fallopian tubes.

A sperm must also be shaped normally (called morphology) to fertilize an egg. All men produce some abnormally shaped and poorly moving sperm; problems arise if too many of a man's sperm are abnormally shaped or move poorly.

The causes of abnormal sperm number, movement (motility), and shape are often unknown. Some known factors that can contribute to infertility in men include:

■ Sexually transmitted diseases (see p.889), such as gonorrhea and chlamydia, which can scar the vas deferens and prohibit the passage of sperm to the urethra.

■ Hormonal disorders, such as diabetes, which can cause nerve damage and impotence.

■ Inflammation of the testicles (see Orchitis, p.1089).

■ Varicose veins in the scrotum, called varicoceles (see p.1090).

■ Surgery, such as prostate surgery, that can cause scarring, nerve damage, or a blockage in the sperm's path to the urethra.

■ Impotence (see p.1092).

■ Retrograde ejaculation, in which sperm travel backward into the bladder.

■ Cystic fibrosis (see p.1003).

■ Using alcohol, tobacco, or illegal drugs, which can reduce the number of sperm produced or the motility of sperm.

Improving Fertility, Naturally: Dr Domar's Advice

There are simple things you and your partner can do to improve fertility:

■ **Exercise moderately** While regular exercise is good for everyone, in women, an exercise regimen that is too vigorous can actually diminish estrogen levels needed for ovulation and progesterone needed for the embryo to implant in the uterus. Women who engage in regular strenuous exercise should slow down to a more modest level (such as a 2-mile stroll each day). In men, vigorous exercise may reduce sperm production. Also, there is some evidence that sitting for long periods on hard bicycle seats can contribute to infertility in men.

■ **Avoid hot tubs** Extreme heat to a man's genitals—which are directly exposed to the high temperatures of hot tubs, whirlpools, saunas, and long hot baths—is thought to reduce production of viable sperm.

■ **Eat a nutritious and healthy diet** (see p.37) Good nutrition is particularly important in maximizing your fertility.

■ **Take vitamins** There is some evidence that taking the recommended daily amount of zinc improves a man's fertility. Women should take 400 micrograms of folic acid (folate) daily.

■ **Gain weight** If you are a thin woman, with a body mass index (BMI) of less than 17 (see p.51), you are less fertile. It will probably improve your fertility if you try to gain enough weight to have a BMI of at least 20.

■ **Lose weight** If you are an overweight woman and have a BMI over 27, your weight may make you less fertile. You will probably improve your fertility if you lose weight to reach a BMI of below 27.

■ **Avoid alcohol** If you are a woman, even moderate drinking (one drink a day) has been associated with lower fertility—as well as spontaneous miscarriages and fetal alcohol syndrome (see p.975). A man's fertility may be reduced by drinking more than two drinks a day, but this is still controversial.

■ **Give up smoking** In women, smoking is associated with decreased ability to become pregnant and an increased chance of stillbirths. In men, smoking may cause impotence (see p.1092).

■ **Avoid herbal supplements** Several, including St John's wort, may reduce fertility in both men and women.

■ **Review your medications** The following prescription and nonprescription (legal and illegal) drugs can interfere with your fertility: cimetidine, digitalis, antidepressants, hypertension medications, body-building steroids, marijuana, and cocaine.

■ **Reduce stress** Stress-reduction techniques (see p.90) can be very helpful for some couples. If you are having symptoms of depression (see p.395), you should get treatment for the depression before you try to get pregnant.

ALICE DOMAR, PHD
BETH ISRAEL DEACONESS MEDICAL CENTER
HARVARD MEDICAL SCHOOL

Infertility Testing and Treatment for Women

INFERTILITY HISTORY

When you see a physician for an infertility evaluation, he or she will first conduct a complete medical history that includes questions about previous pregnancies with all partners, menstrual periods, and any gynecologic problems, such as endometriosis or fibroids, that can make conception difficult. The doctor will also perform an examination and may order some of the tests described here.

TESTS

At-home ovulation tests These tests help determine whether and when you ovulate. Ovulation occurs about 2 weeks before the start of a menstrual period—defined as the first day of bleeding. Your doctor may recommend that you use one of the following methods to predict ovulation:

■ *Basal body temperature* One approach is to make a chart for several months on which you record your daily temperature immediately after awakening, using a sensitive basal body thermometer. You chart your temperature first thing in the morning every day over the course of several menstrual cycles.

Your temperature rises at the time of ovulation and remains higher for the rest of the cycle. After several months, if your cycles are regular, you will be able to estimate the time each month that you ovulate.

Your most fertile time is in the 5 days before you ovulate. During that time, you should have intercourse every 48 hours at minimum and as often as you wish at maximum. Daily or more frequent intercourse around ovulation is not harmful to the sperm count.

■ *Home urine tests* At-home urine tests for ovulation measure how much luteinizing hormone (LH) is circulating in your system. Large amounts are made in the brain the day before ovulation; they circulate in the blood and enter the urine. Test strips dipped in urine taken at the same time every day for about 5 days around the time of ovulation indicate a rise in LH levels; this means that ovulation is imminent.

Intercourse is recommended every day for several days once the test shows an increase in LH.

■ *Vaginal discharge analysis* Some women know they are ovulating when their vaginal discharge becomes thin and clear, like egg white. The cervical mucus method of predicting ovulation requires that you examine your vaginal discharge daily for changes.

After your period, sticky mucus occurs (during which time some women are fertile but most are not). During the 1- to 5-day period before ovulation, when your cervix produces a copious amount of thin, clear, slippery mucus, you are probably at your most fertile time. The mucus will stretch between your fingers into a thin strand.

Blood tests If the methods above do not clearly indicate you are ovulating regularly, your physician may perform a blood test to measure the amount of the hormone progesterone you produce after ovulation.

The hormones follicle-stimulating hormone (FSH) and estradiol, measured on day 3 of the menstrual cycle, predict (for some women) that success may be limited because of a reduced number of eggs inside an ovary.

Depending on your medical history and the results of your physical exam, your doctor may perform other tests (such as testing the levels of prolactin, thyroid, and testosterone) because abnormal levels of these hormones can cause infertility.

Hysterosalpingogram This test helps detect abnormalities of the uterus and fallopian tubes by outlining internal structures with a dye. It can show whether there is an open channel in the fallopian tubes and can also show if there is scar tissue or fibroids in the uterus.

For this procedure, the gynecologist or radiologist inserts a narrow tube into your cervix and injects a dye that is opaque to x-rays. The dye flows through your uterus and fallopian tubes, showing any irregularities.

To ease cramping and to decrease the risk of infection, you may be given a mild sedative, a painkiller, and/or antibiotics before the procedure.

Ultrasound Your physician may use ultrasound (see p.1042) to look for abnormalities in your ovaries and uterus.

Endometrial biopsy Biopsy, in which a piece of the lining of the uterus is removed and examined under a microscope, can help your doctor determine whether your uterine lining has responded fully to progesterone.

Hysteroscopy (see p.1042) Hysteroscopy may be used as an alternative to a hysterosalpingogram for viewing the uterine cavity.

Laparoscopy Laparoscopy allows your doctor to gain a better look at the outside of your fallopian tubes, uterus, or ovaries and to diagnose endometriosis (see p.1071) and pelvic adhesions (scar tissue).

While you are under general anesthesia, several keyhole-sized incisions are made in your abdomen and a lighted viewing tube with a camera is inserted through one of the incisions. The physician examines the pelvic organs on a monitor. Instruments for performing surgery are inserted through the other incisions.

TREATMENT

If you ovulate irregularly, infrequently, or not at all, your doctor may recommend one of the following drugs to induce ovulation:

Clomiphene citrate, taken by mouth on the fifth through

ninth day of the menstrual cycle to induce ovulation, may be useful for women who have periods infrequently. It stimulates the release of FSH and LH from the pituitary gland, which in turn stimulate the ovaries to release an egg.

Side effects include hot flashes and occasional moodiness. In 6% of women treated with clomiphene, twins (or, rarely, triplets) occur. While clomiphene was developed for women who do not ovulate, today it is commonly used for ovulating women to help them release more than one egg and increase the chance of becoming pregnant.

Bromocriptine is used for women whose pituitary gland releases too much prolactin (see p.861) and thus have irregular ovulation. Bromocriptine limits the amount of prolactin released by the pituitary. Side effects include nausea, dizziness, and headache.

Injectable infertility drugs, which are injected into a muscle or under the skin over 1 to 2 weeks, contain FSH and LH together or FSH only. These hormones stimulate the ovaries to release more than one egg (a process known as superovulation). Side effects include abdominal pain, breast tenderness, and mood swings. In some cases, the drug causes hyperstimulation syndrome, in which the ovaries stay large long after ovulation and excess fluid may collect inside the abdomen.

Other drugs When infertility is caused by endometriosis or fibroids, the drugs leuprolide or danazol may be helpful.

Laparoscopic surgery may be used to open blocked fallo-

pian tubes, release adhesions, remove endometriosis, or cut away an ovarian cyst that is blocking eggs from being released by the ovary. Hysteroscopy (see p.1042) is employed to remove some types of uterine fibroids and some abnormalities inside the uterus. Treatment of endometriosis (see p.1071) depends on the severity and location of growths.

Assisted reproductive technologies (see p.911) may be used when other methods fail. These techniques help the woman produce more eggs and place more sperm or more embryos inside the uterus than would occur in a normal menstrual cycle.

Infertility Testing and Treatment for Men

If your semen analysis reveals abnormalities, you may be referred to a urologist (a specialist in disorders of the male reproductive system). The urologist will take a more complete health history and examine your genitals to look for infection, a varicocele (see p.1090), or immature or abnormally developed testicles, any of which can inhibit healthy sperm production.

TESTS

Semen analysis For this test, you abstain from ejaculation for no fewer than 2 days and no more than 4–5 days, and then masturbate into a sterile cup or tube. The samples are analyzed in a laboratory within an hour.

Because sperm levels vary from day to day, you will need to provide samples on at least two different days. Doctors study the

sperm for several characteristics, including the number of sperm, the consistency of the semen, the percentage of moving (motile) sperm, whether the sperm are moving in a straight line or in circles, the percentage of normally shaped sperm, and other elements such as bacteria or white blood cells (which can indicate infection).

In most laboratories, a normal sperm count is considered to be above 20 million sperm per cubic centimeter, with at least 40% to 50% of the sperm moving.

Blood tests or urethral cultures These tests may be ordered by your urologist to measure levels of the hormones testosterone, follicle-stimulating hormone, and luteinizing hormone as well as to identify any infection.

TREATMENT

Poor movement of sperm or low sperm count may be treated by sperm "washing" (a procedure that collects and stimulates the most rapidly moving sperm to try to fertilize the egg), and intrauterine artificial insemination (see Assisted Reproductive Technology, p.911) or in vitro fertilization (see p.912). For men who do not have enough motile sperm, more advanced assisted reproductive approaches, such as intracytoplasmic sperm injection (see p.912) may be successful.

Absence of sperm due to blockage or abnormality of the ejaculatory ducts can occasionally be circumvented by obtaining sperm directly from the epididymis or from the testicles.

Varicoceles are usually treated by surgery. If there are enough healthy sperm, artificial insemination or intrauterine insemination

Preparing for Conception

Your chances of conceiving and carrying a healthy child to term can be improved by having good health habits before and after you become pregnant. This chart lists steps you and your partner should take several months before you conceive, and afterward as well. The healthier you are when you become pregnant, the healthier your fetus will be in the crucial first weeks of development.

CONCERN	WHY IS IT IMPORTANT?
Smoking	Can make both male and female partners less fertile; can increase rate of pregnancy problems such as miscarriage, placental problems, preterm births, small babies, and sudden infant death syndrome.
Alcohol	Can increase rate of infertility and miscarriages; can cause birth defects, mental retardation, and small babies.
Using illegal drugs	May reduce fertility; can increase risk for miscarriage, premature birth, neonatal drug withdrawal, small babies, and possibly birth defects, depending on the drug.
Being overweight	Can increase the risk of ovulation problems; increases the risk of pregnancy complications such as gestational diabetes, hypertension, cesarean section, infection, and large babies.
Being underweight	Interferes with ovulation; increases risk for small babies and premature birth.
Using medications (prescription, over-the-counter, or high-dose vitamins)	The effect on fertility of most drugs is not known; some are known to be harmful to the fetus.
Domestic violence	Frequency and severity increases during pregnancy.
Folic acid (folate) deficiency	Can cause neural tube defects.
Immunizations for varicella and rubella	Getting either of these diseases may be harmful to the developing fetus.
Exercise	Helps prepare your body for the physical stresses of pregnancy.
Nutrition	Improves chances of delivering a normal weight baby.
Medical conditions such as diabetes, hypertension, and epilepsy	Can affect the health and size of the fetus; may increase the need to induce an early delivery.
Family history	You may carry a gene for an inherited disorder that can affect your fetus (specific ethnic groups are at higher risk).
Environmental exposure	Some chemicals or other substances used at work or in hobbies may be harmful to the fetus.

STEPS TO TAKE

Quit smoking (see p.59).

Stop drinking alcohol (see p.65).

Do not use illegal drugs.

Lose weight under medical supervision.

Gain weight under medical supervision.

Inform your physician about all medications you use and ask if it is advisable to continue taking them.

Avoid pregnancy until you have permanently resolved this problem.

Take a vitamin supplement containing 400 micrograms (0.4 milligrams) each day for 1 month before you become pregnant and during the first 3 months of pregnancy.

If you are not already immune, get immunized at least 3 months before conceiving.

Exercise (see p.50) three or more times a week.

Eat a healthful diet (see p.37).

Discuss your condition with your physician, who may recommend an adjustment in your medicines and help you to improve control of your condition before pregnancy occurs.

See Inherited Diseases (p.128). Discuss with your physician.

Discuss with your physician.

(see Assisted Reproductive Technology, below), in which the most rapidly moving sperm are injected into the uterus at ovulation, may be chosen instead of surgery.

Infections (sexually transmitted diseases or prostate infections) that cause infertility are easily treated; the infertility then usually resolves.

Assisted Reproductive Technology

Assisted reproductive technology (ART) is used by fewer than 5% of infertile couples in the United States. Approximately 40,000 babies are born each year using ART.

ART includes in vitro fertilization (IVF), gamete intrafallopian transfer (GIFT), zygote intrafallopian transfer (ZIFT), intracytoplasmic sperm injection (ICSI), and other infrequently used techniques. The vast majority of ART procedures involve IVF, because it has proved simpler than—and as successful as—the other procedures.

PROCEDURES FOR ART

The first step in all forms of ART is the use of medication to induce the ovaries to produce multiple egg-containing follicles (called superovulation).

Some women are first given gonadotropin-releasing hormone agonists (GnRH agonists) to "turn off" their natural hormones so that the artificial hormones can be more precisely administered. Ultrasound tests and hormonal blood measurements (every day or every other day) identify when the follicles are large enough to contain mature eggs (usually in 8 to 14 days).

Adoption

Adoption is an alternative for many couples who have difficulty conceiving. The majority of adoptions take place through licensed social agencies. Some are open adoptions, in which there is contact between the adoptive parents and the birth parents. Others are closed adoptions, in which the agency maintains the privacy of both couples.

Other options include family adoptions, in which parents adopt the child of a relative, and private adoptions, in which arrangements are made with the birth mother through physicians and lawyers.

The adoption process can be lengthy and expensive and varies according to the laws in each state. Most agencies require some type of interview, in which a social worker comes to your home to evaluate your fitness as potential parents; you may pay a fee for this service.

RESOLVE (see p.1228) and the National Adoption Information Clearinghouse (see p.1228) are sources of information for prospective adoptive parents.

Human chorionic gonadotropin (hCG), the hormone made by the placenta, is then given as an injection to cause ovulation about 36 hours later.

Intrauterine artificial insemination (IUI) is performed once or twice before ovulation and at the time of ovulation. If you will have IVF, GIFT, or ICSI sperm injection, eggs are retrieved from the ovary during a short surgical procedure that requires sedation or general anesthesia.

Using intravaginal ultrasound, the physician inserts a needle through the wall of the vagina and extracts eggs from the ovaries. The eggs are then placed in a laboratory dish under ideal environmental conditions; healthy ones are selected for the fertilization process.

From this point on, the procedures differ, as described below.

IN VITRO FERTILIZATION

In in vitro fertilization (IVF), the man's sperm are added to the dish containing the woman's egg and the dish is placed in an incubator. The dish is observed at 12- to 24-hour intervals to determine how many eggs have been fertilized and whether the embryos are dividing normally.

You will need to make a choice about how many embryos to implant. Usually two to four embryos are used in one treatment cycle; the rest may be frozen for later use. Your doctor will make a recommendation based on the quality of the embryos, your age, and your feelings about selective reduction (see Risks of ART, below right).

A thin plastic tube (catheter) is inserted through the opening of the cervix, into the inside of your uterus, and the embryos are passed through the catheter into the uterus. You then take progesterone for several weeks or months to help an embryo implant and grow in the lining of the uterus.

A conclusive diagnosis of pregnancy cannot be made for about 10 days, when a developing placenta begins to secrete hCG into your bloodstream.

ZYGOTE INTRAFALLOPIAN TRANSFER

Zygote intrafallopian transfer (ZIFT) is very similar to IVF except the embryos are transferred into the fallopian tubes using laparoscopic surgery (see p.142). This outpatient surgical procedure requires general anesthesia.

GAMETE INTRAFALLOPIAN TRANSFER

A gamete is an egg or sperm. Gamete intrafallopian transfer (GIFT) is similar to IVF and ZIFT except the mature eggs are not fertilized by sperm in a laboratory dish. Instead, the eggs and healthy sperm are immediately placed by laparoscopy into the fallopian tubes.

INTRACYTOPLASMIC SPERM INJECTION

Intracytoplasmic sperm injection (ICSI) is a laboratory procedure used when male infertility is caused by low numbers of sperm or by problems with sperm binding to and penetrating the egg.

The fertility specialist uses micromanipulation techniques to insert a single sperm directly into an egg (which was induced and retrieved as in IVF). Any fertilized eggs that grow into embryos are then placed in the uterus.

RISKS OF ART

The risk of miscarriage (22%) and of multiple fetuses (30% to 50%) is increased when using ART. With in vitro fertilization, for example, 50% to 70% of live births are single babies, 25% to

45% are twins, and approximately 5% are triplets (or higher-order multiple births).

Couples may face a decision about reducing the number of implanted embryos by a process called selective reduction, in which a drug is injected into the heart of one or more embryos to stop its beating and give the others a better chance of growing nearer to full term.

Selective reduction is usually performed during the first trimester; most often, there are more than two fetuses trying to grow, and selective reduction is used to leave just two in the uterus. The decision on which fetus or fetuses to inject is made based on their position in the uterus.

Carrying multiple fetuses creates a higher-risk pregnancy. The babies usually have a lower birthweight, are usually born prematurely, and are at greater risk of death during the first 2 weeks after birth.

Complications for the mother include preeclampsia (see p.932), anemia (see p.930), and placenta previa (see p.931). If you have multiple fetuses, your physician may recommend monitoring with periodic ultrasound tests and/or more bed rest.

After delivery, support groups can be helpful in coping with the challenges of caring for more than one infant at a time.

Evaluating a Fertility Program

Look for a program that offers the highest success rates. Consider the following points when evaluating a program:

Live birth rate (versus pregnancy rate) per treatment

cycle Many programs advertise high pregnancy rates, but it is more important to find out the "take-home baby" rate per treatment cycle. Ask also about miscarriage rates and rates of multiple births. High multiple birth rates may reflect the practice of placing more embryos into the uterus than may be necessary, in order to increase the overall pregnancy rate.

Type of people in the program To interpret the live birth rate, you must also consider the profile of the people in the program.

For example, younger couples achieve pregnancy more easily than older couples. In states with mandatory insurance coverage for ART, couples with lower success rates undergo more treatment cycles, thus reducing overall success rates.

Staff experience Select a program with qualified reproductive endocrinologists, technologists, and support staff.

Comprehensiveness of service This is especially important if you are interested in services such as freezing embryos for later use

How GIFT Works

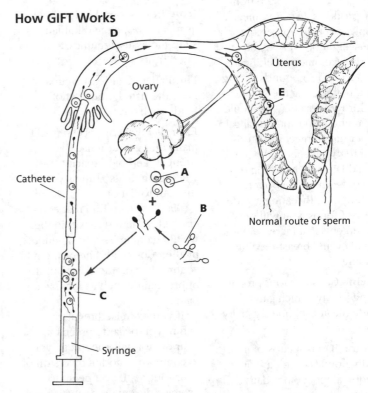

In the gamete intrafallopian transfer (GIFT) procedure for treating infertility, mature eggs are removed from the ovary (A). Sperm are collected and stimulated to be able to penetrate the egg (B). Both the mature eggs and the sperm are injected by a syringe through a catheter into the fallopian tube (C). Fertilization of an egg by a sperm occurs in the fallopian tube (D). If fertilization is successful, the embryos implant in the lining of the uterus (E).

(usually a separate cost), psychological support and counseling, egg and sperm donation, and advanced technologies such as ICSI (see p.912).

Cost of procedure, including drugs, per cycle Ask also about the payment schedule, refunds if the treatment cycle is canceled, and availability and cost of lodging, if necessary.

Accreditation The program should meet standards of the American Society for Reproductive Medicine (ASRM); the lab should be accredited by the College of American Pathologists and ASRM. In addition, most professional programs report results to the Centers for Disease Control and Prevention (CDC).

PREGNANCY

Nutrition and Exercise

Nutrition In general, the demands of pregnancy heighten your need for calories and protein. It is essential that you eat a wide variety of foods, including vegetables, fruits, grains, and protein from dairy products, fish, and meat.

Unless you are extremely underweight or overweight, most experts recommend gaining between 25 and 35 pounds during pregnancy. During the second and third trimesters, you should take in about 300 additional calories per day to meet the nutritional requirements of the fetus.

Read Diet and Nutrition (see p.37) to learn more about a healthful diet. By eating a wide variety of foods, you will satisfy requirements that increase during pregnancy and breast-feeding, including:

Protein Consume four protein servings a day, which can include meat, fish, poultry, dairy, or tofu.

Calcium Drink 4 cups of milk (ideally nonfat) each day, or the equivalent in other dairy products.

Folic acid (folate) Folic acid is found in fresh green, leafy vegetables. Many grain products are also supplemented with folic acid. Because of the risk of neural tube defects (see p.985) caused by a folic acid deficiency, your doctor will prescribe a daily supplement that contains at least 400 micrograms (0.4 milligrams) of folic acid.

Iron Iron is found in foods such as meat, liver, egg yolk, black strap molasses, legumes, and dried fruits.

Fluids Drink at least 8 cups of noncaffeinated, nonalcoholic fluids each day.

Exercise Exercise is essential to maintaining your muscle strength, aerobic capacity, and well-being. It also builds your strength for labor.

Many women find that exercise helps them stay within the weight gain limits recommended by their doctor and helps them to control the common discomforts of pregnancy such as low back pain.

If you exercised regularly before you became pregnant, your doctor will encourage you to continue a modified version of your routine. If you begin to exercise during pregnancy, build up slowly.

Exercise moderately from three to five times a week, but never so intensely that you cannot speak easily while exercising.

Good choices include beginner's yoga, swimming, brisk walking, stationary cycling, calisthenics designed for pregnant women, biking, and dancing.

Many obstetricians do not recommend downhill skiing or vigorous horseback riding after the 20th to 24th weeks of pregnancy. Ask your doctor or midwife for advice about exercise.

Prenatal Care

Prenatal care is a regular schedule of checkups that ensures your health and that of your developing fetus. Women who faithfully follow a prenatal care regimen have a better chance for a safe pregnancy and a healthy infant.

Optimally, prenatal care begins before conception (see Preparing for Conception, p.910). If you become pregnant before you have discussed pregnancy with your doctor, see him or her as soon as possible.

Initial visit During your initial visit, your physician or midwife will conduct a medical history and perform a physical examination—including an internal examination to confirm the pregnancy and detect any abnormalities that could present problems during pregnancy.

Embryonic and Fetal Development

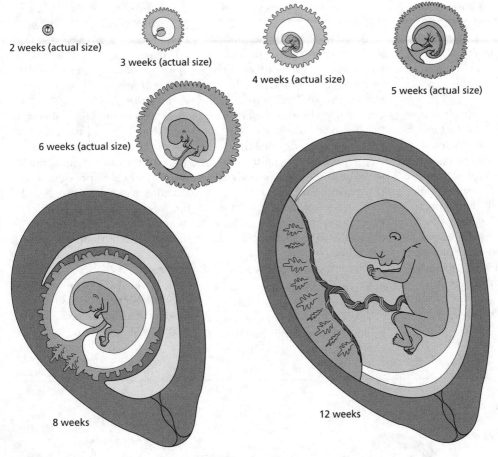

2 weeks (actual size)

3 weeks (actual size)

4 weeks (actual size)

5 weeks (actual size)

6 weeks (actual size)

8 weeks

12 weeks

2 weeks
The embryo has become a sphere of cells that forms the basis for future development of different organs and the placenta. An amniotic sac has grown around the embryo.

3 weeks
The cells assume a pear shape, and the rudiments of a spine have emerged.

4 weeks
Buds of tissue—suggesting the lungs, pancreas, liver, gallbladder, limbs, and back—are now forming.

5 weeks
Facial features begin to take shape and the umbilical cord develops.

6 weeks
From its coiled position, a more human form unfolds, along with the toes and fingers.

8 weeks
The 1-inch-long organism can now officially be called a fetus. Internal organs have formed and blood is circulating. The fetus is moving but it is still too small for the mother to notice the movement.

12 weeks
Now 3 inches long, the fetus has fully formed fingers and toes, complete with nails. It also has external genitals.

Your doctor will ask you about previous pregnancies, any medical conditions (such as diabetes or high blood pressure), any previous surgeries that could affect your pregnancy, any disorders that run in your family, and your use of alcohol, tobacco, or other drugs.

Your physician will also counsel you about the risk factors for the human immunodeficiency virus and offer you testing.

Up to one third of women are struck by violent partners during pregnancy, usually in the breast or abdomen. Ask your doctor for help getting counseling if you are currently in a violent relationship.

Your due date will be established. It is calculated as 40 weeks from the first day of your last period. Ultrasound (see p.919) may be required if there is any uncertainty about when ovulation occurred or if the size of your uterus is larger or smaller than normal for your expected due date.

Blood tests will be performed to check your blood type and Rh factor (see p.157), your immunity to the hepatitis B and rubella viruses, and the absence or presence of syphilis and anemia. The "triple screen" blood test (see p.918) is also performed in women at higher risk for chromosome abnormalities, such as Down syndrome.

Your urine will be tested for infection, sugar (which can indicate diabetes), and albumin (protein), which can be present if you have high blood pressure.

Subsequent visits After your initial visit, the timing of subsequent checkups depends on your health. For uncomplicated pregnancies, the usual schedule is once a month until 28 weeks, after which you will go to the doctor every 2 weeks. If your pregnancy is complicated (see Higher Risk Pregnancy, p.921), you may need to see your doctor more frequently. During the last month of pregnancy, weekly visits are customary.

At subsequent visits, discuss with your doctor or midwife any questions or problems you have. Your doctor will measure your weight and blood pressure, evaluate the size of your uterus and the position of the fetus, and monitor the fetus's heartbeat through a stethoscope or an ultrasound device placed on your abdomen.

You will also have regular tests of your urine. Blood tests for diabetes and anemia are done at 28 weeks' gestation.

If you develop vaginal bleed-

How the Fetus Is Nourished

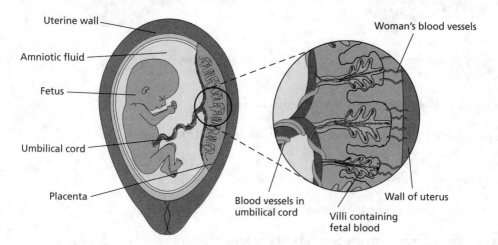

Uterine wall
Amniotic fluid
Fetus
Umbilical cord
Placenta
Woman's blood vessels
Wall of uterus
Villi containing fetal blood
Blood vessels in umbilical cord

Blood from the fetus circulates through the umbilical cord to the placenta, where it is enriched with nutrients such as sugar and oxygen, and where it deposits liquid waste materials from the fetus. Villi (fingerlike projections that enlarge the placental surface) optimize the area for this exchange. In addition to nutrients and oxygen, damaging substances such as alcohol and other drugs can cross the placenta into the fetal blood.

ing, an ultrasound may be performed to help determine the cause. Ultrasound is also done if the uterus is too large or small and to determine if you have twins, if you have a large or small baby, or if there is too little or too much amniotic fluid.

The widespread practice of performing an ultrasound examination at about 18 weeks of pregnancy is of unproven value.

Prenatal Testing and Genetic Disorders

Genetic disorders are those that are passed on to children from one or both parents. You or your partner may carry a defective gene without having the condition or one of you or a family member may have the disorder.

Prenatal tests provide information about your fetus's health. They are generally recommended for women at higher risk of having a baby with a serious abnormality.

However, like all medical tests, they should be performed to enable you and your physician to make a decision based on the result. The choice of whether or not to have a test is yours. Read Who Should Consider Genetic Counseling or Testing? (see p.132) for more information.

The risk of chromosomal abnormalities rises steadily as a woman gets older. For example, the chance of a fetus having any chromosomal abnormality is about 1 of 500 when a woman is age 25, about 1 of 200 at age 35, and about 1 of 20 at age 45. In the United States, many women have a blood test that gives a better estimate of the risk of the most common chromosomal abnormalities.

Many women over age 35 undergo an amniocentesis, which can definitely reveal chromosomal abnormalities.

If a prenatal test reveals that your fetus has a chromosomal abnormality, birth defect, or genetic disorder, you may benefit from genetic counseling to learn more about the condition.

Counseling can help you make an informed decision about terminating the pregnancy or continuing the pregnancy and preparing for a child who will require extra care and support.

AMNIOCENTESIS

In amniocentesis, a small amount of the amniotic fluid, which surrounds the fetus in the uterus and contains skin cells shed by the fetus, is removed with a needle and studied.

Amniocentesis can reveal chromosomal abnormalities such as Down syndrome, or genetic disorders such as Tay-Sachs disease (see p.129) or sickle cell anemia (see p.721). It can detect hundreds of other disorders, but doctors usually test only for genetic conditions for which women are at a high risk (based on their family or personal history).

Amniocentesis

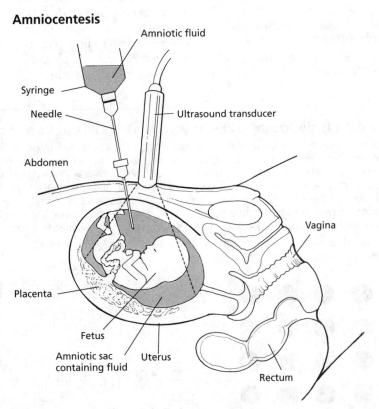

In amniocentesis, a sample of fetal cells is removed, grown in the laboratory, and then analyzed for chromosome abnormalities. Under ultrasound guidance, a needle is inserted through the abdomen into the amniotic sac; amniotic fluid is withdrawn. The fluid contains cells that have been shed from fetal skin.

Genetic amniocentesis is usually performed between the 14th and 18th weeks of pregnancy. Using ultrasound to locate and avoid the fetus, the doctor inserts a long thin needle through your abdominal wall and into the uterus to withdraw 4 teaspoons of amniotic fluid containing fetal skin cells. The procedure takes a few minutes and is not painful.

The cells are permitted to grow for 2 to 3 weeks and their chromosomes are then analyzed. The test results are 99.8% accurate for making a definite diagnosis. In experienced hands, the risk of accidentally terminating a pregnancy from performing amniocentesis is about 1 of 300.

TRIPLE SCREEN (ENHANCED ALPHA FETOPROTEIN) TESTS

A test of the mother's blood for alpha fetoprotein (AFP)—a protein produced by the fetus—along with the hormones human chorionic gonadotropin (hCG) and estriol (a type of estrogen), can estimate the risk of neural tube defect (spina bifida), Down syndrome, and another chromosomal abnormality called trisomy 18.

Blood levels of AFP, hCG, and estriol are entered into a computer program, along with other factors (such as the woman's age, weight, race, whether she has ever had diabetes or a child with a neural tube defect, and how many fetuses she is carrying) that can affect the risk of one of these abnormalities.

The computer program can tell if a woman's chance of having a fetus with a neural tube defect is greater than the average woman's chance of having a fetus with a neural tube defect. The program also determines the chance that the fetus has the two chromosomal abnormalities Down syndrome and trisomy 18.

The test is performed between the 16th and 18th weeks of pregnancy. The test results are not conclusive evidence of any condition. However, the test results can more accurately estimate the risk of having one of the conditions than considering a woman's age alone.

If the test result suggests an increased risk for one of these defects, your doctor will recommend more specific tests, such as ultrasound or amniocentesis.

CHORIONIC VILLUS SAMPLING

In chorionic villus sampling (CVS), a tiny piece of tissue is removed from the placenta to examine it for genetic abnormalities in the fetus. Chorionic villi are minute projections of the pla-

How the Triple Screen Test Helps Determine the Risk of Down Syndrome

The triple screen test measures three substances in a pregnant woman's blood: estriol, human chorionic gonadotropin (hCG), and alpha fetoprotein (AFP). The results of the test can indicate if a woman has a relatively high or relatively low risk of having a child with the chromosomal abnormality Down syndrome. The combination of low estriol, high hCG, and low AFP indicates the highest risk for Down syndrome. If the risk is relatively high (often defined as a risk of more than 1 of 250), your doctor will typically suggest further definitive testing with amniocentesis. The combination of the three screenings is extremely effective in distinguishing high-risk women from low-risk women.

In the example below, a 35-year-old woman can have radically different risks of having a child with Down syndrome based on the test results.

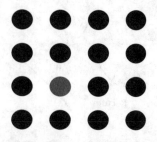

1 OF 16 WOMEN WHO HAVE THE WORST COMBINATION OF RESULTS FROM THE TRIPLE SCREEN TEST WILL HAVE A FETUS WITH DOWN SYNDROME

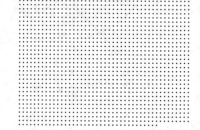

1 OF 1,400 WOMEN WHO HAVE AN INTERMEDIATE COMBINATION OF RESULTS FROM THE TRIPLE SCREEN TEST WILL HAVE A FETUS WITH DOWN SYNDROME

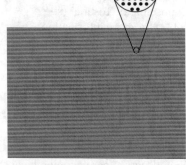

1 OF 52,000 WOMEN WHO HAVE THE BEST COMBINATION OF RESULTS FROM THE TRIPLE SCREEN TEST WILL HAVE A FETUS WITH DOWN SYNDROME

Chorionic Villus Sampling

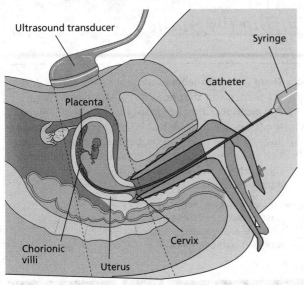

Ultrasound transducer

Syringe

Catheter

Placenta

Chorionic villi

Cervix

Uterus

In chorionic villus sampling, cells from the chorionic villi (minute parts of the placenta) are extracted for laboratory examination. Under the guidance of ultrasound, cells are removed through a catheter inserted through the cervix (via the vagina) or through a needle inserted through the lower abdominal wall.

centa; cells taken from the villi for analysis have the same genetic profile as the fetus.

CVS can be performed as early as the 10th week of pregnancy and test results are available more quickly than amniocentesis, sometimes within 2 weeks.

The cells are obtained by inserting a catheter through the vagina or the abdomen (via a needle) and suctioning out the cells; the cells are grown in a laboratory and analyzed.

CVS performed through the abdomen may carry fewer risks of infection and miscarriage than when performed through the vagina. In experienced centers, the risk of accidentally terminating a pregnancy after CVS is about the same as with amniocentesis (about 1 of 300).

Somewhat more frequently,

CVS causes bleeding or premature rupture of the membranes.

ULTRASOUND

Ultrasound (see p.148) can permit your doctor to evaluate fetal size, development, and position in the uterus. It is also used to check the position of the placenta, the amount of amniotic fluid, and, late in pregnancy, the condition of the fetus.

The ultrasound can detect abnormalities of the bones of the nose and spinal cord that indicate an increased risk for certain genetic conditions, such as Down syndrome.

The procedure can be performed through the abdomen or vagina. For an abdominal ultrasound, a conduction gel is spread across your abdomen and a microphonelike probe called a

transducer is moved across it, producing an image of the fetus on a monitor.

For a vaginal ultrasound—which can give a better view of the cervix or a very early pregnancy—the transducer (which is about the size of a large tampon) is inserted through your vagina.

FETAL HEART RATE MONITORING

The fetus's heart rate reveals much about its health. Your doctor may perform a nonstress test, in which a fetal monitor records the fetus's heart rate over a 10- to 60-minute period. A healthy fetus older than 30 to 32 weeks of age will have a faster heartbeat when it moves than when it is still.

If the nonstress test raises questions about the health of the fetus, your doctor may want to perform a test called a biophysical profile, in which ultrasound is used to evaluate fetal movement, muscle tone, breathing, and amniotic fluid volume.

The results of this test, when evaluated with information from the nonstress test, give your doctor an even clearer idea of the health of the fetus and whether or not more information is needed.

Alternately, your physician may perform a contraction stress test. In this test, you are given the drug oxytocin to stimulate gentle contractions of your uterus. Fetal monitoring (see p.938) is used to see if the fetus responds normally (indicated by no drop in heart rate after contractions) to the stress of impending labor and delivery.

A fetus that does not respond normally may need an earlier delivery or more monitoring the next day.

Moderate Drinking During Pregnancy: Dr Haas's Advice

Q A friend and I are having a disagreement on how much alcohol is safe to drink during pregnancy. She says that having a drink every day or two will not hurt the baby. I learned at my childbirth classes that any amount of alcohol is too much and that pregnant women should not drink. Can you give us the facts?

A You said it best. Any amount of alcohol during pregnancy is too much. Alcohol is the leading preventable cause of mental retardation in newborns. It causes fetal alcohol syndrome (FAS), a group of irreversible neurological, behavioral, and physical problems. Babies born with FAS can have abnormally formed organs, mental retardation, and small brains.

There is no safe level of alcohol consumption during pregnancy, but that does not mean that drinking any alcohol during pregnancy will always damage the fetus. If you have just learned you are pregnant, had not been planning on becoming pregnant, and had some alcoholic drinks in recent months, discuss this with your obstetrician. Chances are that no damage occurred.

SUSAN T. HAAS, MD, MS
BOSTON MEDICAL CENTER, BOSTON UNIVERSITY
BRIGHAM AND WOMEN'S HOSPITAL
HARVARD MEDICAL SCHOOL

GROUP B STREPTOCOCCI TESTING

Group B streptococci (GBS) are bacteria found in the vagina of about one third of women. If undiagnosed and untreated, the bacteria can cause an infection that leads to severe complications or death in about 1 of 1,000 babies.

Your doctor may test for GBS by performing a vaginal culture about 1 month before your baby is due. If the test shows that you carry GBS, you will be treated during labor with penicillin (or another antibiotic if you are allergic to penicillin).

If you are at high risk for GBS infection, your doctor may treat you with antibiotics without obtaining a culture.

RH INCOMPATIBILITY TESTING

Rh factor is a protein on the surface of red blood cells. People have blood that is either Rh positive (85% of the population), meaning their red blood cells have the Rh-factor protein, or Rh negative, meaning their red blood cells do not have the protein.

If you are pregnant and have Rh-negative blood, and the father has Rh-positive blood, your fetus could have Rh-positive blood.

During delivery, some blood cells from your fetus are likely to enter your bloodstream. If the fetus has Rh-positive blood, your immune system will recognize those cells as foreign and produce antibodies against them.

In your first pregnancy, the levels of antibodies are usually low, and do not cause problems. However, in a subsequent pregnancy with another fetus that has Rh-positive blood, the mother's immune system makes large amounts of antibodies that can destroy the fetus's red blood cells and cause anemia in, and even death of, the fetus.

Rh incompatibility is diagnosed during prenatal screening and treated with injections of Rh-immunoglobulin during pregnancy. These injections prevent your immune system from producing the harmful antibodies.

Immediately after delivery, injections are given to prevent antibodies from forming in any future pregnancy.

Choosing a Practitioner

Conventionally, babies are delivered with the help of medical doctors (usually obstetricians or family practitioners) in a hospital setting. However, many communities offer a variety of caregivers for pregnant women.

Obstetricians are medical doctors who specialize in caring for women during pregnancy, labor, and delivery. Most obstetricians also specialize in women's

Higher-Risk Pregnancy

A higher-risk pregnancy is one in which there is a medical condition in the mother, or an abnormality of the fetus or placenta, that could compromise the health of the woman or fetus during pregnancy. Other risk factors include obesity and multiple fetuses. If you know you have any of the common medical conditions listed below, see your physician before you become pregnant and work with him or her during pregnancy to minimize the risk of complications.

CONDITION	POSSIBLE EFFECTS
Asthma (see p.505)	About one third of women with asthma have a worsening of the condition during pregnancy. Other women experience improvement or no change in their condition. Severe asthma that is poorly controlled can reduce the fetus's oxygen supply and increase the chances of premature labor. Therefore, it is important to take medications, as your doctor recommends, during pregnancy.
Diabetes mellitus (see p.832)	Good control of diabetes is critical before attempting pregnancy, as well as during pregnancy, to reduce the risks of fetal birth defects and miscarriage. Diabetes can worsen during pregnancy, and must therefore be treated more intensively.
High blood pressure (see p.644)	Most pregnant women experience a decrease in blood pressure. If you already have high blood pressure, you have an increased risk for developing placental problems, poor growth of the fetus, and preeclampsia.
Epilepsy (see p.375)	Because some drugs used to control seizures in epilepsy can cause birth defects in the fetus, your doctor may change your medication during pregnancy. Having a seizure during pregnancy can be dangerous to you and your baby. Thus, it is important for most women to continue taking anticonvulsants during pregnancy.
Infection (such as rubella, varicella, cytomegalovirus, toxoplasmosis, syphilis, herpes, human immunodeficiency virus, fifth disease, hepatitis, gonorrhea, chlamydia, and group B streptococcus infection)	Risks vary depending on the infectious agent, but may include fetal malformations, infection of the fetus at birth, and higher risk for cesarean section.
Sickle cell anemia (see p.721)	Sickle cell anemia can increase a woman's risk of preeclampsia (see p.932) and anemia. The fetus can be affected by growth retardation or may die if the blood vessels in the placenta are blocked by the sickle cells.
Complications (such as preeclampsia, premature labor, premature rupture of membranes, too much or too little amniotic fluid, fetal abnormalities, incompetent cervix, placenta previa, or multiple fetuses)	A pregnancy may also be higher risk if you develop complications during the pregnancy.

health outside of pregnancy (gynecologists).

Obstetricians have hospital privileges at the institutions where they help deliver babies.

Family practitioners are doctors who are trained to care for people of all ages. Family practitioners have received training in obstetrics and, like obstetricians, have hospital privileges and usually aid in deliveries in a hospital. If complications arise during your pregnancy, your family practitioner may refer you to an obstetrician.

Certified nurse-midwives (CNMs) are registered nurses who have been trained in obstetrics and the care of women whose pregnancies and deliveries are not expected to be complicated. Many hospitals and physician practices offer the services of a CNM.

CNMs are associated with obstetricians on whom they call for advice and to whom they refer women who require the care of a physician.

If you use a CNM, be certain you get to know the affiliated obstetrician and his or her affiliated hospital. The American College of Nurse-Midwives sets standards of care for CNMs.

Doulas are trained to support women physically and emotionally through the birthing process and afterward. Doulas can help explain such things as breathing during labor but do not have any nursing skills and cannot help with delivery.

Choosing a Location for the Birth

Hospitals Most births in the United States take place in a hospital. Hospitals offer advanced medical technology in case of emergency and a staff that is skilled in managing all types of labor and birthing complications.

Most hospitals offer tours of their labor and delivery units to give pregnant women and their partners a sense of the atmosphere and to answer questions about local practices and options.

Freestanding birth centers are more homelike centers that are most suitable for women who are not expected to have complications during labor and delivery. They are usually staffed by certified nurse-midwives, but most also have an obstetrician on call.

If complications arise, the obstetrician takes over or you are transferred to the hospital where the physician has admitting privileges. The centers should be accredited by the Commission for Accreditation of Freestanding Birth Centers.

Home birthing is an option for women who have had normal pregnancies, are expected to have a normal pregnancy and delivery, and are in good physical health. Typically, a certified nurse-midwife or doctor is present.

Because complications can arise without warning, you should plan for the possibility of requiring emergency hospital care. You should also understand that the extra time it takes to get to the hospital may result in harm to you or your baby. Medical insurance companies rarely cover the expenses of home birth.

ABORTION

An abortion is removal of the embryo (before 2 months) or fetus (after 2 months) and the placenta from the uterus, to terminate pregnancy.

Abortion is a safe medical procedure when performed by a trained professional. When performed before the 12th week of pregnancy, it is less risky than carrying a pregnancy to term. After the 12th week of pregnancy, the risk of complications gradually increases.

In the United States, because of the high rate of unintended pregnancy, approximately one third of all pregnancies are terminated in abortion. Since legalization of abortion in 1973, births to teenagers have declined. Most abortions are performed in non-hospital clinics or physician offices during the first trimester.

Women seeking an abortion first have their pregnancies confirmed by a blood or urine test. A blood Rh test (see p.157) is also performed. The number of weeks that you have been pregnant will be carefully determined, using a physical exam and, sometimes, ultrasound. The physician or staff will also take a medical history and offer counseling.

Some state laws require that one or both parents of a girl under 18 be notified before an abortion is performed. The Planned Parenthood chapter in your state can tell you if notification is necessary.

It is recommended that you make a decision on abortion before the 12th week of pregnancy, when the procedure is safest and when, by law, the abortion is still a private decision you make with your physician.

SURGICAL ABORTION

The doctor will first perform a pelvic examination to evaluate the position and size of your uterus. A local anesthetic is injected into the cervix, which is gradually opened (dilated) with a series of progressively larger, smooth rods. You may feel some cramping.

The contents of the uterus are then removed through a thin tube and the wall of your uterus is gently scraped to ensure all tissue is removed.

The contraction-inducing drug oxytocin is sometimes given to cause the uterus to contract and return to its smaller size. For some abortions, intravenous sedation may be used.

With a later pregnancy, the cervix may be dilated for 4 to 24 hours before the procedure with seaweed sticks to reduce the risk of a tear during dilation of the cervix. In contrast to metal rods, which are the original method for dilating the cervix, seaweed sticks are softer and less likely to injure the uterus. They gradually absorb water and swell to two or three times their original size, which results in a very gentle and gradual opening of the cervix.

After the abortion, you may have some cramping and bleeding, both of which will taper off to that of a normal period after several days. Arrange for someone to drive you home an hour or two following the procedure and rest for a day or two.

Your physician will recommend that you not have sexual intercourse for several weeks. You may feel well and think you can skip your scheduled follow-up appointment. It is important to keep the follow-up appointment to make sure your birth-control plan is adequate and to be certain that all the pregnancy tissue has been removed.

If, after an abortion, you experience a fever over 100°F, or bleeding that is more severe than that of a normal period, call your doctor immediately.

NONSURGICAL (MEDICAL) ABORTION USING ABORTION PILLS

Nonsurgical abortions use drugs instead of surgery to terminate a pregnancy. Two drugs are available. Mifepristone (originally called RU-486) is used for inducing abortion before the 49th day of pregnancy. The drug blocks the hormone progesterone, which causes the lining of the uterus to shed—along with the attached, tiny fetus. Typically, mifepristone is used along with a second drug, misoprostol, which causes the uterus to contract and expel the tissue that has been shed. There is bleeding and cramping, as with a menstrual period. Together, mifepristone and misoprostol are 92% to 98% effective.

Another drug, methotrexate, is also used along with misoprostol, but compared to mifepristone, the process is quite prolonged. For this reason, methotrexate is not used as frequently as mifepristone.

COMMON DISCOMFORTS OF PREGNANCY

Even the healthiest pregnancy produces a variety of discomforting symptoms caused by the changes pregnancy produces in your body. While most of the symptoms listed here do not require treatment, talk to your physician about any symptoms that concern you.

Aches and pains are widespread among pregnant women. The hormonal changes of pregnancy, combined with the weight of the uterus, additional fluid, stretching muscles, and poor sleep, create discomfort. The conditions listed here may come and go, or may continue until delivery.

Backache

Lower back pain and sciatica (see p.619) are common during pregnancy, as the weight of the growing fetus in front causes you to compensate by leaning back, which puts stress on the ligaments and muscles of your lower back.

Consult your doctor if your back pain is severe. Otherwise, prevent pain from worsening by gaining only as much weight as recommended and by wearing low-heeled, well-cushioned shoes. In addition, apply an ice pack

Early Signs of Pregnancy

The hormonal changes of pregnancy begin immediately after conception, but the signs of pregnancy occur at different times and vary from woman to woman. If you think you are pregnant, perform a home pregnancy urine test or see your physician for a more sensitive blood test.

SIGN	HOW SOON SIGN MAY APPEAR OR RESULTS MAY OCCUR
Swollen, tender breasts	Within a few days
Positive laboratory blood test result	10 days
Positive office urine test result	10 to 14 days
Positive at-home pregnancy test result	2 weeks
Fatigue	2 weeks
Missed period	2 weeks
Urinating more frequently	6 to 8 weeks
Morning sickness	2 to 8 weeks

Growth of the Uterus

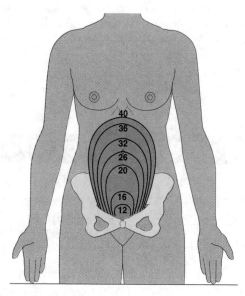

Shown here are the average sizes of the uterus between 8 and 40 weeks of pregnancy. By week 12, your doctor can feel the uterus by gently pressing on the abdomen and will measure its size from the top of your pubic bone to the top of your uterus.

to the aching area. Sleep on a very firm mattress and do low-impact exercises, such as walking and swimming. Learn to lift properly (see p.627).

Performing pelvic-tilt exercises can also be helpful. Stand with your back against a wall and slowly press the small of your back into the wall until it touches. Release and repeat several times each day. See also Preventing Back Pain, p.627.

Bleeding Gums

Bleeding, sore, and swollen gums during pregnancy are caused by inflammation triggered by changing hormones; gums return to their normal state after delivery.

Brush and floss twice daily, and see your dentist if your gums are especially painful or bleed easily. Consider having a professional cleaning and checkup before you get pregnant.

Breathlessness

Breathlessness is common in early pregnancy because the hormone progesterone affects the brain, causing pregnant women to breathe more deeply.

Breathlessness can also occur in the third trimester, when the uterus compresses your diaphragm, which presses on your lungs. During the final weeks of pregnancy, breathing may be easier as the fetus drops in the uterus.

If your breathlessness is severe or is accompanied by rapid breathing or chest pain, call your doctor. Otherwise, help alleviate breathlessness by sleeping and sitting in a comfortable position.

Constipation

Constipation (see p.781) affects more than half of pregnant women, primarily because the hormone progesterone relaxes the muscles and consequently slows the wavelike contractions of the intestinal muscles that move stool through your digestive tract. The iron in prenatal vitamins may also contribute to constipation.

Constipation can be eased by increasing the fiber content of your diet (see p.37), drinking at least eight glasses of water daily, and exercising regularly.

If these measures do not offer relief, consult your doctor, who may recommend a stool softener that is safe to use during pregnancy.

Dizziness

Feeling light-headed or dizzy is common during pregnancy due to a lower overall blood pressure and because the enlarged uterus can compress and block the large vein carrying blood to your heart. Either can cause a reduced supply of blood to the brain.

Brief light-headedness is common, especially when rising from a seated position or when lying on your back. Report repeated dizziness or fainting immediately to your doctor.

To prevent dizziness, rise slowly from seated and lying positions, avoid becoming overheated, and avoid lying flat on your back in the third trimester. During an episode of dizziness, sit down and bend over while breathing deeply, or lie down on your side. Both positions increase blood flow to the brain.

Fatigue

Fatigue is a universal lament during pregnancy as the body's energy is directed toward physically supporting the growing fetus. During the first trimester, your body is undergoing many changes. By the third trimester, you are bearing much more weight. Also, restlessness and interrupted sleep are common.

Alert your doctor if you experience extreme, persistent fatigue. Otherwise, pace your activities, sleep and nap as much as you can, and exercise regularly.

Food Cravings

Up to 90% of pregnant women have food cravings. Hormonal fluctuations during the first trimester are a suspected, though unproved, cause. There is no evidence that cravings signal an underlying nutritional deficiency, and cravings usually abate as the pregnancy progresses.

Consult your doctor if you have cravings for unhealthy foods at the expense of eating important nutrients, or if the cravings are causing excessive

weight gain. Otherwise, the occasional craving can be indulged without harm.

Frequent Urination

The need to urinate more frequently, especially at night, affects many women during the first trimester due to hormonal changes and the added pressure of the growing uterus on your bladder. You may feel the urge to urinate but pass only a small amount of urine.

Frequent urination may recur during the third trimester as the fetus drops in preparation for delivery.

Frequent urination is also a sign of urinary tract infection (see p.804). Notify your doctor if you have pain when urinating. If there is no infection, avoid excessive fluid intake after dinner to prevent disturbed sleep.

Heartburn

Indigestion and heartburn (see p.746) affect almost every pregnant woman. The hormone progesterone relaxes the ringlike sphincter at the base of your

Home Remedies for Leg Cramps

Cramps in the thighs or calves are common during pregnancy and usually occur during the last trimester, often at night. Doctors are not certain of the cause. Try the following home remedies:

- Wear support hose.
- Rest with your feet up.
- During cramping, extend your leg and flex your foot.
- Apply heat or gently massage the cramped area.

esophagus that normally closes off entry to the stomach. As a result, food mixed with digestive enzymes can back up into the esophagus, causing irritation and a burning pain in your chest.

You may also feel full due to the pressure of your expanding uterus on your stomach.

Prevent heartburn and indigestion by staying upright for at least 2 hours after eating and by eating frequent small meals throughout the day.

Notify your doctor if heartburn is persistent or prevents you from eating and gaining weight. Many antacids will relieve heartburn and are safe to take during pregnancy.

Hemorrhoids

Hemorrhoids (see p.795), which are swollen veins in the rectum, affect up to 50% of pregnant women. They develop when the enlarged uterus presses on the veins; they also can worsen if you are constipated or strain during bowel movements.

Symptoms include enlarged veins, painful defecation, and, sometimes, bleeding during a bowel movement.

If you have hemorrhoids, try these approaches:

■ To prevent constipation, eat a fiber-rich diet, drink at least 8 glasses of water daily, and exercise regularly.

■ Apply ice packs.

■ Reduce pressure on anal veins by lying on your side.

■ Improve circulation by doing Kegel exercises (see p.1051).

■ Take warm baths daily.

Incontinence

Incontinence (see p.826), or uncontrolled urination, affects some women during the last trimester. Pressure on the bladder from the growing uterus and relaxation of the pelvic muscles that control urination contribute to the condition.

Symptoms include leakage of urine, especially while laughing, coughing, sneezing, or lifting. Perform muscle-strengthening Kegel exercises (see p.1051) daily and urinate frequently, when you first have the urge.

Morning Sickness

Morning sickness is a misnomer for the nausea or vomiting that can occur at any time during pregnancy, usually during the first trimester but sometimes throughout pregnancy.

It is caused in part by increasing amounts of the hormone estrogen during the first 3 months of pregnancy. Report morning sickness to your doctor if vomiting is extensive, prevents weight gain, or continues after your first trimester. Severe cases may require intravenous feeding and antinausea medication.

Most often, morning sickness can be treated by eating frequent, small meals; eating something, such as a soda cracker, upon awakening in the morning; and eating something light (such as crackers or soup) to minimize hunger and the stimulation of digestive enzymes that can cause nausea.

Many odors, such as greasy foods, household cleaners, and perfumes, can trigger nausea during pregnancy. Try to avoid environments that have odors that make you nauseated.

Skin Changes

Hormonal fluctuations cause darkening of the areola (area surrounding the nipples) and development of a dark line running from the navel to the pubic area.

They also cause a masklike change in skin color on the cheeks, forehead, and above the lips called melasma (see Pigment Changes, p.538). These changes are worsened by exposure to the sun. Some women also have red palms or a blue-tinged, dappled discoloration of their feet.

Changing hormone levels may also cause a short-lived form of

Alternative Medicine: Morning Sickness

Morning sickness is nausea and vomiting that can occur any time of the day or night during pregnancy. It usually goes away by the end of the first trimester. Some women never have it.

Although not proven in scientific studies, some women find relief from drinking raspberry leaf tea, which is high in calcium. Combined with peppermint, it may also ease indigestion.

Childbirth Education

Childbirth education classes are offered at most hospitals and many physician offices to provide new parents with information on pregnancy and childbirth.

These programs are excellent forums for learning about warning signs during pregnancy, ways to stay healthy, and how to prepare for childbirth, breast-feeding, and infant care. Ask your doctor for a recommendation.

acne and a tendency to get heat rash (see p.537).

Stretch marks develop from weight gain and the stretching of the skin over your enlarging breasts and abdomen; this stretching can also cause skin to feel itchy.

Small growths known as skin tags (see p.542) may emerge in areas subject to increased friction. With the exception of skin tags and stretch marks, which may persist, skin changes usually fade after delivery.

If you are concerned about skin changes, see your doctor. Otherwise, keep your skin clean and dry and use cosmetics to cover any changes that annoy you. Moisturizers can ease itchy skin. If your skin itches intensely all over, see your doctor promptly.

Sleep Problems

There are many reasons sleep can be difficult during pregnancy, including the need to alter your sleeping position due to a changing body shape.

Sleeping on your side with your top knee bent and with that knee resting on a pillow may be comfortable and also reduces strain on your back.

Hormonal fluctuations and other discomforts of pregnancy also contribute to interrupted sleep, as can heartburn (see p.746).

Exercise moderately every day and report any severe sleep problems to your doctor.

Stuffy Nose

Nasal congestion during pregnancy can occur when an increased level of the hormone estrogen inflames the mucous membranes of your nose and causes a stuffy feeling. Many women mistake this persistent condition for allergies.

Although stuffiness may worsen as your pregnancy progresses, it usually resolves on its own after delivery. It is made worse by hot air and dry conditions.

Also, the larger volume of blood in your body during pregnancy can cause the tiny blood vessels in your nose to swell and sometimes burst with repeated hard nose blowing, causing a nosebleed (see p.1198).

If your symptoms are severe, see your doctor, who may recommend medications that are safe to take during pregnancy. Keep your environment moist by using a humidifier to ease symptoms and blow your nose gently to avoid bleeding.

Vaginal Discharge

Vaginal discharge commonly occurs because of increased hormone production. However, it is important to distinguish harmless discharge from the symptoms of infection (see Bacterial Vaginosis, p.930).

Vaginal discharge during pregnancy is thin and white with a nonoffensive odor; it may increase in quantity as your pregnancy progresses.

If the discharge is accompanied by itching, burning, or other discomfort, or if it has an unpleasant odor or is green or yellow, see your doctor, who will test the discharge for infection.

Otherwise, reduce the risk of infection by keeping your genital area clean, bathing regularly, drying thoroughly, avoiding tight clothing, wearing cotton underpants, and not using any scented products in your vaginal area.

Varicose Veins

Varicose veins (see p.706) are veins that are swollen and become noticeable through the skin. They may cause your legs to feel heavy and ache.

In pregnancy, they can be caused by pressure from the uterus on the veins in your pelvis and legs, which causes blood to pool there. An increased volume of blood in pregnancy also places pressure on the valves in the veins that normally keep the blood from accumulating.

To help keep blood circulating, take a daily walk, elevate your legs whenever you sit down, and avoid standing in one place for long periods of time. Wearing support hose helps most women.

Water Retention

Swelling of the ankles and feet due to water retention (edema) is caused by an increase in the volume of fluid during pregnancy. Your hands may also swell and rings on your fingers may become tight.

Water retention is usually harmless. However, if you have swelling of the face, blurred vision, or headache, call your physician; you could have preeclampsia (see p.932).

You can relieve the discomfort of water retention by elevating your feet whenever sitting or lying down, wearing support hose, and not standing for long periods.

SERIOUS CONDITIONS OF PREGNANCY

Most serious complications of pregnancy can occur in more than one trimester. This section describes complications under the trimester in which they are most likely to occur.

FIRST TRIMESTER

Miscarriage

Miscarriage (medically known as spontaneous abortion) is elimination of an embryo or fetus from a pregnant woman's body before it is physically able to survive on its own. It occurs in 15% to 30% of all pregnancies.

During the first trimester, it is called an early miscarriage. Between the 12th and the 20th week, it is called a late miscarriage. A delivery after the 20th week and before the 38th week of pregnancy is called preterm birth, even if the fetus is too immature to survive.

If the fetus and placenta are miscarried, it is called a complete abortion. If only part of the tissue is eliminated, it is called an incomplete abortion.

Most early miscarriages are due to chromosomal abnormalities (see p.126) in the embryo or fetus, which cause the woman's body to reject the pregnancy. Using tobacco or cocaine during pregnancy greatly increases the risk of miscarriage.

Rare causes include maternal health problems such as infection, hormonal disorders, or the presence of fibroids or congenital abnormalities of the uterus, which can make implantation in the wall of the uterus difficult.

Having one miscarriage does not reduce your chances of carrying a pregnancy to term when you next conceive. However, if you have more than two miscarriages, there may be a continuing problem that is preventing full-term pregnancy.

Miscarriage

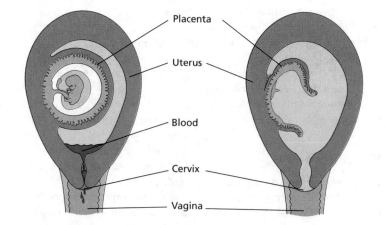

THREATENED ABORTION
(MISCARRIAGE)

INCOMPLETE ABORTION
(MISCARRIAGE)

Threatened abortion or miscarriage (left) is the term for bleeding during the first trimester; the fetus is alive and the cervix is closed. In an incomplete abortion or miscarriage (right), the fetus has died, but some of the placenta and fetal tissue still remain in the uterus. The cervix is open. The remaining tissue must be removed to prevent infection and bleeding.

In this situation, your doctor may order specific tests such as an x-ray of the inside of the uterus and fallopian tubes; blood tests to check for immune system, hormonal, or chromosome problems; or tests for infections.

SYMPTOMS

Symptoms include vaginal bleeding accompanied by uterine cramping and passing of clots or tissue. You cannot prevent an impending miscarriage, but you should save any tissue that you pass and take it to your physician for examination.

TREATMENT OPTIONS

Contact your physician if you have vaginal bleeding or uterine cramping during the first 3 months of pregnancy. A blood sample may be taken to check the level of the hormone human chorionic gonadotropin (hCG), which is released by the placenta during pregnancy.

A falling level of hCG can indicate that the fetus has died. Ultrasound may be performed to try to detect a fetal heartbeat. In many women, miscarriage does not occur until days or weeks after the fetus has died.

If the miscarriage is not complete or if the fetus has died but no tissue has passed, you may require a dilatation and curettage (see p.1077) to remove remaining tissue from your uterus. Your doctor may recommend that you wait until you have one or two menstrual cycles before attempting pregnancy again.

Miscarriage is an emotionally difficult event. It is normal for you and your family to grieve, regardless of how long you were pregnant. A support group can help you cope with the loss; ask your physician to recommend one.

Ectopic Pregnancy

An ectopic pregnancy develops outside of the uterus, usually in one of the fallopian tubes (when it is sometimes called a tubal pregnancy). Occasionally, it occurs in the cervix or abdomen, or on the ovary.

If an embryo growing outside the uterus is not removed, it will continue to grow and ultimately cause life-threatening complications.

Anything that causes scarring and narrowing of the fallopian tube can increase your risk for ectopic pregnancy. Narrowing of the tubes due to pelvic inflammatory disease (see p.1077) is a common cause.

Although some women have no symptoms, many experience pain on one side of the lower abdomen, a missed period, or irregular vaginal bleeding. If there is internal bleeding, you may feel weak, dizzy, and faint.

Your doctor will perform a pelvic examination. If you are in your fifth week of pregnancy or later and if blood tests reveal a low level of human chorionic gonadotropin (hCG), your doctor may suspect that you have an ectopic pregnancy. He or she may order an ultrasound (see p.919) to see if the pregnancy is in the uterus.

If an ectopic pregnancy has occurred, you may need laparoscopic surgery (see p.142) to remove the placenta and embryo from its location outside the uterus. If the fallopian tube has been ruptured, it may need to

Ectopic Pregnancy

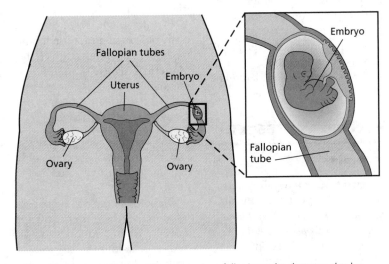

An ectopic pregnancy most often occurs in a fallopian tube, but can also be located in the cervix or abdominal cavity or in an ovary. Usually, a recognizable embryo does not develop. The pregnancy cannot be successfully transplanted to the uterus.

be repaired or removed. Most women can become pregnant with one fallopian tube.

Alternatively, ectopic pregnancy—in certain conditions—may be treated with methotrexate, a drug that causes the tissues of pregnancy to break down and be absorbed by the body.

Bleeding

Vaginal bleeding during the first trimester occurs in 1 of 4 pregnant women; let your doctor know if you have any bleeding. There are several causes.

Implantation bleeding (due to the embryo implanting in the uterus) occurs about a week after conception and does not endanger the pregnancy. It causes a day or two of spotting.

Slight but continuous bleeding for days or weeks with mild cramping or backache can be a sign of impending miscarriage (see p.928). Although many physicians recommend reducing activity, there is no evidence that this practice reduces the risk of miscarriage.

Ectopic pregnancy (see p.929) can also cause bleeding. Ultrasound is often used to determine the cause.

SECOND TRIMESTER

Anemia

Pregnant women require almost double the iron of nonpregnant women—between 30 and 60 milligrams per day—to sustain the fetus's need for iron to make blood cells and for the woman's body's own needs.

If you do not get enough iron, you can become anemic. Your doctor will test for anemia during your pregnancy. Eating iron-rich foods and taking prenatal vitamins helps prevent and treat anemia (see p.713).

Bacterial Vaginosis

Bacterial vaginosis is a common vaginal condition caused by a disproportionately high number of a few types of normal vaginal bacteria.

It can produce a gray or white, fishy-smelling discharge that may be accompanied by irritation of the vulva. Bacterial vaginosis may increase your risk for premature delivery.

If you suspect you have an infection, see your doctor or midwife, who will test a sample of your vaginal discharge for bacteria and for a change in its pH level.

Treatment is with the antibiotic clindamycin, as a pill or in a vaginal cream, in the second trimester, and with the antibiotic metronidazole, as a pill or in a vaginal cream, during the last trimester.

In women who have previously delivered a preterm infant, treatment may reduce the chance of prematurity in a subsequent pregnancy.

Gestational Diabetes

Gestational diabetes mellitus is a form of diabetes that occurs only in pregnancy, usually after 20 weeks.

Diabetes (see p.832) is excess sugar in the blood. In pregnancy, it occurs when hormones increase the amount of sugar in the blood but the pancreas cannot produce enough insulin to transport the sugar into the tissues.

You are at risk for gestational diabetes if you have borne a child who weighed more than 9 pounds, are over 30, are obese, have a close family member who has diabetes mellitus, or have had a stillbirth of undetermined cause.

As part of your prenatal care, you should be screened for diabetes between the 24th and 28th weeks of pregnancy. If the blood screening test indicates probable gestational diabetes, a more specific test, which involves drinking a sugar solution and then having several blood sugar level measurements, may be performed to make a certain diagnosis.

If you have gestational diabetes, your physician will provide a diet for you to follow. Most women do not require insulin to control the condition.

Incompetent Cervix

If the cervix is weak, it may open and give way to the weight of the growing fetus prematurely, a condition called incompetent cervix.

Known factors that can weaken the cervix include previous surgery to the cervix, such as a cone biopsy (see p.1041) or loop electrosurgical excision procedure, which is performed to remove precancerous tissue from the cervix (see p.1071). Exposure to diethylstilbestrol (DES) if your mother took it to prevent miscarriage while pregnant with you can also weaken the cervix. Sometimes no cause can be identified.

Because many women have no symptoms until they miscarry, an incompetent cervix is usually not diagnosed ahead of time. If

Incompetent Cervix

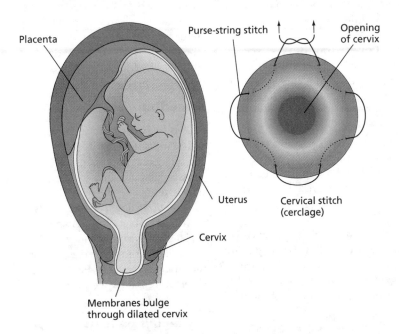

When the opening to the uterus, the cervix, dilates (widens) prematurely, the protective membranes around the fetus can fall through. This condition is called an incompetent cervix. To prevent the membranes from bursting and causing miscarriage, a purse-string stitch is made to tighten the cervix and keep it from dilating. The stitches are removed at about 37 weeks to permit delivery.

you have had a large cone biopsy or DES exposure, your doctor will examine you regularly during pregnancy for signs of cervical opening.

Tell your doctor if you have increased mucus from your vagina or have cramping or a feeling of more heaviness than usual in your pelvis.

Incompetent cervix is sometimes diagnosed by ultrasound. It is treated by cerclage, in which your cervix is stitched closed with a strong thread. Bed rest and abstaining from sexual intercourse may also be recommended. The cerclage is removed during the ninth month so delivery can occur.

Placenta Previa and Abruptio Placentae

The placenta develops inside the uterus to deliver oxygen and nutrients from your bloodstream to the fetus and to take away fetal waste for removal by your kidneys. A healthy placenta is critical to the development of the fetus.

The following placental disorders can occur during pregnancy:

Placenta previa In placenta previa, the placenta is located in an abnormally low position in the uterus, either partially or completely covering the cervix and blocking the route the fetus will take during delivery.

There are three forms. In marginal placenta previa, the placenta is located near the opening of the cervix, but does not block it. In partial placenta previa, the placenta covers part of the cervical opening. In complete placenta previa, the placenta blocks the entire opening of the cervix.

Your doctor may use ultrasound to determine the location of the placenta. In some women, the placenta changes location as pregnancy progresses; your physician may suggest a second ultrasound examination to monitor its location.

A placenta that blocks only a portion of the cervical opening may not inhibit a vaginal delivery; your doctor may recommend only that you rest and not have sexual intercourse.

When the placenta is located over the cervix, bleeding can occur due to mild changes in the cervix when it dilates (opens).

If the bleeding is severe, you may be hospitalized or your doctor may prescribe bed rest. A cesarean section may be required.

Abruptio placentae In this condition, a portion of the placenta detaches itself from the uterine wall, usually causing sudden pain in the abdomen and vaginal bleeding. It usually occurs during the third trimester.

Bleeding is not always noticeable because blood may collect between the wall of the uterus and the placenta. As it accumulates, it can cause the uterus to contract and lead to premature labor.

Because the placenta is the lifeline between you and the fetus, any interruption can cause a life-threatening reduction in circulation to the fetus. Women at risk include those who have high blood pressure, those who have had a direct injury to the abdomen (such as from an auto accident), and those who use cocaine.

Sometimes the bleeding from abruptio placentae can be severe, requiring emergency treatment. More often it is not. If the bleeding is minor and your due date is at least 3 weeks away, your doctor may prescribe bed rest. If the bleeding continues or if too much of the placenta detaches, placing extreme stress on the fetus, delivery, often by cesarean section, is performed immediately.

Urinary Tract Infections

Urinary tract infections (see p.804) in pregnancy, even when they do not cause symptoms, can cause serious kidney infections in the mother and can increase the risk of prematurity or fetal death. It is important to have any urinary tract infection diagnosed and treated. It is important to have a bladder infection treated so that it does not progress to a kidney infection. Kidney infection may require intravenous antibiotics and hospitalization.

LAST TRIMESTER

Amniotic Fluid Disorders

Inside the amniotic sac, which holds the fetus, amniotic fluid bathes and cushions the fetus. The amount of amniotic fluid steadily increases until about 36 weeks of pregnancy, when the volume begins to decline.

Polyhydramnios (too much fluid) and oligohydramnios (too little fluid) can occur late in pregnancy.

Polyhydramnios is excessive accumulation of fluid in the amniotic sac; this rare condition can occur quickly or over a period of time. The cause is often not known, but it occasionally indicates that the fetus has a disorder of the swallowing mechanism, brain, or spine. It can also occur in women who have diabetes and when there are multiple fetuses.

Although polyhydramnios is most often not threatening to the pregnancy, in rare cases it triggers premature labor (see p.934) or premature rupture of membranes.

There may be no symptoms with mild polyhydramnios. More advanced cases may cause breathlessness, indigestion, abdominal pain, and bloating. If you have symptoms, see your doctor, who will arrange for an ultrasound to confirm the excess fluid and to look for malformations in the fetus.

Severe cases may require medications to stabilize the uterus and prevent premature labor. In rare cases, amniocentesis is performed to extract some of the fluid.

Oligohydramnios is an insufficient amount of amniotic fluid. This condition may be caused by preeclampsia (see right), poor function of the placenta, or a urinary or kidney abnormality in the fetus.

Early in the pregnancy, it may cause birth defects in the fetus. Late in pregnancy, the reduced volume of fluid may permit the fetus to push the umbilical cord against the uterus, decreasing

oxygen and nutrition and causing poor growth or even death.

Your physician will monitor the fetus carefully and may deliver the baby before your due date if the oligohydramnios persists.

Bleeding

Bleeding in the third trimester often indicates a problem with the placenta, the organ that passes vital nutrients and oxygen to the fetus.

Call your doctor immediately if you have bleeding. It can signal a serious complication such as placenta previa (see p.931) or abruptio placentae (see p.931) or premature labor (see p.934).

Preeclampsia and Eclampsia

Also called toxemia, preeclampsia is high blood pressure, leaking of protein into urine, and water retention in a pregnant woman. It most often affects women during their first pregnancy.

If preeclampsia is not treated, it can cause seizures. If this occurs, the condition is called eclampsia. Other problems that result from preeclampsia include kidney or liver damage, poor fetal growth, internal bleeding, and fetal death.

Symptoms include sudden weight gain, severe headache, abdominal pain, leg swelling from fluid retention, and blurred vision. Your doctor will test your blood pressure and your urine for protein regularly throughout pregnancy.

Women who have mild preeclampsia may be monitored by nonstress tests (see Fetal Heart Rate Monitoring, p.919) and ultrasound to evaluate fetal growth as well as the amount of amniotic fluid in the uterus. An abnormal test result may indicate that the placenta is not passing enough nutrition to the fetus for proper growth.

If your condition is mild, you may be advised to rest in bed at home. For more severe cases of preeclampsia and for eclampsia, you may need to be hospitalized so your doctor can monitor you closely. Labor may be induced or a cesarean section performed.

High Blood Pressure

Women who have high blood pressure (see p.644) before becoming pregnant should have their blood pressure monitored regularly throughout pregnancy.

Many women can continue to control milder high blood pressure throughout pregnancy with careful attention to diet and exercise, or by taking low doses of blood pressure drugs that are safe to use during pregnancy. Most women with controlled high blood pressure have healthy pregnancies.

Women who have very high blood pressure that is not controlled have more complications during pregnancy, including preeclampsia (see previous article), premature labor (see p.934), abruptio placentae (see p.931), reduced kidney function, and poor fetal growth.

If you have high blood pressure, your physician will test your blood and urine more regularly to ensure that your kidneys are functioning well and that the fetus is developing properly.

Poor Fetal Growth

Poor fetal growth (medically known as intrauterine growth retardation) is defined as a smaller fetus than is normal for the stage of pregnancy. It complicates about 5% of all pregnancies.

In many cases, the placenta is not providing enough nutrients to the fetus. This can be caused by disorders such as high blood pressure (see p.644), preeclampsia (see p.932), or use of alcohol or tobacco by the mother. It can also be caused by multiple fetuses. In some cases, infection or malformation is the cause.

Poor fetal growth is more common among women under 17 or over 35. Without intervention during pregnancy, infants are usually born small for their age, whether premature or not, which makes them vulnerable to complications.

Prenatal checkups are essential to detect poor fetal growth at its earliest stage. The condition may be diagnosed by ultrasound (see p.919). The fetus is then evaluated carefully by periodic ultrasounds or nonstress tests (see Fetal Heart Rate Monitoring, p.919).

Treating the underlying disorder sometimes helps restore the growth rate, but sometimes labor is induced so the infant can be fed and monitored in a neonatal intensive care unit.

Postmaturity

Postmaturity, also called post-term pregnancy, is a condition in which an infant outgrows the nurturing capacity of the placenta and amniotic fluid. A pregnancy is considered to be post-term if it lasts beyond 42 weeks.

Labor may be induced (see p.941) to avoid complications, which occur when the aging placenta can no longer provide enough oxygen and nutrients to the fetus.

Most infants delivered between the 42nd and 44th weeks of pregnancy are healthy, but some experience more stress during delivery. Postmaturity increases the chance of having a difficult labor because of the increased size of the fetus and the poor function of the placenta.

Premature Rupture of the Membranes

Premature rupture of the membranes is bursting of the membranes that make up the amniotic sac surrounding the fetus before labor has started. Symptoms are a slow leak or sudden rush of fluid from the vagina. Call your doctor if this occurs.

When the process occurs before 34 weeks into the pregnancy, your doctor will weigh the risks of prematurity against the risks of prolonging your pregnancy to give your baby a chance to grow and mature further before delivery. Complications, including infection of the uterus and baby, can occur from trying to prolong the pregnancy. Premature rupture can also cause movement of the umbilical cord into the cervix; when the fetus drops down, it can press on the cord, reducing the supply of oxygen.

Bed rest may be prescribed in an attempt to keep the fetus in the uterus for as long as possible so that the lungs can mature. You may need antibiotics to prevent infection or medications to eliminate early contractions.

If you are within a few weeks of your delivery date and it is believed the fetus will have few or no complications, your physician will probably recommend inducing labor.

Premature Labor

Also called preterm labor, premature labor is contractions of the uterus that initiate labor before the 37th week of pregnancy. Approximately 9% of all births in the United States occur prematurely.

Prematurity places an infant at risk of respiratory distress syndrome (a condition in which immature lungs do not permit the baby to get enough oxygen to survive) and death if the lungs have not developed adequately to sustain him or her outside the uterus. Other problems of prematurity include infection, cerebral palsy, stroke, and heart or bowel problems.

In many women, the cause of premature labor cannot be identified. Risk factors include having had a previous premature delivery or premature labor; premature rupture of the membranes (see p.933); polyhydramnios (see Amniotic Fluid Disorders, p.932); multiple fetuses; any surgery that has weakened the cervix (see Incompetent Cervix, p.930); a kidney infection; being under 18 or over 40; or a placental disorder (see p.931).

Women who did not have adequate prenatal care and those who smoke, drink alcohol, or use cocaine are also at higher risk.

SYMPTOMS

You may have no symptoms or you may experience cramps or contractions, pelvic pressure, persistent backache, or a vaginal discharge that is watery or contains blood. Call your physician immediately if you have any of these symptoms or if you have contractions that occur every 10 minutes or more frequently for more than an hour.

TREATMENT OPTIONS

Your doctor will perform a vaginal examination to see if your cervix is dilating (opening) or effacing (thinning). Vaginal secretions, urine, and blood may be tested to identify infection.

Your physician will also determine the position of the fetus. You may be hospitalized if the contractions are strong and regular or your doctor may ask that you keep a record of contractions at home. Your doctor will continue to evaluate your cervix to see if labor is progressing.

Bed rest will probably be prescribed to keep pressure off your cervix. Do not have sexual intercourse.

Occasionally, drugs are given to reduce uterine contractions (especially if you have not reached the 34th week of preg-

nancy) in an attempt to permit the fetus to continue developing. A potent drug is often given to speed up the lungs' maturation if the fetus is under 34 weeks of age.

If the fetus is under stress or if there is a high risk of infection, your doctor may permit labor and delivery to continue. Your infant may need to spend time in an intensive care unit.

Abnormal Presentation

Presentation is the relationship of the fetus to the woman's body. The vast majority of fetuses are in the ideal position—lying with the head down—when labor begins.

Some fetuses are in the proper head-down position, but they face the woman's front. This is called the occipitoposterior position; this position can make passage through the birth canal more difficult.

Some fetuses are in a position in the uterus with their buttocks down. This is called a breech presentation. If your doctor suspects that the fetus is in breech position, it may be confirmed by ultrasound (see p.919).

The doctor may attempt to turn the fetus by gently pushing on your abdomen. In all cases of abnormal presentation, your doctor may let labor begin and, if necessary, deliver by cesarean section (see p.939).

CHILDBIRTH

Signs of Labor

Labor is the term used to describe the process by which the cervix opens and the uterus contracts to push the baby out of the mother's body. Every woman's labor is unique, but usually labor is immediately preceded by one or more of the following signs:

■ **Mucous plug detaches** This blood-tinged mucous discharge, which has sealed the cervix during pregnancy, is disengaged as the weight of the fetus pushes against the cervix and the cervix opens to release the plug. Labor usually occurs within a day or two. Some women do not notice the passage of the plug.

■ **Water sac breaks** In a trickle or a big gush, the amniotic fluid that bathes the fetus during pregnancy is released from the membranes of the amniotic sac (the "bag of water") before labor begins or during its first stage. If the water breaks but labor does not begin, or if the amniotic fluid is dark (because the fetus has had its first bowel movement in the uterus), your physician may recommend inducing labor.

■ **Contractions begin** Contractions that come in regular intervals and get progressively stronger signal labor. Many women have Braxton Hicks contractions during the last 12 weeks of pregnancy. These contractions are not strong or regular and they do not signal labor. Every woman feels contractions differently; some experience them in the lower back while others feel pain in the lower abdomen. Write down the time at the beginning of each contraction. When the contractions begin to occur consistently every 10 minutes, labor is generally beginning.

Stages of Labor

Before labor, the cervix is closed tightly and the uterus, which is a muscle, is not contracting regularly. During labor, the cervix dilates (opens) to 10 centimeters and effaces (thins out). Labor may last from an hour to longer than a day. There are three stages of labor and delivery:

FIRST STAGE

This stage lasts until the cervix is fully dilated, and includes early labor, active labor, and a transition phase into the second stage of labor (delivery).

Early labor Contractions of the uterus cause the cervix to dilate and become thinner (efface), though they may be so mild that you barely notice them.

Contractions will build in intensity and frequency. In addition, you may lose the mucous

Changes in the Cervix During Labor

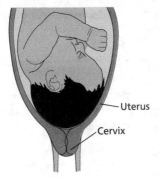

1 Hormones cause cervix to soften

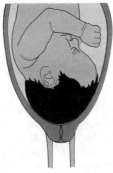

2 Contractions of the uterus pull up and shorten (efface) the cervix

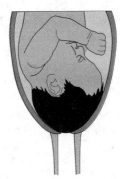

3 Cervix widens (dilates)

The muscular cervix begins to change late in pregnancy and during labor to permit delivery.

Pain Relief During Labor and Delivery

Women cope with the pain of labor and delivery in many ways. Some use one or more prepared childbirth techniques, including focused breathing, distraction, massage and relaxation, and visualization.

Drugs are also available to alleviate pain; discuss pain relief with your physician or midwife and familiarize yourself with the options before labor starts. This chart outlines choices for pain relief during labor and delivery.

PAIN RELIEF/ HOW IT IS ADMINISTERED	EFFECTS	SIDE EFFECTS
Analgesics (painkillers)/ intravenously or intramuscularly	Provide pain relief throughout body and relaxation without interfering with contractions	Drowsiness, nausea, and mildly reduced blood pressure in the woman; drowsiness, reduced sucking reflex, and reduced breathing and tone in the newborn (but only if given close to actual delivery)
Local anesthetics (such as for episiotomy)/injection given into tissue	Block nerve sensation in a particular region of the body but do not cause drowsiness	None
Epidural block (see Regional Anesthesia, p.169)/ injection given in space outside spinal cord by continuous infusion via catheter	Deadens pain below the waist	Occasional drop in woman's blood pressure and occasional slowing of fetal heartbeat; some can block the urge to push, resulting in need for medication to induce contractions (see Inducing Labor, p.941) or forceps or vacuum-assisted vaginal delivery
Pudendal nerve block/injection given inside top of vagina	Blocks pain between vagina and anus; occasionally used for episiotomy (see p.938) or forceps delivery	Rare; occasionally anesthesia of one side of the body does not take full effect
Spinal block/injection by needle into fluid around spinal cord	Makes you unable to move from waist down; used occasionally for forceps delivery and most often for cesarean section	Same as for epidural; occasionally headache the following day
Hypnosis (see p.394)	Changes pain perception	None
General anesthesia (see p.168)/intravenously and as inhaled gases	Makes you lose consciousness; used only when complications occur and quick unconsciousness must be induced (such as for an emergency cesarean section)	None if used immediately before cesarean section

Positions of Twins

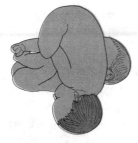

Buttocks down (5 percent)

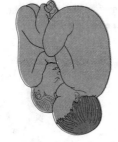

Head down and horizontal (18 percent)

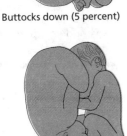

Buttocks down and head down (27 percent)

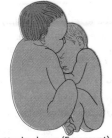

Head down (42 percent)

These are the most common positions of twins in the uterus (the other 8% are in other positions).

Breech Positions

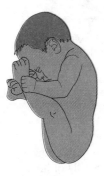

FRANK BREECH

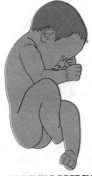

FOOTLING BREECH

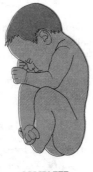

COMPLETE BREECH

There are three common breech positions. In a frank breech position, the baby's hips are flexed and the legs are extended. In some cases, a baby in a frank breech position can be delivered through the vagina. In the footling breech position, one or both feet are positioned over the cervix. When the knees are flexed, the presentation is called complete breech.

plug and your water bag may rupture. Your back may ache and you may have slight cramping in your lower abdomen or anus, along with diarrhea and some nausea.

Unless your membranes have ruptured, there is no need to call your doctor. Relax and reserve your strength for the challenge of active labor.

Active labor Your cervix will dilate from 4 to 8 centimeters and contractions become more intense. Though there is considerable variation, contractions generally last between 40 and 60 seconds and are 3 to 4 minutes apart.

You will experience a steady building of pressure and discomfort, followed by a gradual release.

Breathing exercises during contractions and focused relaxation between them can help minimize pain and reserve your strength. The period of release between contractions will become shorter as labor progresses.

Now is the time to call your physician or midwife, if you have not already, and go to the hospital or birthing center. If the bag of water has not ruptured by the time you are dilated to 3 to 5 centimeters, your doctor or midwife may rupture it manually.

Transition phase This is the most physically and emotionally taxing phase of labor. Your cervix is opening to 10 centimeters and the uterus is contracting strongly. You may enter an emotionally vulnerable state of exhaustion and exhilaration.

The baby moves into your vagina and you may feel a strong urge to push; this must be avoided until you are fully dilated. Get into any position that is comfortable for you.

SECOND STAGE

Pushing and delivery of the baby occur during this stage. When your cervix is fully dilated, you push every time you feel a contraction. Some nurses and midwives massage the area between the vagina and anus to stretch the vaginal opening to avoid the need for an episiotomy.

You may also feel more clear-headed and physically renewed. You will need this energy for the final phase of pushing, which brings your baby into the world after a few minutes or several hours.

Your doctor or midwife will give you instructions on when to push and when to wait. Panting in short breaths may help you to not push when you feel the urge. After your baby is born, your doctor or midwife will quickly evaluate your baby's health and either put the infant on your abdomen or onto a special table with radiant-heat warming lights. Your baby will be wet and naked in a cool room and needs to be dried and warmed promptly.

THIRD STAGE

This stage involves delivery of the placenta (afterbirth). Uterine contractions separate this organ from the uterine wall and expel it from the uterus out the vagina.

Your physician may gently pull on the cord to assist the process. If the placenta does not emerge on its own within 30 minutes, your doctor may need to gently reach inside your uterus and remove the placenta (see Retained Placenta, p.943).

Episiotomy

Episiotomy is an incision made in the tissue between the vagina and the anus (the area called the perineum) to enlarge the vaginal opening while the baby is being born. Many doctors perform it as a routine part of the delivery process to prevent these tissues from tearing raggedly on their own during delivery, which can make repairing the tissues more difficult.

Episiotomies are done less often than they used to be because many doctors think the procedure actually injures more tissue than delivery without episiotomy. Most physicians believe the need for an episiotomy cannot be evaluated until the time of delivery. Ask your doctor about his or her views on the procedure.

Episiotomy

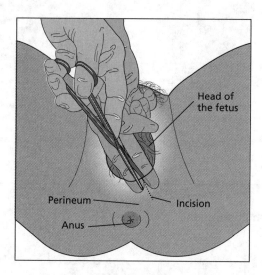

An episiotomy is an incision made in the perineum (the area between the vagina and the anus) to permit passage of the baby during delivery. The doctor administers a local anesthetic to numb the tissues of the perineum and then, protecting the baby's head with the fingers, makes an incision. The cut is stitched closed after delivery.

Fetal Monitoring

Birth and delivery can be physically stressful on the emerging baby. During labor, fetal monitoring is used to check the infant's heart rate and ensure that enough oxygen is available.

The monitor measures the heart rate as well as the response of the heartbeat to the uterine contractions. Fetal monitoring can be done externally or internally.

External monitoring is performed by two small monitors or belts strapped around your abdomen; the monitors measure and record the frequency and length of your contractions as well as the fetal heart rate. The monitors are applied intermittently or continuously throughout the first phase of labor, and continuously or after every contraction during the pushing stage.

Internal monitoring provides more precise evaluation of the fetus and is usually used only when there is a nonreassuring fetal heart rate on the external monitor. In internal monitoring, an electrode is attached to the scalp of the infant via your vagina and cervix to measure the infant's heart rate.

Your doctor may also insert a slender wand into the uterus to measure the frequency, intensity, and length of your contractions.

Cesarean Section

A cesarean section is the delivery of a fetus through incisions in the abdomen and the uterus.

Cesarean section is major surgery performed using anesthesia. About 60% to 80% of women who had a previous cesarean can have safe vaginal deliveries with subsequent pregnancies.

Nearly 25% of American-born babies are delivered by cesarean section. Some surgeries are planned in advance based on medical conditions, such as placenta previa (see p.931), that make vaginal delivery less safe. Most cesareans are performed when the need arises during labor.

Your doctor may recommend cesarean delivery if your contractions are not adequately opening your cervix, and if other methods of encouraging dilation of the cervix (such as administering the

drug oxytocin) have not been effective.

A cesarean section may also be performed if:

- The baby appears to be under too much stress from labor, as indicated by fetal heart rate monitoring.

- The baby is very large compared to the size of your pelvis.

- The baby is in a breech presentation (see p.937), and efforts to turn the baby have not been successful.

- There are triplets or a greater number of multiple births.

For surgery, an intravenous line is inserted to give you fluids, the abdomen is cleansed, and a catheter is placed into your urethra to drain urine during and after surgery. Anesthesia choices include a spinal or epidural block (see p.936), which deadens sen-

sation below the waist and allows you to stay awake during the birth, or general anesthesia, which makes you unconscious.

An incision is made in the abdomen above the pubic bone. The incision is most often horizontal (this is a bikini-line incision, which heals less noticeably) but can be vertical. A second (usually horizontal) incision is made in the uterus.

The baby and placenta are delivered through the incisions. The uterine incision is stitched closed and the external incision is stitched or stapled closed. The surgery takes about 1 hour.

After surgery, you will continue to receive medications for pain. Avoid lifting anything heavier than your baby for several weeks, both while recuperating at the hospital and after you return home. Your scar may itch or feel numb and look red.

Stillbirth

Stillbirth is the term for a fetus born dead after 20 weeks of gestation. An autopsy may be performed (with your permission) to attempt to determine the cause of death.

A fetus that dies in the uterus may be detected through fetal heart rate monitoring or ultrasound, which may be done because you can no longer feel the fetus move or in the course of routine prenatal care. Labor may start on its own after the fetus dies, or it may need to be induced (see p.941).

Stillbirth is relatively rare. The cause is unknown in as many as 30% of stillbirths. Known causes include severe birth defects; multiple fetuses; abruptio placentae (see p.931), high blood pressure, diabetes, or other conditions that affect the placenta's ability to deliver nutrients and oxygen to the fetus; Rh incompatibility (see p.157); and some rare infections acquired during pregnancy.

The emotional effects of having a stillborn child can be as distressing as any other death. Grieving parents may benefit from support groups and professional counseling; ask your physician for a referral.

Complications, which are infrequent, include internal bleeding, pelvic infection, blood clots, bowel dysfunction, and injury to other abdominal organs such as the bowel, bladder, and ureters.

Forceps Delivery

If you have pushed your baby to the opening of your vagina but cannot push the baby out, your physician may use forceps to gently pull at the same time you are pushing.

Forceps are curved, spoonlike metal instruments that are used to grasp both sides of the baby's head and cheekbones. Your doctor will first deaden the area around your vagina by administering a pudendal block or epidural or spinal anesthesia (see p.936), insert the forceps, and perform an episiotomy (see p.938). As you push with each contraction, a gentle pull helps the baby descend and emerge.

Your doctor might also use forceps if your baby is being stressed by labor, as shown on the fetal heart rate monitor.

Vacuum Extraction

Vacuum extraction may be used as an alternative or adjunct to a forceps delivery (see previous article). The vacuum device is a rubber cup that fits onto the crown of the baby's head.

A vacuum is created through a small tube attached to the cup, thus holding it onto the baby's head. While you push, your doctor will gently pull to aid you in pushing out your baby. The baby may have a little swelling where the suction cup was applied.

Vacuum Extraction

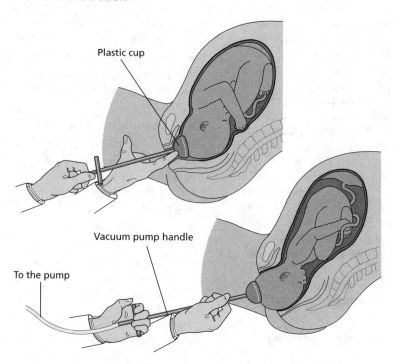

Plastic cup

Vacuum pump handle

To the pump

Vacuum extraction is an alternative to forceps delivery. The extractor is made up of a vacuum pump connected to a soft plastic cup with a handle. During the procedure, the cup is placed on the crown of the baby's head; the vacuum creates a suction that keeps the cup in place. During contractions, the doctor carefully pulls on the handle in the same direction the mother is pushing and, once the head appears through the vagina, removes the cup and assists with the delivery of the baby.

Failure to Progress

Sometimes the steady progress of labor (as evaluated by cervical opening and descent of the fetal head) stops. This may be due to inadequate contractions or disproportion.

Disproportion is a condition in which the woman's bony pelvic outlet is not wide enough to permit passage of the baby's head. It may be due to a large baby or a baby whose head is not in a good position. Most disproportion is not diagnosed until delivery is stalled by the lack of progress of labor.

The other cause of failure to progress is contractions that are not strong enough. The drug oxytocin can be infused to increase the strength of contractions. The strength of contractions is then monitored by a pressure gauge inserted into the uterus.

If labor still does not progress over several hours, a cesarean section is performed.

Apgar Score

The evaluation of an infant's health begins in the minute after birth—and again after 5 minutes—with an Apgar score, which rates heart rate, breathing, muscle tone, reflexes, and color. Each criterion is rated 0, 1, or 2. The maximum total, encompassing all five criteria, is 10. The Apgar score helps the physician evaluate your baby and signals if medical attention is needed. Some infants score low but do not require treatment. A low score should not worry you; it cannot predict your child's long-term potential.

			SIGN		
APGAR SCORE	HEART RATE	BREATHING AND CRYING	MUSCLE TONE	REFLEX RESPONSE*	SKIN COLOR
0	Absent	Absent	Limp	No response	Blue or pale
1	Less than 100 beats per minute	Irregular breathing, weak cry	Some flexing of arms and legs	Grimace	Body pink, extremities blue
2	More than 100 beats per minute	Regular breathing, strong cry	Active motion in arms and legs	Cry, cough, sneeze	Completely pink

*Evaluated by inserting a slender tube into the baby's nose.

Newborn Examination

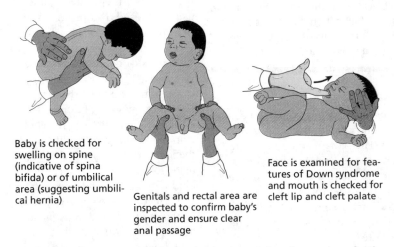

Baby is checked for swelling on spine (indicative of spina bifida) or of umbilical area (suggesting umbilical hernia)

Genitals and rectal area are inspected to confirm baby's gender and ensure clear anal passage

Face is examined for features of Down syndrome and mouth is checked for cleft lip and cleft palate

After examining the heart and lungs, the doctor examines the newborn for the less common abnormalities shown. Feet are also inspected for evidence of clubfoot and the hips for hip dislocation.

Inducing Labor

An induced labor is one that is started by your physician or midwife before it starts on its own. Labor is induced when the risks to the woman or fetus of permitting the pregnancy to continue are judged greater than the risks of inducing labor.

Reasons for inducing labor include preeclampsia (see p.932), postmaturity (see p.933), a low level of amniotic fluid in the uterus (oligohydramnios), infection of the amniotic fluid (see Amniotic Fluid Disorders, p.932), poor fetal growth (see p.933), or placental problems (see p.931).

Labor can be induced in a number of ways, depending on the situation. Rupturing the mem-

What Will My Baby Look Like?

A healthy baby has features that may seem irregular or even alarming (especially babies delivered vaginally) but are perfectly normal.

Head The head's journey through the birth canal can give it a cone or squashed shape. The strange appearance of the head generally subsides within 2 to 4 days as it assumes a rounder form.

Skin Because your baby has spent 9 months bathed in fluid, he or she will emerge with a white coating called vernix that is like a thick lotion. The vernix protects your baby's skin while he or she is in the uterus. Your baby may also have wrinkled, red or pale, blotchy skin, with tiny white spots.

Body proportion Your baby's limbs will be short, the body long and thin, and the head proportionately oversized—overall, your baby may look scrawny. Expect your infant to lose up to 10% of his or her birthweight in the few days following delivery. He or she should regain the weight by 2 weeks of age.

Hair The hair on your baby's head, whether nonexistent, fine, or thick, may fall out within a few weeks or months, to be replaced by new hair. Lanugo, a downy hair on the back, shoulders, and arms, usually sheds within a few weeks.

Genitals Genitals may appear swollen, and girls and boys may have enlarged breasts that leak a milklike substance; girls may have a vaginal secretion or even slight vaginal bleeding. These features are caused by hormones from the mother; they normalize within 2 weeks.

Umbilical stump The stump of the umbilical cord will remain attached to the navel for 1 to 4 weeks, when it usually falls off on its own. It should be washed gently around the edges. Watch for signs of infection (redness and swelling); they should be reported to your pediatrician.

brane that surrounds the fetus to release the amniotic fluid sometimes activates labor.

The drug oxytocin, which is a synthetic form of the hormone that causes spontaneous labor, is given to induce labor. If your cervix is hard, your doctor or midwife may use a vaginal gel or pellet of prostaglandin to soften it before administering oxytocin.

Oxytocin is administered intravenously; the amount is increased progressively until your uterus begins to contract, usually within 60 minutes.

The baby may be monitored while the drug is taking effect to ensure that contractions are not causing too much stress or occurring so frequently that the baby's oxygen supply is inadequate.

Postpartum Infection

Postpartum infection may involve the uterine lining (endometrium) or the tissue in and around the vagina. Symptoms include fever, pain, and a malodorous vaginal discharge.

Infection often gets better with antibiotics but occasionally requires that episiotomy stitches be removed and the wound reopened to drain the infected material.

Postpartum Hemorrhage

All women bleed somewhat after delivery. Postpartum hemorrhage is heavy bleeding after childbirth. It occurs in 2% of births, most often after long labors, multiple births, or when an infection has started in the uterus.

In most women, heavy bleeding occurs when the uterus does not contract adequately after the placenta has been delivered.

In some women, heavy bleeding occurs due to tears of the cervix, vagina, or uterus.

When heavy bleeding starts a week or two after delivery, it is usually caused by a piece of the placenta that has remained in the uterus.

Your doctor will perform a pelvic examination to determine the cause of the bleeding. He or she may massage your abdomen to stimulate contractions (which help stop bleeding), give you the synthetic hormone oxytocin to stimulate contractions, and test your blood for anemia and infection.

If bleeding is excessive, you may require a blood transfusion. If your doctor suspects that placental pieces remain inside the uterus, he or she will perform a dilation and curettage (see p.1077) to remove the tissue.

Retained Placenta

Normally, the placenta separates from the uterine wall and is delivered with the first contractions after delivery, usually within 20 minutes; your doctor will aid the process by gently massaging your abdomen and holding the umbilical cord. If the placenta is not delivered within 30 minutes, it is called a retained placenta.

Because the cervix closes several hours after birth, and the exposed umbilical cord serves as a route for infection to the uterus, a retained placenta must be removed. Nursing your newborn may induce uterine contractions to help deliver the placenta.

Alternately, your doctor may remove the placenta by inserting a hand into the uterus and gently separating the placenta from the uterine wall.

Circumcision

Male circumcision is surgery to remove the foreskin that covers the head of the penis. It is usually performed on newborns within the first 48 hours; when done for religious reasons, it is performed after a week. Complications, which are rare, include infection and bleeding.

Circumcision probably reduces the chance that a child will develop urinary tract infections or, later in life, cancer of the penis. However, since both of these conditions are very rare, the American Academy of Pediatrics no longer recommends that circumcision be performed routinely. Talk to your doctor about the need for circumcision.

During circumcision, babies act in ways that indicate that they feel pain. There is a growing consensus that babies feel less pain when given anesthesia before a circumcision is performed. However, injecting a local painkiller into the penis before circumcision also causes pain.

A painless way of applying local anesthesia to the penis before the circumcision (rather than injecting a local anesthetic) is through the application of creams that contain local anesthetics. However, it has not yet been proven that anesthetic creams are as effective as injections of local anesthetic.

Before circumcision, the genital area is cleaned. The foreskin is then removed using a special circumcision clamp that protects the penis itself.

The edge where the foreskin was removed may appear swollen for several days and a thin, yellow crust will form over the site. Apply petroleum jelly to the raw areas during diaper changes; if the site is red, you may be advised to apply an antibiotic ointment.

Call the doctor if your baby has a rectal temperature higher than 100°F; the circumcision site shows signs of infection (such as redness or swelling) or bleeds; or your baby is fussy and irritable, has a high-pitched cry, or does not urinate for 12 hours.

Common Changes After Labor and Delivery

Most women experience some discomfort after labor and delivery, mostly normal changes that occur as your body recovers.

Some of the most common are outlined here.

Backache The physical challenges of bearing 20 or more pounds of weight and delivering a baby can take their toll on a woman's back, especially when combined with physical and emotional exhaustion. See p.626 for some recommendations for coping with a bad back.

Vaginal bleeding Vaginal bleeding, known as lochia, is normal. It is composed of blood, mucus, and tissue from the uterine lining. Menstrual-like bleeding may be continuous for up to a week after birth, after which it starts to abate and fade in color, eventually turning into a yellow discharge as the uterus returns to its normal size. Continued contractions induced by breast-feeding help the uterus shrink and bleeding diminish.

Breast problems Engorgement is the term for breasts that are swollen, tender, and hard. It can occur any time feeding is delayed, after your milk supply is established (usually in about 3 days).

Your infant can have a difficult time latching on to engorged breasts, so you may need to express a little milk first. To express milk, place your thumb and fingers behind the areola (the darker skin surrounding your nipple) and squeeze as you push toward your chest. Then, squeeze toward the nipple. Move your fingers one quarter turn around the breast and repeat.

Nipple pain and cracking are common among breast-feeding women. Although these symptoms may arise from an improper latching-on position (see p.951), they are also normal ways that nipples adapt to their new roles.

Contact your doctor if pain or cracking persist more than a few days or if skin redness occurs over the non-nipple part of the breast. In the interim, expose your breasts to the air and avoid scented soaps and creams.

The milk ducts are vulnerable to blockage. You may notice a small, tender, red lump on your breast. Pressure on the affected duct may aggravate the problem and lead to infection (see Mastitis, p.1056). Mastitis is best treated by draining the milk ducts as completely as possible, by offering the affected breast first (when your baby is hungriest), and, if necessary, by expressing any remaining milk with a breast pump. If the red lump persists, see your doctor or midwife.

Exercise Women who want to resume exercising can do so within a few days after delivery. Start slowly (perhaps only with brisk walking) and build your routine gradually as your strength increases. Ask your doctor for advice on specific exercises; you may need to avoid doing leg lifts or abdominal exercises for 6 weeks or more.

Hair loss The lustrous sheen that pregnancy brought to your hair may soon go down the drain. Several months after delivery (or when breast-feeding women wean their baby or add solids to the baby's diet), many women are distressed to find they are losing a considerable amount of hair. This change is due to loss of hairs that were not shed during pregnancy because of pregnancy hormones.

Hemorrhoids The pressure of the enlarged uterus and fetus on the veins of the lower abdomen can result in hemorrhoids (see p.795). Sitting on a padded or inflatable ring (called a "donut") can bring some relief. Also, try sitting in warm water for 10 to 15 minutes every day and then applying cold packs to the affected area.

Mood changes or postpartum depression Between 50% and 80% of women are affected by some degree of depression after childbirth. Some researchers believe that dramatic fluctuations in hormones are responsible. Others assert that postpartum depression reflects the reality of how life has changed.

Typically, the symptoms of sadness, anxiety, sleep disorders, hostility, and mood changes disappear within a month of delivery, but may continue for a longer time.

Call your doctor if you have difficulty coping with daily life. You may feel better just talking to someone or, if you suffer from more severe and persistent emotional disturbances, you may benefit from medication and/or counseling.

Pain in the perineum If you delivered vaginally, there are several reasons you may have pain in the area around your vagina. First, the strain of childbirth stretched these tender tissues. Second, any cutting of the area during childbirth—such as tearing or having an episiotomy—takes time to heal.

Your doctor may instruct you in ways to prevent infection, including applying warm water with the help of a squirt bottle or large syringe to the area after urinating or moving your bowels. For pain relief, follow the recommendations given for hemorrhoids (p.795).

Sex Depending on your delivery, you will need to wait at least 4 to 6 weeks before your body heals enough to safely resume sexual intercourse. Although some women feel ready for sex, others find that the fluctuations in hormones, physical exhaustion, and preoccupation with their newborn take a toll on their sexual interest for many months.

When you do have sex, it may be painful due to an episiotomy, tenderness, or lack of vaginal lubrication (caused by hormonal changes, particularly in nursing women). Allow time for your body to heal, for life to resume a predictable pattern, and for you to rebuild intimacy with your partner.

Using a water-based vaginal lubricant can help bridge the gap to a more satisfying sex life.

Stretch marks The red striations around your breasts and hips, caused by hormonal changes and stretching skin, may be more noticeable as your body starts to resume its pre-pregnancy dimensions. Although they will not disappear, they will fade considerably over time.

Health of Infants and Children

Nothing is of more concern to parents and families than the health of their children. Most children are born healthy, develop normally, and become healthy adults. To do so, your child requires good preventive health measures and regular checkups. Your child also needs your help with the most basic functions of life—eating, sleeping, walking, and talking.

When your child develops symptoms, you need to know what to do, including when to call the doctor.

The inability of babies to speak can be difficult for parents. Crying, rash, fever, and changes in bowel movements and behavior can all be signs of sickness, or simply indicate momentary discomfort. While you try to interpret the riddles of your child's signs, symptoms, and behavior, take comfort in the knowledge that these signs and symptoms will become clearer to you with time and experience.

In the meantime, err on the side of caution. Do not hesitate to call your child's doctor with questions that concern you.

How This Chapter Is Organized

This chapter provides information about normal childhood development, and what your child's doctor should be doing to monitor the health of your child. One of the most important aspects of maintaining your child's health—immunizations and the diseases that they prevent—is presented first.

The health of children younger than age 2, including growth, development, and some of their medical problems, is discussed beginning on p.951. The health of children older than age 2 is addressed beginning on p.987.

Physical and Mental Health of Parents

Raising children is a rewarding and challenging responsibility. It is normal for parents to feel a range of emotions—from joy and pride to frustration and even anger.

Doctors Who Care for Children

These are the types of doctors who provide care for children:

- **Pediatricians** receive at least 3 years of training after medical school in the comprehensive primary care of children.

- **Family physicians and internal medicine/pediatric physicians** receive at least 3 years of combined training after medical school in the care of both adults and children.

- **Pediatric subspecialists** receive several additional years of training in specific childhood diseases and conditions. Some concentrate on diagnosis and medical treatment while others can perform surgery. If your child develops an illness that requires the attention of a pediatric subspecialist, your child's doctor can recommend one to you.

Negative feelings toward children rarely occur as isolated events. Certainly, children's behavior can cause frustration, but usually not enough to bring parents to the breaking point unless accompanied by other stresses. Economic struggles and conflicts with partners are other common factors that can shorten a parent's fuse. Many parents feel frustrated by the limits on freedom that their children impose. Others have unresolved psychological problems.

Parents who were physically or sexually abused as children are more likely to abuse their own children. Physical and mental health problems, ranging from fatigue to chronic or severe disease to depression, can also contribute to the stress of parenting. In addition, many parents tend to ignore their own health problems in deference to their children's health and well-being.

For the sake of your children and yourself, it is important to be alert to emotions that may lead you to physically hurt or abuse your child. If you have persistent feelings of frustration or a desire to hurt your child, or have acted on these feelings, seek help.

Talk to your physician, your child's doctor, a trusted friend, or a spiritual counselor about your frustrations and ask for a referral to a counselor or support group in your area. Parents Anonymous (909-621-6184) can also provide a referral to a local support group.

LIFESTYLE CHOICES AND CHILDREN

Parents who engage in destructive health habits—such as overuse of alcohol, tobacco use, or use of (often illegal) street drugs—are not only harming themselves, they are setting poor standards for, and possibly harming the health of, their children.

Secondhand smoke can cause or aggravate childhood respiratory diseases such as asthma and allergies; also, children are more likely to start smoking later in life if their parents smoke.

Alcohol and other drug use makes you less able to cope with the stresses of parenting. Resources to help you with alcohol or drug abuse are listed in the Appendix (see p.1228).

Set a good example by using seatbelts, bike helmets, and other safety gear; it will encourage your child to follow suit.

IMMUNIZATIONS AND THE DISEASES THEY PREVENT

Of all the things you can do to protect your child against ill health, perhaps nothing is more important than immunizations.

Immunizing your child offers him or her protection against a number of potentially deadly infectious diseases. Without immunity to these diseases, exposure to them can cause life-threatening sickness and even death. At one time, thousands of children were disabled or killed every year from infectious diseases. See p.948 for descriptions of childhood infectious diseases for which there are vaccines.

Immunizations work effectively only when given at very specific times in your child's life; most states require proof of immunization for entry into school. The schedule on p.947 shows which immunizations your child needs and at what age. All are given by injection and most combine vaccines against several diseases.

Though side effects are rare, they can occur with any vaccine. The type of reaction and its timing varies with each vaccine. You may be asked to read about these before giving informed consent for your child. If you are concerned about possible side effects, discuss this with your child's doctor before the immunizations are given. In general, the protective effects of immunity far outweigh the risks.

The vaccination schedule outlines when immunizations should be given to a healthy infant and child. If your child has a medical condition, the doctor may recommend adjusting the schedule. You should review the schedule with your child's doctor at each visit to be sure your child's immunizations are up-to-date. Since new vaccines are always being developed, this schedule changes often. The shaded areas indicate when a particular immunization is usually recommended.

Recommended Childhood Immunization Schedule*

VACCINE	BIRTH	1 MONTH	2 MONTHS	4 MONTHS	6 MONTHS	12 MONTHS	15 MONTHS	18 MONTHS	24 MONTHS	4 TO 6 YEARS	11 TO 12 YEARS	13 TO 18 YEARS
Hepatitis B												
1st	▓											
2nd		▓	▓	▓								
3rd					▓	▓	▓	▓				
Diphtheria, Tetanus, Pertussis (Whooping Cough)												
1st			▓									
2nd				▓								
3rd					▓							
4th							▓	▓				
5th										▓		
6th											Tetanus & Diphtheria (Td) only	
***Haemophilus influenzae* Type b**												
1st			▓									
2nd				▓								
3rd					▓							
4th						▓	▓					
Inactivated Poliovirus												
1st			▓									
2nd				▓								
3rd					▓	▓	▓	▓				
4th												
Measles, Mumps, Rubella												
1st						▓	▓					
2nd										▓		
Varicella												
						▓	▓	▓				
Pneumococcal												
1st			▓									
2nd				▓								
3rd					▓							
4th						▓	▓					
Influenza (yearly)												
					▓	▓	▓	▓	▓			
**Hepatitis A **												

▓ Recommended ages for vaccination

* Check the immunizations of all children, including teenagers, at least once a year to insure they are always "up-to-date." Contact your physician for "catch-up" immunization schedules and any special vaccine recommendations for specific populations. Licensed combination vaccines may be given whenever the components of the combination are indicated (and the other components are not contraindicated). Do not forget that more vaccines may be licensed and recommended each year.

** Hepatitis A vaccine is recommended for children and adolescents in selected states and regions and for certain high risk groups (see page 949).

VACCINE-PREVENTABLE CHILDHOOD INFECTIOUS DISEASES

It is essential that your child be vaccinated against the common childhood infectious diseases (see p.947 for the recommended vaccination schedule).

Infectious diseases are spread from person to person by direct contact and by inhaling respiratory secretions from infected individuals. This can occur when an infected person sneezes or coughs droplets in another person's direction, or when hands with secretions on them touch the mucous membranes of the nose or eyes.

Once in the body, the infectious agents go through an incubation period, which varies, depending on the disease. During this incubation period, the germs multiply and spread.

VACCINES UNDER DEVELOPMENT

Already, vaccines are given to adults to protect against meningococcus bacteria, which can cause serious childhood infections. Studies are under way to determine if it would be beneficial to routinely immunize all children with this vaccine.

Likewise, consideration is being given to routinely immunizing all children against the hepatitis A virus (see p.949). A vaccine is also being developed against respiratory syncytial virus, which is a common cause of childhood infections, including bronchiolitis and ear infections.

Chickenpox

(See also Color Guide to Visual Diagnosis, p.568)

Chickenpox is a very contagious infectious disease that is caused by a virus. A vaccine to prevent children from acquiring chickenpox can be given to children beginning at 12 months of age. Keep your child away from any other child who currently has chickenpox.

Within 10 to 21 days after being exposed to a person with chickenpox, your child may start to feel sick, have a fever, and begin to develop a spotty, red rash on the trunk (especially the chest) that spreads to the face, arms, and legs. The rash turns into small, fluid-filled bumps that crust over within several days, and form scabs. Scratching the itchy areas can cause scars. The rash may also affect the inside of the mouth.

The illness lasts about a week from start to finish. Children are contagious a day or two before the rash develops; they stop being contagious after the last sores have crusted over, within about 7 days.

Give your child a fever-reducing drug, such as acetaminophen (not aspirin), in the dose your doctor recommends. Using oatmeal bath preparations (available at the drugstore) and applying calamine lotion to the itchy rash may keep your child from scratching. Keep fingernails short to prevent bacterial infection and scarring of the scratched areas.

Once your child has had chickenpox, he or she will be immune for life. If your child currently has chickenpox, it is all right for the child to play with other children who definitely have had the disease or have been vaccinated, but he or she should be kept away from children who have not.

Diphtheria

Diphtheria is a serious bacterial infection that is most often acquired by traveling to countries where hygiene is poor. It is rare in the United States because children are immunized.

Symptoms of diphtheria include sore throat, breathing difficulties, rapid heartbeat, swollen lymph glands in the neck, and a gray membrane covering the tonsils and throat.

Treatment includes restoring normal breathing and taking antibiotics. The bacteria that cause diphtheria can cause life-threatening damage to the kidneys, heart, and nervous system if the disease is not immediately treated.

Haemophilus Influenzae Type b

Babies are especially vulnerable to *Haemophilus influenzae* type b (Hib). This bacterium can produce ear infections (see p.1005), meningitis (see p.1013), arthritis (see p.605), and other serious infections.

Children should be vaccinated at 2, 4, 6, and 12 months of age against Hib. Properly administered, the vaccine is almost 100% protective.

Hepatitis

Hepatitis is inflammation of the liver. It can cause yellowing of the skin and eyes (jaundice), weakness, listlessness, fever, loss of appetite, nausea and vomiting, and other symptoms. If you think your child may have hepatitis, call the doctor. The different types of hepatitis are discussed on p.758.

In children, hepatitis A (see p.758) is caused by a virus that is transmitted via contaminated water or food, or by direct contact with an infected person. It is also commonly transmitted when caregivers do not wash hands after changing diapers. Many children who have hepatitis A do not have any symptoms or are simply tired for several days. For those children who develop symptoms, hepatitis A infection is almost always temporary; chronic liver disease does not develop.

Immunization against hepatitis A virus is recommended for children traveling to parts of the world where chance of infection is greatest, but immunization is not routinely given to all children.

Hepatitis B (see p.759) can affect newborn babies, who acquire it from infected mothers during delivery. As with hepatitis A, there may be no symptoms, or only temporary symptoms. Unlike hepatitis A, however, hepatitis B infection can produce chronic liver disease, cirrhosis (see p.765), liver failure (see p.764), and liver cancer (see p.766). For this reason, every child should be immunized against this virus. Children should receive three shots during the first year of life (see p.947).

If your child has hepatitis of any kind, talk to your child's doctor before giving the child acetaminophen. In large doses, acetaminophen can cause liver injury. In small doses, if the liver is already injured from hepatitis, acetaminophen (and some other medicines) may be harmful.

Influenza

Influenza (the flu) is a viral infection that can seem to be the common cold, with only nose and throat symptoms, but is often more serious, involving the lungs and other parts of the body. Children, especially those who are young or have medical problems, can get very sick from the flu.

Most cases of the flu can be prevented with the influenza vaccine (flu shot), which is safe for children as young as 6 months of age. As of 2004, the flu vaccine is recommended for all healthy children between 6 and 24 months of age and for those children with certain conditions that put them at risk for serious complications from the flu, including lung disease (asthma, cystic fibrosis), heart disease, sickle cell disease, HIV, and diabetes.

Flu shots must be given every year, usually as early as possible between October and December for maximum protection throughout the winter flu season. For healthy children age 5 and older, a flu vaccine is available that can be sprayed up the nose (instead of a shot). This vaccine contains a weak but "live" form of the virus and cannot be given to children who have problems with their immune system.

Measles

(See also Color Guide to Visual Diagnosis, p.568)

Measles, also called rubeola, is a highly infectious disease caused by a virus. Within about 10 days of exposure, your child will become sick and have a cough, fever (sometimes high), red eyes, and runny nose. Some children get small gray spots inside their mouth before a rash develops.

The flat, pink rash follows within 4 days. It often starts on the face and spreads to the trunk and, eventually, to the entire body. It starts to fade in several days.

Children are contagious beginning several days before the rash appears until the rash and fever subside. In some children, a second infection—such as an ear infection, sore throat, or pneumonia (usually caused by bacteria)—develops along with the measles. Call the doctor for treatment.

Almost all children in the United States are immunized against measles at age 12–15 months and then again when they enter kindergarten. A child who is not immunized and is exposed to a person who has measles should see the doctor. If the child has been exposed within the previous 6 days, the doctor may recommend an injection of an immunoglobulin that has antibodies against the measles virus. Alternately, the child can be vaccinated within 72 hours of exposure.

Other than keeping your child comfortable, there is no specific treatment. Nonetheless, your child should see the doctor so he or she can confirm that your child does indeed have measles. If this is the case, you may be asked to look for signs of pneumonia (see p.496).

Keep your child away from people who have not had measles, and encourage him or her to rest and drink plenty of liquids. Bright light may hurt your child's eyes, so lower the shades at home or provide sunglasses. Ask the doctor for the proper dose of acetaminophen to reduce fever.

Mumps

Mumps is an infection with a virus that causes the salivary glands in the cheeks and under the jaw to swell and become tender. Most children are immunized against mumps at 12–15 months and when they enter kindergarten.

Symptoms of mumps, which occur 2 to 3 weeks after exposure, include swelling of the glands in front of the ear and under the lines of the jaw, problems with chewing due to pain, feeling sick, and having a fever. These symptoms are sometimes accompanied by earache and problems swallowing.

In some children, the joints also swell. Occasionally, the testicles become swollen and painful and, very rarely (if mumps occurs after puberty), this inflammation of the testicles can cause sterility. Meningitis (see p.1013) is another rare complication.

Treatment is to rest, drink plenty of liquids, and take acetaminophen (not aspirin) in the dose recommended by the doctor for pain and fever.

Pertussis

Pertussis, also called whooping cough, is a contagious bacterial infection that causes mucous buildup, inflammation and narrowing of the airways, and bouts of severe coughing alternating with the "whoop" of the child gasping inward for breath. It can cause permanent brain and lung damage and can even be fatal. For this reason, children (starting at 2 months and then again four times over about 6 years) are given a vaccine against pertussis.

Pertussis usually starts like a cold, with nasal discharge and a cough, worsening to severe coughing with the "whooping" for air.

Children less than 1 year old are especially vulnerable because their airways are not fully developed; they may become blue from lack of oxygen and lethargic from coughing. If your infant or child is having difficulty breathing, or you notice a bluish tinge to the lips or nails, call immediately for emergency medical help.

In older children, symptoms also include vomiting after a spell of coughing. The coughing can last from 3 to 10 weeks. Doctors treat pertussis with antibiotics. In serious cases, oxygen and intravenous fluids to prevent dehydration are given.

Do not give any cough-suppressant medicines to your child; he or she needs to cough up the mucus that is clogging the airways.

Pneumococcus

Pneumococcus, also called *Streptococcus pneumoniae,* is a bacterium that can cause serious infections in the lungs (pneumonia), blood (bacteremia), and coverings of the brain and spinal column (spinal meningitis), especially in young children. Pneumococcus is also the most common cause of bacterial infection in the ears (otitis media) and sinuses (sinusitis).

PCV7, a vaccine to protect infants and young children against pneumococcus, was licensed in 2000. Before this vaccine, about 200 children younger than 5 years old died each year as a result of pneumococcal disease and thousands more were left with permanent damage. Four doses of this vaccine are normally recommended for all children younger than 2 years of age, and for children between the ages of 2 and 5 years who are at high risk of complications from pneumococcus infections, including children with sickle cell disease, a damaged or even no spleen, or immune systems that do not always work optimally (for example, children with HIV/AIDS, diabetes, cancer).

Polio

Polio (see p.379) is a viral infection of the brain and spinal cord. Before there was immunization for this infection, children were the prime victims of the disease. Immunization has nearly eradicated polio in the United States and most industrialized countries.

Rubella

(See also Color Guide to Visual Diagnosis, p.568)

Also called German measles, rubella is a mild infectious disease caused by a virus. In many children, it is mistaken for a cold. In others, it causes swollen glands behind the ears and at the back of the neck. It also sometimes causes a fever.

The disease has an incubation period of 2 to 3 weeks, after

which a delicate rash appears, primarily on the trunk. Children are routinely immunized against rubella.

Women who are pregnant or are considering pregnancy should ensure that they are vaccinated against rubella; the virus can cause birth defects in the developing fetus.

Tetanus

Tetanus (see p.880) is a bacterial infection that can cause damage to the brain and nervous system.

Children are immunized against this infection at the same time they receive immunizations for diphtheria and pertussis.

HEALTH AND DEVELOPMENT OF CHILDREN YOUNGER THAN AGE 2

Growth and Development

Healthy children grow physically, emotionally, and intellectually (cognitively) at an astonishing rate during the first 2 years of life. They may double their birthweight by 4 to 6 months of age and triple it by a year.

At each doctor visit, the physician measures how well your baby's head is growing and follows his or her development closely.

The chart called Developmental Milestones (see p.952) presents some of the major developmental steps for children 6 months to 24 months old. Each child is different; do not be concerned if your child has not reached a milestone by the specified age. For example, although the average age at which a child starts walking is between 12 and 13 months, the normal range is from 9 to 17 months. Also, late walking is not an indicator of developmental health. Language skills, though, seem to correlate with later academic achievement; you should talk and read to your baby often, from birth onward.

Failure to gain weight and height, known as "failure to thrive," in an otherwise healthy infant is a serious concern; contact your child's doctor. The signs of failure to thrive in a child under 2 years of age include:

■ Weight below the 3rd or 5th percentile at more than one doctor visit (unless your baby was very small at birth or both parents are small).

■ Abrupt change in weight or height from previous measurements.

■ Loss of weight or height, weight or height that does not change over time, or weight or height that increases more slowly than other children.

Feeding Your Baby

For women who have the option, breast milk (given by breast or bottle) is the ideal food for the first year of a baby's life or for as long as both infant and mother are able to continue. Women who are taking medicine should ask their doctor for advice on breast-feeding because many medicines pass through breast milk and can affect the infant.

The benefits of breast milk are

Latching On

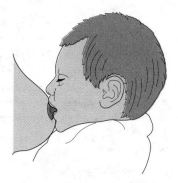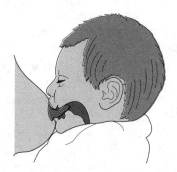

The baby's neck and head are in a straight line with the rest of his or her body and held parallel to the breast (left). In proper latch-on position (right), the baby's mouth should encircle as much of the areola (dark area around the nipple) as possible.

Developmental Milestones

This chart lists some of the major developmental milestones for infants 6 months to 24 months old. Each child is different, so do not be concerned if your child has not reached a milestone by the specified age. Discuss any concerns about development with your child's doctor.

	6 MONTHS	12 MONTHS	18 MONTHS	24 MONTHS
Fine movement skills	■ Reaches ■ Grasps ■ Transfers objects	■ Ambidextrous ■ Takes two objects in one hand ■ Picks up small object with thumb and forefinger ■ Feeds self with fingers	■ Uses objects as tools ■ Uses spoon ■ Drinks from cup ■ Removes socks and shoes ■ Builds tower with blocks	■ Builds tower of cubes ■ Throws ball overhand ■ Uses fork and spoon
Gross movement skills	■ Controls head ■ Pushes up on arms ■ Rolls ■ Sits supported or leaning forward	■ Crawls quickly ■ Takes first steps alone ■ Cruises around furniture	■ Walks ■ Runs stiffly ■ Stoops and stands ■ Climbs up stairs and onto furniture	■ Squats ■ Kicks ball ■ Jumps ■ Removes clothing ■ Tries to dress self ■ Walks up and down stairs using railing
Language skills	■ Babbles ■ May say some words, including simple forms of the words "mother" and "father" by 12 months	■ Says first words ■ Associates words and meanings	■ Babbles in sentencelike rhythm ■ Knows 10 to 25 words	■ Has 50-plus word vocabulary ■ Speaks in two-word sentences
Cognitive development	■ Laughs ■ Shows range of emotions ■ Identifies location of sounds ■ Expresses attachment to parents ■ Tracks objects visually	■ Understands that objects will stay in place ■ Follows commands such as "Please go to the kitchen" ■ Plays alone ■ Shows stranger anxiety ■ Shows separation anxiety	■ Points to body parts ■ Points to objects for parent's attention and naming	■ Sorts objects ■ Matches objects to pictures ■ Performs shape puzzles ■ Follows two-step commands such as "Please go to the kitchen and get a cup"

wide-ranging. It contains all of the nutrients that your baby needs and supplies antibodies for natural immunity against infections. Some studies have shown that breast-feeding significantly reduces the risk of pneumonia (see p.496) and gastroenteritis (see p.976) in the infant's first year.

Breast-feeding costs less than formula feeding, is very portable, and may even help women lose weight after pregnancy. Most important, the close physical contact of breast-feeding encourages bonding between mother and child.

The full-term infant's impulses for nursing are intact at birth. Less than an hour after birth, your baby is physically able to nurse and should be placed at your breast. However, nursing does not always come naturally to the mother. Many women benefit from the advice of family members, perinatal nurses, lactation consultants (see La Leche League, p.1236), their child's doctor, or friends.

When they first start nursing, most women have some discomfort that may be caused by normal nipple tenderness, the need to adjust positions, an infection, or another potentially serious problem. Rather than giving up, ask an expert for guidance.

Your milk may not start flowing steadily until about 2 to 5 days after the birth. In fact, the more your baby nurses, the more milk will flow. Your infant's mouth should encircle as much of the areola, the dark part around the nipple, as possible to stimulate the release of milk.

Nurse 10 to 15 minutes on each breast. If you end a session

Positions for Breast-Feeding

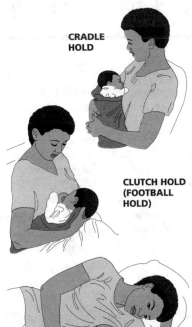

CRADLE HOLD

The baby's head is nestled in the crook of your elbow, the baby's body rests on your forearm, and the baby's buttocks are cradled by your other hand. Ensure the baby is turned on his or her side, with the head, neck, and body aligned, and that the baby's head is brought directly in front of your breast.

CLUTCH HOLD (FOOTBALL HOLD)

Sit up with a pillow beside you and another on your lap. Place the baby on his or her back, with the knees slightly bent and the back of the neck cradled in your hand. Hold your breast up with the opposite hand.

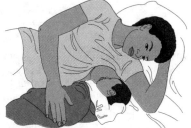

Position two pillows under your head, one behind you, one under your top leg, and another behind your baby. Cradle the baby in the bend of your elbow. Place the baby on his or her side parallel to you.

SIDE-LYING HOLD

with the left breast, start with the right one the next time you nurse.

To establish your milk supply and to get your baby into the rhythm of nursing, breast-feed exclusively for the first 3 to 4 weeks. Avoid using bottles and, unless your baby has a very strong sucking reflex, avoid giving your baby a pacifier.

Your infant knows how much milk he or she needs, and will cry for food as necessary. Some infants are avid and skillful at nursing, demanding meals as often as every 2 hours; others need some coaxing to keep from playing or falling asleep too soon.

To encourage nursing in a sleepy baby, place him or her on your breast and tickle the cheek softly. A diaper change may be stimulating. If your baby does not seem satisfied after nursing, or is not gaining weight, consult your child's doctor.

After your milk starts flowing, you may want to pump it regularly and store it in a bottle in the refrigerator for later feeding. It stays fresh for a few hours at room temperature, 48 hours in the refrigerator, and up to 6 months in the freezer. Many types of pumps are available, ranging in price, variety, style, and ease of use. Pumping per-

The Child Development Touchpoints Model:
Dr Brazelton's Advice

Everyone can benefit from information about child development. Touchpoints are periods during the first 3 years of life during which children's spurts in development may result in pronounced disruption in the family system. Touchpoints are like a map of child development that can be identified and anticipated.

Specific touchpoints have been noted in the first 3 years, beginning in pregnancy. They are centered around caregiving themes, such as feeding or discipline, rather than traditional milestones. The child's negotiation of the points can be seen as a source of success for the family system. Awareness of these touchpoints and strategies for dealing with them can help reduce negative patterns that might otherwise result in problems in the areas of sleep, feeding, or toilet training, for example.

The developmental touchpoints are summarized on the following pages, accompanied by steps you can take to help your child through them. By becoming aware of these expected periods, you can minimize anxiety and seize the opportunity to support your child's growth. Follow your instincts and you will do just fine.

For more information about touchpoints, see my book: *Touchpoints: Emotional and Behavioral Developments*. Reading, Mass: Perseus Books, 1994.

AGE	TOUCHPOINT	WHAT YOU CAN DO
3 weeks	**Feeding:** Your infant will cry when hungry, usually every 2 to 3 hours, but sometimes more often.	Follow your infant's cues about when to feed. Of course, an infant will cry for reasons other than hunger. In particular, from the age of 3 to 12 weeks, expect a certain amount of inconsolable crying at the end of the day.
	Cognitive: Your infant recognizes your face and responds to the sound of your voice.	Talk and sing to your infant often.
	Movement: Your infant may suck his or her thumb, a complex achievement that incorporates arm, hand, and sucking skills.	Do not discourage thumb-sucking; it is a form of self-comfort.
6 to 8 weeks	**Feeding and sleeping:** Most infants can eat and sleep on a schedule of every 3 to 4 hours.	Create a schedule that fits into your day. Allow 5 to 10 minutes of fussing before feedings.
	Cognitive: Your infant may have fussy times that appear predictably at the end of the day.	Recognize fussy periods as necessary ways of working out the day's stimulation (see Colic, p.971).

AGE	TOUCHPOINT	WHAT YOU CAN DO
4 months	**Feeding:** Consider starting to give your infant solid food (see p.958) if he or she suddenly wants to eat every 2 hours.	Be patient; swallowing solids is an important achievement that takes time to learn.
	Sleeping: Your infant's brain is physically mature enough to sleep 6 to 12 hours at night.	Focus on sleep rituals to encourage sleeping skills (see Healthy Sleep Habits in Infants, p.959).
	Cognitive and movement: Your infant will exhibit frustration as he or she tries new skills such as reaching and turning over.	Do not get too involved; frustration is a powerful learning tool.
7 months	**Feeding:** Most infants will use feeding time to practice their manual skills.	Let your baby try to feed himself or herself by presenting two or three soft, bite-sized foods, no matter how messy the foods are.
	Cognitive: Your infant will be acquiring the key skills of playing and learning about the permanence of people and objects.	Play peekaboo and mirror games. Try not to be annoyed when your infant repeatedly drops objects to explore cause and effect.
	Movement: Your infant's movements are more refined and result in greater exploration; any object is a potential toy or something to be put in the mouth.	Scrupulously babyproof (see p.88) your home to provide your infant with a safe environment for exploration.
9 months	**Feeding:** Mealtime is unpredictable as independence is exerted; your infant may refuse most foods unless he or she can pick them up to feed himself or herself.	Let your infant hold spoons and cups while you feed him or her.
	Sleeping: Your infant may use bedtime to practice standing and other skills, which may cause repeated awakenings at night. He or she may prefer practicing skills to sleeping.	Try not to pick up or hold your infant every time he or she cries. Help your baby learn sleeping skills (see p.960).

AGE	TOUCHPOINT	WHAT YOU CAN DO
1 year	**Feeding:** Emerging negativism and independence in your baby may set the stage for food battles.	Present a few finger foods at a time and let your baby feed himself or herself.
	Communication: Your baby may use everything in his or her impressive repertoire to communicate, such as words, skills with objects, or body gestures.	Listen closely for attempts at real speech and "echo" the word. Encourage but do not pressure your baby to vocalize.
	Cognitive: Fear of separation surfaces as your baby recognizes the differences between strangers and friends or family members, and realizes his or her own capacity to leave and return.	Spend extra time together; tell your baby when you are leaving and let him or her know that you will return.
	Movement: Your baby either is walking or will walk soon. He or she both strives for the ability to leave you and fears it intensely.	Create an environment for your baby to explore independently.
15 months	**Feeding:** Your baby may now want to make choices about food, which will be the most important aspect of feeding at this time.	Give foods with a variety of textures and let your baby feed himself or herself small amounts at a time.

mits you to return to work or spend some time away from the house, while your baby continues to receive the benefits of breast milk; it also allows others to share the joy of feeding the baby.

For women who cannot or choose not to breast-feed, formula feeding also has advantages. It is nutritionally complete, though it does not provide antibodies for immunity. It may be easier on the mother (breast-feeding can be physically demanding). And, again, others can share in the joy of feeding the baby. To prepare, follow the directions for the powder, concentrate, or ready-to-feed formula preparations.

Your child needs no supplemental food for at least the first 4 to 6 months. He or she should take up to 4 to 5 ounces of formula at each feeding during the first few months. This amount increases to 6 ounces or more by 4 months, when your baby should be consuming about 1 quart (32 ounces) per day. These are averages and will vary, depending on the size of your baby and the speed of growth.

WEANING YOUR INFANT FROM THE BREAST

When you are ready to wean your baby, replace one nursing session with a bottle of breast milk or formula or, after the age of 1 year, a cup of whole cow's milk. Let a family member other than the mother give the first bottle; the baby associates nursing with the mother and he or she may be more inclined to feed in this new way from another person.

Gradually increase the number of bottles and cups that replace nursing sessions, adding a second bottle-feeding on the third

AGE	TOUCHPOINT	WHAT YOU CAN DO
15 months	**Communication:** Your baby will try to imitate your speech and be frustrated when he or she cannot; however, this will lead to rapid learning.	Do not pressure your baby to speak. Forcing your child to speak may actually delay the process.
	Cognitive: Play is learning. Most babies can find an object hidden under two covers. Your baby also learns that certain actions precede others, such as the sound of keys at the front door signals that Daddy or Mommy is coming home.	Play rhythmic games, and break the rhythm to see whether your child is amused by this sudden break in expectations.
18 months	**Feeding:** Most babies are ready to start eating with a spoon and fork, which helps them practice new skills.	Prepare for messy meals.
	Cognitive: Toddlers begin to learn from other children.	Expose your child to one or two playmates.
	Movement: Your baby probably will try to climb to dangerous heights or run away from you at a moment's notice.	Be careful. Keep padding beneath the crib to break falls. Keep close watch on your exploring toddler.

T. BERRY BRAZELTON, MD
CHILDREN'S HOSPITAL
HARVARD MEDICAL SCHOOL

day and a third bottle-feeding on the fifth day. There is no medical reason to wean your child more rapidly. You can do it over a much longer period of time if you choose.

BURPING, SPITTING UP, AND VOMITING

To help keep their bellies free of air that is swallowed with sucking or swallowing (and which takes up much-needed space for food and can cause discomfort), infants should be burped midway through and after each meal.

To burp your baby, place his or her chest over your shoulder or lie your child facedown on your lap and pat his or her back firmly. Use a cloth diaper over your shoulder or on your lap to catch milk or formula that is spit up.

Most infants under 3 months spit up after meals, some after every feeding. The substance that is spit up is usually milky colored and is sometimes mixed with mucus or a curdled-looking material.

Spitting up usually tapers off when babies start sitting up, after about 6 months. Until then, you can reduce spitting up by calm-

ing your baby before feeding and, if bottle-feeding, by keeping the bottle upside down so your child does not take in too much air. If spitting up continues, or seems to cause your baby discomfort, discuss it with your child's doctor.

Vomiting is different from spitting up. Consult your child's doctor immediately if the vomit is brown or green, has blood in it, or erupts forcefully (this is called projectile vomiting).

These symptoms could indicate overfeeding, an obstruction (see Pyloric Stenosis, p.984),

Three Ways to Burp Your Baby

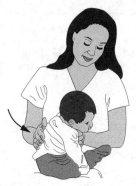 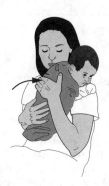 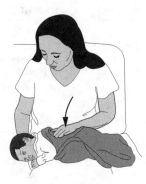

Hold the baby upright and leaning over slightly. While supporting the neck and back, pat or rub the back gently.

Set the baby high on your shoulder with his or her chest over your shoulder and the head draped slightly over. Gently pat or rub the back.

Place the baby stomach-down on your lap or another flat surface. Turn his or her head to one side (make sure it is supported) and gently pat or rub the back with the palm of your hand.

Infant Neck Strength

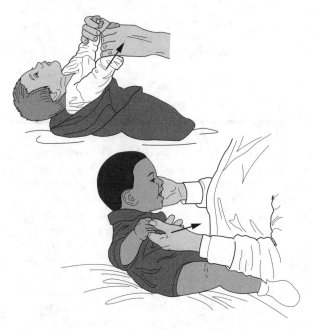

A newborn's neck has not yet developed the muscle strength to hold up the head. Your baby's head always requires support. During the first few months, gently pulling your infant up by his or her hands will result in the head flopping back (top). By about 4 months, muscle strength has developed enough so that your baby can support the head (bottom).

an infection, or a sensitivity to milk protein (see Intolerance to Cow's Milk and Soy, p.959).

STARTING SOLID FOODS

There is no hard-and-fast rule about when to start feeding babies solids, but generally babies are not ready before the age of 4 months. The first solid food should be rice cereal, which is the least likely to cause an allergic reaction. Mix the cereal with breast milk or formula to a soupy consistency, according to the directions. Sit your baby up in your lap or in an infant seat to prevent choking.

Start by giving about ¼ teaspoon at a time. Be prepared for your infant to reject the first few spoonfuls. Take your time. Feeding your baby is essential for nutrition, but equally important is the practice, bonding, and learning of early social skills. It is also guaranteed to be messy. Cultivate your baby's palate for different

Bathing Your Infant

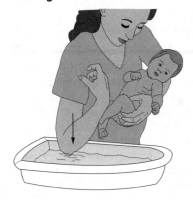

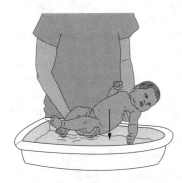

Make sure that the room is warm and draft-free. Put only 2 inches of lukewarm water in a basin (test the water with your wrist or elbow). Support the baby's head with one hand. Use the other hand to slowly and gently place the baby's feet, and then the rest of the body, in the water. Using a hand and a clean washcloth, pour warm water over the exposed body to keep your baby warm. To wash hair, apply a pea-sized amount of tear-free shampoo, lather, and rinse with a cup or two of water.

foods and textures by adding one new food every 5 to 7 days, starting with applesauce, pears, bananas (mashed to a smooth consistency), and other foods that tend not to cause allergies. Specifically, avoid egg whites and dairy products for the first few months. After each addition, look for reactions that might indicate allergy or sensitivity, such as rashes (even sudden diaper rash, see p.973), diarrhea, gas, or other signs of gastrointestinal upset. Follow your baby's lead about the pacing and amount of food in each meal, and give a little breast milk or formula in addition, to ensure adequate nutrition.

When your infant is able to sit up without help, he or she can begin to feed alone. Offer soft foods such as cooked peas, potatoes, and crackers in small pieces that cannot cause choking. Your child should eat about 4 ounces at each of three or more meals per day. This is the amount in a small jar of baby food.

Although there is much water in food, formula, and breast milk, your child may in rare cases also need water, especially in warm weather. Offer it only once or twice a day at most, in addition to the regular feedings of breast milk or formula.

INTOLERANCE TO COW'S MILK AND SOY

Fewer than 7% of infants under 6 months are truly allergic to cow's milk. Soy allergy is even more uncommon. The symptoms of intolerance include colicky behavior (see p.971), diarrhea, vomiting, blood or mucus in the bowel movements, and poor

weight gain. Your doctor may recommend a hypoallergenic formula.

Healthy Sleep Habits in Infants

Sleep—both your baby's and your own—is likely one of your major concerns as a new parent. Sleep disturbances, particularly nighttime awakenings, can strain and exhaust parents. Here is what to expect, and how to handle common problems.

Your newborn may sleep up to 16 hours a day, broken up into short periods. However, soon he or she will start to stay awake—and to sleep—for fewer, shorter periods. In the early weeks, discomfort from colic, acid reflux, or other conditions may cause trouble sleeping. Talk to your doctor if you have concerns.

By about 3 months of age, your baby should be sleeping:

■ About 13 hours total.

■ Mostly at night.

■ In uninterrupted periods for up to 5 or 6 hours at night.

■ With no more than one or two awakenings at night.

As your baby approaches 3 months of age, you should be developing regular routines with your child that lead up to longer periods of sleep. Children vary in the age at which they settle for the night or start sleeping through the night. Some babies are already sleeping through the night by 3 to 4 months; most are doing so by 5 to 6 months.

If, by 4 to 6 months, your child continues to seem to sleep

Teaching Your Baby Sleeping Skills: Dr Ferber's Advice

If your baby is healthy, developing normally, and at least 5 months of age (based on the due date), he or she should have the ability to sleep through the night for at least 9 hours, without the need for feedings, rocking, or other interventions.

If you must return repeatedly to feeding, rocking, or soothing your child, you may be satisfying the baby's expectations more than the baby's needs. If the baby has long awakenings, despite your interventions, the problem may be that he or she is being kept in the crib longer than is needed. For example, you may be keeping your child in the crib for 11 hours when the child may only need 9 hours of sleep.

Babies wake repeatedly during the night, every 1 to 3 hours, as part of normal sleep cycling (adults also awaken briefly during sleep).

Rocking, patting, or feeding a baby at bedtime does not always mean that such interventions will have to be repeated at awakenings, but, if the baby seems to expect them, then it makes sense to help your baby learn to fall asleep without such expectations.

Ask yourself what the conditions will be when your baby is sleeping (and hence when he or she wakes); those are the conditions under which you must let your baby learn to fall asleep at bedtime and back to sleep during the night.

The learning process generally takes 2 to 3 days. Multiple nighttime feedings may have to be eliminated more slowly (for example, by increasing the minimal time between feedings by 30 minutes a night over 1 week).

Since you must let your child fall asleep without the usual contact, there will be crying initially. There is no need to try to change things quickly. The program described here is designed so that you can help your child during the process, in a gradual manner, by checking on the child at increasingly longer intervals.

Each night put your child to bed awake. Let your baby cry at first for a very short time. Then go in to reassure him or her for a minute or two without reestablishing much physical contact, such as rocking, patting, or offering a pacifier. The exception is feedings at the prescribed increasing intervals (the feedings should be eliminated by the end of the first week of the program).

Interactions should be mainly limited to soothing talk and brief positioning of your infant. Each night, the time between visits should be increased until your child begins to fall asleep (and back to sleep) quickly and without interacting with you. You can adjust the number of minutes between reassuring visits to suit your own feelings as long as the times increase progressively.

Day 1 Wait 5 minutes before going in to reassure your child, then 10 minutes, then 15. (If 5 minutes seems too long to you, start with 3 minutes, or even 1 minute, and increase the time from there.)

Day 2 Wait 10 minutes, then 15, then 20.

Day 3 Wait 15 minutes, then 20, then 25.

Day 4 If necessary, wait 20 minutes, then 25, then 30.

Day 5 If necessary, wait 25 minutes, then 30, then 35.

Day 6 If necessary, wait 30 minutes, then 35, then 40.

Day 7 If necessary, wait 35 minutes, then 40, then 45.

If the problem was really one of association, most children will be sleeping well by the end of 3 days, certainly by the end of 1 week. If the problem is not resolving, there may be another cause you have not identified. Discuss this with your pediatrician.

For a more detailed discussion, see my book: *Solve Your Child's Sleep Problems*. New York, NY: Simon & Schuster, 1986.

RICHARD A. FERBER, MD
CHILDREN'S HOSPITAL
HARVARD MEDICAL SCHOOL

less than expected, it is possible that your expectations are too high or that your baby needs less sleep than most. If you are up tending to your child four times a night, it may feel as if your baby never sleeps (even if total sleep time is normal), but it may be you who is not getting enough sleep.

Alternately, something may be interfering with your baby's ability to fall asleep, stay asleep, or go back to sleep. A common cause of such problems in the second half year is an inappropriate sleep schedule.

The ideal sleeping environment for an infant is one that is relatively dark, quiet, and comfortably cool. By 3 months of age, sleep periods should already occur on a regular schedule.

Relaxing, unrushed bedtime routines are helpful. However, for an infant on an appropriate and predictable schedule, these routines should be relatively brief (5 to 10 minutes).

A final feeding, quiet play, songs, and cuddling are all reasonable bedtime activities. As the child gets older, telling stories becomes useful. Security objects, such as a special blanket or stuffed animal, become very important (but do not use these before the child is 1 year of age because they can cause suffocation).

Ideally, your baby should be put to bed awake and allowed to fall asleep in the same crib or bed he or she will remain in the rest of the night. Bedtime should be consistent and at a time you have learned your baby is capable of falling asleep. If it always takes an hour for your baby to fall sleep, bedtime should probably be 1 hour later.

In the early months, sleep tends to be lighter and more broken than later on, and your baby may have difficulty sustaining sleep. Parents may find techniques that seem to help, such as rocking or nursing the baby or giving the baby a pacifier.

However, your baby may come to expect these techniques every time he or she awakens normally between nighttime sleep cycles. In this case, you may want to help your child learn to fall asleep without intervention on your part (see Teaching Your Baby Sleeping Skills: Dr Ferber's Advice, p.960).

Infants and toddlers require a certain amount of sleep. Once they get it, they usually cannot sleep more. They are also capable of sleeping only at certain times of the day and night. So, if your baby is in bed longer at night than he or she can sleep or at times that he or she is not really sleepy (because of being put to bed too early, getting up too late, or napping too much), your child will have periods of wakefulness. Things will get better when you correct the schedule.

Illness, unnecessary feedings, and anxiety can also disrupt sleep. A baby who is awake because of sickness is usually unhappy; simple interventions do not seem to help.

Most full-term babies who are growing normally do not need continued feedings during the night after 4 to 5 months. If the feedings are still given, they may become expected on a learned basis. Gradually decreasing or eliminating the feedings may allow the broken nighttime sleep to consolidate. Separation anxiety, if present, is usually not a

Sleep Positions

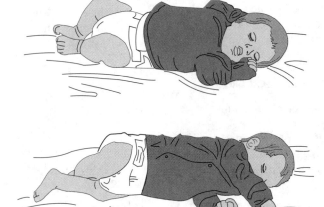

These two sleeping positions—on the back or on the side—are recommended for children under age 1 to prevent sudden infant death syndrome.

problem until toward the end of the first year. Ask your pediatrician for advice.

NIGHTMARES AND CONFUSIONAL AROUSALS

Nightmares are dreams with presumably scary content that may occur in an older infant, particularly during a period of separation anxiety, stress, or illness.

The child will wake fully (usually in the second half of the night), cry, be fully responsive, and calm quickly when comforted. Be attentive and comforting. Your child should promptly return to sleep. Occasional nightmares occur in all children.

Confusional arousals of young children are similar to, but less intense than, the night terrors (see p.989) experienced by older children. Confusional arousals

are partial awakenings (usually within 1 to 4 hours of falling asleep) from deep, nondreaming sleep. During such an event, your child may appear to be upset and confused and is not easily calmed. He or she may even push you away.

An infant may be confused, but is not really experiencing fear. Events end once the child wakes fully.

Your child will have no memory of what happened. Let confusional arousals run their course and simply let your child settle down and go back to sleep. Forceful interventions (such as trying to cuddle or wake your child) may only prolong matters.

Child Safety

Your child's growing independence brings joy—and a higher risk of injury. Most injuries occur because parents are unaware of their children's abilities. One of 4 children is injured each year seriously enough to require medical attention. Each month, nearly 450 children under age 14 die of an unintentional injury, most of which could have been prevented. Follow these safety measures:

GENERAL SAFETY FOR ALL CHILDREN

- Keep emergency phone numbers (such as for police, fire department, and poison control center) posted where family members and baby-sitters can find them easily and quickly.

- Learn cardiopulmonary resuscitation (CPR) for infants and children (see p.1201).

- Never shake or hit a baby.

Kitchen Safety

- Never leave a child alone in the kitchen.

- Turn pot handles inward and out of a child's reach.

- Never lift your child while handling hot food or liquids.

- Keep containers of hot fluids and sharp objects out of a child's reach.

- Prevent scalding by turning down the thermostat on your water heater to 120°F.

BIRTH TO 6 MONTHS

PREVENTING CAR INJURIES

- Always use rear-facing car seats.

- Place the car seat in the center of the backseat (never in the front seat).

- Tightly buckle up the car seat, using a locking clip on lap/shoulder belts with a sliding latch plate.

PREVENTING FALLS

- Never leave your infant on a bed, chair, or changing table.

PREVENTING BURNS

- Never carry hot liquids while carrying your infant.

- Use only fire-retardant sleepwear.

PREVENTING CHOKING OR SUFFOCATION

- Never feed raw vegetables, raw apples, popcorn, or smooth,

Sleep Safety for Infants

Follow these guidelines to keep your child safe during sleep:

- Put your infant to sleep on his or her back or side to reduce the chance of sudden infant death syndrome (see p.986).

- Ensure that the slats of the crib are no more than 2⅜ inches apart.

- Get a larger mattress (or a smaller crib) if you can fit two fingers between the mattress and the sides of the crib.

- Never place an infant on a waterbed, beanbag chair, or pillow; use a firm mattress.

Protecting Our Children's Environment:
Dr Woolf's Advice

Children are sometimes placed at risk of injury from environmental toxins—pesticide residues in foods, a playground built on or near a toxic waste dump, asbestos exposure from the ceiling tiles at school, lead or arsenic contamination of water, environmental cigarette smoke, outdoor air pollution, or residential radon exposure.

Environmental toxin exposure of children differs from that of adults because children breathe faster, are closer to the ground, are more likely to come into contact with and ingest outdoor dust (for example, through a higher frequency of hand-to-mouth activity), tend to choose different foods to eat, and may metabolize specific toxins differently than adults.

You should talk with your children's pediatrician to determine whether your children are at risk for any of these exposures. If so, proper testing should be done to determine if the children have been exposed. If exposure has occurred, the pediatrician and family should discuss whether it might cause harmful health effects now or in the future.

Parents should also learn from their pediatricians how to treat any current toxin-related health problems and how to minimize further exposure.

ALAN D. WOOLF, MD, MPH
CHILDREN'S HOSPITAL
HARVARD MEDICAL SCHOOL

round foods such as peanuts, hot dogs, or grapes to your baby.

■ Never leave rubber balloons or small objects within your infant's reach. An object small enough to fit through a toilet paper tube is a choking hazard.

■ Learn first aid for choking (see Heimlich Maneuver, p.1206).

6 TO 12 MONTHS

In addition to the above:

ENSURING TOY SAFETY

■ Make sure toys have no small (less than 1½ inches) or removable parts.

■ Do not permit your child to play with toys that have strings longer than 12 inches.

■ Never allow your child to play with rubber balloons.

PREVENTING FALLS

■ Replace or cover sharp-edged furniture.

■ Never use baby walkers.

■ Use stair gates at both top and bottom of stairs.

■ Install window guards (screens are not adequate), especially above the first floor.

PREVENTING BURNS

■ Place your child in a high chair or crib while you are cooking.

■ Put protective devices around heating units.

■ Turn pot handles toward back of stove; use back burners when possible.

■ Place all objects, but especially hot liquids, 10 inches or more from the edge of surfaces.

PREVENTING POISONING

■ Store all medicines (including those in a purse or briefcase) and cleansers in a high, locked cabinet.

■ Use safety latches on drawers and cupboards.

■ Keep syrup of ipecac (see p.1214) on hand to induce vomiting (but *only* if inducing vomiting has been recommended by a medical professional).

DROWNING

■ Never leave a child unattended near any amount of water; children can drown in less than 2 inches of water.

■ Install a 4-foot fence around your swimming pool.

■ Empty all standing water (for example, in buckets or kiddie pools) after use.

1 TO 2 YEARS

In addition to the above:

PREVENTING CAR INJURIES

■ Children weighing 40–60 pounds and less than 4'9" tall or younger than 8 years of age should ride in a booster seat in the backseat. Even with tall chil-

In an Emergency

- Dial 911 or your local emergency number. Keep the local emergency number and your local poison control center (800-222-1222) number posted in a prominent place, such as on your refrigerator door.

- Care for the injured child according to the priorities listed on p.1190.

dren or older children, the adult seat belt must always fit correctly. This means the shoulder belt should fit snugly across the chest (not the neck or throat), the lap belt should be low and snug across the thighs (not the stomach), and the child must be able to sit against the vehicle seat's back with his or her legs bent at the knees and feet hanging down.

PREVENTING FIREARM INJURIES

- If you must keep a gun, keep it unloaded, locked away, and separate from ammunition.

PREVENTING FALLS

- Do not allow children to climb on chairs; from chairs, they can easily reach tables, windows, and other high places.

Development of Teeth

Humans produce two complete sets of teeth in a lifetime. The first set is the primary teeth and the second and final set is the permanent teeth.

There are 20 primary teeth (or "baby teeth"), all of which usually emerge by 2 years of age. While the primary front teeth (incisors and canines) are smaller in height and width than their permanent counterparts, the primary back teeth (molars) are larger than the permanent premolar teeth they replace.

The primary teeth are not only important for function but also serve as placeholders for the permanent teeth. Premature loss of a primary tooth as a result of injury or cavities may require the placement of a space-maintaining appliance by a dentist. Keeping a space between the primary incisors helps keep the permanent incisors in proper alignment.

TEETHING

Teething, the process of teeth breaking through the gums, can be painful. Symptoms include drooling and sometimes dryness of the chin and cheeks.

As teeth are emerging, your baby will want to gnaw on objects. Chewing on cold toys or on a piece of frozen bagel can help numb the gums and scratch the itchy discomfort of teething.

Sleep also may be disturbed because of teething pain, which can contribute to fussiness during the day.

There is considerable debate over whether teething causes fever. Many parents report that their baby runs a low-grade fever when he or she is teething. This may be the result of an oral viral infection. A persistent fever should be evaluated by your child's doctor.

Do not apply any anesthetic to your baby's gums. Ask the doctor about the judicious use of acetaminophen during particularly trying periods.

CAUSES AND PREVENTION OF CAVITIES

Cavities (see p.470) are the primary dental health concern for infants. Cavities are caused by the bacteria that gain access to every child's mouth sometime between the ages of 1 and 3. Children of women with high decay rates may be at greater risk of decay.

Some dental offices are able to culture your child's mouth for the presence of these bacteria and

Alternative Medicine: Teething Pain

There are some homeopathic remedies (such as a combination of belladonna and chamomile) that are widely used and felt to be safe for mild, self-limited conditions like teething. Their effectiveness has not been proven in scientific studies. Check with your infant's doctor before using these treatments.

Primary ("Baby") Teeth

This chart shows when primary teeth usually erupt and fall out, although these times vary widely from child to child. Between the ages of 5 and 12, your child will have a mixture of primary and permanent teeth. The 6-year molars are landmarks in tooth development. They are permanent teeth that arrive around the age of 6 years and erupt behind the last primary molars (the second primary molars).

TOP TEETH	COME IN	FALL OUT	BOTTOM TEETH	COME IN	FALL OUT
Central incisors	8 to 12 months	7 to 8 years	Central incisors	6 to 10 months	6 to 7 years
Lateral incisors	9 to 13 months	7 to 9 years	Lateral incisors	10 to 16 months	7 to 8 years
First molars	13 to 19 months	10 to 11 years	First molars	14 to 18 months	10 to 11 years
Cuspids	16 to 23 months	10 to 12 years	Cuspids	16 to 23 months	9 to 11 years
Second molars	25 to 33 months	10 to 11 years	Second molars	23 to 31 months	10 to 12 years

determine the risk for future dental decay. If the risk is high, it is even more important to make sure your child's teeth are brushed regularly.

Prevention should begin even before the first teeth emerge. To prevent nursing bottle cavities, do not permit your child to sleep with a bottle.

Even before your baby's teeth break through the gums, plaque can collect on the gums. To remove it, swab the gums with a clean cloth or gauze after meals. As teeth emerge, brush them with a soft baby toothbrush and, after the first year, a small (pea-sized) amount of toothpaste.

Fluoride (see p.472) in the public water supply helps reduce cavities, but too much can stain teeth. If there is no fluoride in your water supply or you use filtered or bottled water, ask your baby's doctor about supplements.

Some very rare conditions can result in so-called soft teeth, which have a susceptibility to tooth decay. However, tooth decay is more often caused by the presence of decay-causing bacteria, frequent exposure to foods containing sugar, and having teeth with deep grooves and pits that tend to retain food.

DENTAL CARE

The care of the primary (baby) teeth is important, even though they are temporary. The primary teeth are placeholders for the permanent teeth, and their loss from cavities or injury can lead to overcrowding.

It is important to make dental hygiene routine. Brush and floss about a half hour before bedtime; cooperation levels tend to nosedive as bedtime approaches.

Until children can brush their teeth on their own (generally about the time they are able to tie their own shoes), brush your children's teeth daily, especially before bedtime. Use a soft-bristled brush that can reach all tooth surfaces to remove sticky plaque (see p.470).

Emerging Baby Teeth

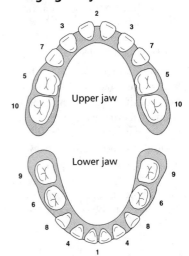

The numbers next to the teeth indicate the sequence in which teeth emerge. The first tooth usually appears in the first year.

The mechanical act of brushing and rinsing is more effective than toothpaste at removing food and plaque. Use only a pea-sized amount of toothpaste; ingesting more than the recommended amount of fluoride can result in defects of the enamel of the permanent teeth, a condition known as fluorosis.

Flossing once a day, preferably before bedtime, should begin when the back teeth are in contact with one another, usually around the age of 4 years. You should floss your child's teeth until about age 8, when he or she will acquire the manual dexterity to perform this task alone.

After brushing and flossing before bedtime, your child should have nothing to eat or drink except water.

THE FIRST DENTAL VISIT

Most children should have their first appointment with a dentist no later than age 3, when their primary teeth have completely emerged and the child is old enough to understand what it means to take care of teeth.

A pediatric dentist is trained in the care of children's teeth and is more likely to be sensitive to their fears and anxieties.

Abnormal Tooth Development

Your infant's teeth can develop abnormally for hereditary reasons and because of poor general health, as outlined in the chart on p.471.

Permanent Teeth

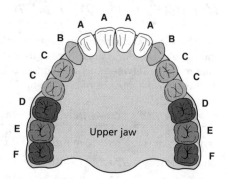

A	Incisors appear at 6 to 9 years
B	Canines appear at 9 to 12 years
C	Premolars appear at 10 to 12 years
D	First molars appear at 6 to 7 years
E	Second molars appear at 11 to 13 years
F	Third molars appear at 17 years or older

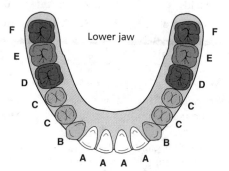

Your child's 32 permanent teeth will emerge starting between age 6 and 7, continuing (as shown above) until about age 17.

Prepare your child for a visit to the dentist by explaining what to expect. Tell your child that the dentist will talk about teeth and then look into his or her mouth and inspect the gums and teeth.

Explain about dental x-rays—that they are pictures of the teeth and that the assistant or dentist may need to put a cardboardlike piece in the mouth.

Avoid fear-provoking words (such as "pain," "painless," "hurt," and "needles"). Pediatric dentists are experts at communicating with children and explaining procedures to children in terms that they will understand. The more

your child knows about what to expect, the more involved and less fearful he or she will be. A fluoride solution may be applied to the teeth to prevent cavities. A fluoride supplement may be prescribed if your water supply does not provide it.

TOOTH DEVELOPMENT

At some point, your child will have some permanent and some primary teeth. There are 32 permanent teeth, and they are designed to last a lifetime.

Continue to monitor brushing and have your child see the dentist regularly after permanent teeth come in, so that any problems can be identified and treated early. You may also want to consider having a sealant (see p.472) applied to your child's teeth to prevent cavities. Fluoride continues to be important as your child grows.

Children who play sports should wear protective mouth guards to prevent injury; they must be worn each time your child plays. Orthodontic braces are discussed on p.479.

Pediatric Well-Child Visits: Birth to 2 Years

During your baby's first 2 years, regular medical evaluation by your pediatrician or family doctor is especially important. Healthy infants generally should see their doctors 11 times for preventive care visits: as newborns, at 2 to 4 days, 1 month, 2 months, 4 months, 6 months, 9 months, 12 months, 15 months, 18 months, and 24 months. Some variation in this schedule may occur depending on your child's needs.

The doctor will vaccinate your child (see p.947) and perform a complete physical examination of your baby during all checkups. This includes evaluating the baby's reflexes, which indicate the health of the nervous system and muscles. The eyes and ears are checked for any problems, and the doctor listens to the lungs and heart. Heart murmurs (see p.980) usually can be detected within the first 48 hours, and, though they most often do not indicate a defect, your doctor may want to see the baby again.

The doctor checks your baby's

Lead Poisoning:
Dr Shannon's Advice

Lead poisoning, a significant cause of abnormal development, is declining. Lead levels in blood are now about 80% lower than they were 25 years ago. This great accomplishment has occurred as a result of public health measures such as the removal of lead from gasoline and paint. Nevertheless, kids still get poisoned by lead.

Lead in the environment Lead enters a child's body when, as a toddler, the child eats peeling lead-based paints (used in homes before 1960), eats soil around homes painted with lead-based paints, or consumes lead from other sources.

Symptoms Lead can damage the growing brain. Lead poisoning is almost always without symptoms in the period during which the child is exposed to the lead. Its consequences appear later in childhood as learning difficulties.

Tests A blood test called blood lead can detect lead poisoning. I advise parents to insist their children get this test in the first 3 years of life if they live in or frequently play in older houses or they have siblings or playmates with lead poisoning. Children of any age should be tested if they live in older houses that are being renovated since lead in paint dust may be in the air.

Treatments Several effective treatments are available. Children with mild lead poisoning can be treated with oral medicine at home. Children with more severe poisoning need to be hospitalized for several days for intravenous treatments.

In addition to these treatments, it is very important to try to locate the source of the poisoning and to eliminate it. Your doctor can help organize a team of experts to help you with this.

MICHAEL SHANNON, MD
CHILDREN'S HOSPITAL
HARVARD MEDICAL SCHOOL

genitalia. In boys, the exam includes making sure the testicles have descended into the scrotum (see Undescended Testicle, p.1019). In girls, the exam includes checking for abnormal vaginal bleeding or discharge (some vaginal bleeding and discharge is normal) and other abnormalities. Your baby's hips will be examined for any sign of abnormality.

The doctor will record growth measurements, perform a screening of hearing and eyesight, and generally examine your child's breathing, heart rate, muscle and joint movement, and skin. At 6 to 12 months, your doctor may draw blood to test for anemia (see p.995) and lead poisoning (see above), depending on whether the homes in your community are likely to be contaminated by lead paint. Your baby's physician is also interested in behavioral and developmental changes.

The office visit is your time to raise any concerns you have. These may include questions about sleeping, eating, movement (such as rolling, crawling, or walking), development, and emotional changes (such as tantrums). The visit is also a time to discuss the physical and emotional health of the family. These issues—such as depression, smoking, alcoholism, family violence, or parental medical concerns—can have a profound effect on your baby's health. Writing your questions down before bringing the baby in for a checkup will ensure that no concern is overlooked.

Child Care

Finding safe and loving child care can be one of the greatest challenges for working parents. Some parents have trusted family members who can care for their children. Many families choose family day care (where an adult cares for children in the caregiver's own home).

Other options include in-home care (in which the caregiver cares for your children in the child's home) and day care centers (which are run by a staff of people in a larger facility and usually involve more children).

Those with flexible work schedules may opt for creative arrangements such as parenting co-ops, where like-minded parents take turns watching the group's children.

The ideal ratio of caregiver-to-child depends on the age of the

child. A good rule of thumb is that it should be one-on-one for infants under age 1, two children per caregiver for 1- or 2-year-olds, and so on. The caregiver should be experienced in child care and the location should be clean and safe. It is extremely important that there be separate areas for napping, eating, and diapering. All caregivers must wash their hands before and after diapering and food service to limit the spread of infectious diseases.

When you are visiting a facility, ask if it is licensed. Request references. Ensure that the caregivers are trained in first aid, and note the cleanliness of the surroundings. Ask about the opportunities for children to play, interact, and have quiet time. Make certain that you are allowed to visit whenever you choose without advance notice. Ask how they manage ill children. Check a sample menu and make sure it is nutritious. Finally, take time to review the contract at home, when you are not rushed. Be sure you understand the details.

Resources for information on child care include friends, your child's doctor, referral and employment agencies, religious institutions, senior citizen organizations, and the local La Leche League.

In selecting a caregiver, make a list of the qualities you desire most, and make a list of questions. Above all, when interviewing a caregiver or deciding to keep your child in a day care center or program, follow your intuition. Once you make a decision, give it a trial period before committing to a long-term arrangement.

Car Safety

Children should ride only in child safety seats approved by the National Highway Traffic Safety Administration (NHTSA). In addition:

■ Never put a child in the front seat of a vehicle with a passenger-side air bag.

■ Infants under 20 pounds and 1 year of age should ride in a rear-facing safety seat in the backseat.

■ Children between 20 and 40 pounds and over 1 year of age should ride in a front-facing safety seat in the backseat.

■ Children between 40 and 60 pounds and less than 8 years of age (or under 4'9" tall) should ride in a booster seat in the backseat.

To check the safety of your car seat, call the NHTSA hotline at 1-800-424-9393.

MEDICAL CONDITIONS

For disorders not listed here, see Medical Conditions starting on p.994.

Autism

Autism is a developmental disability in which children have abnormal communication, impaired social and emotional relationships, and repetitive limited behaviors. This unusual condition affects about 1 of 1000 infants, mostly boys. Current evidence suggests that autism is the result of improper functioning of the brain, not the result of any emotional or environmental influences.

At birth, the autistic child appears normal. Within the first 30 months, however, he or she becomes increasingly unresponsive to the environment. The child may not speak, may develop obsessive routines, may deliberately injure himself or herself, may become very hyperactive, may have seizures, or may respond with severe tantrums to any abrupt changes.

Physically, the autistic child appears normal. Intellectual ability, however, ranges widely. Although many autistic children have developmental delay, some may also be gifted in a specific area. About 20% of autistic children can eventually live independently.

If you suspect a developmental delay in your child, consult your child's doctor, who will conduct tests or refer you to specialists to confirm a diagnosis. Most families of autistic children also learn and get support from parents of other children with autism.

There is no cure, but special schooling, behavior therapy, and medicines for related disorders (such as seizures, hyperactivity, attention disorders, and aggressive behavior) can offer an autistic child the best chance possible. (See also Autism Society of America, p.1230.)

Birthmarks

Birthmarks are areas of discolored skin that are present at birth. Many skin markings, such as freckles, are not actually present at birth, but appear later on your infant's body.

A birthmark may seem very dark and large, but as your baby grows the area often gets smaller and lighter. Sometimes birthmarks disappear entirely.

Café au lait spots These flat brown spots can appear anywhere on your baby's body and may vary in hue (from deep brown to light tan). They usually do not fade over time and may enlarge as your baby's skin grows.

Mongolian spots Darker-skinned babies more commonly have these blue- or dark green–tinged areas of skin that occur on the back or buttocks. These harmless spots usually fade by 5 years of age.

Hemangiomas, including strawberry hemangiomas, port-wine stains, and salmon patches, are malformations of blood vessels.

■ *Strawberry hemangiomas* (see Color Guide to Visual Diagnosis, p.562), commonly known as strawberry marks, are raised, reddish-white blemishes that can be very small or up to several inches in diameter. They can grow quickly in the first year. Most disappear within 5 years without treatment.

■ *Port-wine stains* are flat purple or dark red areas that grow with the child and persist into adulthood. They are rarely associated with problems except in some cases when they are found near the eyelid and forehead. Cosmetic treatment (see Treating Strawberry Marks and Port Wine Stains, p.583) by a plastic surgeon or dermatologist may be possible when your child is older.

■ *Salmon patches,* also called stork bites, are small, flat patches

of pink-red marks located primarily on the lower forehead, upper eyelids, and nape of the neck; they usually become less noticeable within the first year of life.

Bronchiolitis

Bronchiolitis is a common infection that causes inflammation of the bronchioles—the tiny airways of the lungs. It is usually caused by the respiratory syncytial virus (RSV), but other viruses can also lead to bronchiolitis. The virus is usually transmitted person-to-person and frequently causes wheezing.

This infection most often affects infants under 2 years of age because of their immature (and much smaller) airways, which become inflamed and blocked more easily than those of older children or adults.

SYMPTOMS

Bronchiolitis begins like a cold, with sneezing, a runny nose that lasts several days, and a cough. Sometimes the child also has a reduced appetite and low-grade fever (101°F to 102°F).

Within 2 days, the cough worsens and becomes sporadic and wheezy. Your child may be irritable, may breathe rapidly, and may appear breathless. This can cause infants to have trouble feeding.

In mild cases, symptoms disappear within 3 to 5 days. In severe cases, the infant may grunt while trying to take in air because the airways are blocked.

If breathing problems are severe and your child begins to turn blue around the mouth, it is an emergency situation.

TREATMENT OPTIONS

Contact your doctor immediately if your child has trouble breathing. The doctor will examine your child, observe his or her breathing pattern, and listen to his or her lungs. If your infant has a mild form of bronchiolitis, make him or her more comfortable by giving plenty of liquids to prevent dehydration.

Treatment depends on the severity of the illness. Mild illness will go away with rest and quiet activity. At night, elevate the head of the crib to a 30- or 40-degree angle to make breathing more comfortable.

Infants with respiratory distress—inability to breathe well—may be given bronchodilator drugs to open the airways. The effectiveness of these medicines varies from child to child. In severe cases, your infant may be admitted to the hospital to receive extra oxygen, fluid replacement, and, in rare cases, mechanical lung support.

Cleft Lip and Palate

A cleft is a gap that occurs in the top lip (cleft lip) and/or the roof of the mouth (cleft palate). In cleft lip, the split is vertical and usually not centered in the upper lip; it can be a small split or extend to the nose.

Similarly, cleft palate is a gap that runs from behind the teeth to the back of the mouth. Cleft lip and cleft palate can occur individually or together.

This condition affects about 5,000 infants in the United States each year. Heredity plays a role in about 25% of cases; people of Asian and Native American

Cleft Lip and Palate

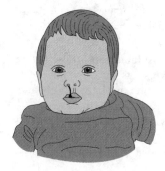
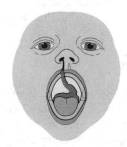

Cleft lip (left) occurs when the lip does not fuse. Cleft palate (right) occurs when the roof of the mouth does not grow together.

descent appear to be more susceptible.

Some cases of cleft palate may be caused by exposure of the fetus to toxins such as alcohol or medicines, or to inadequate nutrition (such as a folic acid deficiency) during fetal development.

Cleft lip or palate is usually first suspected before birth through ultrasound (see p.145). Either condition can be confirmed by a series of sophisticated ultrasound images taken in the later stages of pregnancy.

If your fetus is diagnosed with cleft lip or palate, consult a physician who is experienced in these disorders for counseling and support during delivery.

Infants with a cleft palate must be bottle-fed using a special nipple; some babies with a cleft lip are able to breast-feed. Speech may be delayed, and children with the condition are prone to middle ear infections (see p.457).

Inserting an artificial palate can improve your baby's sucking ability. Surgery for a cleft lip is

performed at about 3 months and is highly successful.

A series of surgeries may be necessary to correct cleft palate (which is more serious), starting at about age 1. A multidisciplinary team usually provides speech therapy, dental care, and braces, as well as psychological counseling. The outcome is usually excellent.

Clubfoot

Clubfoot is a deformity present at birth in which one or both feet turn at an abnormal angle from the ankle. It is more common among boys than girls and affects about 1 of 400 infants.

Researchers suspect that clubfoot arises from a combination of factors during fetal development, such as infection or as a result of medicines taken by the mother.

Untreated, clubfoot can cause abnormal movement and serious damage to skin and underlying tissue.

Clubfoot can take a number of forms. In metatarsus adductus

(the most common form), the front of the foot may turn inward. In other forms, the foot may turn outward at the ankle or inward and downward.

In mild cases, gently exercising the foot and ankle can often restore the foot to its normal position. More severe forms of clubfoot may require manipulation and prosthetic devices, such as a cast or special shoes with braces to retrain the growth of the foot.

Surgery can also be performed to release the tight ligaments and tendons holding the foot in its poor position. The foot is then immobilized in a cast for several months.

Colic

Colic is a catchall term for prolonged crying and discomfort during the first few months of life that cannot be attributed to a specific cause. Doctors diagnose colic in 20% of newborns. It usually begins 2 to 4 weeks after birth and can last for about 3 months.

If your baby is fairly happy at most other times, colic is no cause for concern. Doctors do not know what causes colic.

SYMPTOMS

The typical colicky infant cries inconsolably each day for several hours, usually starting in the late afternoon through early evening. Often the infant swallows air when crying, which causes more gas and discomfort. He or she may pass gas and repeatedly bring the knees to the chest.

Swaddling

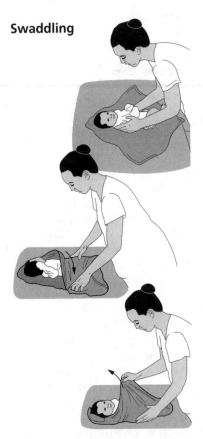

Place your baby in the center of a rectangular blanket, head near the top. Cross your baby's arms over the chest while folding one side of the blanket over and tucking it under your baby's back. Bring the bottom edge of the blanket up. Fold the opposite edge over the other arm, holding it down while crossing the blanket over baby's chest and under his or her back.

TREATMENT OPTIONS

If your infant cries inconsolably for hours on end—and feeding or changing diapers does not help—contact your child's doctor to rule out potentially serious disorders. Never hit or shake an infant; it can cause brain damage or blindness.

If the doctor diagnoses colic:

■ Hold your baby. Studies show that the more you hold your baby, the less the baby cries.

■ Avoid overstimulating environments during the late afternoon (such as busy streets, department stores, or restaurants).

■ Swaddle your baby snugly in a light blanket.

■ Take the baby for a car ride.

■ Provide a steady, rhythmic movement, such as gentle rocking, slow dancing, or walking, as you hold your baby.

■ If you are breast-feeding, avoid foods such as garlic, cabbage, beans, onions, or caffeine or dairy products.

■ Straddle the baby along your forearm with his or her tummy down, place his or her head slightly higher than the feet in the crook of your elbow, and pat his or her back gently. Or place the baby tummy down across your lap while you rub or pat his or her back.

■ If you are nursing, breast-feed more often.

■ Give the baby a pacifier between feedings.

■ Make sure to arrange for time for yourself; colic can be extremely trying for parents.

Constipation

Constipation is a period between bowel movements that is unusually long for your child, with bowel movements that are hard, difficult, or painful to pass.

Streaks of bright red blood may occur on the bowel movement or diaper due to a crack in the skin of the anus. Constipation is rare among breast-fed babies (breast milk softens bowel movements); it is more common in babies who are formula-fed or infants who have started solid foods.

Bowel habits vary from child to child. In general, if your baby appears well and is not having pain and is not vomiting, then long periods between bowel movements are not a cause for concern. On the other hand, if there is a significant change in your baby's normal pattern, with fewer bowel movements, suspect constipation.

Constipation can be caused by an immature or slow digestive tract, an inadequate amount of fiber in the diet, or, in rare cases, a serious disorder such as intestinal obstruction.

Some babies are prone to repeated bouts of constipation. Report constipation to the doctor to rule out a serious disorder. See Home Remedies for Infant Constipation (below) for safe home treatment.

Cradle Cap

Cradle cap appears as scaly red patches on the scalp. It is very common, appearing on many infants within the first weeks of life.

Cradle cap is actually a form of seborrheic dermatitis (see p.551; Color Guide to Visual Diagnosis, p.566), a skin inflammation of unknown cause that does not produce discomfort, but can spread to other areas of the body that contain sebaceous (oil) glands. Cradle cap usually disappears on its own within a few months.

You can treat a mild case of cradle cap yourself by shampooing your baby's head once a day. You can also try massaging your baby's head with a small amount of mineral oil or petroleum jelly, followed by a shampoo or brushing to remove the oil and scales.

For stubborn cases, the doctor can recommend an antiseborrheic shampoo containing sulfur and salicylic acid, though these can occasionally be irritating.

If treatment does not seem to be working, or the rash spreads to other parts of your infant's body, the doctor may prescribe a steroid cream or lotion that should be applied daily.

Crying

All babies cry. Lacking words to communicate their feelings and needs, they cry out of hunger, discomfort, pain, boredom, frustration, fatigue, loneliness, overstimulation, fear, anger, and illness. In the first few months, your baby's cries will serve as signals for feedings and the need for sleep and will help you establish a schedule.

Some babies have fussy periods of crying that do not respond to food or comfort, followed by periods of greater alertness. This type of crying may serve to help infants expel energy and return to a calmer condition.

Most parents learn to diagnose their child's cry by its sound. A hunger cry is often high-pitched and rhythmic; sudden pain is signaled by a few beats of silence followed by an explosive howl.

A high-pitched, screeching cry that does not abate with comforting, feeding, or distraction can be a sign of severe pain (see Ear Infection, p.1005) or a vaccination reaction (see p.946). An infrequent, weak cry may indicate serious illness.

A fussy but persistent cry may be due to teething (see p.964) or, if no cause is apparent, colic (see p.971). If you are ever in doubt

Home Remedies for Infant Constipation

Never give your baby any medicine (prescription or over-the-counter) to treat constipation without your doctor's approval. Try the following home remedies to encourage bowel movements:

■ **For babies not yet eating solids** Add 1 or 2 ounces of apple or prune juice to the diet. If your baby has recently switched from formula to cow's milk, return to formula. Cow's milk can cause constipation in some children.

■ **For babies eating solids** Avoid bananas and white rice. Choose wholegrain instead of white bread. Increase the amount of vegetables and fruits in the diet.

■ **For all babies** Increase water consumption and physical activity. Play "bicycle" with your baby's legs if he or she is not yet crawling.

about the cause of your baby's crying, or feel that you cannot cope with it, contact the doctor.

Developmental Dysplasia of the Hip

Developmental dysplasia of the hip is a general term for a range of abnormalities involving the hip. A dislocated hip is one that is out of the socket in the pelvic bone. An unstable hip is in the correct position but can easily become dislocated. A dysplastic hip is a shallow hip socket that can easily lead to dislocation as the child develops.

Most cases of dysplasia are thought to result from displacement in the uterus of a normally formed hip. A variety of factors may predispose an infant to these problems, including an inherited tendency and a breech (feet-first) birth. First-born females are at higher risk, and the left hip is more often affected, for unknown reasons

The symptoms can be subtle. Dysplasia is often diagnosed by the doctor during an examination of the newborn, but sometimes is diagnosed during well-baby examinations during infancy.

The hip may click when moved. Physical symptoms and pain may become evident as the child grows. To help determine the severity, the doctor may perform ultrasound (see p.148).

The condition is often treated with a brace that repositions the head of the thighbone into the hip socket. The device is worn for a month or two and is usually effective. If treatment is delayed, the child may require traction or a cast to reposition the bones.

Surgery is occasionally necessary if other options fail.

Diaper Rash

(See also Color Guide to Visual Diagnosis, p.568)

Diaper rash is a general term used to describe irritation of the skin beneath the diaper. It affects up to 35% of babies and often occurs repeatedly. Most cases of diaper rash are caused by chafing from the diaper, overexposure to the moisture and irritating chemicals of urine, or overexposure to digestive enzymes in bowel movements.

These conditions can occur when diapers are not changed frequently enough, when infants have frequent bowel movements or diarrhea, and in babies wearing overly tight diapers or diapers covered with rubber pants.

Diaper rash is also more common among infants just starting solid foods and in babies who are taking antibiotics. A yeast (candida) infection can occur in infants taking antibiotics. It may also develop if diaper rash is not treated for several days.

SYMPTOMS

The symptoms of diaper rash vary slightly depending on the cause and type. The affected area is red and sometimes itchy. With seborrheic dermatitis (see p.551; Color Guide to Visual Diagnosis, p.566), there is no itching.

With a secondary yeast (candida) infection, the area is red, may be tender or painful, tends to have small "satellite" sores and seeping pimples, and is often found in the creases of skin.

Cleaning and Diapering Your Baby

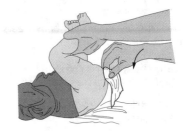

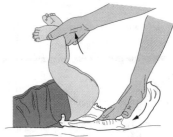

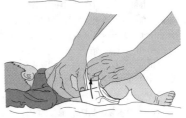

Remove the dirty diaper. Grasp and raise both feet with one hand (top) while you clean the baby's bottom. Check for rash or irritation as you blot or fan the diaper area dry. Place a clean diaper under baby's back (center), aligning the edge with the waist. Bring the bottom portion of the diaper through the baby's legs. Hold the diaper against your baby's stomach (if the umbilical cord stump is still attached, fold the diaper below it). Bring one side of the diaper over the other and pin or tape it (bottom). Do the same on the other side.

Diapers: Cloth Versus Disposable

The type of diaper your baby wears is your choice. There are pros and cons to both, as follows:

ADVANTAGES OF CLOTH	ADVANTAGES OF DISPOSABLE
■ Less expensive, even with a diaper service ■ Softer on baby's skin ■ Does not contribute to landfill waste	■ More convenient ■ More absorbent (less leaking) ■ Less chance of diaper rash (unless left on too long)

TREATMENT OPTIONS

Diaper rash is easily diagnosed by its location. To reduce the risk, change your baby's diaper frequently, and as soon as possible after bowel movements.

Cleanse the area gently with a washcloth or cotton balls and lukewarm water after bowel movements. Another alternative is wipes, although some babies react to the chemicals in wipes. Pat the area dry after washing.

As much as possible, expose the diaper area to air. If using cloth diapers, rinse the diaper in a vinegar-and-water solution (½ cup of vinegar and ½ cup of water) after washing.

If these measures fail, consider switching the type of diaper you use—from cloth to disposable, or vice versa.

A thick ointment can be applied to block urine and bowel movements from direct contact with the skin. Yeast infections may require a prescription medicine from your doctor. If the diaper rash persists, or if it worsens, contact the doctor.

Diaphragmatic Hernia

Diaphragmatic hernia is a congenital (present at birth) condition in which an abnormal opening in the diaphragm—the muscle that separates the chest cavity from the abdomen—permits a portion of the bowel to move into the chest cavity. When it is severe, it causes a life-threatening displacement of the lungs and heart.

Diaphragmatic hernia is rare, affecting 1 of 3,000 infants. It is frequently diagnosed during prenatal ultrasound. The parents of an affected infant are usually referred to a major pediatric center that has specialists skilled in managing the condition.

If the condition is not diagnosed immediately after birth, symptoms can include trouble breathing, blue skin from lack of oxygen, an abnormally fast heart rate, vomiting, and constipation.

In a few children, the hernia is so mild that it causes no symptoms. A suspected diagnosis is confirmed by x-ray. Surgery is performed to repair the hernia.

Esophageal Atresia

Esophageal atresia is a rare birth defect in which the esophagus fails to develop fully. Rather than providing a clear passageway from the throat to the stomach, the esophagus ends blindly. As a result, feeding through the mouth is impossible.

Though rare, this birth defect occurs more commonly among infants who are premature and/or have other birth defects.

Esophageal atresia becomes evident in the delivery or birthing room when an infant who tries to nurse vomits, chokes, turns blue from lack of oxygen, and coughs. Esophageal atresia is diagnosed

Fever: When to Call the Doctor

Call your baby's doctor if:

■ Your infant is younger than 3 months old and has a rectal temperature above 100.3°F.

■ He or she is older than 3 months but has a rectal temperature above 101°F.

■ Your infant's condition concerns or worries you more than usual.

■ He or she has a febrile seizure (see p.1007).

■ The fever is accompanied by lethargy or a rash.

■ You suspect heatstroke (see p.1212).

■ The fever is accompanied by purple dots or spots on your baby's skin.

■ Fever persists for more than 48 hours.

when a tube cannot be passed from the nose to the stomach, and is confirmed by x-ray.

Surgery is always required. After giving general anesthesia and opening the chest, the two closed ends of the esophagus are united. Surgery is usually very successful, but more surgery may be required over time.

Fetal Alcohol Syndrome

Fetal alcohol syndrome is a group of birth defects that can occur when a woman drinks alcohol during pregnancy. The birth defects may range from mild to severe.

Children with fetal alcohol syndrome usually are small and do not grow well during childhood. Their brain size may be abnormal, their development may be delayed, and they may have mental deficiencies and behavior problems.

Children with fetal alcohol syndrome often have unusual facial features such as unusually shaped eyes and small teeth. Their teeth may also have poor enamel. The child may also have heart defects and joint or limb abnormalities.

Since alcohol interferes with the normal growth of the fetus and no safe level of alcohol consumption during pregnancy has been established, talk with your obstetrician about your drinking once you discover you are pregnant.

Fever

Fever is a body temperature above normal. In infants and children, a rectal temperature of 100.3°F or lower, or an oral read-

Taking Your Baby's Temperature

You have several options for taking your baby's temperature. Your child's temperature can be taken rectally, in the armpit, or in the ear (oral thermometers are not recommended until a child is 4 years old).

Taking a rectal temperature is the most accurate method of checking for fever. To take a rectal temperature, shake down the thermometer and apply petroleum jelly to the bulb (the red end). Calm your baby and turn him or her onto the belly, either on a bed or over your lap.

Spread the buttocks with one hand and insert the lubricated thermometer about 1 inch into the rectum at a 90-degree angle. Hold it there for 2 minutes while spreading the anus apart. If your baby becomes very active, remove the thermometer immediately. Electronic digital thermometers are also available for checking rectal temperature.

Tympanic (ear) thermometers are not reliable in infants younger than 3 months or in active toddlers who may be overheated. Axillary (armpit) methods are also not very accurate but can let you know if your child's temperature is rising. For more information on how to take a temperature, see p.1124.

Taking a Rectal Temperature

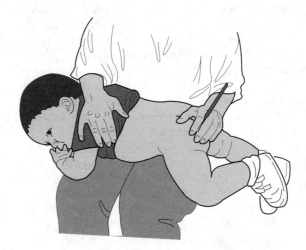

To take a baby's rectal temperature, apply a little petroleum jelly to the end of the thermometer and insert it ½ inch to 1 inch into the anus, holding your baby's lower back to keep the baby from wiggling around too much. Keep the thermometer in place for 2 minutes before reading it.

ing of 99°F or lower, is considered normal. Only temperatures above these levels constitute a fever.

Fever is part of the way that the body's immune system fights infections such as the flu, a bad cold, or an ear infection. In rare cases, it also occurs for other reasons, such as heatstroke (see p.1212).

A child with a fever often has a warm forehead, flushed face, chills, and appears to be trembling. When you suspect a fever, it is best to get an accurate reading with a thermometer.

The doctor may recommend fever-reducing medicines, such as acetaminophen or ibuprofen. Aspirin should not be given to those under 21 years because it can cause Reye syndrome (see p.1017). Be sure to follow the doctor's exact recommendations about the type and dose of medicine. The medicines lower the child's temperature, and often make the child feel better, but they do not treat or cure the infection that might be causing the fever.

Other recommendations for cooling a moderately high fever (below 102°F):

■ Dress your child lightly and keep room temperature cool.

■ In a warm room, sponge him or her with lukewarm water.

■ Make sure your child drinks plenty of fluids, such as water or juice.

Gastroenteritis

Gastroenteritis is inflammation of the stomach and intestines. Just like when it occurs in adults (see

Gastroenteritis and Dehydration: *When to Call the Doctor*

A child is particularly vulnerable to dehydration under certain circumstances. You should contact the doctor if:

■ The soft spot on top of your baby's head is sunken.

■ There are no wet diapers over a 6- to 8-hour period (depending on the child's age).

■ Your child fails to produce tears when crying.

■ Your baby's mouth, eyes, and/or skin are dry.

■ His or her cry is weak or raspy or he or she is significantly less active.

■ Your child has a chronic medical condition.

■ He or she is malnourished.

■ Your infant is less than 2 months old.

■ There is excessive vomiting.

■ There is a significant increase in the usual amount or number of bowel movements each day, or they are bloody or foul-smelling.

p.778), gastroenteritis is usually the result of an infection caused by a virus. It can also be caused by food poisoning from bacteria or parasites, the side effect of a medicine, or a reaction to a new food. Breast-fed infants can get diarrhea from a change in the mother's diet.

Because gastroenteritis often causes vomiting and diarrhea, your child can become dehydrated from the lost fluid. The dehydration is usually mild and easily treated, but can be severe, leading to serious illness and even death.

SYMPTOMS

The most common symptoms are diarrhea, abdominal pain, vomiting, cramping, fussiness, and loss of appetite. Some babies develop

a fever. The symptoms usually come on suddenly (but can appear gradually) and generally last for 2 or 3 days.

Some types of food poisoning can cause shorter-term symptoms. Stomach pain may occur on and off for a week or more with other causes.

TREATMENT OPTIONS

In an otherwise healthy infant, diarrhea usually resolves with little treatment. Make sure your baby drinks plenty of fluids to prevent dehydration. It is best to give your child frequent, small amounts of liquid if a larger amount causes vomiting.

When there are signs of dehydration, or if your child is particularly vulnerable (the younger the child, the greater the risk of dehydration), call your child's doctor (see Gastroenteritis and Dehydration: When to Call the Doctor, see p.976).

If the doctor thinks the dehydration is mild, an oral rehydration solution, available at most drugstores, is the favored treatment. Your baby drinks this solution to help replace lost minerals as well as fluid.

In most cases, milk and solid foods can be continued during the course of the illness. Do not give nonprescription medicines that slow down intestinal movement (antidiarrheal drugs) without the doctor's approval.

If your child has serious dehydration, the doctor may order immediate intravenous (into a vein) fluid therapy in the hospital. Other treatments—such as antibiotics to eliminate bacterial or parasitic infections—may be recommended, depending on the cause of the gastroenteritis. With prompt diagnosis, treatment is effective.

Many cases of gastroenteritis can be prevented. Studies show that breast-feeding reduces the risk by up to 30% by boosting the baby's immunity against infection. Many cases can also be prevented by being scrupulously clean when preparing food (see p.87), including washing hands well.

Gastroesophageal Reflux

Gastroesophageal reflux, characterized by the spitting up of some of the stomach contents after feeding, is common in infants in the first year of life. It is caused by immature function of the valve (sphincter) between the esophagus and the stomach.

The sphincter normally keeps swallowed food in the stomach.

Reflux is effortless and different from vomiting (in vomiting, most of the stomach contents are brought up and sometimes shoot out several feet, as in projectile vomiting).

Call the doctor if you notice that your infant is not gaining weight, is dehydrated, or has pain when spitting up. Otherwise, most infants outgrow reflux as the esophageal sphincter matures.

In the meantime, take these measures to minimize reflux:

■ Avoid feeding your child while he or she is crying.

■ Do not bounce your baby after meals.

■ Feed your child in a calm environment.

■ Burp him or her midway through a feeding and again at the end.

■ Keep your baby in a semi-upright position during and after feeding.

■ If your doctor recommends, place your baby on his or her stomach after feeding (rather than on the back) to avoid choking.

Heart Disorders

Congenital (present at birth) heart defects—abnormalities of the heart's structure—are among the most common and treatable birth defects; about 8 of every 1,000 infants are born with them.

Many heart defects are so mild that they require no treatment. Some heart defects are not even noticed until the child grows. However, several are life-threatening in the first few weeks of life.

Congenital heart defects can be divided into two groups: those that cause an insufficient amount of blood to pass through the lungs and those that cause too much blood to move from the heart to the lungs.

Heart disorders may occur because of exposure of the mother to rubella (see p.950) or another virus. (Because the baby's heart is fully formed by 3 months after conception, a woman may not know she is pregnant at the time of exposure.)

Heart disorders may also occur due to genetic conditions, such as Down syndrome (see p.1004) or Marfan syndrome (see p.129). However, in most cases, there is no known cause for the defect.

Doctors can detect some heart defects before birth through ultrasound (see p.148). Others become apparent when the infant is delivered and turns blue (due to lack of oxygen) or has difficulty breathing. Babies with severe heart problems usually require surgery immediately.

In many children, heart defects repair themselves within 12 months. In others, treatment includes oxygen, rest, and medicine to support the function of the lungs and to improve circulation.

The surgeries recommended for the most common heart defects are described in the chart on p.978. Some are straightforward operations; others are more complex. In rare cases, a heart transplant (see p.688) may be required.

In some babies, a heart defect

Common Heart Defects

This chart describes the most common congenital (present at birth) heart defects and their symptoms and treatment. A healthy heart is shown at right.

NORMAL HEART

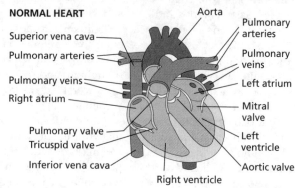

- Aorta
- Superior vena cava
- Pulmonary arteries
- Pulmonary veins
- Right atrium
- Pulmonary valve
- Tricuspid valve
- Inferior vena cava
- Right ventricle
- Pulmonary arteries
- Pulmonary veins
- Left atrium
- Mitral valve
- Left ventricle
- Aortic valve

DISORDER	DESCRIPTION	SYMPTOMS	TREATMENT
PATENT DUCTUS ARTERIOSUS 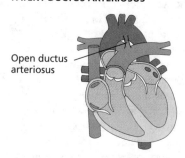 Open ductus arteriosus	Oxygenated blood moves from the aorta through an open duct into the pulmonary artery and mixes with blood going into the lungs. The duct is normally closed near the time of birth.	Often no symptoms. May place strain on the heart and cause: ■ Shortness of breath during exertion ■ Heart murmur (see p.689)	Use of nonsteroidal anti-inflammatory drugs. Surgery, required when the child is 6 or 9 months old, aims at closing the abnormal duct.
VENTRICULAR SEPTAL DEFECT (HOLE IN THE HEART) 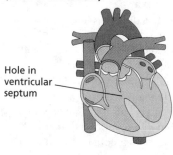 Hole in ventricular septum	A hole in the wall between the pumping chambers of the heart, allowing oxygenated blood to flow from the left to the right ventricle and causing excess blood to go to the lungs. It is the most common congenital heart defect.	No symptoms unless severe. May cause: ■ Fatigue ■ Heart failure (see p.683) ■ High blood pressure in the lungs, as in pulmonary hypertension (see p.515) ■ Poor feeding and poor weight gain	Mild cases resolve on their own. If they do not, surgery may be required when the child is 2 or 3 years old to place a patch over the hole.
COARCTATION OF THE AORTA 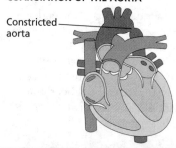 Constricted aorta	A narrowing of part of the aorta—the main artery for blood transport to the body—causing a decrease in blood flow to the body.	Sometimes no symptoms. May cause: ■ Pale complexion ■ Breathlessness ■ Difficulty feeding ■ High blood pressure	Surgery may be required before the child is 2 weeks old to remove the narrowed section of aorta and join the two normal-sized parts. Sometimes surgery is delayed until the child is 2 to 4 years old.

DISORDER	DESCRIPTION	SYMPTOMS	TREATMENT
TRANSPOSITION OF THE GREAT VESSELS 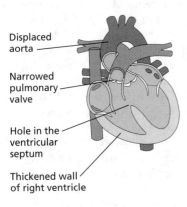 Aorta Pulmonary artery Hole in the ventricular septum	A reversal of the position of the aorta and pulmonary artery (which carry blood from the heart), resulting in return of oxygenated blood to the lungs rather than to the rest of the body.	At birth may cause: ▪ Slowed growth ▪ Blue skin due to lack of oxygenated blood	Surgery is required before the child is 2 weeks old to restore blood flow to the body by creating a hole in the septum (wall between heart chambers). Another operation is needed by age 5 years to reposition (or create artificial) blood vessels.
TETRALOGY OF FALLOT Displaced aorta Narrowed pulmonary valve Hole in the ventricular septum Thickened wall of right ventricle	A combination of the following four defects, causing an insufficient supply of blood to the lungs and resulting in oxygen-poor blood to the rest of the body: ▪ Narrowed valve in pulmonary artery, which takes blood to the lungs, as in pulmonary stenosis ▪ Thickened right ventricle wall ▪ Ventricular septal defect (see p.978) ▪ Displaced aorta	May cause: ▪ Slowed growth ▪ Clubbed fingers and toes ▪ Breathlessness and blue skin and lips due to lack of oxygen	Surgery is required before the child is 1 year old.
HYPOPLASTIC LEFT HEART SYNDROME (not illustrated)	A very rare deformity of the left ventricle and aorta, causing an inability of the blood to reach the aorta except via an extra duct, as in patent ductus arteriosus (see p.978).	Even though the baby may seem healthy at birth may cause: ▪ Trouble breathing after several days due to closing of the duct ▪ Ultimately loss of consciousness and death	A complicated series of operations is required; affected children often die even with surgery.

becomes noticeable only after 12 months, when the child has difficulty breathing or develops a bluish cast to the skin, nails, and lips. If you notice such changes in your child, call the doctor immediately.

HEART MURMURS

Many infants have heart murmurs. Heart murmurs are additional sounds made by the blood rushing through the heart chambers or blood vessels near the heart, in addition to the healthy heartbeat sounds.

Most heart murmurs are not dangerous. If a child has a normal heart structure, the heart murmur is less likely to be something to be concerned about. However, murmurs caused by a structural abnormality such as a ventricular septal defect—a hole between two chambers in the heart—frequently require treatment.

ARRHYTHMIAS

Arrhythmias are abnormalities in the rhythm of the heart (heartbeats). Extra heartbeats are common in healthy children and often go away on their own as the child grows.

Hernia

A hernia is a protruding of the intestine or other organ through a weak spot in surrounding muscles or tissues. In infants, these weak areas are usually caused by incomplete development during fetal growth.

The two most common types of hernias among infants are umbilical hernias and inguinal hernias.

Umbilical Hernia

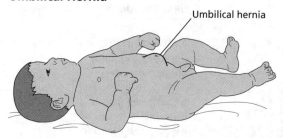

Umbilical hernia

An umbilical hernia is a swelling around the navel. It may push out even farther when your baby cries.

Umbilical hernias are caused by a weakness in the abdominal wall near the navel, which permits the intestine to protrude. The weakness is due to failure of the abdominal muscles to completely form; this normally occurs in the second trimester of pregnancy. Most umbilical hernias heal on their own within a few years. Because there is little risk from an umbilical hernia and because they are usually painless, they are treated primarily for cosmetic reasons, and then only after age 4.

Inguinal hernias account for 75% of all hernias. Boys are far more vulnerable than girls to these types of hernias because they are sometimes born with a weakness in the inguinal canal, the passage through which the testicle descends into the scrotum. An inguinal hernia appears as a bulge in the groin. Because it may result in intestinal strangulation (twisting and constriction that blocks blood flow and may cause tissue death) or blockage, treatment is required. Surgery is described on p.800.

Hirschsprung Disease

This rare disorder results from the absence of nerve cells at the end of the large intestine. This prevents the muscles of the wall of the intestine from moving fecal matter through the intestine. The feces accumulate just above the area where the nerves are missing, causing significant enlargement of the intestine.

The condition is congenital (present at birth) and tends to run in families. It is more common in boys than girls.

Severe constipation (infrequent, hard bowel movements), bloating (a hard, expanded, and tight abdomen), and abdominal discomfort are evident early in life, usually from birth. The infant often does not grow well, and may have anemia (see p.713). Report any of these symptoms to your doctor.

Diagnostic tests for Hirschsprung disease include a barium enema (see p.784), which shows the enlargement of the intestine. To make a diagnosis, the doctor may use a tube to measure the lack of pressure exerted by the intestinal wall muscles. A biopsy of intestinal tissue from the affected area can show if nerve cells are present or missing. Surgery that removes the abnormal portion of intestine and rejoins the healthy parts is usually successful.

Hydrocele

A hydrocele is a fluid-filled sac in the scrotum. It affects up to 50% of newborn boys and usually disappears within 12 months with no treatment. Hydroceles can also occur in older children or adults, often along with an inguinal hernia (see p.980).

A hydrocele causes painless swelling on one side of the scrotum that may lessen when the baby lies down. Your doctor can confirm a suspected hydrocele by shining a light through the scrotum in order to see the fluid.

Surgery is usually not necessary unless there is also pain, fever, or nausea, which can indicate an inguinal hernia.

Call your doctor if your son has any pain or you think he may have a hernia. If necessary, surgery to drain the fluid and repair the hydrocele is performed after age 1.

Hydrocephalus

Hydrocephalus is excess cerebrospinal fluid in the area surrounding the brain. It is caused when the healthy circulation of the fluid is blocked or when an infant is born with an inability to reabsorb the fluid. Because the child's skull bones are soft and pliable to accommodate future growth, the pressure of the accumulating fluid causes the head to enlarge, especially in the front.

Causes of hydrocephalus include spina bifida (see p.985), head injury, infection (see Meningitis, p.1013), or a tumor.

A large head that grows exceptionally fast is the chief symptom, with irritability, seizures, and rigid limbs. In older children, headaches, vomiting, lethargy, or gait abnormalities may occur. Rapidly progressing or long-standing hydrocephalus can cause brain damage and death.

Your child's doctor will arrange for computed tomography (see p.149) to view the brain. Treatment involves draining fluid with a tube (shunt) inserted through a hole in the skull; the shunt may be replaced as the child grows. Infection is a common complication.

Hypospadias

In hypospadias the urethral opening (passageway for urine) is located beneath the penis instead of at its tip. It occurs in about 1 of 500 male infants; 10% of boys born with hypospadias also have an undescended testicle.

Later in life, untreated hypospadias can cause a downward bend in an erection. In rare cases, it can block urine flow.

Hypospadias is readily diagnosed during the newborn's examination. Your physician will recommend against circumcision (because the foreskin may be

---

Fontanelles: a Baby's "Soft Spots"

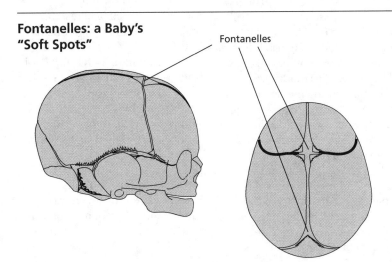

Fontanelles

The anterior (front) fontanelle, or "soft spot" on the top of the baby's head, is an area where the skull bones have not yet grown to cover the brain. It fuses together in the first 18 months as the bones of the skull grow. The soft spot is protected by a tough membrane. Normal handling will not hurt it. The posterior (rear) fontanelle closes by 3 months of age.

needed in later surgery) and refer your baby to a pediatric urologist or surgeon (a specialist in infant male genital disorders).

Surgery is frequently recommended, and is most often performed during the first 12 months. Surgery repositions the urethral opening, closes the defective opening, and straightens the penis, if necessary. Hospitalization is usually not required. The results are usually very successful.

Hypothyroidism

Hypothyroidism is underproduction of thyroid hormone—the hormone responsible for mental and physical growth—due to a genetic defect in the thyroid gland.

About 1 of 4,000 infants is born with this deficiency. If undetected or untreated, it can lead to mental retardation and short stature.

Fatigue and constipation may be the only symptoms until it becomes evident that your child's physical and/or mental development is delayed.

A test is performed on all newborns in the United States to screen for this deficiency. Immediate replacement of thyroid hormone can help ensure normal intelligence and physical development. See also Hypothyroidism, p.848.

Imperforate Anus

An imperforate anus is a closed anal canal, caused either by a membrane that covers the opening or incomplete development of the anal canal that results in a

dead end. An imperforate anus blocks passage of bowel movements from the body.

The first symptom of imperforate anus is the absence of meconium, the infant's first bowel movement after birth. An x-ray or ultrasound (see p.148) may be performed to determine where in the rectum the obstruction lies. Imperforate anus may occur with other birth defects.

In some infants, inserting a series of dilators to widen a narrow anus is all that is necessary. Surgery is required to either remove any tissue covering the anus or open the passageway between the anus and rectum. Surgery is more complex the higher in the rectum the blockage lies; some infants require reconstruction of the anus.

The success of surgery varies according to its extent. Some children are able to achieve bowel control; others have fecal incontinence (see p.794).

Jaundice

Jaundice is yellowing of the skin and whites of the eyes. The most common cause in infants is called physiologic jaundice, and it is important to distinguish it from jaundice due to other causes.

Physiologic jaundice is very common during the first few days of life, occurring in about 60% of healthy newborns. It is the result of excessive blood levels of the pigment bilirubin, which forms when red blood cells are broken down and processed by the spleen and the liver.

Infants are susceptible to this condition because they are often born with higher-than-normal

numbers of red blood cells and their livers are not yet fully mature, resulting in an inability to eliminate the bilirubin.

Less commonly, jaundice can signal a blood or urine infection, an incompatibility with the mother's blood (see Rh Incompatibility, p.157), or another serious metabolic or liver disease. Breast-feeding may also cause jaundice, usually beginning in the second week of life.

If jaundice develops in the first week of life, it is not likely to be caused by breast-feeding, and breast-feeding should be continued. Talk to your doctor before making any changes in how you feed your baby or if you think your baby is dehydrated.

In most infants, jaundice disappears on its own within a few days. However, if it does not subside or is intense, treatment may be necessary to avert a buildup of too much bilirubin, which can damage the nervous system.

The doctor will ask you to watch your baby for signs of deepening yellow tones. If this occurs, he or she will test the baby's blood to monitor bilirubin levels.

Your infant may require light therapy (phototherapy), in which he or she is placed under a lamp or blanket that gives off ultraviolet-B light for several hours a day (light breaks down bilirubin) until the bilirubin level in the blood returns to normal. Additional fluids may also be given. In severe cases, the infant may require a blood transfusion.

Meckel Diverticulum

Meckel diverticulum is a small pouching that pushes out from the wall of the ileum (the last portion of the small intestine). The pouch is often lined with stomach tissue. Meckel diverticulum is a congenital (present at birth) abnormality that affects about 2% of the population.

You may not know that your child was born with a diverticulum unless it begins to bleed from ulceration (blood can be seen in the baby's diaper), becomes infected, or causes blockage of the intestine. Although infection and intestinal blockage can cause pain, the bleeding (even when severe) is usually painless.

To diagnose Meckel diverticulum, the doctor may inject a radioactive dye into the bloodstream; the dye travels to stomach tissue, illuminating the stomach and diverticulum when observed on a nuclear medicine scan (see p.137).

Infections are treated with antibiotics. Transfusions may be needed if bleeding is extensive. The diverticulum should be removed surgically.

Phenylketonuria (PKU)

PKU is an inherited enzyme deficiency that inhibits metabolism of the food-derived chemical phenylalanine, resulting in its buildup and causing severe mental and physical developmental delays. It affects about 1 of 10,000 infants; most have blond hair and blue eyes. Many also have eczema (see p.1006).

Affected infants also have small heads and short stature. PKU is diagnosed in the newborn period by a mandatory blood test taken from the heel. It is treated with a lifelong diet that restricts intake of phenylalanine (which is found in most protein foods) and aspartame, an artificial sweetener. When treated from birth, people with PKU do not experience severe developmental delay.

Prematurity

Prematurity is defined as birth before 37 weeks in the uterus (pregnancy normally lasts about 40 weeks). About 6% of babies in the United States are born prematurely.

Physical problems are common in premature newborns and most require additional medical care after delivery. However, the vast majority of babies born after the seventh month of pregnancy can now survive without serious long-term problems.

Babies born very prematurely (before 32 weeks) usually need help feeding (because they cannot suck well), help maintaining body temperature (due to less body fat), and help breathing (due to underdeveloped lungs). Their skin is red and almost transparent. It is covered with downy hair called lanugo.

Premature infants tend not to cry as often as full-term babies. Their immature internal organs may not function well; therefore, doctors may need to do repeated blood tests to monitor the function of the kidneys and liver.

Many premature infants develop respiratory distress syndrome (RDS) shortly after birth. RDS occurs when the infant's lungs do not produce enough surfactant, a lubricant necessary for the lungs' air sacs (alveoli) to expand and stay expanded in order to permit the child to breathe better. Premature infants with RDS breathe quickly and poorly after birth and, if untreated, may turn blue from lack of oxygen.

RDS usually is most critical during the initial 48 hours after birth and then starts to improve. Mild RDS is treated with oxygen, but many infants are placed on a respirator (see p.520). Frequent blood samples are taken to ensure that the infant is getting enough oxygen and breathing out carbon dioxide. More severe RDS can be treated with supplemental surfactant. Treating premature infants with artificial surfactant lowers the risk of RDS; use of surfactant may also make the course of the disease milder.

Premature babies born before 34 weeks or weighing less than 4 pounds can have rupture and bleeding of the blood vessels in the brain. A severe episode of bleeding can cause hydrocephalus and developmental delays. Very premature babies can also have other complications caused by the immaturity of the intestines (such as necrotizing enterocolitis) and the immaturity of the eyes (such as retinopathy of prematurity).

TREATMENT OPTIONS

Treatment depends on the needs of the baby. Most premature infants are taken out of the normal newborn nursery (and away from the mother), and some may need to be nursed in an incubator, which maintains a constant temperature and shields the infant from infectious organisms.

Some infants are given antibiotic drugs for the first 48 hours to ensure that there is no infection. Many require mechanical ventilation to breathe, artificial feeding, and other supportive therapy.

You may be encouraged to touch your child in the incubator to establish a bond. Although the separation can be stressful for parents and infant, close observation by medical personnel is necessary.

You may be able to express breast milk for your baby, even though you may not be able to nurse him or her right away. Ask the doctor or nurse how active a role you may play in your child's day-to-day life until he or she is strong enough to go home.

OUTLOOK

If supported well during the early months, premature babies who do not have serious complications often develop normally, both mentally and physically.

It is important to view the milestones your child reaches in the context of his or her premature birth date—the child's age calculated from birth minus the weeks born prematurely—until about age 2.

Survival of infants born as early as 23 to 24 weeks of pregnancy is possible, but many of them have very serious problems, both mentally and physically, including blindness, deafness, cerebral palsy, and learning problems.

Pyloric Stenosis

Pyloric stenosis is a thickening of the muscle surrounding the outlet of the stomach, through which stomach contents must pass to reach the small intestine.

Symptoms of pyloric stenosis most often start during the second week after birth. Despite having a good appetite and feeding well, the infant vomits, either shortly after feeding or several hours later. Over several days, the vomiting may become projectile vomiting, shooting out a few feet because of the blockage.

The baby may lose weight and become dehydrated. Bowel movements are limited because an inadequate amount of food is passing through the intestines.

Report projectile vomiting to your baby's doctor immediately. He or she will perform a physical exam and try to feel for a firm mass in the right upper quadrant of the abdomen. To confirm the diagnosis, your child may need an x-ray or an ultrasound (see p.148).

In the meantime, your doctor will prescribe measures to relieve dehydration, either with electrolyte solutions by mouth (which are also commercially available) or by intravenous infusion.

Treatment for pyloric stenosis is by surgery (using general anesthesia) to open the abdomen and cut the thickened muscle to open the passageway.

You will feed your infant soon after the operation, gradually increasing the amount he or she receives while the doctor ensures that the movement of food is occurring normally. Most babies quickly make a full recovery.

Rashes

It takes infants a few months to grow into their legendary, baby-soft complexions. Until then, thin skin and immature body systems render them susceptible to a number of harmless, though unsightly, skin conditions. The most common include:

Milia (milk spots) (see Color Guide to Visual Diagnosis, p.568) are small white cysts that occur when a baby's skin glands begin to secrete oil. They commonly appear across the nose and chin. Milia are not a result of poor hygiene and will not improve with washing or squeezing. They are painless and disappear on their own within a few weeks.

Erythema toxicum is a blotchy, irregularly shaped rash made up of red spots that lighten in the center. This harmless rash requires no treatment and fades on its own within several weeks.

Acne (see Color Guide to Visual Diagnosis, p.562) is not uncommon among newborns. It is caused by hormones from the mother that are still active in the infant. As with milia (see above), undeveloped oil glands may also contribute to the problem. Keep your baby's face clean (wash three times a day with water and a very mild soap, then gently pat dry). The acne will clear on its own within several months.

Infantile eczema (see Color Guide to Visual Diagnosis, p.568) appears as inflamed, weepy, or crusty patches on the baby's face, neck, and groin. It is often itchy, but scratching leads to further skin irritation. It may be caused by an allergy and often can be successfully treated with moisturizing ointment and mild corticosteroid creams. Keep baby's nails short; limit bathtime (and keep bathwater lukewarm); avoid hot, dry air; and replace synthetic materials with natural ones.

Roseola Infantum

Roseola infantum is a mild viral infection that most often affects infants between the ages of 6 months and 2 years. Caused by a type of herpesvirus, roseola follows a very distinct course—high fever with flulike illness, followed by a rash after the fever disappears.

A sudden high fever (up to 105°F) with irritability is the first sign of roseola. The fever may last up to 5 days and may disappear suddenly. But, during this time, flulike symptoms such as sore throat, mild diarrhea, cough, and lethargy appear. A slightly raised rash replaces the subsiding fever, starting on the trunk and spreading up to the shoulders, neck, and face. This rash usually fades within a day or two. Some infants have febrile seizures (see p.1007) due to the sudden high fever.

There is no specific treatment. Your doctor may recommend fever-reducing medicines such as acetaminophen (not aspirin).

Dress your child in lightweight clothes and, if his or her temperature rises above 104°F, give a sponge bath with lukewarm water. Offer fluids frequently and encourage quiet activities. Report any symptoms that concern you to your child's doctor.

Seizures and Epilepsy

A seizure is a sudden, involuntary change in a person's functioning caused by an abnormal electrical discharge from the brain cells. The result is an immediate onset of nervous system symptoms including (depending on the type of seizure) disturbed sensations, uncontrollable jerking movements, change or loss of muscle tone, and loss of consciousness.

A seizure may occur as a result of some acute stress to the brain, such as a head injury, meningitis (see p.1013), encephalitis (see p.374), an electrolyte disturbance, or a tumor. These are called symptomatic, or provoked, seizures.

Seizures that occur spontaneously are called idiopathic, or unprovoked, seizures. Many children have one seizure and never have another.

Seizures may arise from one area in the brain. These are called partial, or focal, seizures. Alternatively, generalized seizures may arise from the entire brain at once.

Febrile seizures (see p.1007) occur only at the time of a fever. They are common in children between the ages of 1 and 5 years old. Febrile seizures occur in about 2% to 5% of children who do not have epilepsy. However, a child who has epileptic seizures may also have febrile seizures, and it is sometimes difficult to differentiate between them. An electroencephalogram (see p.136) can help distinguish an epileptic seizure from a febrile seizure.

Febrile seizures tend to be short (less than 15 minutes) and generalized (occur all over the body, not in just one area).

Febrile seizures are not usually treated with anticonvulsant medicines. The typical age of onset for febrile seizures is 18 months. However, the younger a child is at the time of the first febrile seizure, the more likely a febrile seizure may recur.

Epilepsy (see p.375) is recurring, unprovoked seizures. Epilepsy is a chronic condition, meaning that the seizures recur. A person who has just one seizure is usually not considered to have epilepsy. There are families in which there is a tendency for epilepsy. If a child has a single seizure, or only a few seizures, anticonvulsant medicine may not be needed. However, if the seizures recur, anticonvulsant medicine may be prescribed.

The majority of children with epilepsy respond well to these medicines, but some have epilepsy that is difficult to control. Tests such as an electroencephalogram (see p.136), computed tomography (see p.149), and magnetic resonance imaging (see p.151) may be needed to diagnose epilepsy.

Spina Bifida (Neural Tube Defect)

Spina bifida is a congenital (present at birth) defect of the bones that normally cover the spinal cord. The defect most often occurs in the lower back and affects about 1 of 1,000 newborns.

A baby born with spina bifida has a small pouch pushing out from the spine that contains cerebrospinal fluid and nerves that normally would lead to the lower body.

Pregnant women can greatly reduce the risk of having a child with spina bifida by taking 400 micrograms (0.4 milligrams) of folic acid a day.

Spina bifida in the fetus can be diagnosed by amniocentesis (see p.917) or at birth by physical symptoms. Treatment depends on the severity of the problem.

Usually, surgery must be performed within several days to remove the pouch and close the spinal opening. The defective nerves cannot be treated.

Infants with spina bifida are more prone to infection and hydrocephalus (see p.981). They may also have paralysis and difficulty controlling their bladder and bowels due to the defective nerves. Many children also have learning disabilities and require special education. Some have seizures.

Children with spina bifida are often treated by a multidisciplinary team that includes several specialist physicians, social workers, psychologists, and physical therapists. Contact the organization listed on p.1230 for support and more information.

Sudden Infant Death Syndrome (SIDS)

Sudden infant death syndrome (SIDS) is the sudden death of an otherwise healthy infant under one year of age for unknown reasons. About 1 of 500 children worldwide dies of SIDS, usually during sleep.

Some infants are at higher risk of SIDS than others, including those born prematurely, who are of low birthweight (especially male infants), whose mothers smoke, and who sleep on their stomachs.

Some researchers suspect that infants who die of SIDS have an undetected respiratory, cardiac, or brain abnormality, especially in centers that control breathing.

The striking characteristic of SIDS is the lack of warning signs. Infants are usually healthy in all ways, even when examined during an autopsy.

To reduce the risk of SIDS, put your infant to sleep on his or her back or side. However, if your infant was premature or spits up or vomits regularly during sleep, ask the doctor for advice on what sleep position is best.

Also, to further lower the risk of SIDS, make sure that your child's mattress is firm, and remove all pillows and fluffy toys that could block breathing. Never smoke around your child. If you find that your baby has stopped breathing, perform cardiopulmonary resuscitation (see p.1201) if you have been trained to do so and phone for emergency medical assistance immediately.

Swelling of the Scalp

Caput succedaneum and cephalohematoma are raised areas on the top of an infant's head at birth. Both are caused by delivery through a narrow birth canal in which the head is squeezed or when forceps or suction (see p.940) are used to help deliver the baby.

In caput succedaneum, the result is a swelling on top of the head that can extend horizontally and vertically where the bones of the skull fuse (see illustration on p.981). This swelling subsides after 2 to 3 days without treatment.

Cephalohematoma is bleeding underneath the outermost layer of a skull bone that appears to be raised or swollen, but with no discoloration of the overlying skin. A cephalohematoma may take up to 2 to 3 months to completely resolve.

Thrush

Thrush is a common infection of the mouth that is caused by the fungus *Candida albicans*. This organism is a natural inhabitant of the mouth, where helpful bacteria normally keep it in correct balance with other microorganisms.

When the natural balance of organisms is disrupted—spontaneously or by illness, antibiotics, or other conditions—*C albicans* may proliferate. Unless your baby has an immune disease, thrush is not a serious problem and can be easily treated.

If your baby has thrush, you will see yellow-white, raised patches in the lining of the mouth and throat. If the patches are rubbed off, areas of painful skin are exposed. Thrush may keep your baby from feeding properly, and you may notice him or her turning away from the breast or bottle, or crying in the middle of a feeding.

Most cases of thrush can be easily diagnosed by their appearance. The doctor may recommend an oral antifungal medicine. Babies with thrush can also have a diaper rash from candida, which is treated with an antifungal cream.

Thumb Sucking and Pacifiers

Many infants and children suck their thumbs or use pacifiers. For a long time, some doctors speculated that a child who was impatiently nursed or given a bottle with a poorly designed nipple lost the warmth, security, and feeling of well-being associated with suckling—and therefore sucked the thumb. However, this theory does not explain why ultrasound pictures show fetuses in the uterus sucking their thumbs.

Children have a basic need to suck, a need they are clearly already expressing before they are born. Sucking on pacifiers or thumbs after birth is usually just a natural extension of that basic urge. Most experts agree that

sucking on fingers and pacifiers is generally a harmless habit.

Children usually stop sucking their thumbs on their own by age 3 or 4. There is usually no reason to push them to stop before age 4. Indeed, parents who call negative attention to the habit may cause undue anxiety in their children, making the habit more difficult to give up.

Thumb sucking beyond age 4,

however, may be a red flag for insecurity or other psychological problems. Also, it can cause the teeth to shift or erupt incorrectly; this is often (but not always) temporary and reversible.

There is no evidence that "orthodontic pacifiers" offer protection against dental problems later in childhood. If your child is still thumb-sucking past age 4, talk to his or her doctor.

HEALTH AND DEVELOPMENT OF CHILDREN OLDER THAN AGE 2

Nutrition

When toddlers start eating solid foods as their primary source of nutrition, and no longer rely on breast milk or formula, it is time to think about nutrition.

Over the course of a day, your child should eat a diet with a balance of necessary nutrients (see Understanding the Food Pyramid, p.45). Do not be concerned if your child does not eat well at some meals, or on some days. Take a slightly longer view.

Make sure that your child gets a good variety of wholesome foods, including plenty of fruits and vegetables, over a week-long period.

FEEDING GUIDELINES FOR TODDLERS

Consider these guidelines when preparing foods for your toddler:

■ Feed toddlers meals at least three times a day; offer healthy snacks (such as cheese, vegetables, whole-grain crackers, or yogurt) in between.

■ Serve whole-grain breads instead of refined starches (such as white bread and pasta).

■ Reserve sweets for special occasions—not for regular snacks.

■ Avoid serving processed foods, which can contain high levels of salt (sodium) and hydrogenated fats.

■ Wash fruits and vegetables thoroughly to remove pesticides and bacterial contamination.

Sleep

The bedtime rituals that you established for your infant (see p.960) will help ensure sounder sleep during the years ahead— but new challenges may emerge.

2 TO 3 YEARS

The average 2- or 3-year-old sleeps between 9 and 13 hours a day. By this time, most children need only one long nap at midday, though some need no naps and others require twice-daily naps.

During this developmental period, your child is striving for independence but still has lingering fears of separation from you. This combination can create sleep difficulties for many children, and their parents. After being put to bed, your child may cry out for you or climb out of his or her bed in an effort to continue interaction with the family.

To cope with the problem, continue bedtime rituals (see p.960), but also give your child a sense of independence by offering choices in other areas, such

Nighttime Safety

■ Keep cords from window blinds out of reach (or cut the cord); a child can strangle on the loop of the cord accidentally.

■ Ensure that slats on cribs are no more than 2 3/8 inches apart.

■ Check smoke alarms each month; change batteries twice a year.

as the healthy bedtime snack, pajamas, and stories. It may be especially important at this time for your child to have a security blanket or stuffed animal.

If your son or daughter cries or gets out of bed, return him or her to bed and calmly say that it is time to sleep. Leave the room and let the child cry for several minutes. You may need to repeat this several times a night for many nights before your child learns that you will not change your mind. Being consistent is most important.

4 YEARS AND OLDER

By their fourth year, children want to be part of everything that is going on and may strongly resist going to sleep. Bedtime rit-uals, including quiet activities such as reading stories, are more important than ever.

Your child may still need a security object to get to sleep (and should not be reprimanded or teased about it). There is no evidence that these objects are harmful in any way.

It is best for your child to learn to fall asleep without you

Keeping a Balance of Nutrients

Growing children need a combination of nutrients—carbohydrates, fats, protein, vitamins, minerals. Use this list to review the major nutrients your child requires and the foods that supply them. Supplements are generally not recommended for children, unless required for specific problems as prescribed by your doctor. Vitamins, protein, fats, and minerals from foods provide the best form of nutrition.

NUTRIENT	FOOD SOURCES	
PROTEIN	■ Milk (serve whole milk until age 2)	■ Poultry
	■ Yogurt	■ Fish
	■ Cheese	■ Peanut butter or other nut butter
	■ Meat	■ Legumes (beans, peas, tofu)
	■ Eggs	
VITAMIN C	■ Fruits (citrus, strawberries, melons, kiwi)	■ Tomato
	■ Vegetables (broccoli, green leafy vegetables, red or green pepper)	■ Fortified fruit or vegetable juice
CARBO-HYDRATES	■ Wheat bread (muffin, bagel, pita)	■ Crackers
	■ Wheat pasta	■ Brown or wild rice
FIBER	■ Fruits	■ Whole grains
	■ Vegetables	■ Wheat germ
CALCIUM	■ Milk, yogurt, and other dairy products	■ Broccoli
	■ Canned salmon	■ Calcium-fortified juice
	■ Kale or other leafy greens	
FLUIDS	■ Water	■ Milk
	■ Diluted fruit or vegetable juice	

in the room (see Teaching Your Baby Sleeping Skills: Dr Ferber's Advice, p.960).

(see Teaching Your Baby Sleeping Skills: Dr Ferber's Advice, p.960)

NIGHTMARES, NIGHT TERRORS, AND SLEEP WALKING

As your child grows, sleep disturbances such as nightmares, night terrors, or sleepwalking may become more common.

A nightmare is a bad dream that awakens your child. Nightmares usually occur during rapid eye movement (REM) sleep. Your child may cry, but will be reassured by your presence after a nightmare.

If your child is not old enough to understand the difference between dreams and reality, simply reassure him or her of your protection. If your child knows the difference, remind him or her that it is just a dream and is not real; do not belittle your child for being afraid. He or she may have trouble returning to sleep out of fear and will need your comfort and consolation.

Night terrors are very different from nightmares. They occur during the first hours of deep sleep. During a night terror, your child may thrash and scream, but is unaware of your presence and is actually still asleep. When he or she does wake, there may be fear and confusion. Usually, the child will go back to sleep without a fuss because he or she has never truly awakened. The event will not be remembered the next day. You can help by letting your child experience the night terror with minimal interference, except to ensure safety.

Sleepwalking is very common, affecting about 75% of children, especially boys. It is not linked with psychological problems, although behavior during sleepwalking may seem bizarre, such as talking nonsense, urinating, or returning to the wrong bed.

It is not necessary (and may even be impossible) to wake your child. Just guide him or her safely back to bed. Sleepwalking may be tied to anxiety; examine events that occurred during the day and try to pinpoint any that seem to bring on sleepwalking.

Discipline

Discipline means teaching, not punishment. Setting limits on behavior helps prevent injury. In addition, establishing boundaries through discipline gives your child a sense of security during a time when his or her emotions may feel out of control.

It is important to guide your child toward good behavior and let him or her know what you expect. It is equally important to avoid overloading your child with limits at a time when natural curiosity is peaking. Start by childproofing your house (see Safety, p.990; Child Safety, p.88) to encourage active and safe exploration.

(see Safety, p.990; Child Safety, p.88)

Take time to show extra affection to offset necessary limitations. Defiant behavior usually begins around age 1, when children can emphatically shake their heads and verbalize "no."

Spanking and hitting are discouraged for several reasons. First, hitting teaches children that inflicting physical harm is acceptable. This is confusing to a child when you are teaching him or her not to hit others. Second, you could inadvertently cause serious harm to your child. Finally, it redirects the focus of your child's attention away from his or her behavior and onto you; your child learns to become angry with you rather than to control his or her own actions.

Repetition and calm control are the keys to effective discipline. It is impossible to expect a 2-year-old to remember previous instructions, such as not to touch the stove. Say no, explain why, and, if he or she does not respond, calmly remove your child from the situation. You will need to repeat this sequence often until your child internalizes the instruction and avoids it willingly. This may not happen until your child is 3 or 4 years old. Keep in mind that your child is not trying to defy you; he or she is usually just plain curious.

Developmentally, your toddler is primed for emotional outbursts by the second year of life. The child is simultaneously reaching out for independence and testing your limits. Your child may express this as a temper tantrum, which is a completely normal way for a child to convey frustration and confusion.

By sliding to the ground, kicking and screaming, your child is engaging in a battle to become independent. This battle is most quickly calmed if you do not engage in it.

Explain that you do not like this behavior. Call a time-out and take your child away from all activity. Or leave the child alone until he or she calms down. If the tantrum occurs in a public place, take him or her to the car or a rest room for the time-out.

Safety

Injuries are the leading cause of death among children under age 19, but statistics prove that injury prevention works. The number of children in the United States dying of unintentional injuries has dropped more than 30% since the national SAFE KIDS campaign was launched in 1987.

SAFETY CONCERN	PREVENTION
2 to 4 years	
Falls	■ Use rubber mats on play surfaces when possible. ■ Install gates and window guards. ■ Fence in outdoor play areas, balconies, and porches. ■ Cushion surfaces underneath play equipment.
Firearms	■ If you must keep a gun, keep it unloaded and locked. ■ Lock ammunition in a separate place.
Burns	■ Keep your child away from hot stoves. ■ Turn pot handles inward. ■ Test smoke alarm monthly; replace batteries twice a year. ■ Turn temperature of water heater down to 120°F.
Poisonings	■ Keep household cleansers and medicines tightly capped and in a high, locked cabinet. ■ Keep harmful products in their original containers. ■ Throw away all out-of-date prescriptions. ■ Never call medicine "candy."
Toys	■ Ensure that toys are age-appropriate and have no parts that could cause choking.
Cars	■ Use an approved child safety seat for each car ride.

SAFETY CONCERN	PREVENTION
5 years (in addition to previously listed preventions)	
Bicycles, roller blades, skateboards	■ Make sure your child always wears a helmet and elbow, wrist, and knee guards. ■ Remind him or her not to ride or skate at night. ■ Forbid your child to play in the street.
Streets	■ Have your child play in a playground or park. ■ Teach him or her the proper way to cross a street: to stop at the curb; at only the crosswalk or the corner; and to look left, then right, then left again (and to cross only with an adult). ■ Use a belt-positioning booster seat if your child is over 40 pounds.
Water	■ Encourage swimming lessons. ■ Never allow your child to swim unsupervised. ■ Avoid play around water. ■ Have your child wear a life vest. ■ Have your pool area fenced in.
6 years (in addition to previously listed preventions)	
Fire	■ Devise and practice an escape plan with your child. ■ Teach him or her to stop, drop, and roll if clothes catch fire. ■ Show your child how to crawl low under smoke.

SAFETY CONCERN	PREVENTION
8 years (in addition to previously listed preventions)	
Sports	■ Buy and make sure your child wears the protective equipment recommended by a coach.
Water	■ Make sure your child swims only when an adult is present. ■ Instruct him or her never to swim in fast-moving water.
Cars	■ Have your child buckle up with every ride.

SAFETY CONCERN	PREVENTION
Bicycles, roller blades, skateboards	■ Forbid your child to ride or skate at dusk or at night. ■ Get your child a high-impact helmet.
10 years (in addition to previously listed preventions)	
Firearms	■ Find out if friends carry guns or have them in their homes.

Toilet Training

Toilet training is a complicated skill that requires preparation and readiness on the part of the parents and the child. Until recently, most parents felt it was important to toilet train their children by age 2. Today, experts advocate a more personalized approach.

Some children are ready by 18 months, others are not ready until 3 or 4 years of age. Here are some clues that your child may be ready:

■ Expresses awareness of having defecated or urinated.

■ Understands two-step commands such as "Please go to the hall and get your shoes."

■ Imitates you in the bathroom.

■ Can remove and put on clothing.

■ Shows bladder and/or bowel control (stays dry for 2 to 3 hours).

Until you notice these signs, make your daughter or son aware of bowel and urine activity by pointing out when he or she is defecating or urinating. Also, let him or her observe a parent of the same sex in the bathroom. Avoid any negative

Toilet Training

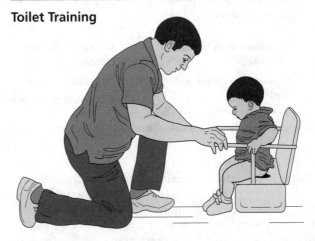

Show your child the potty chair and instruct him or her on how to use it. Your son or daughter may want to sit on it with clothes on at first.

Developmental Milestones

Your 3- to 5-year-old's mental, physical, emotional, and behavioral development will continue to accelerate at an astounding pace. There is a range for reaching each milestone, and each child is unique. Discuss any concerns about your child's development with your doctor.

	3 YEARS	4 YEARS	5 YEARS
Movement skills	■ Puts on clothing without help ■ Prepares cold cereal ■ Swings arms ■ Walks backward ■ Walks alternating arms and legs ■ Jumps with both feet ■ Walks upstairs, alternating feet, without holding onto a rail ■ Walks downstairs, alternating feet, while holding onto a rail ■ Pedals a tricycle	■ Draws person ■ Wiggles thumb ■ Walks downstairs, alternating feet, without holding onto a rail ■ Throws overhand 10 feet ■ Stands on one foot for 6 seconds	■ Jumps over 10-inch-high string ■ Bounces ball ■ Stands on one foot for 10 seconds ■ Walks heel-to-toe
Language skills	■ Uses three- to four-word sentences ■ Uses verbs, adjectives, adverbs, pronouns ■ Knows age and gender; counts to three	■ Uses four- to five-word sentences ■ Uses past tense ■ Describes recent events; sings songs; counts to four	■ Can define words ■ Uses future tense ■ Counts to 10 or above; recognizes letters of alphabet; knows telephone number
Cognitive development	■ Understands two-step commands ■ Identifies seven body parts ■ Knows first and last name	■ Understands three-step commands ■ Names two colors ■ Knows some prepositions	■ Names four colors ■ Knows opposites

responses to bowel movements and urination.

As your child shows awareness of the process, keep a potty chair in the bathroom and talk about its use in a positive, practical manner. Casually put him or her on the potty every so often, or put a favorite doll on it. Your child may want to sit on the potty fully clothed; this is fine.

When voluntarily sitting on the potty, show the child how to keep feet on the floor when moving the bowels. Gradually increase the practice sittings to once a day, eventually leading to

EMOTIONAL AND BEHAVIORAL MILESTONES

Psychologically and behaviorally, your child will also experience
great change. Some of the important steps are outlined in the chart below:

	3 YEARS	4 YEARS	5 YEARS
Social interaction	■ Plays alongside children the same age ■ Offers toys to others ■ Spends up to 20 minutes with friends ■ Shows preference for certain friends	■ Has best friend ■ Plays with others	■ Has a group of friends
Imagination	■ Pretends to feed dolls; imagines monsters	■ Knows fantasy from fact; likes elaborate games ■ May have imaginary friends	■ Dresses up and plays at make believe ■ May have imaginary friends in private
Play	■ Shares ■ Takes turns ■ Exhibits possessiveness ■ Favorite play involves stories and dressing and undressing dolls	■ Follows rules to games ■ Favorite play involves singing, dancing, and stories	■ Follows rules to games

changing his or her diaper in the area of the potty chair.

Finally, let your child play around the potty without a diaper on. When he or she starts to go, remind your child to use the potty. Give a reward if the potty is used correctly, but show no reaction if it is not.

After several successful episodes, switch from diapers to training pants during the day and at night, when your child may not have control of the bladder.

Pediatric Well-Child Visits: 3 to 10 Years

Although the frequency of well-child visits will decrease over the next few years, these visits remain an essential way to monitor your child's health and development (see Developmental Milestones, p.992). Take the opportunity during these visits to discuss any concerns regarding sleeping, eating, exercise, and learning. Your child's doctor may raise these issues as well.

It is also a time for children to begin to form a personal relationship with their doctor. This is an important step in establishing trust for discussing their own concerns and questions as their bodies continue to change.

As a parent, you can help cultivate this relationship. Encourage your child to participate in the exam by asking questions and by discussing the examination before and after it occurs. This will help your child gain a healthy sense of control over his or her health. See also Health of Adolescents, p.1021.

MEDICAL CONDITIONS

For disorders not listed here, see Medical Conditions starting on p.968.

Abdominal Pain

Abdominal pain is a symptom of many different conditions that range in severity from mild to serious. In most children, a "tummy ache" is not serious. However, if your child's stomachache is accompanied by sore throat, fever, or a change in behavior, call the doctor for advice.

In newborns up to about 12 weeks, colic (see p.971) is the most common cause of stomach pain. In children, gastroenteritis (see p.996) is a common cause. Most often, the infection is acquired by eating or drinking contaminated foods. Over age 5, emotional stress is a common cause.

Review the chart Stomachache: Possible Causes, Symptoms, and Treatment (p.996) for information about the most common causes of abdominal pain.

AIDS

Acquired immunodeficiency syndrome (AIDS) (see p.872) is an incurable disease caused by the human immunodeficiency virus (HIV). Infants most often acquire HIV when it is passed from an infected woman to her fetus in the uterus, during delivery, or during breast-feeding.

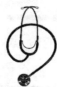

3 to 10 Years: *When You Visit Your Child's Doctor*

This chart shows some of the exams your doctor might perform or topics he or she might discuss when your child sees the doctor for well-child visits. These basic checkups are for all children. Additional visits may be needed if your child has a chronic disease or special needs (see Children With Special Health Care Needs: Dr Palfrey's Advice, p.1014).

3 YEARS

- Medical history
- Measurement of height and weight
- Blood pressure test
- Vision test
- Hearing test
- Developmental assessment
- Physical examination
- Discussion about injury prevention

4 YEARS

Same as above plus:

- Diphtheria/pertussis/tetanus vaccine
- Polio vaccine
- Mumps/measles/rubella vaccine

5 YEARS

Same as for age 3 plus:

- Discussion about school readiness

6 YEARS

Same as for age 3 plus:

- Hearing and vision tests (optional if your child's sight and hearing are fine)
- Discussions about school performance and peers

8 YEARS

Same as for age 6

10 YEARS

Same as for age 8 plus:

- Hearing and vision tests
- Discussions about puberty, sex, and other adolescent issues

It is estimated that HIV develops in approximately 25% of babies born to infected women, although the likelihood of transmitting the virus is lower if the mother is taking medicines to fight HIV. The virus cannot be acquired by hugging, touching, or sharing utensils.

HIV weakens the immune system's disease-fighting ability, causing vulnerability to a wide range of infections. Most infants who acquire HIV at birth get AIDS within 2 years. At first, babies appear to be well, but height and weight soon fall below average. They may also have skin infections, diarrhea, and swollen lymph glands. Common childhood infections can be more severe in HIV-positive children. Otherwise, the course of the disease is similar to that of adults (see p.872). The viral infection progresses and the immune system continues to break down, leading to AIDS.

Though HIV and AIDS cannot be cured, the symptoms can be treated. More important, HIV-infected children need the same level of affection and attention as other children. Playmates, classmates, and caregivers may need to be reminded that HIV and AIDS cannot be acquired through casual contact. Every effort should be made to treat affected children like others and to instill a positive attitude.

If your child is infected with HIV, talk with your physician about helping your child avoid exposure to contagious viruses, bacteria, and fungi. Infections that would cause mild illness in a healthy child can have devastating consequences in an HIV-positive child. Call the doctor if you know your child has been exposed to an infectious disease, such as chickenpox or measles, or if your child has any breathing, swallowing, or skin problems or has a fever or diarrhea.

Some physicians recommend monthly intravenous injections of gamma globulin, a drug used preventively to boost immune defenses and, after exposure to certain infections, to limit their severity. In addition, your child's vaccination schedule may vary depending on the stage of his or her illness.

Allergies

An allergy is a group of symptoms caused by exposure to substances that are usually harmless, but that are perceived by the immune system as being harmful to the body. The immune system overreacts to these substances (called aller-

gens), and mounts an inappropriate defense that involves the release of histamines and other substances that cause symptoms such as runny nose or itchy eyes.

Allergies tend to affect one or more body systems. The most common include the respiratory system (nose, throat, lungs), gastrointestinal system (intestines, stomach), eyes, and skin.

Allergies run in families, but may be expressed differently in family members. If you have respiratory allergies, for example, your child may exhibit skin allergy. Children are vulnerable to the same allergies as adults, though some children outgrow them by adulthood.

Symptoms vary depending on the type of allergy, but can include itchy eyes and a stuffy and runny nose with a clear discharge as in allergic rhinitis (hay fever) (see p.462), asthma (see p.998), and postnasal drip (see p.464). All these symptoms are often mistaken for a cold.

In a food allergy (see p.799), digestive symptoms may include gas, diarrhea, or vomiting. Children with skin allergies may have eczema (see p.1006) or hives (see p.536; Color Guide to Visual Diagnosis, p.562).

Your child's doctor will make a diagnosis based on your reports and, sometimes, blood tests and skin tests (see p.162). Once the cause is known, allergies can best be treated by avoiding the offending substance.

If this is not possible (as in hay fever, for example), your doctor may recommend antihistamines and/or corticosteroid drugs (see p.895) to reduce allergic reactions. Allergy shots may be of help for treating aller-

gic rhinitis or for allergies to insect stings.

Anemia

In anemia (see p.713), the blood does not contain enough red blood cells. The result is low levels of hemoglobin, which is the protein inside red blood cells that delivers oxygen from the lungs to all tissues of the body.

Children most often become anemic because they do not get enough iron (which is essential for making hemoglobin) from their diet. Infants can become anemic if they drink cow's milk (which is very low in iron) before 12 months of age, especially if the infant is not receiving an iron supplement. Infants who drink cow's milk also can have bowel irritation that results in a minute, but significant, loss of blood through the gastrointestinal tract. This can also cause anemia.

The symptoms depend on the cause but, generally, anemic children are pale, easily fatigued, and fussy. They may complain of shortness of breath, and have swollen hands and feet. Developmental delays may also occur. School performance may suffer due to an inability to focus attention.

An uncommon symptom of iron deficiency is pica (the urge to eat dirt, flakes of paint, or other unusual substances), which can result in increased levels of lead in the blood.

Anemia is diagnosed by a blood test. Iron deficiency is treated by supplemental iron in liquid or tablet form. Iron supplements normally can cause the teeth to turn gray, which is reversible. It can also turn the

Stomachache: Possible Causes, Symptoms, and Treatment

It is not always easy to know whether your child's stomach pain requires immediate care. This chart outlines the most common conditions that cause abdominal pain (see p.994), their symptoms, what you should do, and what your child's doctor may do.

CONDITION	SYMPTOMS	WHAT YOU SHOULD DO	WHAT THE DOCTOR MAY DO
Appendicitis (see p.782)	■ Constant abdominal pain that starts around the navel and moves to the lower right side of the abdomen after a few hours ■ Nausea ■ Vomiting ■ Loss of appetite ■ Low-grade fever (100°F to 101°F)	Call doctor immediately.	The doctor may admit your child to the hospital for observation, take x-rays, and consult with a surgeon. Treatment is surgical removal of the appendix (see p.783).
Gastroenteritis (see p.976)	■ Abdominal pain that lasts 2 to 3 days or longer; if caused by food poisoning (see p.881), pain comes and goes and changes location ■ Weight loss ■ Dehydration ■ Loss of appetite ■ Stomach cramps ■ Vomiting ■ Diarrhea (see p.320)	Give your child plenty of liquids. Wash hands frequently and thoroughly to prevent spread to others. Call doctor if symptoms last longer than 5 to 7 days or if condition worsens.	The doctor may give intravenous fluids for dehydration and prescribe antibiotics for some kinds of food poisoning.
Lead poisoning (see p.967)	■ Abdominal pain ■ Sleepiness ■ Poor appetite ■ Crankiness ■ Constipation ■ Learning disabilities at school age ■ Seizures in severe cases	Call doctor for evaluation.	The doctor will perform a blood test to detect poisoning. He or she may prescribe a drug that binds to lead in the body and helps the body eliminate it.

CONDITION	SYMPTOMS	WHAT YOU SHOULD DO	WHAT THE DOCTOR MAY DO
Migraine (see p.355)	■ Severe, regular abdominal pain ■ Headache (main symptom) ■ Vomiting	Call doctor for evaluation.	There is no diagnostic test for migraine. The doctor will rule out other potential causes of abdominal pain and, if migraine is suspected, will treat it using one of the treatments described on p.356.
Milk allergy or intolerance (see p.1011)	■ Abdominal pain ■ Vomiting ■ Diarrhea ■ Blood in bowel movements	Discontinue dairy products. Call doctor for evaluation.	The doctor may perform an examination or wait to see if the abdominal pain improves after dairy products have been discontinued.
Strep throat (see p.1018)	■ Very sore throat (main symptom) ■ Abdominal pain ■ Fever ■ Headache ■ Rash (occasionally) ■ Vomiting (occasionally)	Call doctor for evaluation.	The doctor will order a strep throat test and may prescribe antibiotic treatment.
Stress	■ Intermittent abdominal pain (suspect emotional stress if there are no other symptoms)	Call doctor for evaluation. Consider whether anxiety-provoking events are present.	The doctor will observe the pattern of pain over time and, in some cases, may refer you to a specialist if compassion, reassurance, and talking to your child do not help.
Urinary tract infection	■ Pain in the lower, central part of the abdomen near the bladder ■ Burning pain during urination ■ Need to urinate more often ■ Bed-wetting (when previously dry)	Call doctor for evaluation	The doctor will order a urine test and may prescribe antibiotics.

bowel movements black, which is normal. Treatment for other forms of anemia is described starting on p.713.

Asthma

Asthma is a persistent inflammatory disorder of the airways of the lungs. It causes seasonal or periodic episodes of wheezing and coughing that may lead to sudden and/or severe difficulty breathing. Some asthma attacks can be life-threatening.

Asthma affects millions of children in the United States and is becoming more common. It causes more hospitalizations than any other chronic childhood disease. While it tends to improve in children as they grow and may disappear by adulthood, severe asthma can cause weakened lung function later in life.

Often, the cause of the inflammation in the lungs is an allergy to some inhaled substance in the home. Common allergens (substances that cause inflammation in the airway and trigger an allergic reaction) include dust mites, mold, animal dander, and cockroaches.

Secondhand smoke from a cigarette can irritate the lungs of children with asthma. Exercise and cold air, and especially exercising in cold air, can trigger an attack of asthma.

Respiratory infections, particularly in infants and preschoolers, can bring on an asthma attack. Certain foods (including eggs, shellfish, and nuts) and medicines (particularly aspirin and ibuprofen) can produce the same effects. In about 10% of children, the cause of asthma attacks cannot be traced to any substance or event.

Your child's doctor will recommend a treatment plan that involves avoiding allergens and other triggers, taking medicine to minimize swelling of the bronchial passages, and monitoring lung function using a peak flow meter (see p.510).

It is critical that your child, family members, and doctor work together in the treatment and monitoring of your child's asthma. Most children are able to lead normal lives, participate in activities, and not feel different. See p.505 for a complete discussion of treatment.

Bed-Wetting

Bed-wetting, also called enuresis, is a common and normal occurrence among young children who have just been toilet trained. It may continue to occur a few times a week, gradually declining in frequency, until about age 5.

Many children's bladders are not capable of holding urine for a full night's sleep; in others, the nervous system is not fully developed enough to awaken them from sleep when they have a full bladder.

Less commonly, emotional stress and physical disorders contribute to bed-wetting after age 5. Girls generally achieve control earlier than boys. One of 10 children, mostly boys, continues to wet the bed after age 5, and many have a family history of bed-wetting.

When a child cannot control urinary function during both day and night, there may be a kidney, bladder, or psychological problem.

SYMPTOMS

Bed-wetting is characterized by lack of urinary control during sleep, resulting in a wet bed that often awakens the child.

TREATMENT OPTIONS

If bed-wetting is a problem, consult the doctor, who will examine your child to rule out physical causes that require treatment. This may involve testing urine for infection. If there is no discernible cause, your physician may recommend that your child reduce intake of fluids before bedtime and urinate before going to bed. Some children benefit by being awakened every few hours during the night to urinate.

Bed-wetting can cause considerable shame and fear of punishment. It is essential that you not blame or embarrass your child.

Your doctor may also suggest various behavior modification methods, such as following a urination schedule during the day. This increases your child's awareness of how it feels physically to need to urinate, so that he or she becomes more sensitive to the sensations during sleep.

A more elaborate modification method entails laying a liquid-sensitive pad between the mattress and sheet or attached to the child's underwear. The pad sounds an alarm when wet. This effective method teaches children to awaken as urine is passed.

Medicines such as imipramine and desmopressin may also be used in certain circumstances. Many children simply outgrow bed-wetting.

Cancer

There are many types of cancer (see p.738), but only a few affect children. Children with cancer can be treated, and most survive.

Leukemia is a cancer of the infection-fighting white blood cells produced in the lymph glands; it accounts for half of all childhood cancers. Acute lymphocytic leukemia (see p.724) is the type that most often affects children, primarily those under age 10. The prognosis today is much improved from 20 or 30 years ago. Symptoms, diagnosis, and treatment are discussed starting on p.724.

Brain tumors are the next most common type of cancer in children, most often affecting children 5 to 10 years old. Symptoms, diagnosis, and treatment are discussed on p.357.

Lymphomas are cancers of the lymphatic tissue, the tissue that makes up the lymph glands. A form called non-Hodgkin lymphoma is most common in children. Symptoms, diagnosis, and treatment are discussed starting on p.727.

Neuroblastomas are tumors that occur in the adrenal glands or in the nerves near the spine. These nerves are part of the sympathetic nervous system, which automatically controls some body functions. Neuroblastomas are one of the few cancers that occur only in children, mostly those younger than 4.

The symptoms, which vary by location of the tumor and its spread, include weight loss, an achy feeling, and fussiness. You may feel a lump in your child's abdomen. If the tumor is secreting hormones, your child may have diarrhea, a flushed face, and higher-than-normal blood pressure.

Treatment includes surgery to remove the tumor, followed by radiation and, sometimes, chemotherapy to prevent its spread. Chances for recovery are difficult to project; some tumors are nonthreatening, while others spread quickly.

Wilms tumor is the most common kidney tumor in childhood. More than 75% of cases occur in children under 5 years of age. Most often, the tumor is discovered when a family member or doctor notices a large firm lump in the abdomen. Sometimes the tumor is discovered after a child is examined because of another condition caused by the tumor, such as high blood pressure, blood in the urine, stomachache, fever, or vomiting.

Treatment includes surgery to remove the tumor and to see how far it has spread. Radiation therapy (see p.741) and chemotherapy (see p.741) also are often used. Great strides in treatment have been made in recent years.

COPING WITH CANCER

A diagnosis of cancer in a child raises many difficult feelings for children, parents, siblings, and other loved ones. Guilt, fear, anger, denial, and confusion are common and natural emotions. While it is important to express these feelings, it is equally important to consider their effects on your child.

Children usually can sense that something serious has happened, and tend to fear the unknown more than reality. For this reason, it is best to gently but honestly tell your child as much as he or she can understand about the condition.

For help in coping with the many complex issues concerning cancer in children, ask your physician to suggest a support group that helps families cope with serious illness in children. Most centers that provide treatment of childhood cancer have a multidisciplinary team, including social workers and psychologists that provides support to families. See also The Dying Child, p.1147.

Celiac Disease

Celiac disease is sensitivity of the small intestine to gluten, a protein found in wheat, rye, barley, and possibly oats. It causes an inability to absorb nutrients, due to inflammation and damage to the intestinal lining.

Symptoms include persistent diarrhea, partially digested food in the bowel movements, unexplained weight loss, and irritability. These symptoms often appear soon after introducing cereal. In older children, short stature may be the only sign of celiac disease. See p.774 for a full discussion of celiac disease.

Cellulitis

(See also Color Guide to Visual Diagnosis, p.562)
Cellulitis (see p.532) is a skin infection caused by bacteria. It is often acquired through small scrapes or wounds. The skin is red, warm, swollen, and painful when touched. When it occurs around the eye, which is more common in children than in adults, it can lead to a serious form called orbital cellulitis.

Orbital cellulitis can cause the eyeball to stick out, be painful, and not move well. Vision is impaired.

Cellulitis is a potentially dangerous infection because it can spread to the blood and affect other organs. In infants, whose immune systems are not yet mature, the infection can be particularly dangerous.

Report any symptoms to your child's doctor immediately. Since symptoms of orbital cellulitis resemble conjunctivitis (see p.427; Color Guide to Visual Diagnosis, p.567), your doctor may need to take a sample of the pus or tears for laboratory analysis.

Orbital cellulitis is treated with intravenous antibiotics, and by draining the sources of underlying infection (often the sinuses). Cellulitis of the skin is treated with antibiotics given by mouth, or by intravenous infusion if the cellulitis is more extensive.

Cerebral Palsy

Cerebral palsy (CP) is damage to the parts of the brain that control the muscles; it causes various degrees of lifelong disability. An estimated 6 of 1,000 children in the United States have CP. About 90% are born with it.

CP can be caused by many factors before birth, including lack of oxygen in the uterus, infection that spreads from the woman to her developing fetus, or genetic disorders. In most cases, the cause is unknown.

Infants who are extremely jaundiced (see p.982) may also develop CP. Later in life, children are susceptible to CP due to brain infection (see Meningitis, p.1013), seizures, or head injury.

Although the injury to the nervous system that results in CP does not worsen with age, the muscles may become increasingly tight and not stretch as well unless there is continuing treatment.

SYMPTOMS

At 2 to 3 months of age, you may notice that your baby's limbs are limp or very stiff. When you pick up your child, his or her legs may make a "scissors" motion or the child may arch the neck, pushing away from you. When your baby starts to crawl, he or she does so in an uneven way, or hops on his or her buttocks or knees.

CP falls into one of three categories: spastic (stiff, contracted muscles); dyskinetic or athetoid (uncontrolled thrashing movements); and ataxic (poor gait and coordination). Sometimes, children have a mixture of these different types.

CP can be mild or severe, can affect limbs on one side of the body (hemiplegia), all four limbs equally (quadriplegia), or all four limbs but the legs most severely (diplegia).

Many children with CP have an IQ below normal, but about 25% have normal or above-average intelligence. Feeding, hearing, and/or vision may also be impaired or delayed.

TREATMENT OPTIONS

Symptoms of CP in early infancy may cause developmental delays; report any concerns about your child's development to the doctor. As your child grows, your doctor will watch closely for typical signs. If CP is diagnosed, the physician will recommend a program to help your child make the most of his or her mental and physical potential.

Programs include physical and occupational therapy to train your child to coordinate movements, minimize difficulty with posture, and loosen tight tendons that can lead to shrinking scar tissue. The programs also offer parents access to family counseling so that you can share information with parents who have similar concerns.

Occasionally, medicines can reduce the amount of spasticity. Neurosurgery can also sometimes be helpful in reducing spasticity.

Your involvement at home and at school is essential to help ensure your child's success. Like all children, those with CP thrive with educational opportunity, confidence-building encouragement, and loving support. Some children with mild symptoms recover from CP or grow out of it. See p.1231 for the phone number of the United Cerebral Palsy Association.

Colds

A cold (see Common Cold, p.460) is an infection of the upper respiratory tract—the nose, throat, and upper airways. Colds are usually caused by viruses.

Because children under age 2 are still developing immunity and because there are many different types of viruses, they commonly have as many as eight upper respiratory infections a year. Older children tend to have fewer colds.

SYMPTOMS

Children between 3 months and 3 years of age show symptoms of fever, restlessness, irritability, and sneezing. Within a few hours, the nose starts running, which may interfere with nursing and lead to breathing problems. The ears may also become congested, and some children vomit and have diarrhea.

In older children, nasal dryness and irritation are typically the first symptoms, followed soon by sneezing, muscle aches, and a thin discharge of mucus from the nose. The discharge gets thicker over the next several days and may block the nose, causing mouth breathing; a dry, sore throat; and coughing.

The nasal discharge is initially clear for a couple of days, changes to green or white for 3 to 4 days, and then changes back to clear as the cold resolves (usually by 7 to 10 days). Complications can include ear infection (see p.1005) and, in older children, sinus infection (see Sinusitis, p.464).

TREATMENT OPTIONS

Contact your child's doctor immediately if your child has a high temperature, difficulty breathing, stiff neck, severe headache or cough, persistent earache, or looks ill. Also call the doctor if your child has less severe symptoms but does not show signs of getting better after 3 to 5 days.

There is no cure, but cold symptoms can be eased by having the child drink plenty of fluids and rest. Antibiotics do not work against the viruses that cause colds. The few antiviral medicines that are available either do not kill the viruses that cause colds or are not necessary because the immune system kills them well enough.

Acetaminophen or ibuprofen can help ease symptoms. Do not give your child aspirin because of the possibility of Reye syndrome (see p.1017).

The doctor may recommend nose drops to open up congested nasal passages for children who are having trouble breathing or eating. Never give your child any over-the-counter medicine intended for adults.

There is no need to force children to eat, but they should drink often to replace lost fluids. See p.461 for further recommendations for treatment.

Constipation

Constipation is the infrequent and sometimes painful passing of hard bowel movements. If your child has fewer than one bowel movement every 3 to 4 days and has hard bowel movements, he or she may be constipated. However, patterns of defecation vary in children, just as they do in adults. Sometimes it can be difficult to tell whether your child is truly constipated. See p.971 for a discussion of constipation in infants.

Common causes of constipation include stress, not eating enough fiber (see p.38), or inadequate intake of fluids. Children should drink four to six glasses of liquids a day—more in hot weather.

Constipation is especially common among children between ages 2 and 5, when toilet training and developmental changes are occurring. Fear of using toilets away from home may also lead to constipation.

It is not uncommon for children to withhold bowel move-

ments. Not responding to the urge to defecate can create a chain of events. When a child withholds bowel movements, they remain in the large intestine, where they become more dry, firm, and difficult to pass. If a child withholds one bowel movement, it can make the next one painful. This may encourage further withholding to avoid pain.

If the pattern continues, the bowel movements may eventually stretch the rectum, which can mask the urge to defecate. Sometimes, liquid bowel movements leak out around the hard bowel movements in the rectum.

Your doctor may suggest giving a rectal suppository or stool softener, such as mineral oil, to ease passage of bowel movements and resolve any fear your child has about painful defecation. Never give your child either of these remedies without the doctor's advice.

For milder constipation, adding liquids and more fiber to your child's diet usually resolves the condition.

Encopresis (loss of control of bowel movements) in recently toilet-trained children is not uncommon; it can occur in otherwise healthy youngsters. Instead of using the toilet, they defecate in their clothes or in hidden places. This problem may result from underlying constipation. Ask your physician for advice.

Coughing

A cough is a reflex to remove mucus and other irritants from the air passages such as the throat, nose, windpipe, larynx (voice box), and lungs.

The most common causes of a

Treating Coughs at Home

Some steps you can take at home, regardless of the cause of the cough, include:

- Elevate the head of the bed or crib at night.

- Offer extra fluids.

- Use a humidifier or a cool-mist vaporizer (cool-mist vaporizers are safest, but need to be cleaned daily to prevent colonization by bacteria or fungi).

- For coughing spells in the middle of the night caused by croup (see below right), have your child sit in a steamy bathroom for a few minutes or, if the weather is not too cold, walk outside in the moist, cool air.

---

cough include colds and other upper respiratory illnesses, bronchiolitis (see p.969), pneumonia (see p.1017), and croup (see below).

Allergies (see p.995), teething (see p.964), fumes, smoke, dust, and inhaling objects can also produce a cough. Sinusitis and asthma are the most common causes of a chronic (ongoing) cough.

SYMPTOMS

The sound and duration of a cough vary depending on the cause. A cough that is worse in the early morning may indicate an upper airway infection. Infections of the larynx produce an abrupt, barking cough (see Croup, below right) that worsens at night and causes a hoarse voice. These coughs can linger for days or weeks after the underlying infection goes away.

If there is no fever and the cough is persistent, suspect allergies, asthma, sinusitis, or inhalation of an object.

TREATMENT OPTIONS

Always contact your doctor about a bad cough in a child younger than 2 months. Also call the physician if your older child is having difficulty breathing, breathes rapidly, or turns blue, or if you suspect the child may have inhaled some small object into the breathing tubes. When a cough lasts longer than a week or is accompanied by a fever, call the doctor.

Most coughs are caused by an illness such as a cold or the flu, and will resolve on their own with plenty of fluids and rest.

Tests and x-rays may be performed to rule out pneumonia, tuberculosis (see p.1019), or an inhaled object. Your doctor may recommend specific cough medicines or, if the cause is a bacterial infection, prescribe antibiotics.

Coxsackievirus and Echovirus Infections

Coxsackievirus and echovirus are common viruses that affect children most often in the fall and summer. They spread from mouth to mouth, or from feces to hand

to mouth. All coxsackievirus and echovirus infections take between 3 and 7 days after infection for symptoms to appear.

The viruses can cause rash with fever, hand-foot-and-mouth disease, herpangina, meningitis (see p.1013), and myocarditis (see Cardiomyopathy, p.682).

Your child may have a fever, sore throat (which may cause difficulty nursing or swallowing), blisters in the mouth, rash, vomiting, or diarrhea.

With hand-foot-and-mouth disease, the blisters are few and may be found on the palms, fingers, and soles, and sometimes also on the buttocks, limbs, and face.

In herpangina, painful, gray-white mouth blisters are found in the back of the mouth; they become ulcerated with surrounding redness. Other symptoms of herpangina include vomiting, diarrhea, fatigue, and sore throat.

Older children may complain of headache and muscle pain, as well as nausea and vomiting.

Call the doctor to report the symptoms; a diagnosis can often be made by looking at the sores. There is no specific treatment. The rashes disappear within several days on their own.

Your child should rest and drink plenty of liquids. If necessary, give the child a fever-reducing medicine recommended by your doctor, such as acetaminophen or ibuprofen (not aspirin). For more severe infections of the brain or heart, special treatments are needed.

Croup

Croup is inflammation and subsequent narrowing of the larger airways that produces a sharp, barking cough and may cause difficulty breathing. It is caused by viruses that infect the larynx (voice box), trachea (windpipe), and bronchi (airways).

Croup usually affects children between 3 months and 3 years of age, and boys are more often affected than girls. The virus is acquired by person-to-person contact and most often occurs in the fall. Some children get croup often, a condition called spasmodic croup.

Allergy may play a role in causing repeated episodes of croup; having recurring croup as a child may be related to having asthma later in life.

SYMPTOMS

Cold symptoms usually precede croup. The cough is deep and is often described as sounding like a seal's bark. Laryngitis—loss of the voice, or a raspy, hoarse voice—may also develop. Breathing becomes harsh and noisy, a condition called stridor.

Characteristically, these symptoms wane and peak in intensity from hour to hour. They may almost disappear in the morning, only to worsen as the day progresses, being typically worse at night or following naps. Croup may last 3 to 5 days, but the cough and other breathing problems often persist.

Breathing may become fast and labored, especially at night. Your child's chest and abdominal muscles may move forcefully to help breathing and the skin may take on a bluish tinge because of lack of oxygen. These are signs of respiratory distress; take your child to the emergency department immediately.

TREATMENT OPTIONS

If you suspect your child has croup, keep him or her calm; this can ease breathing. Report croup to your child's doctor, who may want to see the child to rule out serious conditions such as epiglottitis (see p.467).

If breathing is severely impaired (which is rare), your doctor may recommend hospitalization so that your child can be given oxygen and medicines.

Home treatment includes having your child drink plenty of fluids and taking a fever-reducing medicine such as acetaminophen or ibuprofen (not aspirin). Cool-mist vaporizers may help soothe the airway, and some children feel better when taken out into the cool night air.

Corticosteroid drugs (see p.895) may be prescribed to prevent worsening of the symptoms. Hospitalized children may require medicines, such as corticosteroids or epinephrine to open the airways.

Cystic Fibrosis

Cystic fibrosis (CF) is a progressive and often fatal inherited disease in which glands produce abnormally thickened mucus in several different organs, including the pancreas and the bronchi (air passages of the lungs). The liver, intestines, and reproductive organs may also be affected.

The mucus is excessively thick and sticky, clogging the lungs and leading to serious infections, or inhibiting the digestive system from absorbing nutrients.

One of 1,600 white children is born with CF; the incidence in black children is 1 of 17,000 births.

The disease is caused by a defective gene inherited by the child from both parents. Prenatal screening can determine if a fetus is affected. In the United States, 10 to 12 million people are carriers of this genetic defect.

The average life span of a person with CF is 31 years, although mildly affected individuals may live much longer.

SYMPTOMS

The symptoms usually appear within the first year, but may be delayed until adolescence. Early signs of CF may include salty-tasting skin (due to high levels of sodium in the sweat), bulky and foul-smelling bowel movements (due to a deficiency in pancreatic enzymes), and recurring cough or a cough with a thick, difficult-to-cough out mucus.

The cough can lead to bronchitis, pneumonia, and other lung infections. Children with CF usually do not grow and do not gain weight at the normal rate.

TREATMENT OPTIONS

Talk with your child's doctor if you suspect CF. In addition to an examination, he or she will perform a sweat test to measure the amount of sodium in the sweat. Newborns require a blood test to diagnose CF. Other diagnostic measures include x-rays, phlegm (sputum) cultures, and lung function tests (see p.494).

Treatment for CF depends upon the severity and location of the disease. Postural drainage, which involves drumming on the back and chest to loosen mucus from the lungs while the child is in various positions, is often helpful. Lung infections are treated with mucus-thinning drugs; antibiotics are given intravenously, orally, or by inhalation.

Children with digestive problems need to take supplemental digestive enzymes. The excessive salt loss must be replaced. Other treatments are being tested, including gene therapy (see p.133).

It is important to give your child guidance, love, and discipline. You can find support from other families who are coping with the disease by contacting the Cystic Fibrosis Foundation (see p.1232).

Diabetes Mellitus

Diabetes mellitus (see p.832) is a disease that causes an accumulation of glucose (sugar) in the blood and can result in damage to many organs of the body—including the blood vessels, eyes, and kidneys—over several years.

In children, type 1 diabetes is the most common type. In type 1 diabetes, there is a deficiency of insulin, a hormone produced by the pancreas to help the body process glucose (sugar) and other nutrients.

Type 1 diabetes rarely occurs in infants younger than 6 months and most often affects children older than 4 years. Researchers believe that it is the result of two or more related factors, including heredity, an impaired immune system, viral infection, and/or early exposure to cow's milk (breast-fed infants may have a lower risk).

In type 2 diabetes, the body's cells lose their ability to respond to insulin (the cells develop "insulin resistance"). Although type 2 diabetes primarily affects adults (and used to be called

"adult-onset diabetes"), type 2 diabetes is becoming more common in children. While the exact cause is not known, it appears that being overweight and inactive greatly increases the chances of children (and adults) developing type 2 diabetes.

The symptoms of diabetes in children include failure to gain weight and grow, excessive urination, bed-wetting, excessive thirst, fatigue, large appetite, and weight loss. These symptoms may be accompanied by pus-producing skin infections, vomiting, and dehydration.

If you suspect your child has diabetes, take him or her to the physician immediately. The doctor will test a sample of blood and urine to measure the glucose levels. Insulin injections are given once the diagnosis is confirmed.

Treatment is directed at maintaining normal glucose levels, and avoiding fluctuations, to prevent long-term problems. This means vigilant monitoring of blood sugar levels (see p.840).

You and your child will learn how to inject insulin and on what schedule to give the injections. Children as young as 7 can learn to inject themselves. Because this is a treatment your child will require for a lifetime, it is important that you administer the shots calmly and be patient in helping him or her learn how to do it alone.

Eating a proper diet is extremely important in managing your child's diabetes. He or she should eat regular meals interspersed with nutritious snacks (such as yogurt or cheese or peanut butter with bread or crackers) to maintain an appropriate level of sugar in the blood. Candy should be

avoided, though sugarless candy is acceptable. Regular exercise is also essential.

Children who have diabetes can participate in all childhood activities, though coaches and teachers should be informed of the condition so they can provide support and monitor your child's health.

Many families also find it helpful to be involved in a diabetes support group (see p.1232).

Down Syndrome

Down syndrome is a congenital (at birth) disorder caused by an extra chromosome in body cells. It causes varying degrees of mental handicap and physical abnormalities. Down syndrome affects 1 of 800 infants.

Because the likelihood of having a child with this syndrome increases with maternal age, researchers believe that the defect is in the egg, rather than the father's sperm. Amniocentesis (see p.917) or chorionic villus sampling (see p.918) can detect Down syndrome in a fetus.

SYMPTOMS

Characteristic physical features include a small head, short stature, small facial features, a large and protruding tongue, and a head flattened in the back. Hands are often short and wide. Mental disability varies considerably from mild disability to severe retardation.

Emotionally, children with Down syndrome are often open-spirited and affectionate. Other congenital defects often occur, including heart defects, intestinal narrowing, and hearing defects.

TREATMENT OPTIONS

Down syndrome is usually diagnosed at birth by the child's physical features. It is confirmed by a blood test (chromosome analysis). Your doctor will recommend a supportive program for you and your child to learn how to maximize your baby's abilities.

Children with Down syndrome can make the most of their abilities, and many learn to read and live independently with ongoing education and close support. Many families benefit from involvement in a support group (see p.1234).

Ear Infection

Ear infections (see also p.457) are one of the most common medical problems of children. They occur much more frequently in children than in adults. Children get so many more respiratory infections than adults because the very close contact children have with each other makes it easy to spread infections and because, in the growing child, the tube that connects the ears to the back of the nose and throat (the eustachian tube) is more easily blocked.

The symptoms in older children are similar to those in adults. Ear pain and fever are common. Sometimes there is diminished hearing in, or liquid drainage from, the affected ear. In young children, irritability, fussiness, lethargy, or feeding poorly may be the only symptoms. In newborns, even fever may be absent.

Occasionally, the infection involves the nerve that leads to the face, causing one side of the face to droop and making it impossible to fully close the eye.

Are Antibiotics Always Necessary?
Dr Bernstein's Advice

Antibiotics are one of the greatest advances in medicine of this past century. However, if doctors and patients do not use them correctly, more harm than good may result.

Studies show that many antibiotics are prescribed unnecessarily, often for viral illnesses like colds. Other studies show that some people don't take the full course of antibiotics that have been prescribed when antibiotics are necessary, or that they take antibiotics from a bottle in the medicine cabinet for a few days without consulting their doctor.

All of these practices are causing the bacteria in our environment to be increasingly resistant to antibiotics. This means an antibiotic may not work well when truly needed to treat a specific infection.

Educating parents and doctors alike should help to reduce overuse. Both need to understand the role of antibiotics in the treatment of infectious diseases. Good judgment and doctor-patient communication are critical in choosing when and how to use an antibiotic.

When your doctor says that an antibiotic is not necessary, understand that this often is the case, and that unnecessary use of antibiotics could, down the road, cause problems for your family and for society.

HENRY H. BERNSTEIN, DO
CHILDREN'S HOSPITAL
HARVARD MEDICAL SCHOOL

Middle-of-the-Night Care for Ear Pain

It is midnight—a time when earaches seem to happen most often—and your child is howling with pain. Here are some ways to ease the pain until you can get help from your doctor:

■ Give your child the recommended dose of acetaminophen or ibuprofen (not aspirin).

■ Keep your child upright to help drain the eustachian tubes.

■ Apply warm compresses to the affected ear.

■ Offer soothing warm liquids to drink; swallowing will help open the eustachian tubes.

■ Have children older than 5 years chew gum.

■ Have your child suck on an orange.

■ Make a game of yawning.

Rarely, the infection can spread into the bone near the ear, causing osteomyelitis (see p.595), into the tissues of the neck, causing an abscess (see p.877), or into the brain and the lining of the brain, causing meningitis (see p.1013).

Antibiotics are used to treat many ear infections, particularly in children below the age of 2, and probably prevent some of the more serious complications.

Occasionally, in severe infections, the doctor must make a hole in the eardrum to drain the infected fluid from the middle ear. It is important to monitor your child's hearing closely, as ear infections may make it harder for the child to hear, which can interfere with language development.

Eczema and Contact Dermatitis

(See also Color Guide to Visual Diagnosis, p.566)

Two conditions most commonly affect your child's delicate skin— eczema and contact dermatitis.

Eczema (see p.550), also called atopic dermatitis, is a term for skin reactions that cause a rash or inflammation.

In eczema, which can occur in children as young as 2 months old, symptoms include itching, redness, and tiny bumps on the forehead, cheeks, or scalp that sometimes spread to the arms or chest. The sores may ooze.

In older children, the rash consists of scaly, raised, round patches on the face, chest, crook of the elbow, backs of the ankles and wrists, and behind the knees.

The skin may thicken in the affected area. Eczema is sometimes caused by allergy (see p.995); many children who get it

have allergies in the family or have allergies themselves.

Contact dermatitis occurs when an irritating substance— and there are many—comes into contact with the child's skin. The rash does not itch as much as eczema, but nonetheless causes itchy skin and blisters. In contact dermatitis, the location of the affected areas is a clue to the irritant. Poison ivy and poison oak are well-known causes. Lesser-known irritants include laundry detergents and some additives to toothpaste, which can cause a rash around the mouth, as can the child's own saliva.

Acidic beverages, some medicines (including neomycin ointment), rough clothing, and bubble bath ingredients have also been implicated. The best treatment is to avoid any substance that you think may have caused contact dermatitis in the past.

Your child's doctor will diagnose the skin condition and may recommend that you regularly moisturize your child's skin and avoid using harsh detergents. Be sure your child does not take hot baths, which can further dry the skin.

There is no cure for eczema, but the doctor can prescribe an ointment containing a mild corticosteroid drug (see p.895) to reduce the inflammation and thus calm your child's urge to scratch. Antihistamine drugs may also be prescribed to further control itching.

Enlarged Tonsils and Adenoids

Tonsils and adenoids are immune system glands that often become inflamed and infected in young

children. Tonsils are visible on either side of the back of the throat. Adenoids lie between the throat and the back of the nose.

When the tonsils or the adenoids enlarge, your child may experience breathing or swallowing problems, and hearing loss if the adenoids swell.

In both conditions, the swelling usually goes away on its own, often with the resolution of related infections, and requires no treatment. In some children, the glands are swollen without any accompanying infection.

SYMPTOMS

You can see enlarged tonsils by looking in your child's throat. The voice may also seem muffled and he or she may complain of pain while swallowing. Fever, headache, and swollen glands below the jaw may also occur. An abscess (see p.877) sometimes forms in and around the tonsils.

Symptoms of enlarged adenoids include stuffy nose and, in some children, noisy breathing through the mouth, snoring, and altered breathing patterns. Speech may sound like it is being obstructed by a stuffy nose. In severe cases, the symptoms may persist for weeks. Greatly enlarged adenoids can also interfere with hearing if fluid accumulates in the middle ear.

Breathing may be difficult and even interrupted at night, causing restlessness, making it difficult to sleep, and reducing the amount of oxygen in your child's blood. If your child is having breathing problems, call the doctor immediately.

TREATMENT OPTIONS

Ask the doctor for advice if your child's symptoms last for more than several weeks. Unless the symptoms are severe, the physician may recommend that you monitor the condition, waiting to see if the swelling subsides. If it does not, he or she may prescribe antibiotics taken by mouth to eradicate any infection causing the swelling.

Children whose swollen tonsils or adenoids are caused by allergy may benefit from drugs that control allergy symptoms; the glands often shrink as a result.

Operations to remove the tonsils and adenoids (tonsillectomy and adenoidectomy) continue to be common surgical procedures performed on children.

Today, however, surgery is recommended only if the blockage reduces the amount of oxygen in the bloodstream, causes difficulty swallowing, and interferes significantly with your child's ability to sleep, speak, or hear.

Febrile Seizure

A high fever can trigger a febrile seizure in children from 6 months to 5 years. These convulsions most often occur in the first several hours of an illness that has caused a fever in your child. While the seizures may be frightening to witness, they are not harmful in the vast majority of children. Febrile seizures differ from epilepsy (see p.375) in that they occur only during a high fever.

Most febrile seizures occur in conjunction with an upper respiratory infection such as the flu. The chance that your child will have a febrile seizure increases if he or she has a very high fever, has had febrile seizures before, is developmentally delayed, or has family members who have had them.

About a third of children who have had febrile seizures have a recurrence; the younger the child, the greater his or her chances of a recurrence, often within 1 year.

SYMPTOMS

During a febrile seizure, your child stiffens, twitches, and may roll his or her eyes. The child will not respond to any stimuli for several seconds or minutes. Then he or she will be sleepy for a while.

TREATMENT OPTIONS

Let the doctor know if your child has had a febrile seizure. He or she will want to rule out a serious infection such as meningitis (see p.1013) or encephalitis (see p.374). Otherwise, treatment is for the underlying condition.

There is little you can do to stop a febrile seizure in progress or to prevent its recurrence. The best you can do for your child is to follow these steps:

■ Remain calm.

■ Place your child on his or her abdomen or side.

■ Do not force anything between the teeth.

■ Observe your child carefully.

■ If the seizure does not stop after 3 to 5 minutes, call your child's doctor or your local emergency number.

Fifth Disease

(See also Color Guide to Visual Diagnosis, p.568)

Fifth disease (also called erythema infectiosum) is so-named because it is the fifth in the group of common viral infections that affect children—after mumps, measles, chickenpox, and rubella.

There is no vaccine against fifth disease. It is caused by a parvovirus, which spreads from child to child through direct contact.

SYMPTOMS

Fifth disease is a mild illness, and many children who have it feel generally well. It often starts with a sore throat, slight fever, and lethargy. Then, after about a week, comes the characteristic feature—a bright red, possibly warm, rash on the cheeks that gives them the appearance that they have been slapped. Within several days, the rash spreads to the trunk, arms, legs, and buttocks in a lacelike pattern.

The rash usually lasts 7 to 10 days before fading, first on the face and then on the arms, trunk, and legs. In some children, the rash returns over the course of several weeks. In older children and adults, the rash may be accompanied by joint pain.

TREATMENT OPTIONS

Your doctor will diagnose fifth disease based on your report of the symptoms and a physical examination. Your child is infectious while he or she has the sore throat and other coldlike symptoms, but not when the rash is present.

When your child is diagnosed with Fifth disease, he or she is usually no longer contagious.

Nevertheless, to be safe, your child should avoid contact with people who have abnormal immune systems or those who have problems with their red blood cells (such as sickle cell anemia) because parvovirus can cause more serious illness in these types of individuals.

Treatment includes rest, fluids, and fever reduction with acetaminophen or ibuprofen (not aspirin). If the rash itches, apply a bland lotion or ointment. The condition goes away on its own within 10 days. Children who have certain red blood cell disorders, such as sickle cell disease, can develop an unusual type of anemia when they have this infection.

Growing Pains

Growing pains are the vague aches and pains that occur in children, often after exercise and often at night. They are called growing pains because they usually affect the arms and legs—the limbs that show the most obvious evidence of growth.

Most often, they occur in children during the period of dramatic growth between ages 6 and 10. Despite the name of this condition, there is no research to support the idea that the growth process causes pain.

Your school-age child may complain of pains in the legs or arms that range in quality from vague discomfort and aching during times of rest to more severe pain that can make sleep difficult.

If the pain is severe or if your child has other symptoms, report the problem to your doctor, who will rule out other causes. There is no treatment for growing pains; they always disappear on their own.

Let your child know that you believe the pains are real and that you sympathize. Reassure him or her that the pains are very common in children of the same age and that they always go away. You can help your child relax by massaging his or her arms and legs. Practice relaxation therapy and do stretching exercises (see p.55) together.

Growth Problems

"Failure to thrive" is the term doctors use when an infant or child is not gaining weight or growing in height at the normal rate, according to standardized growth charts. Failure to thrive often signals an underlying problem.

A related condition, short stature, is height that is significantly lower than average. Both conditions are based on standardized height and weight measurements for the child's age.

It is helpful for you to record your child's growth, as your doctor does during your child's regular visits. Though infants normally lose a small amount of weight immediately after birth, they should experience a steady upward climb in height and weight thereafter. Illness can cause a brief loss of weight, but any sustained loss of weight or failure to grow in height is cause for concern.

Failure to thrive can occur when a child is not getting enough nutrients to grow and develop, or when a child is sick and unable to digest food. This condition can be caused by not taking in enough breast milk or formula or by difficulty feeding.

The serious digestive condition malabsorption (see p.775)—as well as cystic fibrosis (see p.1003), diabetes (see p.1004), and heart problems—can also lead to inadequate nutrition.

An insidious cause of failure to thrive is lack of emotional nourishment. In the absence of a close relationship with a concerned caregiver, the child's fundamental needs for nurturing remain unfulfilled. Emotional deprivation can lead to depression and lack of appetite. Similarly, not getting enough to eat can hinder the child's emotional development. These causes may require a multidisciplinary approach to treatment.

Short stature can be caused by similar problems, but more commonly is due to an inherited tendency to shortness or, if the parents are at least average height, a temporary delay in growth that disappears in time.

In rare cases, short stature is caused by a growth disorder due to insufficient growth hormone or hypothyroidism (see p.982). It can also signal malabsorption or celiac disease (see p.774), cystic fibrosis (see p.1003), Crohn disease, kidney disease, Down syndrome (see p.1004), or other conditions.

TREATMENT OPTIONS

The diagnosis of both conditions is made based on comparisons with growth charts reflecting national averages for children at various ages. However, since growth problems can be a sign of other conditions, further investigation is always warranted. The doctor will perform a complete physical examination and take a medical history (asking questions about illness in the child and the family).

Sometimes the physician will want to watch how the infant feeds and how he or she behaves afterward. In rare cases, the child's condition will be monitored in the hospital. If there is no evidence of neglect or abuse, parents of children who fail to thrive may need education about nutrition and feeding, along with coaching and support.

In the case of short stature, your child's height will be monitored over several months to see whether the rate of growth is normal. If it is, the doctor may suspect a hereditary factor that has temporarily delayed growth.

Tests may reveal an underlying illness or deficiency that can be treated. For some children who are not producing enough growth hormone, or who fail to grow due to kidney failure, several injectable hormone substitutes have been successful.

Headaches

Children can have the same types of headaches (see p.354) as adults, including migraine and tension headaches. Like adults, serious conditions such as brain tumors (see p.357) or meningitis (see p.1013) may, in rare cases, cause headaches. One cause of headache that is unique to children is hydrocephalus (see p.981).

Children may also complain of headache when they actually have an ear infection (see p.1005); they are more likely than adults to experience a head-ache if they develop heatstroke (see p.1212) or dehydration.

SYMPTOMS

The symptoms of migraine headaches in children are similar to those in adults: pounding or throbbing pain that starts on one side of the head (often behind the eye), sometimes with temporary distortion or blurring of vision and nausea.

More often than in adults, children may develop forms of migraine that do not include headache as the main symptom; indeed, headache may even be absent.

Examples are abdominal migraines, which cause regular bouts of nausea or vomiting; ophthalmic migraines, which cause weakness of the eye muscles (see Crossed Eyes, p.445); and confusional migraines, which predominantly cause confusion or dizziness. Motion sickness is also common with migraines, between headaches.

TREATMENT OPTIONS

Minor tension headaches often go away without any treatment. If your child has regular headaches, if the headache is severe, or if he or she has any symptoms of head injury or meningitis, contact your doctor immediately.

For migraine, acetaminophen is often recommended, either alone or with an antiemetic (a drug to reduce vomiting that may be given in suppository form). If this is not effective, your child's doctor may recommend preventive medications, all of which carry side effects.

Biofeedback (see p.395) is an approach that teaches your child to recognize and control the physical processes that can bring on a headache; it can be very successful in preventing migraine and tension headaches in children. For headache caused by other conditions, treatment is for the underlying disorder.

Head Injuries

Children hit their heads frequently. Most of the time, the injury is minor, and nothing needs to be done. Occasionally, more serious consequences of head injury can occur (see Bleeding, p.1196; Concussion, p.359).

There are a few danger signs after a head injury that should prompt you to call the doctor:

■ Loss of consciousness, even if only briefly

■ Lethargy

■ Vomiting

■ Dizziness

■ Clumsiness

■ Slurring of speech

■ Persistent headache

■ Irritability

■ Unusual behavior

■ Seizures (see p.985)

If loss of consciousness has occurred, or if any of the above symptoms occur, your child should be examined by a physician. No further treatment or tests may be needed if the examination is normal; your child may be sent home and the doctor may ask you to observe him or her.

Check your child periodically during this time, even when sleeping, to be sure that he or she is able to wake up and respond. Contact your doctor again if there is persistent vomiting, lethargy, or irritability, or if seizures occur.

Herpes

Herpes (see p.487) is a common viral illness that produces blisters in the mouth and on the lips.

Also called oral herpes, this highly contagious virus is spread by direct contact with the fluid from open sores. After the infection heals, the virus lies inactive in the nerves until physical or emotional stresses trigger another outbreak.

In rare cases, the virus spreads to a finger, causing a painful swelling called a whitlow. Genital herpes is caused by a different virus that is uncommon in children.

SYMPTOMS

The first symptom is pain and swelling of the gums and other tissues in and around the mouth; there may also be an increase in salivation. On the lips, the area may itch and tingle before becoming painful. After several days, small blisters (commonly called cold sores or fever blisters) form inside the mouth or on the lip and then erupt, ooze, and take 3 to 4 days to heal.

To avoid spreading the virus, your child should not have direct contact with other children during this active phase of the virus. Other symptoms may include swollen glands, irritability, headache, and fever. The first outbreak is usually the most painful; subsequent bouts are milder.

A whitlow is caused when a child puts fingers in contact with the sores in the mouth. This causes a red, swollen, intensely

painful abscess (see p.877) on the fingertip

TREATMENT OPTIONS

Report symptoms of herpes to the doctor. He or she can usually confirm a diagnosis based on visual inspection and a description of the symptoms. Treatment is directed at minimizing discomfort and includes drinking plenty of liquids, avoiding acidic foods and drinks, taking acetaminophen for pain, and sometimes using a special mouthwash to deaden pain in the mouth. Make sure your child gets plenty of rest and sleep.

Some children are treated with an antiviral medicine, but usually the symptoms resolve on their own after a few days. There is no cure for herpes and there is no treatment to prevent future reactivation, which often occurs during times of stress, after the child has been in the sun, or when he or she is overly tired.

Intussusception

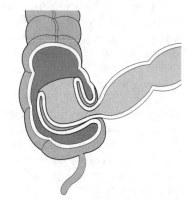

In intussusception, a portion of the intestine folds back on itself. It is most common in young children.

Intussusception

Intussusception occurs when the intestine folds back on itself, causing blockage and severe abdominal pain. It is the most common cause of intestinal blockage in children under age 2.

Researchers suspect that intussusception is most often related to intestinal infection, but it can be due to the presence of a small pouch from the wall of the intestine called a Meckel diverticulum (see p.983).

A child with this disorder may intermittently scream in pain and pull his or her legs up toward the stomach, vomit, and pass blood or mucus in the bowel movements.

Immediately report any severe abdominal pain to the doctor. He or she will perform a physical examination to rule out other conditions and may order an x-ray using air or barium given through the anus (see p.784) or an ultrasound to rule out intussusception. The enema not only can show the abnormal area of the intestine, but frequently unblocks the obstruction.

In some children, however, an operation is necessary to remove the obstruction. The procedure requires general anesthesia (see p.168) and admission to the hospital.

Juvenile Rheumatoid Arthritis

Juvenile rheumatoid arthritis (JRA) causes persistent swelling of the joints and other body organs, often starting between ages 2 and 5. JRA is an autoimmune disorder (see p.870) in which the body mistakenly attacks its own tissues. Researchers believe an otherwise harmless virus is the trigger for the immune system's response.

JRA can affect many joints, or just a few, and can affect other body systems. Its effects can be severe or mild. It usually waxes and wanes, with flare-ups that may last several weeks. JRA may go away at puberty.

Like most autoimmune disorders, girls are more often affected than boys—about four times more often. Children with JRA are also at risk of inflammation of the iris, a condition that can cause scarring and complications such as vision loss and glaucoma.

SYMPTOMS

If your child has JRA, the affected joints become swollen, limited in motion, stiff, painful, and warm. In some children, the area surrounding the eyes becomes painful. System-wide symptoms include swollen lymph nodes in the armpits and neck; a fever that fluctuates from normal to over 103°F at night; a red rash on the arms, legs, and trunk; and abdominal pain.

Your child may lose interest in food, lose weight, and become anemic. Pericarditis, which is swelling of the membrane that surrounds the heart, can cause pain in the chest.

There are no symptoms of inflammation of the iris at first, but it can eventually cause general eye pain or pain in bright light.

TREATMENT OPTIONS

Your child's doctor will make a diagnosis based on symptoms, as well as a physical examination,

blood tests, and x-rays. JRA is treated in much the same way as rheumatoid arthritis in adults (see p.606). Treatment is largely directed toward reducing inflammation.

Regular exercise is essential to maintain the mobility of joints. Your doctor may provide exercises for your child to perform and/or for you to help your child perform. In some cases, physical therapy is also beneficial.

Your son or daughter also needs plenty of rest. Becoming overly tired can trigger a flare-up. Nonetheless, encourage your child to be as active as he or she can. Children with JRA should have a slitlamp eye exam (see p.417) to detect inflammation of the iris.

Kawasaki Disease

Kawasaki disease is a condition of unknown cause that may

result in swelling and obstruction of the coronary arteries, blocking the blood supply to the heart. It mainly affects healthy children under age 8, most of whom recover fully.

Scientists suspect that Kawasaki disease, first identified in the 1960s in Japan, is caused by an unidentified virus or bacterium.

The first symptom is a high fever that lasts for more than 5 days. Within 5 days, other symptoms emerge, including conjunctivitis (see p.427), bright red lips that become swollen and cracked and bleed, red soles and palms, and a rash. The skin then peels on the tips of the toes and fingers.

Other common symptoms include swollen hands and feet, enlarged lymph glands in the neck, and extreme irritability.

Your child's doctor will perform a physical examination. A diagnosis of Kawasaki disease requires immediate hospitaliza-

---

Alternatives to Dairy Products

Dairy products are primary sources of protein and calcium, which are especially important nutrients for growing children. If your child cannot tolerate dairy products, replace the vital nutrients that dairy products contain with these foods:

GOOD SOURCES OF PROTEIN	GOOD SOURCES OF CALCIUM
Eggs	Dark green, leafy vegetables
Poultry	Broccoli
Meat	Canned fish with edible bones
Fish	Citrus fruits
Tofu or other soy products	Calcium-enriched soy milk
Peanut butter	Calcium-enriched orange juice
Legumes (dried peas and beans)	Dried peas
Whole grains, oats, or rice	Beans

tion to monitor the condition of your child's heart. Under the care of a pediatric cardiologist, your child will receive an echocardiogram (see p.665) and intravenous gamma globulin (a substance containing antibodies against many common infections).

If there are no heart problems, your child may leave the hospital a day after the fever subsides. He or she still needs periodic checkups by a pediatric cardiologist.

Lactose Intolerance

Lactose intolerance is a rare congenital (present from birth) disorder in which the body cannot produce lactase, the enzyme needed to digest the sugar, called lactose, that is common in milk and other dairy products.

The disorder may occur because the infant has an inherited deficiency of lactase. Lactose intolerance is much more common in adults (see p.798).

Children with lactose intolerance have diarrhea, abdominal cramping, and gas when they drink cow's milk (including milk-based formulas) or eat dairy products. This is caused by the fermentation of undigested lactose in the small intestine.

If your child shows symptoms, contact the doctor, who will diagnose the problem by putting him or her on a dairy-free diet to see if symptoms disappear. Alternately, your doctor may recommend that you give your child a lactase supplement.

Learning Disabilities

A learning disability is a problem that affects a child's ability to interpret information in the brain.

These limitations may be expressed as specific difficulties in speaking, writing, physical coordination, behavioral impulses, or attention span. They can affect schoolwork (reading, writing, and mathematics), daily routines, or social interactions.

A learning disability is defined as a significant gap between a person's intelligence and the skills the person has achieved at each age. A learning disorder is a broader term that includes anything that causes a continued deficit in the functioning of the developing brain.

.The causes of learning disorders are not fully understood. Evidence suggests that most disabilities arise from problems in bringing information together from different regions of the brain. Some scientists believe that, in many cases, the disturbance begins before birth. Areas under investigation include:

■ Errors in fetal brain development

■ Genetic factors or family environment

■ Smoking, alcohol, and other drugs (such as cocaine) used by the mother during pregnancy

Attention Deficit Hyperactivity Disorder (ADHD):
Dr Rappaport's Advice

Children with attentional problems tend to be hyperactive, impulsive, easily distracted, and unable to complete tasks. These problems often begin before school age and persist into school, although occasionally the first presentation of ADHD is in kindergarten or first grade. ADHD is thought to have a neurological basis and tends to run in families.

If you are concerned that your child may have a significant attentional problem, affecting school and social success as well as interactions at home, talk first to your pediatrician. The pediatrician may refer you to a specialist or, depending on his or her expertise, may manage the problem himself or herself.

The treatment of ADHD usually involves a three-pronged approach—behavioral management, education, and medication. These interventions appear to work better when done together, although studies have suggested that the greatest response is to medication.

A professional with experience in ADHD should monitor your child regularly, providing long-term support and close follow-up, including attention to your child's academic achievement, social success, and sense of self-worth.

Although many children with ADHD have similar problems into adolescence and adulthood (studies suggest between 30% and 70%), the vast majority of children with ADHD do quite well over time.

LEONARD RAPPAPORT, MD
CHILDREN'S HOSPITAL
HARVARD MEDICAL SCHOOL

- Problems of the fetus during pregnancy, such as lack of oxygen
- Environmental toxins

TYPES OF LEARNING DISABILITIES

There are a variety of different classification schemes for learning disabilities. One example divides them into the following three broad categories:

Developmental speech and language disorders Children with these disorders have difficulty making certain sounds (articulation), using language (expression), or understanding language (reception).

Academic skills disorders Children with these disorders lag behind their peers academically. They have a developmental reading (dyslexia), writing, or arithmetic disorder.

Other learning disabilities Attention disorders affect nearly 20% of children with learning disabilities. Affected children tend to daydream often, have difficulty focusing on a task, or are hyperactive. Hyperactive children may have attention deficit hyperactivity disorder (ADHD).

Children with ADHD, mostly boys, do not recognize social boundaries of behavior—they act impulsively, break rules, and interrupt people who are speaking.

All children have periods of heightened activity from time to time. Children with ADHD, however, are clearly more excitable, active, and distracted than other children.

TREATMENT OPTIONS

Learning disabilities are usually first suspected when a child does not reach a critical developmental milestone (see p.992) by the usual age. Your child should be evaluated by a learning specialist if a milestone is long delayed, if there is a history of learning disabilities in the family, or if there are several delayed skills.

Each type of learning disorder is diagnosed in a slightly different way based on specific, medically defined criteria. This includes a complete medical history, physical examination, close communication with school personnel, and laboratory tests if required.

Formal tests may be used in the evaluation along with teacher, guidance counselor, and classroom observation reports. An appropriate, individualized treatment plan requires clear identification of your child's deficiencies.

To give your child the support he or she needs, discuss the learning disorder with school counselors, teachers, your pediatrician, and other experts. Read widely to sort through the sometimes conflicting information about these disorders, and to make sound decisions that are right for your child. This process takes a tremendous amount of time and effort on everyone's part, but the long-term rewards for your child are great.

Meningitis

Meningitis is a serious infection of the coverings of the brain and spinal cord. If caused by bacteria, it can be devastating if not diagnosed early. If caused by viruses, it is usually mild and uncomplicated.

Although the symptoms of meningitis in older children are like symptoms in adults (see p.377), in children less than 2 to 3 years old, the diagnosis may be more difficult, as the only signs may be lethargy, vomiting, or fever.

Mental Retardation

Mental retardation is intelligence that is below average. Retardation often expresses itself in academic limitations as well as developmental and behavioral immaturity. Disorders such as Down syndrome (see p.1004), cerebral palsy (see p.1000), phenylketonuria (see p.983), and hydrocephalus (see p.981) can include some degree of mental retardation.

Some forms of mental retardation, such as those caused by phenylketonuria and hydrocephalus, can be prevented with early diagnosis and treatment.

In many children, the cause is unknown. The severity of mental retardation varies. Some children have impaired body movements, while others appear to have normal physical development.

SYMPTOMS

Developmental delays, such as delays in holding up the head, may be the first indication of mental retardation. However, some children who have mild retardation develop normally during the first few years of life. Later, speaking, movement, and academic skills may lag significantly behind children of the same age.

TREATMENT OPTIONS

If your child shows signs of developmental delay, call the doctor. Any delays should be

Children With Special Health Care Needs: *Dr Palfrey's Advice*

About 20% of children have some illness or condition that requires more than routine health care. These youngsters include those with chronic illnesses such as asthma, diabetes, seizures, cystic fibrosis, sickle cell anemia, and disabilities such as cerebral palsy, birth-related conditions, spina bifida, or traumatic injuries.

Every child with these conditions requires three things. First, each child needs a primary care pediatrician to take care of all of his or her other health needs and to coordinate all medical care—a doctor who will be there 24 hours a day, 7 days a week.

Second, each child needs access to teams of health professionals who have special expertise in caring for the chronic condition. Together, the primary care physician and special teams can coordinate the child's medical, educational, and social services, and can plan (in older children) for the transition to adulthood.

Third, health care professionals need to work closely with parents to define the special health care needs of their children, assuring this care is family centered, culturally appropriate, and comprehensive.

JUDITH S. PALFREY, MD
CHILDREN'S HOSPITAL
HARVARD MEDICAL SCHOOL

interpreted with caution, since children develop at different rates; your doctor may recommend watching and waiting. In the meantime, the physician may perform a physical examination to rule out hearing, vision, or speech problems.

The doctor may also refer you to a specialist in pediatric development or in pediatric neurology, and to a team of people who are expert in evaluating developmental disorders. They will perform tests that identify the nature of the problem and develop a strategy for coping with it.

Based on tests, retardation is classified as borderline (child is able to be educated to a sixth-grade level), mild (fourth-grade level), moderate (first- or second-grade level), or severe (child needs help with daily tasks).

Education is the cornerstone of treatment for children who are mentally retarded. Educational facilities, some within public schools, provide classes for children with special needs.

A diagnosis of retardation can take a toll on family members, who may suffer feelings of guilt or anger. Most parents want to know that their son or daughter will some day be able to function in the world independently. This is possible for many retarded people. Your child will need your love and guidance to reach his or her full potential.

Contact one of the numbers listed on p.1234; these groups offer information on group homes and other supportive living and work arrangements.

Mononucleosis

Infectious mononucleosis ("mono" for short) is an infection, usually caused by the Epstein-Barr virus, that is spread through contact with saliva. Children can easily acquire it, usually through exchanging saliva-contaminated toys. However, mononucleosis is more common in teenagers and young adults than in younger children, and is often acquired through kissing.

In infants, symptoms may be limited to fever and an enlarged spleen. In older children, the symptoms are like those that occur in adults (see p.877).

Affected infants and children should be encouraged to rest and should not attend day care or school until they feel well enough to return. The spleen may remain enlarged for 2 to 4 weeks, placing it at high risk of rupturing, which can occur with any sport or activity where a blow to the abdomen may be received. Ask the doctor how long your child should stay away from contact sports.

Muscular Dystrophy

Muscular dystrophy is a rare genetic disorder that causes progressive muscle degeneration and weakness. Of the several types of muscular dystrophy, Duchenne muscular dystrophy is most common, affecting only boys. Some forms are severe at birth and lead to early death, while others follow a slow, progressive course over many decades.

Women carry the gene for this

disorder and pass it on to half of their male children. A blood test can determine if you are a carrier; prenatal testing can reveal whether a fetus is affected.

SYMPTOMS

Poor head control may be the first symptom of Duchenne muscular dystrophy. Walking is accomplished at a normal age, but toddlers may walk with their feet spread apart wider than normal and may lean to one side. They may fall frequently and have trouble climbing stairs.

The disorder affects the muscles of the hips, thighs, calves, and shoulders first, but eventually muscle weakness spreads throughout the body.

Respiratory infections may result from weakness of the muscles that control breathing and coughing, which helps rid the respiratory tract of bacteria. Most children are able to walk until about age 12 and then are confined to a wheelchair. Heart disease and intellectual impairment are also common. There are other types of muscular dystrophy that may not be as severe.

TREATMENT OPTIONS

If your child's doctor suspects muscular dystrophy, he or she may be able to make the diagnosis based on symptoms and a family history of the disorder. Blood tests, a biopsy of muscle, or a test to see how well the muscles work may be needed to confirm a diagnosis. Treatment includes medicines to prevent or treat heart problems and antibiotics for lung infections.

Good nutrition and weight control are important in less active, infection-prone children.

Gene therapy (see p.133) is being tested, but is still in the early stages.

Nephritis and Nephrotic Syndrome

Nephritis (also called glomerulonephritis; see p.810) and nephrotic syndrome are kidney disorders in which the tiny filters in the kidneys (called glomeruli) are damaged.

When the damage is caused by inflammation, it is called nephritis. Nephritis most often causes blood in the urine, sometimes enough to turn it pink or red. It can occur after an infection of the throat or skin with streptococcal bacteria (see p.879) or as a part of other diseases such as Berger disease (a disease caused by antibodies that attack the kidney), sickle cell anemia (see p.721), or lupus (see p.898).

Nephrotic syndrome occurs when a disorder of the glomeruli results in leakage of large amounts of the protein called albumin from the blood and into the urine. This results in low levels of albumin in the blood and body, and fluid retention, which develops because albumin holds fluid in the blood vessels. When albumin levels in the blood are low, fluid more easily leaks out into body tissues, causing swelling.

Nephrotic syndrome is more common in boys than girls, and most often appears between the ages of 2 and 6, with relapses possible until the early 20s. In the first year of life, congenital (present at birth) nephrotic syndrome may occur due to infection passed from the mother.

Complications include blood

clots, bleeding disorders, and a vulnerability to infections—such as peritonitis (see p.801), urinary tract infection, and pneumonia.

A very common cause of nephrotic syndrome (particularly in children under age 10) is minimal-change disease, a condition in which a biopsy of the kidney reveals minimal damage to the kidney. Most children with minimal-change disease respond well to treatment.

The less common, more serious causes of nephritis and nephrotic syndrome do not respond as well to treatment.

SYMPTOMS

The symptoms of nephritis and nephrotic syndrome vary, depending on the underlying cause. Generally, children with nephrotic syndrome produce a far smaller amount of urine than normal. They also swell and look puffy around the eyes and in the abdomen, hands, and feet. Weight gain (from the extra fluid), abdominal pain, appetite loss, and diarrhea are common. High blood pressure can occur.

Nephritis is characterized by fluid retention, high blood pressure, and low urinary output. Blood in the urine may cause it to look like tea or cola, and it may contain clots. In some cases, the urine looks normal.

Other symptoms may include irritability, fatigue, pain in the side or abdomen, and fever. These symptoms last about a month after the strep infection, but the urinary problems may persist for a year.

TREATMENT OPTIONS

Nephritis and nephrotic syndrome are sometimes detected

during a routine laboratory analysis of blood or urine. If your child appears to be retaining fluid, the doctor will perform a urinalysis (see p.158) and blood tests. Your child may also require a kidney biopsy (see p.161).

Hospitalization is sometimes necessary to monitor and treat high blood pressure. Children with nephritis and nephrotic syndrome are also more prone to infection and to breathing problems caused by the swelling.

Treatment depends on the underlying condition. In nephrotic syndrome, children may be placed on a low-salt, high-protein diet. They may also need to take diuretic drugs to rid the body of fluids and corticosteroid drugs (see p.895) to reduce inflammation.

Depending on the kind of nephritis, different treatments may be recommended, including corticosteroid and immunosuppressive medicines. Protein replacement, in the form of intravenous injections, may also be needed. Many children recover fully.

Despite treatment, some children develop kidney failure (see p.814). If your child does not respond to corticosteroids, or if there are frequent relapses, treatment with other drugs or a kidney transplant (see p.814) may be recommended.

Obesity

Being obese or overweight means having too much body fat for a particular body shape. This is best measured by the body mass index, or BMI (see p.51), which can be calculated using a person's weight and height. As many as 15% of children in the United States are overweight or obese; another 15% are at risk of becoming overweight or obese. Obesity is discussed in more detail on p.853.

Lack of physical activity is a significant factor in many overweight children. Poor eating habits in infancy and childhood can set the stage for weight problems in adulthood, when they are more likely to cause health problems. Even if overweight youngsters do not suffer physical problems in childhood, they often endure anxiety from social isolation and teasing.

Consult the doctor if you think your child is overweight. The doctor will perform an examination, and ask about your family's nutritional habits. Occasionally, urine or blood tests may be performed to look for various unusual hormonal causes of obesity.

Never put your child on a restricted diet without the recommendation of a doctor or dietitian. While adults can benefit from a restricted diet, a growing child can be harmed by the wrong kind of diet.

The doctor may refer you to a dietitian for help in tailoring a diet to your child's needs. To be long-lasting and effective, weight loss should be slow and steady, and physical activity should be a regular part of your child's day.

Overweight children need the support of their families. Have patience, avoid criticism, and show approval for your child's efforts.

Osteomyelitis

Osteomyelitis is an infection of the bone. It is described in more detail on p.595. This rare but serious condition occurs in children most often between ages 5 and 14 and affects more boys than girls. In children, osteomyelitis tends to affect the long bones, such as those in the arms and legs.

The symptoms of acute osteomyelitis include pain, tenderness, and swelling of the area around the infected part of bone, and a decreased use of the affected arm or leg. Fever and fatigue also are common.

If the condition becomes chronic because of inadequate treatment, bone pain can be continuous and the child's limb can stop growing or become deformed.

To confirm a diagnosis, the doctor may perform blood tests, x-rays, a biopsy of the bone, or a bone scan (see p.622). For acute osteomyelitis, antibiotics in intravenous form are prescribed along with bed rest and immobilization of the affected bone.

If surrounding tissue has become infected, or if the condition is chronic, surgical removal of a portion of bone or tissue may be necessary.

Pinworms

Pinworms are an extremely common parasite that inhabit the intestines, usually of children, and cause anal itching. Pinworms are exceptionally transmissible. They enter the body when a child picks up microscopic pinworm eggs on the fingers and puts them in his or her mouth.

The 1/4-inch white, threadlike, adult worms live in the bowel and migrate to the skin outside the anus, where they lay eggs and die. As they hatch, the eggs cause severe itching.

If your child scratches the area and puts unwashed hands into his or her mouth, the eggs travel to the digestive system, mature, and repeat the process. The eggs can also live in soil, house dust, clothing, and bedsheets for several weeks.

SYMPTOMS

The first symptom is itching around the anus and inside the buttocks, often at night. Girls may also experience vaginal itching and pain while urinating. Restlessness and fitful sleep are other common occurrences, though some children have no symptoms.

TREATMENT OPTIONS

You can see the small worms around the anal opening, particularly at night. If you do see them, or if your child complains of anal itching, apply a strip of clear adhesive tape to the affected skin and take it to the doctor, who will examine it under a microscope to establish the presence of pinworms and their eggs.

Your doctor may recommend treating the entire family (because the parasite is so easily spread) with a drug that kills worms.

In addition, trim your child's fingernails, which are a favorite hideout for eggs, and make certain that all family members wash hands frequently, especially after using the toilet or playing with pets. Wash all bed linens in hot water and dry them on high heat to kill any eggs.

Pneumonia

Pneumonia is an infection of the lungs that can be caused by a wide variety of microorganisms. The symptoms of pneumonia in older children are like the symptoms in adults (see p.496)—mainly cough, fever, and a general feeling of weakness and sickness.

The cough is usually worse at night and in the morning and may last up to 10 days. The child may wheeze, make grunting sounds, or have chest pain.

Infants with pneumonia are irritable, less active, and usually cough. They do not always have a fever. They breathe rapidly and with great effort and do not eat as well. If the skin and lips take on a blue tinge, because the child is not getting enough oxygen, get emergency medical help immediately.

Any signs of pneumonia should be reported to your pediatrician. He or she will perform a physical exam using a stethoscope to hear breathing more clearly. A chest x-ray may be taken, but it may not show problems early in the disease, even if the pneumonia is severe. The doctor may recommend fever-reducing medicines such as acetaminophen, plenty of liquids, and bed rest.

Confirmed bacterial infections are always treated with antibiotics taken by mouth. Children who are more seriously ill with pneumonia may need to be hospitalized, and may require intravenous antibiotics and supplementary oxygen.

Reye Syndrome

Reye syndrome is a very rare but serious disorder that may occur after a viral illness, such as the flu or chickenpox. Reye syndrome can damage many different organs, but it most often affects the liver and the brain, sometimes causing brain damage and death.

Researchers suspect that, in some cases (but not all), the disorder is caused by an abnormal response to aspirin given during a viral illness.

Reye syndrome primarily affects children between ages 3 and 12. To prevent it, the safest approach is never to give aspirin-containing medicines to any person under 21. Give acetaminophen instead.

Symptoms start while your child is recovering from the viral illness. He or she vomits every couple of hours over a day or two; may become alternately lethargic, delirious, or angry during this time; and has seizures and difficulty breathing or becomes unconscious.

Report the symptoms immediately to your child's doctor, or go to an emergency department. Diagnosis may require a blood test, lumbar puncture (see p.161) to analyze spinal fluid, or biopsy of the liver (see p.761). Treatment depends on the symptoms.

Rheumatic Fever

Rheumatic fever is an infection that causes inflammation of the joints and sometimes affects the heart. The condition, which usually affects children between ages 6 and 8, usually follows strep throat (see p.467) or another streptococcal illness.

Rheumatic fever is caused when the child's body produces antibodies to fight the strep bacteria, but the antibodies combine with other substances and destroy joint tissue.

SYMPTOMS

Within 6 weeks after a strep throat, your child may have a low-grade fever and symptoms of joint inflammation—pain, swelling, heat, and redness. The elbows, wrists, knees, and ankles are most commonly affected. Inflammation may subside but, if not treated, may recur.

If the infection is affecting only the heart, there may be no symptoms other than feeling generally ill. In severe cases, your child may have trouble breathing, especially when lying down; have a red circular rash on the abdomen, chest, and back; and may have hard bumps underneath the skin over the knuckles, elbows, and knees.

TREATMENT OPTIONS

Consult the doctor if symptoms occur after a strep throat. He or she will take blood tests and an electrocardiogram (see p.135). If the diagnosis is confirmed, your child may be admitted to the hospital for observation. Treatment includes penicillin given orally and/or by injection to eradicate the strep bacteria.

Even if your child shows signs of improvement, be certain that he or she completes the full course of antibiotics. Corticosteroid drugs (see p.895) may be given to reduce inflammation.

Bed rest is extremely important and may be needed for up to 12 weeks, depending on the severity of the infection. Rheumatic fever can be prevented by ensuring that strep throat infections are treated with antibiotics.

Sore Throat

Uncommon under age 1, sore throats are very common from ages 3 through adulthood. A sore throat can be caused by several different conditions, including infection with a virus, such as coxsackievirus and echovirus, or a bacterium, such as streptococcus. It can also occur with many other illnesses, including mononucleosis (see p.1014).

An untreated strep throat can lead to serious conditions, among them rheumatic fever (see p.1017), ear and sinus infections, and nephritis (see p.1015). Children with strep throat also sometimes get scarlet fever, a bright, intense rash that appears first on the upper trunk and neck but soon on the entire body. The rash looks like a mild sunburn and makes the skin feel rough to the touch. The rash fades after a few days and is followed by peeling skin, primarily on the feet, hands, and groin.

SYMPTOMS

With a viral infection, throat pain may be the first symptom or may follow fever and loss of appetite by a day or two. Hoarseness, cough, runny nose, and swollen glands are common.

With strep throat, younger children may have a mild fever, swollen glands, and a minor sore throat. Older children may experience a severe sore throat, fever over 102°F, swollen neck glands, and a coating on the tonsils. Coughing is usually not a symptom of strep throat.

TREATMENT OPTIONS

Strep throat must be eradicated with antibiotics to prevent it from causing serious harm. If you suspect strep throat, your child should see the doctor so that a swab of organisms can be taken from the throat to determine what is causing the sore throat.

Depending on the diagnostic test method your doctor uses (a "rapid test" or a traditional throat culture), results are ready either in a few minutes or within a day. If it is strep, an antibiotic will be prescribed. If the sore throat is caused by a virus, antibiotics are useless; antibiotics are effective only against bacteria. It is very important to complete the prescription, regardless of how well your child feels, to prevent a recurrence or more serious illness. Scarlet fever is treated by treating the strep throat.

There is no treatment for a sore throat caused by a viral infection. Acetaminophen or ibuprofen (not aspirin) may be recommended to relieve pain and reduce fever. Offer your child soft, soothing, room-temperature foods and plenty of fluids.

Stuttering

Stuttering is a speech disorder characterized by repeating syllables or words. Stuttering takes several forms and varies in severity. In mid-sentence, your child may repeat words or sounds, extend the sound of one syllable, or delay speaking words.

Stuttering starts before age 8 in most children and is considered a problem only if the stuttering is prohibiting communication and lasts longer than several months. Many children stutter when they first learn to speak and form sentences. This is perfectly normal.

Stuttering may become worse during times of illness or stress. The causes are not known. During speech development, children may think faster than they can speak and stumble over their words, or they may become distracted and repeat a sound or word until they recapture their train of thought.

The most important thing you can do for your child is to ignore the stuttering. Speak to him or her slowly and clearly, and encourage other family members to do the same. Since anxiety seems to aggravate the problem, never tease your child. Be sure to spend quiet time together every day. Praise him or her for accomplishments and provide encouragement.

Consult the doctor if stuttering is severe or lasts longer than several months. You may be referred to a speech therapist, who will develop a treatment strategy that will include speech therapy.

Swollen Glands

The lymph glands (see p.863) are part of the immune system. They can swell in response to infection, which usually is not serious. However, swollen glands can also be caused by cancer or a drug reaction.

You can often feel the enlargement by gently pressing on the swollen area. The location of the swelling can help direct you to the source of infection (see p.867).

If your child is younger than 3 months and has swollen glands, call the doctor. In older children, swollen glands usually go away on their own as the accompanying infection subsides. More per-

sistent swelling may need to be investigated by the doctor.

Generally, your child should see the doctor if swollen glands are enlarging and are accompanied by a fever for more than 5 to 7 days. Treatment depends on the underlying condition.

Tuberculosis

Tuberculosis (TB) is a potentially life-threatening infection caused by the bacterium *Mycobacterium tuberculosis*. TB is described in more detail on p.504.

The number of children with TB is rising; children may develop it at any age. Most children are infected by contact with an infected adult who spreads the bacteria by coughing. Outbreaks have occurred in schools and child care centers.

When a child first becomes infected, the inhaled bacteria begin to multiply in the child's lungs. Most often, the body's immune system contains the infection and the child may never experience any symptoms of infection. The tiny area of infection may lie dormant in the body for many years; in most people, it remains dormant their whole life.

However, in some people, the infection reawakens years later. In rare cases, when a child first becomes infected, he or she becomes sick and the infection spreads elsewhere in the lungs and to other parts of the body.

Testing for tuberculosis is now performed selectively in children at increased risk for infection, such as those who have close contact with people who are homeless, in jail, infected with HIV, users of injected drugs, or migrant workers.

If your child has had contact

with a person with TB, contact your pediatrician, who will perform a tuberculin skin test, which involves injecting an extract from TB bacteria into the skin.

The skin test should be checked after 2 days; swelling, redness, and itchiness are signs of active disease or past exposure. If the skin test is positive and TB is suspected, a chest x-ray will be performed to determine the extent of the infection. Antituberculosis medicine is prescribed to prevent the disease from progressing.

If your child is infected with TB but is not sick now, he or she will still need to take medicine to treat the infection.

Undescended Testicle

An undescended testicle is one that remains in the abdomen or the groin instead of descending normally into the scrotum before birth or within the first year after birth. The condition occurs more often in premature infants.

The cause of an undescended testicle is not known, but researchers suspect either a hormonal imbalance in the mother during pregnancy or an unusual response by the fetus to hormones. In some cases, a fibrous growth blocks the descent of a testicle.

An undescended testicle increases the risk of infertility (see p.903), inguinal hernia (see p.800), and testicular cancer (see p.1091). In rare cases, the undescended testicle becomes twisted (see Torsion of the Testicle, p.1089), causing pain in the groin. If your child has a severe pain in his groin, call the doctor immediately.

Undescended Testicle

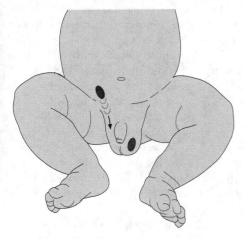

About 8 weeks before birth, testicles descend into the scrotum. A testicle does not descend in about 1 of 30 full-term infant boys. An undescended testicle requires surgery to pull the testicle down into the scrotum.

An undescended testicle is usually monitored carefully for the first year of life. If a testicle remains undescended after 10 months, it usually will not descend on its own and should be brought down surgically, ideally before age 2.

Treatment for some boys, especially those whose testicle has descended part way down the inguinal canal, is by hormonal injections. If this is not successful, surgery is performed to lower the testicle.

Urinary Tract Infections

Infections of the bladder and, sometimes, the kidneys, are common in children. The symptoms, diagnosis, and treatment of urinary infections are discussed in more detail on p.804.

The symptoms in older children are similar to those in adults. In very young infants, however, a urinary tract infection may not produce any outward symptoms except an unexplained fever, vomiting, irritability, lethargy, or failure to thrive (see p.951).

Some children are born with abnormalities in the way their urinary tract is built, some of which can cause obstruction to the normal flow of urine from the kidney into the bladder and out of the body.

Other children are born with a more common defect that causes urine from the bladder to move back up into the kidneys. This condition, called vesicoureteral reflux (see p.821), may require surgical treatment. It often runs in families; a parent or sibling may also have been affected.

Vesicoureteral reflux is diagnosed by an x-ray called a voiding cystourethrogram (see p.805). If the x-ray shows a severe form of the condition, surgery is necessary to prevent recurring infections and scarring of the kidney.

If the x-ray shows that the condition is less severe, there is controversy as to whether surgery is necessary. Some doctors recommend the use of constant low doses of antibiotics (instead of surgery) to keep the urinary tract from becoming infected. If the x-ray shows that the condition is mild, the chances are excellent that it will correct itself without treatment as your child grows. It is very important for your child to be monitored closely by the doctor.

Vulvovaginitis

Vulvovaginitis is inflammation of the vulva (the external female genitals) and vagina that causes itching, redness, and, sometimes, pain when urinating. In some girls, it is caused by masturbation, poor hygiene, or wiping from back to front after a bowel movement so that microorganisms are brought forward.

Chemical irritants (such as cosmetics or laundry soaps) as well as tight-fitting underpants not made of cotton can also cause irritation. In some girls, vulvovaginitis occurs as a result of sexual abuse.

If your child has symptoms of vulvovaginitis, consult the doctor. He or she may recommend a cream be applied each day, after thoroughly washing the area with warm water and then drying the area. Your daughter should not use bubble bath, harsh soaps, or any other irritants in or around the vagina and vulva. She should wear cotton underwear and always wipe from front to back after a bowel movement.

Health of Adolescents

Our bodies are always changing, but seldom are these changes as dramatic as during adolescence. The teenage years chronologically begin at 13 and end at 20. From a health standpoint, however, adolescence starts at puberty, which is defined as the time when girls and boys begin their sexual development and eventually become capable of reproducing.

This period of change and rapid physical growth, which is described starting on p.1026, usually begins earlier in girls than in boys. Puberty comes to an end when full sexual development is reached.

The physical development and growth of puberty is often accompanied by dramatic emotional and mental changes, which can be exciting, exhausting, anxiety provoking, and frustrating for both the adolescent and his or her family. Adolescent health concerns include such normal conditions as acne and body odor, as well as more serious problems such as drug abuse, depression, and eating disorders. This chapter is intended to help both parents (in the first part of this chapter) and adolescents (in the latter half) understand important health issues, gauge their severity, and get them treated.

Your family doctor can answer your questions about the psychological and physical ramifications of adolescence.

FOR PARENTS: KNOWING YOUR ADOLESCENT CHILD

The word adolescence comes from the Latin word "adolescentia," which means "to grow into maturity." Experts look at this stage of life as three major phases (early, middle, and late adolescence) that help mark the progress of physical, emotional, social, and intellectual development.

The boundaries that define normal development are not rigid. Use the information in this section as a general guide. For Teens: Knowing Yourself (see p.1025) provides more information. Ask your son or daughter to read it too. If you are concerned about any facet of your maturing adolescent's development, talk to his or her doctor.

Until this point, your child's life revolved around you. As ado-lescence begins, your child's interests shift from parents to friends. During early adolescence (ages 10 to 13 years), intense friendships with members of the same sex develop. Young teens have an increased need for privacy at this stage and may want to go out with friends instead of being part of the usual family outings.

Early adolescence is characterized by signs of puberty and the rapid increase in height and weight known as a "growth spurt." For boys, puberty usually begins about 1 to 2 years later than it does for girls. Girls usually develop secondary sexual characteristics such as breasts while having their growth spurt.

Teenagers going through this growth spurt can become preoc-cupied with their bodies and concerned about whether they are "normal." They may worry about acne or emerging body hair.

Friendships often take on increasing importance during middle adolescence, which occurs between ages 14 and 17. Interest in romantic relationships and sexual desires usually intensify during this time. Risk-taking behaviors are common in teens during middle adolescence. Teens may experiment with cigarettes, alcohol, or other drugs, or may have unprotected sex; peer pressure becomes an increasingly important issue.

Late adolescence, which is defined as the ages of 18 to 21, paves the way to adulthood. This is often a period of "settling

Guiding Your Child Through the Teenage Years

What you can do:

- Give more independence, when appropriate.
- Establish clear limits.
- Enforce rules; determine appropriate consequences for breaking rules.
- Praise positive behaviors and good choices.
- Keep criticism and demeaning comments to a minimum.
- Respect your teen's need for privacy.
- Encourage decision-making in your teen as he or she matures.

down." Adolescents can begin planning for the future and developing educational goals, career goals, and eventual financial independence. When independence from the family is better established, parental values that were previously rejected may become more easily accepted.

Communicating With Your Adolescent

For many parents, it is an understatement to say that communicating with your child can be difficult during adolescence. It is essential that you keep the lines of communication open. Your child's healthy transition into adulthood can hinge on a trusting and open relationship with a parent or parents. Even if you have different views, you can express your respect and trust in your children, and in this way build their respect and trust in you, by listening to what they have to say. One approach to

differing views is agreeing to disagree.

Try to include adolescents in important decisions that may affect them. Discussing your individual suggestions and sharing responsibility for decisions contributes to the connection you have with your child, and to his or her self-confidence.

One powerful way to influence your adolescent is to be a role model, particularly regarding the use of tobacco, alcohol, and other drugs, but also as it relates to seat-belt use, problem-solving, and respectful resolution to disagreements with others. At the same time, it is important to set limits, especially regarding issues such as curfews, activities at home or school, privileges, and responsibilities.

Even as adolescents outwardly protest your rules and interference, they inwardly rely on the security of the strong base you provide. It is important to act as a parent and not as a peer.

Knowing Your Child's Friends

Because your daughter's or son's peer group plays such a powerful role during adolescence, knowing your teen's friends can illuminate the influences shaping his or her beliefs and actions. Encourage your children to spend time at your house with adult supervision, and be clear and consistent about which activities are restricted. It is also helpful to get to know the parents of your adolescent's friends. You will likely find that you share many of the same concerns and, on a practical level, can speak in a common voice to reinforce curfews and other guidelines for the group.

Helping Adolescents Get the Medical Care They Need

Although teenagers are usually healthy, they should have annual medical checkups (see Teen Checkups: When You Visit Your Doctor, p.1031) to monitor physical and mental health, to assess health concerns and risk behaviors, and to provide guidance about safety, nutrition, family and peer conflicts, school, sexually transmitted disease prevention, birth control, and the use of alcohol, tobacco, and other drugs.

Parents should talk to their child's doctor at least twice during the child's teenage years to obtain guidance on normal development, signs and symptoms of disease and emotional distress, and ways to promote healthy adolescent adjustment.

Discussions About Sex

It is ideal to begin talking about sex as soon as your child starts to ask about it. Before puberty, children need to know what the sex organs are called and how they function, the changes that occur during puberty, and the process of sexual reproduction.

Once they enter their teens, shift your focus to social and emotional aspects of sex, including dating, setting limits on sexual activity, decision-making, resisting peer pressure, sexually transmitted diseases (STDs), birth control, date rape, and masturbation.

These issues can be difficult for many parents to discuss. Schools often have sex education curricula during the early adolescent years. Encourage your adolescent to discuss (with you or other trusted adults) any information learned in these classes and to read the information provided in the section for teens in the latter half of this chapter.

Once a teen starts to have sex, discussions about STDs and pregnancy prevention are essential. Let your children know your values, but make sure they have access to confidential health care.

Problems With Your Teen

It is common for adolescents to be somewhat rebellious. In fact, a certain amount of rebellious behavior is considered healthy because it helps the adolescent establish independence, acquire self-esteem, and learn how to make decisions. Be aware that most teens experiment with new behaviors; those that may appear unusual to you—such as unique haircuts or hair color, or body piercing—may be a form of self-expression.

Sometimes adolescents engage in dangerous, self-destructive behaviors, which can be symptoms of conflict, depression, abuse, school problems, or unhappiness. If you are concerned about your child's behaviors, seek help from your child's pediatrician, school counselors, or a local mental health clinic.

Substance Abuse

Preventing substance abuse is easier than treating it. Prevention starts with positive reinforcement; let your child know how proud you are that he or she is staying away from tobacco, alcohol, and other drugs. Acknowledge that it is a smart, courageous, and healthy choice in the face of many pressures.

Keep the lines of communication open by expressing a willingness to discuss any concerns your teen has about these issues. Read Alcohol, Tobacco, and Other Drugs (p.1036) in the latter half of this chapter. Discuss the dangers of drug abuse and encourage responsible behavior.

Remember, though, that honest dialogue is not a substitute for being a good role model. If you smoke, for example, do not be surprised if your teenager does the same.

It is not always easy to know if your child is using alcohol or other drugs, or the extent of the problem. If you suspect your child has a problem, seek professional help from your physician, the school system, and (for older teens) a support group such as Alcoholics Anonymous or Narcotics Anonymous (see p.1229).

Adolescent Suicide

Suicide is the second leading cause of death among adolescents; studies show that many adolescents have suicidal thoughts. Males are more likely to die than females, but females make more attempts. The most lethal factor in teen suicide is the availability of guns. Clinical depression (p.1037), which should not be confused with normal teen moodiness, can be a precursor to teen suicide.

Be alert to the possibility of depression if your child has a decline in school performance, many physical complaints, family conflicts, abuse of alcohol or other drugs, problems with authorities, or feelings of hopelessness.

Homosexual youth, and teens with depression who have had a close family member who committed suicide, are at even

Body Piercing and Tattoos

Body piercing and tattoos are increasingly popular, particularly among adolescents. While they usually do not cause health problems, they can lead to allergic reactions and infections—some of them quite serious (see p.1035).

greater risk of suicide. Never dismiss a child's mention of suicidal thoughts as an attention-getting device; it is usually a real cry for help. If you are concerned that your teen is suicidal, he or she should see a physician or go to a hospital emergency department.

School Problems

School problems can manifest themselves in a number of ways—poor school performance, skipping classes, or reluctance to go to school. If you suspect your teen is having problems, start by asking him or her about it directly. Sometimes the problem is relatively straightforward, such as falling behind in schoolwork, and can be resolved by talking to teachers, arranging for a tutor, or helping your child organize study hours.

Talking to your child's guidance counselor or physician may also be helpful. They may advise a more complete evaluation to determine if your child's problems are due to depression (see p.395), substance abuse, learning disorders (see p.1012), or attention deficit hyperactivity disorder.

Eating Disorders

Eating disorders are common in adolescents. Obesity (see p.853) is the leading chronic illness in adolescence and can lead to adult obesity. Researchers continue to study obesity, which can be the result of multiple factors, including a genetic propensity to obesity (see Obesity Genes, p.853) as well as unhealthy eating patterns, compulsive overeating, excessive television watching, and/or a lack of exercise.

Anorexia nervosa and bulimia (see p.1037) are serious medical and psychological disorders that are related to a distorted body image, an irrational fear of body fat, and an obsession with food. They can affect up to 10% of teenage girls and women in their early 20s. Boys are affected less often.

Read the section on anorexia and bulimia to learn more about them. Encourage nutritious eating habits, but seek medical help immediately if you suspect your child has anorexia or bulimia. For more information, see the eating disorders listing in the Appendix (see p.1232).

Nutrition

Your child's eating habits can be influenced by your family's eating habits. Try to prepare nutritious meals and snacks at home. The adolescent years are the time when your child builds up bone to its maximum density (mass) and strength. Teenage girls should get 1,200 to 1,500 milligrams of calcium every day, the amount found in 4 cups of milk or about three cartons of yogurt. See p.44 for recommended calcium intake for all people and for the calcium contents of foods.

Anabolic Steroids and Performance-Enhancing Drugs: Dr Grace's Advice

The abuse of anabolic steroids, drug compounds derived from the male hormone testosterone, can be a problem for teens. Young athletes may be seduced into taking steroids or other performance-enhancing drugs by the promise of becoming stronger and bigger without the physical effort required to do so normally. Teens may not be aware of the side effects, which can include increasingly aggressive behavior (sometimes called "roid rage"), impotence, acne, high blood pressure, and high cholesterol, and that these drugs may contain contaminants. If you think your teen is taking steroids, take your child to his or her physician immediately for a checkup.

ESTHERANN GRACE, MD
CHILDREN'S HOSPITAL
HARVARD MEDICAL SCHOOL

Violence

From an early age, children are exposed to violence in the media, and the images they see often present violence in a positive light. Children also may be exposed to violence at home or in their school or neighborhood. Inadequate conflict-solving skills and alcohol and other drug abuse contribute to violent behavior in adolescents. Encourage discussion as a way to resolve conflict and monitor what your teen watches on TV, sees at the movies, and encounters on the Internet. In addition, ensure that your own behavior sets a standard for nonviolent action.

Sports and Physical Fitness

Physical fitness is essential for health and promotes physical and emotional well-being. An inactive adolescence often leads to an inactive adulthood. Your adolescent should have at least 30 minutes of aerobic activity most days of the week. So should you. Make exercise a family activity by planning outings or playing sports together. Supervised organized sports can also promote a positive mental focus, build self-esteem, and help teens learn to cooperate. Participating in sports also helps teens develop friendships.

Separating From Your Child

As children mature, they prepare to leave the security of home and set out on their own. This can be difficult for both you and your child. To make it on their own, adolescents need your help to cultivate the social, emotional, intellectual, and practical skills necessary for independent living; these skills develop with time. You may need to help your child learn the more practical skills of independent living, such as budgeting, laundry, cooking, and cleaning.

FOR TEENS: KNOWING YOURSELF

When you were young, you probably did not notice that your body was growing. This is because children grow so steadily that, to them, change is not readily noticeable. When you start to become aware that your body looks different, you are going through puberty. Puberty means that your body is changing into the body of an adult.

Puberty can start between the ages of 8 and 13 for girls and about 1 to 2 years later, between the ages of 9 and 14, for boys. But everyone develops at his or her own rate and this can vary widely. Do not worry if your body changes in a way that is different from your friends. Chances are that your body will change in the same way as your female relatives if you are a girl or male relatives if you are a boy.

Once puberty begins, it happens quickly over a few years. You will grow taller and put on weight. You will develop secondary sexual characteristics. For boys, this means your testicles and penis will grow, and you will develop underarm hair and thick, curly hair known as pubic hair around your genitals. Girls also develop pubic hair and underarm hair, as well as breasts and a rounder figure; girls also begin to have their periods (menstruate).

Boys will notice their voices getting deeper, hair growing on their face, arms, and back, and increased strength and muscle mass. Boys get their growth spurt between ages $11\frac{1}{2}$ and $15\frac{1}{2}$ (on average at age $13\frac{1}{2}$). Girls get their growth spurts between ages $9\frac{1}{2}$ and 13 (on average at age $11\frac{1}{2}$). For many teens, going through puberty also means getting acne (see p.1038). See Boys Becoming Men and Girls Becoming Women (p.1026) for details of changes during puberty.

As your body changes, it is normal to feel self-conscious or embarrassed. You may be confused about what is happening or worried about what others may be thinking. Talking to a trusted adult about your concerns can be helpful. In addition to the changes that occur to your body, your feelings and attitudes may change. You may prefer to spend more time with your friends or with one special friend of the same sex or opposite sex. All of this is normal, but it can lead to conflicts with your parents, who may not be quite ready for your new need for independence.

After puberty has occurred (it usually takes about 2 to 4 years, but this can vary), you may be less concerned about your physi-

Boys Becoming Men and Girls Becoming Women

There are a number of changes you can expect during puberty, which usually starts between the ages of 9 and 14 for boys and between the ages of 8 and 13 for girls. These changes occur at different ages in different teens. Adolescents of the same age but of different racial or ethnic groups can also develop at very different rates. Read about the stages of development here so you will know what to expect. See your doctor if you are a boy who has not seen any signs of puberty by age 15 or a girl who has not had any breast budding or breast development by age 13.

BOYS

NORMAL CHANGES TO EXPECT	WHAT YOU SHOULD KNOW
STAGE 1	
Your testicles are getting ready to produce more hormones (chemical messengers) but you have no visible changes in your body.	Understand that your body will change.
You may start to have body odor.	Bathe or shower daily and use deodorant and/or antiperspirant. It is normal to sweat more during puberty.
STAGE 2	
Your testicles and scrotum start to get bigger.	
You may start to see pubic hair grow around the base of your penis (or this may start during stage 3). It will be straight and fine hair, not thick and curly.	The amount of pubic hair varies from person to person, depending on your genes (what your biological parents look like).
STAGE 3	
Your penis starts to grow longer but not wider and your testicles continue to grow. Your scrotum may get redder or darker and more wrinkly.	You may experience your first "wet dream," which means that you ejaculate sperm from your penis, usually in the middle of night. You may also feel the impulse to masturbate (to stimulate your penis). All of this is normal.
You are growing taller and are gaining weight. Your muscles start to develop and your body shape starts changing to look more like that of a man.	
Your voice may also start to change, get deeper, and sometime "crack." This is because your larynx (voice box) is enlarging.	Do not be embarrassed. It is a normal part of puberty for your voice to sound deep one moment and squeak the next. This will not last long; soon your voice will be deep all the time.
Your feet and hands may grow bigger.	

NORMAL CHANGES TO EXPECT	WHAT YOU SHOULD KNOW
Breast tissues under your nipples may start to swell and become tender.	Do not worry; this is a temporary condition called gynecomastia that occurs in more than half of all adolescent boys. It is caused by the sex hormones that are creating all the changes in your body. It should go away within 1 to 2 years.

STAGE 4

Your penis grows wider as well as longer. Your testicles and scrotum continue to grow. You develop more pubic hair, which gets curly and coarse. Pubic hair eventually fills the genital area. Most boys start to ejaculate by this time.	If you are having sexual intercourse with a girl, you need to use some form of birth control (see p.1034) to prevent pregnancy and a latex or polyurethane condom to help protect against sexually transmitted diseases (STDs) (see p.1033).
This stage is when most boys get their growth spurt. You may grow about 3 to 4 inches in height in 1 year. Your body shape looks more like a man because your muscles develop more. Your voice is deep and you may have underarm hair.	
You may have more hair on your upper lip and chin.	You may want to start shaving. Early facial hair is fine and fluffy. Later, it becomes thicker. A razor will easily remove hair.

STAGE 5

Your body is now finishing its growth spurt. Your penis reaches its final size. Your testicles and scrotum finish growing. Pubic hair fills the genital area and hair may grow up toward your navel and down your legs. You may have hair on your chest and a lot of facial hair.	Masculine features such as the size of your penis are determined genetically. The size of your penis does not determine how masculine you are.

GIRLS

NORMAL CHANGES TO EXPECT	WHAT YOU SHOULD KNOW

STAGE 1

Your ovaries are beginning to produce hormones (chemical messengers), although you have no visible changes in your body.	Understand that your body will change.
You may develop body odor.	Bathe or shower daily and use a deodorant and/or antiperspirant.

Boys Becoming Men and Girls Becoming Women (continued)

GIRLS

NORMAL CHANGES TO EXPECT	WHAT YOU SHOULD KNOW
STAGE 2	
You will develop a lump under your nipple and the areola (the darker area around the nipple) may grow. This lump may be tender.	The tender area gets less tender as your breasts develop. You can use ibuprofen or other nonaspirin painkillers for tenderness.
You may notice fine pubic hair (hair in the genital area) beginning to grow on your labia—the outer folds of your genital area.	
You will start to grow taller and gain weight. Your hips start to get broader and rounder.	It is normal for your body shape to change.
STAGE 3	
Your breasts continue to grow so that the breast tissue creates a mound.	It is not uncommon for one breast to be larger than the other when you start to develop. This is normal. If the difference in size is dramatic, seek advice from your doctor.
You have your growth spurt and can grow 3 to 4 inches per year. Your weight continues to increase and your hips widen.	
Your pubic hair continues to grow and becomes more curly.	The amount of pubic hair differs from person to person. Some women have very little while others have a lot. Neither pattern is cause for concern.
Your vagina is enlarging and you may start to have a clear discharge from your vagina.	
STAGE 4	
Your breasts continue to grow. You may see that the darker area around your nipple creates a mound separate from that of the rest of the breast.	
Pubic hair fills in the triangle of the genital area. You may get hair under your arms.	
You continue to grow in height and gain weight. This process will continue for 2 years after you start your menstrual period, although at a slower rate.	

NORMAL CHANGES TO EXPECT	WHAT YOU SHOULD KNOW

STAGE 4

Most girls get their period (start menstruation) around this time. Your ovaries may mature and start to produce eggs during some months (ovulation). On average, in the United States, girls get their periods at about age 12½. This can vary depending on your racial and ethnic background and your genes.

Personal hygiene is important during your menstrual period. A daily shower or bath is a good way to prevent odor. You can use sanitary napkins (pads) or tampons (which you put into your vagina) when you have your period. Change them every 2 to 4 hours, depending on your flow. Tampons do not alter virginity.

For cramps (see p.1046), take ibuprofen or another nonaspirin painkiller. Take the amount recommended on the label along with a snack or meal. You can also place a heating pad or hot water bottle on your lower abdomen (make sure it is not too hot). Get plenty of rest if you feel tired. Girls can play sports and do all other activities during their periods. See your doctor if your cramps keep you from doing daily activities.

It may seem like you are losing a lot of blood during your period but it is actually only about 2 to 4 tablespoons (1 to 2 ounces). The average menstrual cycle is 28 days (from the first day of one period to the first day of the next); but most girls and women are more irregular than this, especially during the first few years. Cycles can range from 21 to 45 days in length.

If you have heavy bleeding, or if your period lasts more than 8 to 10 days, contact your doctor. There are many reasons for excessive bleeding and your doctor can help resolve any problems.

STAGE 5

Your breasts reach their final size.

The size of your breasts is determined by your genes, your body type, and your weight. Everyone's breasts look different.

Your pubic hair fills the genital area and may grow onto your inner thighs.

You may ovulate (produce an egg from an ovary) every month.

Once you menstruate, and even in the month before getting your period for the first time, you may be capable of getting pregnant. If you are having sexual intercourse with a boy, you need to use some form of birth control (see p.1034) to prevent pregnancy and a latex or polyurethane condom to help protect against STDs (see p.1033).

You will reach your final height 2 years after you start getting your period and your body shape will stabilize.

cal appearance and more interested in what your friends are doing. You may feel pressure to be like everyone else and to do what everyone else is doing. At times, you may not want to go along with the crowd but fear that if you do not, you will be left out.

Some of the pressures to conform to the group may involve experimenting with alcohol or other drugs or having sex. Most teenagers want to try new things, but it is risky if you are not informed about what will happen as a result.

Never be afraid to say no to something you do not feel comfortable doing or is against your values or your family's values. It is important for you to be able to socialize, meet new friends, and have a good time without using alcohol or other drugs. They alter your ability to make decisions and can contribute to risky situa-

tions, such as driving while drunk or having unsafe sex.

It is also normal to feel sad or moody from time to time. Your life is changing in so many ways, resulting in new choices to make, problems to solve, and issues to consider. The hormones that are causing your body to change can make you more emotional, and this is normal. However, it is not normal to feel miserable for long periods of time such as weeks or months. Sometimes such intense feelings of sadness or anger make it impossible to function and to enjoy life.

You may have particular reasons for such feelings of sadness or you may not be able to pinpoint any reason. Either way, if you feel sad or angry almost every day for more than a few weeks, it is important to get help. Depression is a medical disorder and is nothing to feel embarrassed about; there are medicines

that can help. Ask your parents or doctor for help. If you need to talk to someone other than your parents, speak to a trusted adult such as a relative, parent of a friend, teacher, school counselor, or someone in your religious community.

The next section deals with these issues in more detail. As you read, you will notice that references are made to other parts of the book; this means that more information on the subject can be found by turning to that page. See also Health of Women (p.1039) and Health of Men (p.1086) for more details.

Even You Need a Regular Checkup

You need regular medical checkups to stay healthy (see Teen Checkups: When You Visit Your Doctor, p.1031). Your doctor should see you without your par-

Your Teen Years: Dr Forman's Advice

You are in a really exciting time of life, a time that is full of changes. Sometimes, though, in the middle of all of the change, it is not easy to know what is normal and what is not. Read the introductions to either Health of Women (p.1039) or Health of Men (p.1086) for information on your reproductive system and how to stay healthy. Also, read the section of this chapter written for teens, keeping in mind that, while we all share the same basic parts, each of us is unique. If you are a girl, you may not get your menstrual period at the same time as your friends. If you are a boy, you may have a different amount of facial hair or be a different size and shape than your friends. Remember that comparing yourself to others is not the best way to tell what is normal. Chances are what you are experiencing is completely normal.

The more you know about your body, the more you will feel like you are in control of it and the better you will feel about yourself. You are not expected to be an expert. If you need help, if you have questions—any questions—do not be afraid to ask your doctor, your school nurse, or any other health professional or adult you trust. If you feel you have a serious problem you cannot discuss with anyone you know, check your community for hotlines or teen support agencies. Take control and stay healthy.

SARA F. FORMAN, MD
CHILDREN'S HOSPITAL
HARVARD MEDICAL SCHOOL

Teen Checkups: *When You Visit Your Doctor*

In the past, vaccinations have been a big part of your visit to the doctor. Over the next few years, you can expect to have different types of tests. This box describes some of the tests and procedures your doctor may recommend, and issues and advice he or she will give. This is intended only as a general guide (for example, if you are not sexually active, you can avoid having any of the tests and procedures recommended for people who are sexually active).

PHYSICAL EXAM

At each yearly visit as part of your physical exam, your doctor will check your height, weight, physical development (body changes for puberty), blood pressure, back for scoliosis, and face and back for acne.

If you have had sexual intercourse, your doctor will check you for sexually transmitted diseases such as gonorrhea, chlamydia, or genital warts and, if you are a girl, recommend a Pap smear every year

ISSUES YOUR DOCTOR MAY DISCUSS

Your doctor may discuss fitness; exercise; proper nutrition; safety issues, including driving a car, riding a bicycle, and protecting yourself from violence; making wise choices about alcohol, smoking, and other drugs; sexuality; school; learning problems; and depression or sadness.

BLOOD TESTS

You may need a blood test to check for anemia or a cholesterol test.

If you have had sexual intercourse, your doctor may suggest that you have a test for the human immunodeficiency virus (HIV, the virus that causes AIDS; see p.872) or for syphilis (see p.893).

IMMUNIZATIONS

You will need a tetanus shot every 10 years (probably one time during your teen years).

You will need a second dose of the measles, mumps, and rubella (German measles) vaccine, if they were not given earlier. You may also need two doses of the chicken pox vaccine if you have not had the disease or vaccine before.

All teens should receive three hepatitis B shots if they never received them. Your doctor may also recommend the meningococcal vaccine before starting college, and the hepatitis A vaccine. A skin test is usually done to see if you have been exposed to tuberculosis.

---

ents in the room for some of your visit so that you can discuss any health concerns privately.

Your doctor may ask some general questions, such as how you are doing at school, whether you smoke, or if you use a seat belt, along with very personal questions, such as if you are having sexual intercourse. Try to be honest when answering the questions; the answers will help your doctor advise you about ways to keep healthy, and help him or her decide what treatment, if any, to recommend. Now is a good time to raise any questions you have about the changes you are going through.

PRIVACY

Even though your questions may seem extremely private, do not feel embarrassed. Physicians are trained to discuss these issues and can give you straightforward and clear answers or explanations. Your doctor will keep most private issues confidential. If you are under 18 and you are concerned about your parents' knowing something you need to discuss with the doctor, ask the doctor if the conversation you are having is private. If your doctor feels that your life or the life of someone else is in danger, he or she will help you involve your parents after discussing the situation with you.

Having a Pelvic Exam for the First Time

A pelvic exam is an examination of your vagina and female reproductive organs (uterus, ovaries, and cervix). You should have

Reasons to Have a Pelvic Exam

If you experience any of the following, make an appointment with your doctor for a pelvic exam:

■ Unusual vaginal discharge or a change in the color or texture of vaginal fluids

■ Fishy or other unpleasant odor from the vaginal area

■ Bad cramps, discomfort, pain, or itchiness in the lower abdomen, genital region, or anus

■ Irregular (too little or too much) menstrual bleeding

■ Lack of menstrual periods

your first pelvic exam (in which the doctor checks your sexual organs to make sure they are healthy) if you become sexually active, if you have gynecological problems (see Reasons to Have a Pelvic Exam, above), whenever you are ready, or by age 18. If you are having sexual intercourse, you should have a pelvic exam every year.

Health care providers including gynecologists (doctors who treat women), family physicians, adolescent medicine doctors, pediatricians, internists, and nurse practitioners can perform pelvic exams.

Having a pelvic examination for the first time can be intimidating because you do not know what to expect. It may help to take someone along to keep you company. You may want your

mother, a friend, or a female relative to accompany you. Stay calm during the examination by doing deep breathing or other relaxation exercises (see p.90). Ask your doctor to explain each step before and during the exam.

When you are relaxed, it is more comfortable for you, and easier for the doctor to examine you. Do not worry—going for a pelvic examination is slightly uncomfortable but it does not hurt.

WHAT TO DISCUSS WHEN YOU GO FOR A PELVIC EXAM

Your doctor can help you understand your body and the changes you are going through. If you have any questions (perhaps regarding your breasts or menstrual periods), ask your doctor. He or she is most interested in helping you stay healthy.

If you are having sexual intercourse, even occasionally, you should discuss birth-control options and ways to prevent sexually transmitted diseases (see Contraception and Safer Sex, p.68). Your doctor may raise these issues with you so he or she can help you make smart choices about protection.

WHAT HAPPENS DURING A PELVIC EXAM?

The entire examination takes place in a private examining room and lasts about 10 minutes. You will be asked to take off your clothes, put on a light gown, and lie down on a cushioned examining table. Your doctor will ask you to put your feet in stirrups (which hold your heels) at the end of the table,

and then raise your knees. Your legs will be covered with a sheet. You will be in this position for only a few minutes.

Step 1 The doctor will ask you to spread your knees apart. Wearing gloves, the doctor will examine the outside of your genital area for sores or rashes.

Step 2 The doctor then performs an internal exam, which starts by inserting a speculum into your vagina. A speculum is a metal or plastic device that looks like two large spoons facing each other and is used for opening the walls of your vagina so the doctor can examine it closely. You may feel a slight stretching or pressure inside your vagina. Stay calm and keep breathing deeply; if your muscles are relaxed, the speculum will go in without discomfort.

If the doctor suspects you have an infection, he or she will insert a cotton swab to take a sample of the fluids inside your vagina; most women barely feel this. The sample will be sent to a laboratory to determine what is causing the infection.

Your doctor will also perform a Pap smear (see p.1067), which can indicate a tendency to develop cancer of the cervix. A Pap smear involves taking a small sample of cells from the cervix and sending the sample to a laboratory to check for abnormal cells. Most women barely feel it when the doctor takes cells for a Pap smear.

Step 3 The doctor removes the speculum, puts lubrication on his or her gloved fingers, and inserts the fingers into your vagina, while gently pressing on your abdomen. This allows the doctor to feel the shape and consistency of your uterus, ovaries, and cervix to ensure that their shape, size, and position in your pelvis are normal.

Your doctor may examine your breasts to check for lumps and pain. He or she may also teach you how to examine your breasts on your own (see Breast Self-Examination, p.78). After your examination and after you are dressed, your doctor will discuss any questions or concerns you have.

PAP SMEAR RESULTS

Although the Pap smear is used primarily to detect the early stages of cervical cancer, changes in the cells of the cervix can occur for many reasons, including infections and genital warts (see p.891). If the laboratory reports abnormal results from your Pap smear, your doctor may request that you have another test to confirm the initial results, or to have a procedure called a colposcopy (see p.1041).

Sex

Every human being has sexual desires. The teenage years are a time when you may start to be more aware of your sexuality, your feelings about your body, and your attraction to others. It is important to realize that having feelings about sex does not mean you have to have sexual intercourse or sexual contact.

You have a lifetime ahead during which you may choose to have sexual relationships. If you have a boyfriend or girlfriend, explore other facets of your rela-

tionship, such as friendship; sharing interests in academics, sports, or religion; or just learning about the world together.

Even if some or even most of your friends seem to be having sex, do not be coerced into having it through peer pressure or promises from your boyfriend or girlfriend. Good friends will respect your feelings. Those who have had sex may pressure you to have it because they may be envious that you do not have to worry about pregnancy or about getting a sexually transmitted disease. There are many ways of being sexually intimate (such as kissing or touching) that can be pleasurable but not put you at risk.

Masturbation

One way of releasing sexual tension is through masturbation— stimulating your own genitals to achieve sexual pleasure. There is no risk of either pregnancy or disease with masturbation. You may have heard that masturbation causes blindness or gives you hairy palms, but this is nonsense. It is a common, harmless activity that gives pleasure, reduces tension, and may be a helpful way for you to delay having sex until you feel mature enough to handle the responsibility.

Homosexuality

Being homosexual means having strong sexual feelings for a person of the same sex. Most scientists believe that homosexuality is a normal variation in sexual orientation. During adolescence you may find yourself attracted to a person of the same sex even if

you are heterosexual. This does not necessarily mean that you will be gay.

Even though times are changing, realizing that you are gay can cause a great deal of anxiety. You may feel different and alone and afraid to tell anyone. Our society still shows prejudice against homosexuals. The best thing to do is to find support.

There are many support groups where homosexuals can share their feelings and experiences. Call one of the phone numbers listed in the Appendix under Gay/Lesbian Issues (see p.1233) for help in finding a local support group that can provide an open environment for you to talk about your sexuality with other gay people. Your doctor may also be someone you can talk to.

Sexually Transmitted Diseases

If you choose to have sex, know how to prevent sexually transmitted diseases (STDs) (see p.889) and pregnancy (see Contraception and Safer Sex, p.68). It is essential that you use a condom every time you have intercourse. You can catch all kinds of diseases, some of them deadly, through sexual contact.

Remember that making the choice to have sex is an adult decision, and it comes with responsibility. If you have sex without a condom, you are putting yourself and your boyfriend or girlfriend at risk, no matter how much you trust him or her. Practicing safer sex (see p.76) is always the responsibility of both partners.

Pregnancy and STDs: Dr Emans' Advice

Q A friend of mine says you can't get pregnant if the boy withdraws his penis from your vagina before he ejaculates. Is she right?

A You can indeed get pregnant even if the boy withdraws his penis, because a small amount of semen (which contains millions of sperm) is released even before ejaculation. Also, you can get pregnant even if ejaculation occurs outside of your vagina.

Q My girlfriend takes birth-control pills to prevent pregnancy. I say they also protect us from STDs, but she says we have to use a condom too. Who is right?

A Your girlfriend is. The only way to prevent STDs is to use a latex or polyurethane male condom or a female condom every time you have sex. Birth-control pills only prevent pregnancy. To prevent STDs, you must use a condom.

Q My boyfriend says if I love him I will trust that he does not have any diseases and not make him wear a condom. He will not wear one no matter how often I ask, and I don't want to lose him.

A Your boyfriend is playing Russian roulette with your health and his. A mature sexual relationship includes being informed of the risks of sexual activity and agreeing with your partner on how you will prevent STDs and pregnancy. Many teens have diseases like chlamydia or herpes, but don't know it because they don't have any symptoms. Show your boyfriend the Contraception and Safer Sex section (see p.68). If he still refuses to wear a condom, your only choice is not to have sexual intercourse (and perhaps look for a smarter boyfriend).

Q I've heard more teens are abstaining from sexual relationships. Is that true?

A Many more teens now are postponing having sex until they are older. It is the best way to avoid STDs and pregnancy.

S. JEAN EMANS, MD
CHILDREN'S HOSPITAL
HARVARD MEDICAL SCHOOL

STDs are diseases you can get from having sex without a condom. STDs include gonorrhea, chlamydia, genital warts, herpes, and human immunodeficiency virus (HIV). HIV is the virus that causes acquired immunodeficiency syndrome (AIDS) (see p.872).

STDs can be painful, can affect your fertility without your even knowing it, or can kill you. The best way to prevent getting an STD is to abstain from sexual intercourse.

If you think you might have an STD, or if you have had sex without a condom, get tested by your doctor immediately. It can take months before symptoms appear, and many STDs can have serious consequences if they are not treated. You also need to tell sexual partners if you have an STD so they can be treated.

You must take a complete course of medicine to be cured even if your symptoms go away before you finish your prescription. Do not have sexual intercourse again without a condom. If the person you have sex with does not like using condoms, or if you are shy about bringing up the subject, practice telling him or her. Role-play the discussion with a trusted friend or your doctor, using the exact words you would use to convince your partner. For information on how to use a condom, see p.71.

Contraception

You can get pregnant or get someone else pregnant the very first time you have sex—and any time you have sex. From the beginning of a sexual relationship, you and your partner need to take responsibility for contraception. Contraceptives are methods to prevent pregnancy. Some contraceptives, such as birth-control pills, diaphragms, IUDs (intrauterine devices), or cervical caps, need to be prescribed and/or fitted by a doctor. Hormone injections for birth control are given every 1 to 3 months.

Condoms for both men and women are available in drug-stores. Look under Planned Parenthood in the phone book for another resource for birth-control methods and medical care. See also p.68 for more information on contraception.

Pregnancy

Having a baby is a wonderful event if both parents are capable of raising a child and both have decided this is what they want.

If you become pregnant by accident, the choices you need to make are not easy. This is why not having intercourse, or using birth control to prevent an unwanted pregnancy, is your best course of action.

If you are pregnant, you have three options, as described below. It is wise to discuss them with others (especially your parents or other trusted adults), but the final decision is yours.

See also Abortion (p.922), Pregnancy (p.914), and Childbirth (p.935).

- You can continue with the pregnancy and raise the baby with the baby's father, alone, or with the help of your family. This will be difficult. Plans for your own future are likely to change dramatically because you will need to be available for your child for the next 21 years, minimum, and probably for your lifetime. You may have to drop out of school and get a job to help pay for all the things a child needs, such as diapers, food, clothing, shelter, education, and medical care.

- You can continue with the pregnancy, deliver the child, and give the baby up for adoption. Deciding to put the child up for adoption can be a good idea because you will be helping those who cannot have children of their own. In considering this option, you should keep in mind that giving up your baby after it is born may not be easy.

- You can end the pregnancy by having an abortion. Abortion is an extremely safe medical procedure that will not prevent you from getting pregnant at a later

What You Should Know About Tattoos and Body Piercing

- If possible, discuss it with your parents before you do it.

- States are increasingly requiring parental consent for piercing and tattoos for teens who are under 18; reputable piercers will uphold the law.

- Make sure that piercing is done by experienced personnel who are using clean needles and the appropriate techniques; do not try to do it yourself.

- Painkillers are not usually used before piercing.

- Avoid people who offer to perform body piercing but do not appear to keep surfaces or instruments clean. Antiseptic medicines should always be used to clean the skin before piercing.

- Antibiotic ointments should be applied to outer body-piercing sites, such as the ears or the navel, to help heal the site.

- The metal objects attached through the skin can produce severe allergic reactions and can lead to large scars called keloids (see p.555).

- Body piercing can cause serious bacterial skin infections if not done properly or cared for adequately: 1 of 5 body piercings leads to such infections.

- Serious virus infections such as hepatitis B and hepatitis C can be transmitted if the metal that pierces the skin (or the device that shoots metal through the skin) is infected by the virus. Even the virus that causes AIDS (see p.872) can be passed to the body through unclean equipment.

- Healing can take 3 to 6 weeks for piercing of the tongue, 6 to 8 weeks for piercing of the ears, lips, and eyebrows, 8 to 16 weeks for piercing of the nipples, and up to 9 months for piercing of the navel.

- Consider a tattoo permanent. Removal by laser can take up to 12 treatments, and some tattoos can never be removed.

time. It carries less medical risk than continuing with the pregnancy and going through a delivery. But it, too, can be a difficult decision.

Remember that you do not have to make this decision alone. Talk to your parents, a trusted adult friend, your doctor, or someone at your place of worship to get advice and support.

There are many services and support groups available to help you make the best decision. Planned Parenthood is one organization you can call for help. To find the number of your local Planned Parenthood clinic, look in the phone book or call the national office listed on p.1236.

Peer Pressure

As you grow up and become more independent of your parents, you will find yourself becoming involved with and influenced by your circle of friends. You may feel alienated from your parents, think that they just do not understand you, and be confused about who you are.

Being part of a group can help you feel more secure, but it can be difficult to resist when your friends try to get you to do things that you do not really want to do. You may be afraid that you will lose your friends if you do not go along with what everyone is doing. Good friends will respect you for thinking for yourself; if yours do not, look for a new group of friends whose interests and activities appeal to you. You may also find it helpful to talk to a trusted adult before getting involved in an activity you are unsure of.

Alcohol, Tobacco, and Other Drugs

Many teens start using tobacco or alcohol without thinking of all the consequences. Alcohol affects the entire body, slowing down all functions. It impairs your coordination, judgment, emotional control, and reasoning powers and makes you act in ways that are risky or reckless.

Driving after drinking alcohol can kill you, your friends, and people you do not even know. Even one-time drinkers can endanger themselves or others by making poor choices about their actions.

Drinking alcohol can reduce inhibitions and encourage carelessness, which can lead to unwanted or unsafe sex that results in pregnancy or sexually transmitted diseases (see p.889).

Using large amounts of alcohol causes serious medical problems such as liver damage, changes in the nervous system, and coma. You can also get severe stomach irritation and ulcers. Worse, you can become dependent on alcohol. Dependency means that you will be unable to go without drinking alcohol and may make excuses or break promises just to drink it.

Some people have a genetic predisposition to alcoholism, which means they are born with the potential to become an alcoholic. If you think you may have a problem, read Do You Have a Drug Problem?

Using tobacco in any form—smoking or chewing—can cause health problems. Cigarette advertisements may give the impression that it is cool to smoke, but the advertisements do not tell you that nicotine in tobacco is a highly addictive drug. Some of the short-term effects of smoking include bad breath, wrinkled skin, and chronic coughing. There are other major health problems that can occur after years of smoking, such as cancer and lung disease. Chewing tobacco can cause mouth and throat cancer. The longer you smoke, the more difficult it can be to stop. If you smoke, ask your doctor for help in quitting (see p.59).

Smoking marijuana or doing other drugs (such as LSD, heroin, or cocaine) alters your perception of reality. You can become unmotivated and not put in the effort needed to deal with challenging situations, such as school.

If you feel pressure to use alcohol or other drugs, say you are not interested, you are allergic to them, you cannot take them, or "your parents would kill you." Find a friend who wants to leave the place where drugs are present and go to a movie, out to eat, or anywhere else to remove yourself from the situation.

DO YOU HAVE A DRUG PROBLEM?

If you answer yes to even two of the questions below, you could have a drug problem and may need help. There are many resources that are specifically aimed at helping teenagers cope with addiction.

Talk to your parents, doctor, or school counselor, or contact a support group such as Alcoholics Anonymous or Narcotics Anonymous (see p.1229). The sooner you seek help, the easier it will be for you to control your problem.

- Do you drink or use other drugs to relax, feel better about yourself, or fit in?

- Do you ever drink or use other drugs while you are alone?

- Do any of your closest friends drink or use other drugs?

- Does a close family member have a problem with alcohol or other drugs?

- Does a friend, family member, or other person think you have a problem with alcohol or other drugs?

- Have you ever gotten into trouble drinking or using drugs?

Another question to ask yourself is if you have ever ridden in a car driven by someone (including yourself) who was using drugs or alcohol. If you have, read Driving Safely (below right) for ways to avoid this dangerous situation.

Anorexia and Bulimia

People who have eating disorders feel out of control around food or feel that food rules their life. Eating disorders, which include anorexia nervosa and bulimia (see p.413), often affect teenage girls who want to achieve an impossible degree of thinness. Some adolescents stop eating altogether, literally starving themselves in the process of losing weight. Teens with eating disorders have a distorted body image.

If you have an eating disorder, you see yourself as fat and want to diet even though you may be very thin. You may feel the need to exercise often. Your periods may become irregular or stop completely. You may engage in

secretive behaviors such as hiding food or eating and vomiting in private.

If you have bulimia, you have uncontrollable periods where you eat large amounts of food (bingeing) followed by making yourself vomit or take laxatives (purging).

Eating disorders are extremely serious and require medical treatment. If you or someone you know has an eating disorder, talk to your doctor, your parents, or a school counselor immediately to get help. Eating disorders can kill a person if they are not treated.

Eating Well

During adolescence your body grows so fast that it is important to eat a well-balanced diet to stay healthy. Meat, fresh fruits and vegetables, dairy products, nuts, and grains all make up a balanced diet.

Girls and young women need to be especially sure they get enough calcium (see p.44) to keep bones strong. You should take in 1,200–1,500 milligrams of calcium every day, about the amount in 4 cups of milk or three cartons of yogurt. Eating a nutritious diet is essential for all teens.

Driving Safely

Car accidents are the number one cause of teenage deaths. Prevent them by knowing the rules of the road, driving cautiously, wearing a seat belt, and not driving after using alcohol or other drugs (and not driving with anyone who has).

If you find yourself in a situation where you think you have

no choice but to get into a car with a driver who has been drinking or using other drugs, think again. You do have a choice—call your parents, a friend, or the police to get a ride home. It is best to discuss this with your parents in advance so that your parents or a responsible adult can agree to pick you up at any time, no questions asked, to ensure your safety.

Sadness and Depression

Feeling sad from time to time is normal during adolescence. Sometimes, though, people experience long periods of unhappiness accompanied by physical symptoms. This is called depression (see p.395); it is a medical disorder that can be improved with treatment.

Some of the physical symptoms of depression include sleeping too much or an inability to sleep at night (see Insomnia, p.383), loss of appetite or overeating, fatigue, and irritability. You may also experience deep feelings of hopelessness or worthlessness. It may be difficult for you to concentrate at school, leading to poor grades. You may feel isolated from your family and friends. You may even feel that your life is not worth living.

It is important to get help if you feel this way. Talk to your doctor, your parents, or a school counselor. Although talking to supportive friends or family members can help, depression is best treated by a physician, who is trained to help you through this difficult time.

Acne

Acne is the red bumps, white-heads, or blackheads that break out on the skin, particularly on your face, neck, and back. Hormones that cause the changes during puberty also cause the pores in the skin to produce more oil (called sebum).

Acne occurs when the pores of the skin become blocked with sebum, causing bacteria to multiply and the pore to become red and swollen.

For most adolescents, acne is a normal part of growing up. You may feel unattractive or self-conscious about your appearance when you have acne; however, with treatment, acne is controllable. After a couple of years, acne becomes much less of a problem.

Read the article on p.533 for treatment recommendations. There is no evidence that any activity or food causes acne.

Health of Women

In recent years, medical research has increasingly focused on the health problems of women. There has always been research on conditions that are predominantly or exclusively found in women, such as diseases of the breasts and female reproductive organs. However, there has been relatively less research done to understand the ways in which other important diseases, such as heart disease, affect women.

Women are taking a greater role in their own medical care. In most families, women also take responsibility for the health of children. Overall, women are rightly demanding more and better information about health.

Some diseases—such as osteoporosis, thyroid disorders, systemic lupus erythematosus (see p.898), rheumatoid arthritis (see p.606), and multiple sclerosis (see p.368)—affect women more often than men. Evidence indicates that this is due to the hormonal differences between men and women. In support of that theory, in animals that get diseases very similar to rheumatoid arthritis and multiple sclerosis, it is the female of the species who is most often and most seriously affected.

Other diseases may take a different course in women than in men. For example, before menopause, women are less likely than men to have heart attacks. Studies suggest that it is probably a woman's production of the hormone estrogen before menopause that protects her from developing heart disease.

However, this difference disappears in the years after menopause, when estrogen production stops. By the age of 65, heart attacks become the most common cause of death in women.

A WOMAN'S REPRODUCTIVE SYSTEM

A woman's reproductive system includes both external and internal parts of the body. The visible parts of a woman's reproductive system (the vulva) include:

Mons pubis The skin and tissue that cover the pubic bone. After puberty, the mons pubis becomes covered with pubic hair.

Labia majora and labia minora Labia means "lips" in Latin. The labia majora are liplike folds surrounding the labia minora and the vagina. They are smooth during childhood. After puberty, they become covered with pubic hair, and oil glands develop inside the labia. The labia minora are smaller folds of skin next to the vagina. Increased blood flow during sexual arousal causes them to enlarge.

External Female Genitals

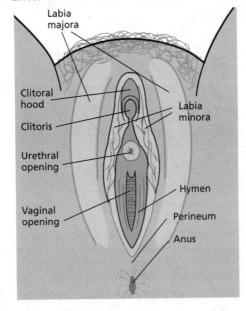

Labia majora

Clitoral hood

Clitoris

Urethral opening

Vaginal opening

Labia minora

Hymen

Perineum

Anus

The external genital structures of the female are called the vulva. Between the vulva and the anus is the perineum.

Internal Female Reproductive System

FRONT VIEW

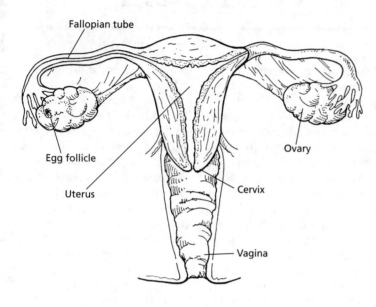

Fallopian tube

Egg follicle

Uterus

Ovary

Cervix

Vagina

SIDE VIEW

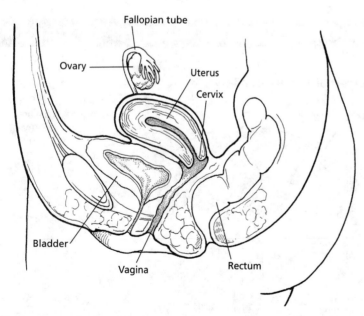

Fallopian tube

Ovary

Uterus

Cervix

Bladder

Vagina

Rectum

The female reproductive system consists of two ovaries (where eggs are stored), two fallopian tubes, the uterus, cervix, vagina, and outer genitals. Each month during menstruation, an egg is released from the ovaries. If fertilized by a sperm cell, the egg begins its journey to the uterus for implantation.

Clitoris A small, round area that becomes firmer and larger during sexual arousal. Orgasm occurs from stimulating the clitoris.

Urethra The urethral opening through which urine passes. It is located below the clitoris.

Hymen A delicate mucous membrane at the opening of the vagina. It helps protect the vagina but is not necessary for health. The hymen is usually broken or torn during a woman's first sexual intercourse, although it may be torn in some women during exercise or from inserting tampons or a diaphragm. It is usually not visible in later life.

Vaginal opening The entrance to a woman's internal reproductive organs; it is also the exit for menstrual blood, vaginal discharge, and a baby during childbirth.

Perineum The skin and tissue between the vagina and the anus.

The internal parts of a woman's reproductive system include:

Vagina The muscular canal, 3 to 5 inches long, that leads from the vaginal opening to the cervix, the entrance to the uterus. The walls of the vagina can stretch tremendously during childbirth to allow a baby to pass. Some discharge from the vagina is normal and is usually made up of secretions that lubricate the walls of the vagina.

The consistency and amount changes according to the hormones present at different stages of your menstrual cycle. This is also why the hormonal changes that accompany menopause, particularly low estrogen levels, can cause a reduction in vaginal lubrication. The vaginal opening is surrounded by strong, elastic muscles. Kegel exercises (see p.1051) help tone these muscles.

Cervix The opening to the uterus at the end of the vagina. The cervix itself is small (about 1 inch in diameter). The opening to the cervix, called the os, is a very small round hole in the middle of the cervix (after pregnancy, it appears as a 1/4-inch slit), which allows the passage of fluids, such as menstrual blood, from the uterus. During the labor of pregnancy, the os opens to 4 to 5 inches to allow the baby to come through.

Uterus A muscular organ about the size of a pear that can stretch enormously to accommodate a developing fetus. The thick inner lining of the uterus, the endometrium, is made of spongy tissue that is rich with blood, which sheds during each monthly menstruation. In pregnancy, the uterus provides a nurturing environment for the growing fetus.

Fallopian tubes Two delicate spaghetti-thin tubes that connect the uterus to the two ovaries. When an ovary releases an egg, tiny fingerlike projections at the tip of the fallopian tubes (fimbriae) help catch and sweep the egg into the tube. The fallopian tubes are critical for reproduction. They provide a passageway for the egg from the ovary to the uterus, often serve as a meeting place for egg and sperm, and move a fertilized egg down to the uterus through continuous contractions.

Ovaries Two oval-shaped organs about 1 inch in diameter that produce hormones and eggs.

TESTS WOMEN MAY HAVE

Cervical Biopsy

There are different ways to remove a piece of tissue from the cervix for analysis under a microscope. In its simplest form, your doctor can scrape some tissue from the cervix by using a curette (a spoon-shaped instrument with a sharp edge).

A punch biopsy involves cutting out a small circle of tissue with a device that looks like a paper punch. A punch biopsy can be performed in the doctor's office without anesthesia. Vaginal spotting and cramping may occur after the biopsy.

In a cone biopsy, which is used not only for diagnosis but to treat some conditions, a cone-shaped section of tissue is removed from the cervical opening. The wound is closed by stitches and by applying heat (a process called cautery) to the area.

This procedure must be performed in the hospital or day surgery unit using local or general anesthesia because the cervix is particularly sensitive to pain. Some vaginal bleeding is the most common side effect.

Colposcopy

A colposcope is a small binocular magnifying glass that helps a doctor see cell changes that could indicate a tendency to develop cancer. A colposcope also helps the physician identify the best sites for a cervical biopsy.

The doctor uses the colposcope to examine the walls of the vagina, the surface of the cervix, and the cervical canal leading into the uterus.

Colposcopy does not usually require anesthesia. Some women experience minor cramping afterward. After inserting a speculum, your doctor will wash the area being evaluated with a special solution to help identify abnormal cells. The colposcope is then used to examine the cells.

Endometrial Biopsy

An endometrial biopsy takes a sample of the endometrium (lining of the uterus).

After making sure that you are not pregnant, the doctor inserts a hollow catheter through the cervical opening until it touches the endometrium. A plunger is gently pulled back so that small pieces of endometrial tissue are sucked inside the catheter.

The biopsy is performed in the doctor's office and takes only a few minutes. The procedure can cause temporary discomfort, but anesthesia is usually not needed. You may have some spotting for a day or two afterward.

FSH and LH Blood Tests

Measuring the levels of follicle-stimulating hormone (FSH) and luteinizing hormone (LH), two hormones in your blood, can help determine the causes of abnormal menstrual cycles, lack of ovulation, and infertility, and can confirm the onset of menopause. (See p.1043 for information on the action of these two hormones in the body.)

Hysteroscopy

A hysteroscope is a thin wand inserted through the vagina and cervical canal to the inside of the uterus. It contains a light source to illuminate the uterus, a lens or video camera to transmit an image, and a device that infuses carbon dioxide or a saline solution to inflate the uterus so that the walls of the organ do not touch.

Tiny instruments such as a scalpel, laser, and scissors can also be inserted into the hysteroscope and used to perform surgery. As a diagnostic procedure, hysteroscopy is usually performed on an outpatient basis. A general or local anesthetic and painkillers may be given to alleviate discomfort.

Mammogram

A mammogram, which takes about 15 minutes, is an x-ray of your breasts. You will disrobe to the waist, put on a loose gown, and stand in front of a machine that has a camera positioned above the breast. A technologist positions one of your breasts on the lower of two compression plates, and then slowly brings the top plate down to flatten your breast.

The technologist will take a side and front view of the breast, then repeat the procedure on the other side. Women with breast implants may require additional views. For recommendations on when to have a mammogram, see p.82.

Pap Smear and HPV Test

The Pap test—short for Papanicolaou (the doctor who invented the test)—examines cells from your cervix for signs of cancer or a precancerous condition. The cells are obtained during a pelvic examination, using a small wooden instrument and a tiny brush that takes samples from inside the opening of the cervix. The cells are examined by specially trained technicians called cytologists and by computerized machines.

Cancer of the cervix is caused by certain strains of human papillomavirus (HPV). When Pap smears have a particular abnormality called ASC-US, adding an HPV test is very useful: If it is positive, you should definitely have a colposcopy examination and possibly a subsequent biopsy, but if it is negative such an examination is not necessary. The value of HPV testing with other slight Pap smear abnormalities (called LSIL and HSIL) has not been established.

The Pap smear should not be done when you are having menstrual bleeding because it can make the test less accurate. Also, you should not douche, use vaginal creams, insert a tampon, or have intercourse for 24 hours before the test. Having a pelvic examination is uncomfortable for some women. You might feel some brief cramping when the cells are being collected, but otherwise the procedure is painless.

Pelvic, Vaginal, and Breast Ultrasound

Ultrasound (see p.148) is a painless imaging procedure that can be used to visualize the internal reproductive organs and breast tissue. For a pelvic or breast ultrasound, the technologist applies a cool, clear gel on the skin and then slides an instrument called a transducer over the area being evaluated.

The transducer sends out sound waves, and receives the reflections of the sound waves, allowing the computer in the ultrasound machine to create a picture of the inside of the body.

For a vaginal ultrasound, a wand-shaped transducer (a little larger in diameter than a high-absorbency tampon) is inserted into the vagina to obtain detailed views of the uterus and ovaries.

Testing for Fungi and Trichomonas

Vaginal infection with yeast (fungus) or with trichomonas (a parasitic infection) can be confirmed by examining vaginal secretions under a microscope.

MENSTRUATION

Menstruation, or having your period, is a process in which the lining of the uterus (the endometrium) is shed. The endometrium passes through the cervix and vagina and appears outside the body as menstrual blood. Menstruation is controlled by an elaborate hormone-signaling system between the brain and the reproductive organs.

The onset of menstruation marks the maturity of a woman's reproductive organs, and the beginning of her ability to bear children. For most women, menstruation occurs about once a month, except during pregnancy and some illnesses, until menopause (see p.1047), when menstruation stops.

The first day of your menstrual period marks the beginning of a new cycle, defined as the

Menstrual Cycle

The menstrual cycle starts when the hypothalamus (a part of the brain) releases gonadotropin-releasing hormone. This stimulates the pituitary gland at the base of the brain to secrete follicle-stimulating hormone (FSH) (1), which stimulates growth of egg follicles in the ovary as well as the production of estrogen by the ovary. Estrogen travels in the blood to the uterus (2) and thickens the lining of the uterus (endometrium).

As estrogen levels rise in the blood (3), the pituitary gland responds by reducing FSH secretion, which lowers estrogen production by the ovary several days later; this is called a "negative feedback" loop, since rising estrogen levels lead to a subsequent fall in estrogen levels. The rising estrogen levels also cause the pituitary gland to produce a surge of luteinizing hormone (LH) (4). High levels of LH cause the release of a mature egg from a follicle (5). The now-empty follicle produces more estrogen as well as progesterone, both of which build up the lining of the uterus in preparation for receiving a fertilized egg (6).

The egg travels (red arrows) to the fallopian tube, where it may be fertilized. If it is fertilized, the egg then travels to the uterus, where it implants in the lining.

If fertilization does not occur, the empty follicle stops making estrogen and progesterone. When the levels of these hormones become too low to maintain the thickened endometrium, menstruation occurs. If fertilization occurs, the empty follicle continues to make estrogen and progesterone and menstruation does not occur during pregnancy.

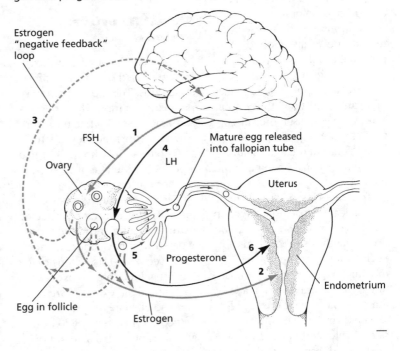

Estrogen "negative feedback" loop

3

FSH

1

4
LH

Ovary

Mature egg released into fallopian tube

Uterus

5

Progesterone

6

2

Endometrium

Egg in follicle

Estrogen

time between the first day of one period and the first day of the next period. The average length of a menstrual cycle is 28 days, but normal cycles can vary from 21 to 35 days. Usually, the length of a menstrual cycle is consistent for an individual woman, but many things can disrupt the cycle (see Irregular Periods, p.1045). Normal menstrual periods vary in length from woman to woman from 3 to 7 days.

Menstrual Hygiene

Menstrual blood is clean and odorless until it comes in contact with bacteria in the vagina and in the air. The bacteria reproduce rapidly in the warm moisture of menstrual blood, causing a disagreeable odor. Bathe or shower daily and change tampons and menstrual pads frequently to keep bacteria from growing and odor from developing.

Tampons are safe to use but require special attention to a few potential problems. If you notice that your vaginal opening is dry and irritated, apply a water-based lubricant to the tip of the tampon. Make sure you insert the tampon well past the vaginal opening so that it does not rub against and irritate the vaginal opening or the urethra.

Toxic shock syndrome (see p.879) is a rare bacterial infection that has been associated with the use of highly absorbent tampons. Such tampons create tiny tears in the lining of the vagina, permitting bacteria and a toxin made by the bacteria to enter the bloodstream. Symptoms include a sudden high fever (over 102°F), a peeling red rash, diarrhea, and

muscle aches. To reduce the chance of this illness, use tampons of the lowest possible absorbency and leave them in your vagina for no longer than 4 hours before inserting a fresh tampon.

Douching is a method of cleansing the vagina, usually by flushing it with water or another preparation. Douching is not necessary and can be harmful. Vaginal secretions naturally clean the vagina and control bacterial growth. Douching upsets the natural balance of bacteria in the vagina, allowing yeast or a type of bacteria to grow. It can irritate the vagina with perfumes and can flush bacteria into the uterus, increasing the risk for infection. Control odor by washing the outside of your vaginal area daily and by changing tampons or pads frequently.

Absent Menstrual Periods

Absent periods, or amenorrhea, can be caused by a variety of conditions. The most common is pregnancy, during which periods stop. Most women begin to menstruate by the time they are 16 years old. A girl who has not had a period by the age of 16 should see her doctor.

Temporary interruptions in the menstrual cycle can occur due to extreme dieting and weight loss. Women who have anorexia nervosa (see p.413) stop menstruating altogether. Intense exercise or sports training, extreme stress, and use of some drugs, such as corticosteroids (see p.895), can also disrupt the balance of hormones that control menstruation,

Charting Your Period

If you have PMS or if your periods are irregular, keep a chart of your periods and your symptoms. Start on day 1 of your period and continue for 4 to 6 months.

Each day, note your physical symptoms (such as bloating or headaches), the amount of menstrual flow (including the presence of clots), your level of pain (low to high on a scale of 1 to 10), and the number of tampons or pads you use. Include information on your emotional state and any food cravings.

The chart can identify patterns or behaviors that you can change and may help you see the benefits of any changes you make, such as a reduction in caffeine before your period. Take the chart to each doctor's appointment so that you and your physician can plan a treatment strategy.

resulting in absent periods. This can interfere with fertility.

Women who are approaching menopause (see p.1047) often miss periods. Hormonal disorders such as hypothyroidism (see p.848), pituitary gland tumors (see p.860), and polycystic ovary syndrome (see p.1081) can also cause absence of periods.

If you are sexually active and miss a period, take a home pregnancy test or see your doctor for a blood pregnancy test, which is more accurate. If you miss two periods and are certain you are not pregnant, see your physician.

He or she will perform a physical exam and may perform blood tests to evaluate your hormone levels. Further tests and medicines may be used to diagnose whether the absent periods are due to another hormonal disorder or to problems with your reproductive hormone levels.

Treatment depends on the underlying cause. Changing medicines, treating a hormonal disorder, or having hormone replacement therapy can return your menstrual cycle. It is important to find the cause of your absent periods and restore the regular menstrual cycle, not only if you want to become pregnant but also to decrease the risk of uterine cancer (see Cancer of the Endometrium, p.1071) and promote health, especially of your bones and heart.

Heavy Periods

Heavy menstrual periods are those that cause more blood loss than usual or last for more than 7 days. Heavy periods are common in girls just starting their periods and in women nearing menopause.

Heavy periods that are also painful may be caused by pelvic inflammatory disease (see p.1077), fibroids (see p.1074), an intrauterine device (IUD) (see p.74), or endometriosis (see p.1073). A heavy period that occurs late in your menstrual cycle can indicate a miscarriage (see p.928).

In some women, heavy periods are caused by failure to ovulate (see Causes of Infertility, p.904). The level of the hormone progesterone is too low to regulate the shedding of the uterine lining, resulting in longer and unpredictable periods.

See your doctor if you think you may have had a miscarriage. He or she may need to perform dilation and curettage (D&C) (see p.1077) to remove any tissue that was not expelled. It is also a good idea to see your doctor if you have several heavy periods. The doctor will do a pelvic examination and may perform a pelvic ultrasound, endometrial biopsy, or hysteroscopy (see p.1042) to examine your uterus for a source of excessive bleeding.

Treatment depends on the underlying cause. Removing an IUD can help relieve bleeding and pain. Iron supplements are often recommended for women with heavy bleeding to prevent iron-deficiency anemia (see p.715).

Irregular Periods

Periods that occur fewer than 21 days apart, or more than 35 days apart, are considered irregular. Irregular periods are a normal part of adolescence and the years preceding menopause, when the hormones that regulate menstruation are changing. Some women have irregular periods most of their adult lives. Others experience changes in their normal pattern with stress, diet, travel, illness, or exercise. Irregular periods do not signal a medical problem for most women but they can cause worry or stress.

Unexpected spotting of menstrual blood is a common type of irregular period. Slight bleeding midway through your period may be caused by hormonal changes that occur with ovulation. Irregu-

lar bleeding accompanied by nipple discharge can occur with pituitary gland tumors (see p.860).

See your doctor if you have irregular periods. He or she will perform a pelvic examination (see p.1069) and possibly blood tests to evaluate levels of the hormones that regulate menstruation and/or the hormones from the pituitary gland, thyroid gland, and hypothalamus.

Higher-than-normal levels of male hormones can also interfere with regular periods, and can cause excessive hair growth and acne. Your doctor will treat any underlying disease or hormonal problem. Birth-control pills can also help regulate periods.

Painful Periods

About 80% of women have some discomfort during their periods. For most, the pain is a normal part of menstruation caused by the release of substances called prostaglandins that induce painful spasms of the uterus (cramping).

Other women have pain that is caused by an underlying condition, such as fibroids (see p.1074), pelvic inflammatory disease (see p.1077), endometriosis (see p.1073), or an intrauterine device (IUD) (see p.74). Some women experience pain during ovulation, halfway through their menstrual cycle. This is caused by the release of an egg from the ovary.

SYMPTOMS

Pain may be felt as cramping in the lower abdomen or aching pain in the back or legs. The pain may be accompanied by vomiting, diarrhea, constipation, headache, dizziness, and fainting. The pain usually begins the day the period starts, and stops by the end of the second or third day.

Painful periods often disappear when a woman reaches her 30s or after pregnancy. If the pain is caused by an underlying disorder, it may be of a different quality and begin after years of not experiencing menstrual pain.

TREATMENT OPTIONS

Most women obtain relief by taking nonsteroidal anti-inflammatory drugs (NSAIDs) such as aspirin or ibuprofen, which work by reducing contractions of the uterus. Take them when you first feel discomfort, and follow the suggestions in Home Remedies for Premenstrual Symptoms and Cramps (see right). Some women find it useful to start taking NSAIDs 1 or 2 days before the expected start of their period.

The birth-control pill can also help prevent pain by preventing ovulation and, therefore, reducing the amount of blood in the endometrium (the lining of the uterus). Periods tend to be lighter and less painful. See your doctor about any menstrual pain that is severe or that you have not experienced before. He or she will perform a pelvic examination (see p.1069). Treating any underlying cause often relieves symptoms.

Premenstrual Syndrome

Premenstrual syndrome (PMS) is a collection of symptoms (including bloating, headaches, mood swings, and depression) occurring during the days between ovulation and menstruation, when the ovaries are making progesterone.

Home Remedies for Premenstrual Symptoms and Cramps

Menstrual cramps can be relieved by a nonprescription painkiller such as aspirin or ibuprofen. The following home remedies can help ease discomfort of premenstrual symptoms and cramps.

To reduce premenstrual symptoms the week before your period:

- Limit your intake of salty and sweet foods.
- Reduce your intake of caffeine-containing drinks and chocolate.
- Avoid alcohol, which can cause the body to retain water.
- Exercise to improve circulation and general well-being.

To reduce the discomfort of menstrual cramps:

- Keep warm. Place a heating pad or hot water bottle over your abdomen, sip warm liquids, and take hot baths.
- Have sexual intercourse. Some women find that orgasm helps decrease menstrual cramps.
- Elevate your legs slightly (over a pillow) while lying down.
- Lie on one side in a fetal position with your knees bent.
- Get a massage or back rub.
- Eat light, frequent meals.
- Relax with meditation or slow, conscious breathing.

At least 75% of women who ovulate experience one or more of the symptoms of PMS. Only about 5% have symptoms severe enough to disrupt their lives and relationships, which constitutes the medical definition of PMS.

The exact causes of PMS are not known. Studies suggest that women with PMS have certain brain chemicals (particularly one called gamma-aminobutyric acid, or GABA) that respond abnormally to fluctuations of sex hormone levels. In the past it was suggested that PMS was an emotional overreaction to normal symptoms and primarily a psychiatric problem. This now seems unlikely.

SYMPTOMS

Fatigue is the most common physical symptom of PMS, followed by cravings for sweet or salty foods, abdominal bloating, swollen hands or feet, headaches, tender breasts, and nausea or other gastrointestinal upsets.

Depression and irritability are the most widely reported psychological symptoms. Some women experience mood swings, tearfulness, and problems with concentration and memory.

Dental and mouth problems, such as gingivitis (see p.474), cold sores, canker sores, swollen salivary glands, and excessive bleeding during dental procedures, can also occur.

Treating PMS: Dr Rigotti's Advice

I generally recommend that a woman suffering from PMS start by paying attention to lifestyle factors. Women spend much of their lives caring for others and need to be reminded how important it is for them to take extra care of themselves, particularly at the time of the month when they feel most vulnerable.

This means simple things like getting regular aerobic exercise; avoiding caffeine, alcohol, salt, and concentrated sweets; eating frequent small meals instead of a few large meals a day; and practicing stress reduction techniques such as the relaxation response. Adding a supplement such as vitamin B_6 to their diet also helps some women.

If several months of following these steps are not enough to control symptoms, I usually recommend trying an SSRI (selective serotonin reuptake inhibitor)–type antidepressant medication as the next step. There is clear evidence that these drugs help, especially with mood swings and other psychological symptoms that are often the most troublesome.

NANCY RIGOTTI, MD
MASSACHUSETTS GENERAL HOSPITAL
HARVARD MEDICAL SCHOOL

TREATMENT OPTIONS

Charting your period and any accompanying symptoms (see p.1044) can help you and your physician determine a treatment plan. Dietary modification and increased physical activity are the first line of treatment of PMS.

Consuming more calcium (taking a calcium supplement of 1,200 milligrams every day may reduce symptoms), magnesium, and vitamins E and B_6, as well as eliminating caffeine, nicotine, alcohol, and salt, may also be recommended.

Some women find that eating five or six small meals a day helps relieve symptoms. Regular exercise can alleviate mood swings by raising the level of endorphins (brain substances that promote a sense of well-being) and reducing bloating.

Prescription drug therapy may include taking selective serotonin reuptake inhibitors (see p.400), which are antidepressants, and prostaglandin (pain receptor) inhibitors, which help relieve some of the physical discomforts of PMS.

For severe PMS, drugs that inhibit estrogen production, called gonadotropin-releasing hormone agonists, have been shown to reduce symptoms. Taking them eliminates your menstrual cycle entirely but can also cause menopauselike symptoms and increase your risk of osteoporosis.

MENOPAUSE

Menopause is not a definitive event like the first time you menstruate. The window in time before periods stop, but after they become irregular, is called perimenopause. It is a gradual process during which periods become irregular and then stop altogether.

Menopause itself is often defined as the absence of menstrual periods for 12 months in a row. It is accompanied by low levels of the female hormone estrogen.

For most women, the process begins in the mid-40s and ends with the last menstrual period at about age 50. However, periods can end at a much earlier or later age. Lifestyle factors play a role in the timing of menopause (for example, cigarette smoking may lead to an earlier menopause). Women who have both ovaries surgically removed (see p.1079) experience menopause immediately.

The changes during menopause are related to changes in the function of the ovaries. At birth, your two ovaries contain a lifetime supply of eggs—over 350,000 per ovary. Around the time of puberty, estrogen production begins in the cells of the follicle (the individual chamber that houses each egg). Estrogen is also produced in much smaller amounts by fat tissue.

In simple terms, menopause marks the end of the reproductive years. The ovaries no longer proceed through the monthly cycle of maturing an egg and preparing the uterus for pregnancy. This causes a decrease in the body's estrogen supply from the ovaries. In a woman, estrogen exerts an effect on the cells of blood vessels, bone, skin, the uterus, breast tissue, the lining of the vagina and urinary tract, and the brain. When estrogen levels decrease, each of these tissues and organs is affected, causing hot flashes, vaginal dryness, and urinary tract irritation in some women.

Fat Distribution Before and After Menopause

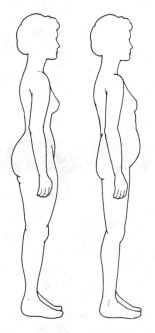

Before menopause, fat tends to concentrate more in the hips and thighs. After menopause, fat tends to concentrate more in the abdomen and above the waist.

The "change of life" during menopause really describes the body's adjustment to a change in estrogen level. Over time, the beneficial effects of estrogen on the bone and on the heart's blood vessels are lost; osteoporosis and heart disease become more common in women who have gone through menopause. Hormone therapy (HT) (see p.1049) is designed to reduce both the short-term symptoms and the long-term health consequences of menopause.

The symptoms of menopause (see p.1049) are sometimes subtle. For this reason, your physician may order blood tests to measure follicle-stimulating hormone (FSH) and luteinizing hormone (LH) levels. These hormones are produced by the pituitary gland in response to stimulation by the hypothalamus, a part of the brain involved in the hormonal signaling process during the menstrual cycle.

During perimenopause, the hypothalamus senses low levels of estrogen and tries to stimulate the ovary with very high levels of FSH and LH. The results of tests for these hormones can help you and your doctor know if you are entering perimenopause.

TREATMENT OPTIONS

Treatment during menopause has had two distinct goals. First, treatment aims to alleviate the symptoms caused by hormonal changes. Until 2002, HT was also prescribed by many doctors for many years following menopause because studies had suggested

Do You Need Tests to Tell If You're Entering Menopause? Dr Gharib's Advice

It can be hard to tell when you're starting menopause. You don't change overnight from a life of regular periods to a life of no periods and hot flashes. Usually, periods become irregular for a couple of years before they stop, and hot flashes can begin even when you're still menstruating.

When you're definitely going through menopause, blood levels of follicle-stimulating hormone (FSH) increase (so doctors sometimes measure FSH level to determine if you're in menopause). However, when you are just entering menopause, FSH levels can be way up one month and down the next (and therefore are not very helpful to measure at this stage).

On the other hand, I use FSH levels to assess how likely it is that a woman in her 30s or 40s will be able to get pregnant. If FSH is at twice normal levels, it is unlikely a woman will be able to conceive.

SOHEYLA GHARIB, MD
BRIGHAM AND WOMEN'S HOSPITAL
HARVARD MEDICAL SCHOOL

Symptoms of Menopause

No two women experience menopause in the same way. Your body is influenced by your overall health, nutrition, stress level, exercise routine, and heredity.

The following chart lists the most common symptoms. Most women do not experience all of them and many women experience only a few.

WHEN	SYMPTOM	DESCRIPTION
Perimenopause	Irregular periods	Menstrual cycle becomes shorter and less regular; you may still be fertile.
Menopause	Hot flashes	Sensation of dramatic changes in body temperature that sometimes begin several years before periods actually stop.
	Insomnia/night sweats	Disturbed sleep, possibly caused by nighttime hot flashes.
Menopause and beyond	Vaginal dryness; urinary irritation or incontinence	Thinning of the vaginal wall and bladder, along with decreased vaginal secretions, can cause vaginal dryness, pain during intercourse, higher risk of vaginal or urinary tract infections, and urinary incontinence (see p.826).
	Sexual problems	May be caused by loss of libido due to low testosterone (produced by the ovary before menopause) levels but can also be a result of vaginal irritation due to vaginal dryness.
	Mood changes	Irritability, anxiety, stress, and depression are not caused by lower estrogen levels, but may occur as a result of disturbed sleep.
Long-term changes	Bone loss (see Osteoporosis, p.596)	Bones become more porous, increasing the risk of breaking a bone.

various health benefits. That has since changed.

Hormone Therapy

Reducing menopausal symptoms For nearly a century, women have taken hormone therapy (HT)—either estrogen alone or a combination of estrogen and progesterone/progestin—to relieve menopausal symptoms in the short term.

(In many women intense menopausal symptoms last only a few years.) There is little doubt that HT effectively relieves such symptoms, although there are other options for achieving the same goal (see "Alternatives to Hormone Therapy").

Long-term use of HT Beginning in the 1950s, women began taking HT for longer periods. Several popular theories held that there were many health benefits

from continued exposure to "youthful" levels of these hormones. By the mid 1970s, it became clear that women whose uterus had not been removed were at greater risk for cancer of the uterus if they took estrogen alone, and so most women took HT preparations that included a combination of estrogen and progestin.

By the mid 1990s, many large, carefully conducted studies had concluded that HT taken for several years or longer probably did have important health effects, some bad but most good. These studies were largely cohort studies (see p.34). In general, they found that long-term use of HT appeared to reduce the risk of heart disease, osteoporosis, and colon cancer, but apparently increased the risk of breast cancer, blood clots, and gallbladder disease. There was weaker evidence that HT might reduce the risk of stroke and dementia. Given the number of women affected by these medical conditions, it seemed as though—for most women—HT was more likely to be helpful than harmful.

In cohort studies, researchers compare the medical records of women who have used hormones with those who have not. Such studies are not regarded as conclusive. It was possible, for example, that the apparent lower risk of heart disease was not caused by taking HT, but rather by something else about the women who chose to take HT—something that the doctors would not have predicted and did not think to measure.

Despite the well-recognized imperfection of cohort studies, the research that had been published involved hundreds of thousands of women followed for several decades, and in general these studies came to similar conclusions. In the mid 1990s this was the best available evidence to guide doctors and patients. And the evidence seemed to say that, for the average woman, the benefits of long-term HT exceeded the risks.

Skin Patch for Estrogen Replacement

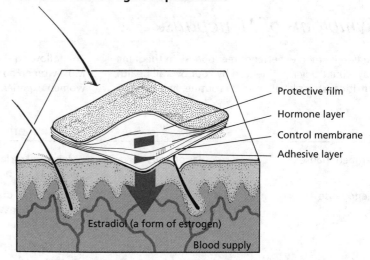

Protective film
Hormone layer
Control membrane
Adhesive layer

Estradiol (a form of estrogen)
Blood supply

This skin patch has four layers. The adhesive layer, the layer closest to the body, holds the patch to the skin. Next is a thin membrane, called the control membrane, through which the estrogen passes at a slow, steady speed. On top of that is a layer that contains the reservoir of estrogen. On the top of the patch is a layer of protective film. A patch containing both estrogen and progesterone was made available in 1999. The patch is changed once or twice a week, depending on the type of patch.

The Women's Health Initiative

Doctors realized, however, that the best available evidence was not the best possible evidence. Experts agreed that the most reliable and conclusive evidence on HT would come from randomized, controlled trials (see p.31). In such a study, researchers randomly assign women to take a medicine (like HT) or a placebo (sugar pill). In such a study, the women who take HT should be identical to the women who take the sugar pill in every respect except one: whether they took HT or the placebo. Therefore, any differences in their medical condition years later are likely to be explained by the one significant difference between them: the kind of pill they took.

The government, through the National Institutes of Health,

began just such a trial in the early 1990s. It was called the Women's Health Initiative (WHI). The WHI was designed to settle once and for all the question of whether long-term hormone therapy could prevent heart disease and other degenerative conditions in healthy postmenopausal women. Women who had a uterus were placed on a specific combination HT pill (Prempro) or placebo. Women who no longer had a uterus were placed on one particular estrogen pill (Premarin) or placebo. Researchers tested Prempro and Premarin because doctors prescribed these HT formulations most often.

In July 2002, the WHI reported the results of the Prempro trial. Just like most of the cohort studies before it, the WHI found that

Alternatives to Hormone Therapy

If you do not want to have hormone therapy (HT), there are other things you can do to achieve some of the benefits. Some involve the use of hormone preparations applied to the vagina; others are nonhormonal.

SYMPTOM	RECOMMENDATIONS
Vaginal dryness	▪ Insert estrogen ointments and creams into your vagina. ▪ Wear a soft estrogen-containing ring in your vagina. ▪ Use water-based lubricants during intercourse. ▪ Remain sexually active, which helps preserve the elasticity of the vaginal wall. ▪ Do Kegel exercises (see right) regularly.
Reduced sex drive	▪ Testosterone in pills, in cream applied to the vulva, or implanted under the skin, helps some women.
Hot flashes / night sweats	▪ Dress in layers so you can remove layers of clothing during a hot flash. ▪ Avoid alcohol and caffeine-containing drinks and food. ▪ Adding soy products to your diet may help some women, but not most. ▪ A blood pressure medicine called clonidine, a seizure medicine called gabapentin, and the SSRI antidepressant drugs all may help some women in dealing with the symptoms.

HT users had *reduced* rates of colorectal cancer, hip fractures, and spinal fractures, and *increased* rates of invasive breast cancer and blood clots in the veins, in particular, those that traveled to the lungs.

However, the WHI Prempro trial found something strikingly different from—indeed the opposite of—the results of many cohort studies: The risk of heart disease *increased*. So did the risk of stroke. The increased risks of heart disease and stroke were seen in the first two years of treatment, and the increased risk of breast cancer shortly thereafter.

Because heart disease and stroke are common and serious health problems, the WHI concluded that the risks of long-term Prempro outweighed the bene-

Kegel Exercises for Pelvic Floor Muscles

The muscles of the pelvic floor are responsible for the strength, tone, and elasticity of the vagina and urethra (the opening to your bladder).

During childbirth, these muscles expand and stretch to deliver the baby; after menopause, they become weaker due to lower estrogen levels. Kegel exercises help restore the tone of these muscles.

Perform the following Kegel exercises to strengthen your pelvic floor muscles and help prevent urinary incontinence:

1 To locate these muscles, stop the flow of urine midstream or squeeze your vagina around your finger or a tampon.

2 Contract and relax the muscle, in quick succession, ten times.

3 Rest for 10 seconds.

4 Contract and hold for 10 seconds, or as long as you can.

5 Rest for 10 seconds.

6 Repeat, working gradually to about 150 contractions a day. Hold the contractions for increasingly longer periods of time.

fits. As a result, the 16,000 women in the study were told to stop taking the medication, and researchers urged the 6 million women on this medication to reconsider their decision with their doctors.

In 2003, the WHI published another report that Prempro did little to improve overall well-

Risks Associated with Taking Prempro

For every 10,000 women who take Prempro, compared with women who do not, each year there will be:

- 8 more cases of breast cancer
- 6 more heart attacks
- 7 more strokes
- 18 more life-threatening blood clots
- 5 fewer hip fractures
- 6 fewer cases of colon cancer

Tips for Tapering Off HT

THE TWO-WEEK PLAN

- Take a full dose every other day (instead of daily) for one week
- Cut back to half doses on alternate days the second week
- Then discontinue completely

F=FULL DOSE   ½ =HALF DOSE

	S	M	T	W	Th	F	S
Week 1	F		F		F		F
2		½		½		½	
3		Discontinue use					

THE SIX-WEEK PLAN

- Skip one dose in the first week
- Skip one additional dose in each following week
- Discontinue use completely in sixth week

	S	M	T	W	Th	F	S
Week 1	F		F	F	F	F	F
2	F		F	F	F		F
3	F		F		F		F
4	F		F		F		
5	F				F		
6	F		Discontinue use				

being or cognitive function above and beyond relieving menopausal symptoms. Worse, it doubled the risk of dementia in women over age 65.

In 2004, the WHI published results from those women that had taken estrogen (Premarin) only. While estrogen did lower the risk of hip fracture, surprisingly it did not affect the risks of heart disease, breast cancer, colorectal cancer, or blood clots in the lungs. It did, however, increase the risk of stroke, and for that reason the women in this study, too, were told to stop taking Premarin.

Putting the risks in perspective Although the WHI demonstrated conclusively that for study volunteers taking Prempro, the risks outweighed the benefits, the *magnitude* of the risks was quite small (see Risks Associated with Taking Prempro).

Were the women in the WHI too old? The WHI trial used the most powerful study design, involved a large number of participants, and was carefully conducted. Yet, the results apply to the type of women who were in the study and to the forms of estrogen and progesterone/progestin tested. It is uncertain if the results apply to women who are different in some important respect, or to alternative hormone preparations.

The average age for women in the WHI was 63. The average age at which women enter menopause in the U.S. is 51. Some critics argue that had the typical woman in the study been in her early 50s the results with regard to heart disease and stroke might have been different. They cite studies in animals

Hormone Therapy:
Dr Col's Advice

The results of the WHI have caused many of my patients to ask me whether they should use HT at all, even for short-term symptom relief as they begin to experience menopausal symptoms. I tell my patients to think about it this way:

If your menopausal symptoms are severe, HT is one option that can help, but there are others. If you take HT, you need to estimate the risks and decide whether you're willing to accept them. Only you can gauge the value of relieving your symptoms, but your doctor can help you estimate the risks.

Hormone therapy (HT) remains the most effective treatment for hot flashes and vaginal dryness, two of the most disruptive menopausal symptoms. But HT does not always do the trick, and sometimes it causes more symptoms (vaginal discharge, uterine bleeding, breast discomfort) than it relieves. Other remedies are less effective than HT, but carry fewer risks. Neurontin (an epilepsy treatment) and certain antidepressants and blood pressure medications can help relieve hot flashes and night sweats. Lifestyle change is definitely an approach worth trying. Exercise and relaxation techniques can help control hot flashes. Many women get relief by avoiding caffeine, spicy foods, and other "triggers."

Does HT make sense for you? The chart titled Weighing Individual Factors (p.1054) summarizes the known risks and benefits. For an average woman, combined HT lowers the risk of osteoporosis and colorectal cancer while increasing the risk of breast cancer, blood clots, heart disease, and stroke. (Stroke is the main hazard of estrogen alone.)

But you are almost surely not the "average woman." If age, family history, or lifestyle makes you especially vulnerable to breast cancer or cardiovascular disease, then HT will carry higher-than-average risks. But HT will pose fewer hazards if you start out at low risk for these conditions.

Whether your own risk is high or low, it makes sense to try lifestyle and nonhormonal strategies first. They're safer than HT and many women find them effective. If that approach doesn't work, and you want to consider HT, look at the risks you face, as summarized in Risks Associated with Taking Prempro (p.1052). As the chart makes clear, most women will not develop breast cancer or cardiovascular disease during any five-year period, whether they take HT or not.

If you start HT, take the lowest effective dose for the shortest possible time. Half the standard dose is often enough. If you experience substantial improvement on HT, stick with the regimen for 6 to 12 months, then gradually taper off (see Tips for Tapering Off HT [p.1052]). If your symptoms return with a vengeance, try another 6 to 12 months of treatment. But if they return in a milder form, try managing them with lifestyle changes or nonhormonal medications. If vaginal dryness is your primary complaint, an estrogen cream or ring may relieve it without affecting the rest of your body.

If your symptoms persist after two years of hormone therapy, you should carefully reevaluate the dangers, for they increase over time. Your doctor can help explain the risks, but only you can decide whether they're worth taking.

NANANDA COL, MD
BRIGHAM AND WOMEN'S HOSPITAL
HARVARD MEDICAL SCHOOL

showing that HT has beneficial effects in younger animals, with less atherosclerosis, whereas it has harmful effects in older animals with more atherosclerosis.

Other doctors counter that there were over 5,000 women (33%) younger than 60 in the WHI, and the results for them were not statistically differ-

ent from those in the older women. Furthermore, none of the previous cohort studies demonstrated any clear difference in HT effect according to

Weighing Individual Factors

Each woman is different and has to make her own decision about HT, taking her whole family and medical history into account.

BREAST CANCER

Factors that raise your risk:

- Advancing age
- Close relatives with breast cancer or ovarian cancer
- Having a first child after 30
- Late menopause (after 55)
- Early menstruation (before 12)
- Alcohol (2 or more drinks a day)

Factors that lower your risk:

- Having a first child before 20
- Breast-feeding
- Late menstruation (after 13)

BLOOD CLOTS

Factors that raise your risk:

- Previous blood clots
- Family history of clotting disorders
- Obesity

CARDIOVASCULAR DISEASE

Factors that raise your risk:

- Cigarette smoking
- High blood pressure
- Diabetes
- Obesity or inactivity
- High cholesterol levels
- Family history of early heart disease (before 55 in males or 64 in females)

Factors that lower your risk:

- Ideal body weight
- Regular aerobic activity

---

the woman's age or years since menopause.

So does age matter? It would take a study like the WHI enrolling younger women to demonstrate for sure that HT has a different effect in younger women than in older women. Such a study would have to be many times the size of the WHI, and therefore very expensive, in order to provide definitive answers, because the number of heart attacks and strokes that occur in younger women is very small, under any circumstances.

No such large studies have been started. However, a randomized, controlled study of HT in younger women is under way. Instead of measuring the rates of heart disease, stroke, and other

diseases, this study is measuring *markers* of atherosclerosis such as the thickness of the wall of the main arteries sending blood to the brain. If this smaller study shows a positive effect on markers of atherosclerosis, it will not prove that HT in younger women actually reduces the risk of atherosclerosis.

Did WHI use the right forms of estrogen and progesterone?
Some argue that the results might have been different had an estrogen and progesterone/progestin preparation other than Prempro and Premarin been used. Others argue that virtually all of the earlier cohort studies that suggested HT prevented heart disease were based on Prempro and Premarin, not on other preparations.

Nevertheless, there are several reasons to think that if the WHI had used different estrogen and progesterone/progestin preparations, the results might have been different. Prempro and Premarin use multiple estrogens collected from the urine of pregnant mares: These are chemically different from the two primary forms of estrogen circulating in a woman's body. Different forms of estrogen can have quite different effects on tissues, such as the lining of blood vessels in the heart.

Prempro also uses a synthetic form of progesterone that is chemically different from that made by a woman's ovaries. As with estrogens, different forms of this hormone can have different effects on tissues.

⊘ *Preventing Breast Cancer*

Women who are at increased risk for developing breast cancer (including women with a mother, sister, or daughter who has had breast cancer or a woman who has already had breast cancer) may be able to reduce their risks by taking an antiestrogen medicine such as tamoxifen. However, tamoxifen can increase the risk of cancer of the endometrium (see p.1070) and pulmonary embolism (see p.512).

Early studies indicate that newer "designer estrogens" such as raloxifene (see Treatment Options, p.1059) may also reduce the risk of breast cancer, but with fewer side effects than tamoxifen. Genetic testing for several breast cancer genes is not recommended for all women. Women who have more than one first-degree relative (such as a mother, sister, or daughter) with breast cancer should discuss screening for breast cancer genes with their doctor.

Most Common Sites for Breast Tumors

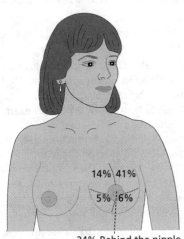

34% Behind the nipple

Cancerous breast tumors occur most often in the upper quadrant of the breast nearest the armpit.

Ductal Carcinoma In Situ

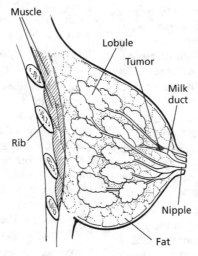

Ductal carcinoma in situ (in situ means "in place") is an early stage of breast cancer that is confined to the breast's milk ducts.

Mammogram

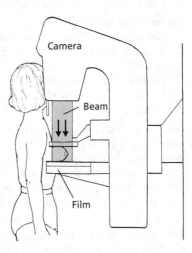

For a mammogram, the breast is pressed between two plates. An x-ray beam passes through the breast to create an image of the inside of the breast.

Finally, most women take HT in pill form. The medication is absorbed in the gut. High concentrations of these hormones travel first from the gut through the liver. Thereafter, much lower concentrations travel through the blood to reach the rest of the body. This is quite different from what happens naturally: The estrogen and progesterone from the ovaries go immediately to all parts of the body. High concentrations do not pass through the liver.

High concentrations of estrogen passing through the liver cause the liver to make increased amounts of certain molecules that may promote atherosclerosis. For this reason, even before the results of the WHI were reported, some doctors recommended that women use an estrogen skin patch rather than an estrogen-containing pill to reduce the risks of blood clots.

Tests for Evaluating Breast Lumps

Diagnosing the cause of a lump in your breast may involve one or more of these tests:

Mammography (see p.1055) can help determine if a lump may be malignant (seen on x-ray film as an irregular mass with tentaclelike appendages and speckles of calcium) and can assist the doctor in mapping the location of the lump for biopsy. Mammography can also identify other areas in both breasts that should be evaluated.

Ultrasound (see p.1042) is sometimes used for mapping the location of a lump for biopsy and is especially good at showing if the lump is solid or filled with fluid (fluid-filled lumps are usually harmless cysts).

Mammography and ultrasound are often followed by further tests to obtain a sample of fluid or breast tissue from the lump for evaluation under a microscope. All of the following tests may be performed on an outpatient basis. Information from your breast examination, mammogram, or ultrasound helps your doctor decide which tests should be performed.

Fine-needle aspiration uses a small needle and syringe to withdraw fluid or tissue from a breast lump. First, the skin above the lump is numbed with a local anesthetic (see p.168). Next, a small needle is inserted into the lump and the plunger on the syringe is pulled back to allow fluid or cells to be collected in the syringe.

If the lump is filled with liquid (which is usually a sign of a harmless cyst), the fluid may be sent to a laboratory, where a pathologist uses a microscope to look for any abnormal cells. Tissue from a solid lump is transferred to a slide and sent to a pathologist. A solid lump is not necessarily cancerous. It can be a benign fibroadenoma (see p.1062).

Biopsy involves removing more tissue from the breast lump than is taken during fine-needle aspiration. There are several types of biopsies:

Needle biopsy involves using a local anesthetic (see p.168) to numb the skin and breast tissue around the lump. A flat needle is inserted into the lump to collect a sample of breast tissue. More tissue is obtained through needle biopsy than through fine-needle aspiration.

Excisional biopsy removes the entire lump. This should not be confused with a lumpectomy (see p.1060), which is an operation to remove a malignant tumor. Lumpectomy removes more tissue than an excisional biopsy. If removing the entire lump would constitute a major operation because of the lump's size or nearby structures, an incisional biopsy (below) can be performed. With either an excisional or incisional biopsy, the cut in the skin is stitched closed and may leave a small scar.

Incisional biopsy involves cutting only a small slice of tissue from the lump.

Wire localization biopsy, also called needle localization biopsy, is used to locate a lump or suspicious breast tissue that was detected during mammography but cannot be felt or is difficult to find during a physical examination. Local anesthesia (see p.168) is used to numb the skin of your breast. A radiologist directs a series of thin wires around the lump (as seen on the mammogram) to outline it for the surgeon. The surgeon then uses the wires as guides to remove a sample of tissue from the area. The wires are removed and the incision is stitched closed, leaving only a small scar.

Stereotactic biopsy uses a computer to locate an area or lump seen on a mammogram that may be difficult to find during a physical examination. You lie face-down on a table that contains an opening for your breast. A mammogram is taken, and the location of the area or lump is plotted by computer. After a local anesthetic (see p.168) is injected, an electronically controlled needle (directed by computer) takes a tissue sample from the mapped area.

BREASTS

Mastitis and Breast Abscesses

Infections of the breast are most common in women who are breast-feeding. Otherwise, breast infections can occur in women who have had surgery on their breasts, particularly when lymph glands have been removed, or in women with compromised immune systems due to chemotherapy or diseases such as AIDS.

Stages of Breast Cancer

The stage of breast cancer (whether it has spread and, if so, how much) is an important factor in making decisions about treatment. A number of tests—including mammography, computed tomography (see p.149) of the brain and abdomen, bone scans (see p.622), and removal of part or all of the lymph glands under the arm—can be used to define the stage. The stages of breast cancer are outlined here. In addition to these stages, breast cancer can be defined in the following ways:

Carcinoma in situ "In situ" means "in place." This is the earliest stage of breast cancer (stage 0), when the cancer has not spread to other parts of the body. Cancer is confined to the milk ducts or the lobules, the glands that produce milk. The abnormality is usually brought to your doctor's attention through mammography (not breast examination).

Inflammatory breast cancer This is a rare type of breast cancer that spreads quickly. The breast looks red and feels warm, and the skin may have ridges, pits, or wheals.

Recurring breast cancer This is cancer that returns (to the breast or to another part of the body) after treatment.

STAGE	LOCATION OF SPREAD	CHANCE OF SURVIVAL 5 YEARS AFTER DIAGNOSIS
I	Cancer is less than 1 inch (2 centimeters [cm]) and has not spread outside the breast.	95%
II	Cancer is 1 to 2 inches (2 to 5 cm) or cancer is smaller than 1 inch (2 cm) but has spread to lymph glands under the arm or cancer is larger than 2 inches (5 cm) but has not spread to lymph glands under the arm.	80%
IIIA	Cancer is larger than 2 inches (5 cm) and has spread to the lymph glands under the arm or cancer is smaller than 2 inches (5 cm), has spread to the lymph glands under the arm, and the lymph glands have grown together or attached themselves to other structures.	50%
IIIB	Cancer has spread to tissues near the breast (such as the chest wall, including the ribs and the muscles) or cancer has spread to lymph glands inside the chest wall along the breastbone.	50%
IV	Cancer has spread to other parts of the body (most often the bones, lungs, liver, or brain) or cancer has spread to the skin or lymph glands inside the neck near the collarbone.	10%

Healthy women may also develop breast infections. Mastitis and abscesses are two types of breast infections.

Mastitis is an inflammation of the breast tissue, usually due to a blocked milk duct in which bacteria multiply. The bacteria normally live on the skin or in the mouth of a nursing infant and are transferred to the breast during nursing.

A breast abscess is an uncommon bacterial infection that produces a pus-filled sac (cyst) in the soft tissues beneath the skin or in a milk duct. It can occur when mastitis is not adequately treated or during the early weeks of breast-feeding if your nipples become cracked and irritated (making it easier for bacteria to infect the breast).

Benefits of Total Mastectomy Versus Lumpectomy and Radiation Therapy

Women diagnosed with stage I or II breast cancer have two options for initial treatment. They can have the affected breast completely removed (total mastectomy) or they can have only the breast lump removed (lumpectomy) along with radiation therapy. Six large randomized controlled trials (see p.31) have found that these two strategies are equally effective. The slight differences shown below are not statistically significant.

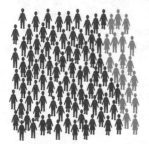

82 OF 100 WOMEN WHO HAVE BREAST CANCER AND HAVE A TOTAL MASTECTOMY ARE ALIVE 5 YEARS LATER

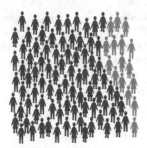

84 OF 100 WOMEN WHO HAVE BREAST CANCER AND HAVE A LUMPECTOMY ALONG WITH RADIATION THERAPY ARE ALIVE 5 YEARS LATER

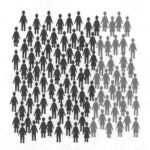

67 OF 100 WOMEN WHO HAVE BREAST CANCER AND HAVE A TOTAL MASTECTOMY HAVE NO RECURRENCE OF BREAST CANCER WITHIN 5 YEARS

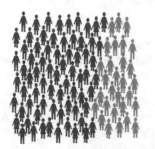

71 OF 100 WOMEN WHO HAVE BREAST CANCER AND HAVE A LUMPECTOMY ALONG WITH RADIATION THERAPY HAVE NO RECURRENCE OF BREAST CANCER WITHIN 5 YEARS

SYMPTOMS

Symptoms of mastitis include breast swelling, redness, tenderness, and a sensation of heat. Fever and fatigue distinguish mastitis (which is an infection) from engorgement or a plugged duct in breast-feeding women.

A breast abscess appears as a red, swollen, tender, painful area of the breast or at the edge of the areola (the darker skin of the nipple). You may have a fever or notice swollen glands in your armpit.

TREATMENT OPTIONS

See your doctor if you have symptoms of mastitis or a breast abscess. He or she will examine your breast to make a diagnosis and will prescribe antibiotics to fight any infection.

It is usually not necessary to

Treating Lymphedema

After a radical mastectomy (in which lymph nodes near the breast are removed along with the breast), the arm on the side of the breast often becomes swollen. This is because lymph, a fluid that travels through vessels that lead to lymph nodes, builds up in the tissues.

Fluid buildup indicates that the mastectomy has damaged the lymph vessels, preventing the fluid from entering the veins. Ongoing tissue swelling can cause the tissues to become hard and the skin dry.

The condition can be painful. About 2 million women in the United States are affected.

There are several treatments for lymphedema:

■ **Massage therapy** by specially trained physical therapists (performed in one or two 45-minute sessions each day for about 4 weeks) pushes the lymph fluid out of the arm tissues and into the blood. Each treatment is followed by wrapping the arm with compression bandages to keep the fluid from returning.

■ **Pneumatic compression sleeves** that rhythmically inflate and deflate are worn for several hours, several times a week, at a hospital.

■ **Compression sleeves** with strong elastic fibers can be worn permanently.

■ **The blood-thinning drug warfarin**, once considered possibly useful, is no longer regarded as beneficial.

Treating Breast Cancer

All forms of breast cancer can be treated, usually starting with surgery to remove the tumor and part or all of the breast. In addition to surgery, there are additional treatments that may be used individually or in combination, depending on the extent of your cancer and other factors such as your overall health, whether you have gone through menopause, and how the cancer cells respond to hormones. Treatment options are listed in this chart.

TREATMENT OPTIONS	DESCRIPTION
Surgery	Surgery involves removing the tumor (lumpectomy) or removing the tumor and part or all of the breast tissue (mastectomy). Most women have some form of surgery to treat breast cancer. See Surgical Treatment of Breast Cancer, p.1060.
Radiation therapy (see p.741)	Radiation is used after surgery to kill any remaining cancer cells.
Chemotherapy (see p.741)	Chemotherapy is the administration of anticancer drugs. It can be used with surgery and/or radiation to eradicate cancer cells and prevent them from spreading or to relieve pain and discomfort if the cancer is incurable. Drugs may be taken as tablets, liquids, injections, or intravenous infusions.
Hormone therapy	Breast cancer cells often have hormone receptors, chemicals that can make the cells grow and divide when exposed to certain hormones. Tamoxifen is a medicine that is like an estrogen that blocks the ability of estrogen to stimulate the growth of breast cancer. Aromatase inhibitors are another new class of medicines that reduce levels of estrogen in the blood. They are of clear use when they are started after a woman has been on tamoxifen for five years, and may prove to be beneficial when used in other ways as well. Raloxifene is a "designer estrogen" that some studies suggest may reduce the risk of breast cancer, although this is unproven.
Biological therapy	Biological therapy is experimental therapy that uses the body's immune system to boost specific types of white blood cells that fight cancer.
Bone marrow transplantation (see p.732)	Higher doses of chemotherapy are better at eliminating cancer cells but usually destroy bone marrow, the site where blood cells are produced. Bone marrow transplantation is an experimental approach that replaces destroyed bone marrow after high-dose chemotherapy. Initial results of this treatment have been disappointing.
Ovarian ablation	Ovaries continue to make estrogen and progesterone, which can stimulate the growth of some cancers. For many years, the ovaries were surgically removed or destroyed with radiation therapy, as part of treatment for breast cancer. More recently, a medicine that causes the ovaries to stop making estrogen and progesterone, goserelin, has proven beneficial.

Surgical Treatment of Breast Cancer

Women with breast cancer often can choose whether to have only the lump (lumpectomy), part of the breast (partial mastectomy), or the entire breast (mastectomy) removed.

Because of additional therapies used in treating breast cancer (see p.1059), many women with breast cancer can achieve the same results (of treatment and prevention of recurrence) with lumpectomy or a partial mastectomy as they would with removal of the entire breast.

You and your physician should discuss all the factors that can affect your decision, such as the stage and predicted course of your cancer, your state of health, and, most importantly, your priorities and concerns. Weigh your options carefully, seek a second opinion, and speak with women who have gone through the different types of surgery.

Lumpectomy removes the smallest amount of tissue. The surgeon takes only the cancerous lump, a section of surrounding tissue, and a portion of the nearby lymph glands. Ask your surgeon what kind of scar will remain, since this depends on many factors, including the location and size of the lump.

Who might consider it? Women whose tests indicate that the cancer is confined to a small area of the breast and is unlikely to spread (usually cancer in stage I or stage II).

How is it performed? Using local anesthesia (see p.168), the surgeon cuts out the cancerous tissue, a small amount of surrounding tissue, and some of the lymph glands under the arm to determine if the cancer has spread.

What happens after surgery? Following a lumpectomy, sometimes patients go home the same day, and usually return to their usual daily routine within two weeks. Surgery is followed by a 6-week course of radiation therapy (see p.1059). You should have a physical examination every 3 months and mammograms every 3 to 6 months.

Mastectomy is the surgical removal of part or all of one or both breasts. It is major surgery that requires general anesthesia (see p.168). Breasts can be reconstructed (see p.1062) during the surgery or at a later date.

In partial mastectomy, the tumor and a surrounding wedge of tissue (but not the overlying skin or nipple) are removed. In a total mastectomy, an oval incision is made and all of the underlying breast tissue, skin, and nipple are removed (but the lymph glands are not). In a modified radical mastectomy, the entire breast, nipple, most of the underarm lymph glands, and the muscle that lies underneath the breast are removed.

Who might consider it? Women whose breast cancer has spread, who have more than one cancerous lump, who have very large tumors, or whose breasts would have a worse cosmetic result after lumpectomy.

How is it performed? Using general anesthesia (see p.168), an incision is made, tissue is removed, and a drainage tube is inserted. Then stitches or clips are used to close the incision. Skin grafts may be necessary to replace the skin removed with the tissue.

What happens after surgery? You usually stay in the hospital for 2–5 days. The drainage tube may be removed 2 or 3 days after the operation. You may be fitted with a temporary prosthetic breast to allow the skin to heal before inserting a more permanent breast implant, or the implant may be inserted during the same surgery. Lymphedema—swelling or puffiness in the region of the surgery or in the arm (see p.1058)—may occur after surgery. It can develop when lymph or other fluid accumulates because the lymph glands that helped drain the fluid have been removed.

Breast reconstruction provides a variety of ways to restore form after breast tissue is removed. A nonsurgical method involves the use of a prosthesis, which is an insert designed to fit your body that can be placed in your bra. If you choose to have surgery, you may have breast reconstruction during the original surgery or you may be advised to wait until radiation therapy is complete.

During reconstructive surgery, either a breast implant (an artificial saline-filled insert) or tissue from another part of your body is used. In the latter case, tissue containing muscle, fat, and its own working blood supply is usually moved from the lower abdomen to the site of the mastectomy. Although it requires more extensive surgery, your own tissue feels more like the original breast tissue, mimics the changes in the other breast that occur with time, and also avoids the risks associated with breast implants.

Total Mastectomy

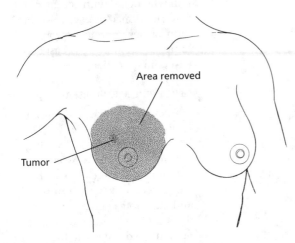

In a total mastectomy, the entire breast is removed, including the nipple, along with the tumor. Lymph glands in the armpit on the same side of the breast may also be removed.

Modified Radical Mastectomy

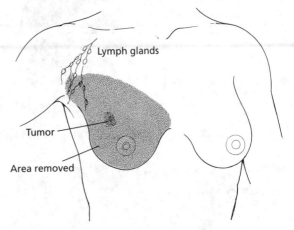

In a modified radical mastectomy, the entire breast is removed, including the nipple and the nearby lymph glands, along with the tumor.

Partial Mastectomy

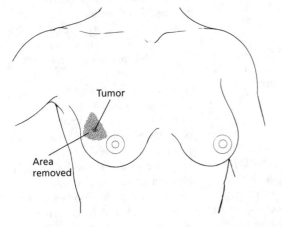

In a partial mastectomy (also called a wedge resection because of the shape of the tissue removed), only the tumor and a wedge of surrounding tissue are removed.

Lumpectomy

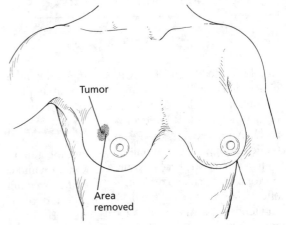

In a lumpectomy, only the tumor and as little surrounding tissue as possible are removed.

Breast Reconstruction After Mastectomy

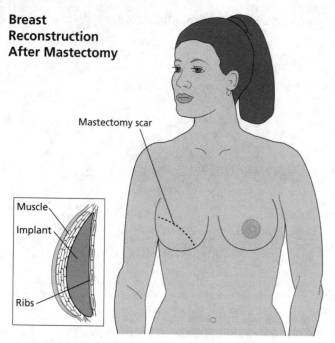

Mastectomy scar

Muscle

Implant

Ribs

The usual site of a mastectomy scar is shown. Immediately after (or anytime after) a mastectomy, a breast implant can be inserted. In the inset at left, it is positioned between the chest muscles and the ribs, though it can be inserted on top of the chest muscle. A new nipple can be constructed from skin taken from the inside of the thigh, and tattooed to obtain a darker skin color.

stop breast-feeding. In fact, with either infection, it is important to continue the flow of milk. The baby is not at risk of infection and may receive some of the antibiotic through the breast milk.

If you have an abscess, your doctor may be able to drain it, often relieving much of the pain and tenderness. After using a local anesthetic, the doctor will make a small incision in the skin and cyst. Some milk may leak from the incision if you are breast-feeding.

You can relieve symptoms by applying warm or cold compresses to the affected area (warmth, in particular, helps open blocked milk ducts) and by taking over-the-counter pain relievers such as acetaminophen or ibuprofen.

Breast Lumps

Finding a lump in your breast is common and can be very frightening. Any lump should be reported to your doctor immediately. However, it is important to remember that up to 85% of lumps are not cancerous. Your physician will perform a breast examination and may ask you to feel for changes in the lump over several menstrual cycles or may perform one or more tests (see Tests for Evaluating Breast Lumps, p.1056).

The only way to tell for certain whether a lump is cancerous is to perform a biopsy. Two common causes of noncancerous lumps are fibrocystic breast disease and fibroadenomas.

FIBROCYSTIC BREAST DISEASE

Fibrocystic breast disease is not really a disease but a group of benign (noncancerous) conditions of breast tissue. Women with fibrocystic breasts may have a lumpy quality to their breasts and may notice an increase in the lumpiness and breast tenderness in the days before their period. Women with multiple and recurring distinct cysts may also be included in this group.

Fibrocystic breast disease describes a kind of breast tissue that is organized into groups that are cystlike or nodular. As breast tissue responds to hormones during the menstrual cycle, these nodules may become more noticeable. You may be told that you have fibrocystic breast tissue after a mammogram or breast biopsy. Women with fibrocystic breast disease do not have an increased risk for cancer.

If you have a large cyst, your doctor may perform needle aspiration (see p.1056) to withdraw fluid from it so it will collapse. If you have fibrocystic breast disease, it is important that you perform a breast self-examination (see p.78) every month so that you can learn to distinguish between harmless lumps in your breasts and any new lumps that develop.

FIBROADENOMAS

A fibroadenoma is a hard, painless, noncancerous lump that may feel rubbery and move when you press on it. Unlike the lumps or nodules that occur with fibrocystic breast disease, fibroadenomas are larger, isolated, and mobile. They also tend to occur in women in the decade after their first period. If you have a large fibroadenoma, your doctor may suggest that you have it removed through excisional biopsy (see p.1056).

Breast Cancer

Breast cancer is the most common cancer in women. Like all cancers, it begins in one spot and grows larger for months or years. It can then metastasize (spread) to other parts of the body via the lymphatic system and bloodstream, ultimately causing illness and death. Early detection of cancerous tumors through self-examination (see p.78) and mammograms (see p.82) is your best defense against breast cancer.

Any of the following factors can increase your risk for breast cancer: being over 40; having a sister, mother, or daughter who has had breast cancer; beginning menstruating at age 12 or younger; starting menopause at age 55 or older; never having carried a pregnancy to term; using hormone therapy for 3 years or longer; being exposed to radiation; or having had breast cancer before.

In addition, certain genes have been discovered that increase a woman's risk of breast cancer. However, the genes identified thus far seem to be responsible for only a small fraction of breast cancers.

In premenopausal women, elevated levels of a hormone called insulinlike growth factor 1 (IGF-1) may indicate an increased risk of breast cancer. However, the value of this test in screening for breast cancer has not yet been proven.

The course of treatment and outlook for recovery depend on several factors, including the type of breast cancer you have, the stage of the cancer (whether it remains only in the breast or has spread to other parts of the body), and whether the cancer is also in the other breast. Your overall health is also an important factor.

SYMPTOMS

The most common outward sign of breast cancer is a hard lump in the breast that is usually not movable and may or may not be painful. The skin over the lump may look dimpled (like the skin of an orange) or indented in areas where the cancer has spread. The nipple may be inverted (turn inward) or leak dark fluid. Any lumps you feel under your arm may be cancer that has spread from breast tissue to the lymph glands under your arm.

TREATMENT OPTIONS

See your doctor immediately if you notice a lump in your breast or armpit or any changes in the outward appearance of your breasts. He or she will perform a breast examination and may recommend a mammogram and biopsy (see Tests for Evaluating Breast Lumps, p.1056). Cancer can be diagnosed only after obtaining tissue or fluid during a biopsy.

If the tissue sample has cancer cells, the cells from the malignant tissue will undergo further testing (through estrogen and progesterone receptor tests). This will determine whether the cells have chemicals called estrogen receptors or progesterone receptors on their surface (most breast cancer cells do). Having these receptors means that the cancer can be stimulated to grow by being exposed to estrogen or progesterone.

Medications that block estrogen receptors—such as tamoxifen and raloxifene—prevent the estrogen from encouraging the cancer to grow. (Progesterone-blocking medicines have not yet been tested.) The most positive experience with estrogen-blocking drugs has been with women over age 50, but there is evidence of effectiveness in women under 50 as well.

Breast cancer cells that do not have hormone receptors on their surface do not respond to hormone-blocking treatments. Determining whether or not your cancer cells are hormone responsive can help you and your doctor evaluate the outlook for your disease and can influence the choice of treatment (see Treating Breast Cancer, above).

A genetically engineered antibody called trastuzumab, which attacks a protein in breast cancer cells, has been proved to slow the growth of the cancer for at least a year. A medicine used to prevent osteoporosis, clodronate, may slow the growth of metastases (tumors that have spread from the original tumor) to the bone and even reduce the number of new metastases.

Nipple Disorders

The nipples of the breast contain small passageways through which milk flows after pregnancy and during breast-feeding. The area of darker skin surrounding the breast is called the areola. It is normal for the nipple and areola to become bigger and darker during pregnancy and breast-feeding. Problems with the nipple itself are commonly related to breast-feeding (see Mastitis and Breast Abscess, p.1056; Common Changes After Labor and Delivery, p.943).

INVERTED NIPPLES

Some women are born with nipples that turn inward, which is no cause for concern. For cosmetic reasons, the retraction can be released in a simple surgical procedure. A normal nipple that becomes inverted can be a sign of breast cancer and should be brought to the attention of your doctor immediately.

PAGET DISEASE OF THE NIPPLE

Paget disease of the nipple is an uncommon type of breast cancer that may first appear as an itchy sore on your nipple. Paget disease of the nipple is a slow-growing cancer that starts in the milk ducts. If you have a sore on your nipple that itches or burns, see your doctor immediately. He or she may take a sample of cells to send to the laboratory to check for cancer. If the cancer is caught early, the chance of a cure is excellent. Depending on how far advanced the cancer is, treatment may include surgery (see Treating Breast Cancer, p.1059).

NIPPLE DISCHARGE

The most common type of nipple discharge is the normal milky fluid that can leak in pregnant or breast-feeding women. Women who are not pregnant or breast-feeding may also have a small amount of watery or milky discharge when they squeeze their breasts or nipples.

A bloody discharge is of some concern because it can be a sign of cancer. However, more often it is caused by the noncancerous condition called intraductal papilloma (see below). Fluid from the nipple that is thicker, yellow or green, or has an odd smell may be pus from an infection such as mastitis (see p.1056).

Milk production is stimulated by a hormone called prolactin, produced by the pituitary gland in the brain. Milk production is normal during pregnancy and breast-feeding but also commonly occurs when taking birth-control pills or medicines that lower blood pressure or stabilize mood.

Tiny noncancerous tumors of the pituitary gland called prolactinomas (see p.860) can also cause a milky discharge by increasing prolactin levels in the blood, which stimulates milk production. High prolactin levels can also interfere with the normal menstrual cycle, cause irregular or absent periods, and be responsible for a treatable form of infertility. In all of these cases, nipple discharge usually comes from both breasts.

If you are not pregnant or breast-feeding and notice a nipple discharge, see your doctor. Bring a list of all medicines you take to your appointment. Your doctor will also want to know whether you have irregular periods. He or she will perform a breast exam, try to express a sample of the discharge, and may check your prolactin level through a blood test. If it is higher than normal, your doctor may order x-rays of your brain to look for a prolactinoma.

CYSTS IN THE AREOLA

Cysts in the areola (the dark area around your nipple) are small, movable sacs filled with fluid or pus. These cysts are most often noncancerous and may be the result of a blocked oil gland in the nipple or a bacterial infection. See your doctor if you have a cyst. Depending on how the cyst looks, he or she may recommend applying heat to encourage the cyst to rupture on its own or may drain it by lancing it. Antibiotics can help eradicate any infection.

INTRADUCTAL PAPILLOMA

An intraductal papilloma is a small, firm growth of tissue in the milk duct of the breast. Although it is often accompanied by discharge from the nipple, which can be a sign of cancer, it is a noncancerous tumor.

If you detect a lump in your breast or have a discharge, see your doctor immediately. He or she may use needle aspiration (see p.1056) to remove fluid from the growth or may remove it and have the fluid or tissue evaluated for the presence of cancer cells. No treatment is necessary for an intraductal papilloma.

VULVA

Bartholin Gland Cysts and Abscesses

The Bartholin glands are located in the labia minora, next to the vaginal opening, and release fluid during sexual arousal. If they become blocked by injury or infection, a painless cyst may develop.

An infected cyst becomes a pus-filled sac called an abscess that can swell and be very painful. If you have these symptoms, see your doctor.

Small abscesses can be treated with hot compresses. Larger abscesses may need to be lanced for drainage and may require the insertion of a temporary drain. A cyst that recurs may be cut open and its edges sewn outward so that it does not heal back into the form of a cyst. All of these procedures can be performed in the doctor's office using local anesthesia (see p.168).

Cancer of the Vulva

Cancer of the vulva can affect any part of the vulva, including the labia, mons pubis, vaginal opening, clitoris, and urethral opening. It may begin as a tiny lump or sore. The majority of vulvar cancers are squamous cell skin cancers (see p.547), although melanoma (see p.543) may also develop in the vulva.

Bartholin Glands

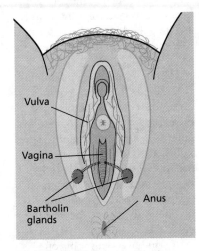

Bartholin glands lie on both sides of the vaginal opening under the skin, where they cannot normally be felt. They can become blocked, develop cysts, and become infected.

SYMPTOMS

The most common symptoms include intense itching or a burning pain anywhere in the vulva, although such symptoms are caused much more often by simple vaginal infections and other less serious conditions than by cancer. In the more advanced, invasive stage, you may notice a large lump or have vaginal discharge or bleeding. Melanomas are black or brown raised areas more commonly found on the labia majora.

TREATMENT OPTIONS

Your doctor will take a sample of tissue from the affected area for examination under a microscope to look for cancer cells. When confined to one area, chances for cure of the cancer are excellent. An anticancer drug can be applied directly to the affected area or a partial vulvectomy can remove only the cancer in the skin and a portion of the underlying tissues. These treatments remove the cancer while preserving as much tissue and sexual function as possible.

A complete vulvectomy is performed when the cancer has spread to surrounding tissue or organs. All affected tissue of the vulva and any affected lymph glands must be removed. Your surgeon will preserve the urethra, vagina, and clitoris as much as possible.

After the surgery, radiation therapy (see p.741) is used for cancers that have spread to the lymph glands.

For large tumors and cancers that have spread to other organs, a combination of radiation therapy and chemotherapy (see p.741) may be used to help shrink the size of the tumor before surgery, thus permitting less extensive surgery.

VAGINA

Vaginal Infections

The vagina is populated by a variety of microscopic organisms that normally live in a delicate balance; none of them proliferate and dominate over the others.

One group of bacteria (lactobacilli) plays a key role in maintaining the appropriate environment by making lactic acid, which keeps other microbes from multiplying out of control and causing an infection. These infections and their symptoms, types of discharge, and treatments are described on p.1065.

Factors that can upset the balance and allow some microbes to proliferate include douching, antibiotics, birth-control pills, diabetes, pregnancy, stress, and inadequate hygiene.

The best way to make a diagnosis of the type of vaginal infection you have and the kind of treatment you need is for your doctor to perform an examination. However, if you are susceptible to getting the same kind of vaginal infection, particularly a yeast infection, repeatedly, and are sure you have a recurrence, treatments are available without prescription.

For women prone to recurring infections, the ways to maintain a healthy vaginal environment are listed in Preventing Vaginitis (see below).

Vaginitis

Vaginitis is inflammation of the vagina. It can be accompanied by uncomfortable symptoms including itching, burning, vaginal discharge, and pain during sexual intercourse. Scratching your genital area can lead to redness and swelling, and blisters may form, seeping clear fluid when they are scratched.

Common causes of inflammation include infections (yeast, protozoa, bacteria, herpes, lice, or scabies), low levels of estrogen (as in atrophic vaginitis, see right), allergies, or exposure to irritants such as soaps, laundry detergents, douches, or scented tampons or pads. In rare cases, itching is a sign of cancer of the vulva (see p.1065).

If you have symptoms of vaginitis, see your doctor for a pelvic examination. He or she will check for infections. Treatment usually depends on the cause. In some cases, a cream containing a corticosteroid drug (see p.895) may be prescribed to ease inflammation and itching.

Atrophic vaginitis Atrophic vaginitis results from the dryness and thinning (atrophy) of vaginal tissues due to low levels of estrogen in women after menopause (see p.1047) or in women whose ovaries have been surgically removed. Lower estrogen levels in women after childbirth (especially in those who are breast-feeding) or in women who use oral contraceptives may also lead to atrophic vaginitis.

Symptoms include genital dryness, itching, burning, or pain during intercourse. Because the vagina's environment is altered by lower estrogen levels and the vaginal tissue is fragile, women with atrophic vaginitis are more susceptible to vaginal infections.

 Preventing Vaginitis

Follow these guidelines to prevent infection and irritation of your vagina:

■ Wear cotton underpants and pantyhose with a cotton crotch. Avoid tight-fitting undergarments that can trap moisture.

■ After using the toilet, wipe from front to back to avoid contaminating your vaginal area with feces.

■ Do not douche or use any scented products, such as scented tampons or pads, in your genital area.

■ Use an unscented soap and water to wash your genitals and anus once a day. Avoid too frequent or vigorous washing; it can be drying and irritating.

■ Use a condom to avoid exposure to infections that are sexually transmitted.

■ If you have symptoms of dryness or pain during sexual intercourse, use a water-soluble lubricant.

Common Vaginal Infections: Symptoms and Treatments

This chart lists the most common vaginal infections, their causes and symptoms, and describes how they are treated.

INFECTION	CAUSED BY	SYMPTOMS	TREATMENT OPTIONS
Vaginosis	Bacteria	Genital itching or burning; gray vaginal discharge with an unusual fishy odor that may be especially noticeable after intercourse	Antibiotics in tablet form taken by mouth or as a cream inserted into the vagina; sexual partner should be treated also
Candida	Yeast-like fungi	Intense burning and genital itching; clumped, white, cottage cheese–like discharge; possible pain during sexual intercourse	Prescription or over-the-counter antifungal cream or suppositories inserted into the vagina soothe the burning and itching for some women; antifungal tablet taken in one dose by mouth
Trichomonas	Protozoa, which are single-celled organisms that are sexually transmitted	Genital itching and burning; possible frothy, gray-green discharge with an unusual odor	Antibiotic in tablet form taken by mouth; sexual partner should be treated also

Rarely, vaginal bleeding or spotting occurs.

If you have symptoms, see your doctor for a pelvic examination. Usually, he or she can make a diagnosis by the appearance of the vaginal tissue alone. At the same time, your doctor may check for any infections. You may be treated with hormone replacement therapy (see p.1049) in tablet form or by placing estrogen cream directly into your vagina (a small amount of estrogen from the cream may be absorbed into your bloodstream).

Women who choose not to take hormones can use nonprescription water-based lubricants to ease symptoms, make sexual intercourse less painful, and make the vagina's environment less favorable for infections.

CERVIX

Abnormal Pap Smear Result

Pap smear (see p.1042) abnormalities range from mild to severe, and do not necessarily mean that you have cancer. Atypical cells, the mildest kind of abnormality, are often caused by simple infections or inflammation. Sometimes they are caused by precancerous conditions that could one day turn into cancer, and start growing into nearby tissue or spreading to other parts of the body. Cervical intraepithelial neoplasia (CIN) is such a precancerous condition. It can show up in the Pap smear. If it appears to be low-grade, a Pap smear result called LSIL, the doctor just keeps a close eye on it, such as by scheduling a repeat Pap test. If it appears to be high-grade (called

HSIL), your doctor may recommend that a more accurate examination of your cervix be performed using colposcopy (see p.1041). In this test, the cervix is examined with a special magnifying scope. If an abnormal-looking area is seen, the physician may perform a biopsy of the cervix, in which a tiny piece of tissue is removed for examination under a microscope to determine the type and extent of cell abnormalities.

Abnormal precancerous areas on the cervix are often treated with an electrical instrument that shaves off tissue (a procedure called LEEP), or treated with a laser. These procedures can be performed in the doctor's office with little or no anesthesia; neither procedure should affect your fertility.

If the abnormal area of CIN involves a lot of cervical tissue, you may need to have a cone biopsy (see p.1041) to remove more tissue. A cone biopsy makes maintaining a pregnancy to term more difficult but not impossible. After treatment, your doctor may recommend more frequent Pap smears to identify any new abnormal cells as early as possible.

Cancer of the Cervix

Cervical cancer is cancer cells in the cervix (the opening to the uterus). It is the third most common type of cancer of the female genital tract and is diagnosed in 15,000 women each year.

This slow-growing malignancy can be detected by Pap smear in its precancerous stage, when it is called cervical intraepithelial neoplasia (CIN) (see Abnormal Pap Smear Result, p.1067). Untreated CIN develops into cervical cancer when it begins to invade neighboring tissue.

Most cases of cervical cancer are thought to be caused by particular strains of the human papillomavirus (HPV) (see Genital Warts, p.891), which can be transmitted sexually. Your risk of cervical cancer increases with every new male sexual partner with whom you have unprotected (without a latex or polyurethane condom) sexual intercourse. Risk is also higher in women who became sexually active early in adolescence. Other strains of the same virus cause genital warts, and cervical cancer is more likely to occur in women with genital warts.

Infection with the human immunodeficiency virus (HIV) (see p.872) increases the risk of

Pap Smear Schedule and Technique

You should have a Pap smear every year after the age of 18, or whenever you become sexually active, whichever occurs first. If your Pap smear is normal for 3 consecutive years, you and your doctor may decide that you can have them less often. If you have a new sexual partner, you should have a Pap smear within a year. If you have an increased risk for having cancer of the cervix (see above), you should have yearly Pap smears.

Try to schedule your Pap smear for the middle of your menstrual cycle, which is the best time to evaluate the cells under a microscope. Do not use spermicides, douches, or any medicines inserted into the vagina for 2 days before your test. These substances can cause inaccurate test results.

Ask your doctor about using newer computerized Pap tests. They are somewhat more accurate, and increasing numbers of doctors recommend them. In these tests, cells from the cervix are spread out in a thinner layer so that a computer can analyze cross-sections of single cells. Cells that appear abnormal are then checked by a human expert.

You can make sure the laboratory used to interpret the Pap smear meets high-quality standards by asking if it is accredited by the College of American Pathologists.

How a Pap Smear Is Performed

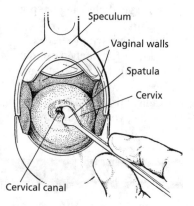

During a Pap smear, the walls of the vagina are held open with a speculum. A small wooden blade (called a spatula) and tiny brush are used to scrape cells from the outside of the cervix and just inside the cervical canal. The specimens can be used for both a Pap smear and HPV testing.

cervical cancer, probably because the weakened immune system allows HPV to more easily cause cancer. Using a condom seems to lower the risk of cervical cancer by preventing the spread of HPV or HIV.

SYMPTOMS

In its early stages, cervical cancer has no symptoms. At later stages, it can be responsible for a bloody, foul-smelling discharge. Vaginal bleeding may occur after sexual intercourse or between periods.

TREATMENT OPTIONS

A Pap smear is the single best means of preventing cervical cancer because it can identify abnormal cells of the cervix (such as in CIN) before they develop into cancer. Early treatment of CIN prevents the development of cervical cancer.

If you have an abnormal Pap smear, your doctor may arrange for colposcopy (see p.1041) to obtain a magnified view of your cervix and take a sample of tissue for evaluation under the microscope.

If CIN is detected, the area will be removed with a cone biopsy (see p.1041). An increasingly used technique for removing the precancerous tissue is called loop electrosurgical excision procedure (LEEP). You are given a local anesthetic. An electrified wire is used to gently cut away the diseased tissue, causing minimal damage to surrounding healthy tissue. Complications are rare.

If cervical cancer is diagnosed, your doctor will identify the stage (how far the cancer has spread) using blood tests; x-rays of the chest, pelvic organs, and lymph

Pelvic Examination

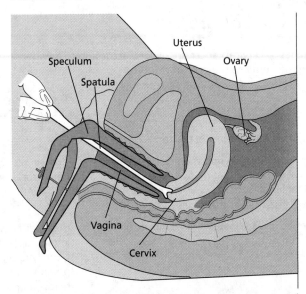

During a pelvic examination, the doctor examines the external genitalia and then inserts a speculum to open the vagina, using a light to view the walls of the vagina and cervix. A Pap smear is performed by inserting a small spatula or brush and gently scraping cells from the cervix.

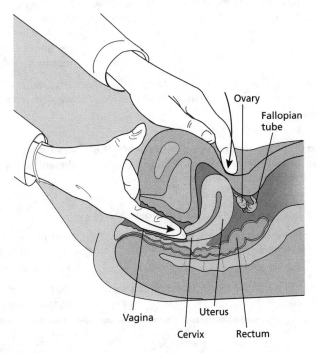

The doctor then gently inserts one or two gloved fingers into the vagina to feel the uterus. At the same time, the doctor presses on the abdomen, feeling between his or her hands for the size and location of the ovaries, uterus, and fallopian tubes.

Stages of Cervical Cancer

The different stages of cervical cancer are divided according to how far the cancer has spread outside the cervix:

STAGE	LOCATION OF SPREAD	CHANCE OF SURVIVAL 5 YEARS AFTER DIAGNOSIS
I	**Cancer is confined to inside the cervix.**	
IA	Cancer has spread beyond the first outer layer of cells of the cervix and measures no deeper than 5 millimeters (mm), with the entire affected area smaller than 7 mm.	After simple hysterectomy (which removes only the uterus)—99%
IB	Cancer has spread deeper than 5 mm or broader than 7 mm but is still inside the tissues of the cervix.	After radical hysterectomy (see p.1070) or radiation therapy—85% if the cancer did not spread to the lymph glands and 50% if the cancer spread to the lymph glands; adding chemotherapy improves survival
II	**Cancer has spread beyond the cervix to nearby areas.**	
IIA	Cancer has spread to the upper two thirds of the vagina.	After radical hysterectomy or radiation therapy—85% if the cancer did not spread to the lymph glands and 50% if the cancer spread to the lymph glands; adding chemotherapy improves survival
IIB	Cancer has spread to the tissue around the cervix or uterus but not to the walls of the pelvis.	After radiation therapy—50% to 60%; adding chemotherapy improves survival
III	**Cancer has spread to the walls of the pelvis, the lower third of the vagina, or the ureters (the tubes that connect the kidney to the bladder).**	After radiation therapy—30% to 35%; adding chemotherapy improves survival
IV	**Cancer has spread to more distant organs.**	
IVA	Cancer has spread to organs closer to the cervix, such as the bladder and rectum.	After radiation therapy or more extensive surgery—10% to 15%; adding chemotherapy improves survival
IVB	Cancer has spread to more distant organs such as the lungs.	After chemotherapy or radiation therapy—less than 10% (death can occur within 1 year)

Diagnosing Cervical Cancer Under the Microscope

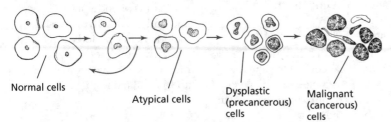

Normal cells

Atypical cells

Dysplastic (precancerous) cells

Malignant (cancerous) cells

When cervical cells are obtained through a Pap smear, the cells are any of the following: clearly normal, atypical but not obviously cancerous, dysplastic (precancerous), or plainly cancerous. Cervical cancer cells clump together and their nuclei (centers) are dramatically enlarged. Atypical cells can progress to malignant cells or return to normal over time.

glands; computed tomography (see p.149); magnetic resonance imaging (see p.151); and a bone scan (see p.622).

Treatment depends on the stage. In the early stages, when cancer is limited to the outer layer of cells in the cervix, a hysterectomy (see p.1072) that removes only the uterus is performed. More advanced cancer often also requires removal of the fallopian tubes, ovaries, and nearby lymph glands (radical hysterectomy).

Radiation therapy (see p.741) may be recommended for women whose cancer has spread to other organs. It is also recommended for women who have large tumors in early stages (to reduce tumor size before surgery)

or for women with other medical problems that might make surgery more difficult. Radiation therapy may be delivered from a source outside the body or via implants put close to the cancer on the inside of the body (called brachytherapy).

In 1999, it was discovered that giving radiation together with chemotherapy (with the anticancer drugs cisplatin or fluorouracil) to women whose cervical cancer had spread to nearby lymph nodes or to other parts of the pelvis improved survival by 30% to 50%. Previously, chemotherapy had been used only for cervical cancer that had spread to more distant parts of the body.

Cervical Polyps

Cervical polyps are noncancerous growths of spongy tissue that look like tiny bulbs attached to the lining of the cervix by a small stem. They can occur singly or in groups and can cause a copious discharge or bleeding between periods, after intercourse, or after menopause.

Very large polyps may block the cervix, causing temporary infertility. An infected polyp can produce a foul-smelling vaginal discharge.

Cervical polyps may cause no symptoms and are usually found during a Pap smear and pelvic examination. They are removed by clipping the polyps from their stem using local anesthesia.

Nabothian Cysts

Nabothian cysts develop from a blocked mucous gland in the cervix. They are more likely to develop after childbirth. A nabothian cyst does not produce symptoms and is usually discovered during a pelvic examination. Treatment is not necessary, but a nabothian cyst can be removed without anesthesia through cryosurgery (the application of liquid nitrogen to freeze the cyst) in the doctor's office.

UTERUS

Cancer of the Endometrium

Endometrial cancer is the growth of malignant cells from the lining of the uterus (endometrium).

Also called cancer of the uterus (or uterine cancer), it is the most common cancer of the reproductive organs among women, and usually occurs after menopause.

Approximately 75% of endometrial cancers have not spread beyond the uterus when they are diagnosed, and most can be cured with treatment.

The stages of endometrial cancer are: stage IA, cancer limited to the endometrial lining; stages IB and IC, cancer that has invaded the muscle wall of the uterus; stage II, cancer that has spread to the cervix; stage III, cancer that has spread to nearby structures; and stage IV, cancer that has spread to other organs.

You have a higher risk for endometrial cancer if you have never had a child. Your risk is also higher if any of the following apply: you are obese; your menopause occurred later than age 51; or you have had long-term estrogen therapy (without progesterone), liver disease, your first period before age 13, or ovarian or breast cancer.

The theory is that these factors all lead to higher levels of estrogen, over a longer period of time, which can stimulate the growth of endometrial cells.

ENDOMETRIAL HYPERPLASIA

Symptoms that can indicate endometrial cancer, such as heavy periods and bleeding between periods or after menopause, can also be caused by endometrial hyperplasia, which is an overgrowth of the cells that line the uterus.

Endometrial hyperplasia is not cancer, but it can turn into cancer, particularly in women who are going through perimenopause or after menopause. In one type of hyperplasia, thumblike projections of tissue called polyps develop; these are not precancerous and do not often recur.

SYMPTOMS

Symptoms of endometrial cancer and endometrial hyperplasia include heavy periods and bleeding between periods or after menopause. Some women have abdominal pain or a vaginal discharge.

TREATMENT OPTIONS

See your doctor immediately if you experience any abnormal bleeding or discharge. Your doctor will perform a pelvic examination (see p.1069) and a Pap smear (see p.1067) and may perform a transvaginal ultrasound (see p.1042) to look for other causes of your symptoms.

He or she will probably also perform an endometrial biopsy to remove a sample of tissue for examination under a microscope. If the biopsy does not provide an

Hysterectomy

A hysterectomy is surgery to remove the uterus. Simple hysterectomy removes the uterus only. A hysterectomy in which the ovaries and tubes are also removed is called hysterectomy and bilateral salpingo-oophorectomy. A hysterectomy in which the cervix is left in place, but the rest of the uterus is removed, is called a supracervical hysterectomy. When there is cancer of the cervix and the uterus, a radical hysterectomy is often performed and the fallopian tubes, ovaries, and lymph glands are removed. This is recommended for more advanced stages of cervical cancer, endometrial cancer, and other cancers involving the uterus.

Hysterectomy is one of the most commonly performed operations. In the past, it was performed not only for cancers involving the uterus, but also for noncancerous conditions, such as fibroids of the uterus (see p.1074), that caused pain and bleeding. In recent years, new medical treatments have reduced the need for hysterectomy in noncancerous conditions.

In rare cases, a hysterectomy is performed in emergency situations, such as when the uterus ruptures during childbirth or when there is uncontrollable, life-threatening bleeding from the uterus.

The two ways hysterectomy can be performed are shown on p.1075 and p.1076. If you are still having menstrual periods and your ovaries will be removed during the hysterectomy, you will go through immediate menopause (see p.1047). Before surgery, discuss your options (including hormone replacement therapy) to treat the symptoms of this surgical menopause.

Hysterectomy is major surgery and ends your ability to bear children. If you have doubts about having a hysterectomy, ask about alternative treatments for your condition, discuss the surgery with other women who have had it, and get a second opinion from another physician.

answer, a dilation and curettage (D&C) (see p.1077) may be required to obtain more tissue.

If you have endometrial hyperplasia, the D&C may treat the symptoms of irregular bleeding by removing the overgrown tissue of the lining of the uterus.

If your doctor suspects your bleeding may be due to polyps, a hysteroscopy (see p.1042), which is the best way to see the polyps, may be performed. In hysteroscopy, a flexible viewing tube containing a light and tiny video camera is inserted through the cervix. The doctor can see the polyps and perform the D&C.

Endometrial cancer is unique in that the stage of the cancer is determined by the results of surgery. After a diagnosis of endometrial cancer, hysterectomy is performed through an abdominal incision (see p.1076). During the hysterectomy, the uterus is opened to determine the depth of cancer spread in the muscle wall, which can change how extensive the remaining surgery will be.

In all cases, the ovaries and fallopian tubes are also removed, and an exploration of the abdomen is performed to find any other sites of cancer spread.

Radiation therapy (see p.741) is usually recommended after surgery. The amount of the pelvic area exposed to radiation depends on the spread, size of tumors, stage, and appearance of the cells. Women with stage IV uterine cancer usually undergo either chemotherapy (see p.741) or hormone therapy with progesterone. The outlook is good for women whose cancer is identified at an early stage; more than

80% are considered cured with no recurrence after 5 years.

Treatment of endometrial hyperplasia depends on your age. Younger women may be prescribed birth-control pills with progesterone; women who have gone through menopause may receive hormone replacement therapy (estrogen and progesterone) or progesterone alone. A hysterectomy is considered only as a last resort.

Endometriosis

Endometriosis is a chronic condition in which cells from the lining of the uterus (the endometrium) also grow on structures outside the uterus. The most common locations for endometrial cell tissue to grow are the ovaries, outer surface of the uterus, ligaments that support the uterus, membranes that line the pelvic cavity, and space between the uterus and the rectum.

Sometimes, the endometrial tissue grows on the bowel or urinary tract. The displaced tissue can also grow into cysts on the ovaries. The cysts are commonly referred to as chocolate cysts because of their color, caused by the dark fluid (consisting of menstrual blood and debris) inside the cyst. Endometriosis is believed to be responsible for 25% of all cases of infertility.

Doctors do not know what causes endometriosis. Some believe that endometrial cells are pushed backward up through the fallopian tubes into the pelvic cavity during menstruation, instead of being pushed out of the body through the vagina. The body's immune system may also

play a role. Eventually, scar tissue from the chronic inflammation may form fibrous webs called adhesions that can trap underlying structures, creating blockages and producing severe abdominal pain.

SYMPTOMS

Symptoms of endometriosis include severe menstrual discomfort, abdominal pain, pain during sexual intercourse, backache, rectal discomfort during bowel movements, diarrhea, constipation, infertility, or recurring miscarriage. The type of pain or problem depends on the location of the displaced tissue or adhesions rather than the extent of the disease.

Symptoms often get worse during the same part of the menstrual cycle each month because the displaced tissue can grow and bleed just like normal uterine lining. For this reason, symptoms of endometriosis usually disappear after menopause.

TREATMENT OPTIONS

Doctors can diagnose endometriosis during laparoscopic surgery. The inside of the abdomen is viewed by making small incisions into the abdomen through which thin tubes are inserted and guided with the use of a video camera attached to the tubes. This allows surgeons to locate the displaced tissue and any adhesions and treat the disease by removing the tissue causing the problems.

Treatment to restore fertility depends on the severity of the disease. Mild endometriosis requires no treatment, and 75%

of the women who have it ultimately are able to conceive. In more advanced cases, the displaced tissue and adhesions can be removed by laparoscopic surgery. About 40% of women who have this treatment are able to become pregnant after treatment. Assisted reproduction (see p.911) may be necessary for those still unable to conceive. Some women experience a temporary time after pregnancy in which they are free from symptoms.

For relief of pain, options include medicines or surgery. Medicines decrease pain by interfering with the normal hormonal changes during the menstrual cycle. They include birth-control pills, the synthetic male hormone danazol, or forms of progesterone. Drugs called gonadotropin-releasing hormone (GnRH) analogs (such as leuprolide) act on the pituitary gland to stop the usual hormonal signals that stimulate the ovaries to produce the hormones of the menstrual cycle. This creates a pseudomenopause with side effects such as hot flashes, headache, vaginal dryness, and osteoporosis. Because of the risk of bone loss, GnRH analogs are not used for long periods of time.

Surgical options depend on the location of the tumors and your desire for fertility. During the laparoscopic surgery for diagnosis, displaced tissue and scar tissue can be removed, which sometimes cures symptoms.

Removing the ovaries, uterus, displaced tissue, and scar tissue relieves pain in 90% of women, but ends your ability to conceive.

Endometriosis

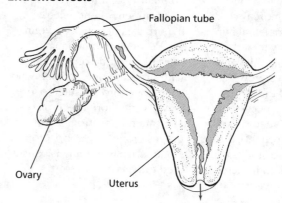

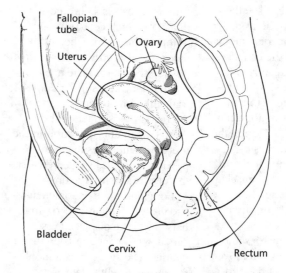

In endometriosis, endometrial tissue (shown in red) is found elsewhere in the body, outside of its normal place in the uterus. Here it is shown on the ovaries, fallopian tubes, cervix, and tissues around the outside of the uterus, rectum, and bladder.

Fibroids of the Uterus

Fibroids are rubbery, noncancerous nodules composed of muscle and fibrous tissue in the wall of the uterus. They affect at least 25% of all women in their 30s and 40s and half of black women in that age group. Their growth is probably stimulated by estrogen; they tend to shrink after menopause when estrogen levels drop.

Fibroids develop from cells in the muscular wall of the uterus that grow slowly and erratically into balls of smooth muscle encased in fibrous tissue. Most grow inside the wall of the uterus, and many cause no symptoms. Women with fibroids usually have more than one. Most fibroids are between the size of a walnut and an orange.

Laparoscopic Vaginal Hysterectomy

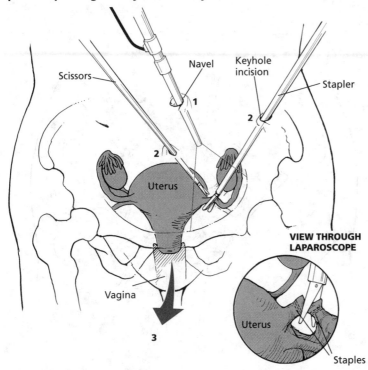

In a laparoscopic vaginal hysterectomy, a laparoscope is inserted through an incision at the navel (1).The laparoscope permits the surgeon to view the procedure and interior organs on a monitor. Next the surgeon inserts slender instruments (such as this scissors and stapler) through two keyhole incisions (2). The surgeon staples the tissue holding the uterus and, inserting a knife through the laparoscope, cuts away the uterus. The staples keep the tissue from bleeding when the uterus is cut away (inset). The uterus is then removed through the vagina (3).

SYMPTOMS

The location of the fibroid in the wall of the uterus usually determines the symptoms. The most common symptom is excessive vaginal bleeding.

Submucosal fibroids grow just beneath the endometrium (the lining of the uterus) and can stimulate excessive bleeding. Pedunculated fibroids dangle from a stalk and either protrude into the uterus (where they may cause cramps as the uterus contracts trying to expel the fibroid) or sit outside the uterine wall.

Subserous fibroids grow against the outer wall of the uterus, where they cause pressure. A fibroid pressing on a pelvic nerve can cause chronic hip and back pain. Large fibroids can press on the bladder and bowel, increasing frequency of urination and causing constipation. If a fibroid blocks a fallopian tube, it can cause infertility. If it presses on the cervix, it can cause miscarriage or premature labor.

Is It Necessary to Have a Hysterectomy?
Dr Schiff's Advice

A hysterectomy is one of the most common surgical procedures in the United States, but it isn't always needed—even when it's been recommended. I always encourage patients to get a second opinion when a hysterectomy has been recommended, often even when I'm the person who recommended it.

At the same time, I also see patients who have avoided hysterectomy, or whose doctors have not recommended hysterectomy, when I think it has the potential to help them enormously.

When a woman has serious symptoms, such as excessive bleeding or pain that interferes with her daily life and activities, medicine is ineffective, and a procedure called hysteroscopic ablation cannot be carried out or is ineffective, a hysterectomy can be the answer.

ISAAC SCHIFF, MD
MASSACHUSETTS GENERAL HOSPITAL
HARVARD MEDICAL SCHOOL

TREATMENT OPTIONS

During a pelvic examination, your doctor may suspect fibroids are present if the uterus feels large and irregular. He or she may obtain a pelvic ultrasound (see p.1042), a transvaginal ultrasound (see p.1042), or magnetic resonance imaging (see p.151) to confirm a diagnosis.

The size of fibroids is sometimes described in terms of the size of the uterus using the nomenclature of pregnancy. A woman may be described as having a "12-week uterus"—that is, her uterus is equivalent in size to the uterus of a woman in her 12th week of pregnancy.

Most fibroids require no treatment. Pain is unusual unless a woman is pregnant, and it can usually be relieved with painkillers such as aspirin, ibuprofen, or acetaminophen. Drugs called gonadotropin-releasing hormone agonists reduce the ovaries' production of estrogen and can make fibroids smaller. However, stopping the medicine allows the fibroids to grow back. These drugs may be used temporarily to shrink fibroids in preparation for surgery. They are not used long-term because they can reduce bone mass and increase the risk of osteoporosis.

Some fibroids can be removed through the vagina using a hysteroscope (see p.1042), a small tube connected to a video camera that is inserted through the cervix into the uterus. A hysteroscope permits the doctor to use a laser or knife to cut out fibroids and heat-seal the endometrium.

Myomectomy is surgery requiring general anesthesia (see

Abdominal Hysterectomy

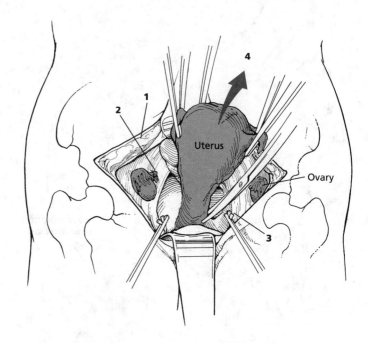

In an abdominal hysterectomy, an incision is made through fat, muscle, and other layers of tissue (1). The fallopian tubes and ligaments (2) and uterine blood vessels (3) are cut and tied and the uterus is freed from its attachments to nearby tissue. Finally, the uterus is removed through the incision (4) and the incision is stitched closed.

p.168) that is performed through an abdominal incision. During myomectomy, the fibroids are cut out of the uterine wall one by one. It potentially saves the uterus for future pregnancy but follow-up surgery is required in 25% of women.

Women who conceive after a myomectomy are more likely to require a cesarean section during childbirth.

Hysterectomy (see p.1072) is the only permanent solution to fibroids. However, because fibroids usually shrink after menopause, many women who are approaching the age of menopause defer surgery.

Prolapse of the Uterus

Prolapse of the uterus is a condition in which the uterus drops into the vagina. In severe cases, it protrudes out of the vaginal opening.

Childbearing and changes that occur with menopause can weaken the walls of the vagina and rectum as well as the ligaments that support the uterus. Without the usual support, the uterus can be pushed out of its normal position by increased pressure in the abdomen during a bowel movement, urination, or a cough.

Symptoms can include heaviness or pressure low in your pelvis, low back pain, urinary incontinence, or pain during sexual intercourse.

Your physician can diagnose uterine prolapse easily during a pelvic examination. Treatment depends on the degree of weakness around the uterus. Estrogen cream inserted into the vagina helps restore the strength of vaginal tissues. Kegel exercises (see p.1051) can help strengthen your pelvic floor muscles. When symptoms are difficult to control, surgery can repair or replace the structures that support the uterus. A hysterectomy (see p.1072) is an option as well.

For women who do not want surgery but have difficulty keeping the uterus in place, a device called a pessary often provides adequate support. A pessary is like a diaphragm; it fits next to the cervix to help prevent the uterus from prolapsing. It needs to be cleaned and checked for correct fit at regular intervals.

Retroverted Uterus

Some women are told they have a retroverted—or tipped—uterus. About 20% of all women have such a uterus, which tilts toward the back rather than tilting forward. Usually, the uterus has been in this position since birth. However, adhesions caused by

endometriosis or surgery can also pull the uterus into a retroverted position, as can large tumors.

Your uterus can move back and forth from retroverted to the usual position and back again during your lifetime.

There is usually no need for concern. Most women do not have symptoms, though some have backaches during their period or notice back pressure or pain with sexual intercourse.

During pregnancy, women with a retroverted uterus tend to have more back pain than others. If there are no symptoms, no treatment is necessary.

Pelvic Inflammatory Disease

Pelvic inflammatory disease (PID) includes any infection or inflammation of the organs of the pelvis, most commonly the uterus, fallopian tubes, or ovaries.

Usually, PID develops from a sexually transmitted disease (STD) (see p.889) such as chlamydia or gonorrhea. It can also develop from an infection related to an intrauterine device (IUD) or diaphragm or after a miscarriage or ectopic pregnancy.

The infection can be acute (with sudden and severe symptoms) or chronic (with less severe, but persistent symp-

Dilation and Curettage

A dilation and curettage (D&C) is the dilation (opening) of the cervix and curettage (scraping) of the lining of the uterus. It is performed on an outpatient basis using either general anesthesia (which induces deep sleep), regional anesthesia (which numbs the region of the body below the waist), or local anesthesia (which numbs only the cervix before dilation).

The physician uses a speculum to hold the vaginal walls apart so he or she can see the cervix. Next, the doctor inserts a series of progressively wider rods into the opening of the cervix. When the opening is wide enough for the instruments, the doctor uses a curette (a thin, long tube with a wire loop or spoon at the tip) to gently scrape away tissue from the endometrium (lining of the uterus). Increasingly, doctors are performing a D&C using hysteroscopy, in which a small endoscope is placed inside the uterus. This measure helps the doctor be sure that all abnormalities have been identified and that all necessary tissue has been removed.

You can go home after the anesthesia wears off. For the next few days, you may have vaginal bleeding like that of a period; avoid sexual intercourse until the bleeding stops. Watch for the following signs of infection or injury to the uterus: fever above 100.4°F, abdominal pain, foul-smelling vaginal discharge, or extremely heavy bleeding. Contact your doctor immediately if you have any of these signs in the first few days after a D&C.

toms). Without early treatment, it can lead to infertility by scarring the ovaries or blocking the fallopian tubes.

SYMPTOMS

In the early stages, you may have no symptoms. This can lead to a chronic infection that causes mild abdominal pain, fatigue, or backaches. An acute infection tends to be diagnosed in an early stage because of high fever and severe pain in the lower abdomen. In either case, you may have very heavy periods, pain during sexual intercourse, or a vaginal dis-

charge that has changed in color or smell.

TREATMENT OPTIONS

Your doctor will perform a pelvic examination and take samples of cervical secretions to send to the laboratory to look for infection. He or she may suspect PID if you have a particularly painful or sensitive cervix or there is pus coming from the cervix.

Infection is treated with antibiotics, usually in tablet form. Any sexual partners you have had within 6 months of the beginning of your symptoms

should also be checked for STDs, even if they have no symptoms. You should not have sexual intercourse until your current partner is treated.

If your symptoms do not improve after 5 to 7 days, or if you have a new high fever or more severe abdominal pain, contact your doctor. You may need to be hospitalized so that you can be given intravenous antibiotics. In severe infections, surgery is necessary to remove scar tissue or pockets of infection (abscesses).

OVARIES AND FALLOPIAN TUBES

Ovarian Cancer

In the United States, ovarian cancer causes more deaths than any other cancer of the genital organs, more than cancer of the cervix and cancer of the uterus combined. There are about 27,000 new cases diagnosed each year.

Cancer of the ovary is very difficult to diagnose at an early stage and, as a result, is more likely to be fatal than cancer of the cervix or endometrium (uterine cancer).

A woman's risk for ovarian cancer increases if she has a family history of ovarian cancer; is over 50; has not had children; has never taken birth-control pills; went through menopause after age 51; or has a history of cancer of the breast, lung, or colon.

Certain genes that increase a woman's risk of getting ovarian cancer have been identified. However, the genes discovered thus

far seem to be responsible for only a small fraction of ovarian cancers.

Certain circumstances protect against getting ovarian cancer, such as the number of children you have had. Taking birth-control pills can decrease your lifetime risk of ovarian cancer by as much as 50%, probably because they prevent ovulation. For this reason, it is recommended that women with a high risk of ovarian cancer take oral contraceptives.

SYMPTOMS

Ovarian cancer is called a "silent" disease because there are often no symptoms until the tumor is large enough for your physician to detect during a pelvic examination or until symptoms occur due to spreading of the cancer to other organs.

In addition, the symptoms—

nausea, vomiting, frequent urination, constipation, or swelling or a sense of fullness in the abdomen—can be similar to those caused by less-serious problems. For these reasons, about 75% of cases are not identified until the late stages of the disease.

Doctors are working hard to find screening tests that will detect ovarian cancer at an early stage, before it causes symptoms. No good screening test has yet been found. Examining the ovaries during a pelvic examination can occasionally detect ovarian cancer at an early stage, but usually does not.

Vaginal ultrasound also can sometimes show ovarian cancer at an early stage, but often does not. Vaginal ultrasound also frequently identifies suspicious areas that turn out to be nothing serious, particularly in women who have not gone through menopause. False positive test results can lead to fear and unnecessary surgical procedures (such as laparoscopy).

TREATMENT OPTIONS

Your doctor may suspect ovarian cancer if a lump is felt on the ovary or seen during a pelvic or vaginal ultrasound. Ultrasound can also differentiate between an ovarian tumor and an ovarian cyst (see p.1080).

Depending on your risk for cancer and how the lump appears, your doctor may recommend that you have another ultrasound in a few months or a biopsy of the lump in the near future so that the tissue can be examined under a microscope for abnormal cancerous cells. A biopsy can be performed through laparoscopy (see p.142), which allows visualization of the ovary and other possible areas of cancer spread in the abdomen.

A cancer antigen (CA-125) blood test can sometimes reveal a protein shed by ovarian cancer cells. However, this test is not highly accurate because the protein level is also high in a large number of noncancerous conditions and can be normal in some women with ovarian cancer. A diagnosis can be made only after examining a sample of tissue from the ovary.

If cancer is diagnosed, the next question is how far it has spread. Your doctor will check for signs of cancer spread; these include a large amount of fluid in the abdomen, other abdominal lumps, swollen lymph glands in the groin, or nodules found during a rectal exam. Computed tomography (see p.149) of the abdomen may be necessary to look for enlarged lymph glands

or other masses that suggest spreading cancer.

To further evaluate the spread of the cancer, and to remove as much cancer as possible, a surgical procedure known as exploratory laparotomy may be performed. In this surgery, the surgeon cuts open the abdomen, examines the inside of the abdomen thoroughly, and takes samples of tissue to be examined in the laboratory for signs of cancer spread. Usually, the ovaries, fallopian tubes, uterus, and sur-

rounding tissue (the omentum) are removed.

If you want to become pregnant, you may choose to have only the affected ovary and fallopian tube removed, leaving the uterus and the other ovary and fallopian tube intact. However, leaving these tissues poses a risk that some small deposits of cancer may not be removed.

Unlike many other cancers where the stage affects the type of surgery performed, the stage of ovarian cancer is determined

---

Family History and Risk of Ovarian Cancer

Ovarian cancer is rare in the general population. However, women with a family history of ovarian cancer are at increased risk of developing the disease in their lifetime.

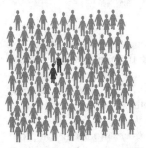

1.75 OF 100 WOMEN DEVELOP OVARIAN CANCER IN THEIR LIFETIME

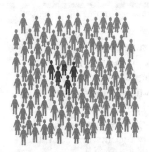

4.5 OF 100 WOMEN WITH ONE RELATIVE WITH OVARIAN CANCER DEVELOP OVARIAN CANCER IN THEIR LIFETIME

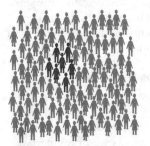

7 OF 100 WOMEN WITH TWO RELATIVES WITH OVARIAN CANCER DEVELOP OVARIAN CANCER IN THEIR LIFETIME

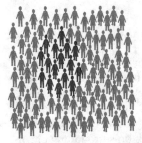

16 OF 100 WOMEN WITH THE BRCA1 OR BRCA2 GENE MUTATION DEVELOP OVARIAN CANCER IN THEIR LIFETIME

Stages of Ovarian Cancer

The different stages of ovarian cancer are divided according to how far the cancer has spread.

STAGE	LOCATION OF SPREAD	CHANCE OF SURVIVAL 5 YEARS AFTER DIAGNOSIS
IA	Cancer is confined to the ovary and no tumor remains after surgery.	After surgery—95%
IB	Cancer is confined to the ovary but some tumor remains after surgery or tumor cells appear to be highly malignant.	After surgery plus chemotherapy and radiation therapy—80%
II	Cancer is confined to the pelvis.	After surgery—70%
III	Cancer has spread to the abdomen.	After surgery plus chemotherapy—30% to 60%
IV	Cancer has spread outside the abdomen	After chemotherapy and (in some cases) surgery—1% to 5%

during surgery. The stage affects the type of treatment you will have after surgery. Because most women have later-stage ovarian cancer, chemotherapy (see p.741) or radiation therapy (see p.741) is usually recommended. If the biopsies of tissue show more extensive spread, further surgery is necessary to remove other organs that may be affected by the cancer.

Ovarian Cysts

An ovarian cyst is a noncancerous sac filled with fluid or semisolid material that grows on an ovary. Cysts are common and usually harmless, although they can push on surrounding organs, twist, or burst, causing severe pain, fever, and nausea. They may also become very large.

Different types of cysts develop from different types of cells. Common cysts known as corpus luteum cysts may develop from follicles in the ovary that normally prepare an egg for release every month. A common cause of cysts is endometriosis (see p.1073). Less frequent are dermoid cysts, known as teratomas, which develop from special embryonic cells that can grow teeth, hair, or fat inside the cyst. Cystadenomas are filled with fluid and tissue.

SYMPTOMS

Many ovarian cysts cause no symptoms. Larger cysts can cause dull or sharp abdominal pain. The symptoms of cysts formed from follicles tend to occur at the same time as symptoms of the menstrual cycle. Cysts may also be responsible for irregular periods or pain during sexual intercourse.

TREATMENT OPTIONS

Your doctor may suspect an ovary is larger than normal during a pelvic examination. An ultrasound can distinguish a cyst from potentially serious conditions such as pelvic inflammatory disease (see p.1077), ectopic pregnancy (see p.929), or ovarian cancer (see p.1078).

Tests may include a blood test to identify infection, the presence of CA-125 (see p.1079) (a protein that can be shed by cancer cells), or a urine test to check for pregnancy. Depending on what the ultrasound reveals, a laparoscopy (see p.142) may be necessary to view the cyst directly, take a biopsy, or remove it. A solid cyst is always removed and analyzed for the presence of cancer cells.

No treatment is necessary unless the cyst is causing intolerable symptoms or appears likely to rupture. Birth-control pills control the growth of some cysts, which improves symptoms and prevents the formation of new cysts.

Ovarian cysts from follicles are very common during the years a woman is menstruating. For this reason, menstruating women usually require only a follow-up examination or an ultrasound, which often shows that the cyst is smaller or has gone away altogether.

Any cyst that occurs after menopause should be removed to check for cancer. If the cyst is large, the entire ovary may require removal.

Polycystic Ovary Syndrome

Polycystic ovary syndrome (PCOS) is a condition in which many cysts develop from ovarian follicles that fail to rupture and release eggs. It is one of the most common hormonal disorders among women, occurring more frequently in women who are obese.

Women with PCOS are often daughters of men who became bald early in life. A defect in a single gene is thought to be responsible for both conditions.

PCOS is the result of abnormally high production of the hormone androgen by the ovaries and adrenal glands. Although androgen hormones are commonly thought of as male hormones, they are also normally produced in smaller amounts in women.

Often, women with PCOS also have a condition called insulin resistance. Insulin resistance helps stimulate the high production of androgens. In a woman with PCOS, the ovaries continue to produce estrogen, which causes the lining of the uterus to grow. However, the high androgen levels prevent ovulation and consequently reduce the production of progesterone. Because of this, the endometrium is not shed, raising the risk of endometrial cancer (see p.1071).

PCOS is a major cause of infertility. It is also associated with a higher risk of diabetes (see p.832). A medicine used to treat insulin resistance and diabetes, metformin, has been found to reduce the production of androgen by the ovaries, to encourage the ovaries to release an egg each month, and to thereby improve fertility in women with PCOS.

SYMPTOMS

Because ovulation does not occur regularly, you may have erratic periods, often with heavy bleeding, or you may not menstruate at all. High levels of the male androgen hormones can be responsible for acne, deepening of the voice, male-pattern baldness, or excess body hair (see Hirsutism, p.557).

Some women notice dark velvety patches (called acanthosis nigricans) on the skin. Other women have no symptoms and are diagnosed only during an evaluation for infertility.

TREATMENT OPTIONS

If you have any of these symptoms, see your doctor for a physical examination. He or she will look for signs of high levels of the androgen hormone and other possible causes. To make a diagnosis, blood tests to measure hormone levels are necessary.

Treatment is tailored to the type and severity of your symptoms. For all women with PCOS, a healthy diet and exercise are especially important because of the tendency toward obesity and diabetes. If you have regular periods, you may only need advice on cosmetic methods to treat the changes in your appearance. There are also medicines

Oophorectomy: Removal of the Ovaries

Oophorectomy is the surgical removal of one or both ovaries. An oophorectomy may be performed to treat certain types of endometriosis or ovarian cysts. You can still have normal menstrual cycles and conceive with one ovary.

When both ovaries are removed, menopause (see p.1047) occurs and it is necessary to start hormone replacement therapy (see p.1049) or discuss with your doctor other ways to prevent the development of osteoporosis and heart disease. The ovaries are also sometimes removed along with the uterus and other pelvic structures during a hysterectomy (see p.1072).

that specifically act against the male androgen hormones that cause the hair growth and acne.

Birth-control pills are useful both for regulating periods and for treating the hirsutism. Women who do not have hirsutism can have regular periods with a tablet form of the progesterone hormone taken 10 days of each month.

Regulating periods decreases the risk for endometrial hyperplasia (see Cancer of the Endometrium, p.1071) and endometrial cancer.

Treating infertility involves the use of clomiphene citrate to induce ovulation; it is very successful in treating women with PCOS. Adding the medicine metformin (used for diabetes) can further increase the chance of becoming pregnant.

Primary Ovarian Failure

Primary ovarian failure is a congenital (from birth) genetic abnormality in which ovaries fail to develop or develop abnormally. About 30% of girls who see a doctor when they have not menstruated by age 18 have abnormal ovaries.

In primary ovarian failure, some or all of the female characteristics (such as breasts) fail to develop due to the absence of the female hormones produced by the ovaries.

The most common form of primary ovarian failure is Turner syndrome, a genetic condition that affects some women more severely than others. In the most severe form, an adolescent girl does not develop breasts, genitals, or hair in the pubic or underarm area, and is small for her age.

SYMPTOMS

Usually, an abnormality is not apparent at birth, and lack of menstruation by the age of 16 is the first sign of primary ovarian failure. Many normal girls do not menstruate until this age or later but still have developed normal physical changes of adolescence.

TREATMENT OPTIONS

If you have not yet had your first period and you are older than 16, see your doctor. He or she will perform a physical examination, including a pelvic examination. Your doctor will also look for other signs of normal adolescent development and check to see if your reproductive organs are present.

Your physician may prescribe the female hormone progesterone to verify that your ovaries are producing estrogen. Taking progesterone will induce menstrual bleeding if the ovaries are operational. A blood test can determine if hormone levels are normal; a pelvic ultrasound (see p.1042) can determine whether ovaries are present.

Treatment with estrogen and progesterone can help women with ovarian failure develop breasts but does not reverse infertility. Some women need plastic surgery to create the appearance of normal female development and may even need to have a vagina constructed to have sexual intercourse.

SEXUALITY

Contraception and Sexually Transmitted Diseases

Having sexual intercourse carries the risk not only of pregnancy, but also of sexually transmitted diseases (STDs) (see p.889). Your risk of STDs is greater if you have more than one sexual partner.

If you do not want to become pregnant, you and your partner must use some form of contraception (see p.68). A latex or polyurethane condom is the only contraceptive method that offers protection against both pregnancy and STDs, but it is not 100% reliable.

The effectiveness of the female condom is not as well proven as that of the male condom, but there is no doubt that using a female condom is much safer than using no condom at all. Anal intercourse and oral sex also can transmit STDs unless a condom is worn.

Sex Therapy

Problems with a woman's sexuality can be related to any of the factors that influence sexuality. Many couples find sex therapy very helpful in identifying and resolving sexual inhibitions and related problems. To locate a reliable sex therapist, ask your physician for a referral or call a hospital and ask to speak to a social worker who can refer you to a therapist.

The American Association of Sex Educators, Counselors, and Therapists (AASECT) can send you a list of certified sex therapists in your area.

Homosexuality and Bisexuality

Men and women who are homosexual or bisexual usually have sensed it from the time they became sexually aware as children. Most scientists believe that homosexuality and bisexuality are normal variations in sexual orientation. Between 5% and 10% of people in all cultures worldwide are homosexual; the statistics on bisexuals are less clear.

Like heterosexuals, homosexuals and bisexuals may require psychotherapy (see p.393) to resolve any of a range of life issues; however, homosexuals and bisexuals do not need psychotherapy because of their sexual orientation.

For friends and family of a gay person or lesbian, Parents and Friends of Lesbians and Gays (PFLAG) (see p.1233) can provide information and support.

PROBLEMS WITH FEMALE SEXUAL FUNCTION

Loss of Sexual Desire

Loss of libido (sexual desire) occurs in both men and women and is a common problem. Sexual desire is influenced by many factors and tends to fluctuate in intensity over a woman's lifetime, with changes in hormonal levels, in child-rearing or job responsibilities, and in the state of her relationship with her partner.

Some women notice a decrease in sexual desire after childbirth. This may be partly due to hormonal changes and partly due to the physical demands of caring for a child. Fatigue or stress can affect any person's interest in sex. Psychological or emotional conflicts can also reduce your sex drive. Depression, conflicts with your partner, and anxiety over finances, self-image, and health can all decrease your interest in sex.

Some women suffer from sexual aversion disorder. After many years of being able to experience sexual desire, they suddenly develop a strong distaste for sexual contact. Other sexual phobias

may be associated with panic disorder (see p.404).

Medicines can also affect sexual desire, including those used to treat high blood pressure, anxiety, and depression. Pain or discomfort during sexual activity is another cause of reduced sexual drive. One common example is pain in the vagina during intercourse (see p.1084). Pain from arthritis in the back, pelvis, or hips is another common example; taking a pain medicine 30 to 60 minutes before sexual relations can be very helpful.

Some women experience diminished sexual drive during perimenopause and menopause. They may benefit from adding androgen (a male hormone) to their hormone replacement therapy. Women normally make androgens, although at levels lower than in men, and androgens normally generate sexual drive in women, as they do in men. Not all women experience increased sexual desire with androgen treatment.

If a change in your desire for sexual activity concerns you, talk to your doctor. He or she will treat any underlying illness or adjust your medicines and can refer you to a sex therapist (see p.1082).

Problems With Orgasm

Some women have normal sexual drive but have difficulty having an orgasm during sexual relations. Orgasm is the climax that occurs during sexual activity. Most women do not reach orgasm through intercourse only; they require stimulation of the clitoris as well.

Problems with orgasm may arise from a variety of sources and often are related to psychological components of guilt, distrust of a sexual partner, conflict in the relationship, and poor self-image. Fatigue or any new medicines can also interfere with your ability to have an orgasm. Your doctor may change your medicines and can refer you to a sex therapist.

One unproven theory is that, in some women, the clitoris does not swell enough to be stimulated ("female impotence"). This theory maintains that treatments for male erectile dysfunction (see p.1092) such as sildenafil (the impotence pill) might help some women who cannot achieve orgasm.

Therapy may include learning how to have satisfying orgasms through masturbation so that you can show your partner how to stimulate you during sex. Therapy can also teach you how to deal with psychological factors, increase communication between you and your partner, experiment, and share involvement in sexual pleasure.

Pain With Sexual Intercourse

Pain during sexual intercourse is a common occurrence among women. Usually it is caused by inadequate vaginal lubrication, either because of insufficient foreplay or vaginal dryness due to lower estrogen levels after menopause. Hormone replacement therapy (see p.1049) or a vaginal cream containing estrogen or nonhormonal water-based lubricants can ease dryness.

If increased lubrication does not resolve the pain, talk to your doctor. He or she will perform a pelvic examination to check for vaginal infections (see p.1066), pelvic inflammatory disease (see p.1077), endometriosis (see p.1071), ovarian cysts (see p.1080), ovarian cancer (see p.1078), fibroids of the uterus (see p.1074), or a prolapsed uterus (see p.1076), all of which can cause painful intercourse.

Another cause of painful intercourse is irritated vaginal tissue, which can result from an allergic reaction. Irritants include soaps, detergents, douches, or feminine hygiene products; a poorly placed diaphragm; or an episiotomy (see p.938). Vaginismus (see below) can also cause painful intercourse.

VAGINISMUS

Vaginismus is a condition in which the muscles of the wall of the vagina contract involuntarily. This condition may be responsible for pain during sexual intercourse or may make it difficult to insert a tampon into your vagina or have a pelvic examination.

Vaginismus is more common in women who have experienced sexual abuse. Other causes can include fear of pregnancy, lack of sexual experience, or fear of pain.

See your doctor if you have symptoms of vaginismus. He or she will check for a physical cause and, if none can be found, may refer you for therapy. Therapy includes discussion to help you overcome any fears, and exercises to help you become familiar and comfortable with your vaginal area. The exercises may involve inserting your finger or tampons into your vagina.

WOMEN AND VIOLENCE

Domestic Violence

Domestic violence is intentional violent or controlling behavior by a person with a past or present close personal relationship with the victim. Most domestic violence (90%) is perpetrated by men against women. Children are also affected. Partner violence is the most common cause of reported injury to women in the United States.

The aim of the abuser is to assert power and maintain control. The abuser may commit any combination of physical, sexual, psychological, verbal, and economic abuse. Many victims are reluctant to disclose information about abuse because of fear (for self or children), economic constraints, social isolation, hope for change, or a sense of failure.

In addition to physical injury, victims of abuse may have symptoms of chronic pain (see p.381), posttraumatic stress disorder (see p.406), anxiety (see p.402), depression (see p.395), and substance abuse (see p.411).

Counseling can help you cope with the profound and long-lasting effects of abuse. Look in the yellow pages of your phone book under "crisis intervention" for a phone number of a hotline or a shelter that can provide counseling, safe quarters, and legal advice. Under the laws of many states, you may obtain a restraining order against the abuser. This means the person is legally forbidden to make contact with you, and you can take legal action for any violation of the restraining order.

Domestic Violence: Dr Sillman's Advice

Domestic violence is a common and serious problem. We doctors often don't suspect it. Many of our patients don't tell us about it—unless we ask.

I ask every one of my female patients if she is in a relationship where she feels threatened or hurt. If her answer is yes, I tell her that she deserves better and that help is available.

An excellent source of help is the National Domestic Violence Hotline (1-800-799-SAFE; TDD: 1-800-787-3224). The hotline staff speaks English, Spanish, and other languages and is available 24 hours a day to counsel callers and inform them about resources near their homes.

If you or a friend is in an abusive relationship and feel there is no one to turn to, call the hotline.

JANE S. SILLMAN, MD
BRIGHAM AND WOMEN'S HOSPITAL
HARVARD MEDICAL SCHOOL

If You Are the Victim of Sexual Assault

Sexual assault, including rape, occurs when any person is forced to engage in sex against his or her will. Rape is a crime; in some states it is also a crime in marriage and between partners of the same sex. In a woman, it occurs when the vagina or any other body opening is forcibly penetrated during sexual intercourse, or with the use of an object.

If you are the victim of sexual assault, phone the police to report the crime, go immediately to a hospital emergency department, and phone a rape crisis hotline or a friend so that someone can accompany you to the hospital.

Because there is evidence of the sexual assault on your body:

- Do not take a bath or shower or wash your hands.

- Do not change clothes.

- Do not brush your teeth or rinse your mouth.

At the hospital, you will be asked to describe the sexual assault. Any loose hairs from your clothes and body will be collected so that they can be matched with those of the assailant. Nail clippings may be taken because there may be skin from the assailant under them.

Next, a physician will examine you. A Pap smear is obtained and samples of vaginal and cervical secretions are collected to test for sexually transmitted diseases and to establish the blood type of sperm, which can help identify the assailant. You will be tested for pregnancy and the human immunodeficiency virus (HIV) as well.

Advocates from a local rape crisis center can guide you to local resources for psychological and legal counseling.

The trauma associated with the sexual assault often leads women to wait hours or days to go to the hospital or the police. By that time, much of the physical evidence of the assault cannot be collected. If you are the victim of a sexual assault, it is important to go to a hospital as soon as possible.

Health of Men

Men are built differently from women. But, then, you knew that. What follows are the details. The male reproductive system is designed to produce sperm and deposit them inside a woman's vagina during sexual intercourse. This requires the coordinated effort of several different glands that are unique to men. Sperm are produced in the testicles and mature in the epididymis, before being expelled through the penis during ejaculation. This all occurs under the direction of hormones made in the brain—follicle-stimulating hormone (FSH) and luteinizing hormone (LH). These brain hormones also direct sexual reproduction in women.

Making sperm At full maturity, each testicle is about 1½ inches long by 1 inch wide. In many men, one testicle is a bit larger than the other; this is normal. Sperm are produced in the testicles by germ cells. Young men produce about 1,000 sperm per second. The Leydig cells in the testicles produce the male hormone testosterone, which is responsible for the male sexual characteristics (see How Hormones Affect Men, p.1087). Coiled behind the testicles is a 20-foot-long tube called the epididymis, a duct where sperm complete their maturation before entering an extension of the tube called the vas deferens.

The testicles and epididymis are contained within a pouch of skin called the scrotum. Because

the scrotum is suspended outside the rest of the body, the temperature of the testicles is about 90°F, about 8° to 9° below the body's internal temperature. The lower temperature helps sperm production. Normal ejaculate contains 2 to 6 milliliters of fluid (about ⅓ to 1 teaspoonful); each milliliter of semen contains 20 million to 200 million sperm. About 50% of men with sperm counts of 20 million to 40 million per milliliter

of semen are unable to make a woman pregnant; virtually all men with counts below 20 million have impaired fertility.

Transporting and nourishing sperm The vas deferens carries the sperm inside the body through an opening called the inguinal canal, a common spot for a hernia (see p.800). Inside the body, the vas deferens continues over and behind the bladder to meet the ejaculatory duct.

Male Reproductive System

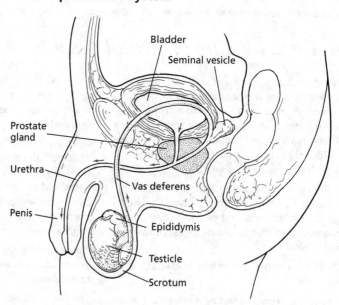

Sperm are produced in the testicles (which are suspended in the scrotum) and move into the epididymis, where they mature. During ejaculation, sperm are transported through the vas deferens to the seminal vesicles, which produce seminal fluid that, along with sperm, makes up semen. The prostate gland secretes a fluid that adds volume to the semen, which moves through the urethra to be ejaculated during orgasm.

How Hormones Affect Men

This chart shows some of the important hormones circulating in a man's body and the effects they have.

HORMONE	WHERE IT IS PRODUCED	WHAT IT DOES
Follicle-stimulating hormone (FSH)	Pituitary gland in the brain	Starts the production of sperm in the testicles
Luteinizing hormone (LH)	Pituitary gland in the brain	Helps the testicles produce testosterone
Testosterone	Leydig cells of the testicles	Helps sperm mature and helps develop the reproductive organs and such male sexual characteristics as facial and body hair, deep voice, and large muscles
Dihydro-testosterone	Tissues (from testosterone)	Mediates various male characteristics, including growth of the prostate and loss of hair in male pattern baldness

The muscular lining of the vas deferens propels sperm during ejaculation.

The sperm require nourishment as they wait to be expelled from the body. That nourishment is provided by semen, a thick fluid produced by three different glands: the prostate gland, the bulbourethral glands, and the seminal vesicles. The ejaculatory ducts are small tracts that receive sperm from the vas deferens and semen from the vesicles. During ejaculation, they empty into the urethra, a tube running through the middle of the penis. The bulbourethral glands and prostate gland also discharge fluid into the semen during ejaculation.

Ejaculating sperm During orgasm, the man ejaculates the mix of sperm and semen. The force of the ejaculation is caused by contractions of the ejaculatory ducts and prostate. The ejaculate travels through the urethra and out the tip of the penis. The urethra also is the passageway for expelling urine from the kidney, but muscles in the bladder neck prevent urine from entering the urethra during ejaculation.

PROTECTING YOUR HEALTH

Most of the things you can do to protect your health are covered in Taking Charge of Your Health (see p.29), including good nutrition, exercise, health checkups, and self-examinations. Self-examinations and good hygiene are important. Wash your penis and scrotum with soap and water every day. If you are not circumcised, pull back the foreskin and clean the head of your penis. This is also a good time to look at your genital area for sores or lumps. If you detect any growths or sores, see your doctor as soon as possible for treatment.

PENIS

Cancer of the Penis

Cancer of the penis is rare; only 1,300 cases are diagnosed in the United States each year. It is probably caused by certain strains of the human papillomavirus (HPV), the same virus that causes cancer of the cervix in women. Poor hygiene under the foreskin of uncircumcised men may increase the risk of this cancer.

The earliest sign of penile cancer is a sore on the penis, usually near the glans (head) or on the foreskin. The sore may be dry and painless, or a painful, moist ulcer. If you have a sore or lump on your penis, see your doctor. Most lumps on the penis are not cancer, but can be caused by other treatable conditions such as genital warts (see Penile Warts, below right), syphilis (see p.893), or another sexually transmitted disease (see p.889).

If the diagnosis is not clear just from looking at the lump, your doctor may perform a biopsy (see p.161). If it reveals malignant (cancerous) cells, more tests may be performed to see whether the cancer has spread to other regions of the body.

Radiation therapy (see p.741) can successfully eradicate the cancer in the early stages. Otherwise, surgery to remove the cancerous part of the penis may be required. Chemotherapy (see p.741) may be necessary in more advanced cases.

Balanitis and Phimosis

Balanitis is inflammation of the glans (head) and foreskin of the penis. The condition is most common in uncircumcised men. The top part of the penis may be red, itchy, and moist from discharge. The most common causes of balanitis are poor hygiene under the foreskin; irritation from condoms, spermicides, or clothing; and infection due to a sexually transmitted disease such as genital herpes (see p.890). Balanitis usually clears up once the underlying cause is corrected; your doctor may prescribe a cream to soothe the inflammation and antibiotic drugs (see p.868) for any infection.

Phimosis is a tightening of the foreskin over the head of the penis that prevents the foreskin from being pulled back. Phimosis can cause balanitis, and it can

make erections painful. In its most extreme form, phimosis can interfere with the ability to pass urine. Phimosis can sometimes be treated by gradually and gently stretching the foreskin every day for several weeks with the aid of warm soapy water or baby oil. If this does not work, call your doctor; a circumcision (see p.943) may be required.

Penile Warts

Warts on the penis are usually caused by human papillomavirus (HPV)—different strains of the virus that cause penile cancer or cancer of the cervix in women. They are similar to the warts that occur on other parts of the body, but they can be spread by sexual contact.

The same virus can cause warts in the anus or the vagina; warts that appears on the penis, anus, or vagina are called genital warts (see p.891). If you have genital warts, it is essential that you inform any sexual partners so they can also be treated.

SYMPTOMS

Penile warts often start out as painless, small, pink or red growths; they reproduce quickly and grow in clumps. The first outbreak can occur up to 18 months after sexual transmission of the virus.

TREATMENT OPTIONS

Always have your doctor check any growth on your penis; growths that look like penile warts may actually be caused by

another sexually transmitted disease (see p.889) or may be cancerous.

Your doctor may take one of several treatment approaches. He or she may paint on a chemical to remove the warts, apply liquid nitrogen to freeze them off, or use an electrical current to cauterize (burn) them off. Other options include scraping, laser surgery, and injections with the drug interferon. Never attempt to treat penile warts yourself with over-the-counter wart preparations; they are not intended for use on the sensitive skin of the penis and can damage it.

There is no cure for the viral infection that causes genital warts. Even after the warts are treated successfully, the virus remains inactive but alive in the skin of the penis. This means that warts can recur at any time. Even without visible warts, the virus can be spread to an unprotected sexual partner. The only sure way to prevent spreading the virus to a sexual partner is to wear a condom.

Injury to the Penis

Injury to the penis is not common. When the penis is not sexually stimulated, it is flaccid, protecting it against injury. A forceful injury to the erect penis, however, can cause a penile fracture (a tear in the erectile tissues), which is a medical emergency. Deep cuts to the penis can cause serious damage to erectile function and are also a medical emergency.

TESTICLES AND SCROTUM

Injury to the Testicles

As every man knows, the testicles are highly sensitive, with even minor injury causing severe pain. However, damage to the structure of the testicles is rare. If you receive a blow to your testicles and you continue to have pain, bruising, or swelling after an hour, call your physician or go to a hospital emergency department. These signs may indicate damage to the internal structure of the testicles that requires prompt treatment. Boys and men should always wear athletic cups when playing contact sports.

Orchitis

Orchitis is inflammation of one or, less commonly, both testicles. It can be caused by a bacterial infection or by the mumps virus; orchitis associated with mumps can be prevented by having the measles, mumps, and rubella (MMR) vaccine (see p.947). Orchitis may also occur with infections of the epididymis (see Epididymitis, p.1090).

Symptoms include swelling and pain in the affected testicle, along with a high fever. If both testicles are involved, inflammation and infection can impair fertility.

If you have symptoms of orchitis, see your doctor as soon as possible. Your doctor will examine your scrotum and prostate and may analyze a sample of your urine to determine the cause of the inflammation. If the orchitis is caused by bacterial infection, your doctor will prescribe antibiotic drugs (see p.868).

Treatment of orchitis due to the mumps virus includes pain medication and ice packs to reduce swelling of the scrotum.

Torsion of the Testicle

Torsion of the testicle occurs when the testicle twists on its spermatic cord, which can cut off the blood supply to the testicle. It is an uncommon but extremely painful condition that requires immediate medical attention to prevent permanent damage to the testicle. Torsion of the testicle is most common between ages 10 and 20, but can occur at any age. The condition can occur after strenuous activity, but it often happens without apparent cause. If the torsion is not treated within a few hours, it can result in infertility or the need to remove the testicle.

SYMPTOMS

Sudden severe pain in a testicle (usually just one) that occurs without injury is the most striking symptom. The pain can be so severe that it produces nausea and vomiting. Your testicle will swell and you may become feverish. If your testicle untwists on its own you will experience immediate relief from the swelling and pain. Although untwisting occurs spontaneously in some cases, you should never postpone medical attention waiting for the testicle to untwist on its own.

TREATMENT OPTIONS

The faster you receive treatment, the better your chances for complete recovery. Your doctor will

examine your testicles to be sure that your symptoms are not caused by another condition, such as epididymitis (see p.1090). He or she may also perform an ultrasound (see p.148), which shows the internal structures of the testicle. The first step in treatment may be an attempt to untwist the testicle by hand. If this is not successful, immediate surgery is needed.

During surgery, your doctor makes an incision in the scrotum and untwists the spermatic cord.

Torsion of the Testicle

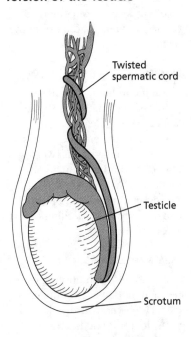

Torsion, or twisting, of the testicle is an uncommon but very painful condition that requires emergency medical care. It occurs when the spermatic cord becomes twisted and cuts off the blood supply to the testicle.

The testicle is then anchored in place with a few stitches. If the testicle has been severely damaged by a lack of blood flow, it may need to be removed. Your doctor may also recommend surgery on the other testicle to stitch it into place to prevent future twisting.

Hydrocele, Spermatocele, and Varicocele

Swelling of the scrotum is the main feature of these usually harmless conditions. In a hydrocele, the swelling is due to an accumulation of fluid between the membranes that surround the testicles. In a spermatocele, the swelling develops in the epididymis. In a varicocele, the swelling results from enlarged (varicose) veins leading from the testicles.

SYMPTOMS

In each condition, you have a painless swelling in the scrotum. With a varicocele, you may be able to feel the enlarged veins through your scrotum; swelling may come and go, usually increasing when you stand up. An inguinal hernia (see p.800) can also produce swelling of the scrotum.

TREATMENT OPTIONS

None of these conditions causes permanent damage to the testicles. However, you should see your doctor if you have any swelling in your scrotum so that he or she can rule out other causes. An ultrasound (see p.148) examination can help your doctor make a diagnosis.

Treatment of hydroceles, sper-

Varicocele

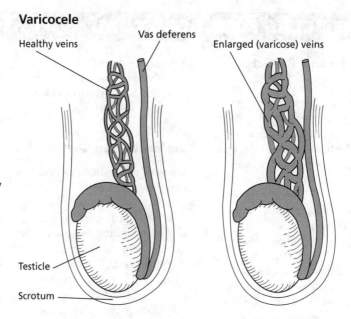

Healthy veins — Vas deferens — Enlarged (varicose) veins

Testicle —

Scrotum —

Varicocele is enlargement of the veins leading from the testicles. It causes swelling of the scrotum and may reduce the number of sperm produced.

matoceles, and varicoceles is needed only when the swelling is uncomfortable. After deadening the area with a local anesthetic (see p.168), your doctor may aspirate (draw out) the excess fluid with a needle and syringe and then inject a substance to prevent the fluid from returning. If a large amount of fluid has accumulated, surgery to remove the fluid and to prevent future accumulation is often required.

The heaviness you may feel with a varicocele can be helped by wearing supportive underwear or an athletic supporter. A varicocele can reduce your fertility because the enlarged veins block the sperm made in the testicles from getting into the ejaculation fluid, but it does not affect your ability to have an erection. If the varicocele is interfering with fertility, ask your doctor to

refer you to a surgeon who will tie off the varicose veins.

Epididymitis

Epididymitis is inflammation of the epididymis, the long coiled tube behind each testicle that carries sperm to the vas deferens (the sperm duct). The condition is usually caused either by an infection with bacteria that are normally present in the intestinal tract (and are not sexually transmitted) or by chlamydia (see p.892), which is sexually transmitted. In some men, the cause of inflammation cannot be found.

SYMPTOMS

Pain in your scrotum and swelling at the back of one of your testicles are the first symptoms of epididymitis, often followed within several hours by fever or chills. Your scrotum may feel hot, tender, and firm to the touch.

TREATMENT OPTIONS

See your doctor immediately if you suspect that you have epididymitis. He or she will examine you to ensure that your symptoms are not being caused by another condition, such as torsion of the testicle (see p.1088). If an infection is suspected, your doctor may take samples of your urine and secretions from your prostate gland to determine the cause. He or she will prescribe antibiotic drugs, which usually clear up the infection.

If the infection is caused by chlamydia, all sexual partners require treatment as well. Your doctor may recommend bed rest and ice packs to relieve the swelling, and analgesic drugs for pain.

Your testicle may remain enlarged for several months after treatment before returning to its normal size; aspirin or other non-steroidal anti-inflammatory drugs (see p.1162) can help control inflammation. In rare instances, surgery may be required to drain an abscess in the epididymis.

Undescended Testicle

In some men, one or both testicles never drop into the scrotal sac before birth, but remain inside the body. This leads to impaired sperm production (by that testicle), an increased risk of infertility, and an increased risk of torsion of the testicle (see p.1089).

Most important, the risk of testicular cancer is 30 to 50 times greater unless the problem is corrected by surgery that pulls the testicle into its normal position in the scrotum. Usually surgery is recommended as soon as the condition is discovered; ideally it is performed before age 2 (see p.1019) but it can also be performed later in life.

Cancer of the Testicle

This uncommon form of cancer most often affects men between ages 15 and 35; it is rare in blacks. It usually affects only one testicle but can affect both. In the vast majority of men, cancer of the testicle is curable if detected (see How to Examine Your Testicles, p.78) and treated early. The risk of this cancer is increased in men who have had an undescended testicle (see above).

SYMPTOMS

Cancer of the testicle appears as a hard lump in the testicle. It usually grows and spreads, which is why regular self-examination is essential. Usually the lump is painless, but it may cause pain and inflammation.

TREATMENT OPTIONS

If you detect a lump in your testicle, report it to your doctor. He or she will examine you and rule out other causes, such as epididymitis (see p.1090). An ultrasound (see p.148) is often the next step in diagnosis. If cancer is suspected, your doctor will perform a biopsy (see p.161). If the biopsy reveals cancerous cells, surgery is required to remove the testicle and nearby lymph nodes. Because it leaves one testicle intact, surgery usually does not affect your fertility or ability to have an erection. In the early stages of some forms of testicular cancer, only surgery is required. In other cases, radiation therapy (see p.741), chemotherapy (see p.741), or both are administered. The results are excellent if the disease is detected early.

SEXUALITY

Contraception and Sexually Transmitted Diseases

Sexual intercourse with a woman or a man carries the risk of sexually transmitted diseases (STDs) (see p.889). Your risk of STDs is greater if you (or your partner) have more than one sexual partner.

If you do not want to father a child, you and your female partner must use some form of contraception (see p.68). A latex or polyurethane condom is the only contraceptive method that offers protection against both pregnancy and STDs, but it is not 100% reliable.

Anal intercourse and oral intercourse also can transmit STDs unless a latex or polyurethane condom is worn. The effectiveness of the female condom is not as well proven as that of the male condom, but there is no doubt that using a female condom is much safer than using no condom at all.

For maximum protection

against pregnancy, couples can combine more secure contraceptive measures, such as the intrauterine device (IUD) or diaphragm, with a condom.

Sex Therapy

Sex therapy can be very successful in helping you overcome sexual inhibitions and related problems. To locate a reliable sex therapist, ask your physician for a referral or call your hospital and ask to speak to a social worker who can refer you to a therapist. It is essential that any sex therapist respect your values. The American Association of Sex Educators, Counselors, and Therapists (AASECT) is a certification organization for sex educators and therapists. This group will send you a list of certified sex therapists in your area.

Homosexuality and Bisexuality

Men and women who are homosexual or bisexual usually have sensed it from the time they became sexually aware as children. There are many theories as to why people are homosexual. Most scientists believe that homosexuality and bisexuality are normal variations in sexual orientation. Homosexuals apparently represent between 5% and 10% of people in all cultures worldwide; the statistics for bisexuals are less clear. Like heterosexuals, homosexuals and bisexuals may require psychotherapy (see p.393) to resolve any of a range of life issues; however, homosexuals and bisexuals do not need psychotherapy because of their sexual orientation. If you need help in accepting a gay or lesbian family member, Parents and Friends of Lesbians and Gays (PFLAG) (see p.1233) can provide support and information.

HEALTH CONCERNS OF GAY AND BISEXUAL MEN

The risk of contracting sexually transmitted diseases (STDs) is increased during anal intercourse. Oral intercourse also carries risk. The single most important preventive measure is to use a latex or polyurethane condom every time you have intercourse. Gay and bisexual men are at increased risk for infection with the herpes virus (see p.890); the human immunodeficiency virus (HIV), which causes acquired immunodeficiency syndrome (AIDS) (see p.872); hepatitis B virus (see p.759); chlamydia (see p.892); and giardiasis (see p.886). Your risk is greater if you or your partner have more than one sexual partner.

PROBLEMS WITH MALE SEXUAL FUNCTION

The Normal Erection

Your whole body—not just your penis—is involved in having an erection. Sexual arousal begins when your thoughts and your senses make you feel sexually excited. Next, nerve endings in your penis release a chemical messenger that widens the blood vessels of your penis. This permits the penis's two erectile chambers, which contain spongelike tissue, to fill with blood and expand, producing an erection.

Impotence

Impotence (also called erectile dysfunction) is the inability to have an erection, an experience that almost every man has at some point in his life. Occasional failure to have an erection is normal, but when a man is unable to have an erection adequate for intercourse on more than 25% of attempts, it is considered abnormal. An estimated 10 million to 20 million men in the United States meet this medical definition of impotence.

About 2% of 40-year-olds are impotent, but the percentage rises with age, exceeding 25% after age 65. Although impotence is more common among older men, it is not an inevitable consequence of aging and it can be treated in men of all ages.

CAUSES OF IMPOTENCE

Any condition that damages the circulatory system—including smoking, drinking alcohol, lack of exercise, and poor nutrition—can contribute to impotence. In men over 60, the leading cause of impotence is atherosclerosis, which narrows arteries throughout the body and restricts blood flow to the penis. Men with diabetes mellitus (see p.832) are at higher risk for impotence because the disease can damage both the blood vessels and nerves involved in erections. Nerve damage is also responsible for the impotence that may occur after surgery for prostate cancer

Erection Problems:
Dr O'Leary's Advice

Erection problems (called erectile dysfunction by doctors) are a very common problem in men and may occur in as many as 25 million U.S. men. It is more common with increasing age, but has been reported in men as young as 40. While we used to believe that the majority of these men had psychological erection problems, we now believe that most erection problems have a physical cause.

Our understanding of what causes the problem, and how to treat it, has improved dramatically over the past 10 years. The most recent advance has been oral sildenafil—the "impotence pill." In properly selected patients, this medicine appears to be highly effective and safe. However, the 20% to 40% of men who do not respond to this medication should not be discouraged; there are a variety of other effective and safe forms of therapy. Today, there is virtually no man who should "suffer in silence" with erectile dysfunction. We have effective forms of therapies for most everyone.

MICHAEL P. O'LEARY, MD, MPH
BRIGHAM AND WOMEN'S HOSPITAL
HARVARD MEDICAL SCHOOL

(see p.1102), or as a complication of neurological conditions including spinal cord injury, Parkinson disease (see p.371), and multiple sclerosis (see p.368).

Prescription drugs can also cause impotence or make it worse. The chief culprits include many medications used to treat high blood pressure, heart disease, and depression. Excessive amounts of alcohol can interfere with erection, as can illegal drugs such as cocaine. Low levels of the male hormone testosterone are responsible in less than 5% of men who are impotent.

About 15% of impotent men have a psychological basis for their impotence, such as anxiety, stress, depression, or problems in the relationship. Sex therapy (see p.1092) can be very successful in helping you overcome sexual inhibitions and related problems.

TREATMENT OPTIONS

If your doctor suspects a prescription drug may be causing your impotence, he or she may recommend that you stop taking the drug (under close supervision).

There are a number of treatments available for impotence.

In the United States, there are now three pills approved for the treatment of impotence: sildenafil (Viagra), tadalafil (Cialis), and vardenafil (Levitra). They all work the same way. Normally, when a man is sexually aroused, the brain sends signals to nerve endings in the penis that release a gas called nitric oxide. This gas stimulates the production of the chemical guanosine monophosphate (GMP). GMP causes blood vessels in the penis to widen, increasing blood flow to the penis and causing an erection. Then, GMP is inactivated by an enzyme.

The impotence pills cause the level of GMP to increase and to last longer. This produces, increases, and prolongs the erection. The pills help most men with impotence, whether it is caused by physical or psychological factors. However, it is not effective in all men who use it and it does not lead to an erection sufficient for intercourse on every attempt. The pills work only if a man is sexually aroused: The drug does not, by itself, increase sexual desire.

In patients with impotence from diabetes or from surgery for prostate disease, the impotence pills are somewhat less effective than in other men. They also have not been proven to enhance sexual performance in men who do not have impotence.

Side effects include headaches, flushing, and gastrointestinal upset in 20% to 30% of men. There are temporary disturbances in color vision in up to 10% of men who take high doses of sildenafil.

The impotence pills should not be taken by any man who is taking a nitrate or an alpha adrenergic antagonist medicine: Serious side effects can occur.

The effects of sildenafil and vardenafil begin within 30 minutes and last up to 4 hours. The effects of tadalafil start as rapidly, but last up to 36 hours. Sildenafil and vardenafil should be taken on an empty stomach.

Diagnosing Impotence

If you experience frequent or consistent impotence, consult your doctor. A specialist is often not required. Your physician will know if you are taking any medicines, have any diseases, or have had any surgery that could cause impotence. The doctor will ask whether you sometimes awaken with an erection or are able to achieve an erection with masturbation. If either is the case, you probably do not have an underlying physical problem but rather a psychological one.

Your doctor will ask you when the problem began, whether it occurs with a specific partner, and how work and stress might contribute. The physical examination will include blood pressure testing, a genital and prostate examination, and tests to check your nerve reflexes and circulation. Your doctor may give you a blood test to check for several physical causes of impotence—including diabetes, thyroid gland disorders, increased levels of the hormone prolactin (see p.860), or decreased levels of testosterone.

A test called nocturnal penile tumescence, in which a small gauge attached to your penis detects erections while you sleep, can be helpful in determining whether the cause of your impotence is physical. During an average night's sleep, healthy men have three to five erections, lasting up to 30 minutes each. If you are able to have erections during sleep, the cause of your impotence is probably not physical. An ultrasound (see p.140) exam may be used to measure both the diameter of the arteries in your penis and the blood flow through them. Alternatively, your doctor can evaluate your arteries by injecting a vasodilator drug directly into your penis; if your arteries are normal, you will develop an erection in 10 to 15 minutes.

All three impotence pills seem equally effective, although there are not enough studies comparing them to one another to say this with confidence.

Other pills Yohimbine and several herbal treatments in pill form appear to help some men, but they have not been tested in large studies or have only limited effectiveness.

Alprostadil Alprostadil is a prostaglandin drug that, like sildenafil, increases blood flow to the penis. Unlike sildenafil, it is not absorbed into the blood in significant amounts and is therefore less likely to produce side effects in parts of the body other than the penis. It can be injected into the base of the penis with a tiny needle or placed inside the urethra of the penis in the form of a soft pellet. Unlike sildenafil, alprostadil can produce erection in a man who is not sexually excited.

When alprostadil is injected (20 minutes before sexual intercourse), it leads to an erection sufficient for intercourse about 90% of the time. The first injection is usually given in the doctor's office so that the dose can be adjusted and you can learn to inject yourself. The most common side effect is pain at the injection site. In some men, it can cause priapism (see p.1096), an uncomfortably prolonged erection that can be reversed by a shot of epinephrine into the penis. The reverse injection should be done promptly (either in the doctor's office or in an emergency department) to prevent permanent damage to the spongy tissue of the penis.

When the alprostadil pellet is inserted into the tip of the penis (5 to 10 minutes before sexual intercourse), it produces an erection that lasts 30 to 60 minutes in about two thirds of men, about two thirds of the time. Brief mild discomfort is experienced by half the men. Prolonged erections, bruising, and scarring are less likely with the pellet than with the injection.

There have not yet been thorough studies of the effects (good or bad) of using alprostadil repeatedly over many years.

Vacuum pump External vacuum therapy is a method of producing an erection without drugs or surgery. The vacuum system consists of a clear plastic cylinder in which the penis is inserted. A pump removes air from the cylinder, creating a partial vacuum that pulls blood into the spongy tissues of the penis; a tension ring applied to the base of the penis traps the blood and maintains the erection. Using the vac-

Comparing Impotence Pills and Alprostadil

This chart compares the advantages and disadvantages of the impotence pills and alprostadil (a drug that can be injected into the penis or placed into the urethra before sexual intercourse). The relative effectiveness of these methods has not been determined because the drugs have not been tested against one another extensively. Preliminary studies indicate alprostadil injection may be most effective.

ADVANTAGE OR DISADVANTAGE	IMPOTENCE PILLS	ALPROSTADIL INJECTION	ALPROSTADIL PELLET
Causes discomfort or pain.	No	Yes (modest discomfort)	Yes (slight discomfort)
Can cause side effects (such as headaches and visual disturbances) in other parts of the body.	Yes	Yes (rarely)	Yes (rarely)
Works even if there is no sexual arousal.	No	Yes	Yes
Restores all men to normal sexual function.	No	No	No
Can work in men with either physical or psychological causes of impotence.	Yes	Yes	Yes (probably)
Has been proven to improve sexual function in men without impotence.	No	No	No
Is dangerous for men taking nitrate drugs, men with very high or very low blood pressure, and men who have recently had a heart attack.	Yes	No	No

uum pump requires a certain amount of dexterity. Side effects include pain, numbness, or bruising of the penis.

Penile prosthesis The success of sildenafil, alprostadil, and the vacuum pump have reduced the demand for surgical treatment of impotence by implanting a semirigid or inflatable penile prosthesis. The simplest implant consists of a pair of bendable silicone rods. With this method, the penis is always erect (and may be difficult to conceal under tight clothing), but can be bent up and down. The principal advantage is its very low failure rate. A more complex inflatable device has cylinders that are inserted in the penis, a fluid reservoir placed in the abdomen, and a pump that is put in the scrotum. Squeezing the pump moves fluid from the reservoir to the cylinders, causing rigidity. Another squeeze reverses this process. Because they have more components, these devices are more likely than silicone rods to malfunction.

Testosterone therapy Testosterone is the male sex hormone (see p.1087). Beyond age 40, the average man's testosterone level falls by about 1% each year. This normal decline does not impair sexual function in healthy men. In about 5% of men, testosterone levels are severely reduced and hormone replacement therapy can help restore potency. Doctors can prescribe injections, a testosterone skin patch, or a testosterone gel for this purpose. The patch and gel provide a more constant and even level of testosterone in the blood. When testosterone treatment is given to men who have measurably low levels of testosterone, it helps restore sexual function and helps build muscle strength and bulk.

Psychotherapy Men suffering from impotence that does not have an underlying physical cause may benefit from therapy with a psychiatrist, psychologist, or sex therapist. Therapy aims to remove inhibitions and to improve the attitudes of one or both partners toward sex by opening communications about sexual needs and by teaching practical techniques. Most often, sex therapy includes both partners.

Priapism and Peyronie Disease

Priapism and Peyronie disease are two different erection abnormalities.

Priapism is a very rare but dangerous condition in which you have a persistent, painful erection without sexual stimulation. In priapism, blood that normally circulates through the penis becomes trapped in its spongy tissue, causing an unrelieved erection. It is a medical emergency; a prolonged erection can cause irreversible damage to the penis and prevent you from having a normal erection. Priapism can be caused by sickle cell anemia, leukemia, injury to the blood vessels that control erection, or an excessive response to alprostadil therapy for impotence (see p.1092). Priapism can also be a side effect of certain medicines such as trazodone and chlorpromazine. Treatment depends on the cause.

Peyronie disease is a curvature of the erect penis that can make sexual intercourse difficult. It primarily affects men from ages 40 to 60 and can be painful. Peyronie disease is caused by scar tissue that forms inside the penis; its cause is not known. The scar tissue does not become engorged with blood during erection, which causes the penis to point toward the side containing the

scar tissue. Peyronie disease is usually mild, usually does not get worse, and often goes away on its own within a few years. If it persists or interferes with sexual activity, see your doctor; surgery can be helpful in some cases.

Premature Ejaculation

Premature ejaculation is a common problem in which ejaculation occurs too early, either during foreplay or just after penetration. Most men experience this problem from time to time, often due to anxiety or overstimulation. Premature ejaculation is not linked to any underlying medical disorder. However, frequent recurrences can foster frustration, feelings of insecurity, and anger between partners.

Many men can learn to control premature ejaculation with the squeeze technique. The method is simple—if you feel an orgasm coming on during foreplay, you or your partner uses a thumb and two fingers to squeeze the area just below the head of your penis for 20 seconds; this inhibits ejaculation and slightly reduces erection.

After about half a minute, resume sexual foreplay to regain your erection. Repeat the squeeze technique when you feel an ejaculation coming on again, and use it as often as necessary until you can enter your partner without

ejaculating. With practice, your body will learn to delay ejaculation without the squeeze.

Delayed Ejaculation

Delayed, or inhibited, ejaculation is an uncommon problem in which sexual stimulation produces a normal erection but does not result in ejaculation. The causes may be psychological or physical. Ask your doctor about potential physical causes before considering psychological help. Diabetes mellitus (see p.832) and some drugs, such as those used to treat hypertension or depression, can inhibit orgasm. If your doctor cannot find a physical cause, sex therapy (see p.1092) may be helpful.

Hemospermia

Hemospermia is the medical term for blood in the semen, which may appear pink, brown, or red. This condition is disconcerting, but is usually harmless. Hemospermia occurs temporarily after a prostate biopsy; it can also result from prostatitis (see below). In most cases, hemospermia goes away on its own. However, if you notice blood in your semen repeatedly, see your doctor so he or she can rule out any serious underlying condition, such as prostate cancer. In most cases, no cause can be found.

PROSTATE GLAND

Prostatitis

Prostatitis is inflammation of the prostate gland and is often the result of a bacterial infection.

Prostatitis is not one disease, but four.

Acute bacterial prostatitis is infection of the prostate caused by bacteria that travel from the

urethra to the prostate. It is the most dramatic form of prostatitis, beginning abruptly with high fever, chills, joint and muscle aches, and profound fatigue. In addition, you may have pain around the base of your penis and behind your scrotum, pain in your lower back, and the feeling of a full rectum. As the prostate becomes more swollen, you may find it difficult to urinate, and the urinary stream may become weak. If you cannot urinate at all, it is a medical emergency—the prostate probably is so swollen that it completely blocks the flow of urine.

If you think you have acute bacterial prostatitis, see your doctor immediately. He or she will examine your prostate (see p.1104) and take urine samples to test for bacteria. A diagnosis can be confirmed by finding numerous bacteria and white blood cells in the urine or in the prostate's secretions. Antibiotics (see p.868), such as a combination of trimethoprim and sulfamethoxazole, or a fluoroquinolone, are highly effective.

Even if you are feeling better, you should keep taking the medication for the full, prescribed course to keep the infection from returning. Other comforting measures include hot baths, stool softeners, and pain medicine such as aspirin or acetaminophen. It is important to drink a lot of fluids to help flush the bacteria from your system.

Chronic bacterial prostatitis is also caused by bacteria. It is more common in older men who have an enlarged prostate (see p.1098) and it can follow a bout of acute bacterial prostatitis. Unlike the acute form, however, chronic bacterial prostatitis is a subtle, low-grade infection that can begin insidiously and persist for weeks or even months.

Typically, an affected man does not have a fever but is troubled by intermittent urinary symptoms such a sudden urge to urinate, frequent urination, painful urination, or the need to get up at night to urinate. Some men have low back pain, pain in the rectum, or a feeling of heaviness behind the scrotum. Others have pain after ejaculation; in some men, the semen is tinged with blood (see Hemospermia, p.1096). These symptoms can wax and wane; because the symptoms are subtle, many men do not know they have it.

If you think you may have chronic bacterial prostatitis, see your doctor, who will examine your prostate (see p.1104) and check your urine and the secretions of your prostate for bacteria and white blood cells. Treatment requires the use of antibiotics in the form of a combination of trimethoprim and sulfamethoxazole, or a fluoroquinolone, for 1 to 3 months. Hot baths may also be recommended to ease discomfort. Even with prolonged treatment, the infection can relapse, but it can usually be controlled with another course of antibiotics.

Nonbacterial prostatitis is the most common form of prostatitis. Its symptoms resemble those of chronic bacterial prostatitis and, in both disorders, white blood cells are found in the urine and the prostate's secretions. In nonbacterial prostatitis, however, bacteria are absent.

Your doctor may prescribe an antibiotic (see p.868) in case bacteria are present. However, because there most often are none, antibiotics usually fail to

reduce the symptoms. For this reason, therapy aims at making you feel better. This includes taking hot baths and emptying the prostate of its secretions, either by your doctor massaging the prostate or through frequent ejaculation. Pain medicines such as aspirin or other nonsteroidal antiinflammatory drugs (see p.1162), which also reduce inflammation, may be recommended. In addition, your doctor may prescribe anticholinergic drugs, which reduce urinary symptoms by decreasing bladder contractions.

Prostatodynia means "pain in the prostate"—the main symptom of the condition. Prostatodynia is a persistent disorder that is often accompanied by depression, anxiety, or sexual dysfunction. Urine flow can also be abnormal, with an interrupted or weak stream, an urge to urinate (even when you can produce little urine), and frequent urination (even of small amounts). Although it can occur at any age, prostatodynia is most common in young to middleaged men.

The condition puzzles doctors because the prostate feels normal when it is examined, the urine is free of infection, and secretions from the prostate do not contain white blood cells. The medications most likely to reduce symptoms are alpha-blocker drugs such as prazosin, terazosin, or doxazosin. These medications relax the muscles at the neck of the bladder, easing the flow of urine, but they must be used with care to prevent excessive reduction in blood pressure.

Enlarged Prostate

An enlarged prostate, also known as benign prostatic hypertrophy or nodular hyperplasia of the prostate, is a noncancerous growth of the prostate that can interfere with urination.

The prostate is tiny at birth and remains small until adolescence. At puberty, testosterone levels rise, and the prostate begins to grow. Testosterone levels decline by about 10% every decade after age 40. But, even as testosterone levels fall, the prostate continues to enlarge and continues to grow into old age. An enlarged prostate is rare in young men, occurring in less than 10% of 30-year-olds. But it affects more than half of men by age 60, with the prevalence rising to about 90% by age 85.

SYMPTOMS

By the age of 85, a quarter of all American men have symptoms of an enlarged prostate that require treatment. About half the men who have an enlarged prostate never develop any symptoms. In the others, the enlarged prostate presses against the urethra (which drains the bladder), somewhat like a foot stepping on a garden hose. The flow of urine is obstructed, forcing the bladder to work harder to push urine through the urethra. In time, the pressure on the urethra can become so severe that you cannot empty your bladder completely, even when you bear down to increase the pressure. As a result, you may feel as though you have to urinate urgently, but have to strain to do

so. You may have a weak urinary stream, or one that stops and starts, or you may dribble after urinating and feel as though you are not emptying your bladder completely. In addition, you may feel the need to urinate frequently and may have to get up often during the night to do so. Some men also experience urinary incontinence, the involuntary discharge of urine.

Certain medicines can make the symptoms worse. For example, diuretics, which increase the amount of urine, often exaggerate the symptoms. Other medicines can cause problems by diminishing the force with which the bladder contracts—primarily medicines with anticholinergic effects. Finally, decongestants such as pseudoephedrine can

---

Normal and Enlarged Prostate Glands

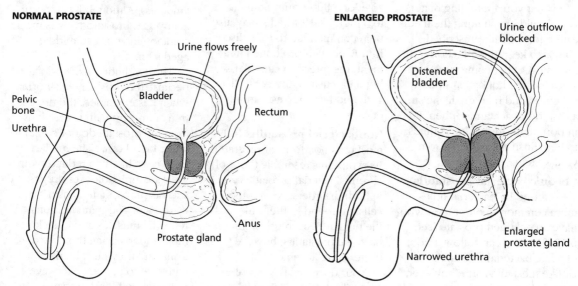

NORMAL PROSTATE

Urine flows freely
Bladder
Pelvic bone
Urethra
Rectum
Anus
Prostate gland

ENLARGED PROSTATE

Urine outflow blocked
Distended bladder
Enlarged prostate gland
Narrowed urethra

The prostate is located just below the bladder in front of the rectum and wraps around the upper part of the urethra. In a man with a healthy prostate gland (left), urine flows freely through the urethra, which runs through the prostate. An enlarged prostate (right) may impede the flow of urine from the bladder by narrowing the urethra.

Relieving the Symptoms of an Enlarged Prostate

- Avoid drinking fluids, particularly alcohol and caffeinated drinks, in the evening. Drinking fluids stimulates urine production, increasing the chance of frequent nighttime trips to the bathroom.

- Reduce stress. Nervous, tense men urinate more frequently.

- Ask your doctor to evaluate any other medications you are taking (to see if they could be contributing to, or aggravating, your symptoms) including diuretics, antihistamines, decongestants, heterocyclic (tricyclic) antidepressants, antispasmodics, and tranquilizers.

- Never pass up a chance to go to the bathroom. The more often you urinate, the less pressure you will have in your bladder. Taking time to empty your bladder completely will reduce the number of trips to the toilet.

---

also make it harder for men who have enlarged prostates to empty their bladders.

An enlarged prostate can produce complications that require medical attention. If the blockage prevents the bladder from emptying completely, you can be susceptible to recurring and serious urinary tract infections (see p.804). The risk of developing bladder stones also increases. As the prostate grows, blood vessels in the urethra can rupture, causing blood to appear in the urine.

If blockage of urine goes untreated for too long, the bladder may become so distended that urine cannot be adequately emptied from the kidney. In the most severe cases, this can lead to kidney failure. However, these major complications are uncommon.

TREATMENT OPTIONS

Your doctor will take your medical history and ask about urinary flow and how long you have had symptoms. He or she will also perform a digital rectal examina-

tion (see p.1104) and possibly a prostate-specific antigen (PSA) test (see p.1104). Treatment depends on your symptoms and on the decisions you and your doctor make together. Options include watchful waiting, medications, and various surgical procedures. Sometimes experimental

treatments such as laser surgery and herbal therapy are tried; all have risks and benefits and none is right for everyone.

Watchful waiting If your symptoms are not particularly bothersome to you, your doctor may recommend doing nothing more than monitoring your condition. Watchful waiting can be a sound strategy for men with mildly to moderately enlarged prostates. Studies show that, without treatment, the conditions of about 40% of men with mildly enlarged prostates improve, 45% have no change in symptoms, and 15% find that their symptoms worsen.

Medication In general, the risks of serious adverse effects are lower with medications than with surgery, leading many men to choose drug therapy as their initial treatment. Finasteride (a drug that shrinks the prostate by reducing androgen levels in the gland) and alpha blockers (medications that relax the muscles in the prostate and bladder outlet)

Alternative Medicine: Enlarged Prostate

The berries of the saw palmetto tree (*Serenoa repens*) have a long history of folk use for disorders of the male reproductive tract, including enlarged prostate. Although many European studies have shown improvement in symptoms, the studies generally have not been up to current scientific standards. More studies are needed to evaluate safety and effectiveness.

Other herbal agents in use in the United States and in Europe include cernilton, a pollen extract derived from plants in Sweden; *Pygeum africanum*, the African plum; and *Radix urticae*. Although some have undergone the rigors of clinical studies, the results are inconclusive.

Keep in mind that, although herbs are "natural," that does not necessarily mean they are safe. Like any medicine, herbs can cause side effects and may be dangerous if taken without your doctor's supervision.

can alleviate the urinary symptoms of an enlarged prostate.

Finasteride can actually shrink the prostate, but acts slowly, often taking 3 to 6 months to improve symptoms; about 4% of men develop impotence as a side effect. It may also reduce levels of PSA, affecting a PSA test's accuracy. Finasteride may be more helpful than alpha blockers (see below) in treating men who have very enlarged prostates.

Alpha blockers—such as doxazosin, tamsulosin, and terazosin—produce partial relief of urinary symptoms in 70% of men, usually within several days to several weeks. The main side effects include dizziness, fatigue, and excessive lowering of blood pressure. Studies indicate that alpha blockers are substantially more effective than finasteride.

Surgery Several different surgeries can help an enlarged prostate:

Transurethral resection of the prostate (TURP) is the most common surgical procedure. In TURP, an instrument called a resectoscope is passed through the urethra in the penis. The enlarged area of the prostate gland that is narrowing the urethra can be viewed through the resectoscope. The instrument also contains an electrical loop that the surgeon can use to burn away the overgrown prostate tissue. A general anesthetic or spinal anesthetic (see p.168) is given for the 90-minute operation, and a hospital stay is required. TURP usually provides more complete relief of symptoms than medication.

The main side effect of TURP is retrograde ejaculation, in which semen flows back into the bladder rather than out the penis.

Treatments for Enlarged Prostate: Dr Barry's Advice

If you're a man who has trouble urinating because of an enlarged prostate, the most important question is how much your symptoms bother you. Two men who have the same symptoms may decide to do different things. If you are not very bothered by your symptoms, you may decide just to wait, and not risk any treatment, until and unless your symptoms do become bothersome. If you are moderately concerned about your symptoms, you may decide to take a medication, which can always be stopped if there are side effects. Finally, if you are really concerned about your symptoms, you may choose surgery, which gives the best chance of symptom relief. It's up to you to make the decision—only you know how bothersome the symptoms are.

MICHAEL J. BARRY, MD
MASSACHUSETTS GENERAL HOSPITAL
HARVARD MEDICAL SCHOOL.

Myths and Facts: Enlarged Prostate

Myth: Too much or too little sexual activity causes or worsens the symptoms of an enlarged prostate.

Fact: There is no evidence that sexual habits affect the development or course of an enlarged prostate—or of prostate cancer.

Myth: Massaging the prostate helps an enlarged prostate.

Fact: In a digital rectal examination, your doctor may massage the prostate to obtain secretions for laboratory analysis. The massage is performed to obtain samples for diagnostic reasons, but has no effect on treatment.

Although this is not harmful to health, it causes infertility. More serious but infrequent long-term side effects include impotence and urinary incontinence as well as short-term problems such as bleeding, infection, and complications related to anesthesia.

Transurethral incision of the prostate (TUIP) involves less tissue damage than TURP. In TUIP only a few small incisions are made in the prostate, which relieves the pressure and allows the urethra to spring open. Overnight hospitalization is not required and the complication rate is low. TUIP can be used only when the prostate is minimally enlarged (weighs 30 grams or less).

Transurethral microwave ther-

Transurethral Microwave Thermotherapy

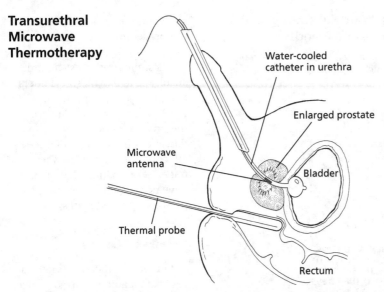

In transurethral microwave thermotherapy (TUMT), a tiny microwave antenna is passed through a catheter in the urethra to the prostate tissue that is impeding urine flow. A thermal probe is placed in the rectum just behind the antenna. It is connected to a computer that regulates the amount of heat directed to the prostate, destroying excess tissue. Cool water circulates through the catheter so that the urethra is not damaged and the heat is not felt.

Transurethral Resection of the Prostate

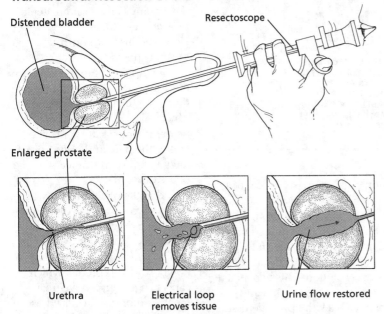

Transurethral resection of the prostate (TURP) is a procedure used to remove overgrown prostate tissue. During TURP, the doctor inserts a resectoscope into the penis to visualize the prostate and manipulate an electrical loop that burns away prostate tissue, relieving blockage of the urethra.

motherapy (TUMT) uses microwave energy to heat the prostate, destroying unwanted tissue. In TUMT, a tiny microwave antenna is inserted into the urethra through a catheter; a computer monitors tissue temperature, delivering just enough energy to heat the prostate to 122°F. TUMT takes about 1 hour and does not require overnight hospitalization or general anesthesia.

TUMT is less expensive than TURP and has fewer complications. About 60% to 70% of men respond favorably, but up to half require additional treatment within 4 years. Men with pacemakers, implanted defibrillators, or artificial hips cannot be treated with TUMT because the microwaves can cause pacemakers to malfunction and can heat the metal and plastic in an artificial hip. The procedure was approved for use in the late 1990s; more time and experience are needed to evaluate its role in treating enlarged prostates.

EXPERIMENTAL TREATMENTS

Burning away overgrown prostate tissue with a laser is less damaging to prostate tissue than the electrical instrument used in TURP. The hope is that laser surgery will prove to be as effective as TURP at relieving urinary obstruction, while producing fewer side effects. There is not enough evidence from long-term studies to determine if the hope will be realized.

Transurethral ultrasound-guided laser-induced prostatectomy (TULIP) visualizes the overgrown prostate tissue by ultrasound, and the excess prostate tissue is cut away by the powerful beam of laser light.

Differences in Outcome Between Watchful Waiting and Surgery (TURP) for an Enlarged Prostate Gland

Differences in outcome between watchful waiting and transurethral resection of the prostate (TURP) in men with moderate symptoms of an enlarged prostate gland.

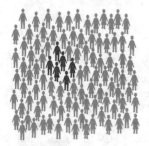

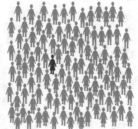

6 OF 100 MEN WHO HAVE MODERATE SYMPTOMS OF AN ENLARGED PROSTATE AND "WATCHFULLY WAIT" DEVELOP SERIOUS SYMPTOMS

1 OF 100 MEN WHO HAVE MODERATE SYMPTOMS OF AN ENLARGED PROSTATE AND UNDERGO TURP DEVELOPS SERIOUS SYMPTOMS

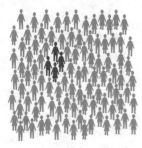

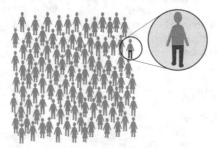

4 OF 100 MEN WHO HAVE MODERATE SYMPTOMS OF AN ENLARGED PROSTATE AND "WATCHFULLY WAIT" ARE UNABLE TO COMPLETELY EMPTY THE BLADDER THROUGH URINATION

FEWER THAN 1 OF 100 MEN WHO HAVE MODERATE SYMPTOMS OF AN ENLARGED PROSTATE AND UNDERGO TURP IS UNABLE TO COMPLETELY EMPTY THE BLADDER THROUGH URINATION

Visualized laser-assisted prostatectomy (VLAP) employs an endoscope (see p.142), rather than ultrasound, to see the overgrown tissue. A laser beam removes the excess tissue, just as in TULIP. Because the tissue is directly visualized, VLAP usually can be done somewhat faster than TULIP, often taking no more than 20 minutes.

Balloon dilatation is a variation on angioplasty (see p.661) in which a catheter with a deflated balloon is inserted through the penis into the constricted urethra. Once there, the balloon is inflated, usually with saline (salt water) solution. This expands the diameter of the urethra and presses back the prostate tissue. The long-term effectiveness of this procedure remains in question; many men feel relief of urinary symptoms immediately after the procedure, but symptoms often return in a few years.

Prostatic urethral stents are small, springlike mesh cylinders that are inserted into the narrowed area of the urethra (via the urethra in the penis), where they are released to widen the channel of the urethra and permit easier urination. The stents have not yet been approved for use in the United States.

Prostate Cancer

Next to lung cancer, prostate cancer is the leading cause of cancer death among American men.

Some prostate cancers grow rapidly and spread to other parts of the body. More often, however, prostate cancer grows slowly and does not spread for many years—even decades. An American man's lifetime risk of developing early, nonthreatening prostate cancer is about 30%. However, his risk of prostate cancer that spreads is only 10%.

A man's risk of dying of the disease is only 3%. That means that 2 of 3 men with prostate cancer will die of something else before their prostate cancer makes them ill, and only 1 of 10 men with prostate cancer will die of the disease.

If doctors could predict which cancers would grow slowly and which would grow rapidly, they could tailor a man's treatment to fit his disease. However, there is no good way to predict which cancers need aggressive treatment. Tumors with cells whose irregular appearance deviates largely from normal prostate tissue (what doctors call poorly differentiated cells) and which have

Living with Prostate Cancer

"After my surgery (a radical prostatectomy) I found the period of recuperation very hard going. The discovery that there was a prostate cancer support group made an enormous difference to my recovery.

At first, I hesitated to go—if there was any subject I didn't want to talk about (or listen to people talk about) it was prostate cancer. But I soon learned that here, at least, was a group of men who had experienced what I had, and to whom such subjects as slow recovery, the possible recurrence of disease, impotence, or incontinence were all too familiar. In fact, they knew a lot more about the difficulties of recovering from prostate cancer than the surgeons did. Most groups also have 'two-by-two' meetings for men and women. These are of enormous help in dealing with the intimate problems that so often accompany this particular disease.

I started going to meetings when I still had a Foley catheter and a bag to collect urine strapped to my leg, and I was so comforted by my fellow support group members that I was soon going to the movies that way. Support groups help you to learn that things *do* get better, that you can learn to live with the problems (and overcome them), and that there are a lot of people who have been through the same thing as you—and a lot of people who are worse off, but still smiling."

Michael Korda, Editor-in-Chief, Simon & Schuster. Author of *Man to Man*. New York, Simon & Schuster.

---

a higher Gleason score (see Staging, p.1107) tend to be more aggressive. However, most cancers have intermediate scores that are uncertain predictors of how they will behave. Researchers are developing genetic tests that may help establish a more accurate prognosis (outlook).

RISK FACTORS

No man is immune to prostate cancer. However, you may have a higher-than-average risk if you are in any of these categories:

Age 55 or older Because prostate cancer is a disease of older men, the risk increases with advancing age. More than three quarters of prostate can-

cers occur in men over age 65. About 40% of men who live to 80 will develop prostate cancer, although most die of other causes.

Family history of prostate cancer A man whose father or brother has had prostate cancer has two to three times the risk for the disease as a man whose father or brother has not had prostate cancer. The risk is ten times greater for a man who has two or more first-degree relatives (father or brothers) with prostate cancer.

African American Black Americans have the highest rate of prostate cancer in the world and have twice the risk of dying of

the disease as white Americans. The death rate may be higher because black men are often diagnosed at a later stage, when cure is more difficult.

High-fat diet Although the relationship between what you eat and prostate cancer has not been proven, evidence increasingly suggests that a diet high in fat, particularly animal fat, increases your susceptibility to the disease. One theory is that a high-fat diet increases the body's production of sex hormones, which in turn raises the risk of prostate cancer.

Tobacco use and alcohol abuse Smoking increases the risk of prostate cancer, as does heavy drinking.

Lower amounts of dietary selenium More recent research has found that men with lower levels of the mineral selenium in their diet may have a higher risk of prostate cancer. There is no proof, however, that taking a selenium supplement is beneficial.

EARLY DETECTION AND DIAGNOSIS

Cure rates for prostate cancer are excellent—about 95%—for malignancies that are treated in the early stages when prostate cancer is confined to the gland itself. However, once the cancer has spread to the lymph nodes, bones, liver, bladder, or rectum, cure rates are extremely low. In its early stages, prostate cancer produces no symptoms, so screening techniques—the digital ("with the finger") rectal examination and the prostate-specific antigen (PSA) test—are the primary means of discovering it.

Digital rectal examination is recommended annually for men over age 40. In this examination, your doctor inserts a gloved and lubricated finger into your rectum to feel the prostate gland in order to determine its size and whether there are lumps or very hard areas in it. The exam takes less than a minute and causes minimal discomfort. The doctor also checks for abnormal lumps in the wall of the rectum and tests the stool for the presence of blood (see Preventing Colon Cancer, p.791).

Prostate-specific antigen (PSA) test The PSA test is an important—but controversial—development in men's health. PSA is a protein produced by the prostate gland. Although most of the protein enters the semen during ejaculation, some also enters the blood, where it can be measured. Many men with prostate cancer have elevated levels of PSA in their blood, but many men with noncancerous prostate conditions also have high PSA levels. In men who are being treated for

Digital Rectal Examination

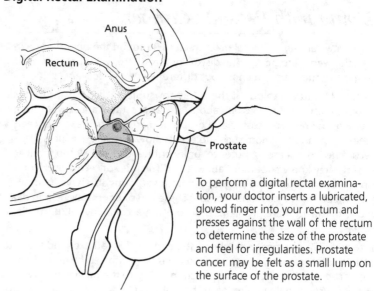

To perform a digital rectal examination, your doctor inserts a lubricated, gloved finger into your rectum and presses against the wall of the rectum to determine the size of the prostate and feel for irregularities. Prostate cancer may be felt as a small lump on the surface of the prostate.

Improving the PSA Test

Your doctor will help you understand your prostate-specific antigen (PSA) score and its importance in light of the results of your rectal exam. Ask him or her to explain any questions you have. Doctors are evaluating several ways to improve the accuracy of the PSA. These still-experimental approaches include taking into consideration factors such as:

Free PSA PSA travels in the blood in two ways: bound to other proteins or free. When the ratio of free PSA to total PSA is less than 25%, the chance of cancer rises. Measuring this ratio may be an improvement on measuring only the total PSA. However, more studies are needed.

PSA velocity Although PSA levels tend to rise with age, an abnormally rapid rise may suggest cancer. The

PSA velocity reflects the rate of change. Many doctors measure PSA levels yearly, and an annual increase of more than 0.75 nanograms per milliliter (ng/mL) is considered worrisome. Although theoretically appealing, the value of the PSA velocity remains unproven.

Age-adjusted normals Since the PSA level rises with age in healthy men, some researchers believe that age should be a factor in interpreting PSA test results. Several age-adjusted standards have been proposed. The following normal ranges have been set forth: ages 40 to 49: 0 to 2.5 ng/mL; ages 50 to 59: 0 to 3.5 ng/mL; ages 60 to 69: 0 to 4.5 ng/mL; and ages 70 to 79: 0 to 6.5 ng/mL. Until these standards are validated by further study, most doctors will still use the single value of 4.0 ng/mL as the upper limit of normal.

Risk of Having Prostate Cancer With Normal and Abnormal Physical Examination Results

Taking a prostate-specific antigen (PSA) test and having a physical examination help your physician determine if you have prostate cancer. However, even if you have these two procedures, more diagnostic tests are necessary to see if you actually have cancer. As shown here, some men with normal PSA test levels and normal physical examination results can have prostate cancer and a substantial number with abnormal PSA test levels and abnormal physical examination results may not. ng/mL indicates nanograms per milliliter.

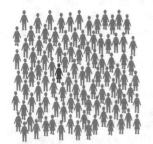

1 OF 100 MEN WHO HAS A PSA LEVEL OF 0 TO 1.9 NG/ML AND HAS NORMAL PHYSICAL EXAMINATION RESULTS HAS PROSTATE CANCER

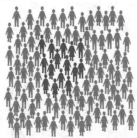

15 OF 100 MEN WHO HAVE PSA LEVELS OF 2 TO 3.9 NG/ML AND HAVE NORMAL PHYSICAL EXAMINATION RESULTS HAVE PROSTATE CANCER

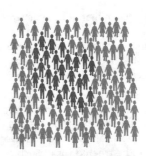

25 OF 100 MEN WHO HAVE PSA LEVELS OF 4 TO 10 NG/ML AND HAVE NORMAL PHYSICAL EXAMINATION RESULTS HAVE PROSTATE CANCER

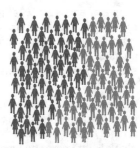

MORE THAN 50 OF 100 MEN WHO HAVE PSA LEVELS OF MORE THAN 10 NG/ML AND HAVE NORMAL PHYSICAL EXAMINATION RESULTS HAVE PROSTATE CANCER

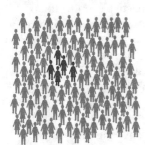

5 OF 100 MEN WHO HAVE PSA LEVELS OF 0 TO 1.9 NG/ML AND HAVE ABNOR-MAL PHYSICAL EXAMINA-TION RESULTS HAVE PROSTATE CANCER

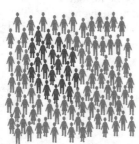

20 OF 100 MEN WHO HAVE PSA LEVELS OF 2 TO 3.9 NG/ML AND HAVE NORMAL PHYSICAL EXAMINA-TION RESULTS HAVE PROSTATE CANCER

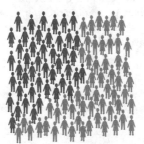

45 OF 100 MEN WHO HAVE PSA LEVELS OF 4 TO 10 NG/ML AND HAVE ABNOR-MAL PHYSICAL EXAMINA-TION RESULTS HAVE PROSTATE CANCER

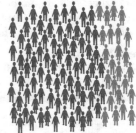

MORE THAN 75 OF 100 MEN WHO HAVE PSA LEVELS OF MORE THAN 10 NG/ML AND HAVE ABNORMAL PHYSICAL EXAMINATION RESULTS HAVE PROSTATE CANCER

prostate cancer, the PSA test is an important way to determine whether the treatment is working.

The role of the PSA test in screening apparently healthy men for prostate cancer, however, is controversial. Some authoritative groups endorse it as an annual test for all men, starting at age 40 for African Americans or men with a family history of prostate cancer, or at age 50 for others. Despite these guidelines, other groups doubt the value of the PSA as a screening test for men who do not have abnormalities or symptoms of prostate cancer that show up on a physical examination.

Why is this? The PSA test is a clear improvement on previous blood tests for prostate cancer and is the best tool for early diagnosis currently available. However, it is still far from perfect. It can be falsely negative—that is, 20% to 40% of men who have prostate cancer have normal levels of PSA. Some opponents of using the test for screening are concerned that men with a "normal" PSA test result (and their doctors) will be falsely reassured.

Prostate Cancer Screening:
Dr Kantoff's Advice

People often ask me whether or not men should be screened for prostate cancer. Unfortunately, no one knows the answer, because there is not yet a study that gives a definitive answer. Most people understand that prostate cancer screening tests—like all tests—are not perfect. Most people also know that prostate cancer is infrequently detected in men below age 50.

What is harder to explain is that many men have a very small, slow-growing cancer restricted to the inside of the prostate that is unlikely to spread. Men in whom such cancers are discovered never needed to know about it, and never needed to be treated for it. Such cancers are more likely as men grow older. These men are more likely to die *with* the disease rather than *from* the disease. In general, I think there is little value in screening men with a life expectancy of less than 10 years.

On the other hand, prostate cancer can be a devastating and lethal disease. So I recommend screening tests for men over age 50 who have a life expectancy of greater than 10 years. Moreover, screening at even younger ages may be justified for men at higher risk, such as African Americans and men who have a father or brother with prostate cancer.

PHILIP W. KANTOFF, MD
DANA-FARBER CANCER INSTITUTE
HARVARD MEDICAL SCHOOL

IGF-I Blood Levels and the Risk of Developing Prostate Cancer

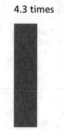

4.3 times

2.8 times

1.9 times

| RISK OF MEN WHO HAVE THE LOWEST LEVELS OF IGF-I IN THEIR BLOOD DEVELOPING PROSTATE CANCER | RISK OF MEN WHO HAVE MODERATE LEVELS OF IGF-I IN THEIR BLOOD DEVELOPING PROSTATE CANCER | RISK OF MEN WHO HAVE HIGHER LEVELS OF IGF-I IN THEIR BLOOD DEVELOPING PROSTATE CANCER | RISK OF MEN WHO HAVE THE HIGHEST LEVELS OF IGF-I IN THEIR BLOOD DEVELOPING PROSTATE CANCER |

Cancers are encouraged to grow by natural body substances called growth factors. Men with high levels of insulinlike growth factor-I (IGF-I) in their blood are more likely to develop prostate cancer. Men with the highest levels of IGF-I have more than four times the risk of developing prostate cancer as men with the lowest levels of IGF-I. The IGF-I blood test is a new test that may help define men at higher risk.

The test also can be falsely positive. As many as 3 of 4 men with elevated levels of PSA do not have prostate cancer but have either prostatitis (see p.1096) or noncancerous enlargement of the prostate gland (see p.1098).

Opponents of using the test for screening note that most men with an elevated level of PSA will live in fear that they have cancer and will have to undergo additional (and, in retrospect, unnecessary) testing before they learn that they do not have cancer. The additional tests involve time, discomfort, and expense, all of which will have been unnecessary in most men with an "abnormal" test result. Finally, since many prostate cancers remain inactive even without treatment, widespread PSA testing may lead to unnecessarily aggressive therapy for many indolent tumors.

Transrectal ultrasound (TRUS) and biopsy If your PSA level is high or if your rectal examination revealed anything suspicious, your doctor may use TRUS to produce an image of the prostate and to pinpoint areas of the prostate that should be explored further with a biopsy. In TRUS (see illustration at left), a probe is inserted into the rectum as you lie on your side. The test is painless and takes only a few minutes. If the biopsy samples of tissue from suspicious-looking areas indicate prostate cancer, computed tomography (see p.149) or magnetic resonance imaging (see p.151) may help your doctor evaluate the spread of malignant cells to surrounding tissues, including the lymph glands. A bone scan can show areas in the bones through-

Imaging the Prostate With Transrectal Ultrasound

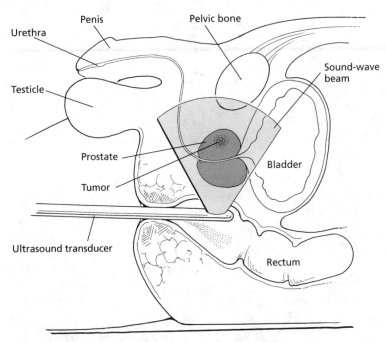

Penis
Pelvic bone
Urethra
Sound-wave beam
Testicle
Prostate
Bladder
Tumor
Ultrasound transducer
Rectum

Transrectal ultrasound (TRUS) is the standard method for imaging the prostate. An ultrasound transducer placed in the rectum beams sound waves at the prostate. Waves reflected back are captured by the probe and electronically converted into images displayed on a screen. TRUS can show small tumors and tumors located deep in the prostate that can be difficult or impossible for the doctor to feel.

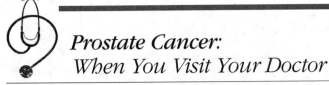

Prostate Cancer: When You Visit Your Doctor

These are some questions you may want to discuss with your doctor if you have been diagnosed with prostate cancer:

- What is your best estimate of the stage of my cancer?

- Can you explain how you reached this estimate?

- Can the volume of the tumor be estimated through a digital rectal examination, biopsy, ultrasound (see p.148), or magnetic resonance imaging (MRI) (see p.151)? How big is the tumor?

- Does digital rectal examination, ultrasound, or MRI suggest any penetration by the tumor of the prostate capsule?

- What is your best estimate as to the cancer's aggressiveness or potential to spread?

- Should I be treated and if so, how?

- How will my condition be affected if I choose not to seek treatment?

out your body to which the cancer may have spread. These tools help doctors identify the stage of the cancer.

STAGING

Prostate cancer progresses in stages. In the first stage, stage T1, the cancer is confined to the prostate and is too small to be felt by the doctor during a digital rectal examination, or to be seen by transrectal ultrasound. In stage T2, cancer is still confined to the prostate but can also be felt by your doctor during a digital rectal examination. In stage T3, the cancer invades nearly the entire gland and breaks through the prostate capsule. In stage M, cancerous cells have spread (metastasized) to the lymph nodes in the pelvis or to other parts of the body, such as bone. This may cause pain in the back, hips, or upper thighs. The prognosis (outlook) and treatment plan depend on the stage of the cancer when it is diagnosed. If detected in stages T1 or T2, it can usually be cured; stage M survival averages only about 3 years.

Doctors also use another assessment scale to predict the progress of prostate cancer. The Gleason tumor grading system is based on the appearance of the cancer cells. If the cells deviate largely from normal prostate tissue, they are called poorly differentiated cells. Doctors examine prostate tissue under a microscope, then assign a grade from between 1 and 5 to the tumor: grade 1 cells look the most normal; grade 5 the most malignant; and grades 2, 3, and 4 lie between the extremes. Since cancer cells from a single biopsy can

Stages of Prostate Cancer

STAGE T1

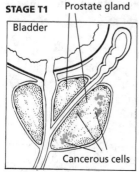

Prostate gland

Bladder

Cancerous cells

A microscopic cancer, too small to be felt during a digital rectal examination (stage T1).

STAGE T2

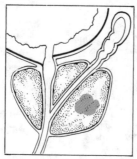

Cancer large enough to be felt during digital rectal examination but confined to one lobe of the prostate (stage T2).

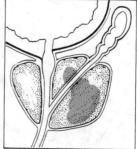

Larger cancerous tumor than the tumor shown at left but one that is still confined to the prostate gland (stage T2).

STAGE T3

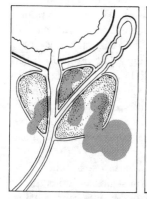

Cancer has grown through prostate capsule (stage T3).

STAGE M

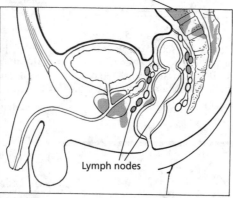

Cancer spread to spine

Lymph nodes

Cancer has spread to adjacent lymph nodes and to the spine (stage M).

The outlook (prognosis) for a man with prostate cancer depends on the stage of cancer when it is diagnosed. A four-point scale, ranging from T1 to M, is often used to describe how far cancer has spread. If cancer is detected in stages T1 and T2, it can often be cured; stage M survival averages about 3 years.

---

vary in appearance, pathologists score the two most representative regions separately, then add them to arrive at a single Gleason score. Tumors with scores of 1, 2, 3, or 4 have the best outlook; those with scores of 8, 9, or 10 have the worst outlook; and those with scores of 5, 6, or 7 carry an intermediate prognosis.

More recent research has identified cancer-related genes that may help your doctor make a more accurate prognosis from biopsy samples.

TREATMENT OPTIONS

Although prostate cancer is a very common disease, doctors are still debating which treatment

is best. That is because studies that compare treatments are not yet complete; until they are, your age, stage of cancer, and Gleason score are used to help determine the best approach to treatment. Discuss the following options with your doctor:

Watchful waiting Also called observation and follow-up, watch-

Worrisome Prostate Symptoms

Most prostate cancers do not cause any symptoms until they have spread beyond the gland itself. In fact, prostate symptoms are usually caused by prostatitis or an enlarged prostate, not cancer. You should make an appointment with your doctor if you:

- Have the urge to urinate frequently, particularly at night.
- Have difficulty starting or stopping urination.
- Have a weak or interrupted urinary stream.
- Cannot urinate.
- Experience pain or burning when you urinate.
- Have painful or blood-tinged ejaculation.
- See blood in your urine.
- Frequently experience pain or stiffness in your lower back, hips, or upper thighs.

ful waiting requires no immediate treatment. It is usually reserved for men whose cancer is at stage T1 or T2 and who have low Gleason scores (which indicate slow-growing cancers), and for men who are older and more likely to die of another condition before prostate cancer becomes dangerous. Older men may also face greater risks from the treatment; the treatment may prove worse than the disease. Physicians usually recommend follow-up PSA tests and regular rectal examinations along with watchful waiting.

Radiation therapy Radiation therapy (see p.741) to destroy cancerous cells is an alternative to watchful waiting or surgery for the treatment of early prostate cancer (stages T1 and T2). It is also a recommended treatment for cancers that have spread beyond the gland and for men who are elderly or in poor health

(and who may not tolerate surgery well).

Your doctor will monitor your response to radiation and, if your PSA tests indicate your level has fallen below 1 nanogram per milliliter (ng/mL), radiation therapy will continue.

There are two approaches to radiation—external beam and brachytherapy:

In *external beam radiation* (the standard approach), rays are aimed directly at the prostate tumor (and sometimes at nearby lymph nodes) from a machine outside the body five times a week for up to 7 weeks. Side effects can include diarrhea, rectal bleeding, impotence, and, rarely, incontinence.

In *brachytherapy* (a newer technique that is promising but less well studied), radiation is delivered by seeds or pellets of radioactive material that are

implanted into the prostate gland via a needle. The radioactive pellets are placed close to the tumor and away from healthy tissue; ultrasound is used during the procedure to help the doctor visualize the location of the cancer. This procedure requires a hospital stay of several days. Because the radiation is placed right next to the tumor (thus sparing healthy tissue the exposure to radiation that is unavoidable with external beam irradiation), there are fewer side effects with this technique.

Radiation is also sometimes used after surgery if surgery has not entirely removed all the cancer cells in or near the prostate gland. The hope is that the radiation will kill the cells that were not removed.

Surgery Radical prostatectomy is surgery to remove the prostate gland. In this procedure, the surgeon removes the prostate and sometimes the lymph glands in the pelvis, usually through an incision in the lower abdomen but sometimes through an incision in the area between the anus and the scrotum.

The best candidates for this surgery are men whose cancer is confined to the gland itself (stages T1 and T2), who are under age 70, and who are expected to live at least another 10 years. The side effects of radical prostatectomy include urinary incontinence (loss of urine control), impotence, and blood loss. In recent years, the surgical technique has improved to reduce the likelihood of these side effects. Ask your surgeon about complication rates involving impotence and incontinence.

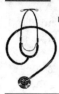

Prostate Removal:
When You Visit Your Doctor

Here is a list of questions to discuss with your doctor after you have had your prostate removed (radical prostatectomy):

- What did the pathologist find? How much of the gland was cancerous?

- Was the cancer confined to the gland?

- Has the cancer penetrated my prostate capsule?

- Is there cancer at the outermost edges of the tissue you cut out? Are my seminal vesicles involved? Are my lymph nodes involved?

- What is my exact pathological stage and grade of cancer?

- Based on all this information, what is my likelihood of cure?

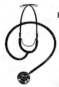

Androgen-Deprivation Therapy:
When You Visit Your Doctor

These are questions your doctor may ask you if you are on androgen-deprivation therapy for prostate cancer:

- Are you losing your sex drive?

- Are you having hot flashes?

- Do you have diarrhea (if taking flutamide or bicalutamide)?

- Do you have back pain that shoots down your leg? Are your legs weak? Have you lost bowel and bladder control? (These can occur if the cancer has spread to the spine, causing a fracture in the vertebrae or compression of the spinal nerves.)

- Do you have pain in your bones that increases with weight-bearing activities? (This could indicate that the cancer has spread to the bones.)

- Do you have swelling in your legs or scrotum? Are you urinating regularly? (The tumor can pinch off the tube that drains the urine from the kidney to the bladder, damaging the kidney.)

Androgen-deprivation therapy

Prostate cells are stimulated by androgens: testosterone and other male hormones. Removing the influence of these hormones slows the growth of these cells, including cancer cells. Hormone therapy in the form of androgen-deprivation therapy is the treatment of choice for men with cancer that has spread beyond the prostate gland and into the lymph nodes or other organs (stage M). It is also being studied as an adjunct to radiation for men with stage T3 disease. Hormone therapy can help slow the course of advanced disease and relieve painful symptoms, but it cannot cure the cancer itself.

Androgen deprivation can be accomplished in several ways. The first is by surgically removing the testicles in a procedure called orchiectomy. Since testosterone is mostly made by the testicles, this approach is generally the surest. However, removing the testicles greatly reduces libido and is for many men an assault on their personal image of masculinity. This causes some men to reject the procedure.

Medications also are effective in reducing testosterone levels. One approach is to use medicines that inhibit the production of luteinizing hormone (LH) by the pituitary gland in the brain. Since LH stimulates the production of testosterone by the testicles, inhibiting LH lowers testosterone levels. Examples of medicines that have this action are leuprolide and buserelin. These medicines have largely replaced use of the female hormone estrogen (which also lowers testosterone levels) because they have fewer side effects.

Another approach is to block the effect of testosterone on prostate cells by blocking the attachment of testosterone to its receptor on the cells. Medicines that do this include flutamide, cyproterone, and bicalutamide.

Side effects of androgen deprivation include impotence, decreased sex drive, hot flashes, and osteoporosis. A combination of hormone therapies, or orchiectomy plus antiandrogen therapy, can slow the progression of disease and improve survival for some men.

Newer approaches Several approaches to prostate cancer are being investigated, notably cryosurgery, which is the application of cold to destroy cancer cells. It is performed using general or spinal anesthesia (see p.168), takes about 1½ hours, and re-

quires a hospital stay of 1 or 2 days. Advocates claim that it is less likely to cause undesirable side effects than prostate removal or radiation therapy. It is not recommended for men whose cancer has spread beyond the prostate or for those with large tumors.

The benefits of cryosurgery are that it seems to spare potency and urinary continence. Side effects can include short-term

soreness, swelling of the scrotum, and painful urination. About 5% to 20% of men have blockage of the urethra, which can be corrected with surgery. Some doctors advocate anticancer chemotherapy (see p.741) for men with advanced prostate cancer when hormones fail to control symptoms and pain. The drugs are given by intravenous injection.

THE AGING MALE

Is There a Male Menopause?

In women, menopause involves an abrupt drop in the production of the sex hormones estrogen and progesterone and an end to reproductive capability. In men, levels of the male sex hormone testosterone also decline with age, but the fall is gradual, amounting to about 10% per decade beyond age 40. Although sex drive declines in many men, most healthy men retain their potency—and even their ability to father children—into old age. Other physiologic changes, although subtler than they are in

women, exist nonetheless: muscles start to weaken and bones give up some of the calcium that keeps them strong.

Hormone Replacement for Men

Hormones decline as men age, and the question arises whether replacing them can slow the aging process and improve health. For most women, there is considerable evidence that hormone replacement therapy (see p.1049) is beneficial.

Is testosterone replacement beneficial for men? Theoretically,

testosterone replacement might increase sexual potency and increase bone density, muscle mass, and strength. Some studies have shown that this can occur. However, concerns exist that increases in testosterone may stimulate the prostate, increasing the risk of an enlarged prostate and prostate cancer. It might also raise cholesterol levels and increase the risk of heart disease.

As with other hormones, more study is needed before supplemental testosterone can be recommended for men whose levels are normal for their age group.

Health of Seniors

Humans are the only species known to live decades past their reproductive years. Other creatures succumb to predators or diseases while still in their prime.

During the 20th century, the average life span of people living in developed countries increased 60%, from about 50 years to 80 years. As a result, the special health problems of aging are being studied.

We know that the major organ systems change in certain ways as a natural consequence of aging. What follows are some of the hallmark changes we all can expect as we age:

Skin Wrinkles, sores, and lack of resilience result mainly from sun exposure, rather than from aging itself.

Nervous system Loss of brain cells and slowing of neurotransmitter production results in somewhat slower responses and less acute sensory perceptions, such as taste and hearing, but the impact is minor.

Cardiovascular system Heart size increases slightly as muscle cells are replaced by scar tissue, causing slightly decreased efficiency in heart function (though the heart functions well even in very old people unless there is also heart disease).

Respiratory system Lungs become less elastic and less able to inflate or deflate completely, and are unable to respond to the coughing reflex effectively, making older people more vulnerable to lung infections.

Musculoskeletal system Loss of bone tissue, called osteoporosis (see p.596), progresses. Muscle strength and mass decline. Strength training (see p.1113) can help improve both conditions.

Digestive system The amount of digestive enzymes declines, causing fewer vitamins and nutrients to be absorbed.

Immune system The primary cells of the immune system, especially the T cells (see What Happens When You Have an Infection? p.864), function less effectively.

Reproductive system During menopause, women's ovaries stop producing estrogen and progesterone, ending their reproductive ability. Some estrogen continues to be produced by the adrenal glands and fat cells (in varying levels in different women). Men's testosterone output diminishes steadily after ages 65 through 70 (but men continue to be able to have erections, make some sperm, and father children).

Urinary system A reduction in blood flow to the kidneys impairs their ability to extract wastes from the blood and to form urine. In most people, this slight impairment has no serious adverse effects. Many people find they need to urinate more frequently as they age, including more than one or two times at night. Also, the urge comes on more suddenly. Leaking urine, however, is not a normal part of aging.

Hormonal system The production of many hormones diminishes somewhat with aging. Except for the reproductive hormones, there are no known significant effects on the body. However, science knows relatively little about this question.

Each body system ages according to its own timetable, and these schedules vary dramatically from person to person. Despite the inevitable toll aging takes on your body, you can slow the process by taking several important preventive steps: avoid exposure to the sun, do not smoke, limit your consumption of alcohol, eat a healthful diet, embrace exercise, and get screening tests for diseases that can be detected early.

Many older people expect that poor health is a natural part of aging. This is not true. Mistakenly believing it is true can lead you to overlook symptoms of disease. At least half the time, older people do not talk to their doctors about important symptoms—symptoms of disorders that are highly treatable. Do not try to self-diagnose; your physician can help you sort out and treat symptoms that are causing you concern.

Read the following section to acquaint yourself with the health issues that particularly concern older adults.

Strength Training for Seniors

Talk to your doctor before starting these exercises. Doctors usually recommend strength training for seniors because it preserves bone density and improves strength and balance. You are never too old to do, and benefit from, these exercises. Even people in their 90s can see improvement. These exercises can be performed in any order. For each exercise, perform eight slow repetitions with each limb, starting with the amount of weight you can comfortably lift. Increase the weights in half-pound increments.

BUILDING ARM AND SHOULDER STRENGTH
Sitting in a chair and using wrist weights

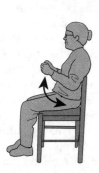 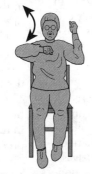 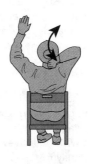 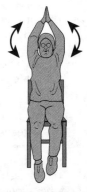

Biceps exercise: Put your arms at your sides. Bend one arm at the elbow, lifting the weight to your shoulder without moving your shoulder or upper arm. Lower your arm slowly. Repeat with other arm.

Triceps exercise I: Bring your hands to the front of your chest with elbows pointing out. Lift one arm at a time over your head until the weight is directly over your head.

Triceps exercise II: Raise your arms straight over your head. Bend one arm at the elbow so that your wrist is resting behind your neck. Lift the bent arm to join the upright arm.

Shoulder exercise: Put your arms at your sides. Raise your arms straight out to the side without bending them. Try to touch your hands over your head. Keeping your arms straight, lower them slowly.

BUILDING LOWER BODY STRENGTH
Standing, holding the back of a chair, and using ankle weights

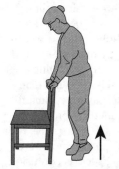 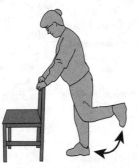 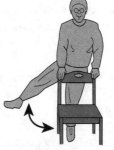 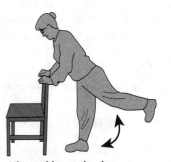

Foot flexibility exercise: Slowly rise up on your toes. Slowly lower your heels to standing position. If this is easy, do the exercise while rising on one leg with the other leg bent at the knee.

Knee exercise: Bend one knee without moving your upper leg. Try to bring your heel to the back of your thigh. Lower your leg slowly.

Hip and thigh exercise: Without bending your knee or waist, move one leg straight out to the side, keeping your toes pointed forward. Lower your leg slowly.

Hip and lower back exercise: Bend forward at the waist about 45 degrees. Lift one leg behind you as straight as you can. Lift your leg as high as possible without bending your knee or moving your upper body. Lower your leg slowly.

How Our Senses Change With Age

Although there is great individual variability in how the senses diminish with age, here are some changes that are common:

SIGHT

Visual acuity, or sharpness of focus, generally deteriorates with age, mainly because of presbyopia (see p.425). Cataracts (see p.430) are relatively common and usually occur later in life. Age-related macular degeneration (see p.440) is a much less common disease that generally occurs later in life.

HEARING

Presbycusis, or hearing loss (see p.451) in both ears, increases with age, beginning between ages 40 and 50. However, many people over age 65 never experience hearing loss that interferes with their lives. If you find yourself asking friends or family to repeat themselves often, or if they suggest you may have a hearing problem, see your doctor. A hearing aid (see p.453) can help considerably.

TASTE AND SMELL

Taste and smell, two interdependent senses that aid in the enjoyment of food, become less sharp with aging. While the number of taste buds remains unchanged, reduced flow of saliva may result in diminished taste sensation. The sense of smell declines rapidly in your 50s; by your 80s, smell detection is almost 50% poorer than it was in your younger years. As these senses become blunted, food flavors and scents may become less appetizing. It is nonetheless important to maintain a varied and sensible diet, adding spices if needed to increase the flavor of foods.

Geriatric Assessment

A geriatrician is a physician trained to treat older people. Geriatric assessment is a multidisciplinary process that evaluates an elderly person's medical, psychological, social, and functional state for the purpose of designing therapy and a follow-up care program. See p.1130 for more information.

Alcohol Abuse

See also:
▶ Alcohol (p.62)
▶ Substance Addiction and Abuse (p.411)

Alcoholism—the continued use of alcohol despite social, occupational, psychological, or physical problems caused by drinking—affects between 2% and 4% of elderly people.

Older men are four times more likely to be affected than women. Age-related changes in the liver and nervous system cause older people to retain higher concentrations of alcohol in their blood than would be present in a younger person. There is also a greater danger of adverse interactions between alcohol and prescription drugs.

There are two categories of alcohol dependence in older people: early onset (before 60) and late onset (60 and older). Between 50% and 75% of elderly alcoholics fall into the early-onset category; there is often also a family history of alcoholism. Late-onset alcoholics represent 25% to 50% of all elderly alcoholics; this form can be triggered by the stresses and losses that occur with aging.

Alcoholism is often not diagnosed in older people, primarily due to other medical problems and medicines that can mask the symptoms. Typical symptoms of alcohol abuse, such as confusion or falling, may be erroneously attributed to the natural progression of aging. Alcoholism in older people may also be accompanied by depression, tobacco dependence, and sleep disorders. See your physician if you have a problem with alcohol.

Cognitive Impairment

See also:

▶ Alzheimer Disease (p.363)
▶ Dementia (p.362)
▶ Confusion and Delirium (p.362)

The ability to think, perceive, and remember are all included in the general term "cognitive function." The natural process of aging means that our minds, like our bodies, slow down somewhat and may not work as efficiently as they once did; this is normal in many people.

In cognitive impairment, a person cannot carry out daily activities, such as conversing, recognizing familiar faces, or attending to personal needs. Most seniors do not have cognitive impairment at any age, although people over 80 are most vulnerable.

If you are concerned about your memory, a physician skilled in caring for older persons can help determine whether your memory problems are part of normal aging or could be something more serious. Read the sections listed at the beginning of this article to gain a clearer understanding of these disorders.

Brain Changes with Aging

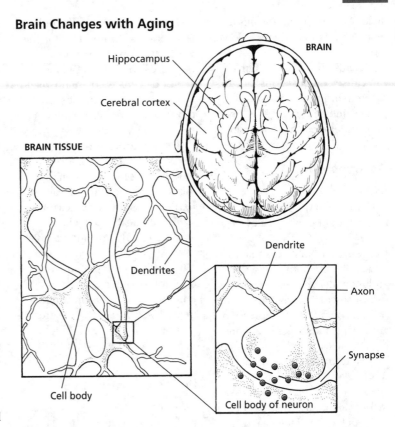

Healthy adult brains shrink with age. Changes in the hippocampus, a part of the brain important in memory, are common. However, experience allows seniors to perform as well as younger persons on most tests. Age diminishes the activity of neurotransmitters (in red), which are chemical messengers that cross the synapse between brain cells. Dendrites, which carry information from one cell to the next, continue growing.

Constipation

See also:

▶ Constipation (p.781)

Constipation is difficulty moving your bowels, passing stools that are hard or dry, or a sense of incomplete defecation. Up to one third of older people report being constipated, although many have daily bowel movements.

There is no normal bowel movement schedule. Healthy seniors can have as many as three bowel movements a day or as few as two a week. What is important is a change in your normal pattern; any change, if it persists, should be reported to your doctor. Treatment includes increasing the amount of fiber in your diet by eating more fruits and vegetables and by using psyllium husk fibers or methylcellulose (available at any drugstore without a prescription).

It is generally a good idea for older adults to drink about eight glasses of fluids each day. However, seniors with congestive heart failure (see p.683) or urinary incontinence (see p.826) or other urinary tract abnormalities should avoid drinking large amounts of liquid to treat constipation. While this is a useful practice in younger people, it can complicate heart and urinary problems.

Try to have a bowel movement about 30 minutes after a meal, especially after breakfast. The intestines are most active in expelling wastes right after a meal. Also, even brief walks (a few blocks) often trigger a bowel movement.

Because the use of laxatives can cause complications, doctors recommend them only when other remedies have failed, and only under medical supervision.

Depression

See also:
▶ Depression (p.395)
▶ Grief and Bereavement (see p.1145)

Depression is an illness that can be debilitating both physically and mentally and carries a high risk of suicide. More than just the "blues," people with depression are incapacitated, generally finding no pleasure in life and often unable to maintain personal or work relationships.

Other symptoms of depression include sleep disorders (sleeping too much or too little), lack of interest, guilt, lack of energy, loss of concentration, and appetite disorders (having too much or too little appetite).

Depression among the elderly is at least as common as it is in younger people. The prevalence of depression is highest among senior citizens who are hospitalized or in nursing homes; 40% of those with dementia experience depression at some point.

Depression can be difficult to recognize and diagnose in elderly people and is commonly mistaken for another disease or part of the natural process of aging. Medical problems such as an overactive or underactive thyroid, poor nutrition, chronic pain, or worsening illness can contribute to depression, as can loneliness. Depression can be treated; see your doctor. Bereavement due to the death of loved ones is a separate condition.

Fecal Incontinence

See also:
▶ Fecal Incontinence (p.794)

Fecal incontinence, the involuntary leakage of stools, is common in people suffering from dementia. However, less than 5% of healthy seniors have fecal incontinence. It can be an extremely embarrassing problem for the person and for his or her family.

One risk factor associated with fecal incontinence is a history of constipation and laxative use, which contributes to weakening of the muscles and ligaments that control defecation. Fecal impaction (see p.794), a mass of immovable stool in the bowel, can result in small amounts of liquid stool leaking around the impaction, causing fecal incontinence.

Less commonly, fecal incontinence is a result of having had a large number of pregnancies, past surgery on the anus or rectum, diabetes (see p.832), infection or inflammation of the bowel, stroke (see p.342), or spinal cord injury or tumor.

Hypothermia

See also:
▶ Hypothermia (p.1212)

While anyone exposed to colder temperatures is at risk for hypothermia—a drop in body temperature of more than 4°F below normal (98.6°F)—older people are especially susceptible. With age, the body becomes progressively less able to sustain an even temperature when exposed to the cold. In addition, the mechanism that senses a decrease in body temperature becomes less sensitive with age, slowing an older person's reaction to cold.

An elderly person need not be exposed to extreme cold to suffer hypothermia; it can happen while sitting in a mildly cool environment. The first signs of hypothermia are drowsiness, weakness, and cold skin over the abdomen,

---

Keeping Mentally Fit:
Dr Marcantonio's Advice

One of the most important factors in successful aging is staying connected to other people and to daily activities. Not only can it enhance the functioning of your immune system, it also helps form new connections in your brain.

People who develop new interests, visit new places, and make new friends seem to be healthier than those who do not. You can help maintain intellectual health by attending classes, reading, working puzzles, or volunteering in your community. Anything that keeps your mind active will help keep you mentally fit.

EDWARD R. MARCANTONIO, MD
BETH ISRAEL-DEACONESS MEDICAL CENTER
HARVARD MEDICAL SCHOOL

followed by stupor, coma, and eventually death.

Hypothermia is treated by slowly rewarming the body in such a way that the vital internal organs receive their blood supply first. The simplest technique is to have the person breathe in heated air. In severe emergencies, blood is circulated outside the body, warmed by a machine, and then infused back into the body.

Medications

See also:
▶ Medicines (p.1148)
▶ Caregiving and Eldercare (p.1120)

Aging changes the way your body absorbs, metabolizes, and excretes drugs, making older people much more vulnerable to their adverse and toxic effects. Elderly people take as many as three times the number of prescription medicines as younger people, and women take twice as many as men. The average senior citizen in the United States receives 18 prescriptions a year. Many also use over-the-counter drugs.

Older people run a much higher risk for adverse drug interactions. In addition, medicines are taken at different dosages and on different schedules. With so many drugs to keep track of, it is easy—and potentially dangerous—to miss a dose, take the wrong dose, or mistakenly overdose.

It is a good idea to periodically take all your medicines to your primary care doctor and review them together. Sometimes drugs can be eliminated or their dosages reduced to make your regimen easier and safer. Read the sections on p.1120 on creating a medication schedule and organizing your medicines.

Sexuality

See also:
▶ Health of Women (p.1039)
▶ Health of Men (p.1086)
▶ Safer Sex (p.76)

While normal aging brings physical changes that can alter sexual response, it is healthy and normal for men and women of all ages to have satisfying sexual relations. Indeed, the majority of older men and women report that sex is as good and satisfying—or better—than when they were younger. Still, changes in sexual desire are normal as you age.

As men grow older, they produce less testosterone, which can reduce sexual desire and activity. Genital sensitivity decreases as well, although erections can continue with adequate stimulation.

For women, the drop in estrogen production that accompanies menopause may reduce the speed and intensity of the sexual response. Although vaginal lubrication may occur more slowly, women can use lubricants or estrogen creams to avoid discomfort.

The degree to which older people desire and enjoy sex is

Medicines Seniors Should Take With Caution

Because older adults metabolize drugs differently than most other people do, some drugs are more likely to cause side effects in seniors. If you take any of the following commonly prescribed medicines, and are experiencing the symptoms described below, check with your doctor to see if the drug may be responsible for your symptoms.

MEDICINE	SYMPTOMS
Alprazolam	Memory problems
Amitriptyline	Irregular heart rhythm, difficulty urinating, blurring of vision
Chlordiazepoxide	Drowsiness, confusion
Diazepam	Drowsiness, confusion
Disopyramide	Heart failure, difficulty urinating, blurring of vision
Doxepin	Irregular heart rhythm, difficulty urinating, blurring of vision
Indomethacin	Confusion, dizziness
Meperidine	Confusion, seizures
Methocarbamol	Difficulty urinating, blurring of vision
Propoxyphene	Drowsiness, confusion

"Ageism" and Drug Side Effects: Dr Avorn's Advice

Older people face a double jeopardy from drug side effects—they are more likely to get them and the side effects are more likely to go unrecognized.

"Ageism" is the tendency to attribute all sorts of problems—such as fatigue, depression, incontinence, forgetfulness, or unsteadiness on the feet—in elderly people to the process of getting old. In fact, not one of these problems is a part of the normal aging process.

However, the new onset of any symptom can be the side effect of a medication and can often be corrected if brought to a physician's attention.

When a new symptom develops, particularly in an older person, it is important not to chalk it up to old age or to the onset of a new disease. Rather, check with the doctor about whether any of the drugs you or a loved one is taking might be the root cause.

JERRY AVORN, MD
BRIGHAM AND WOMEN'S HOSPITAL
HARVARD MEDICAL SCHOOL

closely linked to overall health. Disorders such as arthritis (see p.605), depression (see p.395), incontinence (see p.826), and adverse drug reactions can impair sexual function, but all are treatable.

Skin Disorders

See also:
▶ Color Guide to Visual Diagnosis (p.561)
▶ Skin, Hair, and Nails (p.528)

Aging skin is thinner, drier, more wrinkled, and less elastic than it was in youth. All of these conditions can be worsened by a previous pattern of excessive sun exposure.

Common skin diseases in the elderly include:

Seborrheic dermatitis (see p.551) Characterized by redness and scaly skin on the creases of the face and scalp.

Rosacea (see p.535) Causes a persistent flush of the cheeks, nose, chin, forehead, or eyelids.

Intertrigo Inflammation in the folds of the skin caused by fungi (see p.530) that often affects areas under the breast and in the abdominal folds and groin.

Shingles (see p.537) Caused by the same virus as chickenpox, it is characterized by severe pain along a nerve root on your body or face and is followed by a blistering rash that lasts 4 to 5 days. The rash may be followed by persistent pain. Since the risk of pain with shingles is higher in older adults and can be decreased with early preventive treatment, contact your doctor as soon as possible if you think you have shingles.

Stasis dermatitis (see p.551) Characterized by a chronic redness of the legs related to poor circulation, which predisposes

the skin to ulcers and bacterial infection.

Bedsores (see p.555) Slow healing, moist, open, and extremely uncomfortable wounds caused by prolonged pressure from being bedridden. They usually affect weight-bearing parts of the body such as the hips, shoulder blades, elbows, and heels.

Skin cancer (see p.543) Older people are particularly susceptible to all forms of skin cancer related to sun exposure and should be vigilant about avoiding the sun.

Sleep Changes

See also:
▶ Sleep and Sleep Problems (p.383)

Disturbances in sleep are a common problem in older people. Sleep changes can include nighttime awakenings, a decrease in deep restful sleep, and increased napping during the day.

Sleep disturbances can be caused by a number of medicines as well as underlying medical disorders such as sleep apnea (see p.387) or the need to urinate frequently.

For many older people, initiating a regular bedtime and waking schedule is the first step toward getting a good night's sleep. Other tips include exercising early in the day, keeping naps to a minimum, avoiding spicy foods and caffeine in the evening, keeping your bedroom temperature on the cool side, and reserving the bedroom only for sleep or sex.

In general, pharmaceutical sleep aids are not recommended as a solution for sleep disturbances; if used regularly, they

Trigeminal Neuralgia

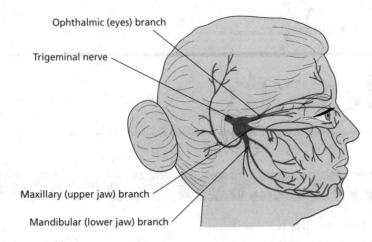

Ophthalmic (eyes) branch

Trigeminal nerve

Maxillary (upper jaw) branch

Mandibular (lower jaw) branch

Trigeminal neuralgia is a disorder of the trigeminal nerve, which extends into several parts of the face. Trigeminal neuralgia causes sudden, severe, stabbing pains that are brief but sometimes excruciating.

lose their effectiveness. Worse, their use has been linked to falls, hip fractures (see p.629), and driving accidents. Two new sleeping pills, eszopiclone and indiplon, are in late stages of development but are not yet approved for use in the United States. The early evidence indicates that these drugs are safe for use in older people. When these—and similar drugs—are used widely, it will become clear if they are truly safer. Your physician may refer you to a sleep clinic (see p.386) for evaluation if your sleep disturbances are severe and persistent.

Trigeminal Neuralgia

See also:
▶ Trigeminal Neuralgia (p.381)
Trigeminal neuralgia, also called tic douloureux, is a disorder of the fifth cranial nerve (trigeminal nerve) that causes severe piercing pain on one side of the face

in the eye, lips, gums, cheek, or chin. The periods of intense pain can be disabling and can last from several seconds to several minutes.

Although the condition usually affects people over 70, it can also occur in younger people with multiple sclerosis (see p.368).

The pain may be triggered by touching a certain area of the face or occur for no apparent reason. The underlying cause of the condition is not known.

Treatment includes painkillers to suppress pain, and surgery (see p.382).

Urinary Incontinence

See also:
▶ Urinary Incontinence (p.826)
Urinary incontinence, the involuntary leakage or loss of urine, is more common among people over age 60 but is not an inevitable result of growing old

(although aging and dementia contribute to it).

There are several different types of incontinence: stress, urge, and overflow. Stress incontinence occurs when urine leaks while coughing, sneezing, lifting, or otherwise putting pressure on the bladder. Stress incontinence becomes more likely for women after childbirth and for men after surgery for prostate cancer.

Urge incontinence occurs when the bladder suddenly contracts and expels urine with little or no warning.

Overflow incontinence is much less common but affects some men who have prostate enlargement. As a result of a partial obstruction, the bladder cannot empty completely, and urine dribbles nearly all the time.

Urinary tract infections (see p.804), depression, some medicines, and other treatable factors also can be responsible for urine leakage.

Incontinence can also result from diseases that do not directly affect the urinary tract, particularly in older people. For example, people with arthritis (see p.605) or Parkinson disease (see p.371) may have mobility problems that prevent them from getting to the toilet in time.

Incontinence is almost always treatable. It is often curable at any age, usually without surgery. Treatment for incontinence depends on the cause of the disorder and what treatment you prefer. Choices include performing exercises to strengthen the urinary sphincter and pelvic muscles (Kegel exercises; see p.1051), retraining the bladder, taking medicines, or, in some cases, undergoing surgery.

Caregiving and Eldercare

CAREGIVING IN YOUR HOME

Families—not health care professionals—provide 80% to 90% of the care for older people. Although about 75% of all caregivers are women, the demands of caregiving can affect the entire family. In a time when people with long-term illnesses are living longer, many families have experienced the stress of taking care of an aging parent. An estimated 25 million adults provide a significant amount of care for older family members, including short-term care for acute illness and long-term care for chronic illness. Current estimates are that, by the year 2020, one third of people in the workplace will have the responsibility of caring for an elderly mother, father, or other elderly family member.

While nurturing skills come naturally to some people, many of us require guidance. This section reviews the basics of caring for a sick or elderly person. The person you are caring for may require measures that are specific to his or her medical condition. Call the doctor if you do not clearly understand any instructions he or she has given you.

Setting Up a Room

If you have a choice, select a room that is bright and cheerful or one that has a view of the yard or the outside. Arrange the room so that there is seating for visitors. Position a good reading lamp and a bedside table next to the bed to hold a telephone, reading material, and water glass.

A television set paired with a remote control that is easy to read and operate will give the person you are caring for the freedom to make viewing choices. Place a bell or a baby monitor next to the bed so he or she can call for help. If the person is very ill or incapacitated, or you expect that person to need help for some time, consider setting up a room on the first floor, ideally near a bathroom. If this is not possible, you may wish to purchase or rent a portable bedside toilet known as a commode. Commodes can also be useful if the person has difficulty getting in and out of the bathroom.

If the sick person is able to sit up in bed, find a large, supportive pillow that helps him or her sit up comfortably. You can rent or purchase many types of equipment (see Assistive Devices, p.1128) to make it easier to care for someone who is ill. The cost of some equipment is covered by Medicare (see p.27). Depending on your patient's condition, the doctor, physical therapist, occupational therapist, or visiting nurse can be helpful in suggesting other useful additions to the room.

Medicines

As caregiver, one of your most important tasks is to give medicines on an appropriate schedule. It is essential that both prescription and nonprescription drugs be given as the doctor prescribes; the effectiveness of many drugs is tied closely to how and when they are taken. If you are uncertain about your loved one's medication schedule, call his or her doctor or bring all the medicines with you to the next appointment and ask about each drug. Or, make a copy of the Sample Medication Schedule on p.1121 and take it to the doctor's office.

If the schedule given by the doctor is difficult for the elderly

Sample Medication Schedule

More than half of older people fail to take their medicines as prescribed by their doctors. If you are taking several drugs, a medication schedule is a helpful tool in remembering which drug should be taken at what time and with what restrictions (such as with or without food). Make a chart or use the sample here to get started. Fill in the name of the drug, the dosage to be taken, and the time of day it should be taken; add any notes. It is helpful to take your medication schedule to all doctor appointments so that all of your physicians are informed of the drugs you are currently taking.

NAME OF MEDICATION		MON	TUES	WED	THURS	FRI	SAT	SUN
	Morning							
	Afternoon							
	Evening							
	Morning							
	Afternoon							
	Evening							
	Morning							
	Afternoon							
	Evening							

or sick person to follow, ask whether adjustments can be made. For example, long-acting medicines taken once a day can sometimes be substituted for short-acting ones taken several times a day. If the person is taking several medicines on different days, purchase a pill box with multiple compartments that correspond to the days of the week. These pill boxes are inexpensive and available at most pharmacies.

Never stop giving a medicine without the doctor's approval, even if the patient appears to be getting better. It can be dangerous to stop medicine suddenly or prematurely. Likewise, taking more or less of any medicine can delay improvement in the person's condition and even cause harm.

Make sure the person's doctor is aware of all prescription and over-the-counter drugs being taken. This is especially important if the sick person is seeing more than one physician. Some drugs can cause side effects and some do not mix well with other drugs. Pharmacies often provide a listing of a drug's potential side effects when they fill a prescription; report any side effects to the doctor. In some cases, adjusting the dosage or type of medicine is required to achieve the best results. Call the doctor to resolve any questions or concerns about medicines.

Meals and Nutrition

Mealtime can be a high point of the day for a sick or ailing person. Your efforts can make the meal appealing while still meeting any dietary requirements (such as a high-protein, low-salt, or sugar-free diet) recommended by the doctor. A nutritionist or nurse can provide recipes and tips for creatively preparing restricted diets, such as increasing the amount of spices used in a low-salt meal. Elderly adults, especially if they are ill or weak, can lose interest in eating (see p.1122). However, they require at least—if not more of—the same vitamins, minerals, and nutrients as younger, healthy people.

Common Causes of Loss of Appetite

Loss of appetite most often is brought on by boredom, loneliness, or depression. However, there are several other causes that you should keep in mind:

■ A medicine may cause mild nausea or loss of appetite. Changing the dose or switching to another medication can relieve the problem; ask the doctor for advice.

■ A chronic illness that may not yet have been diagnosed can cause loss of appetite. If there is no other apparent explanation, ask the physician if a check-up is needed.

■ Appetite is stimulated by exercise. Older people with sedentary lifestyles sometimes have decreased appetites.

■ Dental problems (including ill-fitting dentures) can make eating frustrating. If you suspect a dental problem may be causing loss of interest in eating, a dental check-up is needed.

In some cases, a person is so ill or disabled that assistance is required for eating. Make certain the food is the right temperature and finely minced or pureed so that swallowing is not difficult. A flexible straw can help those with limited mobility and dexterity drink fluids. People with profound swallowing problems, or those who need supplements because they have very great nutritional requirements (such as people who have bedsores, see p.1123), may benefit from drinking liquid nutritional supplements. Special formulas, available in drugstores, tend to be extremely expensive and should generally be used only on a doctor's recommendation. An instant breakfast drink may be a good, cheaper alternative.

Maintaining Hygiene

Keeping the body clean is an essential part of good health, especially for a person who is sick. Good hygiene not only helps prevent infection, it can contribute to good mental health.

Helping a mobile person bathe If the person you are caring for is able to take a shower or bath alone, encourage him or her to do so. Even if the person requires help getting into or out of the tub, provide the privacy to bathe alone. Offer assistance with hair washing if needed. Consider buying or renting a stable, slip-proof chair made for the bathtub. You can also install handles on the edges of the tub or on the shower wall to increase stability. Provide washcloths, soap, shampoo, and towels and stay close in case the person needs assistance.

Giving a sponge bath If the sick person is not able to get out of bed, a daily sponge bath is recommended. If you are giving the sponge bath, you will need a basin with warm (not hot), soapy water; a basin with warm, clear water; a soft washcloth; a large rubber sheet; and several dry towels.

Slip the rubber sheet between the person and the bed (for guidance, see Changing Sheets for a Bedridden Person, p.1128) to help keep the bottom sheet dry. Wipe the person all over top to bottom with the washcloth dipped in soapy water, being careful to keep exposed areas of the body warm and covered with a dry towel. Wash folds of skin especially thoroughly; finish by washing the genital and rectal areas. Repeat the same procedure with the clear, warm water and dry thoroughly with a clean towel. Home health aides (see Health Care Services, p.1130) can provide this service, and Medicaid may pay for it on a long-term basis. Medicare may pay for a home health aide on a short-term basis during the recovery period from an acute illness.

Washing hair in bed To shampoo the hair of someone who is

Assistive Devices for the Bath

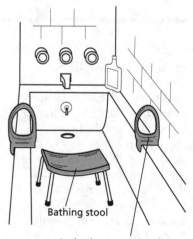

Bathing stool

Bathtub-mounted grab bars

Stability in the bathtub and shower can be improved with a bathing stool, which permits the user to be seated while bathing. Bathtub-mounted grab bars increase stability getting in and out of the tub. Shower wall grab bars are also available.

bedridden, cover the bed sheets with a towel or rubber sheet and move the person so that his or her shoulders are propped up; the head should be positioned over a basin. Wet the person's hair with several cups of warm water, then shampoo, massage the scalp, and rinse with clear water. Dry with a towel and blow dryer (on a warm—never hot—setting) so that the hair is dry enough to be comfortable when the person is situated back in bed. Alternatively, you can purchase a dry shampoo that, when sprinkled on the hair and combed or brushed out, removes oils.

Boosting morale A little makeup for a woman and a shave for a man can boost the person's sense of well-being and optimism. Similarly, a haircut or other hairstyling can increase self-esteem and provide a chance to socialize. Many hairdressers will make house calls.

TOILET NEEDS

If the person you are caring for is able to get to the bathroom un-assisted, make sure you provide night-lights and an unobstructed path to the toilet. Helpful devices for using the toilet include a toi-let safety frame (see above right) and a raised toilet seat, which make getting on and off the toilet easier. Both are available at med-ical supply stores. If the bath-room is too far away for the per-son to reach easily, buy or rent a mobile toilet called a commode to keep in his or her room. If the person is bedridden, consider purchasing an inexpensive bed-pan and, for a man, a handheld urinal. Protect bed sheets with

Assistive Devices for the Toilet

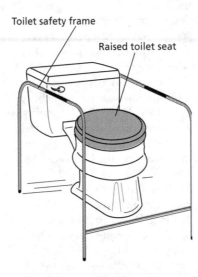

Toilet safety frame

Raised toilet seat

A raised toilet seat elevates the seat of the toilet for those who have diffi-culty lowering themselves onto it. A toilet safety frame provides further stability in the bathroom. Both assistive devices can be rented or purchased from a medical supply store.

---

waterproof liners, which are available at medical supply stores, or use waterproof crib sheets.

If necessary, remind the per-son to empty his or her bladder before napping or going to sleep for the night to avoid wetting the bed. Many elderly people get up to urinate frequently during the night; decreasing fluid intake after dinner can help diminish this need.

Urinary incontinence (uncon-trollable, involuntary urination) (see p.826) is not a normal part of aging. Older people with occa-sional incontinence may be helped by urinating every 2 hours during the day. Following this type of schedule often reduces or

eliminates urinary "accidents." If scheduled urination does not solve the problem, the person's doctor should be notified. Many people with incontinence can be successfully treated. For those who remain incontinent, use of disposable underpads can help minimize the embarrassment of untimely leakage.

Helping with a bed pan If you have ever been in the hospital and had to use a bedpan, you may remember it as a challenging experience, especially if someone else was in the room. Make sure you provide privacy and plenty of time for the person to relax while using a bedpan. First, warm the bedpan in hot water, dry it, and sprinkle the rim with talcum power; this will make it easier to slip the bedpan under the but-tocks. If the person cannot lift his or her buttocks unassisted, lift the person's hips while someone else slips the bedpan under the person's buttocks. If the person cannot maneuver, turn him or her on the side, slip the pan under the buttocks, press the bedpan down into the bed, and turn the person back over on top of it. Wash bedpans and handheld uri-nals thoroughly with a disinfec-tant after each use. Store them under the bed or, if the person can manage unassisted, leave them near the bed for easy access.

Preventing and Treating Bedsores

The most common sites for bed-sores (also known as pressure ulcers or decubitus ulcers) are the hips, heels, knees, shoulder blades, elbows, and spine—all bony prominences that bear the weight of the body against the bed and the bedclothes. If you are caring for a person who is confined to a bed or chair, it is essential that you take steps to keep bedsores from developing.

Frequent exercise is essential and is possible even for the bedridden (see Exercises for the Older Adult, p.1126). In the elderly, bedsores typically occur because the person is not moving, thus reducing the flow of blood. Ask the person's doctor or nurse about isometric and stretching exercises that help keep blood circulating.

Change the position of the person every 2 hours, moving his or her arms and legs as much as possible as you do so. Use pillows generously to raise the person's heels, elbows, and arms and to relieve pressure on the buttocks, hips, and knees. Make sure the person's skin is kept clean and dry, since moisture increases the likelihood of bedsores. Managing incontinence (see p.826) is particularly important, since urine and feces are extremely irritating to the skin.

A bumpy foam mattress (called egg-crate foam) placed on top of the bed mattress may make the bed more comfortable, but has not been shown to decrease the risk of bedsores. Pads and booties made of sheepskin reduce the pressure on elbows, heels, and other ulcer-prone areas. A high-protein diet is helpful in preventing skin breakdown.

Watch for red, inflamed patches of skin—the first signs of bedsores. If not treated, the red, inflamed areas turn purple and the skin breaks down. The open ulcer that follows can become

infected. Bedsores heal very slowly and can be life-threatening. Call the doctor immediately if you see any early signs of bedsores, such as blistered skin or red skin that does not turn white when pressed.

Bedsores are usually treated with special dressings, which often must be applied by a nurse. Antibiotics may also be required to fight infection; depending on the severity of the bedsores, the drug may be taken in pill form, applied directly to the ulcers, or given intravenously.

Once a bedsore has developed, the sick person must be carefully positioned to keep pressure off the affected area. Air pressure beds have been shown to help heal bedsores, but they are extremely expensive and are used primarily in hospitals for people who have severe ulcers. There is some evidence that vitamin E supplements and zinc supplements, available over the counter, can promote healing of

bedsores. Protein supplementation, usually in the form of liquid nutritional supplements, may be necessary for healing to take place.

Taking a Temperature

Normal body temperature is about 98.6°F, but may vary by 1° to 2° during the day. An increase is generally not considered dangerous unless body temperature exceeds 101°F, at which point you should call the doctor. The exception is for a child; a temperature higher than 102°F should prompt a call to your child's physician.

Shaking chills or excessive sweating can alert you that the person you are caring for has a fever. Other symptoms that are cause for concern include listlessness, extensive vomiting, headache, and stiff neck.

You can take a person's temperature with a thermometer placed under the tongue, held in

How to Take a Temperature

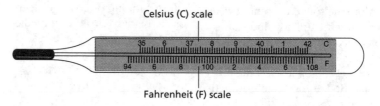

Celsius (C) scale

Fahrenheit (F) scale

Be sure the person is sitting or lying down and that he or she has not smoked or had anything hot or cold to drink for 15 minutes. Grasp the end of the thermometer and shake down the mercury until it is below 96° Fahrenheit (F) (35.6° Celsius [C]). Place the thermometer under the person's tongue and leave it in place for at least 3 minutes. Remove the thermometer and tilt it slightly to see where the mercury ends; this is the temperature reading. Wipe the thermometer with rubbing alcohol or wash it with soap and water, rinse it in cool water, and place it in its container.

Exercise and Recovery From Illness

Keeping the body active when convalescing from an illness or injury improves blood flow, stimulates the appetite, and can contribute to an overall sense of well-being. Exercise can also help a sick person regain a previous level of function. Research has shown that simple weight-lifting exercises (see p.1113) performed regularly by older people can increase mobility and decrease the likelihood of falling and breaking bones. Ask the person's doctor if exercise is appropriate.

A person confined to bed may not be able to lift weights, but he or she can stretch the arms and legs, flex the feet, and rotate the neck. A number of video exercise programs are available for elderly people confined to a wheelchair and for those recovering from a stroke. People who have lost substantial physical conditioning after a long illness or who have specific disabilities such as paralysis can benefit from working with a physical therapist. The patient's doctor must make a referral for the service to be covered by insurance.

For people who are bedridden or convalescing, mental stimulation is important as well. As caregiver, try to make available videotapes and books from the library, or hobby or craft projects that the person you are caring for enjoys doing. Games, music, and books on audiotape can help stimulate thought during long hours in bed. If the person is well enough, encourage short visits from friends, neighbors, and children.

Caring for a Sick Child

Many adults choose to be alone and resting in bed when they are sick, but most children, if they feel well enough, prefer to be up and around and close to the caregiver to get medicine and juice, soothing strokes, and companionship. If you are caring for a child who has an illness such as a fever, headache, or stomachache, he or she may want to stay in bed. However, there is no reason to force the child to remain in bed unless the doctor has recommended it. Try to provide quiet activities; read books, play a game, or watch a video or television program together.

Coping with fever In general, you should call the doctor if your child's temperature is higher than 102°F or is accompanied by troubling symptoms, such as lethargy, seizures, or a rash (see Fever: When to Call the Doctor, p.974). It is important to give a feverish child plenty of fluids, such as water or juice, and keep him or her lightly covered. Give acetaminophen or ibuprofen to help relieve the fever. Do not give aspirin to those under 21 years old; it has been linked to a life-threatening condition called Reye syndrome (see p.1017). If the child's temperature rises or persists for several days, call his or her doctor.

Feeding a sick child You need not be overly concerned if your sick child does not feel like eating. Unless the doctor has provided a special diet, follow your child's cues and offer small amounts of food. If the child has a fever or diarrhea or is vomiting, it is essential that he or she drink plenty of clear liquids, such as water, juice, broth, or carbonated beverages. When your child begins to feel better, offer bland foods, such as toast or crackers, or whatever is tempting.

the armpit, or placed gently in the rectum; some digital thermometers are designed to be inserted into the ear. Do not take a person's temperature after he or she has had a hot or cold drink or after a hot bath; the reading will not be accurate. Oral mercury thermometers are designed to be placed under the tongue, but they can also be used in the armpit (though they give a slightly less accurate reading). Rectal thermometers are designed for use only in the rectum, and are the only thermometers that should be used in the rectum.

Thermometers come in many forms—from the old, mercury thermometer to the quicker, digital types, which can be easier to read. To use a mercury thermometer, grasp it at the top and flip your wrist once or twice to shake the mercury down to the bulb. Position the bulb under the tongue, ask the person to close his or her mouth, and leave the thermometer in place for 3 minutes. Remove the thermometer and tilt it until you can see where the mercury stops. This is the temperature reading. There are many different models of electronic thermometer. To use an electronic thermometer, place the thermometer under the tongue or in the ear and leave it there until it beeps or flashes.

Exercises for the Older Adult

These exercises are geared to different levels of physical ability. Before starting any exercise program, talk to your physician to ensure that exercise will not exacerbate any current medical condition. See also Exercise and Fitness, p.50.

IF BEDRIDDEN:

- Lift legs straight off the bed. Flex arms and ankles.
- Lift head off the pillow and turn from side to side.
- Pull up on a bar above head (pull bars are available at medical supply stores).
- Breathe deeply and exhale completely several times, taking in as much air as possible each time.
- Squeeze a ball or sponge.
- Repeat each exercise, gradually increasing the repetitions.

IF IN A WHEELCHAIR:

- Kick legs. Flex ankles and arms.
- Breathe deeply and exhale completely several times, taking in as much air as possible each time.
- Wheel wheelchair around the house or outside.
- Throw a ball.
- Lift light weights (such as soup cans).

IF ABLE TO GET AROUND INSIDE:

- Walk around the house as many times as possible.
- Throw and kick a large rubber ball.
- Sit down and stand up. Repeat several times.
- Stretch and bend legs, arms, and back.
- Lift light weights (such as soup cans).
- Hold on to the back of a chair and raise and lower each leg.
- Lift weights attached to legs.

IF ABLE TO GET AROUND OUTSIDE:

- Take walks.
- Ride a bicycle.
- Walk up and down stairs.
- Work in the garden.

IF ABLE TO GET AROUND THE COMMUNITY:

- Walk to and from the grocery store or appointments.
- Walk indoors at a shopping center in bad weather.
- Engage in a sport, such as swimming or golfing.
- Set goals and keep track of progress.

Safety

If you are a caregiver, the safety of your home is an integral part of preventing injuries. For older adults living on their own, the same safety issues apply. A physical therapist or visiting nurse can help you examine your home for hazards, pointing out potential dangers. The particular needs of the person you are caring for can also be addressed during a safety review of your living quarters.

Remember that older adults are especially vulnerable to falls because their bodies may be weaker. Osteoporosis (see p.596) makes bones more brittle with age, and thus more prone to fracture during a fall. It also takes an older adult longer to heal. Consider the person's eyesight, hearing, and balance as you review your living area, noting the following:

- Remove or rearrange furniture that is difficult to walk around and make sure floors are not slippery.

- Avoid scatter rugs unless they have a rubber backing that makes them secure.

- Look for worn areas in carpets that could catch a foot and cause a fall.

- Direct electrical cords toward walls and secure them there; they should not run through walking areas.

- Make sure the house is well lighted and equipped with nightlights.

- Store medicines in their origi-

Helping a Person From Bed to Chair

Although it is best for two people to move someone who is sick, weak, or disabled, you can do it alone as long as the person is able to stand. Make sure you are wearing nonslip shoes. To move the person back to bed, follow the instructions in reverse order.

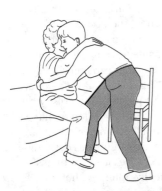

1 Place a chair at a right angle to the bed. Help the person to the edge of the bed to a sitting position, with legs hanging over the side of the bed. Ask the person to place his or her hands on your shoulders in a hugging position.

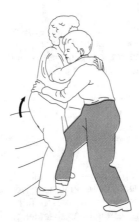

2 Your arms should be wrapped under the person's arms. Stand close to the edge of the bed with knees bent and one foot placed in front of the other so that your right knee is between the person's knees. Ask the person to shift weight forward as you lift. Shift your weight onto your back foot as you pull upward.

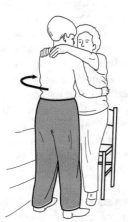

3 As you pull the person up with your arms and hands, shift your feet to a sideways position. Turn the person so that the backs of his or her legs are touching the chair. Ask the person to tell you when he or she can feel the chair.

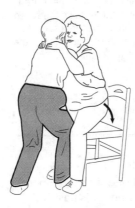

4 With your back straight and knees bent, place one foot in front of the other and between the person's knees. Shift your weight onto your front leg. As you bend your front knee, carefully lower the person into the chair.

nal labeled containers away from the bedroom; do not leave them on a nightstand where they may be taken in the middle of the night accidentally.

■ Make sure light switches are easy to find.

■ Post emergency telephone numbers in large print next to every telephone.

■ Set the hot water heater so the maximum temperature is 120°F. Because of thinner skin and slower reactions, elderly people are more at risk for burning themselves.

■ If the person you are caring for is able to get around, create a medical identification card for his or her wallet that includes your name, address, and phone number and a list of the person's medical conditions. If there is an emergency and you are away, the paramedics will have enough information to start treatment and locate you.

Preventing Falls

Falls are the most common and preventable injury in the elderly. Because nearly all older adults have some degree of osteoporosis (see p.596), which makes bones weak and brittle, they are more susceptible to fractures. People who have dementia (which causes disorientation and poor judgment), poor eyesight, or arthritis (which can cause instability) are at even greater risk of falling. Medicines can also cause dizziness or weakness that can make the user more prone to falls.

Most falls occur at home, and the most dangerous areas are

Changing Sheets for a Bedridden Person

It is easier for two people to change the sheets of someone who is bedridden, but it is possible for one person to do. Some people (such as those with heart failure) cannot breathe easily when lying flat. In such cases, the bedridden person should be lifted into a bedside chair while you change the sheets.

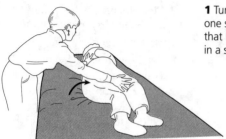

1 Turn the person to the edge of one side of the bed, making sure that he or she is comfortable and in a stable and safe position.

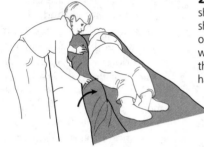

2 Roll up one half of the soiled sheet lengthwise until the rolled sheet is against the person. Roll one half of the clean sheet lengthwise and place it in the center of the bed alongside of the rolled-up half of the soiled sheet.

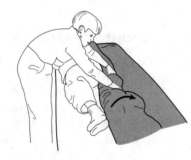

3 Keeping a hand on the person for stability, roll him or her onto the clean sheet and remove the soiled sheet. Then unroll the rest of the clean sheet, stretch it out over the remaining area, and tuck it in securely.

bathrooms and stairways. To prevent falls, apply nonskid strips to the bottom of the bathtub. Handrails can provide stability near the toilet and in the tub and shower. Avoid the use of bath oils; they can make the shower or bathtub floor and other surfaces slippery.

Stairs should have handrails on at least one side; if the person you are caring for is unsteady walking downstairs, there should be handrails on both sides. Some experts recommend painting the edge of each stair a bright color to make it more visible. Place a securely attached rubber strip on

the stair edge to provide even more traction. Finally, make sure there are no loose throw rugs, edges of carpets, or uncovered electric cords on any floor surface.

If, despite your efforts to make the environment safer, the person you are caring for falls frequently, the doctor should check for medical conditions such as heart or neurological problems that can contribute to falls. The doctor may also refer you to a physical therapist who will come to your home, make additional recommendations for improving safety, and determine if an exercise program or assistive device might be helpful. If the person continues to fall, you may want to consider having a personal emergency response system (see p.1129) installed.

Assistive Devices

Assistive devices are aids such as canes and walkers that can make life easier for a person who needs help preparing food, walking, reaching, or using the bathroom. You can buy or rent assistive devices, depending on whether you need them for the short or long term. Medicare (see p.27) covers 80% of the cost of any equipment it deems to be medically necessary. Medicaid (see p.28) covers a greater number of assistive devices but the rules vary from state to state. Here is a partial list of assistive devices that your doctor can order to help:

Canes and walkers Canes and walkers encourage mobility and increase stability. The doctor or, more commonly, a physical therapist fits the device and the person is given specific instructions on how to use it.

Hospital beds Hospital beds (which can be rented or purchased) offer a range of positions and thus can make sitting up more comfortable for a bedridden person. In addition, sitting up can be therapeutic because lung secretions can be more easily coughed up, reducing the chance that fluid will accumulate in the lungs. Hospital beds are available in manual, semi-electric, and fully electric models. Discuss the patient's needs with his or her doctor or physical therapist to choose the most appropriate model. For people who have trouble sitting up in bed (and to provide a means of exercise), an overhead trapeze bar may be recommended so that the person can pull up into a sitting position.

Bathroom aids Because home bathrooms are rarely large enough to accommodate a wheelchair or walker, devices such as grab bars, height-adjustable rails that fit directly over the toilet (see p.1122), and a raised toilet seat are helpful in increasing stability. Toilet paper holders and towel bars should never be used as a substitute for grab bars because they will not support the weight of the average person.

Special-need devices Assistive devices—ranging from washable mattress covers to long-handled reaching devices—are also available for people with special needs. There are long-handled shoehorns, devices that help stroke or arthritis sufferers pull up stockings, and eating utensils for those who have trouble gripping a fork or spoon. These helpful aids are available through medical

Personal Emergency Response System

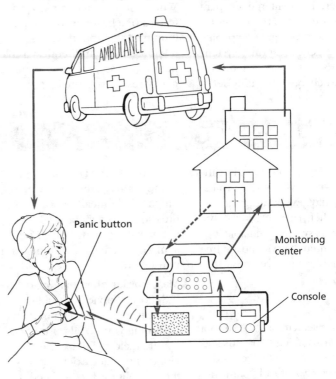

A personal emergency response system allows a frail, homebound person with a medical emergency to push a button and send a call for help to a monitoring center. At the center, the caller is identified by a code and then contacted via phone, two-way intercom, or a previously identified intermediary (such as a neighbor), who will go immediately to the person's home. If an emergency is confirmed, paramedics are sent to the location.

supply stores, rehabilitation departments of hospitals, and special catalogs for the general public. The patient's doctor may provide a referral to an occupational therapist, who specializes in helping people remain independent in their daily activities; the therapist can recommend specific devices to facilitate independence.

Personal emergency response systems For the elderly person living alone, a personal emergency response system provides a way to get help if there is a medical emergency. With these devices, the person wears a "call-for-help" button around the neck or on a bracelet. If the person falls or needs medical help immediately, he or she pushes the button, which relays a call to a monitoring center. At the response center, the caller is identified by a code. The person receiving the alert phones the caller's home and communicates with the person via phone or a two-way intercom attached to the phone. If there is no response or the person confirms that there is an emergency, paramedics are sent to the location immediately. Several companies sell emergency response systems, so prices vary. Some sell the system and charge a monthly ser-vice fee; others lease the system. When choosing a company, try to find one based in your community. Ask about their average response time, and request a trial period to test the system. Emergency response systems can pro-vide reassurance and a greater sense of security to a sick or elderly person who lives alone and to family members. You can learn more about these systems through a visiting nurse association or your local hospital.

SUPPORT SYSTEMS

As a caregiver, you should neither expect—nor try—to be on-call 24 hours a day. Every caregiver needs relief. There are a variety of support systems available in most communities; some are free or available at reduced cost.

How Do I Find Help?

Start your search for local support services by talking to friends and associates who may have used these services. Or call your local senior center and your area's agency on aging to see what services are available. Since agencies on aging are listed under various names, depending on where you live, call the Eldercare Locator (800-677-1116) to find the senior center closest to you. Most senior centers offer free recreation and social programs.

Volunteer helpers Many senior centers offer volunteers who help with chores. The volunteers perform minor repairs and small jobs—such as installing grab bars in a bathroom—for free or on an ability-to-pay basis. Some communities have telephone reassurance and visitor programs that are free or available for a minimal charge. These programs provide volunteers who telephone or visit periodically. They can be helpful in reminding the person to eat meals and take medicine. Companions to the elderly help prepare light meals, assist with dressing, and generally talk to and watch over the elderly person. They usually do not perform housework.

Mail-carrier alert program The U.S. Postal Service offers the mail-carrier alert program. By informing your local post office about an elderly person living alone, the mail carrier will be on the lookout for accumulated mail. If mail stacks up, the carrier will alert a supervisor, who notifies local police.

Meal programs Meal programs are free or available at a minimal charge; they are often located at local community centers, where people eat in a group. Meals-on-wheels delivers meals to the house-bound; the service may be available through a local senior center, religious organizations, or area hospitals. Food delivery volunteers are also trained to observe the general health of the elderly person and will call for assistance if the person appears to need help.

Transportation services Transportation services, usually offered through a community's agency on aging or senior center, provide transportation to the grocery store, doctor appointments, and adult day care (see below). Many of the buses and vans are accessible by wheelchair and most are free or request only a minimal donation to defray expenses.

Adult day care Adult day care is a service that provides elderly people with care, supervision, and activities outside the home (some programs are for people with Alzheimer disease; see p.363). Many families use adult day care programs to provide substantial relief from caregiving responsibilities. In a typical adult day care program, your elderly relative is picked up in the morning by a van, taken to a center where a meal and general care are provided, and then returned home in the early evening. The day is structured with activities, exercise, and a hot lunch; most adult day care centers have a nurse and social worker on staff to dispense medicines and handle emergencies.

Health Care Services

If the elderly person you are caring for is weak, ill, or recovering from surgery, an expansive array of services provided by home health care workers can ease your caregiving responsibilities. This category of services includes

Geriatricians: What They Do and How to Find One

A geriatrician is a doctor experienced in treating the physical and emotional needs of elderly adults, focusing on functioning—the capacity for self-care—rather than just on disease. Geriatricians often work as part of a team that includes a nurse practitioner, a social worker, and sometimes a physical therapist.

Most elderly people receive medical care from an internist or family doctor. However, older people who have complex medical problems that affect their ability to perform daily activities may benefit from a consultation with a specialist in geriatrics or may prefer that the geriatrician serve as their primary care doctor.

Ask friends, relatives, and colleagues if they know a good geriatric doctor or, if you are seeking a consultation, ask your primary care physician to refer you to one. Review the organizations under the heading "Aging" in the Appendix of this book (see p.1228) for assistance. Look for a board-certified geriatrician; this means that the doctor has had special training in geriatric medicine and has passed a rigorous examination in this specialty. Some geriatricians make house calls.

A geriatric doctor will perform a physical examination and test mental and physical function. The physician may ask the patient to bend, reach, turn, sit down, get up, and read a prescription label. A geriatric exam also includes a test of the person's mental state and cognitive abilities. For example, the doctor may ask the person to count backwards from 100 by 7 and give the person three words to memorize and then ask him or her to recall the words several minutes later. The doctor notes any early signs of dementia and asks about the person's housing arrangements, diet, daily habits, and social support systems.

A good geriatrician is interested in understanding diverse aspects of the person's life so that an accurate assessment of health and recommendations for continued care can be made.

home health aides; homemakers; physical, speech, and occupational therapists; social workers; nurses; geriatric case managers; and respite care workers.

If you will be taking care of someone who is coming home from the hospital, the discharge planner at the hospital can often help you make arrangements for continued health care services. However, you can also make arrangements directly with a home health care agency, which offers a full range of services. Most important, Medicare and Medicaid cover the cost of such services if the person is housebound, if the care is prescribed by a doctor, and if a certified agency is used. However, this coverage is for "skilled" care only—that is, the care is provided by nurses and therapists.

In some cases, the cost of home health aides and social workers is covered, but only for as long as their services are needed as an adjunct to the nurse handling the case. It is important that you monitor the quality of care given by all home health care workers.

Home health aides Home health aides are trained to help with bathing, dressing, and toilet needs and occasionally perform light meal preparation and household tasks. Fees vary from $10 an hour to $50 for a 2-hour or 4-hour visit. Medicare and some medical insurance plans cover the cost of home health aides, but usually only for a short time and when the services are needed in addition to nursing care or other therapy.

Homemakers Homemakers help with household chores such as cooking, cleaning, and shopping. Although not strictly health care providers, homemakers often play a critical role in caring for the frail, housebound person. Their services are not covered by Medicare, though in many states Medicaid reimbursement is available.

Occupational therapists, speech therapists, and physical therapists Occupational therapists, speech therapists, and physical therapists make house calls, usually through a hospital or home-care agency. The cost (about $80 for a 1- to 2-hour visit) is often covered by insurance if it is part of a hospital discharge care plan or is ordered by the doctor for short-term rehabilitation. Occupational, speech, or physical therapists often are needed after a person has had an injury, surgery, or stroke.

An occupational therapist helps people with stiff joints or weakness of the upper extremities by working on muscle control and coordination. Occupational therapists also teach the person recovering from an illness greater independence. Speech therapists help people who need to relearn how to speak because of a stroke or other illness. Physical therapists work on improving mobility, strength, and flexibility after an injury or illness.

Nutritionists Nutritionists may be called on to help a person understand a new diet and learn to prepare food according to the diet.

Social workers Social workers provide emotional support for the patient and help the family with referrals for further care.

Nurses Nurses provide a range of medical care, from changing dressings and taking blood to inserting catheters and intravenous lines. They can teach family members how to perform simple but necessary tasks. Nurses typically work for home health agencies and charge an average of $90 a visit. Medicare and Medicaid cover the cost if it is deemed medically necessary and if a doctor orders the care, though only for a short period in most cases.

Geriatric case managers Geriatric case managers coordinate the many services and requirements that may be needed by an elderly person. Geriatric case managers are usually nurses or social workers with special training in geriatrics or elderly care. You can hire a case manager to handle one or all aspects of your loved one's health care, such as housekeeping or nursing care.

A geriatric case manager typically meets with family members to determine what needs must be met; then he or she meets with the elderly person to preliminarily evaluate his or her health and determine daily requirements.

The geriatric case manager then submits a plan that specifies what services will be provided, by whom, and at what cost. The initial assessment can cost from $200 to $300, which does not include the cost of the services themselves. Expect to pay a monthly fee to the case manager; the amount depends on what services are provided. Once you agree to the plan, you should receive a written report or regular phone calls to keep you posted on the person's health.

Respite care caregivers Respite care provides a primary caregiver with a break, for as little as a few hours so you can go

Emotional Help for Caregivers

If you are a caregiver, recognize the importance of finding time for yourself. People who are emotionally and physically exhausted or guilt-ridden cannot provide good care. You may be taking care of a loved one 24 hours a day or you may be stopping at a nursing home every day after work to visit a relative. If you have multiple responsibilities—family, job, children—you may find yourself feeling resentful toward the person to whom you are devoting so much time.

Many caregivers find help through support groups—informal gatherings of people who talk about problems and frustrations and share solutions. Often, the very act of giving encouragement and sympathy to others who are caring for a sick or elderly person can help you feel stronger. Recognize that spending time away from the sick person can help you cope better. Some support groups are designed specifically for the caregivers of those with Alzheimer disease. The

Alzheimer's Association (see p.1229) provides a broad range of services, including caregiver support groups and educational information for families coping with the disease.

Some groups are started by caregivers themselves, while others are established by social service agencies, a local senior center, the area agency on aging, or religious organizations. If you need support but are not comfortable in groups, talk to your doctor, who can refer you to a social worker, psychologist, or psychiatrist.

Many caregivers find it helpful to share the responsibility with other members of the family. Different people have different capacities. For example, a son may find it difficult to provide personal care for his mother but may be able to contribute by handling her financial affairs. Involving grandchildren can help make caregiving a family activity rather than a burden.

Common Mental Health Problems of the Elderly

Depression (see p.395), anxiety (see p.402), and dementia (loss or impairment of mental powers) (see p.362) are common medical conditions in elderly adults.

Depression Many people ignore signs of depression because they consider it an indication of weakness or a character flaw. Depression is a disease and it can be treated. If you know someone who has had several of the following symptoms of depression for more than 2 weeks, call his or her doctor:

- Lack of interest in activities once considered enjoyable
- Sadness and dejection without any apparent cause
- Fatigue and lethargy
- Change in appetite or weight
- Insomnia (inability to sleep) or change in sleep habits
- Feelings of hopelessness, guilt, and worthlessness
- Lack of concentration or muddled thinking
- Increased use of alcohol, tobacco, or other drugs
- Talk of suicide or death

Anxiety As many as 5% of elderly people suffer from a condition known as generalized anxiety disorder (see p.402). A person with anxiety worries about several things at once and usually has a number of physical symptoms, including agitation, shakiness and trembling, nausea, hot and cold flashes, dizziness, shortness of breath, or frequent urination. Anxiety can also be a symptom of depression or dementia, so it is best to encourage anyone with anxiety to talk to his or her doctor about the symptoms. Treatment includes counseling, family support, or learning biofeedback (see p.395). Medication is not often prescribed unless the person is severely anxious because the potential side effects can outweigh the benefits.

Dementia The symptoms of dementia include memory loss, confusion, disorientation, delusions, personality changes, and difficulty with language, math, and visual relationships. Dementia is not a part of aging, but the result of disease. Alzheimer disease (see p.363) is one type of dementia. If a loved one appears increasingly confused or forgetful, he or she should be examined by a doctor. Alzheimer disease and other forms of dementia can be very difficult for both the affected person and family members to accept. Remember that the person's behavior is caused by the disease.

out for dinner, or for as long as several weeks if you need to be away. The fees vary. Some communities have volunteers who provide limited, free respite care. Call a senior center or area agency on aging (see How Do I Find Help? p.1130) in your community. Many religious organizations, even those with which the elderly person is not affiliated, provide help to people of all faiths or can refer you to programs and services in the neighborhood. The United Way is another source of community services; look for your local branch in the telephone book. Also, your employer or your spouse's employer may offer an employee assistance program that provides help with caring for an elderly person.

LIVING ARRANGEMENTS

People are living longer than ever before, increasing the likelihood that a parent or relative will require more care than you alone can give. Perhaps your mother has lived independently for many years but now finds her memory slipping or simply cannot take care of everyday matters. You may have arranged for a home health nurse to care for her for a period of time or perhaps moved her into your home.

Eventually, you may realize that you cannot provide the care or safety she needs. This section reviews the many types of living arrangements available today.

Housing Options for Older Adults

Start by considering your loved one's medical condition. If it is expected to worsen, it may be wise to look at alternatives that offer more care than is needed right now. Some facilities offer two or three levels of care under a single roof, from independent living to full-time nursing care.

If possible, consider living arrangements well in advance of the time they are needed, so that the person who will be moving can participate in the decision-making process. The range of housing options for elderly people is growing. Unless your loved one is very sick or needs full-time nursing care, you probably do not have to face the prospect of placing him or her in a nursing home. There are other housing options to investigate that will give you the reassurance that the person is not alone or without help in an emergency. Your local senior center or area agency (see How Do I Find Help?

p.1130) on aging should have a list of local living arrangements.

Licensing requirements for the following housing options vary from state to state; many facilities are not licensed. Call the health department in your state to determine if it licenses the facility you are interested in.

It may also be helpful to make an unscheduled visit to see how staff members present themselves and to get a feel for the caregiving environment. You may want to ask the administrator for the names of several people who have family members living in the facility so that you can ask

---

Nursing Home Checklist: Questions to Ask

If you believe a relative will require nursing home care, investigate nursing home options in your community before the person needs to be moved. This checklist will help you ask the right questions and can help you locate a home that meets physical, emotional, and financial requirements:

■ What are the credentials of the facility? Does the home have a current state license? Is the administrator of the facility helpful in answering your questions? Is the home certified for Medicare and Medicaid programs? (A nursing home that accepts Medicaid should offer to help arrange for a resident to become eligible.)

■ Do the residents seem content and well taken care of? Are most residents out of their beds and dressed (not in bedclothes)? Is each person clean and well-groomed? Is there an activity going on to occupy the residents? Ask to see a monthly activity calendar and make at least two unannounced visits, one in the evening after dinner.

■ Is the facility welcoming and well-constructed? (Do not be fooled by dramatic foyers with nice furniture and colorful wallpaper.) Is the home in general and the rooms in particular clean, orderly, and reasonably free of unpleasant odors? Are grab bars, handrails, and emergency call buttons located in rooms and hallways? Is the atmosphere warm and friendly? Is the facility accessible to family and friends?

■ What kind of security system is used to keep confused residents from wandering out of the building? Does the building have smoke detectors, sprinkler systems, and emergency lighting?

■ Ask questions about staff and talk to the staff. How many nursing care staff members are permanent employees and how many are from temporary agencies? What is the ratio of nurses to aides? To patients? What is the average length of time staff members have worked in the home? Is a doctor always on call? Is there a nurse on staff during the night? Are staff members friendly and willing to answer questions?

■ What services are offered? Are regular and emergency medical attention assured? What hospital does the nursing home use in an emergency? Does the home offer physical therapy and rehabilitation services? What kind of religious services are available? Ask the administrator for a list of items not covered in the room and board fee. People are often surprised to learn that items such as disposable underpants and facial tissues are not included in the nursing home fee.

■ What are the meals and food services like? Ask to see a sample menu. Are the dining room and kitchen clean? Are meals appealing to look at, nutritious, and tasty? Offer to buy a meal and see for yourself if it is the kind of meal you would enjoy eating.

Organizing Personal Records

Even if you are emotionally close to the elderly person you are caring for, do you know where he or she keeps financial and personal records? This information should be accessible in an emergency. Recommend that the following be stored in a safe place, and that a trusted friend or family member be informed of where they are kept:

- Full legal name and maiden name
- Social Security number
- Legal residence
- Date and place of birth
- Names and addresses of spouse and children
- Names of parents, including maiden or any other names ever used
- Wills, trusts, birth certificates, and death certificates
- Marriage, divorce, and citizenship certificates
- List of employers, with locations and dates of employment
- Education and military records
- Names and addresses of close friends, relatives, doctors, lawyers, and financial advisors
- Arrangements for funeral services and burial
- Living will, health care power of attorney, and other end-of-life documents (see p.1142)

- Financial records that include information about insurance policies, bank accounts, deeds, investments, and other valuables:

  - Sources of income and assets (such as pension funds or interest income)
  - Social Security and Medicare/Medicaid information
  - Investment income (such as stocks, bonds, or real estate)
  - Life, health, and property insurance information and policy numbers
  - Bank account information (such as checking, savings, credit union, IRAs, or certificates of deposit)
  - Location of safe deposit boxes
  - Copy of most recent income tax return
  - Debts and liabilities (what is owed, to whom, and when payments are due)
  - Mortgages (how and when paid)
  - Credit card and charge account names and numbers
  - Property tax info
  - Location of personal items of value (such as jewelry)

---

them for their opinions on the care provided.

Finally, ask if medicines are administered; staff at congregate housing and assisted living facilities may monitor the delivery of medicines, but the facility may not be licensed to administer them.

Shared housing This is a situation in which two or more unrelated people live together in a house or apartment; the cost is typically shared. This type of housing can be suitable for a healthy older adult who wants companionship—someone to share meals, housekeeping, and conversation—and does not want to be (or should not be) alone.

Shared housing offers less privacy than independent living, but it can be a good arrangement for a person who is sociable and in good general health.

Congregate housing Congregate housing is similar to shared housing, but it usually involves more than two or three people. Residents may have their own bedrooms in a large house or separate apartments in a single building. Meals are served in a central dining area and residents may also share a living area for social activities.

Senior apartments This is another option for healthy older adults who are interested in private, fully equipped apartments with optional support services such as on-site group meals, housekeeping, and transportation. Federally subsidized senior apartments are another option, but many have long waiting lists.

Assisted living Assisted living is a term that describes individual apartments in a single building complex with a basic service package. Residents eat meals together in a central dining room. The cost usually includes meals, housekeeping, activities, and a limited amount of assistance with personal care, typically 45 minutes a day. Assisted living is not appropriate for a person who needs constant nursing care or who requires more than a cane or walker to get around. Often there is no medical supervision available.

Continuing care retirement communities Also known as life care centers, continuing care retirement communities offer a range of options, from independent living to nursing home care. These communities are usually expensive (a single large entrance fee plus a monthly rent) and often admit only people who are able to walk or get around by themselves and able to live independently. Once you

become a member, however, you receive whatever care is necessary for the rest of your life.

Nursing homes A nursing home may be the best housing arrangement for people who have advanced dementia (see p.362), are immobile, or have a medical condition that requires frequent nursing supervision.

There are two levels of care offered by nursing homes: intermediate care and skilled care. Intermediate care facilities are for people who require less nursing care. A typical resident may have a chronic (long-term) condition, but does not need intensive nursing care. A skilled care facility provides a registered nurse at all times for elderly people who need constant medical supervision; it also offers rehabilitation services. Both options can be expensive.

INSURANCE

Private insurance and Medicare almost never cover long-term nursing home care. Exceptions include a person who is hospitalized and released to, or back into, a nursing home. In this case, Medicare typically covers up to 100 days of nursing home care, but it is usually offered only for very specific situations. Private long-term care insurance (also called nursing home insurance) covers much of the cost of nursing home care, depending on the policy. Many older individuals start out paying privately for nursing home care (which, on average, costs $30,000 per year) but within 6 months to a year have spent all but $2,000 of their savings. At that point, they are eligible for Medicaid (see p.28). In fact, Medicaid pays for about half of all nursing home care in the United States.

CAREGIVING FOR A PERSON WITH ALZHEIMER DISEASE OR OTHER DEMENTIA

About 90% of people 65 years and older have no significant loss of intellectual capacity. However, 5% to 10% of the elderly experience some loss of mental abilities and 30% to 50% of those over 85 suffer from dementia. To learn more about the normal mental aging process and about more serious conditions, read the articles on Alzheimer disease (p.363) and dementia (p.362).

If you are concerned that a loved one is suffering from serious mental impairment, discuss this with the doctor. See also Emotional Help for Caregivers

(p.1132) and the listing for the Alzheimer's Association (p.1229).

Safety Issues

If your parent or relative has dementia and is living with you, safety is a significant concern. Because dementia can have serious effects on a person's memory, language skills, and sense of judgment, you need to take special precautions.

Begin by reviewing the general safety suggestions on p.1126. Next, turn the temperature on your water heater down to 120°F

to prevent scalding; label all hot-water faucets in large letters to remind the person that the water is hot. Post emergency numbers (such as police, fire, doctor, and 911) near every phone. Install childproof latches on any cabinets that contain medicines, household cleaners, or other potentially dangerous items.

As dementia progresses, people with the disease tend to wander. The affected person may need to wear an identification tag such as a necklace or bracelet in case he or she walks away from home. Place locks very high up on doors that lead outside and remove bedroom and bathroom locks so that your loved one cannot be locked inside.

The stove can be a serious hazard for someone with dementia; remove the knobs to the burners and oven so that the stove cannot be turned on. Smoking is not healthy for anyone, but a person with dementia should never smoke alone; he or she could easily start a fire.

Housing Options

If Alzheimer disease or another form of dementia develops in a loved one living in a retirement village, senior citizens apartment, or assisted living facility, you may find that these living arrangements do not offer the support services required. As the disease progresses and the affected person cannot be left alone, either in your home or where he or she has been living, consider a move to a more supervised environment.

There are many good nursing homes and some assisted living facilities with units dedicated solely to caring for people with dementia. There are also nursing homes that do not have special units but provide good care. Call the Alzheimer's Association (see p.1229) and ask for its booklet entitled "Selecting a Nursing Home With a Dedicated Dementia Care Unit."

While investigating homes, ask to see the wing or other area of the home that is specifically for patients with Alzheimer disease. Be suspicious if the wing proves to be a few rooms with a locked door. Good programs for people with dementia are carefully designed with highly trained staff. The atmosphere should be quiet and calm (people with dementia are easily agitated) and residents should be engaged in small, easy tasks that keep them busy and occupy their time. The unit should be large enough so that residents can wander freely, but secure enough so that no one can leave the unit or the building. Good programs care for all patients without using any physical restraints.

Making Caregiving Promises to Loved Ones: Dr Hesse's Advice

Family members often make promises to each other about future caregiving responsibilities, and later find they cannot fulfill the promises. Spouses promise each other they will never be parted. Children promise they will always be available to provide parents' needed care. Parents promise they will care for severely disabled children at home. The promises cannot always be kept. Caregivers may develop health problems of their own, financial realities may make it impossible, there may be competing family or work obligations, or the patient's needs may be overwhelming.

If a member of your family will need long-term care, I caution you to be careful in your promises—to avoid disappointment and discord over unmet expectations. You should work together with your family to develop a caregiving plan that realistically takes into account the requirements of your loved one and the capacities of those who care about him or her.

KATHERINE HESSE, MSW, MD
MASSACHUSETTS GENERAL HOSPITAL
HARVARD MEDICAL SCHOOL

Planning Ahead

People with dementia, including Alzheimer disease, do not improve; most people eventually deteriorate to a point where they require constant care and may not be able to make decisions for themselves. It is therefore wise to plan for the future with this in mind. Organize important documents (see p.1135) and think about how future medical and living arrangements will be organized and paid for. Advance directives (see p.1142) are important to complete while the person is lucid. These legal documents enable the person to explain in advance his or her wishes regarding medical care and to name someone to make treatment decisions in the event the person is unable to do so.

Death and Dying

National statistics show that most of us will live until our 70s or 80s. While this is encouraging news, many people fear dying or witnessing someone close to them endure a prolonged illness.

There are many questions people ask about dying and death. Will there be physical pain and how will I cope with it? What if I become handicapped or a burden to my family? How will I know when my time is near? How can I make peace with the thought of death? What happens after death?

Medicine can provide answers to some of these questions, though individuals address the reality of impending death and its aftermath in intensely personal ways. People vary in their approach, depending in part on their ethnic or religious background.

If you are caring for a person who is dying, be aware that he or she may be more afraid of the process of dying than of death itself. Some terminally ill people fear being alone at the time of death more than anything else. Your loved one may need to be reassured that you and others will be available until the end.

Families sometimes wish to protect a dying relative from the truth about his or her medical condition; they worry that knowing that not much time is left will make the person depressed or even suicidal.

In fact, the vast majority of people prefer to know the truth. Understanding what the future holds allows a person to say good-bye, to get affairs in order, or to plan realistically for medical treatment.

When people are not told the truth, they may suspect that they have a fatal disease, but their fantasies about their circumstances may be worse than the reality.

Physicians today acknowledge that telling people their diagnosis is an important first step in the dying process. In some cultures, however, people are traditionally not told the diagnosis. If you believe your loved one should

Leading Causes of Death in the United States

This chart shows the major causes of death in the United States in 1994 for different ages. Death in people younger than age 45 is most often due to a single acute medical problem or event, such as a motor vehicle collision, homicide, or cancer. Death in older people is often due to a progressive, chronic problem, such as heart disease, or to a combination of problems such as diabetes, stroke, and pneumonia.

AGES 45 TO 64 YEARS

Cancer

Heart disease

Stroke

Injuries

Chronic obstructive pulmonary disease

Chronic liver disease and cirrhosis

Diabetes mellitus

Suicide

Pneumonia and influenza

Human immunodeficiency virus infection

65 YEARS AND OLDER

Heart disease

Cancer

Stroke

Chronic obstructive pulmonary disease

Pneumonia and influenza

Diabetes mellitus

Injuries

Nephritis, nephrotic syndrome, and nephrosis

Atherosclerosis

Septicemia

not know the nature of his or her illness, discuss the matter with the physician.

Many people who are dying fear pain. Try to make sure the doctor is direct with the person about what to expect and equally reassuring about how the pain can be controlled. Be an advocate for the dying person if pain relief is not effective; ask the doctor for a different or stronger dose of medicine.

Some people are afraid of being a burden as they grow sicker. Provide reassurance that you or other family members are prepared to help them through the final stage of life. Explain that assisting them is meaningful to you and that you will take care of any unfinished personal or financial business.

For many people, facing death prompts a review of what they have done with their lives. Encourage the person to reflect on accomplishments and recall milestones such as children, friends, jobs, and successes.

ISSUES AT THE END OF LIFE

Five Emotional Responses to Impending Death

Dying is the natural, final event in life. Yet, if you or someone you love is terminally ill, there may seem to be nothing natural about it. Five emotional responses are common among terminally ill people.

Elisabeth Kubler-Ross, MD, a pioneer in the field of death and dying, maintained that a dying person (and sometimes those who love him or her) generally experiences the following stages, though these responses to death are not necessarily sequential or universal:

Denial Denial is a common response to the news that the end of life is near. It is a normal, protective response to an unbearable thought. The person may initially feel that he or she could not be nearing death and may sustain this perspective for days, weeks, or months.

Anger Once a person recognizes that death is indeed approaching, he or she may become angry. Anger may be directed inward for becoming ill, at doctors for bringing the bad news, at loved ones who are healthy, or at a higher power for permitting death to happen. Anger may be expressed furiously and loudly or it may be kept inside. Unspoken anger is often acted out through annoyance or irritability at small things that would not usually be upsetting.

Bargaining People who are terminally ill may go through a period of mental bargaining—for time, comfort, good health, or love—often with a spiritual power. Some people bargain for time to make peace with a friend or family member. Others commit to lifestyle changes, such as exercising, as a way to try to gain some control over their destiny.

Depression The realization that there is no escaping death may bring about a period of depression. Kubler-Ross described two types of depression: reactive and preparatory. Reactive depression addresses specific concerns, such as the prospect of suffering pain. In preparatory depression, the person is preparing for death and grieving the loss of life.

Acceptance This last stage is the time when the person accepts that death is approaching. The sick person is no longer trying to bargain, extend life, or get well. There is no anger. The person may be weary or even be glad to stop fighting. This stage may be hardest for family and friends, who may not have accepted the inevitability of death themselves. They may believe that their loved one has given up and could live longer if only he or she would continue to fight.

Talking About Death

Begin by making sure that the dying person understands his or her condition. Encourage the doctor to discuss the best estimate of the course of illness and how symptoms can be controlled.

Doctors are often asked how much time a dying person has left to live. While it is impossible to give a precise answer, an approximate answer such as "a few weeks to several months" may be helpful to the dying person and the family. The doctor's diagnosis is important for establishing a prognosis (outlook) and evaluating treatment.

Many physicians advise a terminally ill person to spend his or her remaining time in a personally meaningful way rather than undergoing frightening, and possibly painful, procedures. Decision-making about care near the end of life should occur as a shared process between doctor and patient, preferably with the involvement of the family.

If you know a person has only a limited amount of time left to live, you may be inclined to avoid any discussion of the future. As difficult as it may be, it is important to broach the subject. There is a very good chance the person may be avoiding the subject for fear of upsetting you.

Both of you may welcome the opportunity to share your sorrow, fears, and love in the last days. Saying "I love you and I will miss you" can be as important for the sick person to say as it is for family and friends.

The dying person is often glad for the opportunity to apologize for any hurt he or she may have caused. Friends and relatives also will appreciate the chance to say "I'm sorry" for any incidents they regret. Speaking honestly will also allow you to discuss any unfinished business, as well as the person's wishes about pain medicine, medical treatment, and hospice care.

Medical Care at the End of Life

Care near the end of life, many physicians believe, should involve a shift in the goals of treatment. Rather than attempting to prolong life or cure disease, both of which may be impossible

to achieve at this stage, the focus of care should be on making the person comfortable, maintaining dignity, enhancing the quality of life, supporting the family, and lessening the burden of illness.

PAIN

Most pain can be managed so that a dying person can be virtually pain-free. Painkilling drugs should be taken around the clock so that the person has a constant level in his or her system. Additional medicine should be available for more intense periods of pain.

Narcotic analgesics, such as morphine, are used for severe pain. These drugs can be given by mouth or via a pump that allows the person to push a button for additional doses when necessary. Strong pain medicine can also be given through a patch on the skin or under the tongue. These routes are especially important to people who have difficulty swallowing or who wish to avoid needles.

Nonnarcotic pain medicine can be used to reduce the amount of narcotic necessary. Other medicines, such as antidepressants, can also enhance the effectiveness of narcotics. If you are caring for a person who is in pain, discuss pain relief with his or her physician.

SHORTNESS OF BREATH

Shortness of breath is common among the elderly who are dying. Oxygen is often helpful. Morphine or another narcotic drug can also relieve shortness of breath and is almost always the preferred method of treatment for the terminally ill.

People with congestive heart failure or lung disease are often helped by more specific medicines such as diuretics (fluid pills) or bronchodilators (asthma inhalers).

AGITATION, ANXIETY, AND DEPRESSION

Agitation and anxiety are common in terminally ill people, as is depression. Agitation may be a reflection of physical problems such as lack of oxygen, it may be a side effect of medicine, or it may result simply from the person's underlying illness. Discomfort and shortness of breath can cause even the calmest person to feel anxious.

Depression can be treated with antidepressant drugs. Many people also find spiritual counseling beneficial. A combination of medicine and reassurance from you and the person's doctor can be very effective in reducing symptoms.

WEIGHT LOSS AND LOSS OF APPETITE

Weight loss occurs almost universally in the last stages of dying. Many people are not hungry or thirsty. The primary goal of feeding should be to satisfy the person's appetite and thirst, rather than provide nutrition. Giving sips of water or ice chips, or just dabbing the mouth with a wet cloth typically alleviates thirst. People who do not experience hunger should not be compelled to eat.

CONSTIPATION

Constipation is common in seriously ill people, who often have an irregular appetite and decreased mobility. It can also be a side effect of some medicines.

The doctor will make dietary recommendations or prescribe a laxative, enema, or stool softener. People whose food intake is minimal have very few bowel movements. As long as they do not experience the sensation of being unable to move their bowels, do not worry if the frequency of bowel movements decreases.

Home Care

You can arrange to care for a person with a serious illness in your home. Many people choose to spend their last days at home, surrounded by the people they love and without the intrusions of hospital life.

Privacy is not without cost, however. Having a terminally ill person at home requires great effort. Family members may need to make meals, dispense medicines, change diapers, and bathe the person.

Visiting nurses and home health aides can provide assistance during part of the day. If it is not possible for you to hire a full-time assistant, someone will have to be on call at night.

When considering home care, think about how you would cope with the physical effort and emotional challenge of having a dying person living with you. Ask the patient's doctor what to expect and what your role will entail.

Social service consultation is available through hospitals, home care agencies, and community programs. A social worker can be very helpful in arranging home care. People who choose to care for a dying family member at home often find enrollment in a hospice program beneficial.

Hospice Care

The focus of hospice care is to make a terminally ill person comfortable and enhance whatever time remains. Most hospice programs care for people with terminal illnesses in their own homes or in a homelike setting. Hospice programs usually accept only those who are diagnosed as having 6 months or less to live.

Hospice programs focus on managing the person's pain rather than trying to cure the terminal disease. The hospice setting allows more privacy and less structure than a nursing home. Hospice organizations typically include a medical director, nurses, home health aides, social workers, psychiatrists, physical therapists, and volunteers. Various members of the hospice team provide the patient and family with medical and psychological support.

Many hospice organizations are affiliated with local hospitals and nursing homes. Your doctor can make a referral to a hospice program in your area.

Hospital or Nursing Home Care

As many as 80% of people die in hospitals, where patients receive 24-hour care by doctors and nurses. Drawbacks of hospital care include the unfamiliarity of a hospital environment and the focus on invasive, curative care. Visiting hours may be restricted and roommates can complicate the opportunities for private conversation or quiet time alone.

Still, some people find that a hospital setting is the right choice for them, especially if the facility has an inpatient hospice unit.

A nursing home offers a setting less clinical than a hospital, and many homes work with local hospice organizations, which provide hospice nurses and volunteers. In this situation, the patient receives meals, medicines, and personal care from nursing home staff and regular visits from a hospice nurse to make recommendations for care.

Decisions About Medical Intervention

At some point, whether you are a patient or a family member, you will probably be faced with deciding how aggressive treatment should be. It is sometimes unclear whether treatment will improve a person's condition.

Many doctors believe that a procedure that cannot improve the quality of the patient's life should be stopped or not given. Generally, people who are dying choose to forgo life-sustaining therapies if given the opportunity to discuss the matter with their physicians.

When starting a treatment of uncertain benefit, it is wise to set a date to reevaluate the benefits and burdens of that treatment. This concept is called a "time-limited trial" of therapy.

DISCUSSING CHOICES

Having a frank discussion about the dying person's wishes can be extraordinarily difficult because it acknowledges that death is approaching. However, it is often useful to ask the person if he or she has specific ideas about medical treatment in the final months of life. Does the person wish to remain at home or go to the hospital? Does the person want potentially reversible illnesses such as urinary tract infections or pneumonia treated, or does he or she favor strictly palliative care?

There are also many non-medical decisions to make. Does the person wish to make advance arrangements for funeral, cremation, or burial? Has the person expressed the wish to donate organs or permit an autopsy?

Advance Directives

Ideally, the dying person will discuss preferences for care with a family member and may choose to write down those preferences using an advance directive.

Advance directives also provide the family with guidance when making health care decisions and reduce the potential for conflict if family members disagree with each other or with the doctor on what the patient's wishes are.

There are three legal documents that are helpful to ensure that you receive the type and amount of treatment you want. These documents are a current will, a living will or other instructional directive, and a durable power of attorney for health care.

A living will (see p.1243) states your wishes in the event that you are close to death and unable to make decisions about medical care. In most cases, a living will requests that you be allowed to die free of pain and aggressive medical treatment if it

is clear that death is inevitable and there is no reasonable chance for recovery. Not all states recognize living wills.

You can make specific requests concerning whether you wish to be put on a respirator or have a "Do Not Resuscitate" order. Cardio-pulmonary resuscitation (CPR) is customarily performed on patients who stop breathing and whose heart stops beating. This procedure involves chest compressions and inserting a tube into the lungs for breathing. Many people regard CPR as very invasive and undignified, given its very low likelihood of success in a person near the end of life.

You can also specify your wishes concerning artificial nutrition and hydration. Fluids given in the dying state increase secretions and urination and prolong life without promoting comfort.

An instructional directive is a more specific document that spells out what medical interventions you would want (such as dialysis, chemotherapy, surgery, or intravenous fluids) under a variety of circumstances, such as irreversible coma, coma with a small chance of recovery, and dementia. Ask your doctor for a form if you are interested in an instructional directive.

A durable power of attorney for health care or health care proxy (see p.1245) permits you to name someone to help make medical decisions if you are incapable of doing so, typically because of confusion due to

severe illness. All states have laws to provide for a durable power of attorney for health care.

Euthanasia and Assisted Suicide

Many people feel that more can be done to provide supportive care to the dying. Make sure you and the terminally ill person fully understand the course of his or her disease and what pain relief, antidepressant medicines, and comfort care are available.

Sometimes those who are dying say that they wish their lives were over and talk about suicide. They may request assistance from their physician. Such requests usually indicate that the person needs reassurance that his family or physician will not abandon him or her. The request for an end to life may be a cry for help, denoting the need for more vigorous treatment of pain or depression.

Some people feel more secure believing that if they ever experienced intolerable pain, they would have the option of physician-assisted suicide.

In 1998, Oregon became the first state in which doctors could legally prescribe lethal drugs for terminally ill people who requested assistance in dying. The law, known as the Death With Dignity Act, provides for a series of safeguards, including mandatory waiting periods after oral and written requests, counseling, and a second medical opinion.

PUTTING AFFAIRS IN ORDER

(See also Organizing Personal Records, p.1135)

Preplanning Funeral Arrangements

Planning ahead for a funeral or memorial service and for burial or cremation can also be useful. If a dying loved one is lucid, ask if he or she has specific wishes. Making arrangements in advance for yourself or for someone else who is dying can be comforting and can help protect survivors from having to make decisions in the hours or days after death.

A traditional funeral may include charges for transporting the body to the funeral home and using the facilities, embalming, cosmetically attending and dressing the body, purchasing the coffin, using the hearse, and providing a guest register and cards of acknowledgment.

There are many more options, which you may choose to decline. Read the contract carefully (and ask a trusted friend or family member to read it as well) to ensure that you are paying only for those services you desire.

Interment or cremation costs are generally separate from funeral services. It is wise to obtain quotes from more than one provider.

Organ and Whole Body Donation

Organ donation should be a consideration for dying and healthy people alike. Many states have formal organ donation cards; some states require only your signature and two witnessing signatures on the back of a driver's license.

You can choose to donate only specific organs or your whole body. Organs from older donors are generally not accepted, but eye banks often accept healthy corneas from a deceased person under the age of 75. Discuss organ donation

---

Coma, Persistent Vegetative State, and Brain Death

There is a medical difference among a coma (see p.373), a persistent vegetative state, and brain death.

When a person is in a coma, he or she is in a state of unconsciousness. Coma occurs when the areas of the brain that control consciousness (including parts of the brainstem and the cerebrum) are damaged. A comatose person appears to be sleeping or under heavy anesthesia and does not respond to most stimuli, although the person may be able to breathe on his or her own. A person in a coma who is not able to breathe but maintains a heartbeat can be kept alive with a respirator and intravenous feedings.

When a person is in a persistent vegetative state, he or she responds to some stimuli. However, he or she does not speak, is not aware of the environment, and cannot think. This state may persist for weeks, months, or even years.

In brain death, there is no function of the part of the brain responsible for thinking or for basic functions such as breathing. The condition is thought to be irreversible. An electroencephalogram (see p.136) is often used to confirm brain death. In the United States, a person who is brain dead and has previously signed an organ donation form may have breathing and heartbeat maintained artificially so that organs can be used for transplantation.

When Death Is Near

The approach of death may be most difficult for the living. As your loved one becomes sicker, he or she will become weaker and probably lose interest in food and drink. Offer to moisten the person's mouth with ice chips or small amounts of water. He or she may be restless or have trouble breathing. The lungs may become congested as the heart fails. The doctor can prescribe medicine to ease any pain or shortness of breath. Assume that the person can hear what you are saying. The moment of death is often quiet and peaceful.

with your family if it is important to you; organ banks require family permission as well as evidence of the wishes of the deceased.

You can also choose to donate your whole body to a medical school. Most medical schools have a need for bodies of any age for medical research and education. In some cases, the body of the donor is returned to the survivors following removal of the donated organs; other medical schools cremate the remains and return them. You may be required to pay transportation costs to the medical institution.

If you are considering organ or body donation, call a local medical school or the National Anatomical Service at 800-727-0700. This private organization can tell you which medical school closest to you has a need for bodies for research.

AFTER DEATH

Autopsy

After death, the doctor may suggest an autopsy—a thorough dissection and examination of the body—for one of two reasons.

The doctor may suggest an autopsy if the death is regarded as suspicious or unnatural. An autopsy is performed by a pathologist to determine the cause of death and determine whether it involved violence, was the result of an injury, or whether it was caused by a transmissible disease that authorities must investigate. Detailed records are kept because the results of this type of medical-legal autopsy are admissible as evidence in court.

The doctor may also suggest an autopsy if he or she thinks the exam would be useful to better understand the cause of death, or if he or she believes that your family would benefit from information about a possible genetic disorder. Many disorders and diseases have been better understood as a result of these types of autopsies, which are performed without charge.

Generally, you must give your permission before an autopsy is performed. If the cause of death is suspicious, the court requires a medical examiner to conduct an autopsy. Feel free to ask the doctor exactly what an autopsy will entail. Sometimes, doctors want to look at only one particular organ or piece of tissue; other times, an autopsy of the entire body is requested. You can designate which parts of the body may be studied.

Discuss the matter with the doctor if you are concerned that the body not be disfigured so that it can be displayed. In the majority of cases, autopsy incisions can be masked with clothing or makeup.

Death Certificate, Funeral, Cremation, and Burial

A medical doctor (or in some instances a nurse practitioner) can certify that someone is dead and state the cause of death. This information is required to obtain a death certificate. Hospitals and nursing homes have death certificates available for physicians to complete. If a person dies at home, the funeral home will generally provide a death certificate to the certifying physician.

Tell the doctor if the person wants his or her body to be used for medical research or organ donation (see p.1143). In the latter instance, arrangements for organ donation must be made before the person is removed from life-support systems or immediately after the person has died.

If you are making the arrangements, you may wish to get an estimate on costs from more than one funeral home. Funerals can range from very simple to elaborate, depending on the type of casket and flowers, whether a grave site must be purchased, or whether the person has requested cremation (in which the body is burned).

You may also face decisions about whether the casket will be open or closed and whether you want a wake before the final services. The funeral director makes these arrangements and will file an obituary with the newspapers you designate, using information you provide.

If the person has requested his or her remains be cremated, you can still hold traditional funeral rites. The person's ashes will be given to you in an urn or other container; the ashes may be buried, placed in a niche at a cemetery, or scattered in a meaningful place. Cremation is generally less expensive than a traditional burial.

Practical Considerations

Request five to ten copies of the death certificate from the funeral director or health department; you will need these when reporting the person's death to insurance companies, the Social Security office, the Internal Revenue Service, and numerous other organizations.

If an executor has been named, this person is responsible for paying outstanding debts and for allocating portions of the estate to beneficiaries. Otherwise, a probate court will designate a person to oversee distribution of the estate.

If you are charged with managing the estate, you will want to:

■ Locate the will (often in a safe-deposit box).

■ Contact the person's lawyer, financial planner, or accountant.

■ Contact the person's bank to close accounts (after all bills have been paid).

■ Notify insurance companies (life, health, mortgage, accident, auto, credit card, employer policies) and ask for help in filing all relevant claims.

■ Contact the person's social security office (and, if applicable, veterans affairs office). There may be death benefits that will help defray the cost of funeral services.

■ Seek out former employers to determine if the person is owed pension benefits, salary, or pay for unused vacation or sick leave.

■ Locate the person's most recent income tax return and make a list of all assets and debts.

Grief and Bereavement

After the death of someone close to you, you may feel numb. You may feel that you are merely going through the motions of life. You may forget that the person is dead and behave as though he or she were still alive. All of these feelings are a part of the grieving process.

Understand that what you feel initially will become more bearable as time passes. The intensity of your grief will lessen over time.

Grief is a necessary and valuable process that allows you to accept your loss, say good-bye to the person you loved, and, finally, move on with your life. Grief is an individual process that cannot be rushed; each person sets his or her own pace.

There are several general phases of grief and, although you may not experience all of them, understanding what they are can help you see that your reactions are normal.

Immediately following the death, you may feel shock, denial, or disbelief. The truth seems real only part of the time; the rest of the time you may feel as if your loved one is with you.

Some people busy themselves with the details of a funeral, memorial service, or financial considerations, while others are unable to do much of anything.

You may experience outbursts of emotion or withdraw from life. You may find yourself thinking that there has been a mistake. All of this is normal.

Once reality settles in, you may feel angry, possibly at the deceased person for leaving you. Or you may be overcome with guilt for things said or not said, or done or not done. You may be highly emotional and experience periods of anger and sadness, swinging from one emotion to another.

Grief often causes physical reactions, upsetting your digestive system, sleep cycle, or even weakening your immune system and leaving you vulnerable to illness. Try to maintain a regular routine of eating a healthful diet, sleeping, and exercising moderately.

Finally, there is a period of decline in intense emotions and the start of your emotional acceptance of the death. You slowly begin to reenter the rhythms of daily life. This is a time during which you learn to live with the loss. You will still mourn, but you will begin to put the death into perspective. You may feel guilt as you cope with the idea that you will continue to live even though your loved one has died.

Many people struggle with the thought of living without the deceased person. This can be a time of great ambivalence as you endeavor to rediscover meaning and purpose in your world.

Occasionally, people have intense and prolonged grief that requires the help of a therapist or other professional counselor. If you find yourself overcome with feelings of sadness or despair, if you are using alcohol or other drugs to deaden the emotional pain, or if intense grief lasts longer than 6 months, ask your doctor or a trusted friend or clergy for help. You may need help with your recovery, possibly by joining a support group where you will meet other people who are also coping with the death of a loved one.

When you are ready, make a point of resuming activities that interest you and meeting with friends, old and new. It is all a part of the recovery process.

Helping a Child Understand Death

Instinct may compel you to protect and shield your child from the painful reality of death, but children—even young ones—are profoundly affected by dying and death. Like adults, children grieve and experience shock, denial, anger, guilt, and, finally, acceptance.

Children react individually to death and some require a great deal of loving support. Tell your child the truth about death. Explain how or why the person died—for example, that the person died from "a serious illness called a heart attack."

Young children need to understand the difference between a serious disease and a routine illness such as the flu. Allow your children to see your emotions; seeing you cry or feel angry lets them know that these emotions are an acceptable part of the grieving process.

Children of different ages generally respond to death in the following ways:

Under age 3, children do not understand death, but they may react to adult emotions and sense the disruption of daily life. Try to maintain the usual routine as much as possible.

Children 3 to 6 may believe that death is reversible and ask when the dead person will come back. They may feel that they played a part in causing the death. Reassure your child that he or she did not cause the death. Explain the death in simple terms—for example, that the person's body did not work any more. Do not tell your child that the dead person "is sleeping" or "has left." Your child may become fearful of sleeping or believe that the person will return.

Children 6 to 9 may need to hear more details about how the person died and may worry that you will die too. Encourage your child to ask questions (you may need to repeat the answers many times) and provide reassurance.

Children 9 to 12 may have feelings of anger or guilt, withdraw from other people, try to hide their emotions, and become aggressive. Reassure your child that it is fine to show emotions, even as you show your own. Encourage conversation about the person who died.

Teenagers may try to hide their feelings, reject conversation about the death, feel guilty or

 ## *Children and Funerals: Ms Missal's Advice*

Q Should I take my 6-year-old son to his grandmother's funeral?

A If your son wants to go, being at the service can make him feel included and reassured. You should prepare him for what will happen. If his grandmother's body will be on view, explain how it will look. He should not be urged to do anything that makes him fearful or uncomfortable.

Whether or not your child attends the funeral, you will want to talk with him about her death, allowing him to ask questions and express feelings. Children 3 to 5 years old cannot understand the finality of death, and older children may understand it intellectually but not emotionally. Children often assume that they are to blame in some way. Otherwise, they think, "Why would Nana leave me?" If these are your son's feelings, reassure him that he did not do anything wrong.

Be honest about your own feelings, too. It is OK for your child to see you cry. Explain that you are sad because you will miss her. Shared rituals such as looking at pictures of grandmother, or visiting places you went together with her, can be very comforting to your son.

SYLVIA M. MISSAL, LICSW
CHILDREN'S HOSPITAL
HARVARD MEDICAL SCHOOL

Death of a Child

Words fail everyone around you. The death of a child at any age produces anger, sadness, and guilt. You may feel a longing for your child and social isolation, question whether you did enough, and experience marital problems. Siblings may experience the symptoms discussed under The Dying Child (see right). Grandparents—sometimes called the "forgotten mourners"—mourn doubly, for their grandchildren and for the sake of their children. A support group for parents who have had a child die can provide understanding and guidance during the grieving process. See p.1230 for more information or ask your doctor for a referral to a group in your area.

angry, or tell you they do not need help. Respect your teen's need for privacy, but reassure him or her that you are available to discuss the death.

The Dying Child

A child who is terminally ill should be told about the illness. The child will fear pain and separation from his or her parents and needs reassurance that the doctors will make him or her as comfortable as possible and that you will be there no matter what happens. While a terminally ill child needs loving support, he or she also needs to lead a normal life for as long as possible.

Siblings may feel that they are receiving little or no attention, and may experience jealousy,

rivalry, and guilt over the situation. They may believe that they must assume a new role as caregiver. Other common responses include sleep disorders, school problems, depression, hostility toward the sick brother or sister, and withdrawal.

As a parent, you may find yourself going through a range of emotions, from unwillingness to accept the diagnosis to feelings of failure and the need to blame someone. Marital problems are also common. Support groups for parents of terminally ill children can be very useful in helping you understand your emotions and those of your family. Ask your doctor for a referral to a group in your area and see Bereavement/Hospice Care (p.1230) for more information.

Medicines

THE BASICS

A medicine can change the course of a disease, alter the function of an organ, relieve symptoms, or ease pain. Your doctor may recommend a medicine such as aspirin to help control a symptom, such as pain and swelling after a muscle strain. Antibiotics (which effectively destroy invading organisms) may be prescribed to treat a bacterial infection, such as a urinary tract infection. In addition, many people take medication as part of a long-term program to manage an ongoing condition such as high blood pressure. Medicines affect your body in complex ways, most of them by changing the way your organs, tissues, or cells function.

Drugs come from a variety of sources, including plants, animals, and microorganisms. Many modern medicines are synthetic versions of substances found in nature. Penicillin, for example, is a synthetic version of a substance discovered on bread mold.

Sometimes, drugs are entirely new chemicals that are not versions of natural substances. For example, scientists combine chemicals to make the over-the-counter medicine cimetidine, which relieves heartburn by reducing the secretion of stomach acid. Genetic engineering has allowed scientists to make certain medicines such as insulin, which once had to be derived from the tissues of animals, in huge quantities.

No matter how a medicine is made, its effect on the human body is far from simple. Drugs differ in how long they stay in the body, how easily they get into different parts of the body, and how they are absorbed and eliminated by the body.

Medicines are available in many different forms: liquids and tablets that are swallowed, tablets that are placed under the tongue, inhalers, lotions, eyedrops, suppositories, and injections.

Some are designed to be released slowly over time, such as nicotine patches, which deliver nicotine to a smoker trying to quit, or estrogen patches, which deliver estrogen to women who need estrogen replacement therapy. Your physician makes a decision on the best method of delivering the drug based on your medical condition.

Most medicines are ultimately absorbed into the bloodstream and carried to the liver—the body's chemical processing plant. There, many drugs are broken down by enzymes. The medicine then travels to its site of action, the place where it does most of its work.

Your body eventually eliminates the drug via urine or by breaking it down in the liver. Many factors influence how effectively a medication works, including what you eat or drink with it, how well you follow your doctor's instructions in taking it, and your age, gender, and metabolism.

How to Read A Prescription

Ask your doctor to explain your prescription before you leave the office. If there is anything you do not understand, ask about it. The first word on the prescription sheet is the name of the medicine, followed by the dosage form (such as liquid, capsule, or tablet) and the strength (such as 150 mg—which stands for milligrams).

Next is the amount you will receive (such as 15 capsules or 5 fluid ounces). The directions for use follow, often written in abbreviations of Latin words (see Decoding Your Prescription, p.1149).

It is the pharmacist's job to translate this information to the label on the container. The prescription also indicates how many times the prescription may be refilled. Ask your doctor whether this is a one-time prescription (such as an antibiotic for an infection or a painkiller for an injury) or whether you can or should continue to refill it.

Pay particular attention to the warning stickers that the pharmacist places on the bottle (for example, "TAKE WITH MEALS" or "AVOID ALCOHOLIC BEVERAGES"). This is vital information that affects how successfully the drug will work and how it interacts with other medicines or with food and drink.

Most pharmacists also provide written information about the medicine being prescribed. Read it completely and ask your physician or pharmacist to clarify anything you do not understand.

Why People Respond Differently to Drugs

People of different ages, genders, and weights and in different states of health respond differently to the same drug. These circumstances can alter the way in which a drug is broken down and processed by your body.

In children, drugs are prescribed according to the child's age and weight. However, children are not simply smaller versions of adults. Their immature organ systems process drugs differently than their mature bodies will in the years ahead. In addition, for ethical and practical reasons, many new drugs are not tested on children, so their effects can be harder to predict.

Never give a child a prescription medicine intended for an adult, even if you administer a smaller dose. Give over-the-counter drugs to children only if the label includes a dose appropriate for the child's age.

Elderly adults can also respond differently to drugs because their kidneys eliminate drugs less effectively and their liver breaks down drugs less effectively. Also, target organs, such as the brain or heart, can become more sensitive to some medicines. These factors can cause an exaggerated effect and/or a prolonged effect in older people.

Women and men may differ in their response to a medicine as well. Women generally have a higher percentage of body fat, while men generally have more muscle tissue. Also, women tend to be smaller than men. There is less water in fat than in muscle, and less total fluid in which the medicines can circulate in a smaller body. This can change the concentration of some drugs in a woman's body, producing an exaggerated or reduced effect as well as side effects or adverse reactions.

Illness can also affect the action of your medicine. If you have liver or kidney disease, the way your medications are broken down or eliminated from your body can change. People who have stomach problems may have impaired absorption of medicines.

Finally, some people metabolize drugs in different ways. This can be due to racial or genetic differences, or other poorly understood reasons. For example, many people of Asian descent have small amounts of a liver enzyme that metabolizes alcohol, and become inebriated easily as a result. Monitor your response to any medicine (even an over-the-counter drug) that you take and report any side effects or unusual responses to your doctor.

Cost

If the cost of your medicine is a concern, ask your doctor if the prescription can be filled with the generic version of the drug or if there is a lower-cost drug that will have virtually the same effect.

When a new drug is approved by the Food and Drug Administration (FDA), it is patented and

---

Decoding Your Prescription

When your doctor writes a prescription, the first word is the name of the drug. Next is the dosage form, the strength, and the amount you will receive. The prescription form also indicates how many times the prescription can be refilled, if at all. The directions for how you will use the medicine follow; they are often abbreviations of Latin words:

ac	before meals
bid	twice a day
daw	dispense as written (no brand name or generic substitutions)
hs	at bedtime
po	by mouth
prn	as needed
qid	four times a day
tid	three times a day
ut dict	as directed by doctor

given a brand name. In exchange for its investment in research and development, the pharmaceutical company is awarded exclusive rights to market the medicine for 17 years, and no generic version is permitted. When the patent expires, other companies may manufacture the drug under another brand name or under the drug's generic name, often at far less expense than the original medicine.

Drug manufacturers must prove to the FDA that the generic drugs they sell are "bioequivalent" to the brand-name drugs—meaning that they have the same purity, strength, and chemical composition; disintegrate at the same rate; and are absorbed by the body at the same rate. There are thousands of FDA-approved generic versions of brand-name medicines.

Occasionally, your doctor may want you to take a brand-name medicine because he or she believes it is more effective than the generic version. However, with only a few exceptions, most generic drugs work as well as brand-name drugs and are much less expensive. Unless a physician requests "no substitutions" on a prescription, pharmacists in all 50 states may dispense generic equivalents for brand-name drugs.

Some people save money on prescription medications by ordering through mail-order pharmacies; this is especially effective for those who have an ongoing medical condition and know that they will need to take a certain medicine daily for an indefinite period. Perhaps the best-known pharmaceutical mail-order service is run by the American Association of Retired Persons (AARP), but several others exist.

Drug Interactions and Citrus Products

Scientists discovered in the 1990s that grapefruit and grapefruit juice increase the levels of some medicines in the blood. This probably occurs because grapefruit inhibits enzymes in the small intestine that break down many medicines. Because this is a relatively recent discovery, doctors do not yet know all of the drugs that might be affected. However, it is known for certain that the interaction occurs with many calcium channel blockers and the sleeping pill triazolam.

Citrus fruits and juices (such as orange and grapefruit juices) contain ascorbic acid, which speeds the absorption of iron from iron supplements. Fruit and vegetable juices with a high acid content can cause some medicines to dissolve in the stomach (where they are more effectively absorbed) instead of in the intestines. A good general rule is to avoid taking medicines within an hour of eating citrus fruits or drinking citrus juices.

There are also programs for people who cannot afford to purchase their medicines. The Pharmaceutical Manufacturers Association (PMA) offers a program for needy people; if you think you might be eligible, you will need the help of your doctor to apply. Call 1-800-PMA-INFO. A representative will describe the eligibility requirements. If your medicines are paid for by insurance or public assistance, you probably do not qualify. Several states provide assistance programs specifically for older people who need medication but cannot afford it. Check with the social services department in your state.

Interactions Between Drugs and Foods

Food can interact with drugs, making them work slower, faster, or even preventing them from working at all. Both the foods you eat and the medications you take are processed and absorbed by your upper gastrointestinal tract.

Some medicines and foods, when taken together, can produce undesirable or even lethal results. For example, a group of antidepressants called monoamine oxidase inhibitors (MAOIs) can cause a potentially fatal rise in blood pressure if taken with foods containing the substance tyramine.

Tyramine is found in aged cheeses, concentrated yeast extracts, aged meats such as salami and sausages, broad beans, sauerkraut, and alcoholic beverages. Before taking an MAOI, ask your doctor what foods and other medicines you should avoid.

Sometimes, a drug is less potent when taken with certain foods. The antibiotic tetracycline becomes less effective or completely ineffective when taken with dairy products or iron supplements. Eating more than two servings of liver and leafy vegetables can hinder the effectiveness

Preventing Problems with Medications

The best way to prevent problems with any medicine is to follow your doctor's or pharmacist's instructions explicitly and phone him or her if you have questions or notice any side effects. Carefully read the medicine label before you take any of the drug. Also:

■ Note whether your medication should be taken on an empty stomach (1 hour before eating or 2 to 3 hours after eating) or whether you should take it with food.

■ Take pills and capsules with a full glass of water. It can decrease irritation of your esophagus and aids absorption by your body.

■ Use all of your medicine, even if you begin to feel better, unless your doctor specifically instructs you otherwise.

■ Do not drink hot beverages with drugs; heat can destroy the effectiveness of some medicines.

■ Take only the recommended dose. Taking more can cause a dangerous reaction; taking less can cause the medication to be ineffective.

■ Never take a prescription drug unless it was prescribed for you.

■ If you take a medication every day, take it at the same time every day.

■ Do not drink alcohol with your medicine if you have been instructed not to do so. It has the potential to seriously interact with both prescription and non-prescription drugs and can make you extremely drowsy.

Storing and Disposing of Drugs

Contrary to common practice, the warm and humid bathroom medicine cabinet is not the best place to store your medicines. A better place is high in a kitchen cabinet or a bedroom closet, away from humidity and temperature extremes and out of the reach of children.

Never keep your medicines near your bedside; in a drowsy state you could mistakenly take another dosage of medication that you took earlier.

Go through your medicines once a year and throw away those that have expired or are more than a year old; some drugs lose their potency and can degrade into harmful substances. Dispose of old drugs by flushing them down the toilet.

It is best to keep your drugs in their original containers. Never keep pills in accessible containers in a purse or briefcase; they can look like candy to children. Wherever you keep your medicines, close lids and caps tightly to prevent accidental poisoning in children.

Childproof caps prevent many poisonings but can be counterproductive if they prevent the user from being able to open them. This sometimes results in leaving the top off altogether, increasing the risk of

poisoning if there are children in the house. If you find your medication container difficult to open, ask your pharmacist for nonchildproof caps, but continue to keep the drugs where children cannot reach them.

Follow these guidelines for disposing of old drugs:

■ Discard any tablets or capsules that are cracked, crumbling, or stuck together.

■ Dispose of ointments, creams, or lotions that are discolored, hardened, or separated or whose containers are punctured.

■ Throw out any medicines that are more than a year old, whose expiration dates have passed, or that have changed odor, color, or consistency.

■ Do not use liquid medications, such as cough syrup, if they are more than a year old; they are especially likely to spoil.

■ Avoid purchasing over-the-counter drugs in very large quantities. It is safer to buy only as much as you will use within 6 months to a year.

■ Never use prescription or nonprescription eyedrops that have been opened and unused for more than 6 months. Bacteria can breed in the vial and can infect your eyes.

of blood thinners because these foods contain vitamin K, which promotes blood clotting.

Chronic use of alcohol can cause changes in your liver that speed up the metabolism of some medicines, such as blood thinners or diabetes drugs. The medicines become less effective because they do not stay in your body long enough. Alcohol abuse can also damage the liver by making it less able to process some drugs, causing them to stay in your system too long.

SAFETY

Side Effects of Over-the-Counter (Nonprescription) Drugs

See also Drug Interactions Chart, p.1167.

Many effective and powerful drugs that once were available only by prescription have become available in any drugstore without a prescription. They are called over-the-counter (nonprescription) drugs.

It is important to remember that nonprescription medicines can have significant side effects. Some of them cause allergic reactions; others interact with prescription or other nonprescription medicines. Still others mask serious symptoms that should be treated by your doctor.

To reduce your risk of drug interactions, be sure to inform your doctor of all the medicines you are taking, both nonprescription and prescription.

Every medication, including nonprescription drugs, has the potential to cause side effects or adverse reactions. Usually these are mild, such as a headache, nausea, or drowsiness. However, anytime a reaction is unexpected or severe (such as a rash or hives, bleeding, weakness, prolonged vomiting, or impaired vision or hearing), call your doctor. Make sure you read the label of any nonprescription medicine be-

fore taking it; contact your doctor if you have any concerns.

Be diligent about monitoring the effects of any nonprescription drug you or a family member is taking. Most nonprescription medications carry a standard warning about restricting use to a short time, but many people overlook or ignore this note of caution. For example, people who have insomnia may get into the habit of taking a nonprescription sleeping pill every night; long-term consequences can be dangerous.

Be especially careful of any nonprescription medicine that contains a mixture of ingredients. The more ingredients in a compound, the greater your risk for side effects or interactions.

Some nonprescription cold remedies contain four or five different ingredients. If you have a reaction, you may not know what ingredient triggered it. In general, it is best to treat your problem with a single effective ingredient or, if necessary, a very small number of single-ingredient products.

Two or more medicines taken at the same time can interact and affect the way one or the other behaves in the body; this applies to both nonprescription and prescription drugs. For example, an antacid can cause a prescription blood-thinning medicine to be absorbed too slowly, while aspirin greatly increases the blood-

thinning effect of such drugs. Antihistamines used to treat colds or allergies can increase the sedative effects of anesthetics, barbiturates, tranquilizers, and some painkillers.

Acetaminophen should not be mixed with alcohol, especially if you have more than two drinks a day. You should not drink alcohol at all if you are taking another central nervous system depressant, such as a cold medicine that can cause drowsiness. Alcohol itself is a depressant of the central nervous system. If you drink alcohol and also take a drug that depresses the central nervous system, your physical performance, judgment, and alertness will be affected.

Side Effects of Prescription Drugs

See also Drug Interactions Chart, p.1167.

Many prescription medicines cause not only the intended beneficial effects but also unwanted side effects in other parts of your body. They occur because the medication affects your entire body, not just the part being treated. For example, some antihistamines for allergies can make you drowsy, and some antidepressants can cause a dry mouth.

Some side effects—such as stomach upset, nausea, dizziness,

Drug Facts Label on Over-the-Counter Drugs

About 100,000 over-the-counter medicines are sold without prescription in the United States. By mid-2001, all such medicines sold in the United States will be required to print the Drug Facts label on their packages. The label is modeled after the Nutrition Facts label (see p.50). The Drug Facts label (like the one shown below) will make it easier to understand important information about the nonprescription drugs you buy.

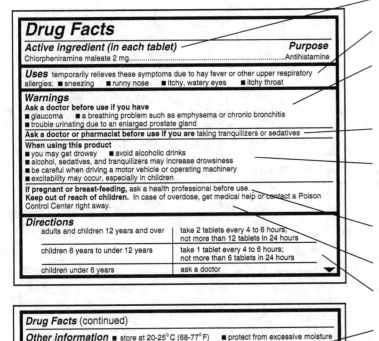

Drug Facts

Active ingredient (in each tablet) — **Purpose**
Chlorpheniramine maleate 2 mg...Antihistamine

Uses temporarily relieves these symptoms due to hay fever or other upper respiratory allergies: ▪ sneezing   ▪ runny nose   ▪ itchy, watery eyes   ▪ itchy throat

Warnings
Ask a doctor before use if you have
▪ glaucoma   ▪ a breathing problem such as emphysema or chronic bronchitis
▪ trouble urinating due to an enlarged prostate gland
Ask a doctor or pharmacist before use if you are taking tranquilizers or sedatives
When using this product
▪ you may get drowsy   ▪ avoid alcoholic drinks
▪ alcohol, sedatives, and tranquilizers may increase drowsiness
▪ be careful when driving a motor vehicle or operating machinery
▪ excitability may occur, especially in children
If pregnant or breast-feeding, ask a health professional before use.
Keep out of reach of children. In case of overdose, get medical help or contact a Poison Control Center right away.

Directions

adults and children 12 years and over	take 2 tablets every 4 to 6 hours; not more than 12 tablets in 24 hours
children 6 years to under 12 years	take 1 tablet every 4 to 6 hours; not more than 6 tablets in 24 hours
children under 6 years	ask a doctor ▼

Drug Facts (continued)

Other information ▪ store at 20-25°C (68-77°F)   ▪ protect from excessive moisture

Inactive ingredients D&C yellow no. 10, lactose, magnesium stearate, microcrystalline cellulose, pregelatinized starch

Active Ingredient Name of the drug(s) in the medicine

Uses Symptoms or diseases that the medicine can treat

Warnings

1 Circumstances when you should definitely not use the medicine (there are none in this example)

2 Interactions with other medicines or with foods

3 Common side effects

4 Serious side effects that indicate you should stop using the medicine (there are none in this example)

5 Potential problems if you are pregnant or breast-feeding

6 Warnings about what to do if children swallow the medicine

Directions How people of different age groups should take the medicine

Other Information Such as how to store the medicine to keep it from deteriorating

Inactive Ingredients Substances used to color or bind the active ingredients

and drowsiness—may gradually disappear as your body becomes accustomed to the medicine; others persist. Not all side effects appear in the first few days after taking a new medicine. Some occur after months or years of use and some do not appear until you stop taking the medicine.

Most side effects are well known by your doctor and pharmacist. Your doctor should ask you if you are taking any other prescription or nonprescription medications before he or she writes a new prescription that could interact adversely with what you are taking. If your doctor does not ask you, show him or her a list of all the medicines you are currently taking.

Potential Drug-Herb Interactions

Herbs have the potential to interact with both prescription and over-the-counter medicines. This list shows some of the interactions that can occur. Drinking large amounts (five or more cups a day) of herbal teas can create some of the same risks as the use of herbal supplements. Talk to your physician about the potential for negative interactions between drugs and herbs before taking any new drug or herbal supplement.

HERBS	INTERACTING DRUGS	DRUG-HERB INTERACTION	WHAT TO DO ABOUT IT
Chamomile	Anticoagulants, iron	Chamomile may interact with anticoagulants. It inhibits iron absorption.	If you are taking an anticoagulant, your doctor should closely monitor your prothrombin time (see p.156). If you are taking iron, do not take chamomile.
Echinacea	Drugs that can damage the liver (such as anabolic steroids, amiodarone, methotrexate, and ketoconazole) and immunodepressants (such as corticosteroids and cyclosporine)	Echinacea can cause liver damage if you take it for more than 8 weeks. It can also stimulate the immune system, negating the effects of immunosuppressive drugs.	Do not take echinacea with other drugs that can damage your liver. If you are taking corticosteroids or cyclosporine, ask your doctor before taking any herbal preparation.
Feverfew	Nonsteroidal anti-inflammatory drugs (NSAIDs), anticoagulants, iron	NSAIDs can negate the benefits of feverfew in treating migraines. Feverfew can also thin your blood; if feverfew is taken with an anticoagulant, bleeding can occur. Feverfew decreases iron absorption.	If you are taking any of these drugs, do not take feverfew.

Your doctor and pharmacist should tell you about the most common side effects you can expect when taking a particular drug. However, remember that people are affected differently by drugs, and that drugs can have many side effects, so all the possible side effects may not be mentioned.

It is important to read the printed material usually provided by the pharmacist with each prescription. If this material is not available, ask the pharmacist about potential side effects and write them down.

It is also important to realize that a side effect may bear no resemblance to the condition the medicine is being used to treat.

HERBS	INTERACTING DRUGS	DRUG-HERB INTERACTION	WHAT TO DO ABOUT IT
Garlic and ginger supplements	Anticoagulants	Garlic and ginger may thin your blood even more if you are taking an anticoagulant; severe bleeding can occur.	If you are taking an anticoagulant, do not take garlic or ginger supplements.
Ginkgo	Anticoagulants, aspirin, heparin, NSAIDs, anticonvulsants	Ginkgo may thin your blood, increasing risk of bleeding if you are taking an anticoagulant, aspirin, heparin, or an NSAID. It may increase your risk of seizures if you are taking an anticonvulsant.	If you are taking any of these drugs, do not take ginkgo. Ginkgo is not recommended if you have a seizure disorder.
Ginseng	Anticoagulants, aspirin, heparin, NSAIDs, corticosteroids, estrogen, digoxin, monoamine oxidase inhibitors (MAOIs), pills that lower blood sugar	Ginseng can interfere with blood clotting, especially if combined with anticoagulants, aspirin, heparin, or NSAIDs. It can increase the effect of corticosteroids and estrogen. It can falsely elevate digoxin levels. If taken with an MAOI, ginseng can cause headache, tremors, and manic episodes. It can also affect blood sugar levels.	If you are taking any of these drugs, do not take ginseng. Ginseng is not recommended if you have diabetes or a history of bipolar disorder or psychosis.
St John's wort	Iron, MAOIs, selective serotonin reuptake inhibitors (SSRIs)	St John's wort can decrease iron absorption from the intestine and may interact with MAOIs and SSRIs.	If you are taking any of these drugs, do not take St John's wort.
Valerian	Barbiturates	If valerian is taken with barbiturates, excessive sedation may occur.	If you are taking a barbiturate, do not take valerian.

For example, you may experience depression from a blood pressure medication or develop a rash from an antibiotic you are taking to treat a urinary tract infection. A new medical problem that crops up shortly after you begin taking a drug is likely to be a side effect of that drug. This is particularly true for older people, in whom symptoms such as confusion, fatigue, instability, or light-headedness may be inappropriately attributed to aging. Consider any new symptom a possible side effect of medication and discuss it with your physician.

If side effects are causing you discomfort or are interfering with your everyday activities, do not stop taking the medicine but do inform your physician. Too often, people wait until the next regularly scheduled visit and suffer needlessly. It may be possible to change your dose or switch you to a different medication.

However, if you have trouble breathing or develop hives after starting a new medicine, stop taking it and call your doctor immediately. You may be having an allergic reaction (see below).

Never take more of a medication than was prescribed without consulting your physician. More medicine will not relieve your symptoms faster and can increase the likelihood of serious side effects.

Drug Interactions

When you take more than one medicine, there can be complications from the interactions of the medicines. This is true whether you are taking prescription or nonprescription drugs. Thousands of drug interactions are possible. Many are not serious but some combinations can be dangerous or even fatal. Most drug interactions are caused by one medicine increasing or decreasing the rate at which your body processes another medicine.

To help you determine if there could be a serious interaction between two or more medicines you are taking, use the Drug Interactions Chart (see p.1167).

Allergies to Medications

Some adverse reactions to medicines are caused by an allergic reaction, in which your body produces antibodies to the drug; the antibodies bind to the drug to rid it from your body.

In the process, the clumps of antibody bound to the drug travel through your blood, and can harm body tissues or interfere with normal body function.

Although allergic reactions are often confined to minor outbreaks of the skin, they may also attack cells in the kidneys, liver, joints, and blood. While allergic reactions are relatively rare, they can be severe.

If you think you are having an allergic reaction, inform your doctor. The most severe type of allergic reaction is anaphylactic shock (see Anaphylaxis, p.894), a life-threatening disorder in which blood pressure drops and your airways become so narrow that you cannot breathe. It requires emergency treatment.

Medication and Sun Exposure

Some drugs can cause your skin to become more sensitive to the sun, a condition called photosensitivity. While taking these medications, you must carefully protect your skin from the sun by using a sunscreen and wearing protective clothing. Without protection, you could get a severe sunburn. Medicines that can cause photosensitivity include antibiotics such as tetracycline and sulfa antibiotics, some birth-control pills, antinausea medicines, and nonsteroidal anti-inflammatory drugs (NSAIDs).

Alternative Remedies

Many health food stores and pharmacies sell herbal and homeopathic remedies over the counter. Although these substances are often grouped under the label "natural remedies," homeopathics and herbals are very different.

Herbals are derived from plants and may contain active ingredients. Homeopathic remedies are highly diluted substances that often have no active ingredient. These products are immensely popular, legal, and in some cases may have value, but they have not been proven to be therapeutically effective through the approval process of the Food and Drug Administration (FDA).

Both types of remedies are regulated by the federal government only as dietary supplements (not medications) and as such are less limited in the kinds of health claims they can make on their labels and package inserts. In the absence of any reasonable standards of accuracy or fairness in such advertising, be particularly cautious about natural products or nutritional supplements that claim to increase mental performance, slow aging, improve alertness, prevent cancer, or cure disease.

It is important to seek information about how to use the products from reliable and knowledgeable sources. It is also essential to tell your physician if you are taking any of these products, as their effects can interact with medications he or she may prescribe.

Most alternative medicines are not harmful. However, if they are used instead of conventional therapies to treat serious diseases, they can cause you to lose precious time that would be better spent fighting a disease with scientifically proven methods and drugs. It is also true that many nutritional supplements taken as an all-around "tonic" to improve vitality are often of no proven benefit.

Drugs and Pregnancy

If you are pregnant, breast-feeding, or planning to become pregnant, ask your doctor about the safety of any drugs you use—both over-the-counter and prescription. In addition, drinking alcohol, using tobacco, or taking any illegal drugs during pregnancy is never safe. Virtually all drugs taken by a pregnant woman travel to the fetus by way of the placenta, in varying quantities. Breast milk can also transmit drugs to a nursing baby. In general, you should not take any medication while pregnant or breast-feeding unless you and your physician have discussed the risks and benefits. One major exception is the vitamins that are essential to prevent birth defects (see Spina Bifida, p.985).

Some herbals can be dangerously toxic if taken in high doses. If you have questions, talk to your doctor, and exercise the same caution in using alternative remedies that you would with any medicine.

Addiction to Prescription Drugs

Many people associate drug abuse with illegal drugs such as cocaine or heroin, but it is far more common to be dependent on prescription medications such as sleeping pills and tranquilizers. Drug dependence (which can be psychological and/or physical) is an uncontrollable desire to experience the pleasurable effects of a drug or to prevent the unpleasant effects of withdrawal.

Your body can build up a tolerance to a drug so that the dose must be increased to achieve the same results. This effect is called drug tolerance and is characteristic of most commonly abused drugs, including alcohol, nicotine, caffeine, and some prescription and over-the-counter medicines.

When a person becomes physically dependent on a prescription medicine, the body has so adapted to the drug that stopping it causes withdrawal symptoms. The drug should be slowly tapered off under your doctor's supervision to prevent severe symptoms of withdrawal.

In a small number of people (particularly those who have addiction problems with other substances), true addictive behavior can develop during treatment with narcotics or tranquilizers. In these circumstances, supportive counseling combined with careful monitoring of prescribed dosages may be necessary to prevent addiction.

Doctors are careful when prescribing medications that can cause the user to become dependent. These drugs include amphetamines, barbiturates, antianxiety medicines for anxiety or sleeplessness, narcotic pain relievers, and nervous system stimulants and depressants.

To avoid becoming dependent, take the medicine as directed, be aware of the signs of dependency, and use the drug only for short-term treatment. Talk to your doctor about other methods of treating the underlying problem, and seek counseling if you think you have become addicted to a prescription drug.

MANAGING YOUR MEDICINES

Having clear and correct information about your medications can make the difference between a safe, therapeutic response to a drug and a severe side effect. In a time of shortened physician office visits and automated pharmacies, you must act as your own advocate, both with your physician and at the pharmacy.

Tell your doctor about all medicines you are taking, including preparations you may not normally think of as medications, such as vitamins, antacids, eyedrops, or aspirin.

Some people find it easiest to take all their medicines to the doctor's office with them or to make a list of all drugs they are taking. Also tell your doctor if you have had an allergic reaction to any medicine (see Allergies to Medications, p.1156).

In addition, tell your doctor if you:

■ Are being treated by another doctor or alternative practitioner.

■ Are pregnant or breast-feeding.

■ Have diabetes, kidney disease, or liver disease.

■ Are on a special diet, or are taking vitamin and mineral supplements.

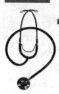

Starting a New Prescription:
Questions to Discuss with Your Doctor

Symptoms that begin shortly after a new medicine is started, or that are described in the printed material, are likely candidates for side effects. Call your doctor if you are concerned about them. He or she may be able to alter the prescription, or suggest a way to minimize the symptoms, such as taking the medicine with food.

When your doctor prescribes a new medication, discuss the following questions with him or her:

■ What is the name of the medicine? (Write it down so you can check it for accuracy against what you receive from the pharmacy.)

■ What is the medicine's intended effect? Will it make pain go away, reduce fever, lower blood pressure, or cure an infection?

■ What side effects might occur? Which should prompt me to phone you?

■ How should I take the medication? Does three times a day mean morning, noon, and night? Should it be taken before meals, with meals, or after meals?

■ Should I get up during the night to take it?

■ What should I do if I miss a dose?

■ How long should I take the medication?

■ Should I take the medicine regularly, or only when I have symptoms?

■ Are there any medicines I should not take while using this one?

■ Are there foods or beverages I should avoid?

■ Can I drink alcohol while taking this drug?

■ Can (and should) the prescription be refilled without seeing you again?

■ Could I use the generic equivalent of the medicine?

■ Use alcohol.

■ Are taking herbal supplements (see p.1154).

Medication Errors

With more than 8,000 medicines available, occasionally a mistake is made when writing or filling a prescription. Generally, though, drug ordering and delivery system safety checks have been put in place to make them even safer and more efficient.

Technology plays an increasing role in improving drug delivery systems. One innovation is the change from prescriptions scrawled in a doctor's handwriting to orders entered into a computer, which eliminates legibility problems and the need for a pharmacist to transcribe the order. Computerized ordering will be even more widely used in the future; a uniform system will probably be universal within the decade.

You need to play a significant role in protecting yourself against errors. Understanding why a particular treatment was selected and knowing the name of the medicine (as well as the dose) when you leave the doctor's office will help you ensure that the pharmacy fills the prescription with the drug your doctor ordered. Read the accompanying printed material from the pharmacist and make sure its effects correspond with what you were told to expect.

Examine a new medication before you take it so you can learn the way it should look and can spot an odd pill. If anything does not look right to you, do not take the medicine; call your doctor or pharmacist. Pharmacies often change from one generic drug manufacturer to another, and this is the most common reason a pill might look odd.

It is best to have all of your family's prescriptions filled at the same pharmacy. A pharmacist who has a complete prescription record of every medicine you are taking can counsel you more effectively and alert you to possible drug interactions or even duplications of drugs prescribed by different doctors.

Following Your Doctor's Instructions

Following your doctor's instructions is called compliance. Studies show that as many as half of prescribed medicines are never taken.

Noncompliance (not taking the medicine your doctor ordered or not following medical direction) is a serious problem with a host of causes. The greater the number of medicines a person is prescribed, and the more complicated the regimen (such as one pill twice a day and another three times a day), the less likely a person is to take his or her medications.

It is not always possible for a doctor to simplify a prescription, but your physician can try if your medication schedule is an impractical combination of drugs that requires you to take them several times a day or at odd hours without food.

Some people fail to take a prescribed medicine because the doctor has not adequately explained the need for it. This is a common problem with conditions such as high blood pressure or elevated cholesterol, which often do not cause symptoms for many years, until they have contributed to a serious condition such as heart disease. Some elderly people do not take their medicines because they are forgetful or confused.

If you have trouble reading your medicine's label or under-

standing your physician's instructions, ask your doctor, nurse, or pharmacist for help. If you are concerned about the number of drugs you are taking or about side effects, discuss this with your doctor. Bring all your medicines with you to the doctor's office in their original containers. Doctors can often make adjustments to the regimen to make it easier for you, or can eliminate medicines that are not absolutely necessary.

Sometimes, people choose not to take a prescribed medicine because it causes intolerable side effects or because they feel it is too expensive. Discuss your concerns honestly with your doctor to see if you can agree on a better and more workable solution.

COMMON DRUG CLASSES

Most medicines you take belong to a class of drugs that includes other medications that have similar actions. It can be valuable to know not only the name of your drug, but also the class it belongs to. Listed here are some of the most frequently used drug classes and their functions.

DRUG CLASS	FUNCTIONS
Amiodarone	Slows heart rate. Used to treat potentially dangerous abnormal heart rhythms.
Androgens	Male hormones. Used to treat various diseases, including endometriosis.
Angiotensin-converting enzyme (ACE) inhibitors	Lower blood pressure. Commonly used to treat high blood pressure and congestive heart failure. Slow progression of kidney disease in diabetics.
Angiotensin-receptor antagonists	Lower blood pressure. Commonly used to treat high blood pressure and congestive heart failure. Slow progression of kidney disease in diabetics.
Antacids containing calcium, aluminum, or magnesium	Counteract acid in the stomach and reduce heartburn and other symptoms aggravated by stomach acid.
Antiadrenergics	Lower blood pressure. Relieve the urinary obstruction that results from an enlarged prostate. Used to treat high blood pressure and an enlarged prostate gland.
Anticoagulants	Blood thinners. Decrease the tendency of the blood to clot after many types of surgery and in people with artificial heart valves, irregular heart rhythms, and blood-clotting disorders.
Anticonvulsants	Prevent seizures in people with epilepsy.

DRUG CLASS	FUNCTIONS
Antifungals	Kill yeast and fungi. Commonly used to treat infections of the skin and nails.
Antihistamines	Alleviate common allergy symptoms (such as itchy red eyes, runny nose, and sneezing) by inhibiting the allergic response.
Antipsychotics	Used to treat hallucinations and other mental disturbances caused by diseases such as schizophrenia.
Antivirals	Inhibit growth of viruses. Used to treat viral infections.
Appetite suppressants containing phenyl-propanolamine or phentermine	Act on the brain to reduce appetite.
Barbiturates	Used to prevent seizures, as sedatives, and to aid sleep. Potentially addicting.
Benzodiazepines	Sedatives. Decrease anxiety and improve sleep.
Beta agonists	Open up tightened breathing tubes in diseases such as asthma and emphysema. Inhaled with a hand-held device called a metered dose inhaler.
Beta blockers	Relax the heart muscle, slow heart rate, and lower blood pressure. Used to treat high blood pressure. Can prolong life in people who have had a heart attack.

COMMON DRUG CLASSES (continued)

DRUG CLASS	FUNCTIONS
Bisphosphonates	Strengthen thin bones. Used to treat osteoporosis.
Bupropion	Antidepressant. Also used to help people quit smoking.
Buspirone	Relieves anxiety.
Calcium channel blockers	Lower blood pressure (some also slow heart rate). Commonly used to treat high blood pressure and angina.
Calcium supplements	Increase the amount of calcium in the body. Can help to strengthen bones.
Cephalosporins	Antibiotics. Used to treat many common bacterial infections of the skin, ears, sinus, throat, and lungs.
Cholesterol-lowering agents (statins)	Reduce cholesterol level. Taken by people with high cholesterol to prevent heart attacks.
Cisapride	Increases the digestive contractions of the stomach and intestines.
Clonidine	Lowers blood pressure.
Contraceptives (oral)	Contain hormones that prevent pregnancy.
Corticosteroids	Inhibit inflammation and the immune system. Used to treat a wide variety of diseases.
Cyclosporine	Inhibits the immune system. Commonly used after organ transplantation to prevent rejection of the transplant.
Dicyclomine	Decreases intestinal spasms. Used to treat irritable bowel syndrome.
Digoxin	Slows heart rate. Used to treat some abnormal heart rhythms. Improves the strength of the heartbeat in congestive heart failure.

DRUG CLASS	FUNCTIONS
Dorzolamide	Used to treat glaucoma.
Epinephrine (adrenaline)	Used to treat life-threatening allergic responses, such as from bee stings.
Ergot alkaloids	Relieve the pain of migraine headaches.
Estrogens	Hormones prescribed after menopause to strengthen bones and decrease hot flashes.
Gemfibrozil	Lowers cholesterol and triglyceride levels.
Histamine$_2$ (H$_2$) blockers	Inhibit the production of acid in the stomach. Used to treat ulcers, gastritis, and acid reflux.
Insulin	Injected by diabetics to lower blood sugar to normal levels.
Iodinated contrast medium	Not a drug, but a substance used for x-ray studies that can interact with certain drugs.
Iron supplements	Increase the amount of iron in the body. Used to treat anemia caused by deficient amounts of iron in the body.
Loop diuretics	"Water" pills. Increase the production of urine. Used to treat congestive heart failure and water retention.
Macrolides	Antibiotics. Inhibit the growth of bacteria. Frequently prescribed to treat many common bacterial infections.
Meperidine	Narcotic painkiller.
Metformin	Lowers blood sugar in diabetics.
Methotrexate	Inhibits the immune system. Used to treat diseases caused by the immune system, such as rheumatoid arthritis, and to treat certain kinds of cancer.

COMMON DRUG CLASSES (continued)

DRUG CLASS	FUNCTIONS
Methylphenidate	Stabilizes mood and improves attention span in people with attention deficit disorder. May be used to treat depression.
Metronidazole	Antibiotic. Used to treat a variety of common infections.
Monoamine oxidase inhibitors (MAOIs)	Antidepressants. Used to treat depression.
Muscle relaxants	Alleviate muscle spasms caused by overuse or minor injury.
Narcotic analgesics	Used to treat pain. Can be addictive.
Nefazodone	Antidepressant. Used to treat depression.
Nitrates	Relieve the pain of angina and heart attacks.
Nitrofurantoin	Antibiotic. Used to treat urinary tract infections.
Nonsteroidal anti-inflammatory drugs (NSAIDs)	Nonaddictive analgesics commonly prescribed for muscle aches, arthritis, and headaches.
Opioids/opiates	Narcotic painkillers.
Penicillin	Antibiotic. Used to treat many common bacterial infections of the skin, ears, sinus, throat, and lungs.
Pentoxifylline	Relieves painful leg cramps caused by blockages in the arteries of the legs.
Potassium-sparing diuretics	"Water" pills. Increase the production of urine. Used to treat fluid buildup and high blood pressure without depleting the body of potassium.
Potassium supplements	Prescribed for those with low blood levels of potassium (most commonly, people taking diuretics).

DRUG CLASS	FUNCTIONS
Progestins	Progesterone hormones commonly prescribed to protect the uterine lining from the growth-promoting effect of estrogen in hormone therapy.
Propafenone	Used to treat potentially dangerous abnormal heart rhythms.
Propoxyphene	Painkiller.
Protease inhibitors	Kill the virus (HIV) that causes AIDS, particularly when used with other antiviral drugs.
Proton pump inhibitors	Inhibit the production of acid in the stomach. Used to treat ulcers, gastritis, and acid reflux.
Quinidine	Used to treat potentially dangerous abnormal heart rhythms.
Quinolones	Antibiotics. Inhibit bacterial growth. Used to treat a variety of bacterial infections.
Rifamycin	Antibiotic. Used to treat bacterial infections.
Salicylates	Include aspirin and related painkillers and anti-inflammatories. Used for relief of minor aches and pains and to prevent or treat many diseases, including arthritis, inflammatory bowel disease, heart attacks, and strokes.
Selective serotonin reuptake inhibitors (SSRIs)	Antidepressants. Increase the level of the hormone serotonin in the brain. Commonly used to treat depression.
Sulfa antibiotics	Inhibit bacterial growth. Used to treat a variety of bacterial infections.
Sulfonylureas	Lower blood sugar. Used by diabetics to lower blood sugar to normal range.
Sumatriptan	Relieves the pain of migraine headaches.
Thyroid hormone	Used to treat low levels of thyroid hormone.

COMMON DRUG CLASSES (continued)

DRUG CLASS	FUNCTIONS
Tamoxifen	Used to treat breast cancer and to decrease the risk of recurrence.
Tetracyclines	Antibiotics. Inhibit the growth of bacteria. Used to treat common bacterial infections.
Theophylline	Improves breathing in people with lung diseases such as emphysema or asthma.
Thiazide diuretics	"Water" pills. Increase the production of urine. Used to treat water retention and high blood pressure.
Thyroid function inhibitors	Used to treat hyperthyroidism (overactive thyroid).

DRUG CLASS	FUNCTIONS
Thyroid hormone	Used to treat low levels of thyroid hormone.
Tramadol	Powerful, nonaddicting analgesic.
Tricyclic antidepressants (heterocyclic antidepressants)	Increase the levels of certain mood-controlling hormones in the brain. Used to treat depression and chronic pain.
Vitamin E	Vitamin supplement that may be useful in reducing the threat of several chronic diseases.
Zinc	Mineral supplement that increases the amount of zinc in the body.
Zolpidem	Sedative. Improves sleep.

DRUG INDEX

TO USE THIS INDEX:

1 Find the medicine's name on the bottle or container (you can use either the generic or brand name).

2 Look for the name of the medicine in the alphabetical listing in the left-hand column.

3 The class to which the drug belongs is shown in the right-hand column.

4 Write down each medicine and its class.

5 Use this information to find out more about the drug class (see Common Drug Classes, p.1160) or to investigate potential drug interactions (see Drug Interactions Chart, p.1167).

MEDICINE	CLASS*
Accupril	ACE inhibitor
Acutrim	Appetite suppressant containing phenyl-propanolamine or phentermine
Adalat	Calcium channel blocker
Alprazolam	Benzodiazepine
Altace	ACE inhibitor
Ambien	Zolpidem
Amiodarone	Amiodarone

MEDICINE	CLASS*
Amitriptylene	Tricyclic antidepressant (heterocyclic antidepressant)
Amlodipine	Calcium channel blocker
Amoxicillin	Penicillin
Amoxicillin-clavulanate	Penicillin
Amoxil	Penicillin
Amphojel	Antacid containing calcium, aluminum, or magnesium
Aspirin	Salicylate

*ACE indicates angiotensin-converting enzyme; NSAID, nonsteroidal anti-inflammatory drug; SSRI, selective serotonin reuptake inhibitor; and MAOI, monoamine oxidase inhibitor.

KEY: Generic name: **boldface**   Brand name: regular type   Nonprescription: *italics*

DRUG INDEX (continued)

MEDICINE	CLASS*
Astemizole	Antihistamine
Atenolol	Beta blocker
Augmentin	Penicillin
Benazepril	ACE inhibitor
Biaxin	Macrolide
Bupropion	Bupropion
Buspar	Buspirone
Buspirone	Buspirone
Cafergot	Ergot alkaloid
Calan	Calcium channel blocker
Calcium	Calcium supplement
Caltrate	Calcium supplement
Capoten	ACE inhibitor
Captopril	ACE inhibitor
Carbamazepine	Anticonvulsant
Cardizem	Calcium channel blocker
Cardura	Antiadrenergic
Cimetidine	Histamine$_2$ (H$_2$) blocker
Cipro	Quinolone
Ciprofloxacin	Quinolone
Cisapride	Cisapride
Citracal	Calcium supplement
Clarithromycin	Macrolide
Clonazepam	Benzodiazepine
Clonidine	Clonidine
Contraceptive (oral)	Contraceptive (oral)
Coumadin	Anticoagulant
Cylosporine	Cyclosporine
Danazol	Androgen
Darvocet	Propoxyphene
Darvon	Propoxyphene
Daypro	NSAID
Delavirdine	Protease inhibitor
Deltasone	Corticosteroid
Demerol	Meperidine
Depakote	Anticonvulsant
Desogen	Contraceptive (oral)

MEDICINE	CLASS*
Dexatrim	Appetite suppressant containing phenyl-propanolamine or phentermine
Diazepam	Benzodiazepine
Diclofenac	NSAID
Diflucan	Antifungal
Digoxin	Digoxin
Dilacor	Calcium channel blocker
Dilantin	Anticonvulsant
Diltiazem	Calcium channel blocker
Doxycycline	Tetracycline
Ecotrin	Salicylate
Enalapril	ACE inhibitor
Epinephrine	Epinephrine (adrenaline)
Ergotamine	Ergot alkaloid
Ery-Tab	Macrolide
Erythromycin	Macrolide
Estrace	Estrogen
Estraderm	Estrogen
Estradiol	Estrogen
Estrogen	Estrogen
Etodolac	NSAID
Ferrous gluconate	Iron supplement
Ferrous sulfate	Iron supplement
Fioricet	Barbiturate
Fiorinal	Barbiturate
Floxin	Quinolone
Fluconazole	Antifungal
Fluoxetine	SSRI
Fluvastatin	Cholesterol-lowering agent (statin)
Fosinopril	ACE inhibitor
Furosemide	Loop diuretic
Gemfibrozil	Gemfibrozil
Glipizide	Sulfonylurea
Glucophage	Metformin
Glucotrol	Sulfonylurea

*ACE indicates angiotensin-converting enzyme; NSAID, nonsteroidal anti-inflammatory drug; SSRI, selective serotonin reuptake inhibitor; and MAOI, monoamine oxidase inhibitor.

KEY: Generic name: **boldface**   Brand name: regular type   Nonprescription: *italics*

DRUG INDEX (continued)

MEDICINE	CLASS*
Glyburide	Sulfonylurea
Glynase	Sulfonylurea
Hismanal	Antihistamine
Humulin	Insulin
Hydrochlorothiazide	Thiazide diuretic
Ibuprofen	NSAID
Imitrex	Sumatriptan
Indinavir	Protease inhibitor
Insulin	Insulin
Iodinated contrast medium	Iodinated contrast medium
K Cl	Potassium supplement
K-Dur	Potassium supplement
Ketoprofen	NSAID
Klonopin	Benzodiazepine
Klor-Con	Potassium supplement
Lanoxin	Digoxin
Lasix	Loop diuretic
Lescol	Cholesterol-lowering agent (statin)
Levaquin	Quinolone
Levofloxacin	Quinolone
Levothyroxine	Thyroid hormone
Levoxyl	Thyroid hormone
Lisinopril	ACE inhibitor
Lodine	NSAID
Loestrin	Contraceptive (oral)
Lo/Ovral	Contraceptive (oral)
Lopressor	Beta blocker
Lorazepam	Benzodiazepine
Lotensin	ACE inhibitor
Lovastatin	Cholesterol-lowering agent (statin)
Lozol	Thiazide diuretic
Maalox	Antacid containing calcium, aluminum, or magnesium
Meperidine	Meperidine
Metformin	Metformin

MEDICINE	CLASS*
Methimazole	Thyroid function inhibitor
Methotrexate	Methotrexate
Methylprednisolone	Corticosteroid
Metoprolol	Beta blocker
Metronidazole	Metronidazole
Mevacor	Cholesterol-lowering agent (statin)
Micronase	Sulfonylurea
Monopril	ACE inhibitor
Mylanta	Antacid containing calcium, aluminum, or magnesium
Nabumetone	NSAID
Naproxen	NSAID
Nardil	MAOI
Nefazodone	Nefazodone
Nelfinavir	Protease inhibitor
Nifedipine	Calcium channel blocker
Niferex	Iron supplement
Norvasc	Calcium channel blocker
Ofloxacin	Quinolone
Ortho-Cept	Contraceptive (oral)
Ortho-Cyclen	Contraceptive (oral)
Ortho-Novum	Contraceptive (oral)
Ortho Tri-Cyclen	Contraceptive (oral)
Oruvail	NSAID
Os-Cal	Calcium supplement
Oxaprozin	NSAID
Parnate	MAOI
Paroxetine	SSRI
Paxil	SSRI
Penicillin	Penicillin
Phenelzine	MAOI
Phenobarbital	Barbiturate
Phenytoin	Anticonvulsant
Potassium chloride	Potassium supplement
Pravachol	Cholesterol-lowering agent (statin)
Pravastatin	Cholesterol-lowering agent (statin)

*ACE indicates angiotensin-converting enzyme; NSAID, nonsteroidal anti-inflammatory drug; SSRI, selective serotonin reuptake inhibitor; and MAOI, monoamine oxidase inhibitor.

KEY: Generic name: **boldface**   Brand name: regular type   Nonprescription: *italics*

DRUG INDEX (continued)

MEDICINE	CLASS*
Prednisone	Corticosteroid
Premarin	Estrogen
Prempro	Estrogen
Prinivil	ACE inhibitor
Procardia	Calcium channel blocker
Propacet	Propoxyphene
Propafenone	Propafenone
Propoxyphene	Propoxyphene
Propulsid	Cisapride
Propylthiouracil	Thyroid function inhibitor
Protease inhibitor	Protease inhibitor
Prozac	SSRI
Quinapril	ACE inhibitor
Quinidine	Quinidine
Ramipril	ACE inhibitor
Relafen	NSAID
Rifamycin	Rifamycin
Ritonavir	Protease inhibitor
Saquinavir	Protease inhibitor
Sertraline	SSRI
Simvastatin	Cholesterol-lowering agent (statin)
Spironolactone	Potassium-sparing diuretic
Sumatriptan	Sumatriptan
Synthroid	Thyroid hormone
Tagamet	Histamine$_2$ (H$_2$) blocker
Tegretol	Anticonvulsant
Temazepam	Benzodiazepine
Tenormin	Beta blocker
Testosterone	Androgen

MEDICINE	CLASS*
Tetracycline	Tetracycline
Theo-Dur	Theophylline
Theophylline	Theophylline
Thyroxine	Thyroid hormone
Timoptic	Beta blocker
Toprol	Beta blocker
Tranylcypromine	MAOI
Tri-Levlen	Contraceptive (oral)
Trimethoprim-sulfamethoxazole	Sulfa antibiotic
Trimox	Penicillin
Triphasil	Contraceptive (oral)
Tums	Antacid containing calcium
Valproic acid	Anticonvulsant
Vasotec	ACE inhibitor
Veetids	Penicillin
Verapamil	Calcium channel blocker
Verelan	Calcium channel blocker
Vitamin E	Vitamin E
Warfarin	Anticoagulant
Wellbutrin	Bupropion
Wigraine	Ergot alkaloid
Xanax	Benzodiazepine
Zestril	ACE inhibitor
Zinc	Zinc
Zocor	Cholesterol-lowering agent (statin)
Zoloft	SSRI
Zolpidem	Zolpidem
Zyban	Bupropion

*ACE indicates angiotensin-converting enzyme; NSAID, nonsteroidal anti-inflammatory drug; SSRI, selective serotonin reuptake inhibitor; and MAOI, monoamine oxidase inhibitor.

KEY: Generic name: **boldface**   Brand name: regular type   Nonprescription: *italics*

DRUG INTERACTIONS CHART

There is not enough space to list all the possible interactions between the thousands of drugs doctors can prescribe. This chart contains only the most commonly used medications and the most potentially serious drug interactions.

Some medicines should not be taken together. Others can be combined if your doctor closely monitors their effects.

Do not be alarmed if you find that you are taking two medicines that may interact; your doctor may have an excellent reason for prescribing the combination. If you are concerned, ask your physician to explain. Many medicines can be combined as long as the effects are monitored.

Never stop taking a medicine without first discussing it with your doctor. Suddenly stopping a medicine can be dangerous.

TO USE THIS CHART:

1 Look up your drugs in the Drug Index on p.1167 to determine what drug classes they belong to.

2 In the left-hand column of this chart, locate the drug class to which one of your drugs belongs.

3 In the second column, look for drug classes that interact with the first class. Does another medicine you are taking belong to one of the classes that interacts with the class of the first medicine?

4 If this chart indicates that two medicines you are taking have a potentially serious interaction, find the effect of the interaction in the third column.

5 The fourth column describes the monitoring your doctor should do (and what you should do) to be sure that the medicines can be used together safely.

MEDICINES IN THIS DRUG CLASS*	MAY INTERACT WITH MEDICINES IN THIS DRUG CLASS*	CAUSING THIS EFFECT	ACTION REQUIRED
ACE inhibitor	NSAID	May make ACE inhibitor less effective in lowering blood pressure.	Your doctor should check blood pressure frequently.
ACE inhibitor	Salicylate	May make ACE inhibitor less effective in lowering blood pressure.	Your doctor should check blood pressure frequently.
Antacid containing calcium, aluminum, or magnesium	Quinolone	May decrease absorption of quinolone from intestine, decreasing its antibiotic effect.	You should avoid taking an antacid at least 6 hours before and 2 hours after taking quinolone.
Antacid containing calcium, aluminum, or magnesium	Tetracycline	May decrease absorption of tetracycline from intestine, decreasing its antibiotic effect.	You should avoid taking an antacid within 4 hours of taking tetracycline.
Anticoagulant	Amiodarone	May increase blood-thinning effect of anticoagulant and can cause bleeding.	Your doctor should monitor prothrombin time (time it takes blood to clot) frequently and adjust anticoagulant dose.

*ACE indicates angiotensin-converting enzyme; NSAID, nonsteroidal anti-inflammatory drug; SSRI, selective serotonin reuptake inhibitor; and MAOI, monoamine oxidase inhibitor.

DRUG INTERACTIONS CHART (continued)

MEDICINES IN THIS DRUG CLASS*	MAY INTERACT WITH MEDICINES IN THIS DRUG CLASS*	CAUSING THIS EFFECT	ACTION REQUIRED
Anticoagulant	Androgen	May increase blood-thinning effect of anticoagulant and can cause bleeding.	Your doctor should monitor prothrombin time (time it takes blood to clot) frequently and adjust anticoagulant dose.
Anticoagulant	Anticonvulsant	May alter effects of both medicines, causing bleeding, clotting, or toxicity from high medicine levels.	Your doctor should check anticonvulsant level in blood and prothrombin time (time it takes blood to clot) frequently and adjust doses if necessary.
Anticoagulant	Antifungal	May increase blood-thinning effect of anticoagulant and can cause bleeding.	Your doctor should monitor prothrombin time (time it takes blood to clot) frequently and adjust anticoagulant dose.
Anticoagulant	Barbiturate	May decrease blood-thinning effect of anticoagulant and can cause blood clots.	Your doctor should monitor prothrombin time (time it takes blood to clot) frequently and adjust anticoagulant dose.
Anticoagulant	Cimetidine (a histamine$_2$ [H$_2$] blocker; see p.1161)	May increase blood-thinning effect of anticoagulant and can cause bleeding.	Your doctor should avoid prescribing these drugs in combination or will monitor prothrombin time (time it takes blood to clot) and adjust anticoagulant dose if necessary.
Anticoagulant	Macrolide	May increase blood-thinning effect of anticoagulant and can cause bleeding.	Your doctor should monitor prothrombin time (time it takes blood to clot) frequently and adjust anticoagulant dose.
Anticoagulant	Metronidazole	May increase blood-thinning effect of anticoagulant and can cause bleeding.	Your doctor should monitor prothrombin time (time it takes blood to clot) frequently and adjust anticoagulant dose.
Anticoagulant	NSAID	May increase risk of bleeding, even if anticoagulant is taken in proper dose.	Your doctor should avoid prescribing these drugs in combination or should monitor prothrombin time (time it takes blood to clot) frequently. Call your doctor if you bruise or bleed easily, see blood in your urine or bowel movements, or observe other signs of bleeding.
Anticoagulant	Penicillin	May increase or decrease anticoagulation level, causing either bleeding or blood clots.	Your doctor should monitor prothrombin time (time it takes blood to clot) frequently and adjust anticoagulant dose.

*ACE indicates angiotensin-converting enzyme; NSAID, nonsteroidal anti-inflammatory drug; SSRI, selective serotonin reuptake inhibitor; and MAOI, monoamine oxidase inhibitor.

DRUG INTERACTIONS CHART (continued)

MEDICINES IN THIS DRUG CLASS*	MAY INTERACT WITH MEDICINES IN THIS DRUG CLASS*	CAUSING THIS EFFECT	ACTION REQUIRED
Anticoagulant	Quinidine	May increase blood-thinning effect of anticoagulant and can cause bleeding.	Your doctor should monitor prothrombin time (time it takes blood to clot) frequently and adjust anticoagulant dose.
Anticoagulant	Salicylate	May increase risk of bleeding, even if anticoagulant is taken in proper dose.	Your doctor should avoid prescribing these drugs in combination or should monitor prothrombin time (time it takes blood to clot) frequently. Call your doctor if you bruise or bleed easily, see blood in your urine or bowel movements, or observe other signs of bleeding.
Anticoagulant	Sulfa antibiotic	May increase blood-thinning effect of anticoagulant and can cause bleeding.	Your doctor should monitor prothrombin time (time it takes blood to clot) frequently and adjust anticoagulant dose.
Anticoagulant	Thyroid function inhibitor	May increase or decrease blood-thinning effect of anticoagulant, causing bleeding or clotting.	Your doctor should monitor prothrombin time (time it takes blood to clot) frequently and adjust anticoagulant dose.
Anticoagulant	Thyroid hormone	May increase blood-thinning effect of anticoagulant and can cause bleeding.	Your doctor should monitor prothrombin time (time it takes blood to clot) frequently and adjust anticoagulant dose.
Anticoagulant	Vitamin E	May increase blood-thinning effect of anticoagulant and can cause bleeding.	Your doctor should monitor prothrombin time (time it takes blood to clot) frequently and adjust anticoagulant dose.
Anticonvulsant	Anticoagulant	May alter effects of both medicines, causing bleeding, clotting, or toxicity from high medicine levels.	Your doctor should check anticonvulsant level in blood and prothrombin time (time it takes blood to clot) frequently and adjust doses if necessary.
Anticonvulsant	Antifungal	May increase blood level of anticonvulsant, causing side effects such as unsteadiness, dizziness, and nausea.	Your doctor should check anticonvulsant level in blood frequently and adjust dose.
Anticonvulsant	Bupropion	May lower level of bupropion, decreasing its effectiveness.	Bupropion generally should not be prescribed for people who have seizures. Your doctor may need to adjust doses of both medicines if anticonvulsant is decreasing effectiveness of bupropion.

*ACE indicates angiotensin-converting enzyme; NSAID, nonsteroidal anti-inflammatory drug; SSRI, selective serotonin reuptake inhibitor; and MAOI, monoamine oxidase inhibitor.

DRUG INTERACTIONS CHART (continued)

MEDICINES IN THIS DRUG CLASS*	MAY INTERACT WITH MEDICINES IN THIS DRUG CLASS*	CAUSING THIS EFFECT	ACTION REQUIRED
Anticonvulsant	Calcium channel blocker	May alter level of either medicine, decreasing effect if level is too low or causing side effects such as unsteadiness, dizziness, nausea, fainting, and swelling of legs if level is too high.	Your doctor should check anticonvulsant level in blood frequently, adjust dose, and monitor blood pressure and heart rate.
Anticonvulsant	Cimetidine (a histamine$_2$ [H$_2$] blocker; see p.1161)	May increase blood level of anticonvulsant, causing side effects such as unsteadiness, dizziness, and nausea.	Your doctor should check anticonvulsant level in blood frequently and adjust dose.
Anticonvulsant	Contraceptive (oral)	May reduce effectiveness of oral contraceptive.	You should use alternative form of birth control.
Anticonvulsant	Corticosteroid	May decrease effectiveness of both medicines.	Your doctor may need to increase corticosteroid dose, monitor anticonvulsant level, and adjust dose.
Anticonvulsant	Cyclosporine	May decrease cyclosporine level, leading to organ transplant rejection.	Your doctor should monitor blood level of cyclosporine frequently.
Anticonvulsant	Estrogen	May increase or decrease level of either medicine, causing side effects if level is too high or lack of effectiveness if level is too low. Symptoms such as hot flashes may indicate low estrogen levels.	Your doctor should check anticonvulsant level in blood frequently and adjust dose.
Anticonvulsant	Macrolide	May increase blood level of anticonvulsant, causing side effects such as unsteadiness, dizziness, and nausea.	Your doctor should check anticonvulsant level in blood frequently and adjust dose.
Anticonvulsant	Propoxyphene	May increase blood level of anticonvulsant, causing side effects such as unsteadiness, dizziness, and nausea.	Your doctor should check anticonvulsant level in blood frequently and adjust dose.
Anticonvulsant	Salicylate	May increase blood level of anticonvulsant, causing side effects such as unsteadiness, dizziness, and nausea.	Your doctor should check anticonvulsant level in blood frequently and adjust dose.
Anticonvulsant	SSRI	May increase blood level of anticonvulsant, causing side effects such as unsteadiness, dizziness, and nausea.	Your doctor should check anticonvulsant level in blood frequently and adjust dose.

*ACE indicates angiotensin-converting enzyme; NSAID, nonsteroidal anti-inflammatory drug; SSRI, selective serotonin reuptake inhibitor; and MAOI, monoamine oxidase inhibitor.

DRUG INTERACTIONS CHART (continued)

MEDICINES IN THIS DRUG CLASS*	MAY INTERACT WITH MEDICINES IN THIS DRUG CLASS*	CAUSING THIS EFFECT	ACTION REQUIRED
Anticonvulsant	Sulfa antibiotic	May increase anticonvulsant effect.	Your doctor should check anticonvulsant level in blood frequently and adjust dose.
Anticonvulsant	Tetracycline	Decreases antibiotic effectiveness of tetracycline.	Your doctor may need to increase tetracycline dose.
Anticonvulsant	Theophylline	May increase or decrease effect of either medicine, resulting in side effects such as unsteadiness, dizziness, nausea, and palpitations.	Your doctor should monitor levels of both medicines and adjust doses.
Anticonvulsant	Tricyclic antidepressant (heterocyclic antidepressant)	May increase blood level of anticonvulsant, causing side effects such as unsteadiness, dizziness, and nausea.	Your doctor should check anticonvulsant level in blood frequently and adjust dose.
Antifungal	Anticoagulant	May increase blood-thinning effect of anticoagulant and can cause bleeding.	Your doctor should monitor prothrombin time (time it takes blood to clot) frequently and adjust anticoagulant dose.
Antifungal	Anticonvulsant	May increase blood level of anticonvulsant, causing side effects such as unsteadiness, dizziness, and nausea.	Your doctor should check anticonvulsant level in blood frequently and adjust dose.
Antifungal	Antihistamine	May increase antihistamine level, which can cause death (in rare cases) due to toxic effect on heart.	Your doctor should not prescribe these drugs in combination.
Antifungal	Benzodiazepine	May increase or prolong effect of benzodiazepine, resulting in excessive sedation and other side effects.	Your doctor should avoid prescribing these drugs in combination or will prescribe a lower dose of benzodiazepine.
Antifungal	Cisapride	May increase cisapride level, which can cause death (in rare cases) due to toxic effect on heart.	Your doctor should not prescribe these drugs in combination.
Antifungal	Cholesterol-lowering agent (statin)	May increase level of cholesterol-lowering agent, which can cause abnormal liver tests and side effects such as muscle aches or weakness.	Your doctor should prescribe these drugs in combination with caution and may need to decrease dose of cholesterol-lowering agent.

*ACE indicates angiotensin-converting enzyme; NSAID, nonsteroidal anti-inflammatory drug; SSRI, selective serotonin reuptake inhibitor; and MAOI, monoamine oxidase inhibitor.

DRUG INTERACTIONS CHART (continued)

MEDICINES IN THIS DRUG CLASS*	MAY INTERACT WITH MEDICINES IN THIS DRUG CLASS*	CAUSING THIS EFFECT	ACTION REQUIRED
Antihistamine	Antifungal	May increase antihistamine level, which can cause death (in rare cases) due to toxic effect on heart.	Your doctor should not prescribe these drugs in combination.
Antihistamine	Macrolide	May increase antihistamine level, which can cause death (in rare cases) due to toxic effect on heart.	Your doctor should not prescribe these drugs in combination.
Antihistamine	Nefazodone	May increase antihistamine level, which can cause death (in rare cases) due to toxic effect on heart.	Your doctor should not prescribe these drugs in combination.
Antihistamine	Protease inhibitor	May increase antihistamine level, which can cause death (in rare cases) due to toxic effect on heart.	Your doctor should not prescribe these drugs in combination.
Antihistamine	SSRI	May increase antihistamine level, which can cause death (in rare cases) due to toxic effect on heart.	Your doctor should not prescribe these drugs in combination.
Appetite suppressant containing phenylpropanolamine or phentermine	MAOI	May cause dramatic elevations in blood pressure, resulting in brain hemorrhage and death.	Your doctor should not prescribe these drugs in combination. MAOI must be stopped for several weeks before appetite suppressant is prescribed.
Appetite suppressant containing phenylpropanolamine or phentermine	SSRI	May cause anxiety, agitation, and tremors.	Your doctor should prescribe these drugs in combination with caution and will advise you to stop taking appetite suppressant if side effects develop.
Barbiturate	Anticoagulant	May decrease blood-thinning effect of anticoagulant and can cause blood clots.	Your doctor should monitor prothrombin time (time it takes blood to clot) frequently and adjust anticoagulant dose.
Benzodiazepine	Antifungal	May increase or prolong effect of benzodiazepine, resulting in excessive sedation and other side effects.	Your doctor should avoid prescribing these drugs in combination or will prescribe a lower dose of benzodiazepine.
Benzodiazepine	Macrolide	May increase or prolong effect of benzodiazepine, resulting in sedation and other side effects.	Your doctor should decrease benzodiazepine dose if side effects or excessive sedation occur.

*ACE indicates angiotensin-converting enzyme; NSAID, nonsteroidal anti-inflammatory drug; SSRI, selective serotonin reuptake inhibitor; and MAOI, monoamine oxidase inhibitor.

DRUG INTERACTIONS CHART (continued)

MEDICINES IN THIS DRUG CLASS*	MAY INTERACT WITH MEDICINES IN THIS DRUG CLASS*	CAUSING THIS EFFECT	ACTION REQUIRED
Benzodiazepine	Protease inhibitor	May increase or prolong effect of benzodiazepine, resulting in sedation and other side effects.	Your doctor should prescribe these drugs in combination with caution.
Beta blocker	Calcium channel blocker	May increase effect of both medicines.	Your doctor should monitor heart rate and blood pressure and decrease doses of both medicines if necessary.
Beta blocker	Cimetidine (a histamine$_2$ [H$_2$] blocker; see p.1161)	May increase effect of beta blocker.	Your doctor should decrease beta blocker dose if slow heart rate or low blood pressure occurs.
Beta blocker	Clonidine	May reverse blood pressure–lowering effect of both medicines, resulting in potentially life-threatening increases in blood pressure.	Your doctor should monitor blood pressure carefully.
Beta blocker	Epinephrine (adrenaline)	May dramatically increase blood pressure.	Your doctor should avoid prescribing these drugs in combination.
Beta blocker	Insulin	May prolong and mask the symptoms of low blood sugar (hypoglycemia) if it occurs.	This combination is frequently prescribed. Diabetics should monitor their blood sugar to avoid hypoglycemic episodes.
Beta blocker	NSAID	May reduce blood pressure–lowering effect of beta blocker.	Your doctor should monitor blood pressure and adjust beta blocker dose if necessary.
Beta blocker	Penicillin	May reduce effectiveness of beta blocker.	Your doctor should monitor blood pressure and may need to increase beta blocker dose or advise you to take penicillin in smaller, more frequent doses.
Beta blocker	Theophylline	May increase theophylline level or decrease effects of both medicines.	Your doctor should monitor theophylline levels frequently and check heart rate and blood pressure.
Bupropion	Anticonvulsant	May lower level of bupropion, decreasing its effectiveness.	Bupropion generally should not be prescribed for people who have seizures. Your doctor may need to adjust doses of both medicines if anticonvulsant is decreasing effectiveness of bupropion.

*ACE indicates angiotensin-converting enzyme; NSAID, nonsteroidal anti-inflammatory drug; SSRI, selective serotonin reuptake inhibitor; and MAOI, monoamine oxidase inhibitor.

DRUG INTERACTIONS CHART (continued)

MEDICINES IN THIS DRUG CLASS*	MAY INTERACT WITH MEDICINES IN THIS DRUG CLASS*	CAUSING THIS EFFECT	ACTION REQUIRED
Buspirone	MAOI	May result in high blood pressure.	Your doctor should not prescribe these drugs in combination or will advise you to wait 10 days after stopping MAOI before starting buspirone.
Calcium channel blocker	Anticonvulsant	May alter level of either medicine, decreasing effectiveness if level is too low or causing side effects such as unsteadiness, dizziness, nausea, fainting, and swelling of legs if level is too high.	Your doctor should check anticonvulsant level in blood frequently, adjust dose, and monitor blood pressure and heart rate.
Calcium channel blocker	Beta blocker	May increase effect of both medicines.	Your doctor should monitor heart rate and blood pressure and decrease doses of both medicines if necessary.
Calcium channel blocker	Calcium supplement	May decrease effectiveness of calcium channel blocker.	Your doctor should prescribe these drugs in combination with caution and monitor heart rate and blood pressure.
Calcium channel blocker	Cimetidine (a histamine$_2$ [H$_2$] blocker; see p.1161)	May increase level of calcium channel blocker.	Your doctor should monitor heart rate and blood pressure and adjust calcium channel blocker dose if necessary.
Calcium channel blocker	Cisapride	May increase level of calcium channel blocker, resulting in side effects such as dizziness, fainting, and swelling of legs.	Your doctor should monitor heart rate and blood pressure and decrease calcium channel blocker dose if necessary.
Calcium channel blocker	Digoxin	May increase digoxin level, causing side effects such as nausea, vomiting, blurry or yellow vision (like looking through yellow-tinted glasses), or abnormally fast or slow heart rate.	Your doctor should monitor digoxin level and adjust dose. Call your doctor if you experience nausea.
Calcium channel blocker	Quinidine	May increase effect of quinidine, resulting in low blood pressure or dangerously irregular heartbeat.	Your doctor should avoid prescribing these drugs in combination or monitor heart rate and blood pressure carefully.
Calcium channel blocker	Theophylline	May increase effect of theophylline.	Your doctor should monitor theophylline level and adjust dose.

*ACE indicates angiotensin-converting enzyme; NSAID, nonsteroidal anti-inflammatory drug; SSRI, selective serotonin reuptake inhibitor; and MAOI, monoamine oxidase inhibitor.

DRUG INTERACTIONS CHART (continued)

MEDICINES IN THIS DRUG CLASS*	MAY INTERACT WITH MEDICINES IN THIS DRUG CLASS*	CAUSING THIS EFFECT	ACTION REQUIRED
Calcium supplement	Calcium channel blocker	May decrease effectiveness of calcium channel blocker.	Your doctor should prescribe these drugs in combination with caution and monitor heart rate and blood pressure.
Calcium supplement	Tetracycline	May bind to tetracycline in intestine, lowering its level in the blood, which may decrease its antibiotic effectiveness.	You should avoid taking calcium within 4 hours of taking tetracycline.
Cholesterol-lowering agent (statin)	Antifungal	May increase level of cholesterol-lowering agent, which can cause abnormal liver tests and side effects such as muscle aches or weakness.	Your doctor should prescribe these drugs in combination with caution and may need to decrease cholesterol-lowering agent dose.
Cholesterol-lowering agent (statin)	Cyclosporine	May result in severe muscle damage.	Your doctor should prescribe these drugs in combination with caution. You should report any unexplained muscle pain or weakness.
Cholesterol-lowering agent (statin)	Gemfibrozil	May result in severe muscle damage.	Your doctor should prescribe these drugs in combination with caution. You should report any unexplained muscle pain or weakness.
Cimetidine (a histamine$_2$ [H$_2$] blocker; see p.1161)	Anticoagulant	May increase blood-thinning effect of anticoagulant and can cause bleeding.	Your doctor should avoid prescribing these drugs in combination or monitor prothrombin time (time it takes blood to clot) and adjust anticoagulant dose if necessary.
Cimetidine (a histamine$_2$ [H$_2$] blocker; see p.1161)	Anticonvulsant	May increase blood level of anticonvulsant, causing side effects such as unsteadiness, dizziness, and nausea.	Your doctor should check anticonvulsant level in blood frequently and adjust dose.
Cimetidine (a histamine$_2$ [H$_2$] blocker; see p.1161)	Beta blocker	May increase effect of beta blocker.	Your doctor should decrease beta blocker dose if slow heart rate or low blood pressure occurs.
Cimetidine (a histamine$_2$ [H$_2$] blocker; see p.1161)	Calcium channel blocker	May increase level of calcium channel blocker.	Your doctor should monitor heart rate and blood pressure and adjust calcium channel blocker dose if necessary.
Cimetidine (a histamine$_2$ [H$_2$] blocker; see p.1161)	Metformin	May increase metformin level.	Your doctor may need to decrease metformin dose.

*ACE indicates angiotensin-converting enzyme; NSAID, nonsteroidal anti-inflammatory drug; SSRI, selective serotonin reuptake inhibitor; and MAOI, monoamine oxidase inhibitor.

DRUG INTERACTIONS CHART (continued)

MEDICINES IN THIS DRUG CLASS*	MAY INTERACT WITH MEDICINES IN THIS DRUG CLASS*	CAUSING THIS EFFECT	ACTION REQUIRED
Cimetidine (a histamine$_2$ [H$_2$] blocker; see p.1161)	Theophylline	May increase theophylline level, resulting in side effects such as nausea, vomiting, and palpitations.	Your doctor should monitor theophylline level.
Cimetidine (a histamine$_2$ [H$_2$] blocker; see p.1161)	Tricyclic antidepressant (heterocyclic antidepressant)	May increase antidepressant level, causing side effects such as abnormal heart rhythm, increased heart rate, and drowsiness.	Your doctor should avoid prescribing these drugs in combination or monitor antidepressant level and lower dose if necessary.
Cisapride	Antifungal	May increase cisapride level, which can cause death (in rare cases) due to toxic effect on heart.	Your doctor should not prescribe these drugs in combination.
Cisapride	Calcium channel blocker	May increase level of calcium channel blocker, resulting in side effects such as dizziness, fainting, and swelling of legs.	Your doctor should monitor heart rate and blood pressure and decrease calcium channel blocker dose if necessary.
Cisapride	Macrolide	May increase cisapride level, which can cause death (in rare cases) due to toxic effect on heart.	Your doctor should not prescribe these drugs in combination.
Cisapride	Nefazodone	May increase cisapride level, which can cause death (in rare cases) due to toxic effect on heart.	Your doctor should not prescribe these drugs in combination.
Cisapride	Protease inhibitor	May increase cisapride level, which can cause death (in rare cases) due to toxic effect on heart.	Your doctor should not prescribe these drugs in combination.
Cisapride	SSRI	May increase cisapride level, which can cause death (in rare cases) due to toxic effect on heart.	Your doctor should not prescribe these drugs in combination.
Clonidine	Beta blocker	May reverse blood pressure–lowering effect of both medicines, resulting in potentially life-threatening increases in blood pressure.	Your doctor should monitor blood pressure carefully.
Clonidine	Tricyclic antidepressant (heterocyclic antidepressant)	May cause dramatic elevations in blood pressure.	Your doctor should avoid prescribing these drugs in combination.

*ACE indicates angiotensin-converting enzyme; NSAID, nonsteroidal anti-inflammatory drug; SSRI, selective serotonin reuptake inhibitor; and MAOI, monoamine oxidase inhibitor.

DRUG INTERACTIONS CHART (continued)

MEDICINES IN THIS DRUG CLASS*	MAY INTERACT WITH MEDICINES IN THIS DRUG CLASS*	CAUSING THIS EFFECT	ACTION REQUIRED
Contraceptive (oral)	Anticonvulsant	May reduce effectiveness of contraceptive.	You should use alternative form of birth control.
Contraceptive (oral)	Corticosteroid	May increase activity and adverse effects of corticosteroid.	Your doctor should decrease corticosteroid dose if side effects occur.
Contraceptive (oral)	Penicillin	May reduce effectiveness of contraceptive.	You should use alternative form of birth control.
Contraceptive (oral)	Tetracycline	May reduce effectiveness of contraceptive.	You should use alternative form of birth control.
Contraceptive (oral)	Theophylline	May increase theophylline level, causing side effects such as nausea, vomiting, and palpitations.	Your doctor should monitor theophylline level and adjust dose.
Corticosteroid	Anticonvulsant	May decrease effectiveness of both medicines.	Your doctor may need to increase corticosteroid dose, monitor anticonvulsant level, and adjust dose.
Corticosteroid	Contraceptive (oral)	May increase activity and adverse effects of corticosteroid.	Your doctor should decrease corticosteroid dose if side effects occur.
Corticosteroid	Estrogen	May increase activity and adverse effects of corticosteroid.	Your doctor should decrease corticosteroid dose if side effects occur.
Corticosteroid	Macrolide	May increase activity and adverse effects of corticosteroid.	Your doctor should decrease corticosteroid dose if side effects occur.
Corticosteroid	Rifamycin	May decrease effectiveness of corticosteroid.	Your doctor may need to increase corticosteroid dose for desired effect.
Corticosteroid	Salicylate	May reduce effectiveness of salicylate and increase risk of peptic ulcer.	Your doctor should tailor salicylate dose as needed for pain control.

*ACE indicates angiotensin-converting enzyme; NSAID, nonsteroidal anti-inflammatory drug; SSRI, selective serotonin reuptake inhibitor; and MAOI, monoamine oxidase inhibitor.

DRUG INTERACTIONS CHART (continued)

MEDICINES IN THIS DRUG CLASS*	MAY INTERACT WITH MEDICINES IN THIS DRUG CLASS*	CAUSING THIS EFFECT	ACTION REQUIRED
Digoxin	Amiodarone	May increase digoxin level, causing side effects such as nausea, vomiting, blurry or yellow vision (like looking through yellow-tinted glasses), or abnormally fast or slow heart rate.	Your doctor should monitor digoxin level and adjust dose. Call your doctor if you experience nausea.
Digoxin	Calcium channel blocker	May increase digoxin level, causing side effects such as nausea, vomiting, blurry or yellow vision (like looking through yellow-tinted glasses), or abnormally fast or slow heart rate.	Your doctor should monitor digoxin level and adjust dose. Call your doctor if you experience nausea.
Digoxin	Cyclosporine	May increase digoxin level, causing side effects such as nausea, vomiting, blurry or yellow vision (like looking through yellow-tinted glasses), or abnormally fast or slow heart rate.	Your doctor should monitor digoxin level and adjust dose. Call your doctor if you experience nausea.
Digoxin	Loop diuretic	May lead to irregularities in heart rhythm if potassium and magnesium levels are lowered by diuretic therapy.	Your doctor should monitor digoxin, potassium, and magnesium levels and may need to prescribe potassium and magnesium supplements if levels are low.
Digoxin	Macrolide	May increase digoxin level, causing side effects such as nausea, vomiting, blurry or yellow vision (like looking through yellow-tinted glasses), or abnormally fast or slow heart rate.	Your doctor should monitor digoxin level and adjust dose. Call your doctor if you experience nausea.
Digoxin	Propafenone	May increase digoxin level, causing side effects such as nausea, vomiting, blurry or yellow vision (like looking through yellow-tinted glasses), or abnormally fast or slow heart rate.	Your doctor should monitor digoxin level and adjust dose. Call your doctor if you experience nausea.

*ACE indicates angiotensin-converting enzyme; NSAID, nonsteroidal anti-inflammatory drug; SSRI, selective serotonin reuptake inhibitor; and MAOI, monoamine oxidase inhibitor.

DRUG INTERACTIONS CHART (continued)

MEDICINES IN THIS DRUG CLASS*	MAY INTERACT WITH MEDICINES IN THIS DRUG CLASS*	CAUSING THIS EFFECT	ACTION REQUIRED
Digoxin	Quinidine	May increase digoxin level, causing side effects such as nausea, vomiting, blurry or yellow vision (like looking through yellow-tinted glasses), or abnormally fast or slow heart rate.	Your doctor should monitor digoxin level and adjust dose. Call your doctor if you experience nausea.
Digoxin	Tetracycline	May increase digoxin level, causing side effects such as nausea, vomiting, blurry or yellow vision (like looking through yellow-tinted glasses), or abnormally fast or slow heart rate.	Your doctor should monitor digoxin level and adjust dose. Call your doctor if you experience nausea.
Digoxin	Thiazide diuretic	May lead to irregularities in heart rhythm if potassium and magnesium levels are lowered by diuretic therapy.	Your doctor should monitor digoxin, potassium, and magnesium levels and may need to prescribe potassium and magnesium supplements if levels are low.
Digoxin	Thyroid hormone	May decrease digoxin level.	Your doctor should monitor digoxin level and adjust dose if necessary.
Ergot alkaloid	Macrolide	May result in decreased blood supply to fingers and toes.	Your doctor should prescribe these drugs in combination with caution and decrease ergot alkaloid dose.
Ergot alkaloid	Sumatriptan	May increase severity of side effects such as flushing, tingling, abnormal heart rhythms, and angina.	You should take these drugs at least 24 hours apart.
Estrogen	Anticonvulsant	May increase or decrease level of either medicine, causing side effects if level is too high or lack of effectiveness if level is too low. Symptoms such as hot flashes may indicate low estrogen levels.	Your doctor should check anticonvulsant level in blood frequently and adjust dose if necessary.
Estrogen	Corticosteroid	May increase activity and adverse effects of corticosteroid.	Your doctor should decrease corticosteroid dose if side effects occur.
Insulin	Beta blocker	May prolong and mask symptoms of low blood sugar (hypoglycemia) if it occurs.	This combination is frequently prescribed. Diabetics should monitor their blood sugar level to avoid hypoglycemic episodes.

*ACE indicates angiotensin-converting enzyme; NSAID, nonsteroidal anti-inflammatory drug; SSRI, selective serotonin reuptake inhibitor; and MAOI, monoamine oxidase inhibitor.

DRUG INTERACTIONS CHART (continued)

MEDICINES IN THIS DRUG CLASS*	MAY INTERACT WITH MEDICINES IN THIS DRUG CLASS*	CAUSING THIS EFFECT	ACTION REQUIRED
Insulin	Salicylate	May increase effect of insulin, causing low blood sugar.	Your doctor should monitor blood glucose level.
Iron supplement	Quinolone	May inhibit absorption of quinolone from intestine, decreasing its antibiotic effect.	Your doctor should avoid prescribing these drugs in combination.
Iron supplement	Tetracycline	May decrease absorption of tetracycline from intestine, decreasing its antibiotic effect.	You should avoid taking iron supplement within 4 hours of taking tetracycline.
Iron supplement	Thyroid hormone	May decrease effect of thyroid hormone, resulting in hypothyroidism.	You should take these drugs at least 4 hours apart. Your doctor should perform thyroid function blood tests regularly and adjust dose if necessary.
Loop diuretic	Digoxin	May lead to irregularities in heart rhythm if potassium and magnesium levels are lowered by diuretic therapy.	Your doctor should monitor digoxin, potassium, and magnesium levels and may need to prescribe potassium and magnesium supplements if levels are low.
Loop diuretic	Thiazide diuretic	May excessively increase urine production, resulting in low levels of magnesium and potassium.	You should monitor yourself for signs of dehydration. Your doctor should monitor potassium and magnesium levels.
Macrolide	Anticoagulant	May increase blood-thinning effect of anticoagulant and can cause bleeding.	Your doctor should monitor prothrombin time (time it takes blood to clot) frequently and adjust anticoagulant dose.
Macrolide	Anticonvulsant	May increase blood level of anticonvulsant, causing side effects such as unsteadiness, dizziness, and nausea.	Your doctor should check anticonvulsant level in blood frequently and adjust dose.
Macrolide	Antihistamine	May increase antihistamine level, which can cause death (in rare cases) due to toxic effect on heart.	Your doctor should not prescribe these drugs in combination.
Macrolide	Benzodiazepine	May increase or prolong effect of benzodiazepine, resulting in sedation and other side effects.	Your doctor should decrease benzodiazepine dose if excessive sedation or other side effects occur.
Macrolide	Cisapride	May increase cisapride level, which can cause death (in rare cases) due to toxic effect on heart.	Your doctor should not prescribe these drugs in combination.

*ACE indicates angiotensin-converting enzyme; NSAID, nonsteroidal anti-inflammatory drug; SSRI, selective serotonin reuptake inhibitor; and MAOI, monoamine oxidase inhibitor.

DRUG INTERACTIONS CHART (continued)

MEDICINES IN THIS DRUG CLASS*	MAY INTERACT WITH MEDICINES IN THIS DRUG CLASS*	CAUSING THIS EFFECT	ACTION REQUIRED
Macrolide	Corticosteroid	May increase activity and adverse effects of corticosteroid.	Your doctor should decrease corticosteroid dose if side effects occur.
Macrolide	Digoxin	May increase digoxin level, causing side effects such as nausea, vomiting, blurry or yellow vision (like looking through yellow-tinted glasses), or abnormally fast or slow heart rate.	Your doctor should monitor digoxin level and adjust dose. Call your doctor if you experience nausea.
Macrolide	Ergot alkaloid	May result in decreased blood supply to fingers and toes.	Your doctor should prescribe these drugs in combination with caution and decrease ergot alkaloid dose.
Macrolide	Theophylline	May increase theophylline level or decrease macrolide level, resulting in side effects such as nausea, vomiting, palpitations, and decreased antibiotic effect of macrolide.	Your doctor should prescribe these drugs in combination with caution and monitor theophylline level and adjust dose.
MAOI	Appetite suppressant containing phenylpropanolamine or phentermine	May cause dramatic elevations in blood pressure, resulting in brain hemorrhage and death.	Your doctor should not prescribe these drugs in combination. MAOI must be stopped for several weeks before appetite suppressant is prescribed.
MAOI	Buspirone	May result in high blood pressure.	Your doctor should not prescribe these drugs in combination or will advise you to wait 10 days after stopping MAOI before starting buspirone.
MAOI	Meperidine	May cause seizures, coma, and death.	Your doctor should not prescribe these drugs in combination.
MAOI	SSRI	May cause altered consciousness.	Your doctor should not prescribe these drugs in combination.
MAOI	Sumatriptan	May increase sumatriptan level and increase chances of coronary artery constriction (low blood flow to heart muscle), heart attack, and death.	Your doctor should not prescribe these drugs in combination.
MAOI	Tricyclic antidepressant (heterocyclic antidepressant)	May cause altered consciousness, seizures, and death.	Your doctor should not prescribe these drugs in combination.

*ACE indicates angiotensin-converting enzyme; NSAID, nonsteroidal anti-inflammatory drug; SSRI, selective serotonin reuptake inhibitor; and MAOI, monoamine oxidase inhibitor.

DRUG INTERACTIONS CHART (continued)

MEDICINES IN THIS DRUG CLASS*	MAY INTERACT WITH MEDICINES IN THIS DRUG CLASS*	CAUSING THIS EFFECT	ACTION REQUIRED
Meperidine	MAOI	May cause seizures, coma, and death.	Your doctor should not prescribe these drugs in combination.
Metformin	Cimetidine (a histamine$_2$ [H$_2$] blocker; see p.1161)	May increase metformin level.	Your doctor may need to decrease metformin dose.
Metformin	Iodinated contrast medium	Increases risk of dangerous acidification of blood (lactic acidosis).	Your doctor should not prescribe these drugs in combination.
Methotrexate	NSAID	Increases risk of methotrexate toxicity.	Call your doctor if you develop fever or signs of infection. Your doctor may order kidney tests and monitor methotrexate level.
Methotrexate	Salicylate	Increases risk of methotrexate toxicity.	Call your doctor if you develop fever or signs of infection. Your doctor may order kidney tests and monitor methotrexate level.
Methotrexate	Sulfa antibiotic	Increases risk of serious bone marrow suppression.	Call your doctor if you develop fatigue, fever, or signs of infection.
Metronidazole	Anticoagulant	May increase blood-thinning effect of anticoagulant and can cause bleeding.	Your doctor should monitor prothrombin time (time it takes blood to clot) frequently and adjust anticoagulant dose.
NSAID	ACE inhibitor	May make ACE inhibitor less effective in lowering blood pressure.	Your doctor should check blood pressure frequently.
NSAID	Anticoagulant	May increase risk of bleeding, even if anticoagulant is taken in proper dose.	Your doctor should avoid prescribing these drugs in combination or should monitor prothrombin time (time it takes blood to clot) frequently. Call your doctor if you bruise or bleed easily, see blood in your urine or bowel movements, or observe other signs of bleeding.
NSAID	Beta blocker	May reduce blood pressure–lowering effect of beta blocker.	Your doctor should monitor blood pressure and adjust beta blocker dose if necessary.
NSAID	Methotrexate	Increases risk of methotrexate toxicity.	Call your doctor if you develop fever or signs of infection. Your doctor may order kidney tests and monitor methotrexate level.

*ACE indicates angiotensin-converting enzyme; NSAID, nonsteroidal anti-inflammatory drug; SSRI, selective serotonin reuptake inhibitor; and MAOI, monoamine oxidase inhibitor.

DRUG INTERACTIONS CHART (continued)

MEDICINES IN THIS DRUG CLASS*	MAY INTERACT WITH MEDICINES IN THIS DRUG CLASS*	CAUSING THIS EFFECT	ACTION REQUIRED
Penicillin	Anticoagulant	May increase or decrease anticoagulant level, causing either bleeding or blood clots.	Your doctor should monitor prothrombin time (time it takes blood to clot) frequently and adjust anticoagulant dose.
Penicillin	Beta blocker	May reduce effectiveness of beta blocker.	Your doctor should monitor blood pressure and may need to increase beta blocker dose or advise you to take penicillin in smaller, more frequent doses.
Penicillin	Contraceptive (oral)	May reduce effectiveness of contraceptive.	You should use alternative form of birth control.
Penicillin	Tetracycline	May reduce effectiveness of penicillin.	Your doctor should avoid prescribing these drugs in combination.
Potassium supplement	Potassium-sparing diuretic	May increase potassium level, which can cause death (in rare cases) due to toxic effect on heart.	Your doctor should avoid prescribing these drugs in combination, unless very low potassium levels are documented, and monitor potassium level frequently.
Propoxyphene	Anticonvulsant	May increase blood level of anticonvulsant, causing side effects such as unsteadiness, dizziness, and nausea.	Your doctor should check anticonvulsant level in blood frequently and adjust dose.
Propoxyphene	Protease inhibitor	May cause dramatic increases in propoxyphene level.	Your doctor should not prescribe these drugs in combination.
Quinidine	Anticoagulant	May increase blood-thinning effect of anticoagulant and can cause bleeding.	Your doctor should monitor prothrombin time (time it takes blood to clot) frequently and adjust anticoagulant dose.
Quinidine	Calcium channel blocker	May increase effect of quinidine, resulting in low blood pressure or dangerously irregular heartbeat.	Your doctor should avoid prescribing these drugs in combination or monitor heart rate and blood pressure carefully.
Quinidine	Digoxin	May increase digoxin level, causing side effects such as nausea, vomiting, blurry or yellow vision (like looking through yellow-tinted glasses), or abnormally fast or slow heart rate.	Your doctor should monitor digoxin level and adjust dose. Call your doctor if you experience nausea.
Quinolone	Antacid containing calcium, aluminum, or magnesium	May decrease absorption of quinolone from intestine, decreasing its antibiotic effect.	You should avoid taking antacid at least 6 hours before and 2 hours after taking quinolone.

*ACE indicates angiotensin-converting enzyme; NSAID, nonsteroidal anti-inflammatory drug; SSRI, selective serotonin reuptake inhibitor; and MAOI, monoamine oxidase inhibitor.

DRUG INTERACTIONS CHART (continued)

MEDICINES IN THIS DRUG CLASS*	MAY INTERACT WITH MEDICINES IN THIS DRUG CLASS*	CAUSING THIS EFFECT	ACTION REQUIRED
Quinolone	Iron supplement	May inhibit absorption of quinolone from intestine, decreasing its antibiotic effect.	Your doctor should avoid prescribing these drugs in combination.
Quinolone	Theophylline	May increase theophylline level, causing side effects such as nausea, vomiting, and palpitations.	Your doctor should check theophylline blood level regularly and adjust dose if necessary.
Salicylate	ACE inhibitor	May make ACE inhibitor less effective in lowering blood pressure.	Your doctor should check blood pressure frequently.
Salicylate	Anticoagulant	May increase risk of bleeding, even if anticoagulant is taken in proper dose.	Your doctor should avoid prescribing these drugs in combination or should monitor prothrombin time (time it takes blood to clot) frequently. Call your doctor if you bruise or bleed easily, see blood in your urine or bowel movements, or observe other signs of bleeding.
Salicylate	Anticonvulsant	May increase blood level of anticonvulsant, causing side effects such as unsteadiness, dizziness, and nausea.	Your doctor should check anticonvulsant level in blood frequently and adjust dose.
Salicylate	Corticosteroid	May reduce effectiveness of salicylate and increase risk of peptic ulcer.	Your doctor should tailor salicylate dose as needed for pain control.
Salicylate	Insulin	May increase insulin effect, causing low blood sugar.	Your doctor should monitor blood glucose level.
Salicylate	Methotrexate	Increases risk of methotrexate toxicity.	Call your doctor if you develop fever or signs of infection. Your doctor may order kidney tests and monitor methotrexate level.
Salicylate	Sulfonylurea	May increase effectiveness of sulfonylurea, resulting in low blood sugar (hypoglycemia).	Your doctor should monitor blood glucose level to avoid hypoglycemia.
SSRI	Anticonvulsant	May increase blood level of anticonvulsant, causing side effects such as unsteadiness, dizziness, and nausea.	Your doctor should check anticonvulsant level in blood frequently and adjust dose.
SSRI	Antihistamine	May increase antihistamine level, which can cause death (in rare cases) due to toxic effect on heart.	Your doctor should not prescribe these drugs in combination.

*ACE indicates angiotensin-converting enzyme; NSAID, nonsteroidal anti-inflammatory drug; SSRI, selective serotonin reuptake inhibitor; and MAOI, monoamine oxidase inhibitor.

DRUG INTERACTIONS CHART (continued)

MEDICINES IN THIS DRUG CLASS*	MAY INTERACT WITH MEDICINES IN THIS DRUG CLASS*	CAUSING THIS EFFECT	ACTION REQUIRED
SSRI	Appetite suppressant containing phenylpropanolamine or phentermine	May cause anxiety, agitation, and tremors.	Your doctor should prescribe these drugs in combination with caution and will advise you to stop taking the appetite suppressant if side effects develop.
SSRI	Cisapride	May increase cisapride level, which can cause death (in rare cases) due to toxic effect on heart.	Your doctor should not prescribe these drugs in combination.
SSRI	MAOI	May cause altered consciousness.	Your doctor should not prescribe these drugs in combination.
SSRI	Tricyclic antidepressant (heterocyclic antidepressant)	May increase level of tricyclic antidepressant, causing side effects such as abnormal heart rhythms, increased heart rate, and drowsiness.	Your doctor should avoid prescribing these drugs in combination or decrease tricyclic antidepressant dose.
Sulfa antibiotic	Anticoagulant	May increase blood-thinning effect of anticoagulant and can cause bleeding.	Your doctor should monitor prothrombin time (time it takes blood to clot) frequently and adjust anticoagulant dose.
Sulfa antibiotic	Anticonvulsant	May increase anticonvulsant effect.	Your doctor should check anticonvulsant level in blood frequently and adjust dose.
Sulfa antibiotic	Cyclosporine	Increases risk of cyclosporine-induced kidney damage and may reduce cyclosporine level, leading to transplant rejection.	Your doctor should prescribe these drugs in combination with caution or monitor kidney function and cyclosporine level with frequent blood tests.
Sulfa antibiotic	Methotrexate	Increases risk of serious bone marrow suppression.	Call your doctor if you develop fatigue, fever, or signs of infection.
Sulfa antibiotic	Sulfonylurea	May prolong effect of sulfonylurea, resulting in low blood sugar (hypoglycemia).	Your doctor should monitor blood glucose level and decrease sulfonylurea dose if necessary.
Sulfonylurea	Salicylate	May increase effectiveness of sulfonylurea, resulting in low blood sugar (hypoglycemia).	Your doctor should monitor blood glucose level to avoid hypoglycemia.
Sulfonylurea	Sulfa antibiotic	May prolong effect of sulfonylurea, resulting in low blood sugar (hypoglycemia).	Your doctor should monitor blood glucose level and decrease sulfonylurea dose if necessary.

*ACE indicates angiotensin-converting enzyme; NSAID, nonsteroidal anti-inflammatory drug; SSRI, selective serotonin reuptake inhibitor; and MAOI, monoamine oxidase inhibitor.

DRUG INTERACTIONS CHART (continued)

MEDICINES IN THIS DRUG CLASS*	MAY INTERACT WITH MEDICINES IN THIS DRUG CLASS*	CAUSING THIS EFFECT	ACTION REQUIRED
Sulfonylurea	Thiazide diuretic	May reduce effectiveness of sulfonylurea.	Your doctor should monitor blood glucose level and increase sulfonylurea dose if necessary.
Sumatriptan	Ergot alkaloid	May increase severity of side effects such as flushing, tingling, abnormal heart rhythms, and angina.	You should take these drugs at least 24 hours apart.
Sumatriptan	MAOI	May increase sumatriptan level and increase chances of coronary artery constriction (low blood flow to heart muscle), heart attack, and death.	Your doctor should not prescribe these drugs in combination.
Tetracycline	Antacid containing calcium, aluminum, or magnesium	May decrease absorption of tetracycline from intestine, decreasing its antibiotic effect.	You should avoid taking antacid within 4 hours of taking tetracycline.
Tetracycline	Anticonvulsant	Decreases antibiotic effectiveness of tetracycline.	Your doctor may need to increase tetracycline dose.
Tetracycline	Calcium supplement	May bind to tetracycline in intestine, lowering its level in the blood, which may decrease its antibiotic effectiveness.	You should avoid taking calcium within 4 hours of taking tetracycline.
Tetracycline	Contraceptive (oral)	May reduce effectiveness of contraceptive.	You should use alternative form of birth control.
Tetracycline	Digoxin	May increase digoxin level, causing side effects such as nausea, vomiting, blurry or yellow vision (like looking through yellow-tinted glasses), or abnormally fast or slow heart rate.	Your doctor should monitor digoxin level and adjust dose. Call your doctor if you experience nausea.
Tetracycline	Iron supplement	May decrease absorption of tetracycline from intestine, decreasing its antibiotic effect.	You should avoid taking iron supplement within 4 hours of taking tetracycline.
Tetracycline	Penicillin	May reduce effectiveness of penicillin.	Your doctor should avoid prescribing these drugs in combination.
Tetracycline	Zinc	May inhibit absorption of tetracycline from intestine, decreasing its antibiotic effect.	You should avoid taking zinc within 4 hours of taking tetracycline.

*ACE indicates angiotensin-converting enzyme; NSAID, nonsteroidal anti-inflammatory drug; SSRI, selective serotonin reuptake inhibitor; and MAOI, monoamine oxidase inhibitor.

DRUG INTERACTIONS CHART (continued)

MEDICINES IN THIS DRUG CLASS*	MAY INTERACT WITH MEDICINES IN THIS DRUG CLASS*	CAUSING THIS EFFECT	ACTION REQUIRED
Theophylline	Anticonvulsant	May increase or decrease effect of either medicine, resulting in side effects such as unsteadiness, dizziness, nausea, and palpitations.	Your doctor should monitor levels of both drugs and adjust doses.
Theophylline	Beta blocker	May increase theophylline level or decrease effect of both medicines.	Your doctor should monitor theophylline level frequently and check heart rate and blood pressure.
Theophylline	Calcium channel blocker	May increase effect of theophylline.	Your doctor should monitor theophylline level and adjust dose.
Theophylline	Cimetidine (a histamine$_2$ [H$_2$] blocker; see p.1161)	May increase theophylline level, resulting in side effects such as nausea, vomiting, and palpitations.	Your doctor should monitor theophylline level.
Theophylline	Contraceptive (oral)	May increase theophylline level, causing side effects such as nausea, vomiting, and palpitations.	Your doctor should monitor theophylline level and adjust dose.
Theophylline	Macrolide	May increase theophylline level or decrease macrolide level, resulting in side effects such as nausea, vomiting, palpitations, and decreased antibiotic effect of macrolide.	Your doctor should prescribe these drugs in combination with caution and monitor theophylline level and adjust dose.
Theophylline	Quinolone	May increase theophylline level, causing side effects such as nausea, vomiting, and palpitations.	Your doctor should monitor theophylline level regularly and adjust dose if necessary.
Theophylline	Thyroid hormone	May increase or decrease theophylline level.	Your doctor should monitor theophylline level and adjust dose if necessary.
Thiazide diuretic	Digoxin	May lead to irregularities in heart rhythm if potassium and magnesium levels are lowered by diuretic therapy.	Your doctor should monitor digoxin, potassium, and magnesium levels and may need to prescribe potassium and magnesium supplements if levels are low.
Thiazide diuretic	Loop diuretic	May excessively increase urine production, resulting in low levels of magnesium and potassium.	You should monitor yourself for signs of dehydration. Your doctor should monitor potassium and magnesium levels.

*ACE indicates angiotensin-converting enzyme; NSAID, nonsteroidal anti-inflammatory drug; SSRI, selective serotonin reuptake inhibitor; and MAOI, monoamine oxidase inhibitor.

DRUG INTERACTIONS CHART (continued)

MEDICINES IN THIS DRUG CLASS*	MAY INTERACT WITH MEDICINES IN THIS DRUG CLASS*	CAUSING THIS EFFECT	ACTION REQUIRED
Thiazide diuretic	Sulfonylurea	May reduce effectiveness of sulfonylurea.	Your doctor should monitor blood glucose level and increase sulfonylurea dose if necessary.
Thyroid function inhibitor	Anticoagulant	May increase or decrease blood-thinning effect of anticoagulant, causing bleeding or clotting.	Your doctor should monitor prothrombin time (time it takes blood to clot) frequently and adjust anticoagulant dose.
Thyroid hormone	Anticoagulant	Increases blood-thinning effect of anticoagulant and can cause bleeding.	Your doctor should monitor prothrombin time (time it takes blood to clot) frequently and adjust anticoagulant dose if necessary.
Thyroid hormone	Digoxin	May decrease digoxin level.	Your doctor should monitor digoxin level and adjust dose if necessary.
Thyroid hormone	Iron supplement	May decrease effect of thyroid hormone, resulting in hypothyroidism.	You should take these drugs at least 4 hours apart. Your doctor should perform thyroid function blood tests regularly and adjust dose if necessary.
Thyroid hormone	Theophylline	May increase or decrease theophylline level.	Your doctor should monitor theophylline level and adjust dose if necessary.
Tricyclic antidepressant	Anticonvulsant	May increase blood level of anticonvulsant, causing side effects such as unsteadiness, dizziness, and nausea.	Your doctor should check anticonvulsant level in blood frequently and adjust dose.
Tricyclic antidepressant (heterocyclic antidepressant)	Cimetidine (a histamine$_2$ [H$_2$] blocker; see p.1161)	May increase antidepressant level, causing side effects such as abnormal heart rhythm, increased heart rate, and drowsiness.	Your doctor should avoid prescribing these drugs in combination or monitor antidepressant level and lower dose if necessary.
Tricyclic antidepressant (heterocyclic antidepressant)	Clonidine	May cause dramatic elevation in blood pressure.	Your doctor should avoid prescribing these drugs in combination.
Tricyclic antidepressant (heterocyclic antidepressant)	MAOI	May cause altered consciousness, seizures, and death.	Your doctor should not prescribe these drugs in combination.

*ACE indicates angiotensin-converting enzyme; NSAID, nonsteroidal anti-inflammatory drug; SSRI, selective serotonin reuptake inhibitor; and MAOI, monoamine oxidase inhibitor.

DRUG INTERACTIONS CHART (continued)

MEDICINES IN THIS DRUG CLASS*	MAY INTERACT WITH MEDICINES IN THIS DRUG CLASS*	CAUSING THIS EFFECT	ACTION REQUIRED
Tricyclic antidepressant (heterocyclic antidepressant)	SSRI	May increase level of antidepressant, causing side effects such as abnormal heart rhythm, increased heart rate, and drowsiness.	Your doctor should avoid prescribing these drugs in combination or decrease antidepressant dose if necessary.
Vitamin E	Anticoagulant	May increase blood-thinning effect of anticoagulant and can cause bleeding.	Your doctor should monitor prothrombin time (time it takes blood to clot) frequently and adjust anticoagulant dose.
Zinc	Tetracycline	May inhibit absorption of tetracycline from intestine, decreasing its antibiotic effect.	You should avoid taking zinc within 4 hours of taking tetracycline.
Zolpidem	Protease inhibitor	May cause severe sedation and respiratory depression.	Your doctor should not prescribe these drugs in combination.

*ACE indicates angiotensin-converting enzyme; NSAID, nonsteroidal anti-inflammatory drug; SSRI, selective serotonin reuptake inhibitor; and MAOI, monoamine oxidase inhibitor.

First Aid and Emergency Care

This chapter provides basic information on first aid and emergency care. Read it thoroughly so that you will be prepared if an emergency occurs.

Preventing emergencies is essential. Your home should be equipped with fire extinguishers and with smoke and carbon monoxide detectors placed strategically on every level. If you have children, make your house safe for them. For more information about preventive measures, see Safety and Preventing Injury, p.86.

Most first aid is direct care: washing a wound, stopping minor bleeding, or applying a bandage. In an emergency, however, you may be required to perform more complex procedures, such as assisting a person who is not breathing.

The basic life-support measures you should follow in an emergency are outlined in this chapter, but many of them, such as performing cardiopulmonary resuscitation (CPR), are best learned in a classroom setting.

In any emergency, it is essential to phone 911 or your local emergency number for expert assistance. You should also keep your local poison control center number readily accessible for family members, guests, babysitters, or caregivers.

EMERGENCY CHECKLIST

This list describes your priorities in an emergency situation. Follow these steps:

1 Evaluate the scene to protect yourself and others from injury or danger.

2 Be calm and reassuring.

3 Do not move the person unless he or she is in imminent danger, or unless you cannot provide assistance without moving the person.

4 Get help. Call out for someone to phone 911 or, if the person does not need immediate assistance, make the call yourself.

5 If the situation is a choking emergency, perform the Heimlich maneuver (see Choking, p.1206).

6 Look, listen, and feel for breathing (see Breathing Difficulties, p.1198).

7 Feel for a pulse to determine if the heart is beating (see step 4, p.1203).

8 Control bleeding with direct pressure (see p.1197).

9 Treat for shock (see p.1216).

10 If the person is unconscious, move him or her into the recovery position (see p.1193).

BASIC LIFESAVING TECHNIQUES

Mouth-to-mouth resuscitation (see p.1198) and cardiopulmonary resuscitation (CPR) (see p.1201) are essential lifesaving techniques. To perform them correctly, you must take classes and become certified. Call your local hospital, fire department, the American Red Cross, or the American Heart Association to locate instruction near you. If you have taken a course previously, make sure your skills are up-to-date.

MEDICAL IDENTIFICATION TAGS

A person with a serious medical condition—such as diabetes, a drug allergy, or a heart condition—should carry information about the condition on a necklace or bracelet, or on a card that can be carried in a pocket or wallet, so that proper care can be given in an emergency.

Be sure to check for a medallion or card if you find yourself in the role of rescuer. If you or a member of your family has a life-threatening medical condition, obtain a medical identification tag or medallion from your local pharmacy and wear it at all times.

EMERGENCY CARE: A TO Z

Allergic Reaction

(See also Bites and Stings, p.1194)
A severe allergic reaction (to food, medicine, or an insect sting), called anaphylaxis, can be life-threatening.

Signs and symptoms include difficulty breathing or swallowing; swelling of the face, neck, and mouth; coughing; wheezing; choking; light-headedness; itching; rash; red tinge to the skin; shock; and unconsciousness.

If the person can talk, ask if he or she is allergic to anything and is carrying epinephrine, which calms the reaction.

Epinephrine may be in the form of an automatic injector or a preloaded syringe. Directions should be included with either device.

Mild allergic reactions (including localized redness, itching, or hives) are irritating, but not serious.

Immediate care Check and open the airway (see Cardiopulmonary Resuscitation, p.1201). Call out for someone to get help, or call 911 yourself if the person does not need immediate assistance.

If the person is carrying epinephrine, help inject it. Administer an antihistamine, if it is available and the person can swallow.

For mild reactions, such as hives, antihistamines may be helpful until assistance can be obtained. Otherwise, help the person get into a position that is most comfortable for breathing. Stay with the person until medical help arrives.

A Well-Stocked First-Aid Kit

A fishing tackle box or a rectangular sealed plastic container makes an ideal first-aid kit. It is wise to keep one in your home, car, boat, or camper. Stock your first-aid kit with the following items:

- One roll of absorbent cotton
- Antihistamine for allergic reactions
- Povidone-iodine antiseptic solution
- Aspirin (for adult use only) and acetaminophen and ibuprofen (in child and adult dosages)
- 1-inch wide adhesive tape
- Bacitracin ointment to treat cuts, scrapes, or puncture wounds
- Bandages in various sizes
- Bar of soap
- Butterfly bandages and thin adhesive strips to hold skin edges together
- Calamine lotion
- Cold pack
- Mouthpiece for protection when performing mouth-to-mouth resuscitation

- Cotton-tipped swabs
- Syrup of ipecac to induce vomiting
- Elastic bandage or wrap
- Eyedropper for irrigating
- Flashlight
- 4-inch x 4-inch gauze pads
- Disposable surgical gloves
- Matches
- Saline eyedrops
- Scissors
- Safety pins
- Sewing needle to help remove a splinter
- Four packets of sugar in a sealed plastic bag to use in case of low blood sugar (see Diabetic Emergencies, p.1207)
- Thermometer
- Two triangular pieces of cloth to use as slings or to cut up as bandages or straps
- Tweezers

Amputation

(See Severed Limbs, p.1215)

Animal Bites

(See Bites and Stings, p.1194)

Asthma

(See also Asthma, p.505)
Asthma is a narrowing of the
bronchial tubes in the lungs. A
person having an asthma attack
may have difficulty breathing
(especially exhaling), wheeze,
become anxious (attempting to
get more air), or turn blue.

Immediate care Ask the person if he or she has asthma and
is carrying an inhaler. Help administer the inhaler. Otherwise,
call out for someone to get help,
or call 911 yourself if the person
does not need immediate assistance. If the person has no history of asthma or heart problems,
treat for a severe allergic reaction
(see p.1191). Help the person
into a position that is comfortable
for breathing (usually sitting
upright). Stay with the person
until medical help arrives.

Back and Neck Injuries

(See also Unconsciousness, p.1217)
Back and neck injuries are always
serious. Broken vertebrae can
damage or sever the spinal cord.
Never move the person unless
the situation is life-threatening
(such as a fire, explosion, or
falling building).

Always suspect back, neck,
and head injuries if you come
upon a person in the water who
is unconscious (the person may
have been in a diving accident);
who has fallen from a height; or
who has been in a vehicle or
bicycle collision.

Moving a Person With a Suspected Back Injury

Unless the person is able to tell you to the contrary, assume that anyone
with a back injury also has a neck injury.

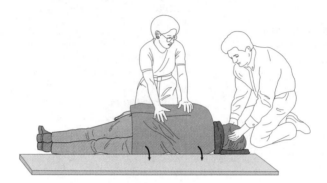

Place a board, such as a door or table leaf, next to the person. The board
should extend below the buttocks (ideally to the feet) and above the
head. Keeping the head aligned with the rest of the body, gently logroll
the person toward you. Move the board under the person and ease him
or her onto it. If the person is vomiting, lay him or her on one side and
continue to support the head.

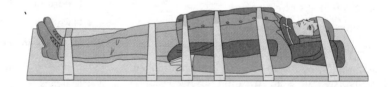

To immobilize the person, tie the person to the board with a rope, shirt,
belt, or strips of cloth at the ankles, legs, chest, and across the forehead.
Tie tightly enough so the person cannot move, but not so tightly that
you cut off circulation or inhibit breathing. Place towels, sweaters, or pillows snugly around the person, especially alongside the head and neck.
Once immobilized, the person can be carefully moved to safety.

If the person is conscious,
symptoms may include neck stiffness or pain, headache, back
pain, tingling sensation in hands
and feet, or inability to move
arms or legs.

Immediate care Call out for
someone to get help, or call 911
yourself if the person does not
need immediate assistance.
Check airway, breathing, and circulation (see Cardiopulmonary

Recovery Position

Adult Recovery Position

This position helps a semiconscious or unconscious person breathe and permits fluids to drain from the nose and throat so they are not breathed in. If the person is unconscious or semiconscious after you have done everything on the Emergency Checklist (see p.1190), move the person into the recovery position while waiting for help to arrive.

Do not use the recovery position if the person has a major injury, such as a back or neck injury (see p.1192).

Infant Recovery Position

Place the infant facedown over your arm with the head slightly lower than the body. Support the head and neck with your hand, keeping the mouth and nose clear. Wait for help to arrive.

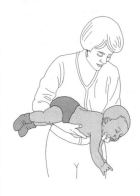

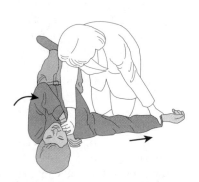

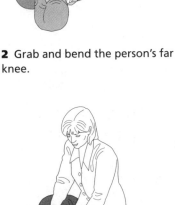

1 Kneel next to the person. Place the arm closest to you straight out from the body. Position the far arm with the back of the hand against the near cheek.

2 Grab and bend the person's far knee.

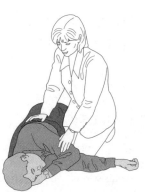

3 Protecting the head with one hand, gently roll the person toward you by pulling the far knee over and to the ground.

4 Tilt the head up slightly so that the airway is open. Make sure that the hand is under the cheek. Place a blanket or coat over the person (unless he or she has a heat illness or fever) and stay close until help arrives.

Emergency Telephone Numbers

Write down important telephone numbers and post them where you can refer to them easily, such as near your telephone or on your refrigerator. List the serious medical conditions (such as asthma or diabetes) of each family member on the back of the list. Teach your children how to call 911 and tell them to show the list to emergency medical personnel.

The list should include the phone numbers of the police, the nearest fire department, ambulance services, a poison control center, and your doctors and the contact numbers for work, other locations, and a nearby relative or friend. You may also wish to include the phone numbers of the gas and electric companies, your children's schools, the local pharmacy, or home health aides.

Resuscitation, p.1201). If you must move the person, follow the steps in Moving a Person With a Suspected Back Injury, p.1192.

Bandages
(See Bleeding, p.1196)

Bites and Stings

A bite from a dog, cat, wild animal, or human can lead to infection. Many animals transmit rabies (see p.380) and tetanus (see p.880). A human bite always requires medical attention to rule out infection. Bee, wasp, or scorpion stings can cause severe swelling and in some cases can lead to a serious allergic reaction (see Allergic Reaction, p.1191).

ANIMAL AND HUMAN BITES

Go to a hospital emergency department for any bite caused by a human, cat, monkey, raccoon, or bat; for any animal bite that is on the face, neck, or hands; or for a bite that is deep or extensive.

Immediate care Wash the wound thoroughly with running water for 5 minutes to remove dirt and bacteria. Gently pat the wound dry and place a sterile bandage on it. Bacitracin ointment will help keep the bandage from sticking. Contact police or animal control if the bite was unprovoked or caused by an unknown or stray animal.

BEE, WASP, AND HORNET STINGS

While the sting of a wasp or hornet is painful, only a honeybee leaves a stinger.

Immediate care If stung by a honeybee, do not wait to remove the stinger. Remove it immediately by pulling it out, using two fingernails. Do not scrape the stinger off with a fingernail or knife. For all stings, put a cold compress (such as ice wrapped in a towel) on the site of the sting. The area may be red, swollen, and painful for several days; taking an antihistamine may alleviate some symptoms. If a severe reaction occurs, treat as for allergic reactions (see p.1191).

JELLYFISH AND PORTUGUESE MAN-OF-WAR STINGS

A sting from a jellyfish or a Portuguese man-of-war is poisonous and causes intense, burning pain at the site of the sting. A Portuguese man-of-war can leave stingers attached to the skin.

Symptoms, which can be serious, include breathing difficulties (see p.1198) and unconsciousness (see p.1217).

Immediate care Apply calamine lotion to a jellyfish sting to help relieve pain or place a cold compress (such as ice wrapped in a towel) on the site. For Portuguese man-o-war stings, call out for someone to get help, or call 911 yourself if the person does not need immediate assistance. Do not attempt to remove stingers that are attached to the skin.

Watch the person for signs of an allergic reaction (see p.1191). Scraping the stingers off can cause further damage. Instead, use vinegar or salt water (not fresh water) to wash the attached stingers (fresh water may cause the tentacles to sting). Place the person in a comfortable position and keep him or her warm until medical help arrives.

SEA URCHIN WOUNDS

Sea urchins are colorful, spiny, hard-shelled animals that live in shallow water along seacoasts. They are a temptation for children to handle and they are easy to step on. Although few are poisonous, a sea urchin spine can puncture the skin and leave a portion of the spine imbedded deep in tissue, causing infection.

Immediate care Do not attempt to remove a spine that is protruding from the skin. It is fragile and may break. Go to a hospital emergency department to have it removed properly.

If the spine is no longer in the skin, pain may be eased by immersion in hot (not scalding) water.

SCORPION STINGS

There are several varieties of scorpions and the stings of some are more poisonous than others. Symptoms include burning, tingling, or numbness at the site of the sting; stomach pain, nausea, and vomiting; muscle twitching (including the jaw muscle); seizures (see p.374); or unconsciousness (see p.1217).

Immediate care Keep the bitten area lower than the person's heart to prevent the spread of venom. Place a cold compress (such as ice wrapped in a towel) on the site of the bite. Take the person to the nearest hospital emergency department.

SNAKEBITES

There are four kinds of poisonous snakes in the United States: copperhead, water moccasin (cottonmouth), rattlesnake, and coral snake. Snakes do not seek out human beings but will strike if provoked. A juvenile poisonous snake can deliver as much venom as an adult. A poisonous snakebite always requires medical attention.

Copperhead The copperhead is found primarily in the southeast and south central areas of the United States. Its light and dark brown markings help it blend in perfectly with forest terrain.

Water moccasin (cottonmouth) The water moccasin is found in the southeast and south central areas of the United States. It is so named because of the white lining in its mouth. This snake's habitat is marshes and rivers.

Rattlesnake Rattlesnakes are found across the United States. A distinctive rattle at the end of the tail warns predators when they are too close. Rattlesnakes prefer dry, rocky surroundings.

Coral snake The coral snake, a member of the cobra family, is the most brightly colored and most deadly of the poisonous snakes in the United States. It has yellow, red, and black rings and a black nose. It can be found in bushes and gardens of the southeastern United States.

Immediate care Move the person away from the snake or area where the bite occurred; a cornered or injured snake can strike several times. Have the person lie down and remain calm. If the bite occurred on a finger, hand, or arm, remove all jewelry. Keep the bitten area lower than the heart, and immediately place a cold compress (such as ice wrapped in a towel) on the bite.

Take the person to the nearest hospital emergency department. Do not use a tourniquet unless you have experience in doing so. Do not suck out any venom. Do not give the person anything to eat or drink. For nonpoisonous snakebites, see Puncture Wounds, p.1215.

If you can do so safely, catch the snake. If you have killed it, keep it as intact as possible so that medical personnel can determine if it is poisonous.

Distinguishing Dangerous Coral Snakes From Safe Look-Alikes: Dr Walls' Advice

There are several species of nonpoisonous snakes that look like the coral snake. How do you tell the dangerous coral snakes from the look-alikes? The difference lies in the placement of the colored rings on the snake's body; coral snakes have red rings next to yellow rings.

Here's the rhyme I recommend to help distinguish poisonous coral snakes from all others: "Red next to yellow, kill a fellow. Red next to black, venom lack." (The rhyme applies only to snakes in the United States and does not hold true in other parts of the world.)

However, if you are bitten by any snake with red, yellow, and black rings, don't take a chance. Kill the snake (be careful not to get bitten again) and take it to the emergency department with you. Symptoms can be delayed and severe, so, unless the snake can be clearly identified, the doctor will likely presume the snake was poisonous and give you an antidote to the poison.

RON M. WALLS, MD
BRIGHAM AND WOMEN'S HOSPITAL
HARVARD MEDICAL SCHOOL

SPIDER BITES

Spiders as a group are nonaggressive and bite only when threatened. However, a bite from a black widow or brown recluse spider is poisonous and always requires medical attention. Both of these spiders live in protected places, such as woodpiles, undisturbed areas of an attic or garage, or under rocks. Bites can be especially dangerous to young children, the elderly, and people who are ill.

Black widow The black widow spider looks like a shiny black button, is about 1½ inches long (including its legs), and has a red hourglass-shaped spot (or two red spots) on its abdomen.

Symptoms of its bite include pain, redness, and swelling at the site of the bite; profuse sweating; stomach cramps; nausea and vomiting; and sometimes breathing difficulties (see p.1198).

Immediate care Keep the bit-ten area lower than the person's heart to prevent the spread of venom. Place a cold compress (such as ice wrapped in a towel) on the site of the bite. Take the person to the nearest hospital emergency department. If possible, carefully catch the spider and take it with you. Do not kill it—you may render it unidentifiable.

Brown recluse The brown recluse or "fiddleback" spider is golden brown, ¼ to ¾ inches long (not including its legs), and has what looks like a fiddle or violin design on its head. The fiddle design may be dark brown or black and shiny.

A brown recluse's bite can lead to severe tissue damage if not treated promptly. Symptoms include burning at the site of the bite, redness, and the formation of a blister, which may look like a bull's-eye. Pain can worsen during the 8 hours after the bite. Fever, chills, nausea and vomit-ing, and sometimes a skin rash may occur within 48 hours.

Immediate care Keep the bit-ten area lower than the person's heart to prevent the spread of venom. Place a cold compress (such as ice wrapped in a towel) on the site of the bite. Take the person to the nearest hospital emergency department. If possible, carefully catch the spider and take it with you. Do not kill it—you may render it unidentifiable.

TICK BITES

If you find a tick attached to the skin, grip it firmly with tweezers pressed flat against the skin, just where the head is attached. (See p.882 for an illustration of proper tick removal.) The head should be firmly gripped as close to the skin as possible and the entire tick removed. Successful removal will result in a brief tugging sensation; the person will feel a small pinch. A tiny piece of skin will remain attached to the tick's mouth parts. If you believe removal has not been complete, see your doctor.

Bleeding

(See also Scrapes and Scratches, p.1215)

While a minor cut will eventually stop bleeding, a severe injury may require elevation and direct pressure on the wound. The goals of first-aid treatment are to control bleeding and prevent infection. If disposable surgical gloves are readily available, use them.

MINOR CUTS

A minor cut damages the outer layer of skin.

Immediate care Wash the skin around the wound with

**Bottom View of
Black Widow Spider**

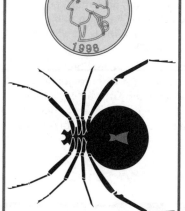
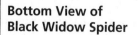

**Top View of
Brown Recluse Spider**

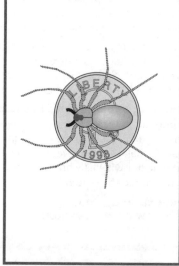

Butterfly Bandage

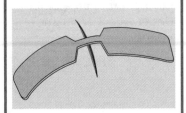

Standard bandages come in a variety of shapes and sizes. The butterfly bandage shown here is used to hold together the edges of a cut.

soap and water. Hold the wound under vigorously running water for 5 minutes to remove all dirt and bacteria. Gently pat it dry, apply bacitracin ointment, and place a sterile bandage over it.

GAPING WOUNDS

If a wound does not come together at its edges or is longer than 1/2 inch, wrap a gauze bandage (or clean T-shirt or sock) around it and go to your doctor's office or a hospital emergency department. Always go to the emergency department for a wound that has glass in it; is on the face, hands, or bottom of the foot; or occurs in a person with poor circulation.

If an object is sticking out of the wound, do not remove it. Being careful to avoid the object, lightly wrap a gauze bandage around the injury and go to the nearest hospital emergency department.

SEVERE BLEEDING

A wound that is deep, bleeding heavily, or has blood spurting from it (caused by bleeding from an artery), may not clot and may

Direct Pressure for Bleeding

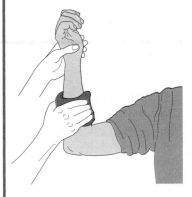
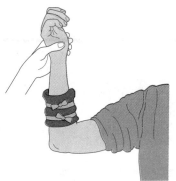

1 Elevate the wound above the heart and apply firm pressure with a clean compress (such as a clean, heavy gauze pad, washcloth, T-shirt, or sock) directly on the wound. Call out for someone to get help, or call 911 yourself. Do not remove a pad that is soaked through with blood; you will disturb any blood clots that have started to form to help stop the bleeding. If blood soaks through, place another pad on top of the soaked one and continue applying direct pressure.

2 When the bleeding slows or stops, tie the pad firmly in place with gauze strips, a necktie, strips of sheet, or a shoelace. Do not tie so tightly that blood flow to the rest of the limb is cut off. Stay with the person and keep the wound elevated until medical help arrives.

Pressure Points for Bleeding

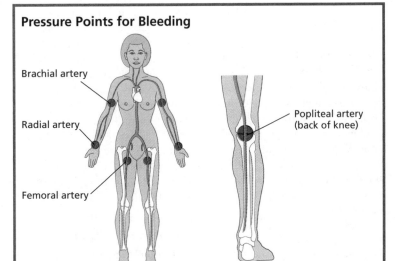

The circles show places to apply direct pressure on an artery in order to stop the flow of blood from an injury.

How to Stop a Nosebleed

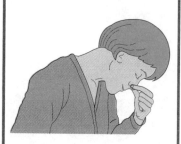

■ Firmly pinch the entire soft part of the nose just above the nostrils.

■ Sit and lean forward (this will ensure that blood and other secretions do not go down your throat).

■ Breathe through your mouth.

Hold this position for 5 minutes. If bleeding continues, hold the position for an additional 10 minutes. If bleeding does not stop, go to the nearest hospital emergency department.

not stop bleeding.

Immediate care Call out for someone to get help, or call 911 yourself. Elevate the wound and apply direct pressure.

PRESSURE POINTS FOR SEVERE BLEEDING

If severe bleeding does not stop with direct pressure and elevation, apply direct pressure to an artery. Use direct pressure on an artery along with elevation and direct pressure on the wound. There are specific major arteries in the body where pressure should be placed (see illustration on facing page).

When you apply pressure to an artery, you stop bleeding by pushing the artery against bone. Press down firmly on the artery between the bleeding site and the

heart. If there is severe bleeding, also apply firm pressure directly to the bleeding site.

To check if bleeding has stopped, release your fingers slowly from the pressure point, but do not release pressure at the bleeding site. If bleeding continues, continue to apply pressure to the artery. Continue until the bleeding stops or until help arrives. After bleeding stops, do not continue to apply pressure to an artery for longer than 5 minutes.

INTERNAL BLEEDING

Suspect internal bleeding if a person has been in a vehicle or bicycle collision, fallen from a height, or suffered a severe blow to the body or head.

Signs and symptoms include coughing up or vomiting blood (or a substance that looks like coffee grounds); pain in the chest, abdomen, or pelvic area; cool, clammy skin; or a rapid or weak pulse.

Immediate care Call out for someone to get help, or call 911 yourself if the person does not need immediate assistance. Check airway, breathing, and circulation (see Cardiopulmonary Resuscitation, p.1201). If a neck or back injury is possible, see Back and Neck Injuries (p.1192) for guidance. If the person is vomiting, turn him or her on one side to prevent choking. Treat for shock (see p.1216). Stay with the person until medical help arrives.

Breathing Difficulties

(See also Cardiopulmonary Resuscitation, p.1201; Asthma, p.1192) Breathing problems can occur for a number of reasons: the person

Mouth-to-Mouth-and-Nose Resuscitation on a Child Under Age 8 or on an Infant

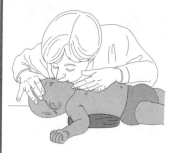

■ Place the child on a hard, flat surface.

■ Look into the mouth and throat to ensure that the airway is clear. If an object is present, try to sweep it out with your fingers. If unsuccessful and the object is blocking the airway, apply the Heimlich maneuver (see p.1206). If vomiting occurs, turn the child onto his or her side and sweep out the mouth with two fingers.

■ Tilt the head back slightly to open the airway.

■ Place your mouth tightly over the nose and mouth. Blow two quick, shallow breaths (smaller breaths than you would give to an adult). Watch for the chest to rise.

■ Remove your mouth. Look for the chest to fall as the child exhales.

■ Listen for the sounds of breathing. Feel for the child's breath on your cheek. If breathing does not start on its own, repeat the procedure.

may have asthma (see p.505) or a sudden lung problem, may be choking (see p.1206), may be having a serious allergic reaction (see p.1191) or heart attack (see p.1212), or may have had a serious injury.

Mouth-to-Mouth Resuscitation on a Child Age 8 or Older or on an Adult

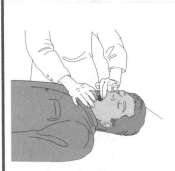

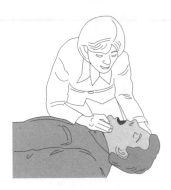

1 Make sure the person is lying on a hard, flat surface. Look into the mouth and throat to ensure that the airway is clear. If an object is present, try to sweep it out with your fingers (wear disposable surgical gloves if they are available). Apply the Heimlich maneuver (see p.1206) if unsuccessful and the object is blocking the airway. If vomiting occurs, turn the person on his or her side and sweep out the mouth with two fingers. Do not place your finger in the mouth if the person is rigid or is having a seizure.

2 Tilt the head back slightly to open the airway. Put upward pressure on the jaw to pull it forward.

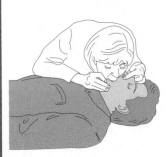

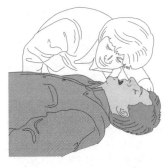

3 Pinch the nostrils closed with thumb and index finger. Place your mouth tightly over the person's mouth. Use a mouthpiece if one is available. Blow two quick breaths and watch for the person's chest to rise.

4 Release the nostrils. Look for the person's chest to fall as he or she exhales. Listen for the sounds of breathing. Feel for the person's breath on your cheek. If the person does not start breathing on his or her own, repeat the procedure.

Immediate care Call out for someone to get help, or call 911 yourself if the person does not need immediate assistance. If you do not see the person's chest rise and fall and you do not hear or feel any breathing, start mouth-to mouth resuscitation (see left and on the previous page) immediately.

Breathing, Lack of
(See Cardiopulmonary Resuscitation, p.1201)

Broken Bones

Broken bones (fractures) are usually not life-threatening. A fracture may not be visible to you through the skin. Symptoms include intense pain, swelling, increased pain when trying to move the injured area, or bleeding. A broken bone always requires medical attention.

Immediate care Call out for someone to get help, or call 911 yourself. Do not move or straighten the broken bone. Splinting is not necessary unless the person needs to be moved without assistance from ambulance personnel, or unless the fracture has blocked blood supply to the limb. If the fracture site is deformed and the skin beyond the site of the fracture is cold, pale, and blue, pull gently lengthwise on the limb to straighten the fracture and then splint the limb.

Burns

A burn can be caused by sunlight, fire, a hot substance or surface, a chemical, or an electric current.

Burns are classified according

How to Make a Sling

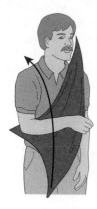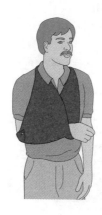

1 To make a sling, cut a piece of cloth, such as a pillowcase, about 40 inches square. Then cut or fold the square diagonally to make a triangle. Slip one end of the bandage under the arm and over the shoulder. Bring the other end of the bandage over the other shoulder, cradling the arm.

2 Tie the ends of the bandage behind the neck. Fasten the edge of the bandage, near the elbow, with a safety pin.

Collar and Cuff Sling

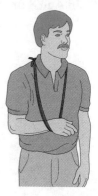

Use a collar and cuff sling for a suspected fracture of the collarbone or elbow when a triangular sling is not available. Wrap a strip of sheet, a pants leg, or pantyhose around the wrist and tie the ends behind the neck.

How to Splint a Fracture

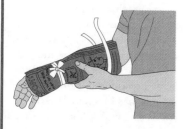

For a lower arm or wrist fracture (left), carefully place a folded newspaper, magazine, or heavy piece of clothing under the arm. Tie it in place with pieces of cloth. A lower leg or ankle fracture (right) can be splinted similarly, with a bulky garment or blanket wrapped and secured around the limb.

A person with a hip or pelvis fracture should not be moved. If the person must be moved, the legs should be strapped together (with a towel or blanket in between them) and the person gently placed on a board, as for a back injury (see p.1192).

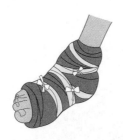

to their degree of severity, with a first-degree burn the least serious and third- or fourth-degree burns the most dangerous.

The risk of infection increases with the amount and severity of the burn. Running cool water continuously on the area of the burn reduces pain and skin temperature, decreasing further tissue damage. Never put butter or ointments on a burn except as described below.

Always seek medical attention if the area of the burn is larger than the palm of your hand; if it occurs on the face, genitals, or hands; or if it was caused by electricity or a chemical.

Any burn can be serious to children under 2 years and the elderly; get medical treatment.

A person who has inhaled fumes, steam, or smoke may have serious internal burns and should see a physician. Any sunburn that blisters requires medical attention.

First-degree burns damage the top layer (epidermis) of skin. The skin may be pink or red, mildly swollen, and painful.

Immediate care Place the burned area under cool running water for 5 to 10 minutes or cover the area with a cool compress (ice wrapped in a towel). Give ibuprofen or acetaminophen to relieve pain and swelling.

Second-degree burns damage two layers of skin, the epidermis and dermis. The skin looks raw and swollen and may be cherry red. There may be intense pain. Blisters may be present or may develop later.

Immediate care Do not break blisters. Do not remove clothing that is stuck to the skin. Place the burned area under cool running water for 5 to 10 minutes or cover the area with a cool compress (ice wrapped in a towel). Then carefully remove any clothing.

Pat the area dry with a clean towel. Elevate the burned area above the heart. Give ibuprofen or acetaminophen to relieve swelling and pain.

Seek medical attention for any second-degree burn from the sun; to the hands, face, neck, or genitalia; or that is larger than the palm of your hand.

If you are not near a medical facility, place bacitracin ointment or honey on the broken blisters to prevent infection and promote healing. This is the only situation in which you should apply anything to burned skin.

Third- or fourth-degree burns damage all layers of skin and may destroy underlying blood vessels and nerves.

A fourth-degree burn is caused by prolonged exposure to the usual causes of a third-degree burn, such as fire or high-voltage electricity. The skin will appear white or charred black. There is less pain because nerves have been damaged.

If the person's skin or clothing is on fire, smother the flames with an article of clothing or roll the person on the ground. Be careful not to burn your hands. The person may have difficulty breathing if he or she also inhaled smoke.

Immediate care Call out for someone to get help or call 911 yourself. Check airway, breathing, and circulation (see Cardiopulmonary Resuscitation, right). Do not remove clothing that is stuck to the skin.

Run cool running water continuously on burned areas to cool the skin. If possible, elevate burned areas above the heart and cover with a clean sheet to help reduce loss of body heat. Be calm and reassuring and stay with the person until medical help arrives.

A burned mouth (from hot food or drink) can be very painful, although the injury usually is not serious.

Immediate care Have the person rinse and gargle with cool water for 5 to 10 minutes to relieve pain and reduce the temperature of the burned area. Give ibuprofen or acetaminophen if necessary for pain. Avoid hot food and drinks for several days. If pain persists, see a doctor.

Corrosive chemical burns can burn through several layers of skin and tissue. (See also Eye Injuries, p.1208.)

Immediate care If possible,

put on disposable surgical gloves, which can protect you against some chemicals. Avoid contaminating yourself or others.

Flush cool running water over the burned area for 15 to 20 minutes.

If there are instructions on the label of the chemical container, follow the instructions. Call out for someone to get help or call 911 yourself.

If the burning sensation returns, flush again with cool running water for 10 minutes. Stay with the person until medical help arrives.

Carbon Monoxide Poisoning
(See Poisonings and Overdoses, p.1213)

Cardiopulmonary Resuscitation

When you perform cardiopulmonary resuscitation (CPR), you are using mouth-to-mouth resuscitation to help the person breathe and chest compressions to help the person's heart pump blood.

The brief review of CPR on the following pages can help you in an emergency; however, this information should not take the place of a certified course in CPR.

Immediate care Assess the situation. Call out for someone to get help, or call 911 yourself if the person does not seem to need immediate assistance. You can determine this by gently shaking the person and asking in a loud voice "Are you OK?" If there is no response, begin CPR and continue until help arrives.

CPR on an Infant

Basic CPR on an infant is five chest compressions and one breath.

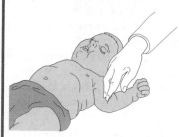 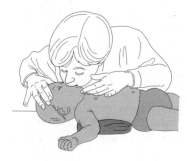 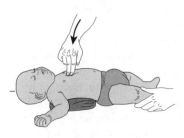

1 To find a pulse, locate the brachial artery in the upper arm. It is located on the underside of the arm between muscle and bone. Use two fingers to feel for the pulse.

2 If the baby is not breathing, tilt the head back slightly to open the airway. Put a washcloth or thin pad of clothing under the baby's shoulders. This keeps the head from assuming its naturally forward position. Form a seal with your mouth over the baby's mouth and nose. Blow one breath (a smaller breath than you would give to an adult), so that the baby's chest rises.

3 If the baby has no pulse, use two fingers to perform chest compressions. Place your fingers one finger width below an imaginary line connecting the infant's nipples. Push down 1 inch with each compression. Count out loud: "1 and 2 and 3 and 4 and 5." You may have to repeat the five compressions and one breath multiple times. You will push down on the chest 120 times per minute. Continue, alternating five compressions and one breath, until help arrives.

CPR on a Child
Under Age 8

Basic CPR on a child is five chest compressions and one breath. You may have to repeat the five compressions and one breath multiple times. You will push down on the chest 100 to 120 times per minute. Continue until breathing begins or help arrives.

■ Kneel next to the child.

■ With the fingers of the hand that is closest to the child's feet, find the bottom of the breastbone.

■ Place the heel of one hand below the nipples and above the

bottom of the breastbone and push down forcefully, 1½ inches with each compression; then let the chest rise. Count out loud: "1 and 2 and 3 and 4 and 5."

■ Then tilt the child's head back slightly and form a seal with your mouth over the child's mouth and nose (see Mouth-to-Mouth-and-Nose Resuscitation on a Child Under Age 8 or on an Infant, p.1198). Blow one breath so that the chest rises.

■ Continue, alternating five compressions and one breath, until help arrives.

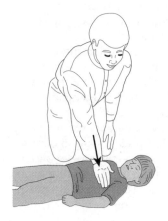

**CPR on a Child Age 8 or Older
or on an Adult**

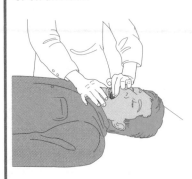

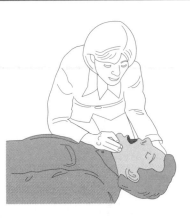

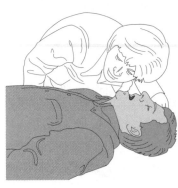

1 Lay the person on a hard, flat sur-face. Look into the mouth and throat to ensure that the airway is clear. If an object is present, try to sweep it out with your fingers. Use disposable surgical gloves if they are available. If vomiting occurs, turn the person on his or her side and sweep out the mouth with two fingers. Do not place fingers in the mouth if there is rigidity or if the person is having a seizure.

2 Tilt the head back slightly to open the airway. Put upward pressure on the jaw to pull it forward.

3 Look for the person's chest to rise and fall. Listen for the sounds of breathing. Feel for the person's breath on your cheek.

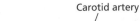
Carotid artery

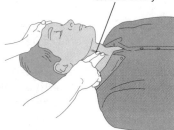

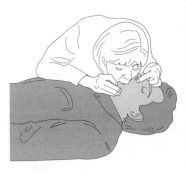

4 If the person is at all responsive (if he or she is moaning, breathing, blinking, or moving any part of the body), his or her heart is beating; do not perform steps 6 or 7.

If the person is not breathing, perform mouth-to-mouth resuscita-tion (see p.1199), even if the heart is beating. If the person is breathing,

cover with a blanket or clothing as for shock (see p.1216).

If the person is not responsive, feel for a pulse on the carotid artery. The artery is in the groove of the neck (see above) off to the side of the Adam's apple. If you do not feel a pulse, go to step 5 immediately.

5 If the person is not breathing, pinch the nostrils closed with your thumb and index finger. Place your mouth tightly over the person's mouth (use a mouthpiece if one is available). Blow two quick breaths and watch for the person's chest to rise. Release the nostrils.

(CONTINUED)

CPR on a Child Age 8 or Older or on an Adult (continued)

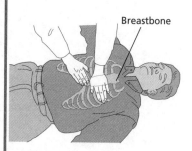

Breastbone

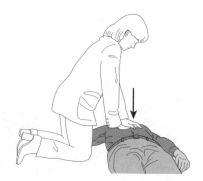

6 If the heart is not beating, kneel at the person's right side. With the fingers of your right hand, find the bottom of the breastbone (in the center where the ribs meet). Place your index and middle fingers side by side, just above the bottom of the breastbone. Place the heel of your left hand just above your fingers, on the breastbone. Move your right hand and place it on top of the left, and interlock the fingers of the two hands.

7 With your elbows straight, push down briskly (about 2 inches) with the heel of your hand 15 times over about 10 seconds. Let the chest rise after each compression.

CPR for an adult includes 15 chest compressions and two breaths. You may have to repeat the 15 chest compressions and two breaths multiple times. Push down on the chest 80 to 100 times per minute. Continue until breathing begins or help arrives. Count out loud: "1 and 2 and 3 and 4 and 5," until you reach 15. Release your hands. Repeat step 5 and watch for the person's chest to fall. Feel for air being exhaled. Repeat, starting at step 5.

Cat Scratches

(See Puncture Wounds, p.1215)

Chemical Burns

(See Eye Injuries, p.1208; Burns, p.1199)

Childbirth

If you are called on to help deliver a baby, remember that childbirth is a natural process and that your role is to assist the woman and offer encouragement. If a woman's contractions are very strong and 2 to 3 minutes apart or the water bag (amniotic fluid) has broken, birth is very near. If the woman tells you that the birth will happen very soon, believe her.

You will see quite a bit of blood, which is normal. You may see bloody fluid coming from the vagina before and during the birth; this is also normal.

Immediate care Call 911 or have someone else call. Put down a large plastic sheet or plastic shower curtain and place sheets and towels or newspapers on top of the plastic to absorb fluids. Help the woman lie down with her legs apart and her back supported by a pillow. Wash your hands. Use disposable surgical gloves if you have them.

During the birth, the woman may wish to lean forward and grab her knees, or she may want to squat or lie on her side. Let her decide which position is most comfortable. When the baby's head is visible in the vaginal opening, the birth is about to occur. Do not try to hurry the birth by pulling on the baby's head. Let the woman push the baby out. Usually, as the baby is born, the face will appear straight down or straight up.

As soon as the head is outside the vagina, put two fingers along the top side of the head and feel around the neck area for a loop of the umbilical cord. It will be about the thickness of your little finger. If you can feel it, hook the loop of cord with your two fin-

CPR on a Child Age 8 or Older or on an Adult

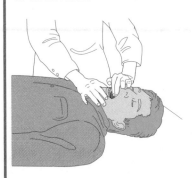

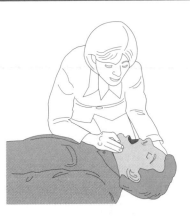

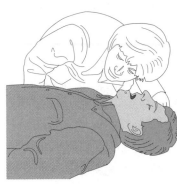

1 Lay the person on a hard, flat surface. Look into the mouth and throat to ensure that the airway is clear. If an object is present, try to sweep it out with your fingers. Use disposable surgical gloves if they are available. If vomiting occurs, turn the person on his or her side and sweep out the mouth with two fingers. Do not place fingers in the mouth if there is rigidity or if the person is having a seizure.

2 Tilt the head back slightly to open the airway. Put upward pressure on the jaw to pull it forward.

3 Look for the person's chest to rise and fall. Listen for the sounds of breathing. Feel for the person's breath on your cheek.

Carotid artery

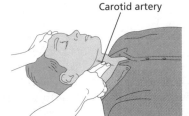

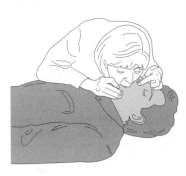

4 If the person is at all responsive (if he or she is moaning, breathing, blinking, or moving any part of the body), his or her heart is beating; do not perform steps 6 or 7.

If the person is not breathing, perform mouth-to-mouth resuscitation (see p.1199), even if the heart is beating. If the person is breathing,

cover with a blanket or clothing as for shock (see p.1216).

If the person is not responsive, feel for a pulse on the carotid artery. The artery is in the groove of the neck (see above) off to the side of the Adam's apple. If you do not feel a pulse, go to step 5 immediately.

5 If the person is not breathing, pinch the nostrils closed with your thumb and index finger. Place your mouth tightly over the person's mouth (use a mouthpiece if one is available). Blow two quick breaths and watch for the person's chest to rise. Release the nostrils.

(CONTINUED)

CPR on a Child Age 8 or Older or on an Adult (continued)

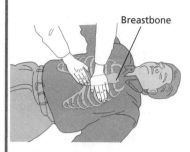

Breastbone

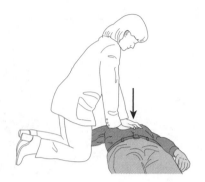

6 If the heart is not beating, kneel at the person's right side. With the fingers of your right hand, find the bottom of the breastbone (in the center where the ribs meet). Place your index and middle fingers side by side, just above the bottom of the breastbone. Place the heel of your left hand just above your fingers, on the breastbone. Move your right hand and place it on top of the left, and interlock the fingers of the two hands.

7 With your elbows straight, push down briskly (about 2 inches) with the heel of your hand 15 times over about 10 seconds. Let the chest rise after each compression.

CPR for an adult includes 15 chest compressions and two breaths. You may have to repeat the 15 chest compressions and two breaths multiple times. Push down on the chest 80 to 100 times per minute. Continue until breathing begins or

help arrives. Count out loud: "1 and 2 and 3 and 4 and 5," until you reach 15. Release your hands. Repeat step 5 and watch for the person's chest to fall. Feel for air being exhaled. Repeat, starting at step 5.

Cat Scratches

(See Puncture Wounds, p.1215)

Chemical Burns

(See Eye Injuries, p.1208; Burns, p.1199)

Childbirth

If you are called on to help deliver a baby, remember that childbirth is a natural process and that your role is to assist the woman and offer encouragement. If a woman's contractions are very strong and 2 to 3 minutes apart or the water bag (amniotic fluid) has broken, birth is very near. If the woman tells you that the

birth will happen very soon, believe her.

You will see quite a bit of blood, which is normal. You may see bloody fluid coming from the vagina before and during the birth; this is also normal.

Immediate care Call 911 or have someone else call. Put down a large plastic sheet or plastic shower curtain and place sheets and towels or newspapers on top of the plastic to absorb fluids. Help the woman lie down with her legs apart and her back supported by a pillow. Wash your hands. Use disposable surgical gloves if you have them.

During the birth, the woman may wish to lean forward and

grab her knees, or she may want to squat or lie on her side. Let her decide which position is most comfortable. When the baby's head is visible in the vaginal opening, the birth is about to occur. Do not try to hurry the birth by pulling on the baby's head. Let the woman push the baby out. Usually, as the baby is born, the face will appear straight down or straight up.

As soon as the head is outside the vagina, put two fingers along the top side of the head and feel around the neck area for a loop of the umbilical cord. It will be about the thickness of your little finger. If you can feel it, hook the loop of cord with your two fin-

Before and After Childbirth

ITEMS TO GATHER:

- Towels, plastic sheet, and newspapers
- Soft blanket for the baby
- Soap and water to wash your hands
- Gloves (ideally disposable surgical gloves), if available

- Thick string, clean shoelace, or sterile tape to tie off umbilical cord
- Plastic bag for placenta

REMEMBER TO...

- Note the time of birth.
- Congratulate the mother!

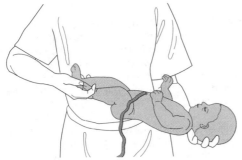

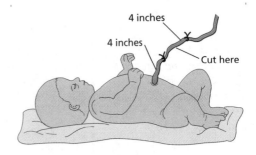

4 inches

4 inches

Cut here

AFTER DELIVERY

After delivery, hold the baby with his or her head slightly lower than the feet to drain fluid from the nose and throat. Do not hold the baby upside down or slap him or her. Gently dry off the baby and wrap him or her in a dry towel or blanket. The baby should start breathing and his or her color should improve as oxygen is breathed in. If the baby does not start breathing, place the baby on his or her back and gently rub the chest or tap the bottoms of the feet. If the baby still does not begin breathing, start mouth-to-mouth-and-nose resuscitation (see p.1198).

CUTTING THE UMBILICAL CORD

The umbilical cord will pulsate during the birth and afterward, indicating that the baby is still receiving blood from the mother. Do not cut the cord until it stops pulsating. After it has stopped pulsating, tie off the cord tightly with heavy string, a clean shoelace, or sterile tape about 4 inches from the baby; tie it again 2 to 4 inches from the first string. Cut between the two ties. Wrap the baby in a soft blanket and place him or her on the mother's stomach.

Birth of the Placenta

The placenta, which has provided the fetus with nourishment, is attached to the umbilical cord and is delivered about 20 minutes after the baby. Do not pull on the cord; delivery of the placenta occurs on its own. You can help by gently massaging the woman's lower abdomen. The uterus will feel like a hard round mass.

Massaging the abdomen helps the uterus contract, which also helps stop bleeding. After the placenta is delivered, place it in a plastic bag to take with the woman and baby to the hospital. It is normal for more bleeding to occur after delivery of the placenta. Continue gently massaging the woman's lower abdomen.

gers and slide it gently over the baby's head.

The baby's head should then turn toward one side and the shoulders should come out. Assist the birth by supporting the baby's head and shoulders, but remember not to pull. Be careful—the baby will be slippery. If there is a membrane covering the baby's mouth and nose, gently wipe it off with a clean cloth. Do not remove the whitish coating on the body.

Choking

A person who is choking will instinctively grab at the throat. The person also may panic, gasp for breath, turn blue, or be unconscious (see p.1217). If the person can cough or speak, he

Heimlich Maneuver on an Adult

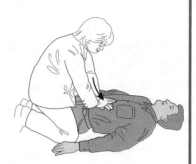

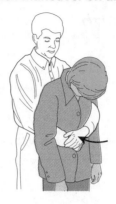

If the person is sitting or standing, stand behind him or her. Form a fist with one hand and place your fist, thumb side in, just below the person's rib cage in the front. Grab your fist with your other hand. Keeping your arms off the person's rib cage, give four quick inward and upward thrusts. You may have to repeat this several times until the obstructing object is coughed out.

If the person is lying down or unconscious, straddle him or her and place the heel of your hand just above the waistline. Place your other hand on top of this hand. Keeping your elbows straight, give four quick upward thrusts. You may have to repeat this procedure several times until the obstructing object is coughed out.

Heimlich Maneuver on a Child

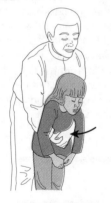

Stand behind the child. With your arms around his or her waist, form a fist with one hand and place it, thumb side in, between the ribs and waistline. Grab your fist with your other hand. Keeping your arms off the child's rib cage, give four quick inward and upward thrusts. You may have to repeat this several times until the obstructing object is coughed out.

Heimlich Maneuver on an Infant

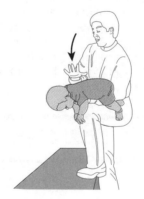

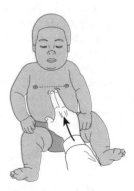

1 Place the infant facedown across your forearm (resting your forearm on your leg) and support the infant's head with your hand. Give four forceful blows to the back with the heel of your hand. You may have to repeat this several times until the obstructing object is coughed out.

2 If this does not work, turn the baby over. With two fingers one finger width below an imaginary line connecting the nipples, give four forceful thrusts to the chest to a depth of 1 inch. You may have to repeat this several times until the obstructing object is coughed out.

or she is getting air. Nothing should be done.

Immediate care If the person cannot cough or speak, begin the Heimlich maneuver (see p.1206) immediately to dislodge the object blocking the windpipe. The Heimlich maneuver creates an artificial cough by forcing the diaphragm up toward the lungs.

If you are choking and alone You can perform the Heimlich maneuver on yourself by giving yourself abdominal thrusts. Or position yourself over the back of a chair or against a railing or counter and press forcefully enough into it so that the thrust dislodges the object.

Cold Exposure

(See Hypothermia, p.1212)

Consciousness, Loss of

(See Unconsciousness, p.1217)

Convulsions

(See How to Help Someone Who is Having a Seizure, p.376)

CPR

(See Cardiopulmonary Resuscitation, p.1201)

Cuts, Deep

(See Bleeding, p.1196)

Cuts, Minor

(See Bleeding, p.1196; Scrapes and Scratches, p.1215)

Diabetic Coma

(See Diabetic Emergencies, next entry)

Diabetic Emergencies

People with diabetes may become ill from either too much or too little sugar in their blood, and either situation can be a medical emergency.

Any diabetic with slurring of speech, confusion, excessive sweating, agitation, weakness, an apparent stroke (see p.1216), seizure (see p.374), excessive sleepiness, unresponsiveness, or coma may have low blood sugar; treat the situation as an emergency.

Immediate care Call 911 immediately. Give the person the most readily accessible source of sugar (such as a glass of juice or water with 2 tablespoons of sugar stirred in, cookies, or a chocolate bar). If, after taking sugar, the person feels much better, then additional food (such as soup or a sandwich) should be given.

If the person does not feel any better, his or her skin is dry, and he or she has been urinating frequently lately and complaining of thirst, the problem may be high rather than low levels of blood sugar. In such a case, the additional sugar you have given will not harm him or her but no additional food should be given. Wait for medical attention.

Dislocations

A dislocation occurs when a bone is forced out of its joint. A sudden impact to the joint, such as a fall or blow, is the usual cause. Dislocations normally occur in a shoulder, elbow, finger, toe, kneecap, or hip. The joint may be noticeably deformed (except in the case of hip and shoulder dislocations, which can be more difficult to see).

There will also be intense pain and swelling. The person will experience severe pain when the affected bone is moved.

Immediate care Call 911 if you suspect the person has a shoulder, elbow, or hip dislocation. Do not try to put the bone back into the joint. Immobilize the joint with a pillow or sling in its current position (see How to Make a Sling, p.1200). Keep the person comfortable and take him or her to the doctor.

Drowning

Drowning can occur in any depth of water. Never leave a child unattended near water—even near a bucket of water. If you see a drowning person, ensure your own safety first.

Always suspect head, neck, and back injuries if you come upon someone in the water who is unconscious; the person may have dived in and struck an object on the bottom (see Head Injuries, p.1211; Back and Neck Injuries, p.1192; Unconsciousness, p.1217).

Immediate care Call out for someone to get help and to call 911. If the drowning person is not breathing, begin mouth-to-mouth resuscitation (see p.1199). If the person's heart is not beating, carefully move him or her to a safe place and begin cardiopulmonary resuscitation immediately (see p.1201).

A person who has been immersed in cold water and whose core body temperature has fallen may need basic lifesaving techniques performed for several hours.

Drug Abuse

(See Poisonings and Overdoses, p.1213)

Ear, Foreign Objects in

A foreign object that enters the ear can damage the delicate structure of the middle ear. Never attempt to remove an object unless it is clearly visible outside the ear canal, because you may push the object in deeper. Do not attempt to flush out the object by putting any liquid in the ear. Follow the steps outlined below:

Insect in ear If the insect is alive (you may hear it buzzing), place several drops of oil (such as cooking oil or baby oil) in the ear to kill it. This is the only situation in which you should put a liquid in the ear. Then seek medical attention to have the insect removed.

Other object in ear If paper or cotton has been stuffed into the ear and is clearly visible outside of the ear canal, carefully remove the object with tweezers or fingers. For all other objects, seek medical attention.

Electric Shock

A shock of electricity can cause breathing to stop or the heart to stop beating. A person who has been shocked by an electric current also poses a serious risk to a rescuer. Do not touch the person with your hand or any object until the current has been turned off or the person is safely away from the source.

With high voltages, the person may have been thrown into the air and may have head, neck, and back injuries (see Head Injuries, p.1211; Back and Neck Injuries, p.1192).

High voltage electricity also can travel through the ground. If you feel a tingling sensation in your feet, walk away from the scene until the power has been turned off.

Immediate care Call out for someone to get help, or call 911 yourself. Do not attempt to touch or move the person in any way until you are certain the power source is off. Then, use a dry wooden object such as a dry board, broom handle, or tree branch to nudge the person away from the electrical source.

Check airway, breathing, and circulation (see Cardiopulmonary Resuscitation, p.1201; Breathing Difficulties, p.1198). Control any bleeding (see p.1196) and stay with the person until medical help arrives. Put dressings on the wound if it is oozing. See also Burns, p.1199.

Eye Injuries

Any injury to the eye is serious and should be seen by a doctor.

CHEMICAL BURNS

A chemical that burns the eye, such as acid, bleach, or an industrial cleaning solution, can cause blindness if not treated promptly. Any chemical in the eye that causes intense irritation or pain should be considered an emergency.

Immediate care Call out for someone to get help. If no one is with you, follow these steps *before*

you call 911 (take a break to call 911 only if the person is capable of flushing the eye alone or after you have helped the person flush the eye for a few minutes).

■ Flush the eye with cool running water by placing the person's head beside a running faucet with the affected eye below the unaffected eye.

■ Using your hand, gently direct water over the eye so that there is a continuous flow of water (you may have to hold the person's eyelid open as you do this).

■ Flush continuously for 2 to 3 minutes. Continue for at least 15 minutes.

■ Do not allow the person to rub the eyes.

If the person is wearing contact lenses Do not try to remove the lens. Flush the eye immediately with water as described above. If the lens has not been flushed out of the eye after several minutes, have the person try to remove it.

CUT EYE

Any cut on the eyelid or in the eye must be seen by a doctor. There may be additional damage inside the eyeball.

Immediate care Cover the eye with a sterile gauze pad and tape. Do not place pressure on the eye. Go to a hospital emergency department.

DIRECT BLOW TO EYE

A direct blow to the eye can cause bruising (a black eye) and possible damage to the eyeball or fracture of the socket.

Immediate care Place a cold compress (such as ice wrapped in a towel) on the eye. Seek medical attention to rule out internal eye damage.

EYE OUT OF SOCKET

An eyeball that has come out of its socket is called an extruded eyeball.

Immediate care Call out for someone to get help or call 911 yourself. Do not handle the eye. Try opening the upper and lower eyelids as widely as possible to see if the eyeball will go back in. Have the person sit or lie down and remain quiet. Cover the eye with a moist cloth or gauze and keep it moist by adding water. Do not place pressure on the eye. Stay with the person until medical help arrives.

FOREIGN BODY IN EYE

An object that is sticking out of the eye, such as a piece of glass or a twig, may have damaged blood vessels and tissue inside the eye. A BB pellet or small chip of stone can penetrate the eye and cause internal damage.

Immediate care Do not remove the object. Keep the person calm and tell him or her not to move the eye. Place a gauze bandage over both eyes (because when one eye moves, the other eye moves) and go to a hospital emergency department.

Minor specks in the eye Occasionally, an eyelash or speck of dirt gets into the eye and causes irritation. If tears that form do not wash out the object, it can sometimes be removed by pulling the upper eyelid down over the lower eyelid. The lashes of the lower eyelid may brush out any foreign object that is caught under the upper lid.

If this does not work, try either of the procedures described in the illustration below left.

Fainting

Fainting is loss of consciousness that occurs when oxygenated blood does not reach the brain. A fainting episode usually lasts no more than a few minutes.

A person who has fallen from a height before or after fainting may be bleeding (see p.1196) or have broken bones (see p.1199), a head injury (see p.1210), or a back or neck injury (see p.1192). If the person does not regain consciousness within a few minutes, see Unconsciousness, p.1217.

Immediate care Have the person lie down for 10 or 15 minutes. Ensure that the airway is open (see Breathing Difficulties, p.1198). Loosen any tight clothing around the neck. Elevate the feet at least 12 inches to help blood reach the brain. Check pulse and breathing; initiate cardiopulmonary resuscitation if necessary (see p.1201).

If the person vomits, turn the head (or his or her whole body) to one side to prevent choking. Stay until he or she feels ready to move. Seek medical attention to rule out a serious cause for the fainting. If the person is pregnant, over 50 years old, diabetic, or has heart problems, chest pain, or shortness of breath, call 911.

FAINTNESS

A person who feels faint may become unsteady and grab onto someone to keep his or her balance.

Immediate care Have the per-

Removing a Speck From the Eye

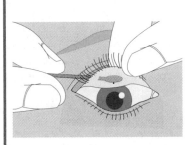

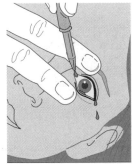

Place a cotton-tipped swab behind the upper eyelid and carefully roll the eyelid back onto it. If you can see the object, remove it with the moistened end of another cotton swab or a facial tissue.

Tilt the person's head to one side. Hold the eyelids open with two fingers and carefully use an eye-dropper or a cup of water to flush water over the eye from the nose outward. If the object cannot be removed, cover the eye with a gauze bandage and seek medical attention.

Removing a Stuck Ring

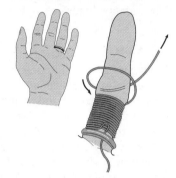

1 Pass an end of fine string or dental floss under the ring. With the other end, begin tightly wrapping the string around the finger. Ensure that the string is wrapped evenly and smoothly past the lower knuckle.

2 With the end that was passed under the ring, begin unwrapping the string in the same direction. The ring should move over the string as the string is unwrapped. If the ring cannot be removed, unwrap the string and go to a hospital emergency department.

son lie down immediately and elevate the feet at least 12 inches. If it is not possible for the person to lie down, have him or her sit forward with the head lower than the shoulders. Loosen tight clothing around the neck. The person should remain lying down or sitting forward for 10 to 15 minutes. Stay close until he or she feels ready to move.

If the person is pregnant, over 50, has heart problems, chest pain, shortness of breath, or still feels faint, consult a physician. A diabetic may feel faint because of low blood sugar (see Diabetic Emergencies, p.1207).

Finger Injuries

A finger that has been caught in a door or hit with a hammer can be very painful. Blood vessels in the finger can break and cause swelling. If the fingertip is injured,

blood may pool under the nail. With a severe injury, a bone may be broken (see Broken Bones, p.1199).

Immediate care Place the injured finger under cold running water or apply ice to help reduce pain and swelling. If the finger is deformed, if there is blood under the nail, or if the nail has been partially or totally torn off, see a physician.

RING REMOVAL

Occasionally, a ring becomes stuck on a finger. If the ring cannot be removed with soap and water, you can attempt to remove it with the method shown in the illustration at left. If you have excessive swelling, go to a hospital emergency department to have the ring cut off.

Fishhook Injuries

Never remove a fishhook that is embedded in the eye or face; seek medical attention immediately to have it removed. A fishhook embedded in skin should be removed by a doctor. If you are in a remote area and a doctor is not available, remove the fishhook following the directions in the illustration below. If the fishhook is

Pulling Out a Fishhook

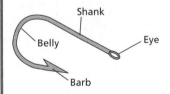

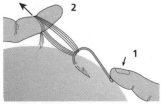

First, make sure that any bystanders are out of the way of the fishhook's path. Next, loop a piece of fishing line several times around the belly of the hook near the skin surface. Press the shank of the hook against the skin with your index finger (1).

Wrap the other end of the string several times around the index finger of your other hand (use your thumb to hold the loose end of the string tightly) (2).

Move your index finger close to the hook to generate slack in the line. Pull on the string suddenly, with a jerk, in line with the hook. Flush the area with water, clean it with soap and water, and bandage it.

embedded deeply in tissue, follow the instructions (below) for a multibarbed fishhook.

A multibarbed fishhook should ideally be removed by a physician. If this is not possible, cut the eye off the shank of the hook, and then push the shank of the hook through the wound, following the path of the hook until the barbs exit and can be grasped with pliers. Flush the area well with running water, clean it with soap and water, and cover it with a bandage.

Food Poisoning
(See p.881)

Fractures
(See Broken Bones, p.1199)

Frostbite

Frostbite occurs when exposed areas of the skin or skin that is not sufficiently protected become frozen from ice crystals forming in tissue. The most commonly affected areas are the ears, nose, face, fingers, and toes. Initially, the skin may be red and painful.

As frostbite develops, the skin turns white and waxy. In severe cases, it turns grayish blue or black and is cold and hard to the touch. There may be no feeling in the affected areas. Any frostbitten area larger than a quarter should be seen by a doctor.

For severe frostbite Call out for someone to get help or call 911 yourself. Help the person to a warm area. Do not warm up or thaw out the frostbitten area if there is a risk of refreezing. Make the person comfortable, taking care not to disturb frostbitten

skin. Stay with the person until medical help arrives.

For mild frostbite Cover affected areas and move the person into a warm area. Do not rub frostbitten areas. Place the frostbitten part in lukewarm water until the skin begins to turn pink and feeling returns. It is normal for the area to feel painful during warming. If water is not available, carefully wrap the frostbitten area in warm clothing. Keep the affected areas elevated above the heart to help prevent swelling.

Fumes, Poisonous
(See Poisonings and Overdoses, p.1213)

Genital Injuries

An injury to the genitals can occur from a fall, a vehicle or bicycle collision, or a direct blow to the genital area.

Immediate care If pain persists after the injury, place a cold compress (such as ice wrapped in a towel) on the area. Give acetaminophen or ibuprofen to reduce pain. If bruising occurs or if the person vomits or pain persists for more than 30 minutes, go to a hospital emergency department.

Gunshot Wounds

A bullet can cause multiple injuries. There may be a small entry wound where the bullet entered the body and possibly no exit wound. If an exit wound is present, it may be larger than the entry wound and may not be directly opposite it.

Immediate care Keep the person very still. Call out for

someone to get help, or call 911 yourself. Time is of the essence. Check airway, breathing, and circulation (see Cardiopulmonary Resuscitation, p.1201). Control bleeding with direct pressure and elevation (see p.1197). If the person is unconscious, see p.1217. Stay with the person until medical help arrives.

Head Injuries

Injury to the head can cause bleeding and swelling inside the brain, which can be fatal. Motor vehicle and bicycle collisions and falling from a height are common causes.

Always suspect head, neck, and back injuries if you find someone unconscious at an accident scene. Never remove a helmet. Never move the person unless the situation is life-threatening. If you have to move a person with suspected back and neck injuries, see p.1192.

Symptoms and signs of a head injury include headache, dizziness, nausea, vomiting, confusion, poor coordination, slurred speech, and unconsciousness. The pupils of the eyes may be different sizes.

Immediate care Call out for someone to get help, or call 911 yourself if the person does not need immediate assistance. Check airway, breathing, and circulation (see Cardiopulmonary Resuscitation, p.1200). Keep the person warm. Stay with him or her until medical help arrives.

SCALP INJURIES

A scalp injury can bleed profusely (see Bleeding, p.1196) but often is not serious. If the person complains of a headache, dizziness, or is vomiting or losing consciousness, have the person lie down and keep him or her comfortable. Call 911. Stay with the person until medical help arrives.

Heart Attack

A heart attack is a life-threatening emergency. The person may have a crushing pressure in the chest that lasts for 10 minutes or longer and/or pain that radiates throughout the chest, face, jaw, shoulders, stomach, or down one or both arms. The pain is often mistaken for indigestion. The person also may sweat heavily, have difficulty breathing, be nauseated, feel light-headed or dizzy, vomit, or lose consciousness.

Immediate care Call out for someone to get help, or call 911 yourself if the person does not need immediate assistance. If the person is unconscious, see p.1216. If conscious, have the person lie down. Loosen any tight-fitting clothing around the neck, keep the person warm, and be reassuring.

Ask if he or she is carrying a heart medicine, such as nitroglycerin. Help the person take the medicine. Have the person chew and swallow an aspirin tablet, followed by a glass of water; this thins the blood, helping the heart get more blood. Do not give anything to eat or drink. Stay with the person until medical help arrives. If supplemental oxygen is available, use it.

Heat Exhaustion

Heat exhaustion can occur after prolonged exposure to high tem-

peratures, high humidity, or both. The person may be dizzy, tired, perspiring heavily, or vomiting and may have pale, clammy skin and/or a headache.

Immediate care Move the person to a cool area and have him or her lie down. Loosen or remove tight-fitting clothing. Give plenty of fluids such as water or a sports drink. Cool the person off in a tub or shower of cool water, with a hose, or with wet cloths. If symptoms persist, or if the person is confused, faints, or has a temperature above 102°F, call 911.

Heatstroke

Heatstroke is a life-threatening emergency. It occurs when the body's core temperature rises—and does not fall—after exposure to a high temperature. The body temperature may be as high as 105°F. The person may feel very hot and have red or flushed skin. Sweating usually does not occur.

The person's mental state also may be impaired or he or she may be unconscious (see p.1217).

Immediate care Call out for someone to get help, or call 911 yourself if the person does not need immediate assistance. Place the person in a bath or shower of cool water to help bring down the temperature or use a hose or bucket to bathe the person in cool water. Continue until the body temperature drops to 101°F. Stay with the person until medical help arrives.

Heimlich Maneuver
(See Choking, p.1206)

Human Bites
(See Bites and Stings, p.1194)

Hypothermia

Hypothermia occurs when the body's core temperature falls below 98.6°F. The person may be shivering, drowsy, numb, confused, or losing consciousness (see p.1217). He or she also may have frostbite (see p.1211).

Immediate care If the person appears confused or has any symptoms other than feeling cold, call out for someone to get help or call 911 yourself. Move the person into a warm area. Remove any wet clothing. Wrap the person in blankets and keep him or her warm. If you are in an isolated area, remove most clothing and huddle inside a sleeping bag with the person. Stay with him or her until medical help arrives or until symptoms subside.

Insect Bites and Stings
(See Bites and Stings, p.1194)

Mouth-to-Mouth Resuscitation
(See Breathing Difficulties, p.1198)

Neck Injuries
(See Back and Neck Injuries, p.1192)

Nose Injuries

An injury to the nose can cause bleeding (see p.1196), bruising, swelling, a displaced septum (cartilage in the nose), or a broken bone (see p.1199).

Immediate care Apply ice wrapped in a towel to the nose.

Seek medical attention if deformity or swelling is significant, if bleeding lasts for more than 1 hour, or if the nose is deformed after 2 days.

Nosebleeds

(See How to Stop a Nosebleed, p.1198)

Overdoses

(See Poisonings and Overdoses, below)

Poisonings and Overdoses

A poison is a substance that disrupts normal functioning of the body. It can be a liquid, solid, or gas that can be swallowed, inhaled, injected, or absorbed through the skin. A nontoxic substance, such as aspirin, taken in large quantities, also can lead to poisoning. Some poisons act quickly in the body; others take more time.

If you suspect poisoning has occurred, contact your local poison control center (see p.1239). Depending on the substance consumed, you may or may not be instructed to induce vomiting. The person handling the call will tell you exactly what to do. For information on how to prevent poisoning, see Safety and Preventing Injury, p.86.

POISONOUS FUMES

Inhaled poisonous fumes can cause breathing difficulties (see p.1198), unconsciousness (see p.1217), and death.

Common poisonous fumes result from a fire occurring in an enclosed space, from a carbon monoxide (CO) leak, or from formation of nitrogen dioxide ("silo gas"), which primarily occurs in rural farming communities. Of these, carbon monoxide is the most common.

Carbon monoxide is a colorless, odorless, tasteless gas. It is present in car exhaust and can also be produced by indoor use of a barbeque or by faulty home heating units, such as kerosene or gas heaters, especially if these units have not been cleaned or serviced regularly. Any fuel-burning product can emit carbon monoxide.

Symptoms of carbon monoxide poisoning include headaches, listlessness, nausea, and vomiting. Disorientation or unconsciousness also may occur. Be especially suspicious of carbon monoxide poisoning if the entire family feels generally sick and has headaches early in the cold weather season (not long after the furnace is reactivated for winter). Sometimes a pet will die suddenly due to carbon monoxide poisoning.

Immediate care Be extremely cautious about entering any area in which there may be poisonous fumes. If you notice a person unconscious in a room and you are certain carbon monoxide is present—and not another type of noxious gas—go in and out of the room quickly and only to remove the person. Take a person who has been overcome by fumes outside into fresh air.

If you are uncertain about the cause, call 911. Paramedics or firefighters will have the appropriate equipment to enter the room.

Check airway, breathing, and circulation (see Cardiopulmonary Resuscitation, p.1201). If the person vomits, turn the head (or the person) to one side to prevent choking. If the person does not respond, call out for someone to

---

Examples of Poisonous Substances

Plants, shrubs, flowers, mushrooms The berry, leaf, flower, or whole plant may be poisonous. Poisonous varieties include aloe (cut leaves), holly or daphne (berries), mistletoe (leaves and stems), and all parts of foxglove, philodendron, and rhododendron. Poisonous wild mushrooms include *Amanita muscaria* (red top with white speckles) and *Amanita phalloides* (looks like an edible mushroom). Call poison control if you suspect any of these substances has been eaten, especially by a young child.

Items in medicine cabinet Any over-the-counter medicines taken in larger than recommended doses; rubbing alcohol; prescription medicines.

Household cleaners Drain, toilet, oven, and general-purpose cleaners; dishwashing and dishwasher detergents and soaps; furniture polish.

Lawn and garden products Weed killers; plant food; slug bait; rat poison; insecticides.

Other Oil-based paints; gasoline; kerosene; automotive fluids.

get help or call 911 yourself. Stay with the person (outside) until medical help arrives.

OVERDOSES

Alcohol Alcohol is a depressant. Any alcoholic beverage consumed in large doses or drunk quickly can be toxic. A person who has consumed dangerous levels of alcohol may be incoherent, belligerent, unable to walk, or unconscious. Small children are especially susceptible to alcohol poisoning.

A person who has passed out after drinking should be taken to the emergency department by ambulance. Call out for someone to get help, or call 911 yourself if the person does not need immediate assistance. In the meantime, treat as for an unconscious person (see p.1217).

Street drugs Depending upon the type of drug taken (a depressant or stimulant), the person may be overly sluggish or hyperactive. In most cases, the person will need medical intervention to counteract the drug's effects.

Ensure your own safety first. A person who is overdosing, especially if hyperactive, may exhibit unusual strength and loss of control and could harm you. Be careful of contaminated needles.

Call out for someone to get help, or call 911 yourself if the person does not need immediate assistance. If you feel you will be safe, stay with the person until medical help arrives. (See also Unconsciousness, p.1217; Breathing Difficulties, p.1198; Cardiopulmonary Resuscitation, p.1201.)

Sleeping pills and tranquilizers Sleeping pills and tranquilizers are depressants. A person who has

How to Induce Vomiting

Syrup of ipecac is a substance used to induce vomiting when certain poisons have been swallowed. If you are instructed by poison control to induce vomiting, follow the poison control instructions. If you do not have syrup of ipecac, have the person drink a large glass of heavily salted water. Then tickle the back of the person's throat with your finger. This will bring on the gag reflex and cause vomiting. Do not induce vomiting if the person is unconscious or looks like he or she might soon lose consciousness. Do not induce vomiting unless instructed to do so by poison control; some poisons do more damage when vomited back up.

overdosed on them may appear to be sleeping but actually may be unconscious (see p.1217).

Symptoms include shallow breathing, weak pulse, and unresponsiveness. Call out for someone to get help, or call 911 yourself if the person does not need immediate assistance. Check airway, breathing, and circulation (see Cardiopulmonary Resuscitation, p.1201). Keep the person on his or her side. Stay with him or her until medical help arrives.

Poison Oak

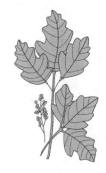

The leaves of poison oak are similar to those of an oak tree. It has white-green flowers and berries. Poison oak grows as a shrub and is common on the west coast from Mexico to British Columbia.

Poison Ivy

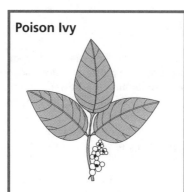

This plant has shiny leaves, small yellow-green flowers, and green-white berries. It grows as a vine, shrub, or bush. It is common throughout the United States, except in the southwest, Alaska, and Hawaii.

PLANTS THAT CAUSE SEVERE SKIN REACTIONS

The plants that most commonly cause skin reactions are poison ivy, poison oak, and poison sumac. Each produces a poisonous sap that is present on the roots, stems, leaves, and berries. Touching the plants easily spreads the poison. If the plants are burned, the smoke may irritate the skin, eyes, throat, and

Poison Sumac

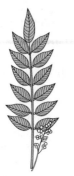

The plant produces yellow-green flowers and white-green berries. The nonpoisonous variety has red berries. It grows as a shrub or tree and is common in the eastern United States and along the Mississippi River.

lungs. In addition, family pets that brush against the plants may carry the irritant on their fur.

The leaves of poison ivy and poison oak grow in groups of three. Remember this saying if you are in doubt about any wild plant: "Leaves of three, let them be."

The leaves of poison sumac grow in pairs, often 7 to 13 pairs on a stem, with a single leaflet at the top.

Reaction to the plants may occur almost immediately or up to 12 to 48 hours after exposure. Symptoms of poisoning include redness, itching, rash, fever, and headache. Small pimple-like blisters may form several days later. The discharge from them will not spread the poison.

Immediate care Protect your skin from exposure by wearing long sleeves and pants. Remove clothing and shoes that have

come in contact with the plant. Wash the affected areas of skin with soap and water as soon as possible after exposure. Avoid scratching, which will spread the poison. Calamine lotion and antihistamines may be used to relieve itching. For more severe reactions, consult a physician.

Puncture Wounds

A puncture wound occurs when a sharp object penetrates the skin and underlying tissue. The injury can be serious because of the risk of infection deep within tissue. The wound may appear as a small hole in the skin and there may be little bleeding.

Immediate care Wash the area with soap and water. Apply bacitracin ointment and place a sterile bandage over the wound. If the puncture wound is on the hands, face, neck, trunk, or feet, or is caused by a bite, go to a hospital emergency department. The person will need a tetanus immunization if he or she has not had one for 10 years.

Ring Removal
(See Finger Injuries, p.1210)

Scalp Injuries
(See Head Injuries, p.1211)

Scrapes and Scratches

A scrape or scratch removes the upper layer of the skin, which helps protect the body from infection. Treat a cat scratch as a bite wound (see p.1194).

Immediate care Wash the injured area with running water

until all dirt is removed. Gently pat the wound dry. You may apply bacitracin ointment and cover the wound with a bandage or sterile gauze pad, but it is better to leave it exposed to the air to help it heal. You will need a tetanus immunization if you have not had one within the past 10 years.

Seizures
(See How to Help Someone Who is Having a Seizure, p.376)

Severed Limbs

A severed limb is a life-threatening emergency. The person may lose a great deal of blood quickly and risks going into shock (see p.1216). Treat the person before attending to the severed limb.

Immediate care Call out for someone to get help, or call 911 yourself. If the person is unconscious, check airway, breathing, and circulation (see Cardiopulmonary Resuscitation, p.1201). Control bleeding as described on p.1196. If the person is vomiting, turn him or her on the side to prevent choking, but only if you do not suspect a back or neck injury (see p.1192). Stay with the person until medical help arrives.

Caring for a severed limb
Place the limb in a plastic bag and seal it. This will keep the limb from drying out. Place this bag in another bag partially filled with ice. Do not place ice or water directly on the limb. Give the bag with the limb to medical personnel. In some instances, the limb can be successfully reattached.

Shock

Shock is a life-threatening medical condition that results when oxygenated blood does not reach tissues and organs.

It can occur with an injury in which a large amount of blood has been lost (internally or externally) or with severe infection, drug overdose, heart conditions, severe allergic reactions, or poisoning. It also can occur after prolonged, severe diarrhea or vomiting.

Signs and symptoms include disorientation, restlessness, trembling, pale or bluish skin, cool or clammy skin, very slow or rapid breathing, and unconsciousness (see p.1217).

Immediate care Call out for someone to get help, or call 911 yourself. Check airway, breathing, and circulation (see Cardiopulmonary Resuscitation, p.1201). Loosen any tight-fitting clothing. Treat the injury or illness that caused the shock.

If you do not suspect back or neck injuries (see p.1192), place the person as flat as possible, and in the most comfortable position based on the injury or illness. Keep the person warm and stay with him or her until medical help arrives.

Snakebites

(See Bites and Stings, p.1194)

Spider Bites

(See Bites and Stings, p.1194)

Spinal Injuries

(See Back and Neck Injuries, p.1192)

Splint

(See Broken Bones, p.1199)

Splinters

A splinter or sliver is a thin piece of wood, glass, metal, or other material that becomes embedded just beneath the skin. Do not attempt to remove a splinter that is lodged deeply in the skin or that is close to the eye (see Eye Injuries, p.1208). Seek medical attention instead.

Immediate care Wash your hands and the area around the wound with soap and warm water. If part of the splinter is visible above the skin, remove it carefully with clean tweezers.

If the splinter breaks, leaving part of it imbedded in the skin, and it is not too deeply imbedded, sterilize a sewing needle by placing its tip in a flame for 10 seconds. Let it cool for a minute and use it to loosen the skin around the splinter. Remove the rest of the splinter with the tweezers. Bleeding from the injury will help wash away bacteria.

After the splinter has been removed, rinse the area thoroughly with running water and pat dry. Apply a small amount of bacitracin ointment.

Leaving the wound exposed to air will help it heal more quickly. Seek medical attention if you are unable to remove the splinter or if infection develops.

Stroke

A stroke occurs when a blood clot or ruptured artery blocks the flow of blood to the brain (see p.342). Emergency medical treatment within the first few hours of a stroke may help diminish any long-lasting effects, such as paralysis.

Immediate care Call out for someone to get help or call 911 yourself. If the person is unconscious, check airway, breathing, and circulation (see Cardiopulmonary Resuscitation, p.1201). If the person is diabetic, immediately administer sugar (see Diabetic Emergencies, p.1207). Otherwise, do not give the person anything to eat or drink. Stay with him or her until medical help arrives.

Teeth, Knocked-Out

A tooth that has been knocked out of its socket often can be reimplanted, provided the tooth is not damaged.

Immediate care Provide care to the person first. Ensure that there are no back or neck injuries (see p.1192). If the person has the tooth and it is clean, immediately and firmly place it back all the way into its socket. Do not touch the root.

If the tooth is dirty, have the person roll it around in his or her mouth with saliva before putting it into the socket. Have the person apply moderate pressure on the tooth.

Alternately, place the tooth under the person's tongue or in milk (not skim milk). Milk has nutrients that will help the tooth survive.

If the tooth is extremely dirty or cannot be found, stop bleeding in the socket by rolling up a small piece of paper towel or gauze and having the person bite on it to apply pressure. Take the person to a dentist or hospital emergency department.

Unconsciousness

Unconsciousness can be caused by an injury (including a fall, accident, or collision) or an illness or medical emergency such as diabetes, epilepsy, heart attack, drug overdose, poisoning, or shock.

The person will be unresponsive to shouts or attempts to rouse him or her.

Immediate care Call out for someone to get help, or call 911 yourself. Check airway, breathing, and circulation (see Cardiopulmonary Resuscitation, p.1201). Loosen any tight-fitting clothing. Treat the injury or illness that caused the unconsciousness. If the person is diabetic and can be aroused, administer sugar (see Diabetic Emergencies, p.1207). If you do not suspect a back or neck injury (see p.1192), place the person in the most comfortable position based on the injury or illness. Keep the person warm and stay with him or her until medical help arrives.

Replaceable Parts of Irreplaceable You

In the recent past, once an organ or other part of the body was diseased, injured, or worn out, people either lived with the reduction in function or died.

Today, doctors can replace an astonishing variety of body parts—from the hip to the heart and many parts in between—with mechanical devices and transplanted organs. Slowly, medical research is learning how to take cells from a healthy person to help heal the sick organ of another person through cell transplantation.

While some new organs, such as corneas, must always come from human donors, other parts of the body can be replaced with devices made of metal or plastic, or from animals. The following pages offer a sampling of the replaceable parts "worn" in the bodies of an increasingly large number of people.

TRANSPLANTS

Bone marrow Transplants of blood-producing bone marrow cells (see p.732) are used to treat conditions such as leukemia, lymphoma, and breast cancer. Primitive blood cells called stem cells (which mature into healthy adult blood cells) are infused into the bloodstream to replace cells affected by disease or high doses of chemotherapy or radiation.

Cells Transplanting cells (rather than organs, such as the heart) taken from aborted fetal tissue is sometimes performed to try to improve degenerative diseases such as macular degeneration (a leading cause of blindness), Parkinson disease, and Huntington disease. Researchers may have discovered a way to grow large amounts of human cells indefinitely, opening the possibility that some day you could obtain a cell transplant—of any kind of cells, from any organ—to restore health to any sick organ.

Cornea More than 35,000 cornea transplants are performed in the United States each year, making this the most common of all transplants. See also p.429.

Heart Heart transplants often receive wide media attention, but they are not frequently performed. Only 2,290 heart transplants were done in 1997 in the United States. See also p.688.

Kidney Kidney transplants are the most common major organ transplant performed today. In 1997, more than 12,000 kidneys were transplanted, included 3,500 from living donors. One reason kidneys are transplanted more often than other organs is that nearly everyone is born with two, and can live on one, so that many healthy people can donate

a kidney. Despite this, some 40,000 people in the United States are still waiting for a kidney. See also p.814.

Liver After kidney transplants, liver transplants are the next most common major organ transplant, with more than 4,000 operations done in the United States in 1997. See also p.767.

Lung The number of lung transplants has increased in recent years. In 1988, 33 transplants were done in the United States. However, in 1997, almost 950 people received a new lung. Fewer than 100 people received both a heart and a lung. See also p.516.

Pancreas The pancreas can be transplanted alone or with a kidney. More than 2,000 pancreata were transplanted alone in 1997 in the United States; about 850 were transplanted with a kidney.

Intestine Transplants of small intestine have increased in the United States from just five operations in 1990 to 67 in 1997. Most recipients are young, either between the ages of 1 and 5 or between 18 and 34 years old.

Stomach Stomach transplants are uncommon and are usually done as part of a multiorgan transplant along with the liver, intestine, or pancreas.

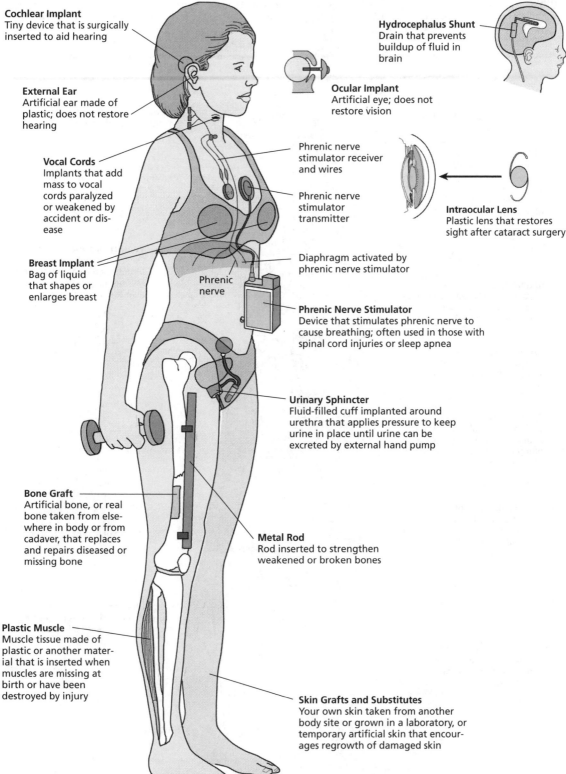

Cochlear Implant
Tiny device that is surgically inserted to aid hearing

External Ear
Artificial ear made of plastic; does not restore hearing

Vocal Cords
Implants that add mass to vocal cords paralyzed or weakened by accident or disease

Breast Implant
Bag of liquid that shapes or enlarges breast

Phrenic nerve

Bone Graft
Artificial bone, or real bone taken from elsewhere in body or from cadaver, that replaces and repairs diseased or missing bone

Plastic Muscle
Muscle tissue made of plastic or another material that is inserted when muscles are missing at birth or have been destroyed by injury

Hydrocephalus Shunt
Drain that prevents buildup of fluid in brain

Ocular Implant
Artificial eye; does not restore vision

Intraocular Lens
Plastic lens that restores sight after cataract surgery

Phrenic nerve stimulator receiver and wires

Phrenic nerve stimulator transmitter

Diaphragm activated by phrenic nerve stimulator

Phrenic Nerve Stimulator
Device that stimulates phrenic nerve to cause breathing; often used in those with spinal cord injuries or sleep apnea

Urinary Sphincter
Fluid-filled cuff implanted around urethra that applies pressure to keep urine in place until urine can be excreted by external hand pump

Metal Rod
Rod inserted to strengthen weakened or broken bones

Skin Grafts and Substitutes
Your own skin taken from another body site or grown in a laboratory, or temporary artificial skin that encourages regrowth of damaged skin

Dental Implants
Implants that are permanently embedded into jaw to replace teeth

Facial Implants
Silicone or plastic objects that give shape to facial features

*Artificial shoulder joint

*Artificial wrist joint

Pacemaker
Electrical device implanted under skin that stimulates regular heartbeat in diseased heart

Spinal Implant
Metal rods and clamps that are attached to spinal column to strengthen or straighten spine

Blood Vessels
Tubes of synthetic material that replace surgically removed arteries

Penile Implant
Tube that is implanted in the penis and inflated by manual pump placed in scrotum when erection is desired

Testicular Implant
Implant in scrotum that restores appearance of surgically removed testicle

Prosthetic Limbs
Legs, feet, and hands made of synthetic materials; prosthetic hands can grasp objects

Titanium Skull and Jaw Plates
Implants that replace or strengthen part of skull or jaw

Artificial Heart Valve
Valve made of metal or plastic, or animal valve, that replaces defective heart valve

Defibrillator
Electrical device, implanted under skin, that shocks heart back into normal rhythm to prevent sudden death

Stents
Tubes of synthetic materials that are placed inside arteries or other natural tubes in body to keep them open

*Artificial elbow joint

Ventricular Bypass Assist
Device that helps heart pump blood; used to ease strain on recuperating heart or in person awaiting heart transplant

*Artificial hip joint

*Artificial knee joint

Artificial Joints*
Synthetic material that replaces surgically removed damaged joints

*Artificial ankle joint

Appendix

MEDICAL TERMINOLOGY

GLOSSARY

abrasion A scraping or rubbing away of the skin or other surface.

abscess A collection of pus that is surrounded by inflamed tissue.

acute Any condition that is characterized by rapid onset, severe symptoms, and short duration.

adhesion Scar tissue that unites two body parts or surfaces that are not normally united—for example, when a loop of intestine adheres to the abdominal wall after surgery.

adjuvant therapy Treatment that enhances a primary treatment. For example, using chemotherapy to treat cancer after a patient has been treated with surgery or radiation.

aerobic Pertaining to processes that require oxygen. Aerobic exercise, for example, requires increased oxygen intake.

allergen A substance—such as fur, pollen, or dust—that produces an allergic reaction.

allergy A reaction—such as a rash, fever, vomiting, sneezing, or headaches—that occurs after exposure to an allergen.

alveoli Tiny air sacs found deep in the lungs, in which inhaled oxygen enters the bloodstream and carbon dioxide leaves the bloodstream to be expelled by the lungs.

ambulatory Able to walk; not confined to a bed.

amnesia A total or partial loss of memory caused by brain damage, emotional trauma, drugs, or disease.

amputation The surgical removal of a limb or other body part.

anaerobic Pertaining to processes that do not require oxygen.

analgesic A drug or other substance—such as aspirin, acetaminophen, or morphine—that is used to relieve pain.

anaphylaxis A severe, abnormal allergic reaction. Anaphylaxis may cause itching and swelling; in rare cases, it causes difficulty breathing, convulsions, shock, and coma.

androgen A hormone, such as testosterone, that is responsible for development of male characteristics such as beard growth. Androgen is produced in the testicles.

anemia A decrease in the body's hemoglobin—the oxygen-carrying component of red blood cells. Anemia typically causes tiredness, breathlessness, and poor resistance to infection.

anencephaly A birth defect in which an infant is born without most of the brain or without the skull bones covering the brain.

aneurysm A bulge or swelling that forms on the wall of a blood vessel. An aneurysm is usually caused by high blood pressure or atherosclerosis.

angina pectoris A temporary pain in the chest that usually occurs when the heart's demand for blood is more than the arteries can supply—for instance, during physical exertion.

anorexia The medical term for loss of appetite that results from illness.

antibiotic A substance that can destroy or inhibit the growth of bacteria and some other organisms that cause disease.

antibody A substance made by the immune system that reacts to and attacks a particular foreign substance. For example, the immune system can produce antibodies that attack germs that invade the body.

anticoagulant A substance that reduces the tendency of the blood to clot.

antigen Any substance that the body sees as foreign, such as pollen, and which causes the immune system to form antibodies.

antihistamine A drug that blocks the action of histamines, which are responsible for allergic symptoms such as sneezing and itching.

antiseptic A chemical that destroys or slows the growth of disease-causing organisms such as bacteria. An antiseptic is usually applied to skin or wounds to prevent infection.

aphasia A disorder that causes problems with speaking and understanding speech and, often, problems with reading and writing. Aphasia is caused by a brain injury.

apnea A temporary halt in breathing.

arrhythmia An abnormal rhythm of the heartbeat.

arthroplasty The surgical rebuilding or replacement of a joint, usually to relieve symptoms of arthritis or to fix an abnormality.

asphyxia A life-threatening lack of oxygen due to drowning or choking or to an obstruction of the airways.

aspiration Suctioning fluid from the body; or the act of breathing in fluid or a foreign body or substance, such as vomit.

asymptomatic Showing no signs or symptoms of disease, whether or not disease is present.

ataxia An inability to control movement, characterized by shaking and an unsteady walk.

atherosclerosis A disease of the arteries in which a buildup of tissue called plaque on the wall of the artery narrows it and reduces blood flow.

atria The upper chambers of the heart.

atrophy Wasting away of an organ or tissue due to undernourishment, disease, or aging.

aura A forewarning of an attack. For example, an aura just before a seizure is sometimes felt as a cold sensation flowing over the body.

autoimmune response A reaction of the body against some of its own tissues. The tissues are incorrectly seen as foreign substances.

autopsy An examination and dissection of the body after death to determine the cause of death or the presence of disease.

avulsion The tearing away of one part of the body from another—for example, a tendon tearing away from a bone.

bacteria Tiny single-celled organisms. Bacteria can cause disease, although many are harmless.

B cell A type of white blood cell. B cells are part of the immune system, come from bone marrow, and produce antibodies to fight off disease.

benign Harmless; or a tumor that is not cancerous and thus usually does not spread.

bile A thick, yellow-green fluid that is secreted by the liver and stored in the gallbladder. Bile is released into the intestine to aid in digestion.

biopsy The removal of a small piece of living tissue from the body for examination under a microscope. A biopsy is often used to diagnose cancer.

bowel The small or large intestine.

brainstem The part of the brain that connects the brain with the spinal cord; it is made up of the medulla oblongata, the pons, and the midbrain. The brainstem controls movement, sensation, and reflex reactions.

bronchiole A small airway in the respiratory system. The bronchiole is a subdivision of the bronchial tube, which leads from the trachea to the lungs.

cancer A general term for a number of illnesses, all of which are characterized by the abnormal growth of cells resulting in tumors that may spread throughout the body.

capillaries The tiniest blood vessels. Capillaries are found in the tissues, connect arteries and veins, and are tiny enough to allow oxygen and other substances to travel from the blood to the tissues.

carcinogen Any substance that can cause cancer.

carcinogenesis The process by which a normal cell becomes cancerous.

carcinoma A malignant tumor that arises in the tissues that line the organs of the body. Carcinomas are found in the skin, large intestine, lungs, stomach, prostate, cervix, ovaries, brain, and breasts.

cardiopulmonary Pertaining to the heart and lungs.

cardiovascular Pertaining to the heart and network of blood vessels.

cartilage The dense connective tissue found in the larynx, trachea, nose, and joints.

catheter A thin, hollow tube that can be inserted into the body to withdraw or insert fluids.

cell The basic building block of living organisms. A cell consists of a cell wall and a fluid called cytoplasm in which numerous structures, such as the nucleus, are suspended.

cerebrovascular Pertaining to the blood vessels in the brain.

chemotherapy The use of chemicals to treat or prevent infections and other diseases. Chemotherapy is often used to destroy cancer cells.

cholesterol A fatlike material found in blood and most tissues, especially in bile, the brain, the liver, the kidneys, and nerves. High concentrations of low-density lipoprotein (LDL) cholesterol in the blood are associated with atherosclerosis. High concentrations of high-density lipoprotein (HDL) cholesterol seem to lower the risk for heart disease.

chromosome A threadlike structure that carries hereditary information in the form of deoxyribonucleic acid (DNA). It is found in the nucleus of a cell.

chronic Any condition that lasts a long time or recurs over time.

cilia Small, hairlike structures on the surface of some cells.

cirrhosis A condition in which the liver forms interlacing strands of fibrous tissue, obstructing blood flow and other functions.

claudication A cramping muscle pain, usually felt in the calf, caused by inadequate blood flow.

clinical Interacting with patients, as opposed to working in a laboratory.

clinical trial Medical research studies that evaluate treatments as well as methods of prevention, detection, and diagnosis. Often, volunteer patients are placed into two groups; one group receives no treatment or the standard treatment and the other group receives a new treatment.

coagulate The process in which a liquid, such as blood, becomes solid or semisolid.

colic Severe abdominal pain caused by spasms in the intestines or in the ureters of the kidneys.

collagen A fibrous material that is a principal component of connective tissue. Collagen is found in skin, bone, cartilage, and ligaments.

colostrum A liquid containing protective antibodies that is made by a woman's breasts shortly after giving birth.

coma A state of deep unconsciousness.

communicable disease Any disease that can be passed from one person or species to another by direct contact, handling an infected object, or breathing in infected droplets that were coughed or exhaled into the air.

conception The start of a pregnancy, when an egg is fertilized by a sperm.

congestion The accumulation of mucus or of blood in an organ.

contracture A shrinking and shortening of a muscle, usually as a result of disease or lack of use. A contracture usually limits the full movement of a joint.

control group In a clinical trial, the group of patients who receive no treatment or the standard treatment. Their response is then measured against the response of the group who received a new form of treatment.

contusion An injury that does not result in a break in the skin but typically causes swelling, discoloration, and pain; a bruise.

convulsion A sudden, involuntary contraction of muscles that results in rhythmic contortions of the body, often accompanied by a loss of consciousness; a seizure.

coronary Pertaining to the arteries that supply blood to the heart.

curettage The scraping of the inside of an organ or body cavity with a spoon-shaped instrument, usually to remove diseased tissue or obtain a specimen.

cyanosis A bluish discoloration of the skin caused by a lack of oxygen in the blood. Cyanosis often accompanies heart failure and lung disease.

cyst An abnormal sac or cavity, usually filled with fluid or semisolid matter, that can occur in many parts of the body.

debility A state of weakness or a loss of physical strength.

degenerative disease Any disease in which the structure or function of tissues deteriorates.

delirium An acute mental disorder characterized by wild enthusiasm or confusion and, frequently, hallucinations.

delusion A false or irrational belief held by a person despite evidence to the contrary.

dementia A progressive mental disorder characterized by confusion, disorientation, and deterioration of intellectual function and memory. Dementia can be caused by drugs, brain tumors, strokes, injury to the brain, or Alzheimer disease.

deoxyribonucleic acid (DNA) The substance that contains the genetic code, found in the nucleus of the cell. DNA is composed of a double strand of tiny units called nucleotides. Strings of nucleotides make up genes, which are the blueprint of the structure of the human body.

detoxification The process of removing poisons from a person.

diastole The period of time between contractions of the heart, when the heart muscle relaxes and the chambers fill up with blood.

digit A finger or toe.

dilate To expand the width of a body opening or cavity, such as the opening of the cervix during labor or the opening of the pupil of the eye in response to decreased light.

dislocation The movement of a bone from its normal position, such as a dislocated shoulder.

diuretic Any drug or substance that increases the volume of urine by increasing the excretion of water and salts from the kidneys.

diverticulum A pouch formed at a weak spot in the wall of the digestive tract, such as in the esophagus, stomach, or intestines.

DNA (see deoxyribonucleic acid)

dominant A gene or its characteristic, such as the gene for eye color, that will be expressed in offspring, regardless of whether its paired gene from the other parent is the same. A dominant gene or characteristic overrides a recessive gene.

dorsal Pertaining to the back of the body or to an organ.

dysplasia An abnormal, sometimes precancerous change in cells of a tissue.

ectopic The abnormal placement of a body part. For example, an ectopic pregnancy occurs outside of the uterus.

edema An abnormal accumulation of fluid in tissues that causes swelling.

effusion The escape of a fluid, such as pus or blood, into a body cavity or joint space.

embolism A condition in which a blood vessel is blocked by a clot of blood, fat, amniotic fluid, or other material that has traveled from another part of the body.

emetic Any drug or other substance that is used to cause vomiting.

emission A discharge or release of a substance, usually a fluid.

endoscopy A process in which a flexible tube with a light is used to look inside a body cavity or organ.

enzyme A substance that speeds up another chemical reaction. For example, digestive enzymes help speed up the digestion of food.

erythema A flushing of the skin due to the dilation (opening) of blood capillaries just below the surface of the skin.

febrile Pertaining to an abnormally high body temperature.

fibrillation An involuntary, repeated contraction of a muscle. When fibrillation occurs in the heart muscle, it causes an irregular heartbeat.

fibroid A noncancerous tumor of connective and muscular tissue that is often found in the uterus.

flatulence The presence of excess gas or air in the stomach or intestines that is expelled from the anus.

fracture A break in a bone. A simple fracture is a clean break with little damage to surrounding tissues; in a compound fracture, the bone usually pierces the skin.

fungus A simple organism that can live as a parasite on plants and animals. Some fungi can cause disease in humans.

ganglion A normal, well-defined mass of nerve tissue; or an abnormal but harmless swelling or cyst that is found in tendon sheaths.

gangrene A disorder in which body tissue decays and dies, usually because of a lack of blood supply to the area.

gastric Pertaining to the stomach.

gastrointestinal Pertaining to all or some of the organs of the digestive tract, from the mouth to the anus.

gene The basic unit of hereditary material. A gene is composed of a particular sequence of nucleic acids and found in a particular spot on a chromosome.

generic drug A drug that is not protected by a company's trademark and is often less expensive than a brand name drug.

gland Any organ or tissue that secretes fluids, such as hormones, for use elsewhere in the body or as wastes.

goiter An enlargement of the thyroid gland that causes swelling in the neck.

hallucination A perception—which may be seen, smelled, heard, tasted, or felt—of something that is not really there.

heart murmur An abnormal sound heard during an examination of the heart, caused by the flow of blood through heart chambers or valves. Many heart murmurs do not indicate heart problems; others do.

hematemesis The vomiting of bright red blood, indicating bleeding in the upper gastrointestinal tract.

hematoma A swelling formed of blood, found in skin tissues or an organ.

hematuria The presence of blood in the urine.

hemodialysis A procedure in which wastes and impurities are mechanically removed from the blood. Hemodialysis is usually performed on people whose kidneys are not working properly.

hemoptysis Coughing up or spitting up blood from the respiratory tract.

hemorrhage Bleeding from a damaged blood vessel.

hirsutism The presence of excessive malelike hair in a female. Hirsutism can be caused by heredity, hormonal imbalances, or other causes.

hormone A chemical that is produced by endocrine glands in one part of the body and regulates the actions of other parts of the body.

hyperglycemia A condition in which there is too much sugar in the bloodstream. Hyperglycemia can occur in any number of diseases, but most often occurs in diabetes when there is not enough insulin in the blood.

hyperplasia The growth of tissues in an organ that results in a larger but still normal appearance, such as the growth of the breasts during pregnancy.

hypertension A condition in which the blood is pumped through the body at an abnormally high pressure; commonly known as high blood pressure.

hypoglycemia A condition in which there is too little sugar in the bloodstream, causing weakness, confusion, sweating, and sometimes coma.

hypotension A condition in which the blood is pumped through the body at an abnormally low pressure; low blood pressure.

hypoxia An inadequate supply of oxygen in the tissues.

iatrogenic Occurring as a result of treatment.

idiopathic A condition or disease of unknown origin.

immobilize To make a limb or other part of the body immovable to help in healing.

immunity The body's ability to resist infection and disease, caused by the presence of antibodies and white blood cells in the bloodstream.

immunization The process by which resistance to a disease is established. Immunization usually occurs in the form of an injection of harmless bacteria or viruses that cause the body to produce its own antibodies to those substances.

impacted Something that is firmly wedged into place and immovable, such as a wisdom tooth.

impotence The inability to maintain an erection or the inability of the penis to become firm enough to have sexual intercourse.

incision A cut made in the skin or soft tissue with a surgical knife.

incontinence The involuntary passing of urine or feces. A common form is stress incontinence, in which urine is passed during coughing.

incubation period The period of time between when a person is exposed to an infection and when symptoms appear.

infarct A section of tissue or organ that has died as a result of an interruption of its blood supply.

infection The invasion of the body by harmful organisms, such as bacteria, that cause disease.

inflammation A condition characterized by swelling, heat, redness, and pain. Inflammation is the body's reaction to an injury or infection.

infusion The slow injection of a fluid into a vein or tissues.

injection The introduction into the body of drugs or fluids by means of a needle inserted into the skin, a muscle, or a blood vessel.

inoperable Any condition that cannot be treated by surgery.

insomnia The inability to fall asleep or remain asleep long enough to feel rested.

intramuscular Pertaining to the inside of muscle tissue. In an intramuscular injection, a needle is inserted into muscle.

intravenous Pertaining to the inside or interior of a vein. For example, an intravenous catheter is inserted into a vein.

ischemia An inadequate flow of oxygenated blood to a part of the body, caused by a blockage in the blood vessels.

jaundice A yellowing of the skin or the whites of the eyes, caused by too much bilirubin (the pigment found in bile) in the blood. Jaundice is associated with several disorders, including diseases of the liver.

keloid An unusually hard or thick scar that forms after surgery or an injury. Most keloids flatten and become less noticeable over time.

laceration A tear in the skin that produces a wound with irregular edges.

laxative A drug or substance that stimulates bowel movements or makes the stool softer or bulkier.

lesion An area of tissue that is not functioning properly because of damage caused by a wound, abscess, tumor, or other abnormality.

ligament A band of fibrous connective tissue that links two bones together at a joint.

ligature Any material that is tied around a blood vessel to stop it from bleeding.

lipoma A noncancerous tumor or growth composed of fat cells.

lymphocyte A type of white blood cell that is essential to the proper functioning of the body's immune system.

malaise A general feeling of illness that can be a sign of disease.

malignant A tumor that has the ability to invade adjacent tissues and spread to other sites in the body; also used to describe any condition that tends to become worse and eventually causes death.

malnutrition A condition caused by a failure to eat or to properly absorb the foods needed to maintain proper health.

melanin A dark brown or black pigment found in the skin, hair, and eyes. Melanin production is increased by exposure to sunlight.

melanoma A cancerous tumor of the skin cells that produce melanin.

membrane A thin layer of tissue that surrounds or lines organs or cavities.

metabolism The total of all the chemical and physical processes that occur in the body to ensure its growth and proper functioning, including the breakdown of food for energy.

metastasis The spread of a malignant tumor from its original location to other sites in the body, usually by means of cells that break off from the tumor and travel through the bloodstream or lymph system.

mucous membrane A thin, moist membrane that lines many structures and cavities in the body, such as the sinuses and mouth.

musculoskeletal Pertaining to the muscles and the skeleton.

myalgia Pain or tenderness in a muscle.

myasthenia An abnormal weakness in a muscle or group of muscles.

necrosis The death of all or some of the cells in an organ or tissues.

neonatal Pertaining to an infant younger than 4 weeks of age.

neoplasm A new and abnormal growth; or any cancerous or noncancerous tumor.

nephritis Inflammation of the kidneys.

neuralgia A burning or stabbing pain that often follows the pathway of a nerve.

occlusion The closing or blocking of a hollow organ or body part.

occult Something that is not visible to the naked eye but can be seen under a microscope or made evident through laboratory testing.

oncogene A gene that, under certain conditions, can cause cancer.

outpatient A patient who receives treatment at a hospital or other medical facility but does not stay overnight.

ovulation The release of an egg from the ovary, at which time it is available to be fertilized by sperm.

palliative care A treatment that will relieve symptoms but is not expected to provide a cure for the disease causing those symptoms.

palpate To examine a part of the body by touching it carefully.

palpitation A pounding or racing of the heart, often caused by emotions or heart disorders.

palsy An abnormal condition characterized by paralysis.

paraplegia Loss of voluntary movement below the waist, including the legs.

paroxysm A sudden, violent attack or convulsion; or the worsening of symptoms or recurrence of disease.

pathogen A tiny organism—such as a virus, bacterium, or parasite—that can invade the body and produce disease.

perforation A hole, such as an ulcer, that erodes an organ or tissue.

peristalsis A wavelike movement along a hollow, tubular body part that serves to move the contents of the tube. Peristalsis in the intestines moves food through the digestive system.

pessary An object placed in the vagina to prevent the uterus or rectum from dropping into the vagina due to weakened tissues.

petechiae Tiny red or purple spots that appear on the skin, indicating tiny hemorrhages in a lower skin layer.

phlegm Mucus or sputum from the sinuses or respiratory tract.

placebo A substance that should have no effect on the body. However, in some instances, a placebo may relieve symptoms because the patient believes it can do so. In clinical trials, new drugs are often tested against placebos.

plaque A layer of bacteria that forms on the surface of a tooth and can cause dental disease; the build-up of deposits on the walls of arteries that occurs in atherosclerosis.

plasma The fluid in which blood cells are suspended.

platelet A colorless, disk-shaped cell in the blood that is necessary for clotting.

polyp A noncancerous growth that is found protruding from tissues. Polyps often occur in the sinuses and in the lining of the colon.

postpartum Pertaining to the period after giving birth.

prognosis A prediction on how a patient's disease will progress in the future.

prolapse The displacement of an organ or other structure from its normal position, usually caused by a weakening in the tissues that normally support the structure. A prolapsed uterus may occur when supporting tissues are weakened by childbirth.

prophylaxis Steps that are taken to prevent a disease or condition, such as taking nitroglycerin to prevent angina.

prosthesis An artificial device—such as a hearing aid, an artificial joint, or dentures—that substitutes for a missing body part.

protocol A plan that lays out the procedures that will be followed in conducting a physical examination, a research study, or the treatment of a disease.

pruritus Itching.

psychogenic Pertaining to symptoms and illnesses that begin in the mind, rather than in the body.

psychosomatic Pertaining to symptoms and illnesses that involve both the mind and the body, such as physical disorders like irritable bowel syndrome, in which psychological stress may cause abdominal pain.

pulmonary Pertaining to the lungs.

purulent Formed of or containing pus.

pus A thick, yellow or green liquid that is composed of dead cells and bacteria, most often found at the site of a bacterial infection.

quadriplegia Paralysis of all limbs, often caused by a severe neck injury.

quarantine To prevent the spread of disease, the period of time in which a sick person is kept away from others.

radiation Energy that is in the form of particles or waves, such as x-rays and gamma rays. Radiation is often used to help make a diagnosis, as in x-rays, or as a treatment for cancer.

recessive A gene that will not be expressed in the offspring unless it is inherited from both the mother and father. A recessive gene from one parent that is paired with a dominant gene from the other parent will be overridden by the dominant gene.

rejection A reaction that occurs when a person's immune system recognizes a transplanted organ as a foreign substance and tries to rid the body of it.

relapse The return of symptoms and disease after a patient seems to recover.

remission A lessening in the severity of a disease and its symptoms. In cancer, a reduction in the size of a tumor and its symptoms.

renal Pertaining to the kidneys.

resection The surgical removal of a part of the body.

respiration The process by which gases enter the body, including external respiration (breathing), and internal respiration, in which oxygen taken in by the lungs is carried by the blood to tissues and carbon dioxide is removed.

resuscitation The process of reviving a person who is not breathing or whose heart is not beating using techniques such as artificial respiration and heart massage.

risk factor Any factor that can cause a person to be more likely to develop a disease. For example, smoking is a risk factor for lung cancer.

roughage The indigestible dietary fiber found in grains, fruits, vegetables, and other foods. Roughage is thought to help prevent conditions such as constipation.

rupture A tear or break in an organ or tissue. Other tissue that protrudes through the opening is known as a hernia.

saline A watery solution that contains a small amount of salt and is often used to administer drugs or as a substitute for plasma.

sarcoma A cancer that arises in the connective tissues that support and separate other tissues or organs. Sarcomas can occur almost anywhere in the body.

secretion The release of chemical substances produced by the body; or the substance that is produced.

sedative A drug or a procedure that has a calming effect and relieves anxiety and tension.

seizure A sudden, involuntary contraction of muscles that results in rhythmic contortions of the body, often accompanied by a loss of consciousness. Also called a convulsion. People with epilepsy have recurring seizures.

sepsis The destruction or infection of tissues by disease-causing organisms, usually accompanied by a fever.

septicemia A condition in which disease-causing organisms have spread to the bloodstream from an infection elsewhere in the body. Also known as blood poisoning.

shock A serious medical condition in which there is not enough blood flowing to the outer portions of the body, resulting in cold, sweaty skin; a weak pulse; irregular breathing; and dilated pupils. Shock can be caused by a loss of blood, severe heart problems, severe infections, allergic reactions, or drug overdoses.

shunt A device that is inserted into the body to redirect the flow of blood or other fluid from one area to another.

side effect An unwanted, and sometimes dangerous, reaction caused by medication or other treatment.

spasm An involuntary muscle contraction.

sphincter A ring of muscle that surrounds an opening and can be contracted to close the opening. For example, the muscles found at the anus and the opening of the bladder are sphincters.

sprain An injury to a ligament caused by suddenly overstretching the ligament.

sputum A mixture of saliva and mucus that is coughed up from the respiratory tract. Sputum may be examined in a laboratory for signs of disease.

staging The process of determining how far a cancerous disease has progressed. Staging is often used to determine the best course of treatment.

stenosis An abnormal narrowing of a passageway, such as a blood vessel, or other type of opening in the body.

sterilization A surgical procedure or other method that results in a person being unable to bear children; or the process by which materials are thoroughly cleaned of all organisms that could cause disease.

stria A line, streak, or band, such as the stretch marks that occur in pregnancy.

stupor A state of lethargy and unresponsiveness.

subacute Pertaining to a disease or condition that progresses slower than an acute condition but faster than a chronic condition.

subcutaneous Beneath the skin.

suppository A solid form of medication that is inserted in the rectum or vagina.

suture The process of sewing tissues together after surgery; or the stitches themselves.

synovial fluid A thick fluid that lubricates the area around a joint.

systemic Pertaining to something that affects the whole body rather than separate organs or parts.

systole The period of time when the heart contracts during a normal heartbeat.

tachycardia An abnormally rapid heartbeat.

T cell A white blood cell that is produced in the bone marrow and is part of the body's immune system.

tendon A light-colored cord of collagen fibers that connect a muscle to a bone.

thoracic Pertaining to the chest.

thrombus A blood clot.

tissue A group of cells that are specialized to do a certain job and are joined together to form a body structure such as a muscle or a kidney.

topical Pertaining to an external surface of the body, such as the skin, mouth, vagina, or anus; often used to describe the administration of medicine that is applied directly to such a surface.

toxic Pertaining to something that is poisonous.

toxin A poison, usually one produced by a living organism.

traction The process of putting a bone or other body part under a pulling tension by applying weights and pulleys to help healing.

transfusion The process of taking blood from a healthy person and injecting it into someone whose own blood has been depleted during surgery or for some reason is not functioning correctly. Transfusions of whole blood or of specific blood cells (such as red cells, white cells, or platelets) are possible.

transplantation The process of removing an organ or other donated body part from one person and implanting it in another person.

tremor A rhythmic, quivering movement of muscles that can be caused by diseases such as Parkinson disease, side effects of medication, or old age.

tumor Any type of swelling or enlargement of tissues; most often used to describe an abnormal growth of tissue, which can be cancerous or noncancerous.

ulcer A break in the skin or other surface that often occurs along with an inflammation, an infection, or a cancerous growth.

vaccination A method of protecting the body against disease by injecting parts or all of a microorganism that will cause the body to develop antibodies against the microorganism and later fight off disease.

vascular Pertaining to a blood vessel.

vasoconstrictor A substance or condition—such as drugs, cold, fear, and nicotine—that causes blood vessels to narrow and decrease the flow of blood.

vasodilator A substance or condition that causes blood vessels to open wider and increase the flow of blood.

venous Pertaining to a vein.

vertigo Dizziness; often a spinning sensation or a feeling that the ground is tilting.

viral Pertaining to or caused by a virus.

virulent A disease or condition that is highly infectious or dangerous or rapidly progressing.

viscera The internal organs, especially those found in the abdomen.

vital signs Measurements that indicate how well the body is functioning, including pulse rate, respiration (breathing) rate, temperature, and blood pressure.

withdrawal A response to danger or stress characterized by apathy, lethargy, and depression; or the physical or psychological response to a sudden lack of an addictive substance such as alcohol or nicotine.

BOARD-CERTIFIED MEDICAL SPECIALISTS

Board-certified physicians have completed additional training in a specialty and passed an examination. Those who have certificates in subspecialties (such as Cardiology) were first certified in a specialty (such as Internal Medicine). You can contact The American Board of Medical Specialties at 1007 Church St, Evanston, IL 60201; 847-491-9091; 800-776-2378; or http://www.certifieddoctor.org to verify that a doctor is board certified. To learn more about what each type of specialist does, see our Web site (address is at the bottom of every index page).

INFORMATION RESOURCES

DISEASES, CONDITIONS, AND ISSUES: PRIVATE ORGANIZATIONS

Adoption

National Adoption Center
1500 Walnut St
Philadelphia, PA 19102
215-735-9988
http://www.nac.adopt.org/nac/nac.html

National Adoption Information Clearinghouse
330 C St SW
Washington, DC 20447
703-352-3488
888-251-0075
http://www.calib.com/naic

RESOLVE, Inc
1310 Broadway
Somerville, MA 02144
617-623-0744
http://www.resolve.org

Aging

American Association of Homes and Services for the Aging
901 E St NW, Suite 500
Washington, DC 20004
202-783-2242

American Association of Retired Persons
601 E St NW
Washington, DC 20049
202-434-2277
800-424-3410

American Geriatric Society
770 Lexington Ave, Suite 300
New York, NY 10021
212-308-1414

American Society on Aging
833 Market St, Suite 512
San Francisco, CA 94103
415-974-9600
http://www.asaging.org

Children of Aging Parents
1609 Woodbourne Rd, Suite 302A
Levittown, PA 19057
215-945-6900
800-227-7294

Eldercare Locator
(referral to senior services)
800-677-1116

Family Caregiver Alliance
425 Bush St
San Francisco, CA 94108
415-434-3388
http://www.caregiver.org/

National Council of Senior Citizens
8403 Colesville Rd, Suite 1200
Silver Spring, MD 20910
301-578-8800
888-3-SENIOR
http://www.ncscinc.org

The National Council on the Aging
409 Third St SW
Washington, DC 20024
202-479-1200
http://www.ncoa.org

AIDS/HIV

American Foundation for AIDS Research
120 Wall St
New York, NY 10005
212-806-1600
http://www.amfar.org

Gay Men's Health Crisis
119 W 24th St
New York, NY 10011
212-807-6664
http://www.gmhc.org

Alcohol and Other Drug Abuse

Alcoholics Anonymous
475 Riverside Dr
New York, NY 10115
212-870-3400

Al-Anon Family Group Headquarters
1600 Corporate Landing Pkwy
Virginia Beach, VA 23454
757-563-1600
800-356-9996
800-344-2666
http://www.al-anon.alateen.org

Adult Children of Alcoholics
ACA World Service
PO Box 3216
Torrance, CA 90510
310-534-1815
http://www.adultchildren.org

Cocaine Abuse Hotline
800-COCAINE

Mothers Against Drunk Driving
511 E John Carpenter Frwy
Irving, TX 75062
214-744-6233
800-438-MADD

Narcotics Anonymous
PO Box 9999
Van Nuys, CA 91409
818-773-9999
http://www.na.org

National Association for Children of Alcoholics
11426 Rockville Pike, Suite 100
Rockville, MD 20852
301-468-0985
888-554-2627
http://www.health.org/nacoa

National Council on Alcoholism and Drug Dependence, Inc
12 W 21st St
New York, NY 10010
212-206-6770
800-622-2255
http://www.ncadd.org

National Drug and Alcohol Treatment Referral Routing Service
800-662-HELP

National Substance Abuse Helplines
164 W 74th St
New York, NY 10023
212-595-5810
800-COCAINE
800-DRUGHELP
http://www.drughelp.org/

Allergies/Asthma

Asthma and Allergy Foundation of America
1125 15th St NW, Suite 502
Washington, DC 20005
202-466-7643
800-7-ASTHMA
http://www.aafa.org

Alternative Medicine

Academy for Guided Imagery
PO Box 2070
Mill Valley, CA 94942
415-389-9324
800-726-2070

American Association of Acupuncture and Oriental Medicine
433 Front St
Catasauqua, PA 18032
610-266-1433
http://www.aaom.org

American Chiropractic Association
1701 Claredon Blvd
Arlington, VA 22209
703-276-8800
http://www.amerchiro.org

American Dance Therapy Association
2000 Century Plaza, Suite 108
Columbia, MD 21044
410-997-4040
http://www.adta.org

American Massage Therapy Association
820 Davis St
Evanston, IL 60201
847-864-0123
http://www.amtamassage.org

Association for Applied Psychophysiology and Biofeedback
10200 W 44th Ave, Suite 304
Wheat Ridge, CO 80033
303-442-8892
http://www.aapb.org

American Association for Music Therapy
8455 Colesville Rd, Suite 1000
Silver Spring, MD 20910
301-589-3300
http://www.musictherapy.org

Alzheimer Disease

The Alzheimer's Association
919 N Michigan Ave, Suite 1000
Chicago, IL 60611
312-335-8700
312-355-8882 (TDD)
800-272-3900
http://www.alz.org

Alzheimer's Disease Education and Referral Center
PO Box 8250
Silver Spring, MD 20907
301-495-3311
800-438-4380
http://www.alzheimers.org

Amputation

The National Amputation Foundation
38-40 Church St
Malverne, NY 11565
516-887-3600

Amyotrophic Lateral Sclerosis

The ALS Association
21021 Ventura Blvd, Suite 321
Woodland Hills, CA 91364
818-340-7500
800-782-4747
http://www.alsa.org

Ankylosing Spondylitis

Spondylitis Association of America
PO Box 5872
Sherman Oaks, CA 91413
800-777-8189

Arthritis

American Juvenile Arthritis Organization
1330 W Peachtree St
Atlanta, GA 30309
404-872-7100
800-283-7800
http://www.arthritis.org/ajao

The Arthritis Foundation
1330 W Peachtree St
Atlanta, GA 30309
404-872-7100
800-283-7800
http://www.arthritis.org

Assistive Devices

The Alliance for Accessible
Technology
2175 E Francisco Blvd
San Rafael, CA 94901
415-455-4575
http://www.ataccess.org

Center for Accessible Technology
2457 Eighth St
Berkeley, CA 95710
510-841-3224
http://www.el.net/CAT/

Autism

Autism Society of America
7910 Woodmount Ave, Suite 650
Bethesda, MD 20814
301-657-0881
800-3AUTISM
http://www.autism-society.org/

Bedwetting

American Enuresis Foundation
PO Box 33062
Tulsa, OK 74153
918-627-8656

National Enuresis Society
7777 Forest Ln, Suite C-737
Dallas, TX 75230
800-NES-8080
http://www.peds.umn.edu/
centers/NES

Bereavement/Hospice Care

Choice in Dying
1035 30th St NW
Washington, DC 20007
202-338-9790
800-989-9455
http://www.choices.org

The Dougy Center
The National Center for Grieving
Children and Families
PO Box 86852
Portland, OR 97286
503-775-5683
http://www.dougy.org

Foundation for Hospice and Home
Care
228 Seventh St NE
Washington, DC 20003
202-547-7424
http://www.nahc.org

The Grief Recovery Institute
PO Box 461659
Los Angeles, CA 90046
213-650-1234
http://www.grief-recovery.com

Hospice Education Institute
190 W Brook Rd, Suite 2
Essex, CT 06426
203-767-1620
800-331-1620

National Hospice Organization
1901 N Moore St, Suite 901
Arlington, VA 22209
703-243-5900
800-658-8898
http://www.nho.org

Pregnancy and Infant Loss Center
1421 E Wayzata Blvd, No. 30
Wayzata, MN 55391
612-473-9372

Birth Defects

American Cleft Palate-Craniofacial
Association
Cleft Palate Foundation
104 S Estes Dr, Suite 204
Chapel Hill, NC 27514
919-933-9044
800-242-5338
http://www.cleft.com

American Genetic Association
PO Box 257
Buckeystown, MD 21717
301-695-9292
http://www.oup.co.uk/jhered

Easter Seals
230 W Monroe St, Suite 1800
Chicago, IL 60606
312-726-6200
312-726-4258 (TDD)
800-221-6827
http://www.seals.org

March of Dimes
1275 Mamaroneck Ave
White Plains, NY 10605
914-428-7100
914-997-4764 (TTY)
888-MODIMES
http://www.modimes.org

National Tay-Sachs & Allied Diseases
Association, Inc
2001 Beacon St
Brighton, MA 02135
617-277-0134
800-906-8723
http://mcrcr2.med.nyu.edu/
murphp01/taysachs.htm

Spina Bifida Association of America
4590 MacArthur Blvd NW, Suite 250
Washington, DC 20007
202-944-3285
800-621-3141
http://www.sbaa.org

Blood Disorders

Leukemia Society of America
600 Third Ave
New York, NY 10016
212-573-8484
800-955-4LSA
http://www.leukemia.org

The National Hemophilia
Foundation
116 W 32nd St
New York, NY 10001
212-328-3700
800-42-HANDI
http://www.hemophilia.org

Cancer

Alliance for Lung Cancer Advocacy,
Support, and Education
1601 Lincoln Ave
Vancouver, WA 98660
360-696-2436
800-298-2436
http://www.alcase.org

American Brain Tumor Association
2720 River Rd
Des Plaines, IL 60618
847-827-9910
800-886-2282
http://www.abta.org/

American Cancer Society, Inc
1599 Clifton Rd, NE
Atlanta, GA 30329
404-320-3333
800-ACS-2345
http://www.cancer.org

The Brain Tumor Society
84 Seattle St
Boston, MA 02134
617-783-0340
800-770-8287
http://www.tbts.org

Cancer Care, Inc
1180 Avenue of the Americas
New York, NY 10036
212-302-2400
800-813-HOPE
http://www.cancercareinc.org

The Candlelighters Childhood
Cancer Foundation
7910 Woodmont Ave, Suite 460
Bethesda, MD 20814
301-657-8401
800-366-CCCF
http://www.candlelighters.org

Corporate Angel Network, Inc
1 Loop Rd
White Plains, NY 10604
914-328-1313
http://www.corpangelnetwork.org

Lymphoma Research Foundation of
America
8800 Venice Blvd, No. 207
Los Angeles, CA 90034
310-204-7040
http://www.lymphoma.org

National Alliance of Breast Cancer
Organizations
9 E 37th St
New York, NY 10016
212-719-0154
888-80-NABCO
http://www.nabco.org

National Brain Tumor Foundation
785 Market St, Suite 1600
San Francisco, CA 94103
415-284-0208
800-934-CURE
http://www.braintumor.org

National Breast Cancer Coalition
1707 L St NW
Washington, DC 20036
202-296-7477
http://www.natlbcc.org

National Coalition for Cancer
Survivorship
1010 Wayne Ave
Silver Spring, MD 20910
301-650-8868
http://www.cansearch.org

Ronald McDonald House Charities
1 Kroc Dr
Oak Brook, IL 60523
630-623-7048
http://www.rmhc.com

Skin Cancer Foundation
PO Box 561
New York, NY 10156
800-SKIN-490

Susan G. Komen Breast Cancer
Foundation
5005 LBJ Frwy, Suite 370
Dallas, TX 75244
972-855-1600
800-462-9273
http://www.breastcancerinfo.com

US TOO International (prostate
cancer)
930 N York Rd, Suite 50
Hinsdale, IL 60521
630-323-1002
800-808-7866
http://www.ustoo.com

Y-Me National Breast Cancer
Organization
212 W Van Buren
Chicago, IL 60607
312-986-8338
800-221-2141
http://www.y-me.org

Cardiovascular Disorders

American Heart Association
7272 Greenville Ave
Dallas, TX 75231
214-373-6300
800-242-8721
http://www.amhrt.org

Caregiving

National Family Caregivers
Association
10605 Concord St, Suite 501
Kensington, MD 20895
800-896-3650
http://www.nfcacares.org

The National Association for Home
Care
228 Seventh St NE
Washington, DC 20003
202-547-7424
http://www.nahc.org

National Federation of Interfaith
Volunteer Caregivers
368 Broadway
Kingston, NY 12401
914-331-1358
http://www.nfivc.org

Visiting Nurse Association of America
11 Beacon St
Boston, MA 02108
617-523-4042
http://www.vnaa.org

Well Spouse Foundation
610 Lexington Ave, Suite 208
New York, NY 10022
212-644-1241
800-838-0879
http://www.wellspouse.org

Cerebral Palsy

United Cerebral Palsy Association
1660 L St NW, Suite 700
Washington, DC 20036
800-872-5827
http://www.ucpa.org

Child Abuse/Domestic Violence

National Center for Missing and
Exploited Children
2101 Wilson Blvd
Arlington, VA 22201
703-235-3900
800-843-5678
http://www.missingkids.com

National Child Abuse Hotline
800-422-4453

National Clearinghouse on Child
Abuse and Neglect Information
330 C St SW
Washington, DC 20047
703-385-7565
800-FYI-3366
http://www.calib.com/nccanch

National Committee to Prevent
Child Abuse
200 S Michigan Ave
Chicago, IL 60604
312-663-3520
800-556-2722
http://www.childabuse.org

National Council on Child Abuse
and Family Violence
1155 Connecticut Ave, NW
Washington, DC 20036
202-429-6695

National Domestic Violence Hotline
PO Box 161810
Austin, TX 78716
512-453-8117
800-799-SAFE
800-787-3224 (TDD)
http://www.ndvh.org

Chronic Fatigue Syndrome

CFIDS Association of America, Inc.
PO Box 220398
Charlotte, NC 28222
800-442-3437
http://www.cfids.org

Cystic Fibrosis

Cystic Fibrosis Foundation
6931 Arlington Rd
Bethesda, MD 20814
301-951-4422
800-FIGHT-CF
http://www.cff.org

Diabetes

American Diabetes Association
1660 Duke St
Alexandria, VA 22314
800-342-2383
http://www.diabetes.org

The Juvenile Diabetes Foundation
International
120 Wall St
New York, NY 10005
212-785-9500
800-JDF-CURE
http://www.jdfcure.org

Digestive Diseases

Crohn's & Colitis Foundation of
America, Inc
386 Park Ave S
New York, NY 10016
212-685-3440
800-932-2423
http://www.ccfa.org

Digestive Disease National Coalition
507 Capitol Ct NE, Suite 200
Washington, DC 20002
202-544-7497

Gastro-Intestinal Research
Foundation
70 E Lake St, Suite 1015
Chicago, IL 60601
312-332-1350

Intestinal Disease Foundation, Inc
1323 Forbes Ave, Suite 200
Pittsburgh, PA 15219
412-261-5888

Disabled Resources

National Spinal Cord Injury Hotline
2200 Kernan Dr
Baltimore, MD 21207
410-448-6623
800-526-3456
http://www.scihotline.org

Clearinghouse on Disability
Information
Office of Special Education and
Rehabilitative Services
330 C St SW
Switzer Bldg, Room 3132
Washington, DC 20202
202-205-8241
http://www.ed.gov/OFFICES/OSERS

Disabled American Veterans
PO Box 14301
Cincinnati, OH 45250
606-441-7300
http://www.dav.org

Federation of the Handicapped
211 W 14th St
New York, NY 10011
212-727-4200

National Information Center for
Children and Youth With Disabilities
PO Box 1492
Washington, DC 20013
202-884-8200
800-695-0285
http://www.nichcy.org

National Spinal Cord Injury
Association
8300 Colesville Rd, Suite 551
Silver Spring, MD 20910
800-962-9629
http://www.spinalcord.org

Paralyzed Veterans of America
801 18th St NW
Washington, DC 20006
202-872-1300
800-424-8200
http://www.pva.org

Eating Disorders

National Association of Anorexia
Nervosa and Associated Disorders
PO Box 7
Highland Park, IL 60035
847-831-3438
http://www.members.aol.com/
anad20/index.html

Environmental Health

Mothers and Others for Pesticide
Limits
40 W 20th St
New York, NY 10011
212-727-2700
http://www.mothers.org

National Pesticide Telecommunica-
tions Network
333 Weniger Hall
Corvallis, OR 97331
541-737-6123
800-858-7378
http://ace.orst.edu/info/nptn

Natural Resources Defense Council
40 W 20th St
New York, NY 10011
212-727-2700
http://www.nrdc.org

Epilepsy

Epilepsy Foundation
4351 Garden City Dr
Landover, MD 20785
301-459-3700
800-EFA-1000
http://www.efa.org

Epilepsy Institute
257 Park Ave S
New York, NY 10010
212-677-8550

Exercise/Fitness

President's Council on Physical
Fitness and Sports
200 Independence Ave SW
Washington, DC 20201
202-690-9000

Women's Sports Foundation
Eisenhower Park
East Meadow, NY 11554
516-543-4700
800-227-3988
http://www.lifetimetv.com/WoSport

Fibromyalgia

Fibromyalgia Network
PO Box 31750
Tucson, AZ 85751
800-853-2929
http://www.fmnetnews.com

Gambling

Gamblers Anonymous
PO Box 17173
Los Angeles, CA 90017
213-386-8789
http://www.gamblersanonymous
.org

Gay/Lesbian Issues

Gay, Lesbian and Straight Education
Network
121 W 27th St, Suite 804
New York, NY 10001
212-727-0135
http://www.glsen.org

!OutProud!
The National Coalition for Gay,
Lesbian, Bisexual and Transgender
Youth
369 Third St, Suite B-362
San Rafael, CA 94901
415-460-5452
http://www.outproud.org

Parents and Friends of Lesbians and
Gays (PFLAG)
1101 14th St NW
Washington, DC 20005
202-638-4200
http://www.pflag.org

Youth Resource
Advocates for Youth
1025 Vermont Ave NW
Washington, DC 20005
202-347-5700
http://www.youthresource.com

Genetic Diseases/Testing

Alliance of Genetic Support Groups
4301 Connecticut Ave NW
Washington, DC 20008
202-966-5557
800-336-GENE
http://www.medhelp.org/
geneticalliance/

A National Center for Genome
Resources
1800-A Old Pecos Trail
Santa Fe, NM 87505
505-982-7840
http://www.ncgr.org

National Society of Genetic
Counselors
233 Canterbury Dr
Wallingford, PA 19086
610-872-7608

Guillain-Barré Syndrome

Guillain-Barré Syndrome Foundation
International
PO Box 262
Wynnewood, PA 19096
610-667-0131
http://www.webmast.com/gbs

Hair Loss

National Alopecia Areata Foundation
710 C St, Suite 11
San Rafael, CA 94901
415-456-4274
http://www.alopeciaareata.com

Head Injuries

The National Brain Injury
Association
105 N Alfred St
Alexandria, VA 22314
703-236-6000
http://www.biausa.org

Health Care

American Medical Association
515 N State St
Chicago, IL 60610
312-464-5000
http://www.ama-assn.org

American Hospital Association
1 N Franklin St
Chicago, IL 60606
312-422-3000
800-242-2626
http://www.aha.org

Federation of State Medical Boards
Federation Place
400 Fuller Wiser Rd
Euless, TX 76039
817-868-4000
http://www.fsmb.org

National Association of Insurance
Commissioners
120 W 12th St, Suite 1100
Kansas City, MO 64105
816-842-3600
http://www.naic.org

Huntington Disease

Huntington's Disease Society of
America
158 W 29th St, Seventh Floor
New York, NY 10001
212-242-1968
800-345-HDSA
http://hdsa.mgh.harvard.edu/

Kidney Disease

American Association of Kidney
Patients
100 S Ashley Dr, Suite 280
Tampa, FL 33602
813-223-7099
800-749-2257
http://www.aakp.org/

American Kidney Fund
6110 Executive Blvd, Suite 1010
Rockville, MD 20852
301-881-3052
800-638-8299
http://www.akfinc.org

National Kidney Foundation
30 E 33rd St
New York, NY 10016
212-889-2210
800-622-9010
http://www.kidney.org

Learning Disabilities

Learning Disabilities Association of
America
4156 Library Rd
Pittsburgh, PA 15234
412-341-1515
888-300-6710
http://www.ldanatl.org

The International Dyslexia
Association
8600 LaSalle Rd
Chester Building, Suite 382
Baltimore, MD 21286
410-296-0232
800-ABCD-123
http://www.interdys.org

Liver Diseases

American Liver Foundation
1425 Pompton Ave
Cedar Grove, NJ 07009
800-GO-LIVER
http://www.liverfoundation.org

Hepatitis Foundation International
30 Sunrise Terr
Cedar Grove, NJ 07009
973-239-1035
800-891-0707
http://www.hepfi.org

Lupus Erythematosus

Lupus Foundation of America, Inc
1300 Piccard Dr, Suite 200
Rockville, MD 20850
301-670-9292
800-558-0121
http://www.internet-plaza.net/lupus

Lyme Disease

Lyme Disease Foundation
One Financial Plaza
Hartford, CT 06103
860-525-2000
800-886-5963
http://www.lyme.org

Medical Identification Tags

Medic Alert Foundation
International
PO Box 819008
Turlock, CA 95381
209-668-3333
800-ID-ALERT
800-344-3226
http://www.medicalert.org/

Mental Health

Depressive and Related Affective
Disorders Association
Johns Hopkins Hospital
600 N Wolfe St
Meyer 3-181
Baltimore, MD 21287
410-955-4647
http://www.med.jhu.edu/drada/

National Alliance for the Mentally Ill
200 N Glebe Rd
Arlington, VA 22203
703-524-7600
800-950-6264
http://www.nami.org

National Depressive and Manic-
Depressive Association
730 N Franklin, Suite 501
Chicago, IL 60610
312-642-0049
800-82-NDMDA
http://www.ndmda.org

National Mental Health Association
1021 Prince St
Alexandria, VA 22314
703-139-9333
800-969-NMHA
800-433-5959 (TTY)
http://www.nmha.org

Mental Retardation

American Association on Mental
Retardation
444 N Capitol St NW, Suite 846
Washington, DC 20001
202-387-1968
800-424-3688
http://www.aamr.org

The ARC of the United States
500 E Border St, Suite 300
Arlington, TX 76010
817-261-6003
http://www.thearc.org/welcome/
htm

Kennedy Child Study Center
151 E 67th St
New York, NY 10021
212-988-9500

National Down Syndrome Society
666 Broadway
New York, NY 10012
212-460-9330
800-221-4602
http://www.ndss.org

Minority Health

National Black Women's Health
Project
1211 Connecticut Ave NW
Suite 310
Washington, DC 20036
202-835-0117

Office of Minority Health Resource
Center
PO Box 37337
Washington, DC 20013
800-444-6472
http://www.omhrc.gov

Neurofibromatosis

National Neurofibromatosis
Foundation
95 Pine St
New York, NY 10005
212-344-6633
800-323-7938
http://www.nf.org

Neurological Disorders

The ALS Association
21021 Ventura Blvd
Woodland Hills, CA 91364
818-340-7500
800-782-4747
http://www.alsa.org

Charcot-Marie-Tooth Association
601 Upland Ave
Upland, PA 19015
610-499-7486
800-606-2682
http://www.charcot-marie-tooth.org

National Aphasia Association
156 Fifth Ave, Suite 707
New York, NY 10010
800-922-4622
http://www.aphasia.org

National Ataxia Foundation
2600 Fernbrook Lane, Suite 119
Wayzata, MN 55447
612-553-0020
http://www.ataxia.org

Tourette Syndrome Association
42-40 Bell Blvd
Bayside, NY 11361
718-224-2999
800-237-0717
http://tsa.mgh.harvard.edu/

Neuromuscular Disorders

Muscular Dystrophy Association of
America
3300 E Sunrise Dr
Tucson, AZ 85718
800-572-1717
http://www.mdausa.org

Myasthenia Gravis Foundation, Inc
61 Gramercy Park N, Room 605
New York, NY 10010
212-533-7005
800-643-0808

National Multiple Sclerosis Society
733 Third Ave
New York, NY 10017
212-986-3240
800-FIGHT MS
http://www.nmss.org

Nutrition

American Dietetic Association
216 W Jackson Blvd
Chicago, IL 60606
312-899-0040
800-366-1655
http://www.eatright.org

Center for Nutrition Policy and
Promotion
1120 20th St NW, Suite 200N
Washington, DC 20036
202-418-2312
http://www.usda.gov/cnpp

International Food Information Council
1100 Connecticut Ave NW
Suite 430
Washington, DC 20036
202-296-6540
http://www.ificinfo.health.org

Obesity

American Obesity Association
1250 24th St NW
Washington, DC 20037
800-98-OBESE
http://www.obese.org

Overeaters Anonymous
6075 Zenith Ct NE
Rio Rancho, NM 87124
505-891-2664
http://www.overeatersanonymous
.org

Weight Watchers International
175 Crossways Park W
Woodbury, NY 11797
(check local listings for phone numbers)
http://www.weight-watchers.com

Organ/Marrow/Blood Donation

American Red Cross
1621 N Kent St
Arlington, VA 22209
703-248-4222
800-HELP-NOW
http://www.redcross.org

Blood & Marrow Transplant Newsletter
1985 Spruce Ave
Highland Park, IL 60035
847-831-1913
http://www.bmtnews.org

Cord Blood Registry
1200 Bayhill Dr, Suite 301
San Bruno, CA 94066
800-588-6377
http://www.cordblood.com

The Living Bank
PO Box 6725
Houston, TX 77265
713-528-2971
800-528-2971
http://www.livingbank.org

National Marrow Donor Program
3433 Broadway St NE, Suite 500
Minneapolis, MN 55413
800-MARROW2
http://www.marrow.org

Transplant Recipients International Organization
1000 16th St NW, Suite 602
Washington, DC 20036
202-293-0980
800-TRIO-386
http://www.trioweb.org

The United Network for Organ Sharing
PO Box 13770
1100 Boulders Pkwy, Suite 500
Richmond, VA 23225
804-330-8500
800-355-7427 (donors)
888-894-6361 (patients)
http://www.unos.org

Osteoporosis

National Osteoporosis Foundation
1150 17th St NW, Suite 500
Washington, DC 20036
202-223-2226
800-223-9994
http://www.nof.org

Ostomies

United Ostomy Association
19772 MacArthur Blvd, Suite 200
Irvine, CA 92612
949-660-8624
800-826-0826
http://www.uoa.org

Paget Disease

The Paget Foundation
120 Wall St, Suite 1602
New York, NY 10005
212-509-5335
800-23-PAGET
http://www.paget.org

Pain Control

American Chronic Pain Association, Inc
PO Box 850
Rocklin, CA 95677
916-632-0922
http://www.theacpa.org

American Council for Headache Education
19 Mantua Rd
Mt Royal, NJ 08061
609-423-0258
800-255-ACHE
http://www.achenet.org

International Association for the Study of Pain
909 NE 43rd St, Suite 306
Seattle, WA 98105
206-547-6409
http://www.halcyon.com/iasp

National Headache Foundation
428 W St James Pl
Chicago, IL 60614
773-388-6399
800-843-2256
http://www.headaches.org

Parkinson Disease

American Parkinson Disease Association
1250 Hylan Blvd, Suite 4B
Staten Island, NY 10305
718-981-8001
800-223-2732
http://www.apdaparkinson.com

National Parkinson Foundation
1501 NW Ninth Ave
Miami, FL 33136
305-547-6666
800-327-4545
http://www.parkinson.org

Parkinson's Disease Foundation
710 W 168th St
New York, NY 10032
212-923-4700
800-457-6676
http://www.parkinsons-foundation
.org

The Parkinson Support Group of America
11376 Cherry Hill Rd, Suite 204
Beltsville, MD 20705
301-937-1545

Psoriasis

National Psoriasis Foundation
6600 SW 92nd Ave, Suite 300
Portland, OR 97223
503-244-7404
800-723-9166
http://www.psoriasis.org

Rare Diseases

National Organization for Rare Disorders
PO Box 8923
New Fairfield, CT 06812
203-746-6518
800-999-6673
http://www.rarediseases.org

Rehabilitation

American Occupational Therapy Association, Inc
PO Box 31220
Bethesda, MD 20814
301-652-2682
http://www.aota.org

National Rehabilitation Association
633 S Washington St
Alexandria, VA 22314
703-836-0850
http://www.nationalrehab.org

National Rehabilitation Information Center
8455 Colesville Rd, Suite 935
Silver Spring, MD 20910
301-588-9284
800-346-2742
http://www.naric.com/naric

Reproductive Health/ Fertility

American Society for Reproductive Medicine
1209 Montgomery Hwy
Birmingham, AL 35216
205-978-5000
http://www.asrm.org

Endometriosis Association
8585 N 76th Pl
Milwaukee, WI 53223
414-355-2200
800-992-3636
http://www.endometriosisassn.org

International Childbirth Education Association, Inc
PO Box 20048
Minneapolis, MN 55420
612-854-8660
http://www.icea.org

LaLeche League International
1400 N Meacham
PO Box 4079
Schaumburg, IL 60168
847-519-7730
800-LA LECHE
http://www.lalecheleague.org

Maternity Center Association
281 Park Ave S
New York, NY 10010
212-777-5000

Planned Parenthood Federation of America, Inc
810 Seventh Ave
New York, NY 10019
212-541-7800
800-829-7732
800-230-7526 (clinic locator hotline)
http://www.plannedparenthood.org

RESOLVE, Inc
1310 Broadway
Somerville, MA 02144
617-623-0744
http://www.resolve.org

Sexuality Information and Education Council of the United States
130 W 42nd St, Suite 350
New York, NY 10036
212-819-9770
http://www.siecus.org

Respiratory Disorders

American Lung Association
1740 S Broadway
New York, NY 10019
212-315-8700
800-LUNG-USA
http://www.lungusa.org

Lung Line Information Service
National Jewish Medical and Research Center
303-355-LUNG
800-222-5864

Second Wind Lung Transplant Association
300 S Duncan Ave
Clearwater, FL 33755
888-222-2690
http://www.2ndwind.org

Sexually Transmitted Diseases

ASHA Resource Center
American Social Health Association
PO Box 13827
Research Triangle Park, NC 27709
919-361-8488 (herpes hotline)
800-230-6039
http://www.ashastd.org

CDC STD Hotline
PO Box 13827
Research Triangle Park, NC 27709
800-227-8922

Sickle Cell Anemia

Sickle Cell Disease Association of America, Inc
200 Corporate Point, Suite 495
Culver City, CA 90230
310-216-6363
800-421-8453

Sleep Disorders

American Sleep Apnea Association
1424 K St NW
Washington, DC 20005
202-293-3650
http://www.sleepapnea.org

The American Sleep Disorders Association
6301 Bandel Rd, Suite 101
Rochester, MN 55901
507-287-6006
http://www.asda.org

Narcolepsy Network
277 Fairfield Rd
Fairfield, NJ 07004
973-276-0115
http://www.websciences.org/narnet/default.html

National Sleep Foundation
729 15th St
Washington, DC 20005
202-347-3471
http://www.sleepfoundation.org

Restless Legs Syndrome Foundation
4410 19th St NW, Suite 201
Rochester, MN 55901
507-287-6465
http://www.rls.org

Young Americans With Narcolepsy (YAWN)
1451 W 31st
Minneapolis, MN 55408
612-824-1355
http://www.yawn.org

Smoking Cessation

Action on Smoking and Health
2013 H Street NW
Washington, DC 20006
202-659-4310
http://www.ash.org

American Lung Association
1740 S Broadway
New York, NY 10019
212-315-8700
800-LUNG-USA
http://www.lungusa.org

Smokenders
666 11th St NW, Suite 200
Washington, DC 20001
800-828-4357
http://www.smokenders.com

Speech and Hearing Disorders

Alexander Graham Bell Association for the Deaf
3417 Volta Pl NW
Washington, DC 20007
202-337-5220
http://www.agbell.org

American Hearing Research Foundation
55 E Washington St, Suite 2022
Chicago, IL 60602
312-726-9670

American Speech-Language-Hearing Association
10801 Rockville Pike
Rockville, MD 20852
301-897-5700
800-638-8255
http://www.asha.org

American Tinnitus Association
PO Box 5
Portland, OR 97207
503-248-9985
800-634-8978
http://www.ata.org

Cleft Palate Foundation
104 S Estes Dr, Suite 204
Chapel Hill, NC 27514
919-933-9044
800-24-CLEFT
http://www.cleft.com

Deafness Research Foundation
575 Fifth Ave
New York, NY 10017
212-599-0027
800-535-3323
http://www.drf.org

Dogs for the Deaf
10175 Wheeler Rd
Central Point, OR 97502
541-826-9220
800-990-3647
http://www.dogsforthedeaf.org

International Hearing Society
16880 Middlebelt Rd
Livonia, MI 48154
734-522-7200
800-521-5247 (hearing aid helpline)
http://www.hearingihs.org

National Association of the Deaf
814 Thayer Ave
Silver Spring, MD 20910
301-587-1788
301-587-1789 (TDD)
http://www.nad.org

National Information Center on Deafness
Gallaudet University
800 Florida Ave NE
Washington, DC 20002
202-651-5051
202-651-5052 (TDD)
http://www.gallaudet.edu/~nicd

Stuttering Foundation of America
PO Box 11749
Memphis, TN 38111
901-452-7343
800-992-9392
http://www.stuttersfa.org

Stroke

American Paralysis Association
500 Morris Ave
Springfield, NJ 07081
973-379-2690
800-225-0292
http://www.apacure.org

National Aphasia Association
Murray Hill Station
PO Box 1887
New York, NY 10156
800-922-4NAA

National Stroke Association
96 Inverness Dr E, Suite I
Englewood, CO 80112
303-649-9299
800-STROKES
http://www.stroke.org

Sudden Infant Death Syndrome

American Sudden Infant Death Syndrome Institute
6065 Roswell Rd, Suite 876
Atlanta, GA 30328
404-843-1030
800-232-SIDS
http://www.sids.org

National Sudden Infant Death Syndrome (SIDS) Resource Center
2070 Chain Bridge Rd, Suite 450
Vienna, VA 22182
703-821-8955
http://www.circsol.com/sids

Sudden Infant Death Syndrome Alliance
1314 Bedford Ave
Baltimore, MD 21208
410-653-8226
800-221-7437
http://www.sidsalliance.org

Thyroid Disorders

Thyroid Foundation of America
Ruth Sleeper Hall, RSL 350
40 Parkman St
Boston, MA 02114
800-832-8321

Travelers' Health Information

AEA SOS
(emergency evacuation assistance)
PO Box 11568
Philadelphia, PA 19116
215-244-1500
800-523-8930

Centers for Disease Control and Prevention
1600 Clifton Rd NE
Atlanta, GA 30333
404-639-8100
http://www.cdc.gov/travel/index.htm

The International Association for Medical Assistance to Travelers
417 Center St
Lewiston, NY 14092
716-754-4883

Urinary Tract Disorders

American Foundation for Urologic Disease
1128 N Charles St
Baltimore, MD 21201
410-468-1800
800-242-AFUD
http://www.afud.org

American Urological Association
1120 N Charles St
Baltimore, MD 21201
410-727-1100
http://www.auanet.org

Simon Foundation for Continence
PO Box 813
Wilmette, IL 60091
847-864-3913
800-23-SIMON
http://www.simonfoundation.org

Vision Disorders

American Council of the Blind
1155 15th St, Suite 720
Washington, DC 20005
202-467-5081
800-424-8666
http://www.acb.org

American Foundation for the Blind
11 Penn Plaza
New York, NY 10001
212-502-7600
800-232-5463
http://www.afb.org

Associated Blind, Inc
135 W 23rd St
New York, NY 10011
212-255-1122

Associated Services for the Blind
919 Walnut St
Philadelphia, PA 19107
215-627-0600
http://www.libertynet.org/~asbinfo

Association for Macular Diseases, Inc
210 E 64th St
New York, NY 10021
212-605-3719
http://www.macula.org

Eye Bank Association of America
1001 Connecticut Ave NW
Suite 601
Washington, DC 20036
202-775-4999
http://www.restoresight.org

Glaucoma Research Foundation
200 Pine St
San Francisco, CA 94104
415-986-3162
800-826-6693
http://www.glaucoma.org

Guide Dogs for the Blind, Inc
PO Box 151200
San Rafael, CA 94915
415-499-4000
800-295-4050
http://www.guidedogs.com

Guiding Eyes for the Blind, Inc
611 Granite Springs Rd
Yorktown Heights, NY 10598
914-245-4024
800-942-0149
http://www.guiding-eyes.org

Lighthouse International
111 E 59th St
New York, NY 10022
212-821-9200
800-334-5497
http://www.lighthouse.org

National Association for Visually Handicapped
22 W 21st St
New York, NY 10010
212-889-3141
http://www.navh.org

National Federation of the Blind
1800 Johnson St
Baltimore, MD 21230
410-659-9314
http://www.nfb.org

Prevent Blindness America
500 E Remington
Schaumburg, IL 60173
847-843-2020
800-331-2020
http://www.preventblindness.org

Retinitis Pigmentosa International
PO Box 900
Woodland Hills, CA 91365
818-992-0500
800-FIGHTRP
http://www.rpinternational.org

The Seeing Eye, Inc
PO Box 375
Morristown, NJ 07963
973-539-4425
http://www.seeingeye.org

DISEASES, CONDITIONS, AND ISSUES: FEDERAL AGENCIES

For a listing of additional federal agencies, see our Web site (address is at the bottom of every index page).

National Institutes of Health (NIH) Agencies

http://www.nih.gov

AIDS Clinical Trials Information Service
800-TRIALS A

AIDS Treatment Information Service
800-HIV-0440

Clinical Trials Information at NIH
Patient Recruitment Line and Public Liaison Office
800-411-1222
http://www.cc.nih.gov

Other Agencies

Centers for Disease Control and Prevention
National AIDS Information Clearinghouse
PO Box 6003
Rockville, MD 20850
800-458-5231
http://www.cdcnac.org

Centers for Disease Control and Prevention
AIDS Hotlines
800-342-AIDS
800-334-7492 (Spanish)
800-243-7889 (TDD)

Centers for Disease Control and Prevention
Public Inquiries
1600 Clifton Rd NE
Atlanta, GA 30333
800-311-3435
888-232-3228 (fax information service)
http://www.cdc.gov

Food and Drug Administration
Department of Health and Human Services
Office of Consumer Affairs
5600 Fischers Ln
Rockville, MD 20857
888-INFOFDA
http://www.fda.gov

Medicare
Department of Health and Human Services
Medicare Hotline
800-MEDICARE (for general Medicare questions; for billing questions, check your Medicare statement for local phone number)

National Health Information Center
Department of Health and Human Services
PO Box 1133
Washington, DC 20013
301-565-4167
http://nhic-nt.health.org.
(referrals to government agencies and private organizations)

MEDICAL INTERNET RESOURCES

See our Web site (address is at the bottom of every index page), which will direct you to other health Web sites.

NATIONAL CANCER INSTITUTE– DESIGNATED CANCER CENTERS

For a listing of specific cancer centers in the United States, contact the National Cancer Institute by phone or at the following Web site: http://www.nci.nih.gov/cancercenters/centers1.htm

Alternatively, see our Web site (address is at the bottom of every index page).

National Cancer Institute
Office of Cancer Communications
9000 Rockville Pike
Bethesda, MD 20892
800-4-CANCER (Cancer Information Service)
301-402-5874 (CancerFax [information by fax])
http://www.nci.nih.gov

POISON CONTROL CENTERS

Alabama

Birmingham
Regional Poison Control Center
The Children's Hospital of Alabama
1600 Seventh Ave S
Birmingham, AL 35233
205-939-9201
800-292-6678 (calls from Alabama only)
205-933-4050

Tuscaloosa
Alabama Poison Center
2503 Phoenix Dr
Tuscaloosa, AL 35405
800-462-0800 (calls from Alabama only)
205-345-0600

Alaska

Anchorage Poison Control Center
Providence Hospital Pharmacy
PO Box 196604
Anchorage, AK 99516
800-478-3193 (calls from Alaska only)
907-261-3193

Arizona

Phoenix
Samaritan Regional Poison Center
Good Samaritan Regional Medical Center
Ancillary-2
1111 E McDowell Rd
Phoenix, AZ 85006
602-253-3334

Tucson
Arizona Poison and Drug Information Center
Arizona Health Sciences Center
1501 N Campbell Ave, Room 1156
Tucson, AZ 85724
800-322-0101 (calls from Arizona only)
520-626-6016

Arkansas

Arkansas Poison and Drug Information Center
University of Arkansas for Medical Sciences
4301 W Markham St, Slot 522
Little Rock, AR 72205
800-376-4766

East Arkansas
Southern Poison Center Inc
847 Monroe Ave, Suite 230
Memphis, TN 38163
901-528-6048
800-288-9999 (calls from Tennessee only)

California

California Poison Control System
Valley Children's Hospital
3151 N Millbrook, IN31
Fresno, CA 93703
800-876-4766 (calls from California only)

Colorado

Rocky Mountain Poison Center
8802 E Ninth Ave
Denver, CO 80220
800-332-3073 (calls from Colorado only)
303-739-1123

Connecticut

Connecticut Poison Control Center
UCONN Health Center
263 Farmington Ave
Farmington, CT 06030
860-679-3456
800-343-2722 (calls from Connecticut only)

Delaware

The Poison Control Center
3600 Sciences Center, Suite 220
Philadelphia, PA 19104
215-386-2100

Poison Information Center
Medical Center of Delaware
Wilmington Hospital
501 W 14th St
Wilmington, DE 19899
302-655-3389

District of Columbia

National Capital Poison Center
3201 New Mexico Ave NW
Suite 310
Washington, DC 20016
202-625-3333
202-362-8563 (TTY)

Florida

Jacksonville
Florida Poison Information Center
University Medical Center
University of Florida Health Science Center
655 W Eighth St
Jacksonville, FL 32009
904-549-4480
800-282-3171 (calls from Florida only)

Miami
Florida Poison Information Center
University of Miami School of Medicine
Department of Pediatrics
PO Box 016960, R-131
Miami, FL 33101
800-282-3171 (calls from Florida only)

Tampa
The Florida Poison Information Center and Toxicology Resource Center
Tampa General Hospital
PO Box 1289
Tampa, FL 33606
813-253-4444
800-282-3171 (calls from Florida only)

Georgia

Georgia Poison Center
Grady Memorial Hospital
80 Butler St SE
PO Box 26066
Atlanta, GA 30335
800-282-5846 (calls from Georgia only)
404-616-9000

Hawaii

Hawaii Poison Center
Kapiolani Medical Center for Women and Children
1319 Punahou St
Honolulu, HI 96826
800-362-3585 (calls from the outer islands of Hawaii only)
800-362-3586
808-941-4411

Idaho

Rocky Mountain Poison Center
8802 E Ninth Ave
Denver, CO 80220
800-860-0620

Illinois

Normal (and nearby counties)
BroMenn Poison Control Center
BroMenn Regional Medical Center
Franklin at Virginia
Normal, IL 61761
309-454-6666

Chicago and northeast counties
Chicago & Northeastern Illinois Regional Poison Control Center (Rush Poison Control Center)
Rush-Presbyterian–St Luke's Medical Center
1653 W Congress Pkwy
Chicago, IL 60612
312-942-5969
800-942-5969 (calls from northeastern Illinois only)

Central and southern Illinois
Regional Poison Resource Center
St John's Hospital
800 E Carpenter St
Springfield, IL 62769
800-252-2022 (calls from Illinois only)
217-753-3330

Interstate Center–Cardinal Glennon Children's Hospital
Regional Poison Resource Center
1465 S Grand Blvd
St Louis, MO 63104
800-366-8888 (calls from western Illinois only)

Indiana

Indiana Poison Center
Methodist Hospital of Indiana
1701 N Senate Blvd
Indianapolis, IN 46206
800-382-9097 (calls from Indiana only)
317-929-2323

Iowa

Western Iowa
St Luke's Poison Center
St Luke's Regional Medical Center
2720 Stone Park Blvd
Sioux City, IA 51104
712-277-2222
800-352-2222

Interstate Center–The Poison Center
Children's Memorial Hospital
8301 Dodge St
Omaha, NE 68114
800-955-9119

Kansas

Mid-America Poison Control Center
University of Kansas Medical Center
3901 Rainbow Blvd, Room B-400
Kansas City, KS 66160
913-588-6633
800-332-6633 (calls from Kansas only and the Kansas City area)

Interstate Center–Cardinal Glennon Children's Hospital
Regional Poison Center
1465 S Grand Blvd
St Louis, MO 63104
800-366-8888 (calls from Topeka only)

Kentucky

Kentucky Regional Poison Center of Kosair Children's Hospital
Medical Towers S, Suite 572
PO Box 35070
Louisville, KY 40232
502-589-8222
800-722-5725 (calls from Kentucky only)

Louisiana

Louisiana Drug and Poison Information Center
Northeast Louisiana University
Sugar Hall
Monroe, LA 71209
800-256-9822 (calls from Louisiana only)

Maine

Maine Poison Control Center
Maine Medical Center
Department of Emergency Medicine
22 Bramhall St
Portland, ME 04102
207-871-2950
800-442-6305 (calls from Maine only)

Maryland

Maryland Poison Center
20 N Pine St
Baltimore, MD 21201
410-528-7701
800-492-2414 (calls from Maryland only)

Massachusetts

Massachusetts Poison Control System
300 Longwood Ave
Boston, MA 02115
617-232-2120
800-682-9211 (calls from Massachusetts only)

Michigan

Detroit
Poison Control Center
Children's Hospital of Michigan
4160 John R St, Suite 616
Detroit, MI 48201
800-764-7661 (calls from Michigan only)
313-745-5711

Grand Rapids
Blodgett Regional Poison Center
1840 Wealthy SE
Grand Rapids, MI 49506
800-764-7661 (calls from Michigan only)

Minnesota

Hennepin Regional Poison Center
Hennepin County Medical Center
701 Park Ave
Minneapolis, MN 55415
612-347-3141
800-POISON1 (800-764-7661) (calls from Minnesota and nearby areas only)

Minnesota Regional Poison Center
8100 34th Ave S
PO Box 1309
Minneapolis, MN 55440
800-POISON1 (800-764-7661) (calls from Minnesota only)
612-221-2113

Mississippi

Mississippi Regional Poison Control Center
University of Mississippi Medical Center
2500 N State St
Jackson, MS 39216
601-354-7660

North Mississippi
Southern Poison Center Inc
847 Monroe Ave, Suite 230
Memphis, TN 38163
901-528-6048
800-288-9999 (calls from Tennessee only)

Missouri

Missouri Regional Poison Center
Cardinal Glennon Children's Hospital
1465 S Grand Blvd
St Louis, MO 63104
314-772-5200
800-366-8888

Montana

Rocky Mountain Poison and Drug Center
8802 E Ninth Ave
Denver, CO 80220
800-525-5042 (calls from Montana only)

Nebraska

The Poison Center
8301 Dodge St
Omaha, NE 68114
402-354-5555
800-955-9119 (calls from Nebraska only)

Nevada

Clark and Nye Counties
Rocky Mountain Poison Center
8802 E Ninth Ave
Denver, CO 80220
702-732-4989
800-446-6179

New Hampshire

New Hampshire Poison Information Center
Dartmouth-Hitchcock Medical Center
1 Medical Center Dr
Lebanon, NH 03756
603-650-8000
603-650-5000 (between 11 PM and 8 AM only)
800-562-8236 (calls from New Hampshire only)

New Jersey

New Jersey Poison Information and Education System
201 Lyons Ave
Newark, NJ 07112
800-764-7661 (calls from New Jersey only)

New Mexico

New Mexico Poison and Drug Information Center
University of New Mexico
Health Sciences Library, Room 125
Albuquerque, NM 87131
505-843-2551
800-432-6866 (calls from New Mexico only)

New York

Mineola
Long Island Regional Poison Control Center
Winthrop University Hospital
259 First St
Mineola, NY 11501
516-542-2323

New York City
New York City Poison Control Center
NYC Department of Health
455 First Ave, Room 123
New York, NY 10016
212-340-4494
212-POISONS
212-VENENOS (Spanish)

North Tarrytown
Hudson Valley Regional Poison Center
Phelps Memorial Hospital Center
701 N Broadway
North Tarrytown, NY 10591
800-336-6997 (calls from New York only)
914-366-3030

Rochester
Finger Lakes Regional Poison Center
University of Rochester Medical Center
601 Elmwood Ave, Box 321
Room 1-3360
Rochester, NY 14642
800-333-0542 (calls from New York only)
716-275-3232

Syracuse
Central New York Poison Control Center
SUNY Health Science Center
750 E Adams St
Syracuse, NY 13203
315-476-4766
800-252-5655 (calls from New York only)

North Carolina

Carolinas Poison Center
PO Box 32861
Charlotte, NC 28232
704-355-4000
800-848-6946 (calls from North Carolina only)

North Dakota

North Dakota Poison Information Center
MeritCare Medical Center
720 Fourth St N
Fargo, ND 58122
701-234-5575
800-732-2200 (calls from North Dakota, Minnesota, and South Dakota only)

Ohio

Cincinnati
Cincinnati Drug and Poison
Information Center and Regional
Poison Control System
2368 Victory Pkwy, Suite 300
Cincinnati, OH 45206
513-558-5111
800-872-5111 (calls from Ohio
only)

Columbus
Central Ohio Poison Center
700 Children's Dr
Columbus, OH 43205
614-228-1323
800-682-7625 (calls from Ohio only)

Oklahoma

Oklahoma Poison Control Center
Room 3N118
940 NE 13th St
Oklahoma City, OK 73104
405-271-5454
800-522-4611 (calls from Oklahoma
only)

Oregon

Oregon Poison Center
Oregon Health Sciences University
3181 SW Sam Jackson Park Rd,
CB550
Portland, OR 97201
503-494-8968
800-452-7165 (calls from Oregon
only)

Pennsylvania

Hershey
Central Pennsylvania Poison Center
University Hospital
Milton S. Hershey Medical Center
Hershey, PA 17033
717-531-6111
800-521-6110 (calls from Pennsyl-
vania only)

Philadelphia
The Poison Control Center
3600 Sciences Center, Suite 220
Philadelphia, PA 19104
215-386-2100
800-722-7112 (calls from Pennsylvania only)

Pittsburgh
Pittsburgh Poison Center
3705 Fifth Ave
Pittsburgh, PA 15213
412-681-6669

Rhode Island

Lifespan Poison Center
Rhode Island Hospital
593 Eddy St
Providence, RI 02903
401-444-5727

South Carolina

Palmetto Poison Center
University of South Carolina
College of Pharmacy
Columbia, SC 29208
803-765-7359
800-922-1117

South Dakota

McKennan Poison Center
800 E 21st St, Box 5045
Sioux Falls, SD 57117
800-952-0123 (calls from South
Dakota only)
800-764-7661
800-POISON-1

Southeast South Dakota
St Luke's Poison Center
St Luke's Regional Medical Center
2720 Stone Park Blvd
Sioux City, IA 51104
712-277-2222
800-352-2222

Tennessee

Middle Tennessee Poison Center
The Center for Clinical Toxicology
Vanderbilt University Medical
Center
1161 21st Ave S
501 Oxford House
Nashville, TN 37232
800-288-9999 (calls from Tennessee
only)
615-936-2034

Texas

Dallas
North Texas Poison Center
5201 Harry Hines Blvd
PO Box 35926
Dallas, TX 75235
800-764-7661 (calls from Texas
only)

El Paso
West Texas Regional Poison Center
4815 Alameda Ave
El Paso, TX 79905
800-764-7661 (calls from Texas only)

Galveston
Southeast Texas Poison Center
The University of Texas Medical
Branch
301 University Ave
Galveston, TX 77550
409-765-1420
800-764-7661 (calls from Texas
only)

San Antonio
South Texas Poison Center
University of Texas Health Science
Center at San Antonio
7703 Floyd Curl Dr
San Antonio, TX 78284
800-764-7661

Temple
Central Texas Poison Center
Scott and White Memorial Hospital
2401 S 31st St
Temple, TX 76508
800-764-7661 (calls from Texas
only)

Utah

Utah Poison Control Center
410 Chipeta Way, Suite 230
Salt Lake City, UT 84108
801-581-2151
800-456-7707 (calls from Utah only)

Vermont

Vermont Poison Center
Fletcher Allen Health Care
111 Colchester Ave
Burlington, VT 05401
802-658-3456

Virginia

Blue Ridge Poison Center
Box 437, Blue Ridge
University of Virginia Health System
Charlottesville, VA 22908
804-924-5543
800-451-1428 (calls from Virginia
only)

Washington

Washington Poison Center
155 NE 100th St, Suite 400
Seattle, WA 98125
206-526-2121
800-732-6985 (calls from Washington only)

West Virginia

West Virginia Poison Center
3110 MacCorkle Ave SE
Charleston, WV 25304
800-642-3625 (calls from West
Virginia only)
304-348-4211

Wisconsin

Eastern Wisconsin
Poison Center of Eastern Wisconsin
PO Box 1997
Milwaukee, WI 53201
414-266-2222
800-815-8855 (calls from Wisconsin
only)

Western Wisconsin
University of Wisconsin Hospital
Regional Poison Center
600 Highland Ave, Room E5/238
Madison, WI 53792
608-262-3702
800-815-8855

Wyoming

The Poison Center
8301 Dodge St
Omaha, NE 68114
402-390-5555
800-955-9119 (calls from Wyoming
only)

Animal Poison Control

ASPCA National Animal Poison
Control
800-548-2423
888-4ANIHELP
(above numbers, $30 per call on
credit card)
900-680-0000
(above number, $30 per call on
phone bill)

MEDICAL FORMS AND CHARTS

LIVING WILLS

Information About the Living Will Declaration, Health Care Proxy, and Five Wishes Living Will

The following form is supplied to patients in facilities affiliated with Harvard Medical School in Massachusetts. Your state may require a different form.

Brigham and Women's Hospital recognizes the right of individuals to make decisions about their treatment, including if and when to withhold or withdraw life support. In the event you become unable to make decisions, there are two ways to insure that your wishes are carried out. One is a living will declaration that gives you the opportunity to specify your wishes. The second is a document called a health care proxy that allows you to designate in writing a person who can make medical decisions on your behalf. Under state law, a proxy form may be completed by anyone 18 years of age or older, providing he or she is competent.

You may complete either form or both. You may also submit your own forms, which the hospital will honor as long as they do not conflict with current law. Be assured that in the absence of a living will or health care proxy, Brigham and Women's Hospital staff will provide all appropriate medical care, pain relief, and comfort. Nevertheless, we recommend that you complete these forms so that your wishes may be known and followed should you become physically or mentally unable to express them.

Before filling out these forms you should discuss your wishes with your doctor as well as the individual you plan to appoint to make decisions on your behalf. You may also wish to appoint an alternate should the first person you have chosen be unavailable. Please sign the health care proxy form in the presence of two witnesses (persons at least 18 years of age, who are not designated to act for you) and give a copy of the form to your doctor, to persons you have desig-

nated, and to close family or friends if you wish.

You may revoke or change these documents at any time by notifying your doctor or sending in a replacement. We recommend that you periodically check to be sure your health care agents remain available and willing. The hospital shall keep these documents in your medical record to consult if necessary.

Your primary care provider will ask you about your living will or advance directive on an annual basis. In addition, he or she will keep an electronic record of your discussions, which will be used to update other practitioners who might care for you.

You will find that if you are admitted to the hospital, a nurse will ask about your living will or health care proxy. If he or she finds that you have different ideas than what appears in your medical record, the nurse will be in touch with your primary care provider so that you can have further discussion. The nurse can also offer you health care proxy and living will declaration forms.

The Brigham and Women's Hospital is committed to offering living will and health care proxy forms to every patient, and to discussing care at the end of life with patients.

Patients have told us they appreciate this opportunity.

If you have any questions regarding these documents, please ask your doctor.

Living Will Declaration

The following form is supplied to patients in facilities affiliated with Harvard Medical School in Massachusetts. Your state may require a different form.

To my family, doctors, and all those concerned with my care:

I, _____, residing at _____, make this statement to express my wishes regarding the withholding or withdrawal of life support should a time come when, as determined by my doctor, I am unable to participate in decisions regarding my health care.

Should a time come when there is no expectation of my recovery from physical or mental disability or disease, I direct that I be allowed to die with dignity, and that my doctor withhold or withdraw treatment that merely prolongs life and is unlikely to offer a cure or remission of the disease. I direct that my treatment be limited to measures that will keep me comfortable and relieve pain.

These directives are made after careful consideration and in accordance with my strong convictions and beliefs. I expect my family, doctor, and others concerned with my care to abide by my wishes and in doing so, to be free of any legal or moral liability.

Additional instructions/comments: _____

_____

Signature: _____

Date: _____

Health Care Proxy

The following form is supplied to patients in facilities affiliated with Harvard Medical School in Massachusetts. Your state may require a different form.

I, _____, residing at _____, appoint _____, residing at _____, telephone _____, as my health care agent with the authority to make all health care decisions on my behalf. This authority becomes effective if my attending physician determines in writing that I lack the capacity to make or communicate health care decisions myself. My health care agent shall have the same authority as I would to make these decisions

except (list the limitations, if any, you wish to place on this authority):

_____

I direct my health care agent to make decisions based on his/her assessment of my personal wishes, including those expressed in my living will declaration I have signed. Should my wishes be unknown, my agent shall make decisions based on his/her assessment of my best interests. Photocopies of this proxy form shall have the same force and effect of the original.

If the person I have named is unavailable, unwilling, or not competent to serve, I designate the following person as his or her alternate:

Name: _____

Address: _____

Telephone: _____

Note: Generally, you may not choose as your health care agent an employee or member of the medical staff of a hospital or other health care facility unless you are related to that person by blood, marriage, or adoption.

Patient's signature: _____ Date: _____

WITNESS STATEMENT

This form requires two witnesses 18 years of age or older:

We, the undersigned witnesses, each declare that we have witnessed the signing of this document and that the person appears to be at least 18 years of age, of

sound mind, and under no constraints or undue influence. Neither of us is named as the health care agent or alternate.

Witness One

Name (print): _____

Address: _____

Date: _____

Signature: _____

Witness Two

Name (print): _____

Address: _____

Date: _____

Signature: _____

Five Wishes Living Will

The Five Wishes Living Will, produced by the Commission on Aging with Dignity, provides loved ones with very specific information on how you want to be treated—such as whether or not you want a breathing tube, if necessary, and whether or not you would like family members to be at your bedside. It covers five areas:

■ The kind of medical treatment you want or do not want.

■ How comfortable you want to be.

■ How you want people to treat you.

■ What you want your loved ones to know.

■ Who you want to make health care decisions for you when you cannot make them.

The Five Wishes Living Will is not legally valid in every state. However, it may help you think about end-of-life issues. It can be ordered from:

Five Wishes Living Will
Commission on Aging With Dignity
PO Box 11180
Tallahassee, FL 32302
850-681-2010
888-5-WISHES

MEDICAL RECORD SUMMARY

When you see a new doctor, it is very important to bring with you a summary of your medical history. If you are uncertain about any information, check with the offices of doctors who have cared for you in the past. Use this form as a guide to create your personal medical record.

Personal Health Record

	Yes	No	Not sure
Have you signed a living will?	____	____	_____
Have you signed an organ donor card?	____	____	_____
Have you signed a document designating a health proxy*?	____	____	_____

Name of health proxy: _____

Phone no. of health proxy:_____

*A health proxy is someone who makes decisions about your medical care if you are incapacitated and unable to make them.

- List all chronic conditions/diseases you have.

- If you have stayed in a hospital overnight, list the reason, the name of the hospital, and the date (year) for each stay.

- If you have had surgery, list the kind of surgery, the name of the hospital, and the date (year) for each surgery.

- List all medicines (prescription and over-the-counter) you currently take.

- List all medicines to which you have an allergy.

Have you had any of these illnesses? List the year of each one.

	Yes	Year
Measles	____	_____
Chickenpox	____	_____
German measles (rubella)	____	_____
Polio	____	_____
Mumps	____	_____
Hepatitis	____	_____

Have you had any of these immunizations? List the year of the last one.

	Yes	Year
Measles	____	_____
Tetanus	____	_____
German measles (rubella)	____	_____
Polio	____	_____
Mumps	____	_____
Hepatitis B	____	_____
Diphtheria	____	_____
Haemophilus influenzae type b	____	_____
Pertussis	____	_____
Chickenpox	____	_____
Pneumococcus (pneumonia)	____	_____
Influenza (flu shot)	____	_____

Have you had any of these screening tests? List the year of the last one.

	Yes	Year
Mammogram (if a woman)	____	_____
Pap smear (if a woman)	____	_____
Polio	____	_____
Test for blood in bowel movement	____	_____
Hepatitis A or B	____	_____
Sigmoidoscopy	____	_____
Haemophilus influenzae type b	____	_____
Colonoscopy	____	_____
Chickenpox	____	_____

TYPE OF ACTIVITY AND CALORIES BURNED

CALORIES EXPENDED BY A 140-POUND PERSON FOR 1 HOUR:

ACTIVITY	NO. OF CALORIES	ACTIVITY	NO. OF CALORIES
basketball	528	running	792
bowling	84	sitting quietly	78
cycling (10 miles per hour)	384	skating, ice or roller	414
dancing, aerobic	516	skiing, cross country	528
dancing, social	198	skiing, water or downhill	396
gardening	354	swimming	540
golf (no cart)	324	tennis	414
golf (power cart)	150	walking	456
hiking	312	weight training	456
jogging	648		

CALORIE, FIBER, AND FAT CONTENT OF COMMON FOODS

FOOD ITEM	PORTION SIZE	CALORIES	FIBER (GRAMS)	FAT (GRAMS)	FOOD ITEM	PORTION SIZE	CALORIES	FIBER (GRAMS)	FAT (GRAMS)
Baked Goods					cola	1½ cups	151	0	0
bagel	1	200	1	2	ginger ale	1½ cups	124	0	0
Italian bread	1 slice	83	<1	<1	orange soda	1½ cups	177	0	0
rye bread	1 slice	65	2	1	coffee	1 cup	2	0	0
white bread	1 slice	65	1	1	lemonade from concentrate	1 cup	100	<1	<1
whole-wheat bread	1 slice	70	3	1	tea	1 cup	2	0	0
angel food cake	1 piece	125	<1	<1					
Boston cream pie	1 piece	260	<1	8	**Dairy**				
coffee cake	1 piece	230	1	7	shredded cheddar cheese	1 cup	455	0	37
devil's food cake	1 piece	235	<1	8	large-curd cottage cheese	1 cup	235	0	10
chocolate chip cookies	4	180	<1	9	cream cheese	1 oz	99	0	10
oatmeal raisin cookies	4	245	<1	10	Monterey Jack cheese	1 oz	106	0	9
vanilla wafers	10	185	<1	7	part-skim mozzarella cheese	1 oz	80	0	5
graham crackers	2	60	1	2	parmesan cheese	1 tbsp	23	0	2
cake doughnut	1	210	<1	12	provolone cheese	1 oz	100	0	8
glazed doughnut	1	235	<1	13	half-and-half	1 tbsp	20	0	2
bran muffin	1	140	1	5	heavy whipping cream	1 tbsp	51	0	6
corn muffin	1	145	2	6	sour cream	1 tbsp	30	0	3
Beverages					whole milk	1 cup	150	0	8
beer	1½ cups	146	1	0	skim milk	1 cup	86	0	<1
light beer	1½ cups	100	<1	0	chocolate milk shake	1¼ cup	360	<1	10
90-proof gin, vodka, or whiskey	1.5 oz	110	0	0					
club soda	1½ cups	0	0	0					

FOOD ITEM	PORTION SIZE	CALORIES	FIBER (GRAMS)	FAT (GRAMS)
Eggs				
raw	1	79	0	6
white	1	16	0	<1
yolk	1	63	0	6
fried in butter	1	95	0	6
scrambled	1	95	0	7
Fats and Oils				
butter	1 tbsp	100	0	11
regular margarine	1 tbsp	100	0	11
60% fat margarine	1 tbsp	75	0	8
corn oil	1 tbsp	125	0	14
olive oil	1 tbsp	125	0	14
sunflower oil	1 tbsp	125	0	14
Italian dressing	1 tbsp	80	<1	9
thousand island dressing	1 tbsp	60	<1	6
mayonnaise	1 tbsp	100	0	11
Fish and Shellfish				
canned crab meat	1 cup	133	0	2
fish sticks	2	155	0	7
canned salmon	3 oz	118	0	5
smoked salmon	3 oz	100	0	4
breaded scallops	6	200	<1	10
fried shrimp	3 oz	206	<1	10
trout	3 oz	129	0	4
tuna in oil	3 oz	169	0	7
tuna in water	3 oz	111	0	<1
Fruit				
2 3/4-inch-diameter apple	1	80	4	<1
mashed avocado	1 cup	370	6	35
banana	1	105	3	<1
blueberries	1 cup	82	5	1
chopped dates	1 cup	489	16	1
white grapefruit	1 half	39	1	<1
seedless grapes	10	35	1	<1
orange	1	60	3	<1
peach	1	73	4	<1
raisins	0.5 oz	41	1	<1

FOOD ITEM	PORTION SIZE	CALORIES	FIBER (GRAMS)	FAT (GRAMS)
Grain Products				
instant cream of wheat	1 cup	140	1	1
instant oatmeal	1 cup	145	9	2
macaroni	1 cup	190	1	1
egg noodles	1 cup	200	<1	2
chow mein noodles	1 cup	220	<1	11
plain air-popped popcorn	1 cup	30	1	<1
cooked brown rice	1 cup	232	4	1
cooked white rice	1 cup	186	1	<1
spaghetti	1 cup	190	1	1
toasted wheat germ	1 cup	431	3	12
Meat and Meat Products				
fatty beef	3 oz	325	0	26
lean beef	2.8 oz	173	0	8
ground beef	3 oz	246	0	18
fatty rib roast	3 oz	324	0	27
steak	3 oz	238	0	16
broiled lamb loin chops	2.8 oz	235	0	16
bacon	3 pieces	109	0	9
ham	3 oz	207	0	14
pork chops	3.1 oz	275	0	19
fried chicken thighs	1	238	<1	14
roasted chicken thighs	1	153	0	10
roasted light-meat turkey	3 oz	133	0	3
bologna	1 piece	89	0	8
sausage links	1	50	0	5
hot dogs	1	145	0	13
salami	2 pieces	145	0	11
Nuts and Seeds				
dried whole almonds	1 oz	167	3	15
roasted cashews	1 oz	163	2	14
roasted macadamia nuts	1 oz	204	1	22
roasted peanuts	1 oz	163	2	14
peanut butter	1 tbsp	94	1	8
shelled dried pistachio nuts	1 oz	164	1	14

FOOD ITEM	PORTION SIZE	CALORIES	FIBER (GRAMS)	FAT (GRAMS)
Vegetables and Legumes				
cooked black beans	1 cup	227	15	1
cooked snap beans	1 cup	44	3	<1
navy beans with pork	1 cup	247	19	3
bean sprouts	1 cup	32	2	1
chopped broccoli	1 cup	24	3	<1
chopped cabbage	1 cup	16	2	<1
carrot	1	31	2	<1
cauliflower	½ cup	12	1	<1
celery	1 stalk	6	1	<1
corn	1 ear	83	4	1
cooked eggplant	1 cup	45	6	<1
cooked garbanzo beans	1 cup	269	9	4

FOOD ITEM	PORTION SIZE	CALORIES	FIBER (GRAMS)	FAT (GRAMS)
canned kidney beans	1 cup	208	20	1
cooked lentils	1 cup	231	10	1
mushrooms	½ cup	9	1	<1
chopped onions	1 cup	54	3	1
canned peas	½ cup	59	5	<1
cooked pinto beans	1 cup	235	19	1
baked potato with skin	1	220	4	<1
french fries	10	158	2	8
hash brown potatoes	1 cup	340	2	18
refried beans	1 cup	270	22	3
raw spinach	1 cup	12	2	<1
sweet potatoes	1	118	3	<1
tomatoes	1	24	2	<1

Index

Page numbers in **boldface** refer to the primary discussion of a topic.

Heat:
and brain/nervous system, 338
and children, 298, 327
and diet and nutrition, 37
first aid/emergency care for, **1212**
intolerance to, 172
symptom charts about, 172, 195, 298
Heat exhaustion, **1212**
Heat sensitivity and hormone disorders, 846, 847, 849
Heatstroke, 765, **1212**
Heat therapy, 383, 607, 615, 624, 626, 639

Heavy menstrual periods, symptom chart, 268–70

Heberden nodes, 605
Heel pain, **638–39**
and plantar fasciitis, **640–41**
Heel spurs, **641**
Height, 80, 82
Heimlich maneuver, 1190, **1206**
Helicobacter pylori, 752, 753, **754–55,** 756, 757
Hemangiomas, **969**
Hematemesis. *See* Vomit/vomiting: blood in
Hematocrit test, **155**
Hematologists, 724, 729
Hematoma, 352, 459, 577
Hemochromatosis, 717, 765
Hemodialysis, 815, **816–17**
Hemoglobin electrophoresis, **155,** 721–22
Hemoglobin tests, **155, 841**
Hemolytic anemia, 713, 715, 718, **719–20,** 721, 723
Hemophilia, 129, 156, 218, 711, **735,** 737, 763
Hemorrhage, **351, 352**
see also types of hemorrhage
Hemorrhoids, 79, 372, 542, 715, 784, **795–97, 926, 944**
symptom charts about, 256, 258, 259
Hemospermia, **1096,** 1097
Heparin, 344, 349, 514, 515, **667,** 737, 1155
Hepatic vein thrombosis, 767
Hepatitis, 866, **947, 948–49**
acute, **758–59, 762**
and addictions/abuse, 65, 67, 68
alcoholic, 765

autoimmune, 762, 764
and behavioral and emotional disorders, 412
causes of, 735
chronic, 759, **762, 764,** 765, 767
and diagnosing disease, 153, 154
and digestive disorders, 765, 767, 768
from drugs or toxins, **758**
and eye disorders, 429
and pregnancy, 921
prevention of, 93, **763**
risks of, **764**
symptoms of, **759, 762**
treatment options for, **759, 762, 764**
see also types of hepatitis
Hepatitis A, **94,** 762, 764, 1031
Hepatitis B, **94,** 160, 711, 722, 758, 762, 764, 810, 1031, 1035, 1092
Hepatitis C, **84,** 711, 758, 762, 764, 810, 1035
Hepatitis D, 764
Hepatitis E, 764
Hepatoma, 766
Herbs, 400, 789, 854, **907,** 1094, 1099, 1158
medicine interactions with, **1154–55**
Hernias, 247, 789, **800–801, 974, 980,** 1086
see also types of hernias
Herniated disk, 613, 619, 620, 621, **622–25**
symptom charts about, 212, 226, 229
Herpes virus:
and adolescents, 1033
and brain/nervous system, 374, 379, 381
in children, **1010**
and cosmetic and reconstructive surgery, 583
and digestive disorders, 764
and eye disorders, 427, 429, 430, 444
and men's health, 1092
and mouth disorders, 469, 487
and pregnancy, 921
simplex, 374, 381, 429, 430, 444, 487, 764
and skin conditions, 537
symptom charts about, 209, 231

zoster, 379, 444, 537
see also Genital herpes
Heterocyclic antidepressants, 384, **843**
see also Tricyclic antidepressants
Hiatal hernias, 241, 242, 246, 250, **747, 748**
Hiccups, **522,** 786
High blood pressure. *See* Hypertension

Hip pain, symptom chart, 216–17

Hips, **628–32**
arthritis of, **628**
artificial, 1101
and aseptic necrosis, **628**
bleeding in, 216
of children, **973**
developmental dysplasia of, **973**
exercise for, **1113**
fractures of, 85, 216, **629,** 1119
inflammation of, 628
and joint disorders, 605, 606, 629
and men's health, 1107, 1109
pain in, 214, **216–17,** 628, 1107, 1109
replacement of, 628, **629–32**
of seniors, **1113,** 1119
sprain/strain of, 216
surgery on, 628, 630
swelling in, 628
symptom charts about, 214, **216–17**
treatment options for, 217
Hirschsprung disease, **980–81**
Hirsutism, **558–59,** 857
Histamine blockers. *See* H2 (histamine) blockers
Histoplasmosis, **503–4,** 866
HIV (human immunodeficiency virus), **872**
and addictions/abuse, 67, 68
in adolescents, 1031, 1033
and blood disorders, 721, 730, 736
and blood donation/transfusions, 711
and brain/nervous system, 354, 363, 374, 377
and cervical cancer, 1068–69
and contraception, 76
and digestive disorders, 748

Medical instruments, When you visit/call your doctor, 122
